Oncology Nursing

Oncology Nursing

SHIRLEY E. OTTO, MSN, CRNI, AOCN
Clinical Nurse Specialist
Via Christi Regional Medical Center: St. Francis Campus
Wichita, Kansas

THIRD EDITION
with 110 *illustrations*

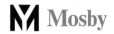 Mosby

St. Louis   Baltimore   Boston
Carlsbad   Chicago   Naples   New York   Philadelphia   Portland
London   Madrid   Mexico City   Singapore   Sydney   Tokyo   Toronto   Wiesbaden

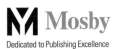
Mosby
Dedicated to Publishing Excellence

A Times Mirror
Company

Vice President and Publisher: Nancy L. Coon
Editor: Jeff Burnham
Associate Developmental Editor: Lisa P. Newton
Project Manager: Patricia Tannian
Project Specialist: Betty Hazelwood
Book Design Manager: Gail Morey Hudson
Manufacturing Manager: David Graybill
Cover Designer: Teresa Breckwoldt
Cover Image: © Contributor/Custom Medical Stock Photo, Inc.

THIRD EDITION

Copyright © 1997 by Mosby–Year Book, Inc.

Previous editions copyrighted 1991, 1994

A NOTE TO THE READER
The author and publisher have made every attempt to check dosages and
nursing content for accuracy. Because the science of pharmacology is continually
advancing, our knowledge base continues to expand. Therefore we recommend
that the reader always check product information for changes in dosage or
administration before administering any medication. This is particularly important
with new or rarely used drugs.

Printed in the United States of America
Composition by Clarinda Company
Printing/binding by Maple-Vail Book Mfg. Group

Mosby–Year Book, Inc.
11830 Westline Industrial Drive
St. Louis, Missouri 63146

Library of Congress Cataloging in Publication Data

Oncology nursing / [edited by] Shirley E. Otto.—3rd ed.
    p.   cm.
   Includes bibliographical references and index.
   ISBN 0-8151-8955-9
   1. Cancer—Nursing.   I. Otto, Shirley E.
   [DNLM: 1. Neoplasms—nursing. 2. Neoplasms—therapy.   WY 156
05748 1996]
RC266.053 1996
610.73′698—dc20
DNLM/DLC
for Library of Congress   96-23227
                              CIP

96 97 98 99 00 / 9 8 7 6 5 4 3 2 1

TO ALL THE NURSES
who challenge themselves to
make a difference
in the quality of life for the
patient and family with cancer.

Contributors

Joyce Alexander, MSN, RN, OCN (Chapter 4)

Clinical Nurse Specialist
Oncology/Bone Marrow Transplant
Halifax Medical Center
Daytona Beach, Florida

Linda Anderson, MS, RN, CS, AOCN (Chapter 28)

Oncology Nurse Practitioner
Oakwood Hospital and Medical Center
Dearborn, Michigan

Margaret L. Barnett, MSN, ARNP, AOCN (Chapter 26)

Cancer Care/Pain Management
Clinical Nurse Specialist
Department of Nursing
University of Kansas Medical Center
Kansas City, Kansas

Cynthia F. Brodgon, MSN, RN, AOCN (Chapter 12)

Clinical Nurse Specialist
Amgen
Thousand Oaks, California

Kathleen R. Bulson, RN, OCN (Chapter 14)

Office Nurse
Medical Oncologist
Grand Rapids, Michigan

Jane C. Clark, MSN, RN, OCN, AOCN (Chapters 10 and 16)

Clinical Nurse Specialist
Emory University Hospital
Atlanta, Georgia

Frances H. Cornelius, MSN, RN (Chapter 27)

Clinical Faculty: Community Health
Holy Family College and Widner University Schools of Nursing
Philadelphia, Pennsylvania

Rebecca Crane, PhD(c), RN, AOCN (Chapter 6)

Doctoral Candidate
University of California, Los Angeles;
Clinical Nurse Specialist
Joyce Eisenberg Keefer Breast Center
John Wayne Cancer Research Institute
Saint John's Hospital and Health Center
Santa Monica, California

Betty Thomas Daniel, MSN, RN, OCN (Chapters 8 and 15)

Clinical Nurse Specialist
The University of Texas M.D. Anderson
Cancer Center, Houston, Texas;
Doctoral Student
University of Texas
Austin, Texas

Susan Brennan Giacalone, MSN, RN, OCN (Chapter 25)

Manager Cancer Center Clinical Trials Core
Karmanos Cancer Institute
Wayne State University
Detroit, Michigan

Karen Goldman, MSN, RN, OCN (Chapter 2)

Director Oncology Patient Services
Karmanos Cancer Institute
The Detroit Medical Center
Detroit, Michigan

Mary Magee Gullatte, MN, RN, CNP, AOCN (Chapter 3)

Director of Nursing
Oncology and Transplant Services
Emory University Hospital
Atlanta, Georgia

Andrea Sampson Haggood, MSN, RN, CS, ANP (Chapter 11)

Nurse Practitioner Oncology Patient Services
Karmanos Cancer Institute
The Detroit Medical Center
Detroit, Michigan

Ryan Iwamoto, MN, ARNP (Chapter 21)

Clinical Nurse Specialist
Department of Radiation Oncology
Virginia Mason Medical Center
Seattle, Washington

Claire Keller, MSN, RN, OCN (Chapter 24)

BMT Clinical Nurse Specialist
Karmanos Cancer Institute
The Detroit Medical Center
Detroit, Michigan

Martha Langhorne, MSN, RN, OCN (Chapter 22)

Clinical Nurse Specialist
Oncology Services
United Health Services Hospitals
Johnson City, New York

Noella Devolder McCray, MN, RN, OCN (Chapter 31)

Patient Education Coordinator
St. Joseph Health Center
Kansas City, Missouri

Mary E. Murphy, MS, RN, OCN (Chapters 5 and 7)

Home Care Team Coordinator
Hospice of Dayton
Dayton, Ohio

Rosanne Lucy Eble Ososki, MSN, RNC (Chapter 13)

Nurse Practitioner
Karmanos Cancer Institute
The Detroit Medical Center
Detroit, Michigan

Shirley E. Otto, MSN, CRNI, AOCN (Chapter 17 and Appendixes)

Clinical Nurse Specialist
Via Christi Regional Medical Center: St. Francis Campus
Wichita, Kansas

Jeanne Parzuchowski, MS, RN, OCN (Chapter 9)

Clinical Faculty, Department of Urology
Wayne State University;
Genitourinary Cancer Coordinator
Karmanos Cancer Institute
The Detroit Medical Center
Detroit, Michigan

Karen A. Pfeifer, PhD(c), RN, CNA, OCN (Chapters 1 and 20)

Doctoral Candidate
Graduate Research Assistant
Texas Woman's University
Denton, Texas

Paula Trahan Rieger, MSN, RN, ANP, CS, OCN (Chapter 23)

Nurse Practitioner
The University of Texas M.D. Anderson Cancer Center
Houston, Texas

Susan Tobin Rumelhart, MA, RN, CPNP, CPON (Chapter 18)

Pediatric Nurse Practitioner
Pediatric Center, P.C.
Cedar Rapids, Iowa

Sandra Lee Schafer, MN, RN, AOCN (Chapter 19)

Clinical Nurse Specialist in Cancer Care
Shadyside Hospital
Pittsburgh, Pennsylvania

Suzanne Shaffer, MN, ARNP, AOCN (Chapter 30)

Cancer Care Clinical Nurse Specialist
Nursing Services
University of Kansas Medical Center
Kansas City, Kansas

Judith A. Shell, MS, MA, RN, AOCN (Chapters 14 and 32)

Oncology Clinical Nurse Specialist
Butterworth Hospital
Grand Rapids, Michigan;
Doctoral Student
Marriage and Family Therapy
Michigan State University
Lansing, Michigan

Carol J. Swenson, MS, RN, AOCN (Chapter 29)

Program Director
Swedish American Health System
Regional Cancer Center
Rockford, Illinois

Linda F. VanderLugt, RN, OCN (Chapter 14)

Office Nurse
Medical Oncologist
Grand Rapids, Michigan

Michelle Wallace, BSN, RN, OCN (Chapter 9)

Nurse Specialist
Radiation Oncology Center
Karmanos Cancer Institute
The Detroit Medical Center
Detroit, Michigan

Deborah Ward, MSN, RN, CS, OCN (Chapter 28)

Oncology Nurse Practitioner
Karmanos Cancer Institute
The Detroit Medical Center
Detroit, Michigan

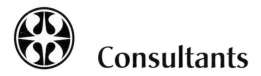

Consultants

Doris Bartlett, BSN, RN, MS

Assistant Professor, Bethel College
Mishawaka, Indiana;
Oncology Staff Nurse, Memorial Hospital
South Bend, Indiana

Carolyn Harvey, PhD, RN

Assistant Professor
University of Texas at Tyler
Tyler, Texas

Mary Beth Kiefner, MS, RN

Nursing Faculty
Illinois Central College
East Peoria, Illinois

Maureen E. O'Rourke, PhC, RN, OCN

Doctoral Candidate
University of North Carolina—Chapel Hill
Chapel Hill, North Carolina

Susan Sturgeon, BS, RN, OCN

Vice President, Professional Development
Community Cancer Care, Inc.
Indianapolis, Indiana

Victoria R. Ullemeyer, MSN, RN, OCN

Director, Oncology Services
Meridia South Pointe Hospital
Warrensville Heights, Ohio

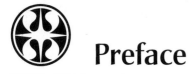

Preface

Oncology Nursing's first and second editions were designed to provide the most current and relevant information needed for nursing care of patients with cancer. The books' strong clinical focus made them a valuable resource for nurses in a variety of settings, including major cancer centers, local hospitals, clinics, physicians' offices, and patients' homes. Based on the many excellent comments received, the books met the varied practice needs:

"Someone wrote an oncology book with the staff nurse in mind. I can read, interpret, and incorporate the concepts into my nursing practice."

"It was the book of choice to prepare/review for the oncology nursing certification exam."

"The book is an excellent resource for the clinical nurse specialist, nurse practitioner, academia, or advanced practice nurse preparing informal/formal educational programs."

Other health care professionals stated that they found the book to be an excellent resource enabling them to become more knowledgeable in cancer care.

The *third edition* of *Oncology Nursing* could be subtitled *Making a Difference.* Multiple positive comments have been received from the previous editions. The consistent theme of comments is that "*Oncology Nursing* has made a difference for me and my oncology practice." These comments and suggestions such as "have you thought about adding multiple choice questions/answers to the book" have been incorporated into this *third edition.* The original format has stayed the same, and the book continues to expand with more disease, treatment, and supportive care chapters and an additional appendix on clinical pathways. Multiple choice questions have been added at the end of each chapter, and all answers are at the end of the book.

Each chapter received major revisions, and features such as geriatric considerations, patient teaching priorities, expected patient outcome goals, disease- and treatment-related complications, future directions, and advances in therapy were incorporated throughout all the chapters.

Unit I opens with a chapter on cancer pathophysiology that gives a fundamental explanation of carcinogenesis, neoplastic classification systems, cell cycle properties, hereditary and genetic issues, and the metastatic process. Chapters covering epidemiology; prevention, screening, and detection; and diagnosis and staging complete the unit. The most recent guidelines, recommendations, and statistics from the National Cancer Institute, the American Cancer Society, and the American Joint Committee on Cancer Staging are incorporated throughout the book. Updated information regarding chemoprevention trials for prevention of breast, prostate, and colorectal cancer; environmental and hereditary cancers and genetics in cancer prediction; and socioeconomic factors of poor, underserved, and uninsured Americans will be of interest to many nurses.

The chapters in Unit II cover clinical management of the most common cancers (brain/CNS, breast, colorectal, gastrointestinal, genitourinary, gynecologic, head and neck, HIV-related cancers, leukemia, lung, lymphoma, myeloma, and skin cancers) and oncologic complications. An additional chapter included in this section is pediatric cancers. This chapter features the most common pediatric cancers (leukemia, lymphoma, Hodgkin's disease, Wilms' tumor, neuroblastoma, rhabdomyosarcoma, osteogenic sarcoma, and Ewing's sarcoma). All the disease chapters examine the epidemiology, etiology, prevention, screening, and detection of the particular type of cancer being discussed. Information on how the disease is classified, diagnosed, and staged, its clinical features, and the metastatic process precedes sections that explain the most prevalent treatments and prognosis for each type of cancer. Nursing diagnosis, interventions, and patient expected outcomes are presented in nursing management sections incorporated in each chapter. Additional features include geriatric considerations, patient teaching priorities, and disease- and treatment-related complications.

The chapter on oncologic complications defines the major complications that may occur as a result of cancer or its treatment. Etiology, incidence and risk factors, pathophysiology, clinical features, diagnostic evaluation, treatment modalities, and nursing management are covered for each of the following complications: disseminated intravascular coagulation, hypercalcemia, malignant pleural effusion, neoplastic cardiac tamponade, septic shock, spinal cord compression, superior vena cava syndrome, and syndrome of inappropriate antidiuretic hormone secretion. Algorithms for decision tree assessment and management of the varied oncologic complications have been updated.

Unit II, which discusses cancer treatment modalities, includes chapters on surgery, radiation therapy, chemotherapy, biotherapy, bone marrow transplantation, and cancer clinical trials. These chapters examine the principles and roles of each therapy. The surgery chapter explores preoperative, perioperative, and postoperative nursing assessment and interventions. The most recent concepts related to laser therapy options, videothoroscopy, and intraoperative surgery with radiation therapy have been added to this chapter. Radiation therapy issues such as whole body, fractionated dose schedule, hyperthermia, photodynamic therapy, radiation sensitizers, and intraoperative therapies are included. The chapters on biotherapy and chemotherapy detail what the agents are and how they work, provide administration guidelines, and explain safe handling, storage, and disposal. The bone marrow transplantation chapter provides pretransplant and posttransplant conditioning, dose-intensity regimens, transplantation options, intervention, and follow-up medical/nursing treatment protocols. Peripheral blood stem cell transplantation issues include the catheter placement, pheresis process, costs, diseases most commonly treated, and survivorship issues. The cancer clinical trials chapter contains updates on all the current and upcoming disease prevention and treatment trials. Additional information includes ambulatory care setting and home care considerations and future directions and advances in all these therapies.

Unit IV, which features chapters on fatigue, home care and cancer resources, nutrition, pain management, protective mechanisms, and psychosocial/survivorship and sexuality issues, is intended to equip the nurse to better support and care for the patient and family regardless of the type of cancer or method of treatment. Fatigue, the most frequently experienced symptom of cancer and cancer treatment, has become an oncology practice priority. Definition, pathophysiology, etiology, and cancer therapies with nursing assessment and interventions for fatigue are addressed. The home care/cancer resources chapter provides many resources and guidelines to assist the nurse in discharging the patient from the acute care, ambulatory care, and/or extended care setting to the patient's home. Checklists for caregiver and home care/extended care assessment are provided. Multiple professional and public national and local resources are profiled (e.g., indigent patient drug resources). An excellent table describing the ambulatory infusion pumps' features used in multiple settings has been added.

The nutrition chapter addresses the impact of cancer on nutritional status; assessment parameters are identified, and interventions for oral, enteral, and parenteral nutrition are suggested. Additional features include geriatric and ethical considerations. The chapter on pain management discusses analgesics, nonanalgesics, and nonsteroidal drugs, as well as drug administration principles specific to route, dose titration, schedule, and side effects. Noninvasive pain management strategies are presented. Invasive pain management modalities are defined, rationales for the procedures are given, and potential outcomes are discussed. New pain management guidelines from the American Pain Society and Agency for Health Care Policy and Research—Cancer Pain Management have been incorporated throughout the chapter; multiple professional and pain management resources are listed.

Protective mechanisms, such as skin, mucous membrane, and bone marrow, are defined, and parameters of nursing assessment with effective interventions are provided. Information regarding *Clinical Practice Guidelines on Pressure Ulcers in Adults: Prediction and Prevention* from the Agency for Health Care Policy and Research and specialty bed placement/reimbursement issues are discussed. The psychosocial chapter has incorporated these timely topics, including quality of life, disability issues, hospice care, survivorship, ethics, advance directives, right-to die legislation information, and the well-being of the professional and lay caregiver. The sexuality chapter discusses the impact of cancer and its therapy on sexuality. Many sensitive issues are explored, and strategies intended to help the patient enhance self and sexual images are provided.

About one in three, or 85 million, Americans will eventually develop cancer. The vast majority of nurses in all practice settings feel the impact of the disease personally or professionally at some time during their career. Because we believe the nurse is vital in providing high-quality care for patients with cancer, the nurse's role is interwoven throughout each chapter and then focused in nursing management sections. These sections include nursing diagnoses, interventions, and expected patient outcomes to provide the nurse with concrete guidelines to ensure the best quality care throughout the course of the disease. Now, more than ever, during all the changing practices in cancer care, compassionate, competent, and conscientious nursing care is the right of the patient and family with cancer. What we say and do does make a difference in the quality of life for these individuals.

ACKNOWLEDGMENTS

I wish to express my sincere appreciation to the many people who made this publication possible: the contributing authors, Karen P., Karen G., Mary G., Joyce, Mary M., Becky, Betty, Jeanne, Michelle, Jane, Andrea, Cynthia, Roseanne, Judy, Linda V., Kathleen, Susan T.R., Sandy L.S., Ryan, Martha, Paula, Claire, Susan G., Marge, Fran, Linda A., Deborah, Carol, Suzanne, and Noella who, despite their personal, family, educational, and professional responsibilities, provided excellent chapters; to all the Mosby staff; and to all my oncology peers who continually encourage and support me. Thank you.

Shirley E. Otto

Contents in Brief

Contents

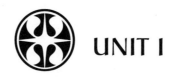 UNIT I

CLINICAL ASPECTS OF THE CANCER DIAGNOSIS

CHAPTER 1
Pathophysiology

KAREN A. PFEIFER

Cancer, the second most common cause of death in the United States, kills approximately 555,000 persons each year. Cancer is the primary cause of death from disease in children up to 14 years of age, and approximately 60% of all cancer deaths occur among individuals older than 65 years.[1,41]

Medical researchers have identified approximately 100 different types of cancers. Each cancer cell within these various diseases has an altered morphology and biochemistry from the normal cell. Cancer is not a disorderly growth of immature cells, but rather a logical, coordinated process in which a normal cell undergoes changes and acquires special capabilities.[27]

THE NORMAL CELL

The basic unit of structure and function in all living things is the *cell.* Approximately 60,000 billion cells are in the adult human body, and although there are many different types of cells, all of them have certain common characteristics. For example, all cells need nourishment to maintain life, and all cells use almost identical nutrients. All cells use oxygen (O_2); the O_2 combines with fat, protein, or carbohydrates (CHO) to release the energy needed for cells to function. The mechanisms for changing nutrients into energy are generally the same in all cells, and all cells deliver their end-products of chemical reactions into nearby fluids. Most cells have the ability to reproduce. Whenever cells are destroyed, the remaining cells of the same type reproduce until the correct number has been replenished. This orderly replacement of cells is governed by a control mechanism that stops when the loss or damage has been corrected. Dynamic, active, and orderly, the healthy cell is a small powerhouse, laboratory, factory, and duplicating machine—perfectly copying itself over and over.[5,19] Figure 1-1 shows the phases and characteristics of *mitosis* (cell division).

PROLIFERATIVE GROWTH PATTERNS

Cancer cells are not subject to the usual restrictions placed by the host on cell proliferation. However, proliferation is not always indicative of cancer. Abnormal cellular growth is classified as *nonneoplastic* and *neoplastic.*[12,19,32,38,42]

Nonneoplastic Growth Patterns

The four common nonneoplastic growth patterns are as follows: hypertrophy, hyperplasia, metaplasia, and dysplasia.[12,19,32,38,42]

Hypertrophy is an increase in cell size. It commonly results from increased workload, hormonal stimulation, or compensation directly related to the functional loss of other tissue.[42]

Hyperplasia is a reversible increase in the number of cells of a certain tissue type, resulting in increased tissue mass. Hyperplasia commonly occurs as a normal physiologic response at times of rapid growth and development (e.g., pregnancy, adolescence). It is abnormal when the volume of cells produced exceeds the normal physiologic demand.[12,19,38,42]

In *metaplasia,* one adult cell type is substituted for another type not usually found in the involved tissue (e.g., glandular for squamous). The process is reversible if the stimulus is removed, or metaplasia may progress to dysplasia if the stimulus persists. Metaplasia can be induced by inflammation, vitamin deficiencies, irritation, and various chemical agents. A common area for metaplasia to occur is the uterine cervix.[12,19,38,42]

Dysplasia is characterized by alterations in normal adult cells in which the cell varies from its normal size, shape, or organization or one mature cell type is replaced with a less mature cell type. The common stimulus creating a dysplasia is usually an external one (e.g., radiation, inflammation, toxic chemicals, chronic irritation). Dysplasia is possibly reversible if the stimulus is removed.[19,38,42]

Hyperplasia, metaplasia, and dysplasia are not neoplastic conditions but may precede the development of cancer.[42]

Interphase
- Cell grows in size
- Chromosomes elongate
- DNA replicates

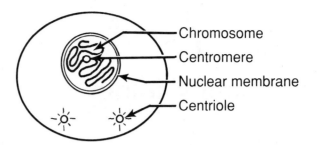

Chromosome
Centromere
Nuclear membrane
Centriole

Prophase
- DNA coils
- Centrioles move to opposite poles

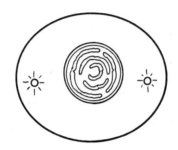

Metaphase
- Chromosomes align across cell equator
- Nucleoli and nuclear membrane disappear

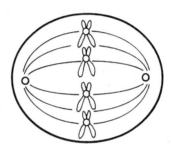

Anaphase
- Chromosomes divide
- Chromosomes move to opposite poles

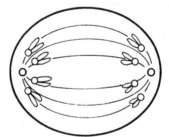

Telophase
- Chromosomes elongate
- Nuclear membranes reappear and enclose chromosomes
- Cytokinesis occurs
- Centrioles replicate

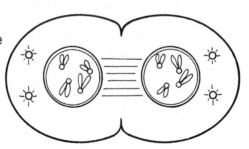

Figure 1-1   Mitosis: phases and characteristics. *DNA*, Deoxyribonucleic acid. (From Griffiths M, Murray K, Russo P: *Oncology nursing: pathophysiology, assessment, and intervention*, New York, 1984, Macmillan.)

Table 1-1 Comparison of Benign and Malignant Tumors

Characteristic	Malignant tumor	Benign tumor
Encapsulated	Rarely	Usually
Differentiated	Poorly	Partially
Metastasis	Frequently present	Absent
Recurrence	Frequent	Rare
Vascularity	Moderate to marked	Slight
Mode of growth	Infiltrative and expansive	Expansive
Cell characteristics	Cells abnormal and become more unlike parent cells	Fairly normal; similar to parent cells

From Bender CM, Yasko JM, Strohl RA: Cancer. In Lewis SM, Collier IC, Heitkemper MM, editors: *Medical-surgical nursing: assessment and management of clinical problems,* ed 4, St Louis, 1996, Mosby.

Neoplastic Growth Patterns

Anaplasia means "without form" and is an irreversible change in which the structures of adult cells regress to more primitive levels. It is a hallmark of cancer. Anaplastic cells lose the capacity for specialized functions and are positionally and cytologically disorganized.*

Neoplasm means "new growth" and describes an abnormal tissue mass that extends beyond the boundaries of normal tissue, failing to fulfill the normal function of cells in that tissue. Neoplasms are characterized by uncontrolled functioning, unregulated division and growth, and abnormal motility. Some neoplasms are potentially harmful to the host because they occupy space and compete for essential nutrients. Neoplastic growths are referred to as *benign neoplasms* or *malignant neoplasms.* Benign neoplasms include papillomas or warts. Malignant neoplasms include solid tumors and leukemia; these have the ability to destroy the host. *Cancer* is the common term for all malignant neoplasms.† Table 1-1 summarizes the differences between benign and malignant growths.

CHARACTERISTICS OF CANCER CELLS
Microscopic Properties

Microscopic examination of cancer cells shows certain structural changes that are described in pathologic terms, as follows:[20,42,44]

- *Pleomorphism.* Cancer cells vary in size and shape. Some are unusually large, whereas others are too small to be detected microscopically. Multiple nuclei may be seen.

- *Hyperchromatism.* Nuclear chromatin, the major component of genes, is more pronounced on staining.
- *Polymorphism.* The nucleus is larger and varies in shape.
- *Aneuploidy.* Unusual numbers of chromosomes are seen.
- *Abnormal chromosome arrangements.* A variety of possibilities exist, including translocations, the exchange of material between chromosomes, deletions, loss of chromosome sections, additions, extra chromosomes, and *fragile sites,* weak sections on chromosomes.

Kinetic Properties

Cancer cells possess certain kinetic characteristics, as follows:

- *Loss of proliferative control.* All cancer cells possess this characteristic. The need for cell renewal or replacement is the usual stimulus for cell proliferation. Cell production stops when the stimulus is gone, producing a balance between cell production and cell loss. In cancer, proliferation continues once the stimulus initiates the process, and cancer cells progress in continued, uncontrolled growth. The host's normal control mechanisms fail to stop this proliferation.[12,19]
- *Loss of capacity to differentiate.* Differentiation is the process by which cells diversify and acquire specific structural and functional characteristics. In cancer, *differentiation* refers to the extent to which cancer cells resemble comparable normal cells. Cancer cells vary in their ability to retain the original tissue's morphologic and functional traits. Cells that closely resemble the normal cell but form slow-growing, usually encapsulated tumors are *well differentiated.* These cells have recognizable specialized structures and functions. Cells that grow rapidly and do not have the original tissue's morphologic characteristics and specialized cell functions are termed *undifferentiated.* These cells have lost the capacity for specialized functions. The process by which cells lose characteristics of normal cells is called *dedifferentiation.* The more undifferentiated a malignant cell, the more virulent it is believed to be. It is possible to cause cells at one level of differentiation to transform into less well-differentiated cells by exposing them to cancer-causing agents.[12,19,20,38,42]
- *Altered biochemical properties.* Because of the cancer cell's loss of the capacity to differentiate, certain biochemical properties may be missing because of the cell's new immature state, or cells may acquire new properties because of enzyme pattern changes or alterations in deoxyribonucleic acid (DNA). Examples of these altered biochemical properties include production of tumor-associated antigens marking the cancer cell as "nonself"; continued reproduction despite diminished concentrations of growth hormones; higher rates

*References 18, 19, 20, 34, 38, 42.
†References 12, 19, 20, 22, 41, 42.

of anaerobic glycolysis, making the cell less dependent on O_2; loss of cell-to-cell cohesiveness and adhesiveness; and abnormal production of hormones or hormonelike substances that induce paraneoplastic syndromes. In the latter, cancer cells may inappropriately secrete hormones in an organ or tissue that does not normally produce or release those hormones, resulting in signs and symptoms not directly related to the local effects of the tumor. For example, in bronchogenic carcinoma, antidiuretic hormone (ADH) is produced, resulting in hyponatremia (Table 1-2).[10,12,20,42]

- *Chromosomal instability.* Cancer cells are less genetically stable than normal cells because of the development of abnormal chromosome arrangements. Chromosomal instability results in new, increasingly malignant mutants as cancer cells proliferate. These mutant cells can create a surviving subpopulation of advanced neoplasms with unique biologic and cytogenetic characteristics that are highly resistant to therapy.*

- *Capacity to metastasize. Metastasis,* the spread of cancer cells from a *primary* (parent) site to distant secondary sites, is aided by the production of enzymes on the surface of the cancer cell. Cancer cells become increasingly malignant with each mutation, and an asso-

ciation exists between a cell's degree of malignancy and its ability to metastasize.[12,19,20,42]

CELLULAR KINETICS

The field of *cellular kinetics* is the study of the quantitative growth and division of cells.[7,12,42]

Cell Cycle

The *cell cycle* is the sequence of events involved in replication and distribution of DNA to the daughter cells produced by cell division. All cells, nonmalignant and malignant, progress through the five phases of the cell cycle: G_0, G_1, S, G_2, and M (Figure 1-2).[3,12,19,42]

G_0 **phase (postmitotic resting phase).** The G_0 phase encompasses that period of the cell cycle when normal renewable tissue is not actively proliferating. In this phase, cells perform all functions except those related to proliferation. This category includes nondividing cells and resting cells. Normal cells in the G_0 phase are activated to reenter the reproductive cycle only by certain stimuli (e.g., death of a cell of the same type).*

G_1 **phase (growth or postmitotic/presynthesis period).** The G_1 phase, which lasts from 12 to 14 hours,

---

*References 11, 12, 16, 21, 42, 44.

---

*References 3, 12, 19, 20, 38, 42.

Table 1-2 Paraneoplastic Syndromes

Clinical syndrome	Underlying cancers	Causal substance
Cushing's syndrome	Bronchogenic (small cell) carcinoma Pancreatic carcinoma Neural tumors	Adrenocorticotropic hormone (ACTH) or ACTH-like substance
Hyponatremia	Bronchogenic carcinoma Intracranial neoplasms	Antidiuretic hormone (ADH) or ADH-like substance
Hypercalcemia	Bronchogenic squamous cell carcinoma Breast carcinoma Renal carcinoma Adult T-cell lymphoma	(?) Parathyroid hormone–like substance Transforming growth factor (TGF)–α
Hyperthyroidism	Blood dyscrasias Bronchogenic carcinoma Prostatic carcinoma	Thyroid-stimulating hormone (TSH) or TSH-like substance
Hypoglycemia	Fibrosarcoma Other mesenchymal sarcomas Hepatocellular carcinoma	Insulin or insulin-like substance
Carcinoid syndrome	Bronchial adenoma (carcinoid) Pancreatic carcinoma Gastric carcinoma	Serotonin, bradykinin, (?) histamine
Polycythemia	Renal carcinoma Cerebellar hemangioma Hepatocellular carcinoma	Erythropoietin
Venous thrombosis	Pancreatic carcinoma Bronchogenic carcinoma Other cancers	(?) Hypercoagulability

From Volker DL: Pathophysiology of cancer. In Clark JC, McGee RF, editors: *Core curriculum for oncology nursing,* ed 2, Philadelphia, 1992, Saunders.
Modified from Cotran RS, Kumar V, Robbins SL: *Robbins pathologic basis of disease,* ed 4, Philadelphia, 1989, Saunders.

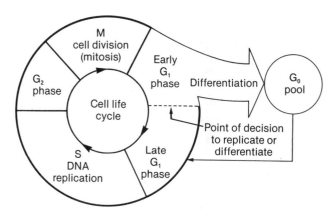

Figure 1-2   Cell generation cycle. (Courtesy Adria Laboratories, Columbus, Ohio.)

extends from the completion of the previous cell division to the beginning of chromosome replication. This is a period of decreased metabolic activity. Cells carry out their designated physiologic functions, synthesizing proteins needed in the formation of ribonucleic acid (RNA). The G$_1$ phase is primarily a stage of readiness, as cells prepare for entry into the S phase.*

S phase (synthesis). In the S phase, which lasts approximately 7 to 20 hours, RNA is synthesized, which is essential for the synthesis of DNA. DNA synthesis is limited exclusively to this phase. *Histones,* the basic protein of chromatin, are also synthesized in the S phase. Cells are most vulnerable to damage during the S phase.*

G$_2$ phase (postsynthetic/premitotic phase). The G$_2$ phase, which lasts from 1 to 4 hours, is one of relative hypoactivity, as the cells await entry into the mitotic phase. This phase encompasses the interval from the termination of DNA synthesis to the beginning of cell division. Some additional protein synthesis occurs during G$_2$, but it is mostly synthesis of structural proteins versus enzymes. Some additional RNA synthesis also occurs.[3,12,19,38,42]

M phase (mitosis). In the M phase, which lasts from 40 minutes to 2 hours, mitosis and cell division occur. Protein synthesis continues but is drastically reduced. Duplication of DNA must be complete before cells enter the mitotic cycle. This phase is further subdivided into four stages: *prophase, metaphase, anaphase,* and *telophase* (see Figure 1-1). *Interphase* encompasses all events before mitosis (i.e., G$_1$, S, and G$_2$). After mitosis the daughter cells either return to the G$_0$ phase and stop dividing or, if a stimulus for cell division exists, enter the G$_1$ phase and begin the cell reproductive cycle again.*

Cancer cells are able to complete the cell cycle more quickly by decreasing the length of time spent in the G$_1$ phase. They are also much less likely to enter or remain

in the G$_0$ phase of the cell cycle than are normal cells; thus cancer cells divide continuously.[3,12,27,38]

The number of cells in the body "in cycle" is only a small fraction of the total number of cells, and this is true of cancer cells as well. The duration of the M, G$_2$, and S phases is relatively constant, whereas the time a cell spends in G$_1$ varies from a few hours to several days. This determines the overall length of the cell cycle. The *cell cycle time* (T$_c$) is the sum of M, G$_1$, S, and G$_2$:

$$T_c = TM + TG_1 + TS + TG_2$$

Those cells in the late G$_1$ or early S phase of the cell cycle are the most vulnerable to dedifferentiation.[3,12,19,20,42]

TUMOR GROWTH

In normal cell proliferation, cell birth approximates cell death. The body's demand for an increase in the number of cells and for cell replacement is initiated by loss of cells of the same type or by extra tissue function demands. All elements of normal tissue growth are found in cancer cell growth and reproduction. However, progressive failure of intrinsic normal growth mechanisms produces the growth common to cancer.[29,32,38]

A common misconception is that cancer is a population of cells that reproduces much faster than normal cells. In fact, many cancers are rather slow growing compared with some normal cells (e.g., cells of the epithelial lining, bone marrow cells). Not all cancer cells can proliferate indefinitely, but every neoplasm contains cells that fail to abide by the restraints placed on proliferation. This results in cell growth beyond normal margins and pressure on other organs and may contribute to the tendency of cancer cells to invade neighboring tissues and structures.[20]

Tumor Growth Properties

In general, cancer cells possess the following properties[22,35]:
- *Immortality of transformed cells.* Cancer cells are capable of passing through an infinite number of population doublings if sufficient nutrition and growth factors are available.[22]
- *Decreased contact inhibition of movement.* Normal cells adjust to the proximity of neighboring cells by halting growth. They arrest movement when another cell is encountered and symmetrically arrange themselves around each other. Cancer cells invade others without respect to these constraints.[20,22]
- *Decreased contact inhibition of cell division.* Normal cells stop dividing because of full contact with other cells, not because nutrients become depleted or because of accumulated wastes. When normal cells are surrounded, they simply stop dividing. Cancer cells lack

or exhibit decreased contact inhibition of growth, continuing to divide and even piling atop one another.[20,22]

- *Decreased adhesiveness.* Cancer cells are less adhesive, resulting in increased cell mobility. This is possibly caused by the loss of extracellular fibronectin. *Fibronectin,* a *l*arge *e*xternal *t*ransformation-*s*ensitive glycoprotein (LETS), facilitates intercellular adhesion by collagen and elastin links.[22,24,27,42]
- *Loss of anchorage dependence.* Cancer cells do not need a surface on which to attach and proliferate. This property affects cells' shape and adhesiveness because the cell assumes a more rotund shape.[22]
- *Loss of restrictive point control.* In the normal cell, several environmental growth conditions (e.g., high cell density or depletion of essential amino acids, glucose, and lipids) cause the cell to be blocked in G_1. This is called the *restriction point of G_1,* or the point where the cell is blocked from continuing the cell cycle. Cancer cells lose this stringent restriction point control and continue to proliferate despite suboptimal nutrition and high cell density.[22]

Tumor Growth Concepts

Normal cells are divided into three major categories of cell growth: *static* (nondividing), *expanding* (resting), and *renewing* (continuously dividing). Static cells do not continue to divide after the postembryonic period. If these cells are damaged or destroyed, they cannot be replaced. Examples are nerve and brain cells. Expanding cells temporarily stop reproduction on reaching normal size, but they can reenter the cell cycle and divide during times of physiologic need. Examples are liver, kidney, and endocrine gland cells. Renewing cells have the highest level of reproductive activity. These cells have a finite life span and continuously replicate to replace dying cells. Examples are germ cells, epithelial cells of the gastrointestinal mucosa, and blood cells. Likewise, not all cancer cells participate in active proliferation. Tumors are composed of mixtures of nondividing, resting, and continuously dividing cells.[12,19]

In the simplest model for cell growth, a cell divides to produce two daughter cells, each of which then divides, producing four cells, eight cells, and so on. Thus, cell numbers increase in powers of two *(exponential growth).*[7,42]

The growth rate of tumors is expressed in doubling time. *Tumor volume-doubling time* (DT) is the time needed for a tumor mass to double its volume. Tumor cells undergo a series of doublings as the tumor increases in size. The average DT of most primary solid tumors is approximately 2 to 3 months, with a range of 11 to 90 weeks. In general, a tumor must progress through approximately 30 doublings before becoming palpable. The minimum clinically detectable body burden of tumor *(tumor volume)* is 10 billion cells (1 g). Tumor masses are usually 100 billion cells or 10 g at detection. Death of the host usually occurs when the body burden of tumor equals or exceeds 1 trillion cells or 1 kg of tumor. This growth from 1 g to 1 kg of tumor requires only 10 more doublings.[7,12,19,29,42]

Because not all tumor cells divide simultaneously, *growth fraction* (GF) is an important concept in the determination of DT. GF is the ratio of the total number of cells to the number of proliferating cells. Tumors with larger GFs increase their tumor mass more quickly.[12,20,42] As tumor volume increases, GF decreases. In the latter stages of tumor growth, the tumor usually has only a small proportion of actively proliferating cells. The tumor loses cells by differentiation, death, or desquamation. Cell growth usually continues only at the periphery of the tumor, with the center becoming increasingly dormant and eventually turning necrotic. Finally, the tumor reaches a point where cell death approximates cell birth, and a plateau is reached. The rapid proliferation of tumor cells followed by this continuous, but slowed, proliferation is called the *Gompertz function.* The Gompertz function can be expressed by the *Gompertz growth curve* (Figure 1-3). The growth curve illustrates the initial exponential growth of cancer cells, followed by the steady and progressive decrease in the GF because of a decrease in the fraction of proliferating cells and an increase in the rate of cell death.*

CARCINOGENESIS

Carcinogenesis is the process by which normal cells are transformed into cancer cells. Although numerous theo-

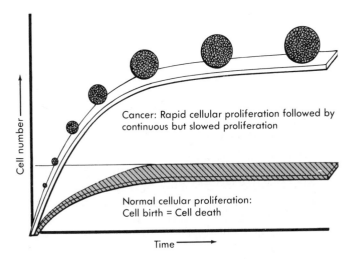

Figure 1-3   Gompertz function as viewed by growth curve. (From Goodman M: *Cancer: chemotherapy and care,* part I, 1990, Bristol Laboratories, Division of Bristol-Myers Co, Evansville, Ind.)

---

*References 7, 12, 19, 28, 29, 42.

ries have been proposed to explain it, no single unifying hypothesis has been offered or accepted. The exact cause of most human cancers is still unknown today.[12,20,42]

An understanding of the following terms is necessary before theories of carcinogenesis can be discussed:

• *Initiating agent (carcinogen).* An initiating agent is a chemical, biologic, or physical agent capable of permanently, directly, and irreversibly changing the molecular structure of the genetic component (DNA) of a cell. This predisposes the cell to transformation when exposed to a prolonged or continuous promoting agent. An initiating agent may cause (1) complete division of the DNA chain in one or more places, (2) elimination of one of the component parts of the DNA chain (e.g., sugars, bases), or (3) errors in DNA repair. It may act at the initial point of contact, in the organ where carcinogens have accumulated, or at the site of metabolism or excretion. *Viral, environmental or life-style,* and *genetic factors* have all been identified as initiators of carcinogenesis.[36,38,42]

• *Promoting agent (cocarcinogen).* A promoting agent alters the expression of genetic information of the cell, thereby enhancing cellular transformation. Examples include hormones, plant products, and drugs. Promoting agents do not directly react with a cell's genetic material and cannot mutate DNA by themselves. Although they work in conjunction with initiating agents to promote neoplastic change, promoting agents themselves do not cause cancer. The effects of promoting agents are temporary and reversible.[12,38,42]

• *Complete carcinogen.* A complete carcinogen possesses both initiating and promoting properties and is capable of inducing cancer on its own. The ability to act as a complete carcinogen may be dose related. Radiation is an example of a dose-related complete carcinogen.[12,20,27,36]

• *Reversing agent.* A reversing agent inhibits the effects of promoting agents by stimulating metabolic pathways in the cell that destroy carcinogens or altering the initiating potency of chemical carcinogens. Examples include drugs, enzymes, and vitamins.[20,42]

• *Oncogene.* An oncogene is a gene that has evolved to control growth and repair of tissues. It is the genetic code that functions as the "off" and "on" signals that cells send and receive to control reproduction. Oncogenes include *proto-oncogenes,* the portion of DNA that regulates normal cell proliferation and repair, and *antioncogenes,* the portion of DNA that stops cell division. Oncogenes are the targets of carcinogens, producing mutations that may leave proto-oncogenes permanently in the "on" position and prevent antioncogenes from exerting the "off" signal at the appropriate time.[20,42]

• *Progression.* As tumor cells proliferate, they undergo changes in their microscopic structures. This is referred to as *progression,* or the change in a tumor from a preneoplastic state, or low degree of malignancy, to a rapidly growing, virulent tumor. Tumor progression may be characterized by changes in growth rate, invasive potential, metastatic frequency, morphologic traits, and responsiveness to therapy. Progression occurs as a result of a cell type that grows more rapidly or metabolizes at a faster rate than other cells in the tumor mass. This cell then becomes the dominant cell type. Also, cytotoxic treatments may enhance tumor progression by their mutagenic effects, hastening the appearance of increasingly malignant variants.[12]

• *Heterogeneity.* The concept of heterogeneity is closely related to progression. It refers to differences among individual cells within a tumor. As mentioned earlier, cancer cells have a higher frequency of random mutation because of their genetic instability. These mutations produce clones whose acquired genetic variability results in heterogeneity within a tumor. Cells within a tumor can be heterogeneous with respect to ability to invade surrounding tissue, genetic composition, growth rate, metastatic potential, hormone receptors, and susceptibility to antineoplastic therapy. The degree of heterogeneity increases as the tumor increases in size.[11,12,15,21]

• *Transformation.* Transformation is a multistep process by which cells become progressively dedifferentiated after exposure to an initiating agent. There is probably more than one way to transform a cell. Transformation, however, generally results from a genetic alteration in the cell, which deregulates the control of cell proliferation. The controversy centers around the question of what stimuli induce the needed transformation in a cell's DNA. Many authorities believe that as many as 80% of known human cancers are the direct result of an individual's exposure to environmental carcinogens.[12,20,42]

Theories of Carcinogenesis

Carcinogenesis is believed to involve two or more steps. The *Berenblum theory,* first proposed in 1947, states that cancer occurs as the result of two distinct events: *initiation* and *promotion.* Initiation occurs first and is usually believed to be rapid and mutational. The change is brought about by an initiating agent (e.g., a chemical substance). The second event involves a promoting agent, and its effect is generally believed to include changes in cell growth, transport, and metabolism. Without promotion, initiation will not result in a truly transformed cell. Promotion may occur shortly after initiation or much later in an individual's life. Initiation produces a change in the cell, but cancer will not develop until the cell is affected by one or several promoting agents (Figure 1-4).[4]

Over the years, Berenblum's theory has evolved into

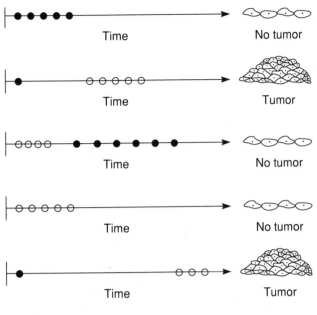

● Introduction of initiator

○ Introduction of promoter

Figure 1-4 Interactions of initiation and promotion.

the *three-stage theory of carcinogenesis*. This theory proposes that the process of transforming a normal cell into a cancer cell consists of three distinct phases with several substages, all of which occur in the cell's DNA.

In the first stage, *initiation,* a carcinogen damages DNA by altering a specific gene. This gene (1) undergoes repair, and no cancer results, (2) permanently changes but causes no cancer unless subsequently exposed to the action of a cocarcinogen at a later date, or (3) transforms and produces a cancer cell if the initiator is a complete carcinogen.[20,42]

In the second stage, *promotion,* cocarcinogens are subsequently introduced, resulting in either reversible or irreversible damage to the proliferating mechanism of the cell. Irreversible damage results in cancer cell transformation. Cocarcinogens' effects may be inhibited by cancer-reversing agents (e.g., vitamin C; certain host characteristics, such as an effective immune system; limited time or dose exposure to the cocarcinogen).[20,42]

In the final stage, *progression,* both mutagenic and nonmutagenic events occur, leading to morphologic changes within the cell and increased grades of malignant behavior (e.g., invasion, metastasis, drug resistance). This process is irreversible.[20,42]

Carcinogenesis is a process that can occupy the better part of a person's life. In humans, carcinogenesis is more complex than any researcher-induced laboratory model. The distinction between the three stages is often blurred and complicated by the presence of a *latent period* between the initial exposure to a carcinogen and the actual development of a clinically detectable malignancy. This latent period is not characterized by particular clinical or subjective signs or symptoms, and no tests have been developed to detect latent transformed cells. It is therefore impossible to predict whether certain segments of a population are at risk for developing cancer. Tumors might not appear for 20, 30, or 40 years in these at-risk groups. Also, most persons diagnosed with cancer have no obvious history of exposure to a carcinogen. This phenomenon, known as the *multiple factor effect,* plays a significant role in human carcinogenesis.[20,42]

Medical researchers have not been able to prove definitively that the initial event in carcinogenesis is a mutation. Whatever causes cancer, the final result is an irreversible change in the cellular genetic code. This leads to cell clones that eventually give rise to clinically detectable cancer.[20,27,42]

Hormonal Carcinogenesis

Changes in a person's hormonal environment most likely result from an overproduction of endogenous hormones or an excessive administration of exogenous hormones. Four main types of human cancer (i.e., cancer of the prostate, brain, breast, and endometrium) occur in hormone-responsive tissues *(target tissues).* Although target tissues require hormones for normal growth and function, there is little evidence that hormones produce any direct carcinogenic effects. Hormones do not interact with or exert an effect on nucleic acid. Rather, hormones promote the carcinogenic process by sensitizing a cell to the carcinogenic insult or modifying the growth of an established tumor.[19,25]

Chemical Carcinogenesis

Despite more than 6 million chemicals having been identified and registered with the Chemical Abstracts Service and more than 50,000 estimated to be used regularly in business and industry, probably fewer than 1000 chemicals or exposures have been examined as to their potential to cause cancer. Even so, the literature for even this small fraction of known exposures is massive. Since the early 1970s, an extensive effort has been made to systematize available data on cancer risks attributed to chemical carcinogens.[39]

Chemical carcinogens include compounds or elements that alter DNA. The relationship between chemical carcinogens and cancer has been documented for several centuries, beginning with the high incidence of scrotal cancer observed among chimneysweeps. However, chemical carcinogens are not confined solely to the occupational arena. Environmental chemical carcinogens range from food preservatives to atmospheric pollution. The list of known human chemical carcinogens is short; the list of suspected human chemical carcinogens is longer and grows yearly. Table 1-3 provides examples

Table 1-3   Chemicals and Mixtures Carcinogenic or Probably Carcinogenic in Humans

Agent	Site
LIFE-STYLE/PERSONAL CHOICE EXPOSURE	
Tobacco	Lung, pancreas, oral cavity and pharynx, larynx, urinary tract
Tobacco quids and betel nut	Oral mucosa
Ethanol with smoking	Esophagus
INDUSTRIAL EXPOSURE	
Arsenic compounds	Skin, lungs
p-Biphenylamine and *o*-nitrobiphenyl	Urinary bladder
Asbestos	Pleura, peritoneum, lung
Asbestos with cigarette smoking	Synergistic increase in lung
Benzidine (4,4′-diaminobiphenyl)	Urinary bladder
Bis(chloromethyl)ether	Lung
Bis(2-chloroethyl)sulfide	Respiratory tract
Chromium compounds	Lung
2(or β)-Naphthylamine	Urinary bladder
Nickel compounds	Lungs, nasal sinuses
Soots, tars, oils	Skin, lungs
Vinyl chloride	Liver mesenchyme
Radon gas (radiation)	Lung
Radon gas with cigarette smoking	Synergistic increase in lung
DRUGS AND THERAPEUTIC EXPOSURE	
N,*N*-Bis(2-chloroethyl)-2-naphthylamine (Chlornaphazine)	Urinary bladder
Cancer chemotherapy regimens (alkylating agents)	Leukemias, lymphomas, solid tumors
Diethylstilbestrol	Vagina
Estrogen	Breast, uterus
Phenacetin	Renal pelvis
Psoralen with ultraviolet radiation	Skin

From Damjanov I, Linder J, editors: *Anderson's pathology,* ed 10, St Louis, 1996, Mosby.

of known or suspected chemicals and mixtures that act as carcinogens.[10,20,27,42]

The International Agency for Research on Cancer (IARC) has developed a comprehensive method for assessment of human cancer risks as related to chemical carcinogens. The IARC classifies chemical exposures into four categories: sufficient, limited, inadequate evidence of carcinogenicity, or evidence suggesting lack of carcinogenicity. *Sufficient evidence* of carcinogenicity implies that a causal relationship has been established between exposure to the chemical and human cancer and that chance, bias, and confounding evidence have been ruled out with reasonable confidence. *Limited evidence* implies that a positive association has been observed between exposure to the chemical and cancer for which a causal interpretation is considered to be credible, but chance, bias, or confounding evidence cannot be ruled out with reasonable confidence. *Inadequate evidence* of carcinogenicity means that the available research is of insufficient quality, consistency, or statistical power to permit a conclusion regarding causal association or that no data on cancer in humans are available. *Evidence suggesting lack of carcinogenicity* means that several

adequate studies have covered the full range of exposure levels in humans and are mutually consistent in not showing a positive association between exposure to the chemical and the studied cancer at any observed level of exposure.[39]

Chemical carcinogens may be divided into two categories regardless of origin. The first category, *direct-acting chemical carcinogens,* acts directly on nucleic acids and proteins. These carcinogens form reactive ions that mutate DNA and do not require metabolic activation by the host. Examples include busulfan and nitrogen mustard. The second category involves *procarcinogens,* which are not directly effective as carcinogens but can mutate DNA after metabolic activation. These must be activated by carcinogen-activating enzymes attached to cells. Most chemical carcinogens are procarcinogens. Examples include soot, coal tar products, and cigarette smoke. Once metabolized, procarcinogens become *ultimate carcinogens.*[19,20,42]

Viral Carcinogenesis

Although evidence of viral carcinogenesis in animals has existed for many years, the connection between viruses and human cancers has been a fairly recent development. Viruses are thought to contribute to human carcinogenesis by infecting the host DNA, resulting in proto-oncogenic changes and cell mutation. Viral carcinogens may be *slow acting* (adenoviruses, herpesviruses) or *fast acting* (human T-cell leukemia/lymphoma [lymphotrophic] virus, or HTLV) and are *tissue specific,* infecting tissue selectively. Age and immunocompetence are believed to interact with and affect a person's vulnerability to viral carcinogens.[12,20,38,42]

The link between the Epstein-Barr virus (EBV) and Burkitt's lymphoma and nasopharyngeal cancer as well as the association between hepatitis B virus (HBV) and hepatocellular cancer has been firmly established. The herpes simplex type 2 virus (HSV-2) is believed to be linked to the development of cervical cancer, but the evidence is inconclusive. Cytomegaloviruses (CMVs) have been linked to Kaposi's sarcoma and are found in the tissues of persons with different cancers. Table 1-4 provides additional information on oncogenic viruses.[19,27,38]

Time-space clusters of persons with leukemia and Hodgkin's disease suggest an infectious etiology. However, other environmental factors may be equally significant in both these conditions. In the past the importance of viruses in carcinogenesis was considered minimal; however, as more information is uncovered about these relationships, this is changing.[19,27]

Radiation Carcinogenesis

Radiation is a carcinogen and has the potential to be a complete carcinogen. Damage to the cell by this source may give rise to cancer when damage affects proto-oncogenes or antioncogenes. The first documented evidence of radiation carcinogenesis was shown when skin cancer occurred as a result of chronic exposure to radioactive chemicals, x-rays, and other radioactive materials (e.g., paints). Radiation appears to initiate carcinogenesis by damaging susceptible DNA, producing changes in the DNA structure. These changes may be single- and double-strand breaks or cross-linking of spiral changes. Cell death may result, or the cells may become permanently altered and escape normal control mechanisms.[12,19,27,42]

Both *ionizing radiation* and *electromagnetic radiation* have been known to cause cancer in animals and humans. Sources of ionizing radiation exposure include radioactive ground minerals, diagnostic or therapeutic x-rays, and synthetic radioactive materials (e.g., radioisotopes). Factors that apparently influence the risk of carcinogenesis by ionizing radiation include the following:

Table 1-4 Oncogenic Viruses

Family	Virus	Associated tumors	Other risk factors
DNA VIRUSES			
Hepadenovirus	Hepatitis B virus group (HBV)	Liver cancer	Alcohol Smoking Fungal toxins Other viruses
Papovavirus	Human papillomavirus (HPV)	Genital, laryngeal, and skin warts Skin cancers in clients with epidermodysplasia verruciformis In situ and invasive cancers of the vulva and uterine cervix	Sunlight Genetic disorders possibly affecting immunity
Herpesvirus	Epstein-Barr virus (EBV)	Burkitt's lymphoma Immunoblastic lymphoma Nasopharyngeal carcinoma	Malaria Immunodeficiency Histocompatibility antigen genotype
	Herpes simplex virus type 2 (HSV-2)	Cancer of uterine cervix	
	Cytomegalovirus (CMV)	Kaposi's sarcoma	Immune deficiency Histocompatibility antigen genotype
RNA VIRUSES			
Type D	Human T-cell leukemia/lymphoma (lymphotrophic) virus 1 (HTLV-1)	Adult T-cell leukemia/lymphoma	

From Fernoglio-Preiser CM and others: *New concepts in neoplasia as applied to diagnostic pathology,* Baltimore, 1986, Williams & Wilkins.

- Host characteristics—these include level of tissue oxygenation, genetic makeup, age, and degree of stress.
- Cell cycle phase—cells in G_2 phase are more sensitive than cells in S or G_1 phase.
- Degree of differentiation—immature cells are most vulnerable.
- Cellular proliferation rate—cells with high mitotic rates are most vulnerable.
- Tissue type—gastrointestinal and hematopoietic tissues are extremely sensitive to radiation.
- Rate of dose and total dose—the higher the dose rate and total dose, the greater is the chance for mutation to occur.

Less than 3% of human cancers have been related to ionizing radiation.[12,27,38,42]

Sources of *ultraviolet light* (UVL) radiation include the sun and certain industrial sources (e.g., welding arcs, germicidal lights). The risk of developing skin cancer from sunlight is well documented. Sunlight is responsible for most cases of squamous and basal cell carcinomas of the skin. UVL from the sun has little ability to penetrate body tissues, leaving the skin most vulnerable to its effects. The longer and more intense the exposure to the sun, the greater is the chance of developing skin cancer. Persons at greatest risk are fair-skinned white individuals (Irish, Scotch, Welsh, albinos, those with xeroderma pigmentosum) and those who work outdoors. UVL increases the risk of basal cell epithelioma and melanoma.[19,27,38,42]

The long latency period between exposure and tumor growth has hindered the evaluation of radiation as a carcinogen, but several types of human cancers have been associated with previous exposure to radiation. Leukemia, particularly acute myelogenous leukemia (AML) and chronic myelogenous leukemia (CML), lymphoma, skin cancer, osteosarcoma, and cancers of the lung, thyroid, and breast have all been shown to occur at varying lengths of time after radiation exposure.[20,42]

Immune System in Carcinogenesis

The immune system normally controls the proliferation of potential cancer cells. Potentially cancerous cells constantly arise within the human body but are continuously screened by the immune system and eliminated before a tumor can be established. Human immunity to malignant disease is a function of *humoral factors* (tumor-specific antibodies) and *cellular factors* (sensitized lymphocytes and macrophages). Cancer cells often possess antigens that differ from the person's own antigens and therefore are recognized as foreign cells by the immune system and are destroyed.[38]

Cancer should arise only when the immune system is overwhelmed, as in malnutrition, chronic disease, advancing age, and stress. Support for this theory comes from the recognition that immunosuppressed or immunodeficient persons have a much higher chance of developing cancer than persons with normal immune system function. When evaluated at the time of initial diagnosis, persons with cancer often have abnormal immune function. However, not all types of cancer are increased by immunodeficiency.[38]

Heredity and Carcinogenesis

Knowledge about the role of genetics in the process of carcinogenesis is expanding at a rapid rate, partly because of the worldwide *Human Genome Project.* This project, which began in 1990 and is scheduled to be completed in 2005, seeks to locate, map, and sequence the more than 100,000 genes that comprise the human genome. This research has the potential to identify and locate defective genes that play a role in individuals' inherited predisposition to developing cancer.[13,31]

Some genetic markers are available for clinical use to identify individuals who have a genetic susceptibility to cancer. However, many of the specific locations for defective genes are unknown. Frequently, clinical data and family history are the primary means used to identify those individuals and families with a potential hereditary predisposition to cancer (otherwise known as *hereditary cancer syndrome,* or HCS). Families with HCS include individuals at high risk for developing cancer and those who previously have had cancer and are at high risk for developing a second malignancy.[31]

A basic understanding of HCS is necessary to understand how it differs from sporadic cancers. *Sporadic cancers* are more common than HCS cancers. Variations in presentation and the lack of easily available laboratory diagnostic methods make it difficult to identify the exact number of cases of HCS. It is estimated that 5% to 10% of all cancers result from hereditary predisposition. An inherited predisposition to cancer may be suspected when families have more cases of cancer than one would expect to occur by chance. As noted in Table 1-5, HCS is characterized by diagnosis of the same cancer in multiple family members across multiple generations, an earlier age of onset than one would expect, unique tumor site combinations, an increased number of bilateral cancers in paired organs, and the presence of precancerous syndromes and rare cancers.[31]

HCS results from mutations within germ cells. These mutations occur in the egg or sperm and are inherited by subsequent generations through *mendelian transmission* (the basic laws of inheritance described by Gregor Mendel in 1865 that describe autosomal dominant and autosomal recessive transmission of traits). In *autosomal recessive transmission,* the trait is expressed only if both gene loci are abnormal. Therefore both parents must have the gene in order for it to be expressed in their offspring.

Table 1-5 Comparison of Sporadic and Hereditary Cancers

Characteristic	Sporadic	Hereditary
Age of onset	As normally expected for site	10 to 15 years earlier
Cancer in paired organs	Seldom bilateral	Often bilateral
Number of relatives	Seldom have first- or second-degree relatives with the same cancer(s)	Often have two or more members of one generation with the same cancer(s)
Number of generations	Seldom have two or more generations with same cancers	Transmission usually seen across three or more generations
Unique tumor site combinations	Seldom seen	Often seen, particularly breast, colon, ovary, and uterus
Presence of precursor symptoms	Seldom seen	Often seen; examples include colorectal cancer (multiple polyps) or malignant melanoma (dysplastic nevus syndrome)

From Mahon SM, Casperson DS: *Oncol Nurs Forum* 22(5):763, 1995.

In *autosomal dominant inheritance,* disease can be manifested when only one gene of the pair is abnormal. Most commonly, HCS is transmitted through the autosomal dominant route, leaving offspring with a 50% chance of carrying the gene for HCS.[31]

In HCS the fertilized egg contains an imperfect copy of a gene. As this egg divides, each new cell receives the imperfect gene. However, although every cell in the body has a copy of the imperfect gene, cancer occurs in only one or two organs. Also, because multiple mutations are necessary, even individuals with a germ cell mutation may never develop the cancer associated with the mutated gene. It is important to remember that the trait being genetically passed to subsequent generations is a *predisposition* to developing cancer, not an actual cancer.[31]

TUMOR NOMENCLATURE
Histogenetic Classification System

Tumors are grouped according to the tissue from which they originate and are described by the *histogenetic classification system.* In this classification system, tumors are described by Latin and Greek terms (Table 1-6).[5]

Benign tumors usually end in the suffix *oma,* the Greek root for *tumor.* When the suffix *oma* follows a prefix designating a specific tissue, a benign tumor can be identified. For example, fibromas and adenomas are benign tumors of fibrous and glandular tissue, respectively. Exceptions to this rule include hepatomas and melanomas. By name, these cancers should be benign. However, melanomas are malignant neoplasias of melanocytes, and hepatomas are malignant neoplasias of the liver.[18,20,37,42]

Malignant tumors also use the suffix *oma* to designate the presence of a tumor. However, malignant tumors of epithelial origin are designated by the root *carcin* (crab-like), and those of connective tissue origin are designated by the root *sarc* (flesh).[37,42] *Sarcomas* comprise about 10% of human cancers. Prefixes that describe specific connective tissue sarcomas include the following[5,19,20,37,42]:

Osteo—sarcomas arising in the bone
Chondro—sarcomas arising from cartilage
Lipo—sarcomas arising from fat
Rhabdo—sarcomas arising from skeletal muscle
Leiomyo—sarcomas arising from smooth muscle

Carcinomas comprise about 80% of human cancers. Certain prefixes are used to describe the type of epithelial tissue from which carcinomas originate. For example, *adeno* describes tumors originating from glandular (columnar) epithelium. *Squamous* describes tumors arising from squamous epithelial tissue.[20,37,42]

Blastoma is a suffix used for neoplasms with histologic features suggesting origin in embryonal tissue. Examples include neuroblastoma, hepatoblastoma, nephroblastoma, and retinoblastoma (i.e., tumors that arise in the adrenal gland, liver, kidney, and retina, respectively). *Mixed tumors* contain more than one neoplastic cell type. *Teratomas* are a special type of mixed tumor and may be benign or malignant. These tumors arise from totipotential (germ) cells and may be composed of several differentiated tissue types. Teratomas arise from three germ layers: endoderm, ectoderm, and mesoderm.[18,20,42]

Hematologic Malignancies

Leukemia is a cancer of the hematologic system and is a diffuse rather than a solid tumor. This disease is characterized by the abnormal proliferation and release of leukocyte (white blood cell, WBC) precursors. Leukemia is classified as either *lymphoid* or *myeloid* according to the predominant cell type and as *acute* or *chronic* according to the level of maturity shown by the predominant cell. Acute leukemia is characterized by the proliferation of primitive WBCs; chronic leukemia is characterized by the proliferation of mature cells. The prefix *lympho* describes a leukemia of lymphoid (lymphatic system) origin. The prefix *myelo* or *granulo* describes a leukemia of myeloid (bone marrow) origin. The suffix *blastic* describes immature WBCs, whereas the suffix *cystic* describes the presence of more mature cells. For example, acute lymphoblastic leukemia describes a WBC disease

Table 1-6 Classification of Neoplasms by Tissue of Origin

Tissue of origin	Benign	Malignant
Connective tissue		Sarcoma
Embryonic fibrous tissue	Myxoma	Myxosarcoma
Fibrous tissue	Fibroma	Fibrosarcoma
Adipose tissue	Lipoma	Liposarcoma
Cartilage	Chondroma	Chondrosarcoma
Bone	Osteoma	Osteogenic sarcoma
Epithelium		Carcinoma
Skin and mucous membrane	Papilloma	Squamous cell carcinoma
Glands	Polyp	Basal cell carcinoma
		Transitional cell carcinoma
	Adenoma	Adenocarcinoma
	Cystadenoma	
Pigmented cells (melanoblasts)	Nevus	Malignant melanoma
Endothelium		Endothelioma
Blood vessels	Hemangioma	Hemangioendothelioma
		Hemangiosarcoma
Lymph vessels	Lymphangioma	Lymphangiosarcoma
		Lymphangioendothelioma
Bone marrow		Multiple myeloma
		Ewing's sarcoma
		Leukemia
Lymphoid tissue		Malignant lymphoma
		Lymphosarcoma
		Reticulum cell sarcoma
		Lymphatic leukemia
Muscle tissue		
Smooth muscle	Leiomyoma	Leiomyosarcoma
Striated muscle	Rhabdomyoma	Rhabdomyosarcoma
Nerve tissue		
Nerve fibers and sheaths	Neuroma	Neurogenic sarcoma
	Neurinoma (neurilemoma)	
	Neurofibroma	Neurofibrosarcoma
Ganglion cells	Ganglioneuroma	Neuroblastoma
Glial cells	Glioma	Glioblastoma
		Spongioblastoma
Meninges	Meningioma	Malignant meningioma
Gonads	Dermoid cyst	Embryonal carcinoma
		Embryonal sarcoma
		Teratocarcinoma

From Matassarin-Jacobs E, Petardi LA: Basic concepts of neoplastic disorders. In Black JM, Matassarin-Jacobs E, editors: *Luckmann and Sorensen's medical-surgical nursing: a psychophysiologic approach,* ed 4, Philadelphia, 1993, Saunders.

that involves immature cells of lymphoid origin.[38,42] For additional information on leukemia, see Chapter 13.

Malignant lymphoma is a cancer of the lymphoid tissue. Both non-Hodgkin's lymphoma and Hodgkin's disease are classified according to four primary features: cell type, degree of differentiation, type of reaction elicited by tumor cells, and growth patterns. If a nodular growth pattern is observed, the term *nodular* is used after the cell type. If no mention of growth pattern is made, the lymphoma is of a *diffuse* type.[38,42] For additional information on lymphoma, see Chapter 15.

Multiple myeloma is a cancerous proliferation of plasma cells (B lymphocytes). It is characterized by bone marrow involvement, bone destruction, and the presence of a homogeneous immunoglobulin in the urine or serum.[20,42] For additional information on multiple myeloma, see Chapter 16.

ROUTES OF TUMOR SPREAD

Cancer may remain a locally invasive process, or it may spread to nonadjacent areas by hematogenous or lymphatic channels. Some tumors exhibit an orderly pattern of progression. Initially, they grow locally, and as tumor growth continues, tumor cells spread to and colonize regional nodes. Finally, distant metastases occur. Other tumors metastasize to distant organs before or with their spread to regional nodes. Because there are different patterns of tumor spread, it is important to determine the extent of disease in the cancer patient.[21]

The spread of cancer depends on a series of events that occur at the surface of the tumor cell and in the vascular bed of the person with cancer. The spread of cancer cells from a primary tumor occurs by two major processes: *direct spread* to contiguous areas or *metastatic spread* to nonadjacent tissues. Dissemination of cancer cells may not be limited to only one process, since spread by one route may permit entry into another.[12,23,43]

Direct Spread

Direct invasion is the ability of a tumor to penetrate and destroy adjoining tissue. Factors believed to enhance this process include the following[12,20,42]:

- *Tumor angiogenesis factor.* This substance, when secreted by cancer cells, stimulates new capillary formation. Once a tumor becomes vascularized, its growth rate increases and its ability to invade local tissue is enhanced.[12,23]
- *Mechanical pressure and rate of tumor growth.* Rapid tumor growth creates an intratumor pressure that forces fingerlike projections of cancer cells into adjacent tissues. Uncontrolled replication produces densely packed and expanding tumor masses that exert pressure on adjacent tissues. Tumors extend into normal tissue along natural fracture lines that part in response to mechanical pressure.[11,23]
- *Cell motility and loss of cellular adhesiveness.* Cancer cells have a propensity for locomotion, and this, coupled with the slippery nature of cancer cells, promotes tumor cell dispersion.[19]
- *Tumor-secreted enzymes.* Recent research documents a strong association between the invasive potential of some tumor cells and the intracellular levels of specific enzymes (e.g., *plasminogen activator*). These enzymes may play a role in the destruction of normal tissue barriers, allowing invasion of cancer cells.[20]

Direct spread of tumor cells also occurs by *serosal seeding.* After tumor cells spread locally into tissue and penetrate body cavities, these cells can embolize, attaching to the serosal surfaces of organs within the cavity. Serosal seeding commonly occurs with lung and ovarian tumors. Although tumor cells implant on the surface of organs in the pleural and peritoneal cavities, tumor cell infiltration into the parenchyma of the organ is uncommon.[12]

Surgical instrumentation also provides a direct pathway for the spread of cancer cells. Contamination of normal tissue can occur during the course of surgical procedures (e.g., diagnostic biopsy, paracentesis). Tumor cells may be seeded by needles as the needles are withdrawn, or manipulation of the tumor during surgery may release cells into the circulation.[12]

Metastatic Spread

Metastasis is derived from the Greek prefix *meta,* indicating a change. This process permits the release of cells from the primary site and subsequent spread and attachment to structures in distant sites (Figure 1-5). A cancer cell's ability to invade adjacent tissues and metastasize to distant sites is its most virulent property. This is an important characteristic of cancer. Benign tumors do not metastasize. Approximately 30% of patients with solid tumors have clinically detectable metastasis at the time of initial diagnosis. An additional 20% to 30% of patients have occult micrometastases at the time of initial treatment of the primary tumor. As many as 75% of those persons with cancer who die have metastatic lesions in the liver, and it is estimated that liver failure is the direct cause of death in 40% of persons with liver involvement. Anorexia and cachexia secondary to metastatic disease are also frequent causes of death.[12,19,30,38,43]

The sequence of events in the metastatic process by *hematogenous channels* (dissemination of tumor cells through veins or arteries) is as follows:

- *Growth and progression of the primary tumor.* The first requirement for metastasis is rapid growth of the primary tumor. Most tumors must reach 10 billion cells or 1 cm in size before metastasis is possible.[19,23]
- *Angiogenesis at the primary site.* As in direct invasion, release of tumor angiogenesis factor stimulates new capillary formation. An avascular tumor is rarely metastatic. It has been shown experimentally that tumor cells do not enter the bloodstream until after the primary tumor has been vascularized.[2,23]
- *Detachment.* Cancer cells are more motile than normal cells. The period of least cellular adhesiveness is during mitosis; a tumor with a high mitotic index might be able to detach more cells than normal tissue. In the advancing tips of a tumor's capillaries, wide gaps exist between these endothelial cells, and there is no basement membrane in the foremost part of the capillaries. This may explain the apparent ease with which tumor cells can enter the bloodstream from a vascularized tumor.[2,23]
- *Circulation of tumor cells.* Tumor cells have been found in the bloodstream of both patients and animals with vascularized tumors. In some animal tumors, cancer cells are shed into the circulation continuously—as many as 1 million cells per day. However, most of these cells usually die. Only about 1% or fewer survive to become a viable metastatic lesion. It seems that the circulatory system itself is cytotoxic. The longer tumor cells circulate in the bloodstream, the higher their death rate. Factors that inhibit coagulation also keep tumor

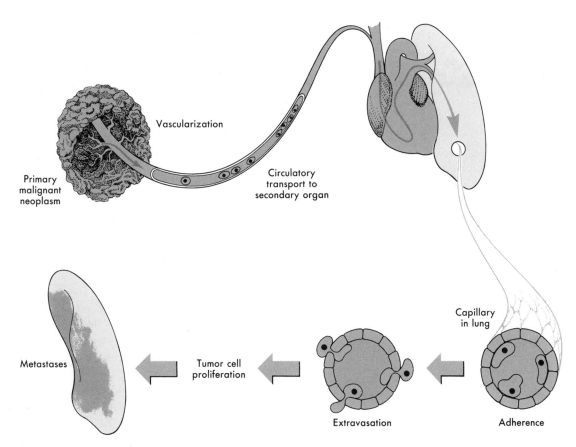

Figure 1-5 Lymphatic-hematogenic spread. (From Beare P, Myers J: *Principles and practice of adult health nursing,* ed 2, St Louis, 1994, Mosby.)

cells circulating and reduce the number of tumor emboli that attach to the vascular bed. Other causes of cell death have been proposed (i.e., immunologic destruction of circulating tumor cells).[6,9,19,23]

- *Arrest of tumor cells on vascular endothelium.* After entering the bloodstream, tumor cells aggregate with lymphocytes, platelets, or other tumor cells and form a fibrin-platelet clot. This protects the tumor cells from the hostile environment and promotes metastasis by enhancing their ability to adhere to the capillary walls of the target organ.[12]
- *Site predilection.* Site predilection does not depend on the anatomy of the circulation as previously believed. Tumor cells flow through the circulatory system based on venous drainage from the primary tumor. However, the site and survival of disseminated tumor cells depend on the *qualities and properties unique to the tumor cell* itself. Certain tumor cells possess an affinity for specific organs. The metastatic process is not random.[14,19,23,26,33]
- *Escape from the circulation.* Once implanted into the vessel wall of the chosen organ, tumor cells must exit the organ's circulation and penetrate its tissue in order

to proliferate *(extravasation)*. This process is complex. Arrested tumor cells appear to damage the intact endothelium of the blood vessel by compression. Once the endothelium is damaged, tumor cells escape through the vessel wall and invade the organ tissue itself (Figure 1-6).[8,12,23]

- *Angiogenesis of metastatic implant.* Once tumor cells arrive in the extravascular tissue, they continue to grow as a small cluster up to about 10 million cells. Continued growth, however, requires the induction of new capillaries. Without an adequate blood supply, tumor cells remain dormant and harmless, receiving only enough diffused nutrition to maintain viability. New blood vessels, induced again by the tumor's release of tumor angiogenesis factor, are needed for the continued growth of the new metastatic lesion.[12,17,23]

Lymphatic spread occurs when the cancer cells penetrate lymphatic channels draining the affected site. Much less is known about this mechanism versus spread of cancer cells by hematogenous channels. In many cancers the first evidence of spread of disease is a mass in the lymph nodes that drain the area or region of the body carrying the tumor. Previously it was thought that the fil-

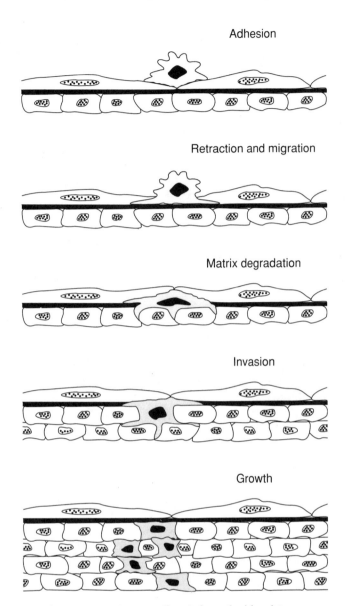

Adhesion

Retraction and migration

Matrix degradation

Invasion

Growth

Figure 1-6 Cancer cells exit from the bloodstream.

tering action of lymph nodes was responsible for nodal metastasis, but recent research shows that filtration is a relatively minor factor. The physiochemical changes on the cancer cell's surface and lymph node interaction may also be important in determining whether and where cancer cells become lodged in lymph nodes. Conventional thinking also asserts that lymph nodes become positive primarily for anatomic reasons, since the lymph nodes that drain the primary tumor are often positive first. This is a naive assumption, however, for the same reason it is now realized that hematogenous metastases are not random or completely directed by anatomy. In some instances, metastatic tumor cells bypass local lymph nodes and seed in more distant nodes in the lymph chain.[20,42]

Several outcomes await those cancer cells that do become lodged in lymph nodes. They may die as a result

of local inflammation or the encountered environment; they can grow into a lump; or they can remain dormant for unknown reasons. A significant feature of the lymphatic system is that the main lymphatic trunk enters the venous system just before the veins enter the heart. Therefore the lymphatic and circulatory systems are interconnected, and cancer cells that enter the lymphatic system are able to enter the bloodstream as well.[20,42]

Carcinomatosis, the extensive dissemination of tumor cells by gravity, may also be a causal factor of metastasis. During the spread of cancer over the serous membranes of larger cavities (e.g., pleural, peritoneal), cancer cells may break away and gravitate to the lower reaches of the cavity.[20]

Host and Treatment Factors as Modifiers of Metastasis

Several factors and conditions modify the frequency of metastasis. Factors known to *increase* the likelihood of metastasis include a primary tumor of long duration; a high mitotic rate; trauma, including biopsy and tumor massage; heat; radiation; and chemotherapy. Factors known to *decrease* the likelihood of metastasis include those that reduce tumor cell adherence to endothelial cells, retard intravascular coagulation, and kill tumor cells.[20]

Although the search continues for the key cellular factors that determine metastatic potential, all that is known to date in regard to clinical application is that undifferentiated tumors are more likely to metastasize than differentiated tumors. Even with histologically similar tumors, however, individuals can exhibit different metastatic disease patterns. This suggests that host factors, such as hormonal environment and age, are important in determining how, and whether, tumors will metastasize.[20]

Other Aspects of the Metastatic Process

Metastases from metastasis. Because a metastatic tumor is penetrated by new blood vessels in the same manner as a primary tumor, the secondary implant itself may release cells in the circulation, leading to tertiary implants. This is an important clinical concern. The decision about when, or whether, to remove metastatic lesions surgically depends partly on the threat of further metastases from a metastasis.[20,23]

Inhibitory effect of primary tumors. Remarkable evidence indicates that a primary tumor can inhibit the growth of already established metastatic lesions and in some cases can inhibit implantation. The strength of this inhibition is directly related to tumor mass. This may explain the increased growth rate of existing metastatic lesions observed after a primary tumor is removed. It also provides further substantiation for initiating adjuvant chemotherapy after surgical resection of an advanced primary tumor instead of waiting for the first metastasis to appear.[20,23,40]

Dormancy. Metastatic growth may appear in persons many years after apparent cure of a primary tumor. For example, in breast cancer, metastases can appear in the vertebrae 30 years after the original diagnosis. Presumably, metastatic tumor cells remain dormant for periods far beyond what would be expected based on logarithmic division of cells. Investigators do not know what causes metastatic tumor cells to go into a dormant stage and remain dormant or what causes them to eventually reemerge. Of all aspects of metastasis, this is the least understood.[20,23]

CONCLUSION

The essential features of the cancer cell that distinguish it from the normal cell are its ability to reproduce uncontrollably, invade normal tissue, disseminate to distant body sites, and destroy the host. These factors constitute the essence of the transformed cell.[19]

The nurse involved in the care of cancer patients must comprehend the principles of normal and abnormal cellular physiology. These principles form the basis for defining the essential concepts related to the nursing care of the individual with cancer (e.g., teaching about health promotion and prevention, diagnosis, treatment, and follow-up) and determining implications for the professional development of the oncology nurse (e.g., use of appropriate terminology and nomenclature necessary for teaching and interdisciplinary communication; understanding rationale for treatment protocols, timing of treatment, follow-up, intensity of initial treatment protocols, current research and trends in care, and disease prognoses; initiating cancer nursing research; enhancing participation in discussion of ethical issues related to cancer and treatment).[42]

_____ CASE STUDY _____

Your patient, Mrs. H., a 68-year-old white female, is admitted for a radical vulvar excision and bilateral inguinal node dissection. The patient initially presented 2 weeks ago with a 4-year history of unremitting vulvar pruritus and the recent finding of a wart on her vulva. Initial biopsy revealed squamous cell carcinoma of the vulva. Mrs. H.'s Pap smear results were within normal limits 6 months ago. The family history reveals a sister diagnosed with endometrial cancer 8 years ago, who is now doing well.

Discuss how you would answer this individual's questions relative to why she has developed cancer.

■ CHAPTER QUESTIONS

1. A leiomyosarcoma arises from:
   a. Bone
   b. Smooth muscle
   c. Skeletal muscle
   d. Cartilage
2. *Pleomorphism* means that many cancer cells:
   a. Contain unusual numbers of chromosomes
   b. Have large nuclei
   c. Vary in size and shape
   d. Contain abnormal chromosome arrangements
3. DNA synthesis is limited exclusively to which phase of the cell cycle?
   a. G_0
   b. S
   c. M
   d. G_2
4. The loss of restrictive point control allows a cancer cell to:
   a. Invade neighboring tissues
   b. Adhere to other cancer cells
   c. Assume a more rotund shape
   d. Continue to divide
5. The minimum clinically detectable tumor volume is:
   a. 1 g
   b. 10 g
   c. 0.1 g
   d. 1 kg
6. Cancer cells within a tumor can be heterogeneous with respect to:
   a. Ability to invade neighboring tissues
   b. Growth rate
   c. Susceptibility to chemotherapy
   d. All the above
7. A malignant tumor that originates in epithelial tissue is a:
   a. Sarcoma
   b. Adenoma
   c. Carcinoma
   d. Fibroma
8. Metaplasia:
   a. Is an increase in the number of cells within tissue
   b. Is an increase in cell size
   c. Occurs when one cell type is substituted for another not usually found in the involved tissue
   d. Occurs when a mature cell is replaced with a cell that is less mature
9. In cancer, *differentiation* refers to the:
   a. Extent to which cancer cells resemble normal cells
   b. Change in a tumor from a premalignant state to a malignant tumor
   c. Differences among individual cells within a tumor
   d. Process by which normal cells are transformed into cancer cells
10. Hyponatremia is a clinical symptom resulting from the paraneoplastic syndrome in which antidiuretic hormone (ADH) is produced in:
    a. Pancreatic carcinoma
    b. Prostatic carcinoma
    c. Bronchogenic carcinoma
    d. Fibrosarcoma

BIBLIOGRAPHY

1. American Cancer Society: *Cancer facts and figures—1996,* Atlanta, 1996, The Society.
2. Ausprunk DH, Folkman J: Migration and proliferation of endothelial cells in preformed and newly formed blood vessels during tumor angiogenesis, *Microvasc Res* 14:53, 1977.
3. Bender C: Implications of antineoplastic therapy for nursing. In Clark JC, McGee RF, editors: *Core curriculum for oncology nursing,* ed 2, Philadelphia, 1992, Saunders.
4. Berenblum I: Established principles and unresolved problems in carcinogenesis, *J Natl Cancer Inst* 60:723, 1978.
5. Black JM, Matassarin-Jacobs E, editors: *Luckmann and Sorensen's medical-surgical nursing: a psychophysiologic approach,* ed 4, Philadelphia, 1993, Saunders.
6. Butler TP, Gullino PM: Quantitation of cell shedding into efferent blood of mammary adenocarcinoma, *Cancer Res* 35:512, 1975.
7. Calabresi P, Schein PS, Rosenberg SA, editors: *Medical oncology: basic principles and clinical management of cancer,* ed 2, New York, 1993, McGraw-Hill.
8. Chew EC, Josephson RL, Wallace AC: Morphologic aspects of the arrest of circulating cancer cells. In Weiss L, editor: *Fundamental aspects of metastasis,* Amsterdam, 1975, North-Holland.
9. Clifton EE, Agostino D: The effects of fibrin formation and alterations in the clotting mechanism on the development of metastases, *Vasc Dis* 2:43, 1965.
10. DeVita VT Jr, Hellman S, Rosenberg SA, editors: *Cancer: principles and practice of oncology,* ed 4, Philadelphia, 1993, Lippincott.
11. Dexter DL, Calabresi P: Intraneoplastic diversity, *Biochim Biophys Acta* 695:97, 1982.
12. Donehower MG: The behavior of malignancies. In Johnson BL, Gross J, editors: *Handbook of oncology nursing,* New York, 1985, Wiley & Sons.
13. Engelking C: The human genome exposed: a glimpse of promise, predicament, and impact on practice, *Oncol Nurs Forum* 22(2 suppl):3, 1995.
14. Fidler IJ: Selection of successive tumor lives for metastases, *Nature New Biol* 242:148, 1973.
15. Fidler IJ: The evolution of biological heterogeneity in metastatic neoplasms. In Nicholson GL, Miles L, editors: *Cancer invasion and metastasis: biologic and therapeutic aspects,* New York, 1984, Raven.
16. Fidler IJ, Hart IR: Biological diversity in metastatic neoplasms: origins and implications, *Science* 217:998, 1982.
17. Folkman J, Cotran RS: Relation of vascular proliferation to tumor growth. In Richter GW, Epstein MA, editors: *International review of experimental pathology,* New York, 1976, Academic.
18. Goldfarb S: Pathology of neoplasia. In Kahn SB and others, editors: *Concepts in cancer medicine,* New York, 1983, Grune & Stratton.
19. Griffiths MJ, Murray KH, Russo PC: *Oncology nursing: pathophysiology, assessment, and intervention,* New York, 1984, Macmillan.
20. Groenwald SL and others, editors: *Cancer nursing: principles and practice,* ed 3, Boston, 1993, Jones & Bartlett.
21. Haskell CM, editor: *Cancer treatment,* ed 4, Philadelphia, 1995, Saunders.
22. Holland G: Pathophysiological features of cancer: clinical knowledge for nurses. In McIntire SN, Cioppa AL, editors: *Cancer nursing: a developmental approach,* New York, 1984, Wiley & Sons.
23. Holland JF, Frei E III, editors: *Cancer medicine,* ed 3, Philadelphia, 1993, Lea & Febiger.
24. Hynes RO: Fibronectins, *Sci Am* 254:42, 1986.
25. Jordan VC: Hormones. In Kahn SB and others, editors: *Concepts in cancer medicine,* New York, 1983, Grune & Stratton.
26. Kinsey DL: An experimental study of preferential metastases, *Cancer* 13:674, 1960.
27. Kirkpatrick CS: *Nurse's guide to cancer care,* Totowa, NJ, 1986, Rowman.
28. Laishes BA: Local growth of neoplasms. In Kahn SB and others, editors: *Concepts in cancer medicine,* New York, 1983, Grune & Stratton.
29. LaRocca JC, Otto SE: *Pocket guide to intravenous therapy,* ed 2, St Louis, 1993, Mosby.
30. Lydon J: Metastasis. Part I. Biology and prevention, *Oncol Nurs* 2(5):1, 1995.
31. Mahon SM, Casperson DS: Hereditary cancer syndrome. Part 1. Clinical and educational issues, *Oncol Nurs Forum* 22(5):763, 1995.
32. Marx J: Cell growth control takes balance, *Science* 239:975, 1988.
33. Nicolson G: Organ specificity of tumor metastasis: role of preferential adhesion, invasion and growth of malignant cells at specific secondary sites, *Cancer Metastasis Rev* 7:143, 1988.
34. Potter VR: The cancer cell. In Kahn SB and others, editors: *Concepts in cancer medicine,* New York, 1983, Grune & Stratton.
35. Ruddon R: *Cancer biology,* New York, 1981, Oxford University Press.
36. Sirica AE: Pathogenesis. In Kahn SB and others, editors: *Concepts in cancer medicine,* New York, 1983, Grune & Stratton.
37. Sirica AE: Classification of neoplasms. In Sirica AE, editor: *The pathobiology of neoplasia,* New York, 1989, Plenum.
38. Snyder CC: *Oncology nursing,* Boston, 1986, Little, Brown.
39. Stellman JM, Stellman SD: Cancer and the workplace, *CA Cancer J Clin* 46(2):70, 1996.
40. Sugarbaker EV, Thornthwaite J, Ketcham AS: Inhibitory effect of primary tumor on metastasis. In Day SB, editor: *Cancer invasion and metastasis,* New York, 1977, Raven.
41. Thompson JM and others: *Mosby's clinical nursing,* ed 3, St Louis, 1993, Mosby.
42. Volker DL: Pathophysiology of cancer. In Clark JC, McGee RF, editors: *Core curriculum for oncology nursing,* ed 2, Philadelphia, 1992, Saunders.
43. Wolberg WH: Metastasis. In Kahn SB and others, editors: *Concepts in cancer medicine,* New York, 1983, Grune & Stratton.
44. Yunis JJ, Hoffman WR: Fragile sites as a mechanism in carcinogenesis, *Cancer Bull* 41:283, 1989.

CHAPTER 2
Epidemiology

KAREN GOLDMAN

The science of epidemiology studies the variations in disease frequencies among human population groups and the factors influencing these variations. The goal of epidemiology is to identify the cause of disease so that the causative agent may be removed and ultimately that the disease can be prevented. Unlike basic research, the emphasis of epidemiology is on humans rather than animals, and unlike clinical medicine, epidemiology studies groups or populations rather than individuals. In addition, epidemiology focuses on the events occurring before the illness rather than the treatment after disease diagnosis. The endpoint of therapeutic research is to discover the cure for cancer: the endpoint of epidemiologic research is to *prevent* cancer. Epidemiology was initially associated with the study of infectious diseases. In the 1940s, however, scientists began to notice an increasing number of deaths from chronic causes, such as cancer and heart disease. One of the earliest and best known cancer epidemiologic studies was performed by the British surgeon Percival Pott in 1775. Pott first described occupational carcinogens by noting the high incidence of scrotal cancer in chimneysweeps. The astute observation of Dr. Pott preceded the laboratory discovery of the carcinogenic properties of polycyclic hydrocarbons, such as coal and soot, by decades. Cancer epidemiology became a refined research discipline partly as a result of oncology becoming a distinct subspecialty and the beginning of the computer age.

In addition to epidemiologic principles, demography and the natural and social sciences are used to help discover causes of cancer. Examples of these fields include geographic variations in the occurrence of cancer, the relationship of cancer incidence to social habits and environmental agents, the comparison of populations with and without cancer, and results after removal of suspected cancer-causing agents.

A basic understanding of epidemiologic terminology and techniques assists oncology nurses to interpret literature about cancer patterns and causation. This knowledge is useful in targeting populations for education, prevention, and screening programs.

This chapter presents the terminology most frequently found in epidemiologic literature. The terms are defined, and examples of their use are illustrated. Basic information about the types of epidemiologic studies are presented. This chapter lays the foundation for the subsequent disease chapters of this text, which present epidemiologic information specific to that disease site.

Etiology, the cause of cancer, is described only briefly here, since this information is presented more extensively in the subsequent disease chapters.

TERMINOLOGY

Many terms are associated with the science of epidemiology. This chapter limits discussion to four terms that help to describe the cancer problem and are commonly used in cancer literature: incidence, prevalence, mortality, and survival.

Incidence

The number of newly diagnosed cases of cancer in a specified period of time in a defined population is called the cancer *incidence*. It is defined as follows:

$$\frac{\text{Number of persons developing cancer in a specified period of time}}{\text{Total population living at that time}}$$

Usually the period is 1 year and the rates are expressed per 100,000 persons. For example, in 1995 for the Metropolitan Detroit tricounty female population of 2,006,867, there were 2564 cases of invasive breast cancer diagnosed. Using the formula, the incidence rate for breast cancer is 127.76:

$$\frac{2564}{2,006,867} \times 100,000 = 127.76$$

In the United States in 1995, there were 182,000 newly diagnosed cases of breast cancer in women and the incident rate was 110 per 100,000.[1] The advantage of expressing incidence as a rate is that it allows comparison of rates among different populations. The fact that in 1995 Utah had 850 new cases of breast cancer and California had 17,600 new cases of breast cancer has little meaning because of their population differences. If the rate of incidence per 100,000 population in Utah was 72.3 and in California it was 93.8, however, one could investigate what differences were responsible for the higher incidence rate in California. In addition, when the incidence rate is age adjusted, it also takes into account population age differences, which can influence the rate. Important epidemiologic questions may arise when comparing incidence rates around the United States and around the world.

The longest ongoing population-based resource is the Connecticut Tumor Registry, which has been collecting incidence data since 1935. Before 1973, cancer incidence data were collected through several periodic surveys in selected U.S. areas. These surveys, coordinated by the National Cancer Institute (NCI), were conducted in 1937-1939, 1947-1948, and 1969-1971. In 1973 the NCI established and funded the Surveillance, Epidemiology, and End-Results Program (SEER) to gather information on cancer incidence, mortality, and survival. The registries located in Atlanta; Detroit; San Francisco/Oakland; Seattle/Puget Sound; the entire states of Connecticut, Hawaii, Iowa, New Mexico, and Utah; and Puerto Rico represent about 10% of the U.S. population with considerable geographic and ethnic variations.

In addition to SEER data, incidence information is also collected in individual hospital cancer registries. Individual tumor registries are certified by the American College of Surgeons (ACS). These registries abstract demographic and disease-related information from the charts of newly diagnosed cancer patients. All patients are followed for survival data. The registries also conduct disease-specific studies as requested by the ACS.

Incidence data collection focuses on two specific areas: demographic and medical. *Demographic* information extrapolates age, gender, race, marital status, and place of residence. *Medical* data on the same individual report onset of illness, location of tumor, stage, histology, treatment, and survival over time. These data assist epidemiologists in describing the current cancer problem in terms of geographic distribution, age and race of patients, and increase or decrease in specific types of cancer.

Care must be exercised when deriving conclusions from incidence data. For example, there has been a slight but steady increase in the overall cancer incidence over the past decade. This information does not necessarily mean cancer is on the rise. Consider this hypothesis: more than half of all cancers are diagnosed after age 65; with the "graying of America," a greater portion of the population is over 65, and therefore this expanding aged population accounts for some of the increase in new cases. Apply this theory to these data: there were 142,900 new cases of breast cancer in 1989 compared with 182,000 in 1995. These figures would seem to indicate

an increasing rate of breast cancer incidence, but in fact they reflect population growth because there were more women alive over the age of 50 in 1995 with the potential to develop breast cancer. Concomitantly, marked increases in mammography utilization, allowing for early detection of breast cancers, have also influenced the rising incidence rate.

Prevalence

The measurement of all cancer cases, both old and new, at a *designated point in time,* is called cancer *prevalence.*[6] The prevalence rate is defined as follows:

$$\frac{\text{Number of persons with cancer at a given point in time}}{\text{Total population living at that time}}$$

These data are not routinely collected by the SEER registries and must be determined by conducting a special survey. This is expensive and is further prohibited by the difficulty in determining who actually has been cured of the disease and should not be counted in the prevalence survey. Also, any cancer therapy that improves survival would actually increase the prevalence of cancer.

The prevalence rate provides useful information for health care planning, including physical facilities, manpower, and the design and implementation of screening programs.[12]

Mortality

The number of deaths attributed to cancer in a specified time period and in a defined population is the cancer *mortality.*[6]

The mortality rate is defined as follows:

$$\frac{\text{Number of persons dying of cancer in a specified period of time}}{\text{Total population living at that time}}$$

The 1996 estimated number of cancer deaths in the United States is 554,740 persons.[1] Unlike incidence data, mortality data have routinely been collected in the United States since 1930. The National Death Index is a centralized source for death information and can be accessed by investigators. Mortality data of comparable quality are available throughout the world and can be used for comparison of death rates. The shortcoming of mortality data, however, is accuracy. Death certificates routinely assign a single cause of death to each patient. A patient with colon cancer that metastasized to the liver may be reported to have died from liver failure rather than colon cancer.

Mortality figures are actually only a variable reflection of the cancer incidence. Therefore, when epidemiologists try to determine causes of cancer, the incidence figures are usually more helpful. Mortality data enable us to determine trends over time in the magnitude of cancer as a cause of death among members of the U.S. population.[8,9] It is also useful in evaluating the impact of advances in cancer treatment.

Survival

The link between incidence and mortality data is *survival analysis,* the observation over time of persons with cancer and the calculation of their probability of dying over several time periods.[13] Survival data historically have not been as available as incidence or mortality data, and it is difficult to prove how representative the existing data are.[9]

Despite these difficulties, survival data are a useful measure of the end result of cancer treatment and can indicate improvements over time in the management of cancer. Survival data can provide a baseline for individual institutions to compare their local survival rates with national rates. Major discrepancies may indicate the need for education of community physicians regarding cancer management or more intense community education regarding early detection.[9] The disadvantage of survival data, however, is that the data are influenced by measures unrelated to treatment efficacy, such as earlier detection and changes in disease classification systems. These factors appear to lengthen survival without actually changing the natural course of the disease.[4] The 5-year survival rate has become almost a standard term, although there is no specific biologic significance about having survived 5 years. Myers and Ries[10] studied 10-year follow-up data from the SEER program to analyze the outcome of 5-year survivors and to determine the chance of long-term survival in cancer patients. For most cancers the chances of surviving the second 5 years are greater than surviving the first 5 years. However, one must consider the natural history and biology of each cancer. Very few pancreatic cancer patients survive the first 5 years, but those who do generally survive the following 5 years. Conversely, many breast cancer patients may survive the first 5 years after diagnosis but will not ultimately survive their cancer. The chronicity of some forms of cancer emphasizes the need for continued long-term disease follow-up beyond any arbitrary point such as 5 years.

Identification of Trends

The ultimate value of incidence, prevalence, mortality, and survival data is the identification of trends. This is the root of epidemiologic studies. A particular trend is identified that raises the question "why?" From that point, a study is designed to determine the possible cause of the trend. Why have lung cancer deaths exceeded breast cancer deaths in women? Why has the incidence of melanoma increased 1000% over the past 50 years? Why is cancer mortality higher in blacks than in whites?

The trends found in monitoring cancer incidence and mortality statistics have significant implications for cancer education and prevention. For example, the incidence of lung cancer in women increased dramatically every year this past decade. Epidemiologic studies reveal this

was caused by the acceptance of and subsequent increase in women smoking after World War II. This was an impetus for education and smoking cessation interventions targeting women. Likewise, the alarming increase in the incidence of malignant melanoma resulted in nationwide public education about the risks of sun exposure. Industry responded to both medical research and public concern by marketing more effective sunscreen products and including "sun-sense" education in their advertising campaigns.

The box, p. 24, lists some examples of current trends in cancer incidence, mortality, and survival.

TYPES OF STUDIES

The epidemiologic method is composed of an orderly progression of three types of studies: descriptive, analytic, and experimental. *Descriptive studies* are observational in nature and record the existing patterns of disease. Identified trends generate a hypothesis as to the possible cause of the cancer trend. The intermediate step, *the analytic study,* tests the hypothesis and tries to identify the causal relationship. The final step, the *experimental study,* removes the suspected cause and evaluates the effect on the population (Figure 2-1).

Descriptive Studies

Descriptive studies form the body of data within which the hypothesis may be sought. The disease of cancer can be described in many ways. One method of description might be evaluating the *frequency* of a cancer. This is the purpose of incidence, prevalence, and mortality data.

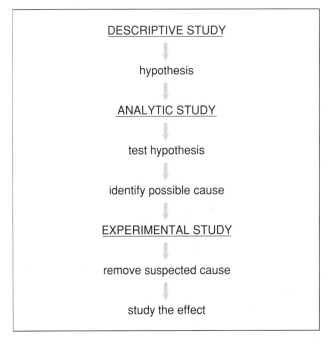

Figure 2-1 The epidemiologic method.

CURRENT TRENDS IN CANCER INCIDENCE, MORTALITY, AND SURVIVAL

INCIDENCE

More than 1,359,150 new cases of cancer were diagnosed in the United States in 1996.

Higher rate of incidence is seen in males than females.

Overall incidence is highest in Hawaiians and lowest in Native Americans.

Prostate cancer incidence rates are 32% higher for black men than white men.

Leading sites of incidence in males are prostate, lung, and colon.

Leading sites of incidence in females are breast, lung, and colon.

Melanoma incidence has increased 1000% in the past 50 years.

MORTALITY

More than 554,740 cancer-related deaths occurred in the United States in 1996.

Lung cancer accounts for 32% of male cancer deaths.

Lung cancer accounts for 25% of female cancer deaths.

Risks of dying of lung cancer are 22 times higher for male smokers and 12 times higher for female smokers.

Leading causes of male death are cancers of the lung, prostate, colon, and pancreas and leukemia.

Leading causes of female death are cancers of the lung, breast, colon, pancreas, and ovary.

Cancer is the leading cause of death in women from ages 35 to 74.

For all ages, cancer is the second most common cause of death, following heart disease.

For children under age 15, cancer is the fourth most common cause of deaths.

SURVIVAL

Overall 5-year relative survival rate for all cancer is 54%.

Larger survival increases are seen in Hodgkin's disease, melanoma skin cancer, and cancer of the testes, prostate, and bladder.[11]

Survival depends on extent of disease at diagnosis.

Less favorable survival rates are seen in blacks.

Five-year survival for all types of childhood cancer increased from 28% in the early 1960s to 63% in the early 1980s.[11]

Data from American Cancer Society: *Cancer facts and figures*—1996, Atlanta, 1996, The Society.

Specific methods are available to describe the *classification* of the cancer: site of the tumor, morphology and grade, and the stage of the disease. This information is found in the medical record at the time of diagnosis and can be extrapolated by the epidemiologist. Person, place, and time are classic descriptive epidemiologic variables that serve as a major source of clues to cancer etiology.

Person. Age, gender, and racial differences account for fundamental differences in cancer rates.

Age. With a few exceptions, cancer becomes more prevalent in older individuals. Epidemiologists previously explained the increase of cancer incidence with advancing age as an increased susceptibility problem or perhaps an impaired immune system. It is now believed, however, that the increased incidence reflects the importance of duration of carcinogen exposure and of long induction periods of some cancers.[3] More than half of all cancers are diagnosed after age 65.

Gender. More men develop cancer than do women, and more men die from cancer than do women. As women adopt roles and habits in society similar to men, the rates of non-gender-linked cancers would become similar, if the current differences are related to environmental and occupational causes.[13]

Race. There are striking racial and ethnic variations in cancer incidence in the United States. The male incidence of cancer is highest in blacks, followed by whites, and then Hawaiians. In females, however, the exact opposite is true: Hawaiians have the highest incidence, followed by whites, and then blacks.[16] There is also a significant variation in the kinds of cancer seen in different races. Compared with other races, whites have especially high rates of melanoma, Hodgkin's disease, non-Hodgkin's lymphomas, and leukemia. Blacks have elevated rates of multiple myeloma and cancers of the oral cavity, esophagus, and colon. Hispanics have especially high rates of cervical cancer, and Native Americans have a remarkable prevalence of stomach cancer. Chinese people have more liver cancer diagnosed, and Japanese people have a high percentage of stomach cancers. Hawaiian women develop lung and breast cancer more frequently than others.[11] Racial and ethnic populations present unique opportunities for studying environmental and host differences.

Other factors. Other "person" or host factors such as general health and wellness status—including nutritional status, cultural and socioeconomic variables, marital status, psychologic factors, and susceptibility factors—help to describe the cancer situation. These variables add to the body of information and may help define the hypothesis of a particular cancer cause.

Place. The evaluation of incidence and mortality statistics for various geographic locales has led to the identification of major international differences in the cancer burden. Japan exemplifies a unique cancer spectrum when compared with 24 other countries. The Japanese population has the lowest international death rate for breast cancer and the highest international mortality rate for stomach cancer.[6] Differing genetic constitutions and social habits may be possible explanations. Japanese women who migrate to Hawaii or California and adopt new habits develop cancer risks similar to American

---

DESCRIPTIVE EPIDEMIOLOGY FACTORS

FREQUENCY	DISEASE	PERSON	PLACE	TIME
Incidence	Site	Age	Physical environment	Changes in frequency patterns over speci-
Prevalence	Morphology	Gender	Biologic environment	fied periods of time
Mortality	Grade	Race	Geographic location	
	Stage	Marital status		
		Nutritional status		
		Cultural differences		
		Socioeconomic variables		
		Psychologic factors		
		Susceptibility factors		

---

women, with an increase in their breast cancer incidence and a decrease in stomach cancers.

In addition to a specific location, the category of place in descriptive studies also involves physical and biologic environmental variables such as geologic structure, water sources, flora, weather, climate, plants, and animals. "Place" descriptions also include the socioeconomic environment: urban versus rural, waste disposal systems, industrialization, pollution, and so forth. Epidemiologists may study changes in the environment that coincide with changes in cancer incidence to develop a hypothesis about the potential causative agent.

Time. Evaluating the incidence of cancer over time may indicate significant trends. The alarming increase in melanoma over the past several decades reflects societal attitudes regarding the healthy appearance of a suntan. The well-recognized time trend of mounting lung cancer deaths led to the extensive series of studies that ultimately incriminated cigarette smoking as a principal cause.

Studying descriptive data and incidence trends raises obvious questions regarding environmental, geographic, dietary, and sociocultural variables of affected populations. Sources of variability and even sources of nonvariability may serve as an element of hypothesis formulation. See the box above for factors used in descriptive epidemiologic study.

Analytic Studies

Descriptive epidemiologic studies generate possible causes of disease. These etiologic hypotheses are then tested in the second investigative phase, the analytic study. Analytic epidemiology also assists in further defining risk factors. This type of study is observational in nature, and its purpose is to elucidate which type of exposure causes which kind(s) of cancer.[12] The three types of analytic studies are cross-sectional studies, case-control studies, and cohort studies. The element of *time* distinguishes these types of studies. A cross-sectional study occurs in the present, case-control studies are based on subjects with past exposure *(retrospective),* and cohort studies examine populations who have been exposed to see if they develop the disease in the future *(prospective).*

Cross-sectional studies. These studies may also be called *prevalence surveys.* The purpose is to canvas a population of subjects to ascertain a relationship between the disease and variables of interest as they exist in the group at a specific time. The drawback of such a survey is that the causal nature of a relationship cannot be established because the design does not allow accounting for the time sequence of events.[15]

Cohort design. This type of study examines over time a population or group of individuals with or without a specific exposure to determine their disease incident rate and/or health outcome. When the study is conducted prospectively, it may also be referred to as a *concurrent study.* People selected for a cohort study all have been exposed to the suspected cancer-causing factor. These subjects are followed into the future to evaluate the possible development of cancer. For example, to test the hypothesis that tanning in a tanning parlor causes skin cancer, two groups of people are followed: a group who tanned in parlors and a group who did not. All subjects are followed over a period of years to determine if the exposed group had a higher incidence of skin cancer. The disease incidence or mortality rates for various levels of exposure (high, medium, low, none) are then compared. If a causal relationship exists between tanning booths and skin cancer, one would expect to see the highest incidence of skin cancer in the sample with the most frequent exposure to tanning beds.

A second type of cohort study is the *historical cohort design,* also called the *historical prospective study.* This design is frequently used in occupational studies because both the exposure and the onset of cancer have already occurred. Information is collected by reviewing records of the sample under study and reconstructing the disease history.

It is important in a cohort or prospective study that the time the study begins is clearly identified, that all of the participants are free of cancer when enrolled in the study, and that all participants are followed the same way. Complete long-term follow-up of all the participants in a cohort study, using medical records, death certificates, and other available resources, is crucial. Prospective studies have the disadvantage of being very large and expensive trials that take an extended period of time to complete.

Case-control design. This method evaluates a case group of persons diagnosed with the cancer under study who have exposure to the suspected cancer-causing agent. This group is compared with a control group chosen from the general population. The case-control design is a retrospective study that evaluates the outcome of past events. This type of study is frequently used because it is quickly implemented and can be performed with even small numbers of cases.[12]

An example of a case-control study is the evaluation of two groups of women—one group with a diagnosis of endometrial cancer and one group without. Both groups are interviewed to determine prior use of estrogens to test the hypothesis that estrogen use causes endometrial cancer. The percentage of women with endometrial cancer who used estrogens is referred to as the *exposure frequency*. If the exposure frequency is greater in the case group than the control group, the incidence of endometrial cancer after estrogen use is greater than the incidence of endometrial cancer without estrogen use.

Study analysis. The endpoint of an analytic study is the determination of risk. *Risk* refers to the likelihood that people who are without a disease but who come in contact with certain factors thought to increase the disease risk will acquire the disease.[15] Factors associated with an increased risk of acquiring cancer are *risk factors*. Risk factors may be associated with the environment (e.g., ultraviolet radiation, toxins), personal behavior (e.g., tobacco and alcohol use, sexual practices), or personal history (e.g., genetic changes).

Risk can be calculated as either relative or attributable. *Relative risk* estimates how much the risk of acquiring cancer increases with exposure to a risk factor.[15] Relative risk can also be thought of as the ratio of the rate of cancer between exposed and unexposed individuals. The higher the relative risk, the stronger is the association between the risk factor and the cancer. A relative risk of 1.0 means the risk is the same for both groups. Thus a relative risk factor of 10 implies that the risk of acquiring cancer is 10 times greater for an exposed person than an unexposed person. Relative risk ratios are a useful tool for identifying factors that increase risk for developing a particular kind of cancer. Early age of sexual intercourse, multiple sexual partners, and cigarette smoking are known risk factors for developing cervical cancer; women with these behaviors show several times the rate of cervical cancer than women without these behaviors.

Attributable risk describes the expected or normal number of unexposed people who acquire cancer, such as the number of nonsmokers expected to develop lung cancer in a year. Attributable risk is calculated by simply subtracting the rate of incidence in the exposed population from the rate of incidence in the nonexposed population. If a nonsmoking population develops lung cancer at a rate of 200 per 100,000 and a smoking population develops lung cancer at a rate of 543 per 100,000, then 343 cases of lung cancer per 100,000 population were caused by smoking and could have been prevented.

Experimental Studies

An experimental study modifies host characteristics, makes life-style changes, or uses screening to prevent disease. Experimental studies are prospective and often take the form of a randomized clinical trial. Experimental studies may also be called *intervention studies, clinical trials,* or *prophylactic studies.* A randomized clinical trial is an experiment involving volunteers that determines which intervention is superior among various alternatives. An example of the experimental study design is the chemoprevention trial, in which an agent is given to achieve regression of a precursor lesion, to prevent cancer recurrence, or to prevent the development of cancer in a high-risk population. The Breast Cancer Prevention Trial, initiated in 1992 by the NCI and the National Surgical Adjuvant Breast and Bowel Project (NSABP) is a prospective randomized chemoprevention trial. The study will enroll 16,000 female volunteers determined to be at high risk for developing breast cancer either because of age or personal and family history. The chemopreventive agent under investigation is tamoxifen, an antiestrogen known to be beneficial in treating both early and advanced stages of breast cancer. The objective of the study, which is double blind and placebo controlled, is to determine if tamoxifen prevents high-risk women from developing breast cancer. The population will also be assessed for lipid levels and bone density to evaluate additional potential benefits from tamoxifen. An experimental study that is *double blind* involves keeping the assignment to either the control or the intervention group unknown to the researcher and subject to prevent biasing.

CAUSES OF CANCER

Because one of the primary purposes of epidemiology is to discover the causes of cancer, the concept of "cause" must be understood. *Sufficient cause* is one that produces the effect.[14] In other words, if sufficient cause existed and were removed, the event would not occur. Because cancer is a complex and multifactorial disease, there is no single sufficient cause, the removal of which will prevent the disease. What must be examined then are various components of sufficient causes. The presence of a component increases the probability of the effect but requires other components to produce it. Components may

Table 2-1   Environmental Causes of Human Cancer

Agent	Type of exposure	Site of cancer
Aflatoxin	Contaminated foodstuffs	Liver
Alcoholic beverages	Drinking	Mouth, pharynx, esophagus, larynx, liver
Alkylating agents (melphalan, cyclophosphamide, chlorambucil, semustine)	Medication	Leukemia
Androgen-anabolic steroids	Medication	Liver
Aromatic amines (benzidine, 2-naphthylamine, 4-aminobiphenyl)	Manufacturing of dyes and other chemicals	Bladder
Arsenic (inorganic)	Mining and smelting of certain ores, pesticide manufacturing and use, medication, drinking water	Lung, skin, liver (angiosarcoma)
Asbestos	Manufacturing and use	Lung, pleura, peritoneum
Benzene	Leather, petroleum, and other industries	Leukemia
Bis(chloromethyl)ether	Manufacturing	Lung (small cell)
Chlornaphazine	Medication	Bladder
Chromium compounds	Manufacturing	Lung
Estrogens	Medication	
Synthetic (diethylstilbestrol)		Vagina, cervix (adenocarcinoma)
Conjugated (Premarin)		Endometrium
Steroid contraceptives		Liver, cervix
Immunosuppressants (azathioprine, cyclosporine)	Medication	Non-Hodgkin's lymphoma, skin (squamous carcinoma and melanoma), soft tissue tumors (including Kaposi's sarcoma)
Ionizing radiation	Atomic bomb explosions, treatment and diagnosis, radium dial painting, uranium and metal mining	Most sites
Isopropyl alcohol production	Manufacturing by strong acid process	Nasal sinuses
Leather industry	Manufacturing and repair (boot and shoe)	Nasal sinuses, bladder
Mustard gas	Manufacturing	Lung, larynx, nasal sinuses
Nickel dust	Refining	Lung, nasal sinuses
Parasites	Infection	
Schistosoma haematobium		Bladder (squamous carcinoma)
Clonorchis (Opisthorchis) sinensis		Liver (cholangiocarcinoma)
Pesticides	Application	Non-Hodgkin's lymphoma, lung
Phenacetin-containing analgesics	Medication	Renal pelvis
Polycyclic hydrocarbons	Coal carbonization products and some mineral oils	Lung, skin (squamous carcinoma)
Tobacco chews, including betel nut	Snuff dipping and chewing of tobacco, betel, lime	Mouth
Tobacco smoke	Smoking, especially cigarettes	Lung, larynx, mouth, pharynx, esophagus, bladder, pancreas, kidney
Ultraviolet radiation	Sunlight	Skin (including melanoma), lip
Viruses	Infection	
Epstein-Barr virus		Burkitt's lymphoma, nasopharyngeal carcinoma
Hepatitis B and C viruses		Hepatocellular carcinoma
Human immunodeficiency virus		Kaposi's sarcoma, non-Hodgkin's lymphoma
Human papillomavirus		Cervix, other anogenital tumors
Human T-cell leukemia/lymphoma (lymphotrophic) virus type I		T-cell leukemia/lymphoma
Vinyl chloride	Manufacturing of polyvinyl chloride	Liver (angiosarcoma)
Wood dusts	Furniture manufacturing (hardwood)	Nasal sinuses (adenocarcinoma)

From Fraumeni JF and others: Epidemiology of cancer. In DeVita VT, Hellman S, Rosenberg SA, editors: *Cancer: principles and practice of oncology,* ed 4, Philadelphia, 1993, Lippincott.

be active or passive. Personal susceptibility factors (e.g., genetics, environment, immunity) are *passive components;* carcinogens are *active components.* Each of these component causes is not "complete"; blocking the action of a component cause can make an otherwise sufficient cause become insufficient to produce the effect.[14] The box on p. 25 lists descriptive epidemiology factors.

The various theories of carcinogenesis are discussed extensively in Chapter 1. To review, initiators are early stage sequences of limited exposure and are irreversible, whereas promoters occur at a later stage, involve repeated exposures at frequent intervals, and are reversible. Therefore limiting or eliminating the promoter may prevent the occurrence of cancer or reverse malignant changes. The promoter, or carcinogen, may be the active component cause. By removing this agent, sufficient cause cannot exist.

Chapter 1 also describes the various groups of carcinogens: chemicals, hormones, viruses, and radiation. In addition, specific cancer etiologies are presented in Chapter 3 and each of the disease chapters. This chapter does not repeat a discussion of these agents, but Table 2-1 lists a number of environmental causes of cancer, the type of exposure, and the kind of resulting cancer. Some of these carcinogenic agents were identified by laboratory research; others were identified by the epidemiologic methods detailed in this chapter.

An excellent historic example of an epidemiologic study is the Argonne Radium Study. In the 1920s, many people worked as "luminators" in watch factories. Their job was to apply radium paint to the numerals on watch dials. This obviously detailed work required a paintbrush with a very fine tip. This pointed tip was achieved by touching the end of the brush to the lips or tongue. This practice transferred a considerable amount of the sticky radium paint to the mouth. In a few years a luminator may have ingested 5 mg or more of radioactive substances, which would be deposited in their bones, spleen, and liver. It would remain in these organs, emitting a steady stream of radioactivity to the surrounding tissues.

By 1924, nine young women working in the same New Jersey factory died within 3 years. Other workers developed gingivitis, osteomyelitis, and anemia. The Argonne Radium Study was initiated to study the luminators as well as chemists and patients treated with radium. This became one of the largest epidemiologic studies to evaluate the health effects of ionizing radiation on humans. The Argonne study produced an undeniable link between radiation exposure and certain forms of cancer, including osteosarcomas, paranasal sinus cancers, and mastoid cancers.[7,12] Even more than 65 years later, this study continues as epidemiologists identify, interview, and even arrange for the exhumation of additional subjects.

An impressive contribution of the Argonne study is that it served as a basis for plutonium exposure guidelines during the Manhattan Project of the World War II era.

CONCLUSION

Examples of cancer-causing agents highlight the role of epidemiology in the cancer problem. Once a cancer-causing agent is identified, steps must be taken to eliminate or limit exposure. This involves public health and government agencies at the local, state, and national levels. Nurses must be knowledgeable about environmental carcinogens not only to answer patient questions, but also to take more accurate health histories and adequately assess high-risk exposures. Oncology nurses can use their knowledge of epidemiology, cancer patterns, and trends to develop educational programs to increase awareness and prevention activity. Screening and detection efforts can be targeted to populations that are at great risk for specific cancers. Familiarity with terminology and epidemiologic methods enables the nurse to interpret medical literature more accurately; new information can be more easily understood and therefore integrated into the personal knowledge base. Nurses can develop a more acute awareness in their practice setting, allowing possible observations of clusters or trends. Curiosity and observation may lead to nursing research questions.

■ CHAPTER QUESTIONS

1. In the Metropolitan Detroit tricounty area the black female population is 516,963 and there were 524 cases of invasive breast cancer in 1995. The 1995 breast cancer incidence rate for black females living in this area is:
   a. 986 per 100,000
   b. 101.36 per 100,000
   c. 0.001 per 100,000
   d. 1 of every 100
2. The likelihood that a certain factor is strongly associated with causing a specific cancer is called:
   a. Relative risk factor
   b. Prospective risk
   c. Attributable risk
   d. Exposure risk
3. To prevent investigator biases, a study design may be:
   a. Experimental
   b. Cohort design
   c. Random selection
   d. Double blind
4. The advantage(s) of a retrospective study is (are):
   a. Study is usually less expensive.
   b. Medical records are used for data collection.
   c. The study uses a previously defined cohort.
   d. All the above are correct.
5. Cancer prevalence is defined as:
   a. Likelihood cancer will occur in a lifetime
   b. Number of persons with cancer at a given point in time
   c. Number of new cancers in a year
   d. All cancer cases over 5 years old

6. Individuals participating in a cohort study:
   a. Are of similar age, race, and economic status
   b. Must have already been diagnosed with cancer
   c. Must be related
   d. Have all been exposed to a certain factor
7. The science of epidemiology focuses on:
   a. Curing cancer
   b. Natural progression of the cancer
   c. Groups or populations
   d. None of the above
8. The Surveillance, Epidemiology, and End-Results Program (SEER):
   a. Gathers information on cancer incidence, mortality, and survival
   b. Is performed in only large university-affiliated hospitals
   c. Does not represent the minority populations
   d. Represents 25% of the world population
9. Which of the following statements is *true* about incident rates?
   a. They are more useful for comparisons when age adjusted.
   b. They are expressed per 1 million population.
   c. They determine relative risk.
   d. They are determined every 5 years.
10. The purpose of a randomized clinical trial is to:
    a. Follow subjects over time
    b. Determine causation
    c. Determine which intervention is more effective
    d. None of the above

BIBLIOGRAPHY

1. American Cancer Society: *Cancer facts and figures—1996,* Atlanta, 1996, The Society.
2. Boring CC, Squires TS, Tong T: Cancer statistics, 1992, *Cancer* 43(1):7, 1993.
3. Doll R, Peto R: The causes of cancer, *J Natl Cancer Inst* 66:1191, 1981.
4. Feinstein AR, Sosin DM, Wells CK: The Will Rogers phenomenon: stage migration and new diagnostic techniques as a source of misleading statistics for survival in cancer, *N Engl J Med* 312:1604, 1985.
5. Fraumeni JF and others: Epidemiology of cancer. In DeVita VT, Hellman S, Rosenberg SA, editors: *Cancer: principles and practice of oncology,* ed 4, Philadelphia, 1993, Lippincott.
6. Hutchison GB: The epidemiologic method. In Schottenfeld D, Fraumeni JF, editors: *Cancer epidemiology and prevention,* Philadelphia, 1982, Saunders.
7. Merz B: Studies illuminate hazards of ingested radiation, *JAMA* 258(5):584, 1987.
8. Mettlin C: Trends in years of life lost to cancer, 1970-1985, *CA Cancer J Clin* 39(1):33, 1989.
9. Myers MH, Hankey BF: Cancer patient survival in the United States. In Schottenfeld D, Fraumeni JF, editors: *Cancer epidemiology and prevention,* Philadelphia, 1982, Saunders.
10. Myers MH, Ries LG: Cancer patient survival rates: SEER Program results for 10 years of follow-up, *CA Cancer J Clin* 39(1):21, 1989.
11. Newell GR and others: Epidemiology of cancer. In DeVita VT, Hellman S, Rosenberg SA, editors: *Cancer: principles and practice of oncology,* ed 3, Philadelphia, 1989, Lippincott.
12. Oleske DM: Epidemiologic principles for nursing practice: assessing the cancer problem and planning its control. In Baird SB, McCorkle R, Grant M, editors: *Cancer nursing: a comprehensive textbook,* Philadelphia, 1991, Saunders.
13. Oleske DM, Groenwald SL: Epidemiology of cancer. In Groenwald SL, Frogge MH, Goodman M, editors: *Cancer nursing: practice and principles,* ed 2, Boston, 1990, Jones & Bartlett.
14. Rothman KJ: Causation and causal inference. In Schottenfeld D, Fraumeni JF, editors: *Cancer epidemiology and prevention,* Philadelphia, 1982, Saunders.
15. Valanis B: Epidemiology in nursing and allied health, East Norwalk, Conn, 1986, Appleton-Century-Crofts.
16. Young JL, Pollack ES: The incidence of cancer in the United States. In Schottenfeld D, Fraumeni JF, editors: *Cancer epidemiology and prevention,* Philadelphia, 1982, Saunders.

CHAPTER 3
Prevention, Screening, and Detection

MARY MAGEE GULLATTE

Approximately 85 million Americans alive today will eventually have cancer, or about one in three according to present rates, striking approximately three of four families.[11] Cancer continues to be the second leading cause of death in the United States. The American Cancer Society (ACS) estimates that more than 1 million new cancer cases will be diagnosed in 1996.[47]

Prevention, screening, and early detection are among the best strategies available in the quest to conquer cancer. The United States' goal in cancer control, as identified by the National Cancer Institute (NCI), is to reduce the cancer death rate by 50% for all Americans by the year 2000, saving about 230,000 lives each year.[52] These reductions are to be achieved by smoking cessation, diet modification, early detection through screening programs, and state-of-the art cancer treatments.[23] Further reductions may be achieved through elimination of occupational and environmental risks and changes in lifestyle, focusing on healthy choices in diet and exercise. Early diagnosis is crucial to reducing the morbidity and mortality associated with cancer. Table 3-1 shows the positive impact of early detection on survival for the four most prevalent cancers.

Prevention of human cancers is a major focus in education and research as America moves toward the year 2000. Despite advances in the treatment of cancers, overall mortality statistics greatly exceed desired outcomes.

Neoplastic transformation is a multistep process in the development of human cancers involving three sequences of events: initiation, promotion, and progression. Goals of prevention, risk reduction, and early detection are aimed at eliminating and/or modifying neoplastic transformation of human cells.

The ACS and NCI are promoting nationwide cancer education, screening, and early detection initiatives, targeting black, Hispanic, Asian-Pacific, and Native Americans and the underserved or socioeconomically disadvantaged (SED) populations. The differences in cancer incidence, mortality, and survival among minority Americans is disproportionately high for most sites when compared with nonminority Americans. Tables 3-2, 3-3, and 3-4 depict the cancer incidence, mortality, and survival rates by race and ethnic group. The rates presented in each table depict differences in neoplastic growth that appear to result from ethnic, cultural, environmental, economic, or hereditary differences within each group.

Cancer incidence rates are nearly twice as high or higher for blacks compared with whites for cancers of the esophagus, uterus, cervix, liver, stomach, prostate, and multiple myeloma.[50] Cancer mortality is higher in blacks than in all races for several reasons, including higher rates of new disease, later stage at diagnosis, and poor survival experience.[3,8,12]

CANCER PREVENTION GUIDELINES

The focus of prevention of cancer in this chapter is two dimensional: *primary prevention* aimed at measures to ensure that the cancer never develops and *secondary prevention* aimed at detecting and treating the cancer early while in its most curable stage.

The ACS estimates that 80% of all cancers may be associated with environmental exposures and are potentially preventable.[17] Smoking accounts for the highest overall health risk in the United States. Cigarette smoking is the major cause of lung cancer and is estimated to cause 83% of lung cancer deaths.[11]

Major factors placing humans at risk for developing cancer include tobacco, diet, life-style, and occupational and environmental exposures. Table 3-5 presents site-specific guidelines related to cancer risk factors, signs and symptoms, screening, and early detection. Health promotion, cancer prevention, and risk reduction guidelines of selected life-style, occupational, socioeconomic status (SES), and environmental factors are reviewed next.

TOBACCO

The link between cigarette smoking and lung cancer was first suspected in the 1920s and 1930s.[14] The ACS estimates that cigarette smoking is responsible for 85% of lung cancer deaths among men and 75% among women.[11] Over the past few years the gap between the number of lung cancer deaths caused by smoking in men and women is narrowing. Lung cancer now exceeds breast cancer as the leading cause of cancer death in women. Passive exposure to cigarette smoke (side stream and exhaled smoke) appears to increase risk of lung cancer in nonsmokers who live with smokers.[35] Smoking is associated with cancers of the mouth, pharynx, larynx, esophagus, pancreas, uterine cervix, kidney, and bladder.[11,16]

Racial differences in smoking habits between blacks and whites in the United States have also been identified. Black adolescents are less likely than white adolescents to smoke; however, black adults are more likely than white adults to begin smoking after adolescence.[12,15,19,34] Tables 3-6 and 3-7 depict differences in smoking trends by age and race. The data in these tables correlate with recent studies that indicate an overall decline in cigarette smoking in the United States.[51]

One of the national health objectives for the year 2000 is to reduce the initiation of cigarette smoking among youth. Among current smokers, more than 80% started smoking before age 21 and about half started before age 18.[12] The goal is that no more than 15% of youth become regular smokers by the age of 20 years.[15,19,54,56]

Table 3-1 Five-Year Survival Rates for Four Most Prevalent Cancers and Leading Causes of Cancer Deaths, Localized and Metastatic, Diagnosed between 1979 and 1984 in the United States*

Cancer	Stage at diagnosis†	5-Year survival rate (%)
Female breast	Localized	90
	Distant	17
Lung	Localized	32
	Distant	2
Colorectal	Localized	84
	Distant	6
Prostate	Localized	84
	Distant	29

From Surveillance and Operations Research Branch, National Cancer Institute. In *Cancer facts and figures—1989*, Atlanta, 1989, American Cancer Society.
*Adjusted for normal life expectancy.
†Distant stage refers to disease that has spread to other parts of the body from the primary site.

The following measures have been identified to achieve this goal[15,56]:
1. Offer health education classes on tobacco use in schools.
2. Establish tobacco-free environments in schools.

Table 3-2 Cancer Incidence Rates* Per 100,000 Population by Race/Ethnic Group, 1977-1983

Cancer site	White	Black	Chinese	Japanese	Filipino	Native American	Mexican American	Native Hawaiian
All sites	**345.1**	**382.8**	**247.6**	**242.5**	**212.4**	**137.6**	**245.1**	**346.5**
Oral cavity	11.3	15.0	15.4	4.8	8.9	2.1	6.6	9.0
Esophagus	3.0	11.6	3.3	2.8	3.4	1.0	1.6	7.3
Stomach	7.9	14.5	10.5	26.6	7.8	15.1	15.3	27.0
Colon/rectum	50.1	50.3	40.4	48.8	30.3	9.6	26.2	31.7
Liver	1.8	3.6	9.6	3.6	5.4	2.1	3.1	5.5
Gallbladder	1.3	1.0	1.0	1.5	1.4	10.0	4.6	1.3
Pancreas	9.1	13.8	6.3	7.1	4.9	3.7	11.0	8.0
Lung	51.8	69.8	40.6	27.1	27.3	6.3	23.4	66.9
Melanoma (skin)	9.2	0.8	0.7	1.2	1.0	1.9	1.9	1.1
Breast (female)	88.8	75.2	57.8	55.0	41.3	21.3	52.1	106.1
Cervix uteri	8.7	19.7	10.3	5.9	8.6	19.9	16.1	15.2
Corpus uteri	25.7	15.0	18.0	17.7	11.3	7.2	11.3	28.2
Ovary	13.8	10.2	9.2	8.8	9.7	7.5	11.3	14.4
Prostate	77.9	125.5	29.6	43.8	44.0	31.0	76.3	56.1
Urinary bladder	17.0	9.6	9.0	8.0	4.4	1.4	7.9	8.5
Kidney	7.1	6.8	3.5	3.6	3.1	5.7	6.4	4.2
Brain/CNS	6.1	3.4	2.4	2.4	1.9	1.2	3.7	3.0
Hodgkin's disease	3.0	1.8	0.6	0.5	1.2	0.2	2.6	1.0
Non-Hodgkin's lymphoma	10.9	7.2	8.5	7.2	8.3	2.8	6.7	8.4
Leukemia	10.6	9.1	4.8	5.7	7.1	4.6	6.9	8.2

From American Cancer Society: *Cancer facts and figures for minority Americans*, Atlanta, 1991, The Society.
*Age adjusted to 1970 U.S. standard population.
CNS, Central nervous system.

Table 3-3 Reported Cancer Deaths by Race and Ethnicity, United States, 1992, 10 Leading Sites of Cancer Death and Percent of Total Cancer Deaths

White	Black	Native American*,†	Asian and Pacific Islander†	Hispanic‡
All sites **454,516** **100.0%**	**All sites** **58,401** **100.0%**	**All sites** **1473** **100.0%**	**All sites** **6173** **100.0%**	**All sites** **15,218** **100%**
Lung 128,704 28.3%	Lung 15,472 26.5%	Lung 381 25.9%	Lung 1371 22.2%	Lung 2674 17.6%
Colon/rectum 50,516 11.1%	Colon/rectum 6073 10.4%	Colon/rectum 119 8.1%	Colon/rectum 668 10.8%	Colon/rectum 1466 9.6%
Breast (female) 37,797 8.3%	Prostate 5485 9.4%	Breast (female) 105 7.1%	Liver/other biliary 653 10.6%	Breast (female) 1297 8.5%
Prostate 28,430 6.3%	Breast (female) 4779 8.2%	Liver/other biliary 87 5.9%	Stomach 523 8.5%	Liver/other biliary 913 6.0%
Pancreas 22,519 5.0%	Pancreas 3180 5.4%	Prostate 87 5.9%	Breast (female) 387 6.3%	Stomach 885 5.8%
Lymphoma 20,074 4.4%	Stomach 2213 3.8%	Stomach 67 4.5%	Pancreas 309 5.0%	Prostate 873 5.7%
Leukemia 17,405 3.8%	Esophagus 1897 3.2%	Pancreas 63 4.3%	Lymphoma 263 4.3%	Lymphoma 851 5.6%
Ovary 12,142 2.7%	Leukemia 1587 2.7%	Leukemia 55 3.7%	Prostate 238 3.9%	Pancreas 850 5.6%
Liver/other biliary 11,283 2.5%	Multiple myeloma 1543 2.6%	Kidney 53 3.6%	Leukemia 225 3.6%	Leukemia 739 4.9%
Brain/CNS 11,132 2.4%	Liver/other biliary 1476 2.5%	Ovary 41 2.8%	Oral cavity 156 2.5%	Ovary 454 3.0%

From Parker SL and others: *CA Cancer J Clin* 46(1):20, 1996.
NOTE: Since each column includes only the top 10 cancer sites, site-specific numbers and percentages do not add up to the all-sites totals.
*Includes American Indians and Native Alaskans.
†Numbers are likely to be underestimates because of underreporting of Asian, Pacific Islander, and Native American races on death certificates.
‡Persons classified as of Hispanic origin on death certificates may be of any race. Hispanic origin is reported for all states except New Hampshire and Oklahoma. In 1990 the 48 states from which data were collected accounted for about 99.6% of the Hispanic population in the United States.
CNS, Central nervous system.

3. Enact and enforce laws prohibiting sale and distribution of tobacco products to minors (including smokeless tobacco).
4. Reduce or restrict tobacco advertising where youth are likely to be exposed.
5. Plan to unify all 50 states to reduce tobacco use, especially among youth.

A number of organizations offer smoking cessation programs and are reporting successes in the campaign toward a smoke-free America. Cessation of smoking reduces the risk of death from lung cancer; after 15 years, former smokers have lung cancer death rates only about two times greater than nonsmokers.[14]

DIET

Research continues into the connection between diet, cancer causation, and prevention. At this time the only consensus recommendations related to cancer, diet, and nutrition are to reduce the intake of fat, both saturated

Table 3-4 Trends in Cancer Survival by Race and Years of Diagnosis United States, 1960-1991

	Relative 5-year survival rates (%)									
	1960-1963*		1970-1973*		1974-1976†		1980-1982†		1986-1991†	
Site	White	Black	White	Black	White	Black	White	Black	White	Black
All sites‡	**39**	**27**	**43**	**31**	**50**	**39**	**52**	**40**	**58**	**42§**
Oral cavity/pharynx	45	—	43	—	55	36	55	31	55	33
Esophagus	4	1	4	4	5	4	7	5	11§	7§
Stomach	11	8	13	13	15	16	16	19	19§	20
Colon	43	34	49	37	50	45	56	49	62§	53§
Rectum	38	27	45	30	49	42	53	38	60§	52§
Liver	—	—	—	—	4	1	4	2	6§	5§
Pancreas	1	1	2	2	3	3	3	5	3§	5§
Larynx	53	—	62	—	66	58	69	59	68	52
Lung/bronchus	8	5	10	7	12	11	14	12	14§	11
Melanoma of skin	60	—	68	—	80	66	83	60‖	87§	70¶
Breast (female)	63	46	68	51	75	63	77	66	84§	69§
Cervix uteri	58	47	64	61	69	64	68	61	71	56§
Corpus/unspecified uterus	73	31	81	44	89	61	83	54	85§	56
Ovary	32	32	36	32	36	40	39	38	44§	38
Prostate	50	35	63	55	68	58	74	65	87§	71§
Testis	63	—	72	—	79	76¶	92	90‡	95§	86¶
Urinary bladder	53	24	61	36	74	47	79	58	82§	59§
Kidney/renal pelvis	37	38	46	44	52	49	51	55	59§	54
Brain/CNS	18	19	20	19	22	27	25	31	28§	31
Thyroid gland	83	—	86	—	92	88	94	95	95§	91
Hodgkin's disease	40	—	67	—	71	69	75	71	81§	70
Non-Hodgkin's lymphoma	31	—	41	—	47	48	52	51	52§	45
Multiple myeloma	12	—	19	—	24	27	28	29	28§	29
Leukemia	14	—	22	—	35	31	39	33	41§	32

From Parker SL and others: *CA Cancer J Clin* 46(1):21, 1996.
*Data from End-Results Group, 1960-1973. Data were collected from a series of hospital registries and one population-based registry.
†Data from NCI Surveillance, Epidemiology, and End-Results Program, 1995.
‡Excludes basal and squamous cell skin cancers and in situ carcinomas except bladder.
§Difference in rates between 1974-1976 and 1986-1991 is statistically significant ($p < 0.05$).
‖Standard error of the survival rate is greater than 10 percentage points.
¶Standard error of the survival rate is between 5 and 10 percentage points.
—Valid survival rate could not be calculated.
CNS, Central nervous system.

and unsaturated, and to increase the amount of daily intake of natural fiber (components that are not broken down during the digestive process) in the diet.

Specific dietary recommendations, related to macronutrients and micronutrients, chemoprevention, and sources of mutagenic and carcinogenic chemicals used to preserve, protect, or cultivate food sources, remain clouded in uncertainty. Estimates are that 30% to 60% of all cancers in men and women, respectively, are related to diet.[18,65] Foods high in fat have been associated with an increased incidence of colon, prostate, and breast cancer. Dietary fat acts as a cancer promoter. Table 3-8 depicts the median intake frequency per week for selected foods, by race and gender. As much as 40% of food energy in the American diet is provided by fat.[40] Studies indicate that obesity (40% or more overweight)

is a risk factor in the development of cancer of the colon, breast, endometrium, and prostate.[14,17] In a cancer prevention study conducted by the ACS from 1960 to 1972, women 40% over their ideal body weight had a 55% greater mortality from cancer than those of normal weight; overweight men had a 33% greater mortality.[4,47]

Although the exact mechanism(s) of action is unknown, dietary fiber appears to offer a protective effect in relation to colon cancer. Fiber can be found in fresh fruits and vegetables, legumes, and whole-grain breads and cereals. Several functions are believed to account for the protective effect of dietary fiber. Fiber reduces the concentration of fecal bile acids, dilutes colonic content, reduces the level of fecal mutagens, and decreases transient time of fecal material in the gut.[30,31,49,69]

Text continued on p. 39.

Table 3-5 Site-Specific Cancer Risk, Screening, and Early Detection Guidelines[14,17,24]

Site	Associated risk factors	Signs and symptoms	Screening and detection
Biliary tract (gallbladder and bile ducts)	Older Americans (ages 60s-70s) Female predominance Higher in white females than black females Chronic infection with liver parasites *(Clonorchis sinensis)* Eating raw or pickled freshwater fish from Southeast Asia Chronic ulcerative colitis	Pruritus Jaundice Abdominal pain Nausea and vomiting Fever Malaise Enlarged liver Palpable mass in upper right quadrant Lower extremity edema Ascites	Physical examination Ultrasound
Bladder	Occupational exposure (e.g., textile, rubber) Cigarette smoking Chronic bladder infections	Microscopic or gross hematuria Dysuria Bladder irritability Urinary urgency, frequency, and hesitancy	Urinalysis Urine cytology Physical examination
Brain	Environmental exposures (e.g., vinyl chlorides) Epstein-Barr virus	Persistent generalized headache Vomiting Seizures Loss of fine motor control Unsteady gait Change in personality Lethargy Slurring of speech Loss of memory Impaired vision	Physical examination Prompt follow-up with onset of signs and symptoms
Breast	Previous history of cancer (colon, thyroid, endometrial, ovary, breast) Obesity High fat intake Family history of breast cancer Exposure to ionizing radiation before age 35 Early menarche Late menopause Nulliparity First pregnancy after age 30	Painless mass or thickening in breast or axilla Skin dimpling, puckering, or nipple retraction Nipple discharge or scaliness Edema (peau d'orange) Erythema, ulceration Change in size, contour, or shape of breast	Consist of three modalities[2]: 1. *Breast self-examination* monthly at age 20 and older 2. *Clinical examination* ages 20-40: every 3 years; over 40: every year 3. *Mammography* ages 40-49: every 1-2 years; ages 50 and over: every year Baseline mammogram at age 25 recommended for genetically predisposed women Fine-needle aspiration Ultrasound

Central nervous system	Unknown etiology
	Speculation related to genetic disorders
		Headache
		Nausea and vomiting
		Edema
		Loss of fine motor coordination
		Unsteady gait
		Seizures
		Vision and speech problems
			No effective screening measures
			Family history
			Computed tomography scan of brain
			Magnetic resonance imaging
			Cerebrospinal fluid analysis
			Tumor markers
			  α-Fetoprotein
			  β-Human chorionic gonadotropin

Table 3-5   Site-Specific Cancer Risk, Screening, and Early Detection Guidelines—cont'd

Site	Associated risk factors	Signs and symptoms	Screening and detection
Cervix	Early age at first intercourse (before age 20) Multiple sex partners Smoking Human papillomavirus infection (condylomata acuminata, warts) Herpes simplex virus type 2 Diet	Abnormal vaginal bleeding Persistent postcoital spotting	Papanicolaou (Pap) test Pelvic examination
Colon and rectum	Colorectal polyps(s) Diets high in fat Diets low in fiber Genetic component: 　Familial polyposis 　Gardner's syndrome 　Peutz-Jeghers syndrome 　Inflammatory bowel disease 　Crohn's disease 　Ulcerative colitis	Depend on location of tumor: *Right colon* 　Anemia 　Gastrointestinal bleeding 　Persistent lower abdominal pain 　Right lower quadrant mass *Left colon* 　Gross blood in stool 　Decrease in stool caliber 　Change in bowel habits, constipation, diarrhea *Rectum* 　Hematochezia 　Tenesmus 　Feeling of incomplete evacuation 　Rectal pain (late sign) 　Prolapse of tumor	Digital rectal examination, annually after age 40 Stool occult blood testing, annually age 50 and older Flexible sigmoidoscopy (See Table 3-10 for frequency of these tests/procedures)
Endometrium	Postmenopause High socioeconomic status Nulliparity Obesity: >50 pounds over ideal body weight Prolonged use of exodgenous estrogen without supplemental progesterone High fat intake Diabetes Hypertension Stein-Leventhal syndrome (failure to ovulate and infertility—polycystic ovaries) Menstrual aberration	*Early sign* 　Abnormal vaginal bleeding *Late signs* 　Pain in pelvis, legs, or back 　General weakness 　Weight loss	Annual pelvic examination ages 40-49 Aspiration curettage At menopause, endometrial tissue in high-risk women
Esophagus	Elderly men (70-80 years old) Nitrosamines and ethanol consumption Cigarette smoking Precancerous lesions Achalasia (failure of lower esophagus to relax with swallowing) Combined smoking and drinking Barrett's esophagus (chronic gastric reflux)	*Early* 　Dysphagia 　Weight loss 　Regurgitation 　Aspiration 　Odynophagia (pain on swallowing) 　Gastroesophageal reflux *Advanced* 　Cervical adenopathy 　Chronic cough 　Choking after eating 　Massive hemoptysis 　Hematemesis 　Hoarseness	Esophagoscopy with staining techniques Brush biopsy Radioisotopes in tumor scanning

Continued.

Table 3-5 Site-Specific Cancer Risk, Screening, and Early Detection Guidelines—cont'd

Site	Associated risk factors	Signs and symptoms	Screening and detection

Head and neck	Tobacco (inhaled or chewed)
	Ethyl alcohol
	Combination of tobacco and alcohol
	Poor oral hygiene
	Wood dust inhalation
	Nickel exposure
	Leukoplakia
		Mouth and oral cavity
		  Swelling
		  Ulcer that does not heal
		Nose and sinuses
		  Pain
		  Swelling
		  Bloody nasal discharge
		  Nasal obstruction
		Salivary glands
		  Painless swelling
		  Unilateral facial paralysis
		Hypopharynx
		  Dysphagia
		  Persistent earache
		  Lymphadenopathy
		Nasopharynx
		  Double vision
		  Hearing loss
		  Loss of smell
		  Hoarseness
		  Adenopathy
		Larynx
		  Hoarseness
		  Difficulty breathing
			Semiannual dental/oral examination
			Awareness of signs and symptoms (cancer's seven warning signs)

Human immunodeficiency virus/acquired immunodeficiency syndrome (HIV/AIDS) related (Kaposi's sarcoma [KS])	All age-groups
	Homosexual or bisexual men highest risk
	Intravenous drug users
	Unprotected sexual contact
	Multiple sex partners
		Multifocal, widespread lesions on skin (face, extremities, torso)
		Persistent intermittent fever
		Weight loss, diarrhea
		Malaise, fatigue
		Severe cellular immune deficiency
		Generalized lymphadenopathy
		Respiratory infections:
		  Pneumocystis carinii
		  Tuberculosis
		Difficulty breathing
		Oral lesions
		Enlarged liver and spleen
			High-risk group
			Appearance of skin lesions
			HIV serum testing
			Oral examination

Leukemia *Acute*	Men higher risk than women Whites higher risk than blacks Exposure to radiation Exposure to toxic organic chemicals (e.g., benzene) Drugs (e.g., alkylating agents, chloramphenicol)	Low-grade fever Anemia, pallor Lymphadenopathy Generalized weakness Frequent infections Easy bruising Bleeding (nose, gums) Petechiae on lower extremities Bone and joint pain	Complete blood count Platelet count Physical examination
Chronic	Benzene exposure High-dose radiation Philadelphia chromosome	Lymphadenopathy Splenomegaly Weight loss Night sweats Malaise, weakness Recurrent infections, fever Early satiety	

Table 3-5   Site-Specific Cancer Risk, Screening, and Early Detection Guidelines—cont'd

Site	Associated risk factors	Signs and symptoms	Screening and detection
Liver	Exposure to aflatoxin Environmental exposures Viral hepatitis More frequent in males Alcoholic cirrhosis Parasitic infestation Chronic venous obstruction Paraneoplastic syndromes Anabolic steroid use	*Early* Bloating Abdominal pain Fever Weight loss Decreased appetite Nausea *Advanced* Jaundice Ascites Extreme weight loss Anorexia	Annual physical examination Awareness of risk factors Ultrasound
Lung	Cigarette smoking (active, passive) Increase in age Asbestos Occupational exposure among miners Air pollution (e.g., benzopyrenes, hydrocarbons) Genetic predisposition Vitamin A deficiency	Nagging cough Dull ache in the chest Recurrent or persistent upper respiratory infection Wheezing Dyspnea Hemoptysis Change in volume, color, and odor of sputum	None
Lymphoma *Hodgkin's*	Epstein-Barr virus Higher socioeconomic status Small family	Persistent swelling or painless lymph nodes (neck, axilla) Recurrent fevers Night sweats Weight loss Pruritus Cough, shortness of breath Leukocytosis	Physical examination Complete blood count
Non-Hodgkin's	Occupational exposure (flour and agricultural industries) Abnormalities of immune system HIV Exposure to radiation or chemotherapy	Lymphadenopathy Fatigue Fever, chills Night sweats Decreased appetite Weight loss	
Multiple myeloma	Older Americans High levels of immunoglobulin (B cells) Blacks at significantly increased risk than whites (14:1)	*Early* Anemia Fatigue Bone pain (back, legs) Weakness Unexplained bleeding (nose, gums) Recurrent upper respiratory infection *Advanced* Hypercalcemia Pathologic fractures	Annual physical examination Radiologic tests
Ovary	Familial disposition Late menopause Nulliparity First pregnancy after age 30	*Early* Vague abdominal discomfort Dyspepsia Flatulence Bloating Digestive disturbance *Advanced* Abdominal distention Pain Abdominal and pelvic masses Ascites Lower extremity edema	Pelvic ultrasonography (with vaginal probe) Elevated serum markers: Carcinoembryonic antigen (CEA) CA-125 antigen

Continued.

Table 3-5   Site-Specific Cancer Risk, Screening, and Early Detection Guidelines—cont'd

Site	Associated risk factors	Signs and symptoms	Screening and detection
Pancreas	Older men Smoking Chronic pancreatitis Ethanol consumption Diabetes	*Early* Hypoglycemia Weight loss, anorexia Abdominal pain Cramping pain associated with diarrhea Pruritus *Advanced* Jaundice Ascites Lower extremity edema	Blood glucose test Physical examination
Prostate	Occupational exposure Cadmium, heavy metals, chemicals Age (median age of incidence, 70 years) Increased fat intake	*Early* Difficult starting urinary stream Unexplained cystitis Urinary bleeding Dribbling Bladder retention *Advanced* Bladder outlet obstruction Urinary retention Ureteral obstruction with anuria Azotemia Uremia Anorexia Hematuria Bone pain	Digital rectal examination Biochemical markers Prostate-specific antigen (PSA) Transrectal ultrasound
Skin (nonmelanoma)	Fair-skinned, freckles Blonde hair, blue eyes Sun exposure Severe sunburn in childhood Familial conditions Previous skin cancers History of dysplastic nevi	Changes in wart or mole Sore that does not heal *ABCDs* of skin cancer: *A*—Asymmetry (change in size and shape) *B*—Border irregularity *C*—Color (change in color) *D*—Diameter (> than 6 mm)	Extensive skin examination Mole mapping
Soft tissue sarcoma (bone or muscle)	Familial and genetic syndromes (e.g., von Recklinghausen's disease) High-dose radiation Toxic chemical exposure (e.g., Agent Orange)	Swelling of extremity Painless mass Fever Malaise Weight loss Occasionally hypoglycemia Functional difficulty or pain in joints Pathologic fractures	Annual physical examination Awareness of cancer's early warning signs
Stomach	Dietary carcinogens (e.g., smoked, salt-cured, and charcoal-cooked foods) Familial and genetic disposition Persons with type A blood (15%-20% increase incidence) Benign gastric ulcers	Feeling of fullness Weight loss Loss of appetite Anemia (iron deficiency) Malaise Complaints of indigestion Gastrointestinal bleeding Abdominal pain Persistent epigastric distress	Occult blood testing Complete blood count

Table 3-5   Site-Specific Cancer Risk, Screening, and Early Detection Guidelines—cont'd

Site	Associated risk factors	Signs and symptoms	Screening and detection

Testis	Cryptorchid testes
	Young white males have rate four times that of blacks
		Early
		  Painless mass
		  Gynecomastia
		  Heavy sensation in scrotum
		Advanced
		  Ureteral obstruction
		  Abdominal mass
		  Pulmonary symptoms
		  Elevated human chorionic gonadotropin
			Testicular self-examination (monthly) beginning in adolescence
			Testicular ultrasound

Vulva	Postmenopausal History of genital warts Human papillomavirus Other sexually transmitted diseases Lower socioeconomic status Multiple sex partners Precancerous or cancerous lesions of cervix	Lump or ulcer Itching Pain Burning Bleeding Discharge	Visual and manual inspection of external genitalia Colposcopic exam in women with human papillomavirus

Table 3-6   Prevalence of Tobacco Use Among High-School Students, 1990

Race/Sex	Cigarette use*	Frequent cigarette use†	Smokeless tobacco use
White	36.4	15.9	12.6
Male	36.8	15.2	23.9
Female	36.0	16.6	1.5
Black	16.1	2.3	1.9
Male	16.8	3.0	3.1
Female	15.7	1.8	0.8
Hispanic	30.8	7.4	5.7
Male	34.7	9.6	10.9
Female	27.2	5.5	1.0

From Centers for Disease Control and Prevention: *Youth Risk Behavior Survey*, Atlanta, 1990, The Center.
*Smoked at any time during the 30 days preceding the survey.
†Smoked on more than 25 of the 30 days preceding the survey.

Table 3-7   Trends in Smoking Prevalence, 1965-1987, Adults Ages 20 and Older[8]

Race	1965	1976	1987
Blacks	43.0%	41.2%	34.0%
Whites	40.0%	35.6%	28.8%

The *food guide pyramid* (Figure 3-1) is now widely used to increase public awareness about healthier eating. The pyramid reinforces the principles of good nutrition, balance, and variety in daily food choices. The food guide is also consistent with the dietary guidelines from both the ACS and NCI.[4]

Several micronutrients have been profiled as having a protective effect in reducing cancer risk. Naturally occurring vitamin A in the form of β-*carotene*, found in yellow and green vegetables and fruits, and *retinol*, occurring in foods of animal origin, dairy products, eggs, and liver, are associated with a protective effect against cancer. Inverse associations have been found in studies relating vitamin A precursors and cancers of the lung, larynx, esophagus, stomach, and prostate.[27,28,31]

The protective action of vitamin C hinders the formation of nitrosamines by blocking the reaction between nitrite and amines. Historic studies have shown an inverse association between vitamin C and cancers of the stomach, esophagus, larynx, and cervix.

Another micronutrient is *selenium*. Animal studies involving selenium indicate a protective role against chemically induced cancers. A fine line exists between therapeutic and toxic levels of selenium, however, and the evidence does not support its use as an anticancer compound.[14,40]

Table 3-8 Median Intake Frequency per Week for Selected Foods,* by Race and Sex

Food	White		Black		Hispanic	
	Male	Female	Male	Female	Male	Female
High-fiber bread or cereal	3.0	3.0	0.5	1.0	1.0	1.0
All fruit	3.0	3.9	2.5	3.2	3.4	4.2
Fruit, juice	7.5	9.0	8.0	9.0	9.1	10.2
Dried legumes, chili	0.7	0.5	1.0	0.5	2.0	1.0
Garden vegetables	4.9	5.4	5.0	5.2	6.2	7.0
Potatoes	4.0	3.0	3.0	2.7	3.2	3.0
Salad	2.0	3.0	1.0	1.2	2.0	3.0
Hamburger, beef, pork	3.3	2.5	3.2	2.7	4.0	3.2
Chicken, fish	1.6	1.7	3.0	2.9	2.3	2.0
Bacon, sausage, hot dogs, lunch meats	3.5	2.1	5.0	3.6	3.4	2.2
Beer, wine, liquors	1.9	0.2	1.3	0.0	2.6	0.1

From American Cancer Society: *Cancer facts and figures for minority Americans,* Atlanta, 1991, The Society; data from National Health Interview Survey, 1987.

*Estimates are weighted to reflect U.S. census population estimates for 1987.

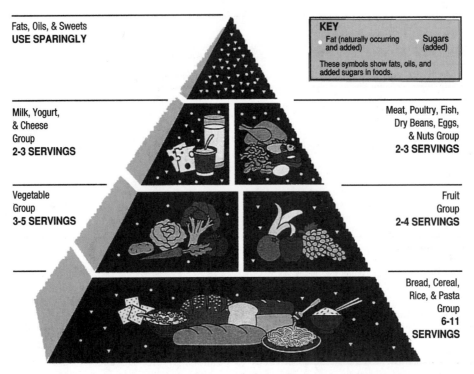

Figure 3-1 A guide to daily food choices. (From US Department of Agriculture: USDA's food guide pyramid, USDA Human Nutrition Information Pub No. 249, Washington, DC, 1992, US Government Printing Office. In Potter PA, Perry AG: *Fundamentals of nursing: concepts, process, and practice,* ed 3, 1993, St Louis, Mosby.)

The NCI estimates that dietary modifications could save 30,000 lives by the year 2000.[23] The NCI is currently sponsoring human chemoprevention and diet and nutrition trials in an effort to answer questions and update earlier studies related to the diet and cancer connection. Cancer prevention trials are aimed at behavior modification or deliberate and planned intervention designed to interfere with carcinogenesis. These trials may be either nutritive or nonnutritive. Two nonnutritive hormonal agents are presently being inves-

DIETARY RECOMMENDATIONS FOR CANCER PREVENTION

1. Reduce the amount of saturated and unsaturated fats in the diet from 40% to 30% of total daily caloric intake.
2. Increase the amount of fiber in the diet by eating fresh fruits, vegetables (especially cruciferous vegetables), and whole-grain breads and cereals.
3. Drink alcoholic beverages in moderation (one or two drinks daily) or not at all.
4. Eat limited amounts of broiled, charcoaled, smoked, and salt- or nitrite-cured foods.
5. Maintain ideal body weight.

Modified from American Cancer Society: *Cancer facts and figures—1996,* Atlanta, 1996, The Society.

tigated. The NCI and the National Surgical Adjuvant Breast and Bowel Project (NSABP) are conducting placebo-controlled tamoxifen trials for women at increased risk of developing breast cancer and a trial involving finasteride, a 5-α reductase inhibitor for prostate cancer prevention.[4] The ACS, NCI, and other organizations with an interest in health promotion through dietary modifications have developed dietary guidelines to reduce cancer and other health risks. These dietary recommendations have many similarities and are summarized in the box above.

ALCOHOL

Excessive consumption of ethyl alcohol can lead to cancers in the head and neck, larynx, and possibly the liver and pancreas.[9,39,52,68] The synergistic effects of alcohol and tobacco can be a lethal combination. The lethal effects of alcohol and tobacco may involve the direct action of alcohol on epithelial tissues or the ability of alcohol as a solvent to increase the delivery of smoke-derived chemicals, including formaldehyde, arsenic, tar, and many others, to cause cancer.

GENETIC PREDISPOSITION

The genetic or family factor associated with cancer risk and causation is recognized but not well understood. There are two approaches in the study of familial clustering: epidemiologic and genetic. The *epidemiologic approach* examines the frequency of the disease among relatives; the *genetic approach* studies the pattern of disease expression among relatives.[1,29,43] These approaches help to provide evidence of familial aggregation but do not answer why a particular cancer expresses itself. The greatest known cancer risk exists when there is a primary

relative of a patient with an autosomal dominant inherited cancer.[42-44] A thorough and complete family history can be invaluable in identifying relative risks (RRs) and traits within a family aggregate.

The first report of familial aggregation of breast cancer was in Roman medical literature in 100 AD.[42] Studies in the 1930s revealed that the RR for developing breast cancer if a first-degree relative had the disease was twofold to threefold. Although the role of genetics is not completely clear in human oncogenesis, it is certain that the environmental carcinogens in the tissue is modified by the host-genetic makeup.[35] No known genetic basis exists to explain the major racial differences in cancer incidence and outcome.[26] Continued research into the genetic/hereditary factor in the development of human cancers represents another edge in the fight toward cancer prevention and risk reduction.

SOCIOECONOMIC FACTORS

Issues related to barriers to primary prevention and health care access have been reported as major factors in the differences in cancer incidence, delayed diagnosis, poor survival statistics, and increased mortality from cancer in minority and SED populations. Figure 3-2 reviews the 5-year relative survival rate for all cancers diagnosed between 1986 and 1991. There is a marked difference in overall survival for blacks and whites; the rate is 58% for whites and 42% for blacks.[10-12,47] The estimated numbers of cancer cases and deaths for blacks in 1992 were 115,000 and 58,401.[7,10,47]

The ACS, in collaboration with the NCI and the Centers for Disease Control and Prevention (CDC), in May and June 1989 sponsored national hearings on cancer and the poor. The objective of the hearings was to determine the magnitude of unmet cancer prevention and control needs among poor and underserved Americans. The most profound findings came from the ACS's report to the nation in June 1989. Freeman,[26] then president of the National ACS, reported the following five critical issues related to cancer and the poor:

1. Poor people endure greater pain and suffering from cancer than other Americans.
2. Poor people and their families must make extraordinary personal sacrifices to obtain and pay for health care.
3. Poor people face substantial obstacles in obtaining and using health insurance and often do not seek care if they cannot pay for it.
4. Current cancer education programs are culturally insensitive and irrelevant to many poor Americans.
5. Fatalism about cancer is prevalent among the poor and prevents them from seeking health care.

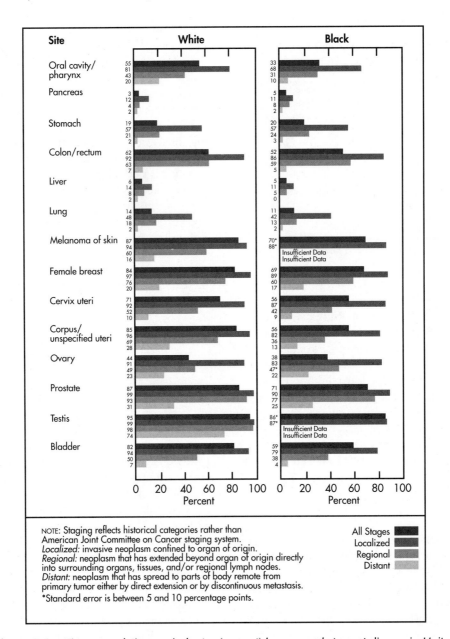

Figure 3-2   Five-year relative survival rates (percent) by race and stage at diagnosis, United States, 1986-1991. (Redrawn from: Parker SL and others: Cancer statistics, 1996, *CA Cancer J Clin* 46(1):20, 1996.)

Freeman further reported other findings about the poor: there are 39 million poor Americans (living below the poverty level of $11,200 a year for a family of four); two thirds of the poor are white, and nearly one third are black; and a total of 37 million Americans have no health insurance.[26] Poverty is a proxy for other elements of living, including lack of education, unemployment, substandard housing, inadequate nutrition, risk-promoting behaviors and life-style, and limited or no access to health care.[5,10,12,26] Freeman remarked that to be poor and black and to have cancer is a double-jeopardy

situation.[26] Differences in survival for blacks and SED populations largely result from the late stage of cancer diagnosis.

In a study of socioeconomic factors and cancer incidence among blacks and whites, Baquet and others[5] found that when age-adjusted incidence data were correlated with SES, the comparative risks changed: whites showed an elevated risk of cancer at all sites combined. These findings, presented in Table 3-9, conclude that the disproportionate distribution of blacks at lower socioeconomic levels accounts for a large percentage of their ex-

Table 3-9 Incidence Rates* by Race, Income, and Educational Level, Ages 25 and Older, 1978 to 1982

	White	Black
EDUCATIONAL LEVEL		
<12 years of school	385.9	383.0
High-school graduate	352.6	324.4
Some college	342.1	339.8
College graduate	338.3	270.6
TOTAL	350.5	328.7
INCOME LEVEL (ANNUAL)		
Less than $15,000	403.2	371.7
$15,000-$24,999	352.7	341.9
$25,000-$29,999	348.1	285.8
$30,000 and over	336.8	326.6
TOTAL	349.3	323.4

From Boring CC, Squires TS, Heath CW: *CA Cancer J Clin* 43(1):7, 1993.
*Rates are per 100,000 and are age adjusted to the 1970 U.S. standard population.

cess cancer burden. It is therefore imperative for health care professionals to target SED and minority populations with culturally sensitive and relevant educational information on cancer prevention, risk reduction, and early detection and to legislate for changes in health care policies to facilitate access to health care for all Americans. In the words of the great civil rights leader, the Reverend Martin Luther King, Jr., "Of all the forms of inequality, injustice in health is the most shocking and inhumane."[26]

ELECTROMAGNETIC FIELDS

The public continues to express concern about cancer risk and exposure to electromagnetic fields (EMFs). The presence of electric power lines, running through and surrounding residential and industrial areas where one lives and works, is the basis of this growing concern. Epidemiologic studies have been in progress since the late 1970s attempting to document a possible link between EMF exposure over time and the development of certain cancers in humans. In a review of the literature by Heath,[36] at present no form of electromagnetic energy at frequency levels below those of ionizing radiation (x-rays) and ultraviolet radiation has been shown to cause cancer.

SUNLIGHT

The sun is the primary source of natural ultraviolet (UV) light exposure that is known to cause skin cancer. The three types of skin cancers are basal cell, squamous cell, and melanoma. Of the three types of skin cancer, *mela-*

noma is the most potentially lethal and is increasing in incidence at a rate of 4% per year.[11]

At highest risk for developing skin cancer are persons who work outdoors, who are fair-skinned, and with occupational exposure to coal tar, arsenic compounds, and radium. Among blacks the incidence of skin cancer development is low because of heavy skin pigmentation. UV rays of the sun are strongest between 10 AM and 3 PM. Sun exposure should be limited during those hours and/or protective clothing (hats, scarves, long sleeves) worn to offer some protection from the UV rays. Children should be especially protected because of the possible link between severe sunburn in childhood and greatly increased risk of melanoma in later life.[11] Sunscreens should be worn when deliberate sun exposure is expected (i.e., when pool side or on the beach). A sunscreen with a sun protection factor (SPF) of 15 or higher should be worn on all sun-exposed skin surfaces. Sunscreens protect against a spectra of UV rays and should be applied before sun exposure and reapplied after being in the water. Suntanning parlors, which are increasing in popularity among Americans, should be avoided.

Early detection of skin cancers is crucial to saving lives and reducing the extent of surgical intervention. Basal and squamous cell cancers of the skin usually appear over areas of the body chronically exposed to the sun, including the nose, cheeks, and ears. These cancers appear as pale, waxlike nodules or a red, scaly patch that tends to bleed. Melanomas are small, molelike eruptions on the skin that can appear anywhere on the body, including the soles of the feet and palms of the hand. Melanomas change in color, shape, and size and can ulcerate and bleed.

A simple *ABCD* rule outlines the warning signs of melanoma: *A* is for asymmetry; *B* is for border irregularity; *C* is for change in color or pigmentation; and *D* is for diameter greater than 6 mm.[11] Adults should practice skin self-examination and mole mapping monthly and report any suspicious indicators to a member of the health care team.

SEXUAL LIFE-STYLES

Sexual beliefs, attitudes, and practices are no longer private and unassuming. The sexual mores of the 1980s and 1990s have thrust the association between sexual activity and cancer risk from obscurity to the front lines. The advertising slogan "sex sells" has almost prompted an attitude of "anything goes." Sexually transmitted diseases (STDs), genital cancers, and acquired immunodeficiency syndrome (AIDS) have a documented direct relationship to sexual life-styles and practices. The association between sex and genital cancer has been known for more than 150 years.[37] Research indicates an association between sexual life-styles and cancer of the cervix, vulva, vagina, and AIDS. Risk factors common in women with cervical cancer include a high rate of STDs, early age at first coitus, multiple sexual partners, and exposure to high-risk sexual partners. Several viruses have been implicated in the etiology of cervical neoplasia, including herpes simplex virus (HSV) and human papillomavirus (HPV). Penile HPV (genital wart or condyloma acuminatum) infection in a male partner places the woman at risk of cervical cancer.

The incurable and deadly disease AIDS has cast a shadow over the American sexual revolution and sexual freedom as has no other disease or health threat. Sexual behaviors considered to be high-risk factors associated with AIDS include unprotected vaginal or anal intercourse, internal "water sports" (urinating into a body cavity such as the vagina or anus), "fisting" (inserting a finger, fingers, or fist into the anus), and oral-anal sex, also known as "rimming."[37] Sharing of dirty needles by intravenous (IV) drug users is also a high-risk factor. Male homosexuals and IV drug users are at greatest risk for acquiring AIDS and other related neoplasms; however, the CDC reports a growing rate of human immunodeficiency virus (HIV) and AIDS cases among the hetero-

sexual population.[63] The mortality rate for AIDS is greater than 40% within the first year of diagnosis.[37,63] Reducing the cancer risk related to sexual life-styles can be effected by safe sexual practices.[33,62]

EARLY DETECTION AND SCREENING RECOMMENDATIONS

Americans are adopting more health-conscious behaviors, including diet modification, physical fitness, smoking cessation, and overall healthier life-styles. Heightened awareness of health-promoting activities and early detection techniques related to cancer continue to be a focus of many cancer information agencies (e.g., ACS, NCI) and professional organizations (e.g., Oncology Nursing Society). In 1996 the ACS updated screening and early detection guidelines (Table 3-10).

A number of socioeconomic barriers to screening and early detection exist, such as lack of health insurance, poverty, unemployment, and lack of education. Empowering people to overcome some of these barriers is key to the success of reducing cancer related deaths by the year 2000. Overall cancer survival can be increased through

Table 3-10 Summary of American Cancer Society Recommendations for the Early Detection of Cancer in Asymptomatic People

	Population		
Test or procedure	Sex	Age	Frequency
Sigmoidoscopy, preferably flexible	M & F	50 and over	Every 3 to 5 years
Fecal occult blood test	M & F	50 and over	Every year
Digital rectal examination	M & F	40 and over	Every year
Prostate examination	M	50 and over*	Every year
Papanicolaou (Pap) test	F	All women who are or have been sexually active or who have reached age 18 should have an annual Pap test and pelvic examination. After a woman has had three or more consecutive satisfactory normal annual examinations, the Pap test may be performed less frequently at the discretion of her physician.	
Pelvic examination	F	18-40	Every 1-3 years with Pap test
		Over 40	Every year
Endometrial tissue sample	F	At menopause, women at high risk†	At menopause
Breast self-examination	F	20 and over	Every month
Clinical breast examination	F	20-40	Every 3 years
		Over 40	Every year
Mammography‡	F	40-49	Every 1-2 years
		50 and over	Every year
Health counseling and cancer checkup§	M & F	Over 20	Every 3 years
	M & F	Over 40	Every year

From Fink DJ, Mettlin CJ: Cancer detection: the cancer related checkup guidelines. In Murphy G, Lawrence W, Lenhard R, editors: *ACS textbook of clinical oncology,* ed 2, Atlanta, 1995, American Cancer Society.
*Annual digital rectal examination and prostate-specific antigen (PSA) testing should be performed on men age 50 and older. If either is abnormal, further evaluation should be considered.
†History of infertility, obesity, failure to ovulate, abnormal uterine bleeding, or estrogen therapy.
‡Screening mammography should begin by age 40.
§To include examination for cancers of the thyroid, testes, prostate, ovaries, lymph nodes, oral region, and skin.

NURSING MANAGEMENT

Patient and family education in the prevention, screening, and early detection of cancer lays the foundation for overcoming ignorance and fear of cancer related to health beliefs, practices, and attitudes. Nurses can take active roles in sharing knowledge, skills, and expertise with those Americans who have limited access to health care and who are at a higher risk for developing certain cancers. Nurses can work through neighborhood outreach groups and legislators to advocate for reduced-cost or no-cost cancer screening tests for the underserved and high-risk population. Nurses can involve at-risk youth by facilitating health education programs, conducting risk appraisals, and providing information on nutrition and life-style choices and changes for health promotion and disease prevention. (See box below.)

Overall, professional nurses can have the greatest impact on the public by "walking the talk," that is, by practicing good health habits, weight reduction, smoking cessation, and self-examination and by facilitating public and professional education programs. The nurse can take a proactive role by coordinating screening projects and participating in health fairs.[48,66,67]

By eliciting the aid of church, social, and civic organizations, nurses can reach many of those individuals who have limited or no access to health care and who are at greatest risk for cancer morbidity and mortality.[32]

NURSING DIAGNOSIS

- *Knowledge deficit related to prevention and early detection of site-specific cancers (see Table 3-5)*

OUTCOME GOALS

Patient/significant other will be able to:
- State the seven warning signals of cancer.
- Demonstrate site-related self-examination related to breast, oral, skin, vulva, penile, and testicular cancers.
- Recognize cancer-related signs and symptoms that require follow-up in the health care system.
- Identify cancer information sources (e.g., ACS, Leukemia Society, NCI).
- Identify his or her relative risk for cancer development.

ASSESSMENTS

Assess the following:
- Patient education level
- Literacy level
- Cultural/ethnic perspectives of patient/significant other
- Beliefs and attitudes toward cancer
- Patient/family history and relative risk of cancer development

INTERVENTIONS

- Discuss site-specific cancer risk factors.
- Identify signs and symptoms of site-specific cancer.
- Implement health teaching related to diet, nutrition, and life-style choices.
- Provide appropriate and culturally sensitive printed information to patient.
- Provide a list of cancer information and support agencies.
- Instruct patient in self-examination of breast, mouth, skin, cervix, vulva, penis, and testes, as appropriate.
- Review ACS screening guidelines.[6,20,25]
- Assist patient with access to health care issues for cancer screening and early detection.
- Identify signs and symptoms that warrant access to the health care system.
- Identify community resources available to help patient
  —Stop smoking
  —Reduce stress
  —Control weight and diet
- Identify occupational and environmental risk factors and reporting agencies: OSHA (Occupational Safety and Health Administration), EPA (Environmental Protection Agency), NRC (Nuclear Regulatory Commission), and FDA (Food and Drug Administration).
- Provide mechanism for necessary referral and follow-up.[55,59]

 PATIENT TEACHING PRIORITIES
Cancer

Ensure that printed teaching materials are literacy appropriate at or below the fifth-grade reading level.

Include culturally sensitive and relevant content and visual aids with printed materials and presentations.

Seek out or develop translated printed materials appropriate to the target population.

In reaching out to diverse communities with cancer prevention, screening, and detection strategies, consider the following:

Assessment of cultural and community needs

Community volunteers in the program planning process

Collaboration with community volunteers on time, location, and length of the program

Ease of access by the target population

Partnerships with community leaders and other organizations with similar health promotion and disease prevention goals to maximize resources early detection. Regular breast, cervical, and prostate screening techniques are validated by scientific evidence of their effectiveness in detecting cancers early. The public should be educated to individual risk factors and screening recommendations.[20,21]

CONCLUSION

Cancer mortality will not be reduced without heightened public awareness and a multidisciplinary approach involving health care professionals, epidemiologists, and researchers. Agencies such as the ACS, Leukemia Society, and NCI play a vital role in cancer control efforts through funding and support of all aspects of cancer research and public and professional education. These agencies and organizations also must increase activity and involvement in social and political decisions influencing health care policy, cancer research, and treatment. A positive example of such efforts by the American public and support agencies is the ban on cigarette smoking on all domestic airline flights.

Because cancer is predominantly a disease of older adults, many signs and symptoms can mimic the normal aging process and are ignored and undetected by older persons and their significant others. Nurses can play a vital role in cancer prevention, screening, and risk reduction by identifying high-risk individuals and assessing life-style, personal and family history, and occupational or environmental exposure to carcinogens. Nurses' efforts should also include promoting follow-up and surveillance of those identified as high risk.

Underserved Americans offer the greatest challenge to nurses and other health care professionals. The underserved and SED populations make up a significant percentage of the American public and often bear the greatest burden of cancer risk and mortality. This is reflected in poorer overall survival, most frequently because of a later stage at which the cancer is detected. Millions of Americans are uninsured or underinsured, and this number is escalating with the climbing unemployment rate. Another barrier for this population is limited access to health care because of lack of health insurance, unemployment, homelessness, transportation issues, and inability to wait 6 to 8 hours in a overcrowded health care facility because of family and job responsibilities. Screening and early detection have little significance but to imply a "death sentence" to someone who has no access to health care intervention and follow-up and for whom the situation seems hopeless.[22,41,58,60,61]

To offer public health teaching and support, the nurse and other health care professionals must be sensitive to social, cultural, ethnic, and religious beliefs, values, and attitudes that can affect an individual's receptivity to health promotion and disease prevention strategies. Nurses can best prepare to meet the public education needs through sensitivity training sessions, development of printed materials that reflect cultural diversity and are at an appropriate literacy level, and thorough "train-the-trainer" programs for volunteers. Train-the-trainer programs facilitate contact with previously difficult-to-reach groups by training a volunteer from within the community or group to deliver the message of cancer prevention, risk reduction, and health promotion. Cancer prevention efforts should be aimed at improved agricultural and grain storage techniques, safe sexual practices, reduced occupational and environmental exposure to carcinogens, health promotion activities, and education.[53,57]

■ CHAPTER QUESTIONS

1. Neoplastic transformation in human cancers involves the following sequence of events:
   a. Stimulus, response, and initiation
   b. Risk, exposure, and progression
   c. Initiation, promotion, and progression
   d. Irritation, promotion, and susceptibility
2. Goals of prevention, risk reduction, and early detection are aimed at:
   a. Ensuring access to care to economically disadvantaged persons
   b. Finding a cure for the most preventable human cancers
   c. Reducing cancer mortality by 50% by the year 2000
   d. Eliminating and/or modifying neoplastic transformation
3. Major factors placing humans at risk for developing cancer include:
   a. Tobacco, diet, life-style, and occupational or environmental exposures
   b. Fatty foods, ozone depletion, alcohol, and age
   c. Sexual orientation, obesity, ethnicity, and poverty
   d. Occupation, age at first intercourse, HIV exposure, and hepatitis
4. In addition to lung cancer, smoking is associated with which of the following cancers?
   a. Multiple myeloma, esophagus, bladder, stomach, sarcoma, and leukemia
   b. Pharynx, oral, larynx, esophagus, pancreas, uterus, kidney, and bladder
   c. Oral, uterus, pancreas, colon, rectum, bone, and skin
   d. Endometrium, lymphoma, ovary, kidney, stomach, bladder, and pancreas
5. According to the American Cancer Society guidelines, women should have a mammogram every 1 to 2 years at the following ages:
   a. 20 to 29 years
   b. 30 to 39 years
   c. 40 to 49 years
   d. 50 to 60 years
6. Differences in increased cancer risk and poor survival are more pronounced among which racial/ethnic group?
   a. Native Americans
   b. Blacks
   c. Asians and Pacific Islanders
   d. Hispanics and Latinos

7. Poor survival statistics, delayed diagnosis, and increased mortality among minority populations stem from barriers related to:
   a. Primary prevention and lack of access
   b. Socioeconomic status and secondary prevention
   c. Lack of access and illiteracy
   d. Secondary and tertiary prevention
8. Differences in survival for minority and underserved populations is a result of:
   a. Illiteracy among the high-risk group
   b. Fatalism about cancer diagnosis and treatment
   c. Lack of concern about health practices
   d. Late stage of cancer diagnosis
9. The nurse teaching about skin cancer prevention should advise the patient to avoid sun exposure between:
   a. 12 noon and 4 PM
   b. 11 AM and 2 PM
   c. 10 AM and 3 PM
   d. 9 AM and 3 PM
10. Reducing the cancer risk related to sexual life-styles can *best* be accomplished by:
   a. Avoiding homosexuality
   b. Engaging in safe sexual practices
   c. Practicing abstinence
   d. Avoiding intravenous drug use

BIBLIOGRAPHY

1. Albright LA and others: Genetic predisposition to cancer. In DeVita VT Jr, Hellman S, Rosenberg SA, editors: *Important advances in oncology,* Philadelphia, 1991, Lippincott.
2. American Cancer Society: Guidelines for the cancer related checkup: update, January 1992, *CA Cancer J Clin* 42:44, 1992.
3. *Annotated bibliography of cancer-related literature on black populations,* NIH Pub No 89-3024, Public Health Service, US Department of Health and Human Services.
4. Bal DG and others: Cancer prevention. In Murphy G, Lawrence W, Lenhard R, editors: *ACS textbook of clinical oncology,* ed 2, Atlanta, 1995, American Cancer Society.
5. Baquet CR and others: Socioeconomic factors and cancer incidence among blacks and whites, *J Natl Cancer Inst* 83:551, 1991.
6. Bell I: Testicular self-examination, *Nurs Times* 86:38, 1990.
7. *Black and minority health: report of the secretary's task force,* Washington, DC, 1985, US Department of Health and Human Services.
8. Boring CC, Squires TS, Heath CW: Cancer statistics for African Americans, *CA Cancer J Clin* 43(1):7, 1993.
9. Bridford K: Pathogenesis and prevention of hepatocellular carcinoma, *Cancer Detect Prev* 14:191, 1989.
10. *Cancer among blacks and other minorities: statistical profiles,* NIH Pub No 86-2785, Washington, DC, 1986, Public Health Service, US Department of Health and Human Services.
11. *Cancer facts and figures—1996,* Atlanta, 1996, American Cancer Society.
12. *Cancer facts and figures for minority Americans—1991,* Atlanta, 1991, American Cancer Society.
13. *Cancer prevention and detection,* Atlanta, 1989, American Cancer Society.
14. *Cancer rates and risks,* NIH Pub No 85-691, Washington, DC, 1985, US Department of Health and Human Services.
15. Cigarette smoking among youth—United States, 1989, *MMWR* 40:712, 1991.
16. Cook-Mozaffari P: The epidemiology of cancer of the esophagus, *Nutr Cancer* 1:51, 1979.
17. Croghan IT, Omoto MK: cancer prevention and risk reduction. In Baird SB, editor: *A cancer source book for nurses,* Atlanta, 1991, American Cancer Society.
18. *Diet, nutrition and cancer prevention: a guide to food choices,* NIH Pub No 85-2711, Washington, DC, 1984, US Department of Health and Human Services.
19. Differences in age of smoking initiation between blacks and whites—United States, *MMWR* 40:754, 1991.
20. Dodd GD: American cancer society guidelines on screening for breast cancer: an overview, *CA Cancer J Clin* 42:177, 1992.
21. Drago JR: The role of new modalities in the early detection and diagnosis of prostate cancer, *CA Cancer J Clin* 39:326, 1989.
22. Faulkenberry JE: Cancer in men: a case for cancer prevention and early detection, *Dimens Oncol Nurs* 2:17, 1988.
23. Fighting cancer in America: achieving the "year 2000 goal," *Cancer Nurs* 12:359, 1989.
24. Fink DJ, Mettlin CJ: Cancer detection: the cancer related checkup guidelines. In Murphy G, Lawrence W, Lenhard R, editors: *ACS textbook of clinical oncology,* ed 2, Atlanta 1995, American Cancer Society.
25. Fitzsimmons ML and others: Hereditary cancer syndromes: nursing's role in identification and education, *Oncol Nurs Forum* 16:87, 1989.
26. Freeman HP: Cancer in the socioeconomically disadvantaged, *CA Cancer J Clin* 39:266, 1989.
27. Graham S, Mettlin C, Marshall J: Dietary factors in the epidemiology of cancer of the larynx, *Am J Epidemiol* 113:675, 1981.
28. Graham S, Schotz W, Martino P: Alimentary factors in the epidemiology of gastric cancer, *Cancer* 30:927, 1972.
29. Graves PL, Thomas CB, Mead LA: Familial and psychological predictors of cancer, *Cancer Detect Prev* 15:59, 1991.
30. Griffiths EK, Schapira DV: Serum ferritin and stool occult blood and colon cancer screening, *Cancer Detect Prev* 15:303, 1991.
31. Gullate MM: *Cancer prevention and early detection in black Americans: prostate, in touch* 9:4, 1988, American Cancer Society, Atlanta, Ga.
32. Gullate MM: Cancer prevention and early detection in black Americans: colon and rectum, *J Natl Black Nurses Assoc* 3:49, 1989.
33. Hahn RA and others: Prevalence of HIV infection among intravenous drug users in the United States, *JAMA* 261:2677, 1989.
34. Headen SW and others: Are the correlates of cigarette smoking initiation different for black and white adolescents? *Am J Public Health* 81:854, 1991.
35. Heath CW: Cancer prevention. In Holleb AI, Fink DJ, Murphy GP, editors: *ACS textbook of clinical oncology,* Atlanta, 1991, American Cancer Society.
36. Heath CW: Electromagnetic field exposure and cancer: a review of epidemiologic evidence, *CA Cancer J Clin* 46(1):29, 1996.

37. Holmes BC: *Sexual lifestyles and cancer risk,* Atlanta, 1988, American Cancer Society.

38. Increasing breast cancer screening among the medically underserved—Dade County, Florida, September 1987-March 1991, *MMWR* 40:261, 1991.

39. Knopp JM, Croghan IT: Screening, detection, and diagnosis. In Baird SB, editor: *A cancer source book for nurses,* Atlanta, 1991, American Cancer Society.

40. Kritchewsky D: Diet and cancer. In Holleb AI, Fink DJ, Murphy GP, editors: *ACS textbook of clinical oncology,* Atlanta, 1991, American Cancer Society.

41. Littrup PJ, Lee F, Mettlin C: Prostate cancer screening: current trends and future implications, *CA Cancer J Clin* 42:198, 1992.

42. Lynch HT: *Genetics and breast cancer,* New York, 1981, Van Nostrand Reinhold.

43. Lynch HT, Lynch JF: Familial factors and genetic predisposition to cancer: population studies, *Cancer Detect Prev* 15:49, 1991.

44. Lynch HT: The family history and cancer control: hereditary breast cancer, *Arch Surg* 125:151, 1990.

45. Miller AB: Role of early diagnosis and screening: biomarkers, *Cancer Detect Prev* 15:21, 1991.

46. Murphy GP, Lawrence W, Lenhard RE: *ACS textbook of clinical oncology,* ed 2, Atlanta, 1995, American Cancer Society.

47. Parker SL and others: Cancer statistics, 1996, *CA Cancer J Clin* 46(1):5, 1996.

48. Post WJ and others: Nutrition and cancer: educating the public through a health fair, *Oncol Nurs Forum* 16:115, 1989.

49. Reddy BS, Sharma C, Simi B: Metabolic epidemiology of colon cancer: effects of dietary fiber on fecal mutagens and bile acids in healthy subjects, *Cancer Res* 75:791, 1987.

50. Reis LA and others: *Cancer statistics review, 1973-1988,* NIH Pub No 91-2789, 1991, National Cancer Institute, Bethesda, Md.

51. Resnicow K, Kabat G, Wynder E: Progress in decreasing cigarette smoking. In DeVita VT Jr, Hellman S, Rosenberg SA, editors: *Important advances in oncology,* Philadelphia, 1991, Lippincott.

52. Rosenbaum EH, Dollinger M, Newell GR: *Risk assessment, cancer screening and prevention: everyone's guide to cancer therapy,* Kansas City, 1991, Somerville House.

53. Schuman LM, Mandell JS, Radke A: Some selected features of the epidemiology of prostate cancer: Minneapolis-St. Paul case control study 1976-79. In Magnus K, editor: *Trends in cancer incidence: causes and practical implications,* Washington, DC, 1982, Hemisphere.

54. Smoking—attributable mortality and years of potential life lost—United States, 1988, *MMWR* 40:62, 1991.

55. Stromborg MF, Olsen SJ: *Cancer prevention in minority populations: cultural implications for health care professionals,* St Louis, 1993, Mosby.

56. Tobacco use among high school students—United States, 1990, *MMWR* 40:617, 1991.

57. Tubiana M: Trends in primary and secondary prevention, *Cancer Detect Prev* 15:1, 1991.

58. Underwood SM: African-American men: perceptual determinants of early cancer detection and cancer risk reduction, *Cancer Nurs* 14:281, 1991.

59. Underwood SM: Testicular self-examination among African-American men, *J Natl Black Nurses Assoc* 5:18, 1991.

60. Underwood SM: Cancer risk reduction and early detection behaviors among black men: focus on learned helplessness, *J Community Health Nurs* 9:21, 1992.

61. Vainio H, Hemminki K: Use of exposure information and animal cancer data in the prevention of environmental and occupational cancer, *Cancer Detect Prev* 15:7, 1991.

62. Vlahov D and others: Trends of HIV-1 risk reduction among initiates into intravenous drug use: 1982-1987, *Am J Drug Alcohol Abuse* 17:39, 1991.

63. Volker DL: Acquired immune deficiency syndrome: an overview, *Dimens Oncol Nurs* 2:22, 1988.

64. Watkins MC: Computerized cancer information sources, *J Med Assoc Ga* 81:143, 1992.

65. White K: Diet and cancer, *Med World News* 52, August 1982.

66. Wholihan DJ: Incorporating cancer prevention interventions into the home health visit, *Home Healthcare Nurse* 9:19, 1991.

67. Willis MA and others: Inter-agency collaboration: teaching breast self-examination to black women, *Oncol Nurs Forum* 16:171, 1989.

68. Wogan GN: Dietary risk factors for primary hepatocellular carcinoma, *Cancer Detect Prev* 14:209, 1989.

69. Ziegler RG, Devesa SS, Fravmeni JF Jr: Epidemiologic patterns of colorectal cancer. In DeVita VT Jr, Hellman S, Rosenberg SA, editors: *Important advances in oncology,* Philadelphia, 1991, Lippincott.

CHAPTER 4
Diagnosis and Staging

JOYCE ALEXANDER

The diagnosis of cancer involves many members of the health care team, including the attending physician, specialists, radiologists, surgeons, oncologists, pathologists, technicians, and nurses. Treatment decisions are based on the histology (tumor type) and the assessed extent of disease. New techniques to diagnose and stage cancers have facilitated development of sophisticated plans of treatment, which have produced improved patient survival rates, as well as cures for some malignancies.

DIAGNOSIS
History and Physical Examination

A patient's past medical history and physical examination (H&P) and presenting signs and symptoms provide important data toward diagnosing a malignancy. In addition to the thorough H&P by the physician, the nurse takes a nursing history and performs a complete systems assessment, documenting variations from normal. Carefully listening to the patient's experience of symptoms provides vital information. In young children the parents' report of behavior changes can also provide important clues. From this database, a potential diagnosis can be made and testing initiated to rule out various reasons for the patient's problem. The medical history and family history provide valuable information regarding a patient's cancer risk factors. For example, a previous diagnosis of Crohn's disease (regional enteritis) in a patient with bloody stools raises the index of suspicion that a malignancy might be present in the colon. Thorough and complete histories help guide the initial diagnostic work-up.

The physical examination is a systematic assessment of major body sites: head, ears, nose, throat, cardiovascular system, chest, abdomen, genitourinary system, extremities, lymph nodes, and nervous system. Positive and negative findings are documented and evaluated in terms of the patient's medical history. An enlarged liver may cause the physician to suspect metastatic disease if the patient has a past history of colon or breast cancer.

A cancer diagnosis may be easily determined or difficult. The diagnostic work-up, planned from the patient's symptoms and H&P, may yield a presumptive malignant diagnosis. That diagnosis must be confirmed through histologic and cytologic examination. Staging completes the necessary information for planning treatment.

Diagnostic Work-up

A diagnostic work-up is initiated to determine the cause of a patient's symptoms. A wide range of diagnostic procedures may be used in the individualized work-up for each patient. Testing begins with less invasive procedures but may include highly technical innovations. After the diagnosis of malignancy is established, further diagnostic tests may be done to determine the stage of the cancer. Knowledge of symptoms, a high index of suspicion for malignancy, and knowledge of biologic behavior of a particular cancer are all useful in reaching a diagnosis.

Radiologic studies. A work-up often begins with a basic chest x-ray film. A mammogram, a flat plate of the abdomen, or x-ray films of the extremities may also add information. Barium studies of the gastrointestinal tract, an intravenous pyelogram (IVP) to evaluate the urinary tract, and a myelogram to assess the spinal canal are added when indicated. Computed tomography (CT) combines computer technology with radiology to produce multiple cross-sectional depictions of internal structures. CT images are based on varying density of tissues. Contrast solutions containing iodine may be used to improve images.

Magnetic resonance imaging (MRI). MRI provides sensitive images of soft tissues without interference from bone. Images are produced by placing the patient within a strong magnetic field, causing alignment of certain atoms within cellular molecules. Pulsed radio waves cause absorption and release of energy as the atomic nuclei change orientation. Energy differences are detected and measured by antennae, and the information is used by the MRI computer to produce images. MRI is superior for visualization of tissues obscured by bone in other diagnostic techniques, including central nervous system, mediastinal, and hilar areas. MRI may also be used to visualize abnormal vascular states, edema, and other tumors.[18] MRI is the preferred test in the diagnosis of pediatric brain tumors.[2]

Ultrasonography. High-frequency sound waves may be used to visualize internal structures. Abdominal, pelvic, or peritoneal masses may be detected by ultrasound. This technique is sometimes used to evaluate masses in the breast, thyroid, and prostate.

Nuclear medicine scans. Radioactive isotopes may be injected and tracked to those tissues for which the isotope has an affinity. Concentrations of the isotope in focal points indicate greater activity of cells, which may be caused by disease, infection, or malignancy. Areas of decreased uptake may also be significant in tissues that normally take up an isotope. A bone scan is often done to detect areas of possible bony metastasis. Other scans, including thyroid, brain, and liver, are done to evaluate possible primary or metastatic disease in those organs. Radiolabeled monoclonal antibodies specific to tumor antigens may be used to produce gamma camera images of tumors through a process called *immunoscintography.*[19]

Positron emission tomography (PET). PET measures physiologic and biochemical processes. Images are provided by the selective uptake of or concentration of radiolabeled compounds by malignant cells. Through computed cross-sectional images, PET provides information about the biologic activity of tumors, differentiates benign from malignant processes, and tracks response to treatment.[12]

Radioimmunoconjugates. Radioimmunoconjugates are used in the detection and evaluation of a variety of tumors, including colorectal, head and neck, breast, and ovarian tumors; lymphomas; and melanomas. Antibodies against different cancers have been identified and, when labeled with a radioisotope, are administered to the patient to assist in the staging of the disease. The antibodies aggregate at the tumor site(s) and, with scanning, identify sites of occult disease.[14]

Visualization. Advances in endoscopy techniques have made visual examination of many tissues possible. Colonoscopy and flexible sigmoidoscopy are used in the diagnosis of colorectal cancer; bronchoscopy is often useful in diagnosis of cancer of bronchogenic or lung origin; gastroscopy can differentiate causes of gastric symptoms; and laparoscopy is now being used to view and biopsy abdominal tissues. These techniques are used not only to visualize the tissues, but also to obtain samples for pathologic examination.

Laboratory studies. Each patient's work-up includes a battery of common laboratory procedures: complete blood count (CBC) with differential analysis of white blood cells, blood chemistries, liver function tests, renal function tests, and urinalysis. Additional laboratory studies, such as serum electrophoresis, calcium and magnesium levels, and levels of tumor markers, are ordered as indicated by the patient's symptoms. Table 4-1 lists some common laboratory studies used in a diagnostic work-up.

Tumor markers. Tumor markers are hormones, enzymes, or antigens produced by tumor cells and measurable in the blood of persons with malignancies. Tumor markers are measurable by chemical analysis or more recently by monoclonal antibodies designed to identify specific antigens in a sample of blood. *Bence-Jones protein,* produced by myeloma cells, was the first known tumor marker.[21] Hormonal tumor markers include *human chorionic gonadotropin* (HCG) and *α-fetoprotein* (AFP), produced by germ cell tumors.

Usefulness of a tumor marker in diagnosis and tracking of malignancy depends on the marker's *sensitivity* and *specificity*. The most sensitive marker would always be identifiable in the presence of a malignancy. The most specific marker would never be positive in the absence

Table 4–1 Selected Laboratory Studies

Examination	Detects or assesses
Bone marrow aspiration/biopsy	Hematologic abnormalities Presence of metastatic disease in marrow
Chemistry profile: bilirubin, calcium, uric acid, blood urea nitrogen (BUN), creatinine, electrolytes, lactate dehydrogenase (LDH), serum aspartate aminotransferase (AST, glutamic-oxaloacetic transaminase), alkaline phosphatase, serum alanine aminotransferase (ALT, glutamic-pyruvic transaminase), magnesium	Liver, kidney, and bone abnormalities secondary to cancer, therapy, and certain chronic illnesses May be used to monitor response to treatment
Complete blood count (CBC)	Bone marrow abnormalities Toxicity of therapy
Creatinine clearance	Kidney function; especially important when giving nephrotoxic drugs
Hemoccult test	Presence of blood in stool; not specific for cancer
Papanicolaou (Pap) smear	Cervical cancer or premalignant changes
Serum electrophoresis	Serum protein and immunoglobulin levels (e.g., multiple myeloma)
Urine catecholamines	Neuroblastoma, pheochromocytoma

of disease. Tumor markers vary in sensitivity and specificity. For example, *CA-15-3,* a human breast tissue antigen, has a low sensitivity in early disease but is useful for monitoring and identifying metastatic spread.[24] Combinations of tumor markers may overcome sensitivity and specificity problems. *Carcinoembryonic antigen* (CEA) is an antigen identified in colorectal, lung, and breast cancer. The addition of a second marker, *CA-72-4,* produces a more sensitive test that may prove useful in detecting colorectal, gastric, and ovarian carcinoma, as well as in tracking spread of disease.[11]

Prostate-specific antigen (PSA) is a tumor marker now being used in screening for prostate cancer. Although elevations may occur in benign prostatic disease, elevation of PSA indicates a need for further evaluation.

The significance of tumor marker levels must be assessed according to the patient's symptoms and other work-up data. Table 4-2 lists some commonly used tumor markers.[15]

Grade

Grade is a classification of tumor cells based on cellular *differentiation,* or resemblance to normal cells in structure, function, and maturity. Actual tumor cells must be obtained and examined by the pathologist before a clinical diagnosis of cancer or a determination of the grade of the malignancy can be made. Cells may be obtained by cytologic examination techniques, biopsy, or surgical excision of a suspected mass.

Cytology. Cytology is the examination of cells obtained from tissue scrapings, body fluids, secretions, or washings. *Pap smears* (named for Dr. George *Papanicolaou,* who developed the technique) use scrapings from the cervix to identify abnormal cervical cells. A new reporting scheme, the *Bethesda system,* provides improved Pap smear reporting. The Bethesda system reports infectious or reactive changes as benign cellular changes. Epithelial cell abnormalities include squamous or glandular cells, ranging from atypical cells to carcinoma. Fluids aspirated by thoracentesis, paracentesis, or lumbar puncture may yield cells for examination. Fine-needle aspiration may also be used to obtain cells for evaluation. Once procured, cytology specimens must be evaluated by a skilled pathologist. False-positive results are possible, and negative results indicate only that no cancer cells were found in the sample.

Biopsy. A portion of tissue, generally obtained by surgical procedure, is examined in a biopsy specimen. Biopsy is often done as part of an endoscopic procedure or under the guidance of CT to ensure that suspicious areas are sampled. *Bone marrow biopsy,* which uses a special needle to aspirate bone marrow tissue, is included in the work-up for hematologic disorders, including lymphomas, and when bone marrow metastasis is suspected.

Excision and analysis. Whenever a mass is surgically removed, whether or not a definitive diagnosis has been made, the tissue removed must be examined by a pathologist. The pathologist uses a number of techniques to determine the tissue type and the degree of differentiation (grade) of the tumor. *Frozen section* is a procedure by which a small amount of tissue is quickly frozen, thinly sliced, and stained for immediate examination. A permanent section is prepared using tissue preserved in formalin, thinly sliced, stained, and prepared for microscopic examination. The pathologist begins the examination of the tissues with an overview and measurement of the gross specimen and then examines prepared slides using light microscopy. Careful attention is paid to the margins of the excised specimen to determine if margins are free of malignancy.

Table 4-2   Commonly Used Tumor Markers

Marker	Elevations may indicate	Useful for
CEA (carcinoembryonic antigen)	Breast, colorectal, and lung cancers	Monitoring or management of patients with known disease
PSA (prostate-specific antigen)	Prostate cancer, benign prostate enlargement	Prostate cancer screening when combined with rectal examination; monitoring response to treatment and recurrence
HCG (human chorionic gonadotropin)	Germ cell tumors (testicular, certain types of ovarian, others), pregnancy	Differentiation of germ cell tumors
AFP (α-fetoprotein)	Germ cell tumors, liver cancer, benign liver disease, pregnancy	Differentiation of germ cell tumors
CA-125 (antigen)	Ovarian, colorectal, and gastric cancers	Monitoring response to treatment
CA-15-3 (two antigens)	Metastatic or recurrent breast cancer	Monitoring recurrence of disease
CA-19-9 (antigens)	Pancreatic, colorectal, and gastric cancers; inflammatory bowel and biliary disease	Monitoring response to treatment
CA-72-4 (antigens)	Ovarian, colorectal, and gastric cancers	Detection of primary disease and monitoring of treatment progress[11]
CA-242	Pancreatic cancer	Monitoring disease progress when combined with CA-19-9

Immunoperoxidase staining identifies specific cell types using monoclonal or polyclonal antibodies against cellular antigens. PSA can be stained using a monoclonal antibody and suggests that tissue is of prostatic origin. Leukocyte common antigen can be used to identify non-Hodgkin's lymphomas.[8] Electron microscopy may be used when light microscopy and special stains fail to differentiate the cell type.

Polymerase chain reaction (PCR) identifies specific genetic changes or chromosomal abnormalities. PCR can be used to determine risk of certain inherited cancers but is more often used in the identification of malignant cells in tissue, blood, or body fluid. Hematologic and other malignancies can be differentiated on the basis of PCR data; effectiveness of therapy can be tracked; and early relapse can be identified.

In addition to determining the definitive diagnosis of cancer and the tissue of origin, the pathologist must determine the grade. As noted, grade is a classification based on the differentiation of the malignancy. The more unlike normal tissue and less differentiated or less mature the cells, the higher is the grade. Behavior of a malignancy can be predicted on the basis of grade. Table 4-3 lists grade classifications.

Table 4-3 Grades of Tumors

Grade	Differentiation	Definition/cells
X	Cannot be assessed	
I	Well differentiated	Mature cells resembling normal tissue
II	Moderately differentiated	Cells with some immaturity
III	Poorly differentiated	Immature cells with little resemblance to normal tissue
IV	Undifferentiated	No resemblance to normal tissue

Classification of lymphomas. A simple grading system does not provide sufficient information about the behavior and prognosis of lymphomas to be useful. The *Working Formulation,* published in 1982, subdivided three grades of lymphoma (low grade, intermediate grade, and high grade) into specific cell types based on the microscopic appearance of the cells (morphology). As new information develops from immunologic and genetic examinations, this formulation is also proving to be inadequate. A new classification system proposed by the International Lymphoma Study Group, the *Revised European-American Classification of Lymphoid Neoplasms* (REAL), combines information from immunologic, histologic, and genetic features.[13] Lymphoid leukemias have also been included in this classification as lymphoid neoplasms. The REAL classification provides more information regarding prognosis and clinical behavior of disease than did previous systems. However, lymphomas range in aggressiveness within REAL classifications. Table 4-4 provides a partial listing of the REAL classification.

STAGING

Once a cancer diagnosis is confirmed by pathology, information from previous tests and scans is combined with additional work-up studies to determine the stage of the malignancy. *Stage* is a classification system based on the apparent anatomic extent of the malignancy.[3] A universal system of staging allows comparison of cancers of similar cellular origin. Classification assists in determination of a treatment plan and prognosis for the individual patient, evaluation of research, comparison of treatment results between institutions, and comparison of worldwide statistics.

A comprehensive staging system was developed by the American Joint Committee on Cancer (AJCC), a coalition sponsored by the ACS, NCI, College of American

Table 4-4 Partial Listing of Revised European–American Classification of Lymphoid Neoplasms (REAL)

B-cell lymphomas	T-cell lymphomas	Hodgkin's disease*
PRECURSOR B CELL	**PRECURSOR T CELL**	**I** Lymphocyte predominant
B-Lymphoblastic leukemia/lymphoma	T-Lymphoblastic leukemia/lymphoma	**II** Nodular sclerosis
PERIPHERAL B CELL	**PERIPHERAL T CELL**	**III** Mixed cellularity
Chronic lymphocytic leukemia/small lymphocytic lymphoma	T-cell chronic lymphocytic leukemia	**IV** Lymphocyte depleted
Mantle cell lymphoma	Cutaneous T-cell lymphoma	
Follicular center lymphoma	Peripheral T-cell lymphoma	
Marginal zone lymphoma	Angioimmunoblastic T-cell lymphoma	
Diffuse, large, B-cell lymphoma	Intestinal T-cell lymphoma	
Burkitt's lymphoma	Anaplastic, large, T-cell lymphoma	

*Recommendations on classification of Hodgkin's disease coincide with the Rye classification.

Pathologists, American College of Physicians, American College of Radiology, and American College of Surgeons. This group published the first staging manual in 1977. The International Union Against Cancer later joined the group, and the system became international. The fourth edition, published in 1992, included recommendations of the International Federation of Gynecology and Obstetrics (FIGO) to broaden the international scope.[3]

The *TNM system* outlined by AJCC involves assessment of three basic components: the size of the *primary tumor (T)*, the absence or presence of regional *lymph nodes (N)*, and the absence or presence of distant *metastatic disease (M)*. General definitions used throughout the system are included in Table 4-5.[3]

Information from the TNM classification is combined to define the stage. Stage classifications have been determined for most cancer sites and are published in the *Manual for Staging of Cancer.*[3] Examples for selected disease sites are included in Table 4-6. The stage is determined before beginning treatment and is the basis for treatment decisions. The stage is often changed after surgery, however, when pathologic measurements more accurately define tumor size and nodal involvement. Stage determined before treatment is termed the *clinical stage* (cTNM or TNM). When stage is changed after surgery, the term *pathologic stage* (pTNM) is used.

Before 1992, gynecologic cancers were typically classified using a separate system developed by FIGO. Information from the FIGO system has been incorporated into the staging system published in the *Manual for Staging of Cancer,*[3] and a separate system is no longer necessary. Table 4-7 provides examples.

Staging of cancers of the central nervous system (CNS) varies from that for other disease sites. Important prognostic indicators in brain cancer are the biologic behavior, or rate of growth, and the location and size of the tumor (see Chapter 5). Staging for brain cancer, therefore, considers grade *(G)* and tumor size and location *(T)*. A higher grade is a more malignant tumor; a grade 3 tumor *(G3)* is classified *stage III* unless the tumor crosses the midline. Any tumor that crosses the midline *(T4)* or any CNS tumor with metastasis is classified *stage IV.* The brain is not supplied with lymphatic drainage; therefore "N" is not used.

Hematologic malignancies cannot be classified using the TNM system. Leukemias are classified according to cell type and differentiation but are not staged further. Leukemia research compares patients on the basis of remission or first, second, or third relapse, and prognosis can be determined on that information. Myeloma may be staged on the basis of clinical manifestations, including hemoglobin, serum calcium, presence of lytic bone lesions, and serum protein levels. A patient with a hemoglobin level less than 8.5 g/dl, calcium level greater than 12 mg/dl, or several lytic bone lesions would be expected to have a large mass of myeloma cells and would be classified stage III.[20] After pathologic classification, lymphomas, both Hodgkin's disease and non-Hodgkin's lymphoma, are staged according to the Ann Arbor system. Under the *Ann Arbor system,* lymphomas are staged *I, II, III,* or *IV* based on the area or region of lymph nodes involved. Stages are subdivided into A or B—*A* indicating absence of systemic symptoms and *B* indicating presence of systemic symptoms.[3] Table 4-8 outlines general principles of the Ann Arbor system.

In addition to TNM staging, colorectal tumors may also be classified by the *Duke's system,*[3] outlined as follows:

Stage A   Carcinoma limited to mucosa
Stage B1   Carcinoma invades muscle but is confined to bowel wall
Stage B2   Carcinoma penetrates muscularis propria into serosa and connective tissue
Stage B3   Same as B2 with adherence or invasion into adjacent organs, but with negative nodes
Stage C1   Lymph nodes positive for metastatic disease, but main tumor confined to bowel wall
Stage C2   Lymph nodes positive for metastatic disease, and tumor completely penetrates bowel wall
Stage C3   Same as B3, with positive nodes
Stage D   Distant metastasis

Duke's stage in comparison to TNM is included in Table 4-6.

The prognosis for patients with malignant melanoma largely depends on the depth of penetration of the original lesion. Two classification systems, *Clark's* and *Breslow's,* have been used to classify melanomas on the

Table 4-5   General TNM Definitions

	Stage designation	Definition
T	Primary tumor	Size, extent, and depth of primary tumor
	TX	Primary tumor cannot be assessed
	T0	No evidence of primary tumor
	Tis	Carcinoma in situ
	T1 to T4	Increasing size or extent of primary tumor
N	Nodal metastasis	Extent and location of involved regional lymph nodes
	NX	Regional lymph nodes cannot be assessed
	N0	No regional lymph node metastasis
	N1 to N3	Increasing numbers and size of involved regional lymph nodes
M	Metastasis	Absence or presence of distant spread of disease
	MX	Distant disease cannot be assessed
	M0	No distant spread of disease
	M1	Distant spread of disease

Table 4-6 Selected TNM Staging Guidelines

Stage	Lung	Breast	Bone
Occult	**TX-N0-M0** TX: primary tumor proved only by cells (sputum)		
0	**Tis-N0-M0** Tis: carcinoma in situ	**Tis-N0-M0** Tis: carcinoma in situ	
I	**T1 or T2-N0-M0** T1: tumor ≤3 cm T2: >3 cm and/or involving main bronchus or pleura	**T1-N0-M0** T1: tumor ≤2 cm	**G1 or G2-T1 or T2** **N0-M0** G1: well differentiated G2: moderately differentiated T1: within cortex T2: outside cortex
II	**T1 or T2-N1-M0** N1: peribronchial or hilar lymph node metastasis; same side as tumor	**T0 or T1-N1-M0** **T2-N0 or N1-M0** **T3-N0-M0** T2: tumor 2-5 cm T3: tumor >5 cm N1: metastasis to movable axillary lymph node(s); same side as tumor	**G3 or G4-T1 or T2** **N0-M0** G3: poorly differentiated G4: undifferentiated
IIIA	**T1 or T2-N2-M0** **T3-any N-M0** N2: mediastinal or subclavian node metastasis; same side as tumor T3: tumor invades chest wall, diaphragm, mediastinal pleura, pericardium	**T0, T1, or T2-N2-M0** **T3-N1 or N2-M0** N2: metastasis to fixed axillary lymph nodes; same side as tumor	**Not defined**
IIIB	**Any T-N3-M0** **T4-any N-M0** N3: metastasis in lymph nodes; opposite side from tumor T4: tumor invades other organs (heart, mediastinum, etc.) or pleural effusion	**T4-any N-M0** **Any T-N3-M0** T4: tumor invades chest wall or skin N3: internal mammary node metastasis; same side as tumor	
IV	**Any T-any N-M1** M1: distant metastasis	**Any T-any N-M1** M1: distant metastasis	**Any G and T-N1-M0** **Any G and T-Any N-M1**

Stage	Larynx	Colorectal/Duke's
0	**Tis-N0-M0** Tis: carcinoma in situ	**Tis-N0-M0** Tis: carcinoma in situ
I	**T1-N0-M0** T1: tumor limited to vocal cord with normal mobility	**T1 or T2-N0-M0/Duke's A** T1: tumor invading submucosa T2: tumor invading muscle layer
II	**T2-N0-M0** T2: tumor extends to supraglottis and/or subglottis with impaired cord mobility	**T3 or T4-N0-M0/Duke's B** T3: tumor invades through muscle layer into subserosa T4: tumor directly invades other organs or perforates visceral peritoneum
III	**T3-N0-M0** **T1, T2, or T3-N1-M0** T3: tumor limited to larynx with vocal cord fixation N1: single, same-side node <3 cm	**Any T-N1, N2, or N3-M0/Duke's C** N1: 1-3 pericolic or perirectal lymph node metastases N2: ≤4 pericolic or perirectal lymph node metastases N3: any nodal metastasis along vascular trunk or apical node
IV	**T4-N0 or N1-M0** **Any T-N2 or N3-M0** **Any T-any N-M1** T4: tumor invades thyroid cartilage and/or tissues beyond larynx N2: single node, same side, 3-6 cm N3: any node >6 cm M1: distant metastasis	**Any T-any N-M1/Duke's D** M1: distant metastasis

Modified from Beahrs O and others: *Manual for staging of cancer*, ed 4, Philadelphia, 1992, Lippincott.

Table 4-6 Selected TNM Staging Guidelines—cont'd

Stage	Gastric	Prostate
0	**Tis-N0-M0** Tis: carcinoma in situ	**T1a-N0-M0 (G1)** T1a: incidental finding <5% of tissue G1: well differentiated
IA	**T1-N0-M0** T1: tumor invades lamina propria or submucosa	**T1a, T1b, or T1c-N0-M0** T1b: incidental finding >5% of tissue T1c: identified by needle biopsy
IB	**T1-N1-M0** **T2-N0-M0** T2: tumor invades muscle layer or subserosa N1: perigastric node within 3 cm of primary site	
II	**T1-N2-M0** N2: perigastric node >3 cm from primary or any other nodes	**T2-N0-M0** T2: tumor confined within prostate
IIIA	**T2-N2-M0** **T3-N1-M0** **T4-N0-M0** T3: tumor penetrates visceral peritoneum without invasion of other structures T4: tumor invades other adjacent structures	**T3-N0-M0** T3: tumor extends through prostatic capsule
IIIB	**T3-N2-M0; T4-N1-M0**	
IV	**T4-N2-M0** **Any T-any N-M1** M1: distant metastasis	**T4-N0-M0** **Any T-N1, N2, or N3-M0** **Any T-any N-M1** T4: tumor fixed and invades adjacent structures N1: single node ≤2 cm N2: single node 2-5 cm N3: 1 or more nodes >5 cm M1: distant metastasis

Stage	Soft tissue sarcoma	Pancreas	Liver
0			
I	**T1 or T2-N0-M0** T1: tumor <5 cm T2: tumor >5 cm	**T1 or T2-N0-M0** T1: tumor limited to pancreas T2: direct extension into duodenum, bile duct, or peripancreatic tissues	**T1-N0-M0** T1: single tumor 2 cm or less
II	**T1 or T2-N0-M0 (G2)** G2: moderately differentiated	**T3-N0-M0** T3: tumor extends directly into stomach, spleen, colon, or large vessels	**T2-N0-M0** T2: single >2 cm or multiple <2 cm without vascular invasion or single >2 cm with vascular invasion
III	**T1 or T2-N0-M0 (G3 or G4)** G3: poorly differentiated G4: undifferentiated	**Any T-N1-M0** N1: regional lymph nodes involved	**T1 or T2-N1-M0** **T3-N0 or N1-M0** T3: single >2 cm with vascular invasion; multiple in one lobe N1: regional lymph nodes involved
IV	**Any T-N1-M0** **Any T-any N-M1** N1: lymph nodes involved M1: distant metastasis	**Any T-any N-M1** M1: distant metastasis	**T4-any N-M0** **Any T-any N-M1** T4: multiple, more than 1 lobe or major blood vessels M1: distant metastasis

Continued.

Table 4-6 Selected TNM Staging Guidelines—cont'd

Stage	Small bowel	Esophagus
0	**Tis-N0-M0** Tis: carcinoma in situ	**Tis-N0-M0** Tis: carcinoma in situ
I	**T1 or T2-N0-M0** T1: tumor invades lamina propria T2: tumor invades muscularis	**T1-N0-M0** T1: tumor invades lamina propria or submucosa
II	**T3 or T4-N0-M0** T3: tumor invades through muscularis T4: tumor perforates peritoneum or invades other organs	**T2 or T3-N0-M0** T2: tumor invades muscularis T3: tumor invades adventitia into pancreas **T1 or T2-N1-M0** N1: regional lymph nodes involved
III	**Any T-N1-M0** N1: regional lymph nodes involved	**T3 or T4-N1-M0** T4: tumor invades adjacent structures
IV	**Any T-any N-M1** M1: distant metastasis	**Any T-any N-M1** M1: distant metastasis

Table 4-7 Staging of Ovarian Cancer: Comparison of TNM and International Federation of Gynecology and Obstetrics (FIGO)

Stage	TNM	FIGO
0	**Tis-N0-M0** Tis: carcinoma in situ	
I	**T1-N0-M0** T1: tumor confined to corpus uteri	I
II	**T2-N0-M0** T2: tumor invades cervix but not extending beyond uterus	II
III (A and B)	**T3-N0-M0** T3: tumor involves serosa or adnexa	IIIA and IIIB
IIIC	**T1, T2, or T3-N1-M0** N1: regional lymph node metastasis	IIIC
IVA	**T4-any N-M0** T4: tumor invades bladder or rectal mucosa	IVA
IVB	**Any T-any N-M1** M1: distant metastasis	IVB

Modified from Beahrs O and others: *Manual for staging of cancer,* ed 4, Philadelphia, 1992, Lippincott.

Table 4-8 Ann Arbor Staging System for Lymphomas

Stage	Description
I	Single lymph node region involved or localized involvement of single organ
II	Two or more lymph node regions on same side of diaphragm involved or localized involvement of a single organ plus regional lymph nodes
III	Lymph nodes on both sides of diaphragm involved; may include localized involvement of single organ and/or spleen
IV	Disseminated involvement of extralymphatic organs or isolated organ involved plus distant lymph nodes
A	No systemic symptoms
B	Presence of systemic symptoms

Modified from Beahrs O and others: *Manual for staging of cancer,* ed 4, Philadelphia, 1992, Lippincott.

Table 4-9 Melanoma Staging*

Stage	TNM	Clark's
I	**pT1-N0-M0** pT1: tumor <0.75 mm thickness and invading papillary dermis	Level II
	pT2: tumor 0.75-1.50 mm and/or invades papillary-reticular dermal boundary	Level III
II	**pT3-N0-M0** pT3: tumor 1.5-4.0 mm thickness and/or invades reticular dermis	Level IV
III	**pT4-N0-M0** **Any pT-N1 or N2-M0** pT4: tumor >4 mm thickness and/or invades subcutaneous tissue and/or satellite lesions	Level V
IV	**Any pT-any N-M1**	

Modified from Beahrs O and others: *Manual for staging of cancer,* ed 4, Philadelphia, 1992, Lippincott.
*Breslow's staging system incorporates measurements of tumor depth now incorporated into the TNM system.

basis of depth of penetration. Information from these systems has been incorporated into the TNM system, using a pathologic (after-excision) T staging.[3] Table 4-9 compares the classifications for melanoma.

Staging of pediatric rhabdomyosarcoma has followed the *clinical grouping system,* based partly on resectability of the tumor. A site-specific TNM system is being evaluated in current studies.[22]

NURSING MANAGEMENT

The word "cancer" has frightening connotations for individuals who may associate a diagnosis of cancer with death or pain. Virtually all diagnostic work-ups involve periods of waiting for information. Time may be perceived as endless and may be extremely anxiety provoking for the patient and family awaiting an unknown or feared diagnosis. The family of a child with a potential cancer diagnosis may find this time especially stressful. Regardless of the patient's age, the family shares this experience with the patient and frequently is the patient's major support system. Families must be an integral part of the care of oncology patients, especially during the stressful time of diagnosis and staging. Responses of the patient and family are influenced by social and cultural factors, which must also be considered. This section describes nursing assessments, diagnoses, and interventions for both patients and families during the difficult period of diagnosis and staging.

Initial nursing assessments during the diagnosis and staging phase include assessment of the patient's and family's feelings and beliefs about the diagnostic process and about cancer; cultural and social influences on beliefs about cancer and healing and on coping styles; knowledge of the diagnostic process; ability to understand information presented; support systems available and used in past crisis situations; and effectiveness of coping styles. The nurse must establish rapport before the patient and family can feel comfortable sharing this information. Sitting with them, maintaining eye contact when eye contact is culturally appropriate, demonstrating respect for the individual, listening, and arranging uninterrupted time can be helpful in establishing rapport. The following responses may be experienced by the patient and family during this phase and may be identified as nursing diagnoses from a successful interview: fear related to a possible diagnosis of cancer; anxiety related to uncertainty about a diagnosis of cancer; ineffective individual coping; ineffective family coping; spiritual distress; knowledge deficit regarding procedure; knowledge deficit regarding cancer, disease, and treatment; anticipatory grieving; and health-seeking behaviors. Other nursing diagnoses may be identified depending on presenting symptoms, prior conditions, and individual and family responses.

One result of recent changes in health care is the movement of most diagnostic and staging procedures to the outpatient setting. In addition to the previously described responses, patients and families experience problems unique to the outpatient setting. There is an increased potential for delays in diagnosis, staging, and treatment because appointments may be scheduled weeks rather than days apart, appointments may be missed, or results may be lost within the system. The nurse can advocate for the patient by coordinating scheduling and following up on tests and evaluations. Transportation may also present a problem and should be included in the nursing assessment. The nurse must also contribute to development of systems that facilitate procedures and allow time for patient and family assessment, questions, teaching, and support. Nursing input in the development of *care maps* for outpatient diagnosis and staging is one means of accomplishing this goal.

Nursing interventions depend on identified nursing diagnoses. Basic information about the diagnostic process, what test is to be done (do not assume the patient understood the physician's explanation), what may be learned, and how that information fits into the total picture is needed by most patients and families. When providing patient teaching materials, the nurse should evaluate and select material that is appropriate to the patient's reading level and that is culturally sensitive. Nurses can also correct misconceptions and provide reassurance. Some cancers can be cured and others can be controlled for many years, with treatment based on appropriate staging information. The nurse can present information about the treatment plan once a diagnosis has been determined. The patient and family will be asked to participate in the decision-making process at this point. Patients often feel pressured and turn to the nurse for assistance. Further clarification of options and potential outcomes is one possible intervention. The nurse should show respect for individual and cultural decision-making styles in any intervention at this time. Information about support groups and interaction with cancer survivors may also be helpful after a diagnosis has been confirmed.

Continued.

NURSING DIAGNOSIS

• *Fear related to possible cancer diagnosis*

OUTCOME GOALS

Patient/significant others will be able to:
• Acknowledge validity of feelings.
• Identify effective means of dealing with diagnosis and treatment.

ASSESSMENTS

• Emotional response
• Knowledge base and misconceptions, support systems

INTERVENTIONS

• Establish rapport.
• Acknowledge validity of feelings.
• Correct misconceptions and provide information.
• Encourage use of support systems.

NURSING DIAGNOSIS

• *Anxiety related to uncertainty/diagnosis of cancer*

OUTCOME GOALS

Patient/significant others will be able to:
• Identify source of anxiety.
• Utilize effective skills for dealing with the perceived threat.

ASSESSMENTS

• Uncertainty of diagnosis, situation, or prognosis
• Perceptions of individual about the situation
• Psychosocial responses to the situation
• Physical responses (sweating, flushing, hyperactivity, sighing respirations or shortness of breath, rapid heart rate, elevated blood pressure)
• Speech patterns (pressured speech, blaming, returning to a single topic, refusing to talk about cancer)

INTERVENTIONS

• Limit time waiting for information.
• Provide information about disease and treatment.
• Encourage exploration and verbalization of feelings.
• Explore previous effective responses.
• Encourage use of effective responses.
• Teach behavioral interventions, including relaxation and distraction.[7]

NURSING DIAGNOSIS

• *Knowledge deficit related to procedure*

OUTCOME GOAL

Patient/significant others will be able to:
• Verbalize knowledge of procedure, rationale, and information to be obtained.

ASSESSMENTS

• Knowledge of procedure
• Cognitive level and reading ability
• Stress level

INTERVENTIONS

• Explain procedure and rationale.
• Explain what information may be gained.
• Provide culturally sensitive, written information appropriate to patient's cognitive and reading level.
• Repeat and simplify information for those persons under stress.

NURSING DIAGNOSIS

• *Ineffective family coping*

OUTCOME GOAL

Family/patient will be able to:
• Utilize effective coping strategies.

ASSESSMENTS

• Coping styles
• Family communication patterns
• Support systems
• Community and cultural expectations

INTERVENTIONS

• Identify and encourage effective coping strategies.
• Encourage effective family communication.
• Encourage use of support systems, including community support.
• Consult social worker, chaplain, and other support services as appropriate.[8]

NURSING DIAGNOSIS

• *Health-seeking behaviors*

OUTCOME GOAL

Patient/significant others will be able to:
• Identify effective health-seeking behaviors.

ASSESSMENTS

• Behaviors and questions aimed at seeking health
• Effectiveness of those behaviors
• Cultural beliefs about health

INTERVENTIONS

• Encourage behaviors that are effective in prevention of cancer or maintenance of a healthy life-style (stopping smoking, low-fat diet, increased exercise).
• Answer questions openly and provide information.

CONCLUSION

The diagnostic period can be confusing and frightening for both the patient and the family. Overwhelmed patients and family ultimately look to the nurse to be their advocate and educator. Competent and confident delivery of nursing care can help reduce the anxiety experienced during this period.

■ CHAPTER QUESTIONS

1. Magnetic resonance imaging (MRI) is most useful for which of the following?
   a. Suspected osteosarcoma of the femur
   b. Suspected lung metastasis in a woman with breast cancer
   c. Suspected brain tumor in a child
   d. Suspected colon cancer in an elderly man
2. Mrs. S., a patient with breast cancer, is being evaluated for presence of metastasis. She can expect to have which of the following tests?
   a. Abdominal ultrasound
   b. Myelogram
   c. Intravenous pyelogram
   d. Bone scan
3. A patient asks, "Why can't they measure a CA-15-3 on everyone instead of doing a mammogram? Couldn't they find breast cancer earlier that way?" The correct answer is:
   a. CA-15-3 has a low sensitivity in early breast cancer, so it would not be useful for screening.
   b. It would be too expensive to screen many women with a blood test.
   c. CA-15-3 is a sensitive screening test for colon cancer, not for breast cancer.
   d. CA-15-3 is more specific than a mammogram and cannot be used for screening because too many unnecessary biopsies would be done.
4. Mr. J. has an elevated prostate-specific antigen (PSA) level. What additional information is needed for a diagnosis of prostate cancer?
   (1) Blood levels of carcinoembryonic antigen (CEA)
   (2) Physical examination, including rectal
   (3) Presence of blood in the urine
   (4) Biopsy with pathology report positive for malignancy
   a. (1) and (2)
   b. (1) and (3)
   c. (2) and (4)
   d. All the above
5. Grade is a classification system based on:
   a. Anatomic location of a tumor
   b. Size of the original tumor
   c. Resectability and location of a malignancy
   d. Differentiation of the cells
6. The REAL classification of lymphomas uses information from:
   a. Location of the lymphoma cells
   b. Size of the original lymphoma
   c. Immunologic, histologic, and genetic features of lymphoma cells
   d. Aggressiveness of the lymphoma cells
7. Staging is necessary for:
   a. Comparison of treatment results and research data among facilities
   b. Planning of treatment and prognosis for the individual patient
   c. Comparison of worldwide statistics
   d. All the above
8. A reference on a patient's chart to a "T1-N0-M0" stage malignancy means the patient:
   a. Has a small tumor with negative lymph nodes and no metastases
   b. Has a large tumor and status of lymph nodes and metastases is unknown
   c. Has expressed a wish that NO one be Told about the malignancy
   d. Has a small tumor with multiple lymph nodes involved and widespread metastases
9. Mr. J. is an elderly smoker; a chest x-ray film is positive for a suspicious lesion. He has been scheduled for outpatient evaluation with a CT scan. In preparing Mr. J. for this test, the nurse should assess:
   a. Age; ability to walk about his home; compliance with medical instructions
   b. Medications currently taken; age; smoking history; complete physical assessment
   c. Knowledge of lung cancer; preparation for receiving chemotherapy
   d. Understanding of the test and preparation; knowledge of the scheduled time; transportation to and from the test site
10. Mrs. Y. tells the nurse that she is fearful of the outcome of her breast biopsy. The nurse should:
    a. Tell Mrs. Y. that there is nothing to be afraid of; everything will be all right
    b. Acknowledge the validity of Mrs. Y.'s feelings and allow her to verbalize them further
    c. Tell Mrs. Y. that since 80% of breast cancer biopsies are negative, she has nothing to fear
    d. Provide Mrs. Y. with printed information about breast cancer, the various forms of treatment, and the side effects of treatment

BIBLIOGRAPHY

1. *Acta Cytologica:* The Bethesda system for reporting cervical/vaginal cytologic diagnoses, *J Clin Cytol Cytopathol* 37(2):115, 1993.
2. Albright A: Pediatric brain tumors, *CA Cancer J Clin* 43:272, 1993.
3. Beahrs O and others: *Manual for staging of cancer,* ed 4, Philadelphia, 1992, Lippincott.
4. Borg S, Rosenthal S: *Handbook of cancer diagnosis and staging—a clinical atlas,* New York, 1984, Wiley & Sons.
5. Bragg D, Putnam C, Hendee W: Oncologic imaging: state of the art and research priorities, *Am J Clin Oncol* 11:394, 1988.
6. Bristol-Meyers Oncology Division: *The basics of cancer treatment,* vol 2, Oncology: programmed modules for nurses, New York, 1995, LP Communications.
7. Clark J, McGee R, Preston R: Nursing management of responses to the cancer experience. In Clark J, McGee R, edi-

tors: *Core curriculum for oncology nursing,* ed 2, Philadelphia, 1992, Saunders.

8. Dufault K and others: Ineffective family coping. In McNally J and others, editors: *Guidelines for oncology nursing practice,* ed 2, Philadelphia, 1991, Saunders.

9. Flam T and others: Diagnosis and markers in prostate cancer, *Cancer* 70:357, 1992.

10. Greco F, Hainsworth J: Tumors of unknown origin, *CA Cancer J Clin* 42:96, 1992.

11. Guadagni F and others: CA 72-4 serum marker—a new tool in the management of carcinoma patients, *Cancer Invest* 13(2):227, 1995.

12. Gupta N, Frick M: Clinical applications of positron-emission tomography in cancer, *CA Cancer J Clin* 43:235, 1993.

13. Harris N and others: A revised European-American classification of lymphoid neoplasms: a proposal from the International Lymphoma Study Group, *Blood* 84(5):1361, 1994.

14. Harrison KA, Tempero MA: Diagnostic use of radiolabeled antibodies for cancer, *Oncology* 9:625, 1995.

15. Heberman RB: *Tumor markers,* Alameda, Calif, 1991, American Association for Clinical Chemistry, National Cancer Institute, Triton Diagnostics.

16. Hellman S, Jaffe E, DeVita V Jr: Hodgkin's disease. In DeVita V Jr, Hellman S, Rosenberg S, editors: *Cancer: principles and practice of oncology,* ed 4, Philadelphia, 1993, Lippincott.

17. Markel D: Introduction to classics in oncology: "Spectrophotometer: new instrument of ultrarapid cell analysis by Kamentsky, Metamed, & Derman," *CA Cancer J Clin* 42:57, 1992.

18. Newman F, Ogburn-Russell L, Rutledge J: Magnetic resonance imaging: the latest in diagnostic technology, *Nursing '87*:44, 1987.

19. Perkins A, Pimm M: *Immunoscintography: practical aspects and clinical applications,* 1987, New York, Wiley-Liss.

20. Salmon S, Cassady R: Plasma cell neoplasms. In DeVita V Jr, Hellman S, Rosenberg S, editors: *Cancer: principles and practice of oncology,* ed 4, Philadelphia, 1993, Lippincott.

21. Schwartz M: Markers in diagnosis and screening. In Ting S, Chan J, Schwartz M, editors: *Human tumor markers,* New York, 1989, Excerpta Medica.

22. Strohl R: Implications of diagnosis and staging on treatment goals and strategies. In Clark J, McGee R, editors: *Core curriculum for oncology nursing,* ed 2, Philadelphia, 1992, Saunders.

23. Wexler L, Helman L: Pediatric soft tissue sarcomas, *CA Cancer J Clin* 44:211, 1994.

24. Wojtacki J and others: Evaluation of CA 15-3 tumor marker in the diagnosis of breast cancer: a pilot study, *Neoplasma* 41(4):213, 1994.

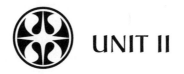

UNIT II

CLINICAL MANAGEMENT OF MAJOR CANCER DISEASES

CHAPTER 5

Cancers of the Brain and Central Nervous System

MARY E. MURPHY

Cancer of the central nervous system (CNS) includes primary and metastatic tumors of the brain and spinal cord. Despite a relatively high ratio of primary tumors in the pediatric population, adult CNS tumors represent only 2.2% of all cancer deaths. Metastatic lesions continue to present symptom and treatment management concerns. This chapter deals with adult CNS tumors. Additional readings are recommended for the pediatric population.[5,7,15,16]

EPIDEMIOLOGY

Cancer of the CNS accounts for less than 2% of all malignancies, with 17,900 diagnosed cases in 1996. Peak incidence occurs from birth to 6 years and after age 45. CNS tumors are the fourth leading cause of cancer death in persons ages 15 to 34. Incidence is slightly higher in males. Race differences have not been documented. Metastatic lesions represent 20% to 40% of all CNS neoplasms, with most arising from lung and breast cancers. Sarcomas, melanomas, and tumors may arise from the kidney and the colon.[10,15]

ETIOLOGY AND RISK FACTORS

Specific causes and risk factors have not been identified. Chemical carcinogens and some oncologic viruses have induced CNS tumors in laboratory animals. Genetic factors have been linked with neurofibromatosis, tuberous sclerosis, familial polyposis, von Hippel-Lindau disease,[20,22] Turcot syndrome, and family syndromes of breast cancer, soft tissue sarcoma, and leukemia.

Chemical exposures that have been implicated include vinyl chloride, radiation, petrochemicals, inks, acrylonitrile, lubricating oils, and solvents.[22] Viruses have also been implicated, including the Epstein-Barr virus genome. Traumatic causes and environmental carcinogens have not been indicated at this time. Ongoing investigation is in progress.

PREVENTION AND SCREENING DETECTION

At this time, no screening or prevention methods exist for CNS and brain cancer. Symptoms appear gradually and do not lend themselves to diagnostic prescreening methods.

CLASSIFICATION

To provide a simplistic understanding of the complexity of CNS tumors, a variety of systems have been developed. Tumors of the CNS include both brain and spinal cord tumors. CNS tumors are classified as primary and metastatic in nature. *Primary tumors* may exist as intracerebral or extracerebral. Major *intracerebral tumors* include those within the brain, neuroglia (Figure 5-1), neurons, and cells of the blood vessels of the connective tissue. *Extracerebral tumors* originate outside of the brain and include meningiomas and acoustic nerve, pituitary, and pineal gland tumors. *Metastatic tumors* may exist either inside or outside the body. The classification of benign versus malignant is not differentiated, since surgical accessibility determines the ultimate prognosis.

Within each specific location the classification of CNS tumors is based on all types of differentiation and location.[7] Detailed classifications were developed by the World Health Organization (WHO) in 1979 and are available for reference.[10] Table 5-1 provides an outline and a modified system of common CNS tumors, cell type, occurrence, and malignant state.[3]

Glial tumors represent two thirds of all types of CNS tumors, with *glioblastomas* representing the largest subclass. *Schwannomas* and *meningiomas* represent the largest classification of spinal cord tumors. CNS *lymphomas* are seen among immunosuppressed patients, particularly patients diagnosed with acquired immunodeficiency syndrome (AIDS). Metastatic brain tumors may be present in as many as 35% of all cancer patients, with the largest representation among patients with lung tumors.[10,14,20]

Ependymal cell   Astrocyte

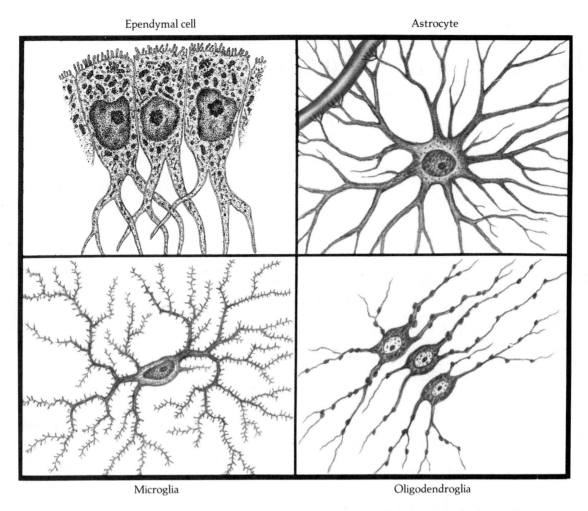

Microglia   Oligodendroglia

Figure 5-1 Types of neuroglia cells. (From McCance KL, Huether SE: *Pathophysiology: the biological basis for disease in adults and children*, 1990, Mosby. From Thompson JM, McFarland GK, Hirsch JE, Tucker SM: *Mosby's clinical nursing*, St Louis, 1993, Mosby.)

CLINICAL FEATURES

The clinical features manifested by CNS tumors vary according to their size and specific location. The most common symptoms are headache and seizure activity. Headaches are typically bifrontal and bioccipital and occur on awakening. Episodes of nausea and vomiting may also occur with the complaints of headache. Seizure activity is seen in 20% to 50% of all patients with brain tumors and are most common in parietal and temporal tumors.[20-22,25] As tumor bulk increases in size, cerebral edema accumulates and increased intracranial pressure (ICP) and brain tissue hemorrhages may be seen. Displacement of cerebral structures may result in brain herniation, an emergency and often lethal complication of increased tumor size and local invasion.[7,10,11,15]

Structural changes, memory defects, and speech, motor, and visual changes are also displayed and vary depending on tumor location and size. Figure 5-2 demonstrates the principal functional subdivisions of the cerebral hemisphere and the functions of specific cortical ar-

eas. Figure 5-3 illustrates common sites of intracranial tumors. Tumor-related side effects can be expected and understood with knowledge of tumor type, location of tumor, and approximate size of tumor at diagnosis.

Spinal cord tumors are also related to the site and size of the lesion. Pain is the most common presenting symptom. Weakness, sensory loss, muscle spasms, and loss of bowel and bladder control occur as the tumor invades local tissue causing nerve destruction.[25,27] The box, p. 67, summarizes common clinical features of CNS tumors.

DIAGNOSTIC AND PATHOLOGIC STAGING

An initial assessment of a suspected CNS tumor would include a physical and neurologic assessment. Pertinent data on emotional and physical changes may need to be obtained from family members. Computed tomography (CT) and magnetic resonance imaging (MRI) are the two most common and valuable diagnostic tests used to di-

Table 5-1 Brain and Spinal Cord Tumors

Neoplasm	Percent of tumors	Location	Characteristics	Cell of origin
Gliomas				
Astrocytoma	20	Anywhere in brain or spinal cord	Grade I and II Slow growing, invasive	Supportive tissue, astrocytes, glial cells
Glioblastoma multiforme	30	Common in cerebral hemispheres	Grade III, IV Highly invasive and malignant	Thought to arise from mature astrocytes
Oligodendrocytoma	4	Common in frontal lobes deep in white matter; may arise in brain stem, cerebellum, and spinal cord	Avascular, tends to be encapsulated; more malignant form called *oligodendroblastoma*	Oligodendrites, glial cells
Ependymoma	5	Intramedullary; wall of ventricles; may arise in caudal tail of spinal cord	Common in children, variable growth rates; more malignant, invasive form called *ependymoblastoma;* may extend into ventricle or invade brain tissue	Ependymal cells
Neurilemoma	4	Cranial nerves (most often vestibular division of cranial nerve VIII)	Slow growing	Schwann cells
Neurofibroma		Extramedullary: spinal cord	Slow growing	Neurilemma, Schwann cells
Pituitary tumors	8	Pituitary gland; may extend to or invade floor of third ventricle	Age linked, several types slow growing, macroadenomas and microadenomas may be secreting or nonsecreting	Pituitary cells, pituitary chromophobes, basophils, eosinophils
Pineal region tumors	1	Pineal region; pineal parenchyma, posterior or third ventricle	Several types (e.g., germinoma, pineocytoma, teratoma)	Several types with different cell origin
Blood vessel tumors				
Angioma	3	Predominantly in posterior cerebral hemispheres	Slow growing	Arising from congenitally malformed arteriovenous connections
Neuronal cell tumors				
Medulloblastoma	1	Posterior cerebellar vermis, roof of fourth ventricle	Well demarcated, rapid growing, fills fourth ventricle	Embryonic cells
Mesodermal tissue tumors				
Meningioma	20	Intradural, extramedullary; sylvian fissure region, superior parasagittal surface of frontal and parietal lobes, olfactory groove, wing of sphenoid bone, superior surface of cerebellum, cerebellopontine angle, spinal cord	Slow growing, circumscribed, encapsulated, sharply demarcated from normal tissues, compressive in nature	
Choroid plexus tumors				
Papilloma	1	Choroid plexus of ventricular system; lateral ventricle in children, fourth ventricle in adults	Usually benign; slow in expansion, inducing hemorrhage and hydrocephalus; malignant tumor is rare	Epithelial cells
Cranial nerve and spinal nerve root tumors				
Hemangioblastoma	2	Arises from blood vessels, predominant in cerebellum	Benign, slow growing	Embryonic vascular tissue
Lymphoma	1	Cerebral hemispheres	Metastasis common	B cells
Metastatic tumors	35 of all cancer patients	Cerebral cortex diencephalon	Malignant spread	From lung, breast, colon, kidney, thyroid, prostate

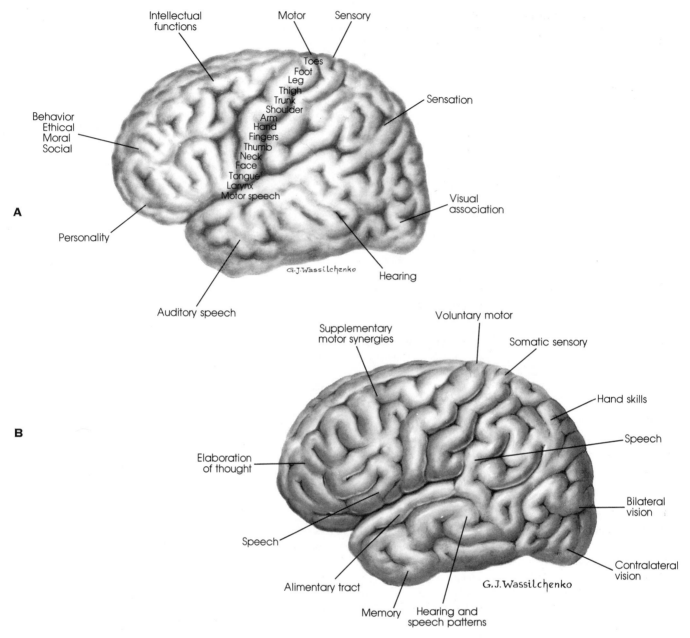

Figure 5-2   **A**, Principal functional subdivisions of the cerebral hemisphere. **B**, Functional areas of specific cortical areas. (In McCance KL, Huether SE: *Pathophysiology: the biologic basis for disease in adults and children*, St Louis, 1990, Mosby. From Rudy E: *Advanced neurological neurosurgical nursing*, St Louis, 1984, Mosby.)

agnose CNS tumors. CT is the most useful in low-grade astrocytomas and small diameter tumors because of their increased visibility for tumor location and size. CT is also useful for spinal cord tumors and evaluation of tumor recurrence and treatment response.[4]

MRI provides exquisite detail to tumor location and reconstruction of images at three views at right angles: axial, sagittal, and coronal.[4,12] MRI also has the ability to detect edema but does not differentiate between edema and tumor (Figure 5-4).

Positron emission tomography (PET) uses CT to detect the emission of positive electrons and some radioactive substances. Chemical substances such as glucose are distributed in tissues to evaluate the tumor response and activity. These metabolic activities are produced in a series of color pictures. Until now, PET has only been used as part of research protocols.

Cerebral angiograms and radionuclide (RN) angiograms are x-rays used to evaluate cerebral blood vessel flow near the tumor. These x-rays should only be used

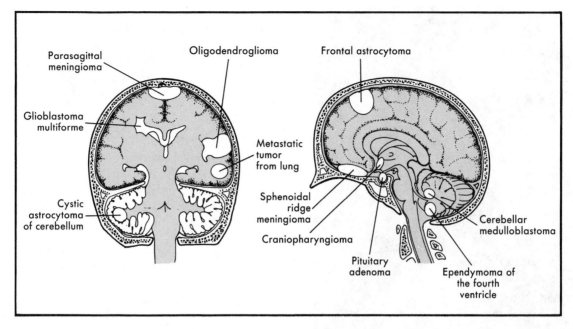

Figure 5-3   Common sites of intracranial tumors. (From McCance KL, Huether SE: *Pathophysiology: the biologic basis for disease in adults and children,* ed 2, St Louis, 1994, Mosby.)

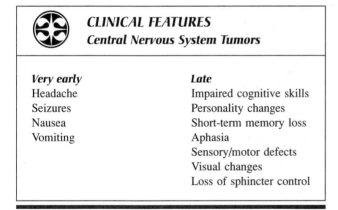

CLINICAL FEATURES
Central Nervous System Tumors

Very early	*Late*
Headache	Impaired cognitive skills
Seizures	Personality changes
Nausea	Short-term memory loss
Vomiting	Aphasia
	Sensory/motor defects
	Visual changes
	Loss of sphincter control

after CT and MRI. RN angiograms show various concentrations of injected material in the brain. Additional examinations that may be ordered include skull and spinal films and evoked potentials. Evoked potentials measure the electrode activity of nerves and may be important at the time of surgical removal of tumors that surround nerves.[12]

Electroencephalography (EEG) is a rare test with little diagnostic ability. Tumor markers have only demonstrated usefulness in embryonal tumors in the pineal area. α-Fetoprotein and β-human chorionic gonadotropin (HCG) are found in cerebrospinal fluid (CSF).[6,10] Lumbar puncture (LP) examinations should be performed only when risk of increased ICP has been ruled out and after MRI and CT. An LP is useful in the diagnosis of meningeal involvement, periventricular tumors, and CNS lymphomas. Results from CSF analysis that may indicate tumor involvement include increased spinal pressure readings, elevated white blood cell (WBC) and protein count, and glucose level.

Diagnostic examinations are only tentative; a definitive diagnosis can be made only when the specific tumor type is identified. The identification of tumor cell type can be done only by a biopsy of tumor tissue. This can be accomplished by either open biopsy, such as a craniotomy, or through stereotactic needle biopsy, which is a closed system into a burr hole opening. A biopsy probe in a three-dimensional space is used to visualize the tumor. Simple needle biopsies yield inadequate specimens and may result in bleeding complications. When biopsy specimens are not available because of tumor location, interpretation must be done with only diagnostic examinations. Metastatic CNS tumors are evaluated in a similar manner with the primary focus on the discovery of the tumor's primary site.

Pathologic staging is based on histology, grade, and the completeness of tumor removal. The TNM (tumor, nodes, metastatic disease) staging system is used to stage CNS tumors. Tumor locations are divided into supratentorial (above the tentorium cerebelli), intratentorial (below the tentorium cerebelli), and infratentorial. Category N (node) is not applicable because lymph nodes do not exist in CNS tumors. Tumor grading is based on cell differentiation. Stages I through IV exist with subcategories A and B (see box, p. 69).[3,29]

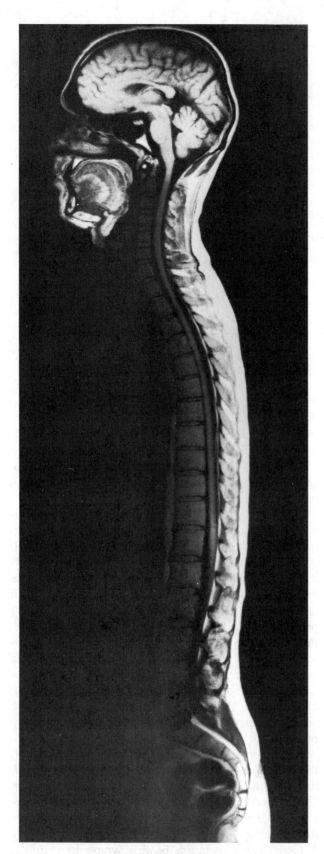

Figure 5-4 Midsagittal MR image demonstrating the extraordinary anatomic detail possible with this technique. (From McCance KL, Huether SE: *Pathophysiology: the biologic basis for disease in adults cind children*, ed 2, St Louis, 1994, Mosby.)

METASTASIS

The spread of primary CNS tumors beyond the brain and spinal cord is rare. Seeding is the most common method of spread within the CNS and spinal cord. Medulloblastoma tumors have the greatest potential to develop metastatic lesions within the CNS.[2,7,15]

TREATMENT MODALITIES

Surgery remains the treatment of choice for all CNS tumors. Nonresectable or partially resectable tumors may require additional treatment modalities such as radiation, chemotherapy, biotherapy oncogenes, and use of steroids and anticonvulsant therapy to treat tumor or treatment side effects.

Pretreatment techniques involve use of steroids such as dexamethasone (Decadron) that are administered to assist with the reduction of cerebral edema, which may cause personality changes, altered level of consciousness, and sensorimotor defects. Anticonvulsant therapy may also be administered for those patients with focal changes that result in seizure activity. Steroidal and anticonvulsant therapy may be continued after surgery or radiation to minimize potential side effects.[5,19,22]

Surgery

Surgery serves as a diagnostic and treatment modality. Surgical intervention provides tissue sampling for histology, decreases the tumor burden for further treatment, and can provide a cure for low-grade tumors. The ability for complete resection varies with size and tumor location. Various types of surgical procedures may be performed depending on the ability to access the tumor and the patient's overall ability to tolerate the surgical procedure without gross neurologic defects. A craniotomy is the most common surgical procedure performed to remove tumor mass or debulk the largest portion of the tumor. Additional surgical procedures may include stereotactic biopsy for the removal of smaller tumors and placement of radioactive substances to treat nonresectable tumors.[5,13]

Metastatic tumors may also lend themselves to surgical removal if benign lesions exist or favorable prognosis from the original primary tumor exists.

Radiation Therapy

Tumors that are inoperable or have only partial tumor resection may respond to radiation therapy if the tumor histology is radiosensitive. Tumors that are radiosensitive include medulloblastomas, high-grade astrocytomas, metastatic brain tumors of the breast and lung, and sarcomas.[2,5,10,15]

Radiation treatments may be administered in a variety of doses and methods. Conventional dose therapy is usually given over a series of weeks, allowing normal tissue to heal and hypoxic tumor cells to become more sus-

TNM CLASSIFICATION OF BRAIN TUMORS

PRIMARY TUMOR (T)

TX: primary tumor cannot be assessed

T0: no evidence of primary tumor

SUPRATENTORIAL TUMOR

T1: tumor 5 cm or less in greatest dimension; limited to one side

T2: tumor more than 5 cm in greatest dimension; limited to one side

T3: tumor invades or encroaches on ventricular system

T4: tumor crosses midline, invades opposite hemisphere, or invades infratentorially

INFRATENTORIAL TUMOR

T1: tumor 3 cm or less in greatest dimension; limited to one side

T2: tumor more than 3 cm in greatest dimension; limited to one side

T3: tumor invades or encroaches on the ventricular system

T4: tumor crosses midline, invades opposite hemisphere, or invades supratentorially

REGIONAL LYMPH NODES (N)

This category does not apply to this site.

DISTANT METASTASIS (M)

MX: presence of distant metastasis cannot be assessed

M0: no distant metastasis

M1: distant metastasis

HISTOPATHOLOGIC GRADE (G)

GX: grade cannot be assessed

G1: well differentiated

G2: moderately well differentiated

G3: poorly differentiated

G4: undifferentiated

STAGE GROUPING

Stage IA:	G1-T1-M0
Stage IIB:	G1-T2-M0
	G1-T3-M0
Stage IIA:	G2-T1-M0
Stage IIB:	G2-T2-M0
	G2-T3-M0
Stage IIIA:	G3-T1-M0
Stage IIIB:	G3-T2-M0
	G3-T3-M0
Stage IV:	G1, G2, G3-T4-M0
	G4-any T-M0
	Any G-any T-M1

From Beahrs OH and others: *Manual for staging of cancer,* ed 4, Philadelphia, 1992, Lippincott.

ceptible to treatment. Doses may also be given to the entire brain and spinal cord when there is risk of metastasis to surrounding tissue.

Additional methods of radiation may be given at the time of surgery and include interstitial implants of radioactive seeds directly to the tumor. Radiation may also be administered via the stereotactic route during surgery. This method allows a single dose of radiation to be administered to one area of the brain.[1,5]

Other methods of radiation administration include *hyperthermia,* a local treatment done during surgery that uses catheters implanted into the tumor. These catheters administer heat throughout the tumor. Tumor cells are more sensitive to heat, and therefore hyperthermia may enhance radiation therapy to the tumor site. Experimental treatment modalities include radioactive sensitizers, hyperfractionation, heavy particle radiation therapy, photodynamic therapy, and neutron capture therapy.[1,6,8,9,27]

Stereotactic Therapy

Therapy is delivered with the use of a gamma knife, linear accelerator, and heavy beam particles. Heavy beam particles are used because they can be adjusted without causing damage to surrounding tissues. Stereotactic surgery offers alternatives to craniotomy surgery for tumors under 30 mm in size. Complications include nausea and

vomiting, radiation necrosis, and intracranial neuropathies. Use of this technique is limited because of the complexity of medical knowledge needed to provide treatment, technical considerations, and added cost for treatment and equipment. As technology develops, the future of stereotactic surgery remains hopeful as an alternative to current therapy.[1,2,7]

Photodynamic Therapy

Of all the treatments just listed, photodynamic therapy (PDT) may have the greatest potential. PDT is an oxygen-dependent, photochemical oxidative process in which retention of the photosensitizing agents in the tumor tissue results in entrapment of tumor tissue because of the inability to eliminate the chemical. The therapy then impacts the tumor's neovasculature, resulting in tumor necrosis. The most widely used substance is hematoporphyrin derivative (HPD) (Photofrin). Photofrin has photodynamic properties that are activated by 30 nm light therapy, producing cytotoxicity. HPD can be administered intravenously or via the artery. Surgically, HPD may be administered and external illumination done to the resected area. Limitations exist for tumors reaching sizes of 0.5 to 1.0 cm, since HPD is unable to reach infiltrating gliomas. Side effects include edema resulting in increased ICP. PTD refinement and development of more chemical oxidative substances hold the potential for future control of malignant brain tumors.[8,17]

Table 5-2 summarizes other experimental treatments.[1,6,8,9,27]

Chemotherapy

Chemotherapy may be used in combination with surgery and radiation for the treatment of gliomas and medulloblastomas. Response rate remains as low as 20% to 40% because of the blood-brain barrier mechanism.[6] The most frequently used drugs are the nitrosoureas (BCNU, CCNU). Additional agents are the alkylating (cisplatin, cyclophosphamide, nitrogen mustard) and antitumor antibiotics (bleomycin), plant alkaloids (vincristine, etoposide), antimetabolites (methotrexate), and procarbazine.[2,6,9]

Common routes of administration include oral and intravenous. Additional methods include intraarterial into the carotid or vertebral artery via timed-release biodegradable wafers impregnated with chemotherapy and into the spinal column. Shunting of fluids or circulation may be done by use of a surgical technique such as superficial temporal artery to middle cerebral artery (STA-MCA), a microneurosurgical bypass procedure to improve circulation, or placement of a ventricular shunt to treat hydrocephalus. Placement of an Ommaya reservoir

EXPERIMENTAL BIOTHERAPY
Interferon
Growth factors
Tumor necrosis factors
Interleukins
Colony-stimulating factors
Monoclonal antibodies
Lymphokine-activated killer cells
Tumor-infiltrating lymphocytes
Immunotoxins
Bacterial derivatives
Retinoids
Cellular transfer

into the ventricles allows for easy access of CSF administration of chemotherapy and reduces the need for LPs (see Figure 20-1.)[24]

The box above lists experimental uses of biotherapy.[6]

Metastatic Brain Tumors

Brain metastases represent a continued concern because of the frequency of a majority of cancer metastases occurring to the brain from the "end-artery" pattern, where 20% of the blood flow from the heart allows trapped cancer cells to multiply and form metastatic deposits. Thirty percent of all brain tumors are the result of metastatic disease. Common sites of metastasis include lung, breast, melanomas, and unknown primary sites. Most patients have multiple lesions, which significantly alters the treatment potential. Treatment is based on location, size, and prognostic factors. Prognosis is 3-6 months survival from time of metastatic diagnosis. Table 5-3 summarizes these characteristics and the nursing management.[10,13,15]

SPINAL CORD TUMORS

Spinal cord tumors represent a rare primary malignancy and only 1% of all cancers. Secondary tumors from metastatic disease are documented as high as 40%. Tumors

Table 5-2   Investigational Treatments with Radiation Therapy

Type	Definition
Radiosensitizer	Uses radiosensitized drugs to substitute ingredient to repair cells
Fractional radiation therapy	Doses of radiation are given in fractional increments closer apart to allow for cell cycle vulnerability
Heavy particle therapy	Changed particles are superior to external rays by decreasing damage and increasing tumor cell kill
Neutron capture therapy	Nonionizing radiation with a drug concentrates in tumor cells; radiation activates tumor cells and kills them

Table 5-3   Characteristics of Metastatic Brain Tumors

Disease	Clinical features	Nursing management
Lung	Headache	Note time, duration, and location of headache; medicate per orders.
Breast	Weakness	Monitor for increased intracranial pressure (wide pulse pressure, irregular respirations, bradycardia); elevate head of bed.
Melanoma	Seizure activity	Institute seizure precautions (note time, duration, and site of seizure).
Urinary organs	Blurred vision	Monitor for altered level of consciousness; orient; perform cranial checks.
Colon/rectum	Gait disturbance	Institute safety precautions with ambulation; assist with activities of daily living.
	Altered sensorium	Explain tests, procedures, and treatment modalities.
	Personality changes	Offer support to patient/caregiver if terminal prognosis.

may grow in or around the spinal column, with neurilemomas, meningiomas, and sarcomas representing the major histologic types. Presentation of tumor is highest in the thoracic and cervical areas. Metastasis is likely to occur from primary sites of breast, lung, thyroid, kidney, and prostate cancer.

Patients' chief complaints are back pain, weakness, and sensorimotor alterations as well as bowel and bladder dysfunction. The diagnosis is made using enhanced MRI, myelography, and CT. Treatment modalities include steroid therapy, partial or complete resection of the tumor followed by radiation therapy, and hormonal therapy for breast and prostate cancer patients.

Nursing management is similar to the preoperative and postoperative care of the patient experiencing a brain tumor, with a focus on early detection and management of complications. Rehabilitation is indicated in individuals with residual neurologic deficits.[11]

DISEASE-RELATED COMPLICATIONS

Major disease-related complications include increased ICP from cerebral edema and displaced brain structures resulting in brain herniation. A major complication of

spinal cord tumors is spinal cord compression (see Chapter 19).

ICP is caused by an increase in intracellular volume from the expanding tumor mass and edema. The box below lists clinical features of ICP and brain stem herniation. Cerebral edema results in tissue hypoxia and acidosis (Figure 5-5). If left to progress, brain stem com-

---

 CLINICAL FEATURES
Increased Intracranial Pressure (ICP) and Brain Stem Herniation

Headache
Vomiting
Mental acuity changes
Seizures
Alterations in motor or sensory responses
Changes in vital signs
Ocular changes
Wide pulse pressure
Irregular respirations
Bradycardia

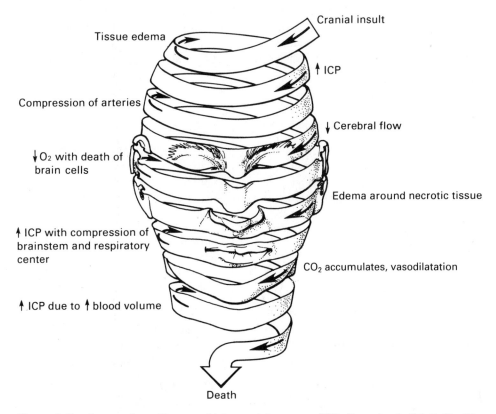

Figure 5-5 Progression of increased intracranial pressure (ICP). (From Lewis SM, Collier IC: *Medical-surgical nursing: assessment and management of clinical problems,* ed 3, St Louis, 1992, Mosby.)

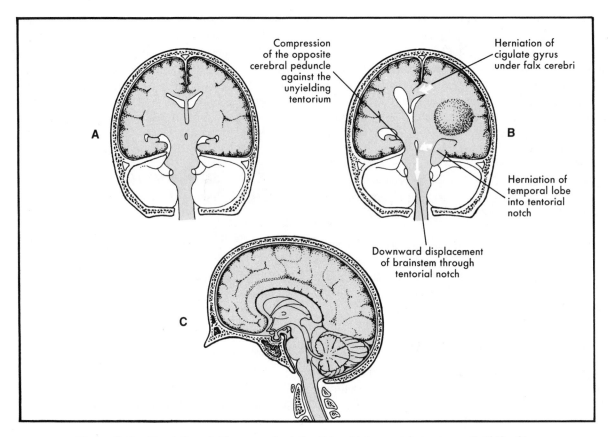

Figure 5-6 Herniation. **A,** The normal relationship of intracranial structures. **B,** Shift of intracranial structures. **C,** Downward herniation of the cerebellar tonsils into the foramen magnum. (In Lewis SM, Collier IC: *Medical-surgical nursing: assessment and management of clinical problems,* ed 3, St Louis, 1992, Mosby. From McCance KL, Huether SE: *Pathophysiology: biologic basis for disease in adults and children,* St Louis, 1990, Mosby.)

pression occurs and herniation of the brain results. Ultimately, respiratory arrest will follow. Management includes surgical removal and supportive therapy with diuretics and corticosteroids. Close nursing observation is required to monitor a potentially fatal outcome (Figure 5-6).[10,20,25]

TREATMENT-RELATED COMPLICATIONS
Radiation Therapy

Radiation treatment–related side effects are based on the dose and location of treatment. Local and long-term side effects can be experienced (see box at right). Most side effects are temporary and related to local irritation or disruption of myelin formation. Radiation doses are cumulative, and retreatment in the same manner is not recommended.[20,28]

Chemotherapy

Major side effects related to chemotherapy are based on the combination of drugs and their specific dose. Major

RADIATION THERAPY SIDE EFFECTS

EARLY

Hair loss
Skin changes (redness, darkness, itching)
Nausea
Inflammation around the ear
Edema (increased intracranial pressure)
Anorexia
Lethargy

LONG TERM

Decreased intellect
Altered motor and sensory functions
Pituitary dysfunction

SPINAL CORD

Radiation myelopathy

Table 5-4   Chemotherapy Drugs and Related Side Effects

Drug	Side effects
BCNU	Bone marrow suppression
CCNU	Nausea, alopecia, pulmonary fibrosis
Cisplatin	Ototoxicity, renal dysfunction, bone marrow depression, anorexia, nausea/vomiting
Cyclophosphamide	Nausea/vomiting, diarrhea, alopecia, bone marrow suppression
Nitrogen mustard	Nausea/vomiting, anorexia, alopecia, diarrhea, bone marrow suppression, hepatic/neurologic dysfunction
Bleomycin	Nausea/vomiting, stomatitis, hepatic/neurologic dysfunction, pulmonary fibrosis
Vincristine	Nausea/vomiting, anorexia, alopecia, neurologic dysfunction
Etoposide	Nausea/vomiting, anorexia, hypotension, bone marrow suppression
Methotrexate	Bone marrow suppression, renal tubular necrosis, stomatitis, diarrhea, hepatic dysfunction
Procarbazine	Nausea/vomiting, diarrhea, alopecia, myelosuppression, hepatic and neurologic dysfunction

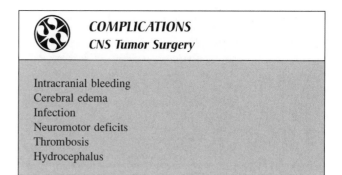

COMPLICATIONS
CNS Tumor Surgery

Intracranial bleeding
Cerebral edema
Infection
Neuromotor deficits
Thrombosis
Hydrocephalus

STEROID THERAPY SIDE EFFECTS

Hyperglycemia
Irritability
Insomnia
Psychotic reactions, mood swings
Hypokalemia
Hypernatremia
Depressed immune response
Elevated lipid and cholesterol levels
Fluid retention
Cataract formation
Osteoporosis
Thrombophlebitis
Steroid-induced gastric ulcers
Relocation of fat deposits (round face and thick trunk)
Cutaneous striae
Withdrawal symptoms (doses must be reduced from intravenous to oral and then in amount and frequency)

BIOTHERAPY SIDE EFFECTS

Flu-like symptoms (headache, fever, chills, arthralgia, myalgia)
Nausea/vomiting (varies with individual and amount of dose)
Weight loss (amount depends on amount of side effects)
Altered neurologic functioning (decreased short-term memory concentration and attention)
Alopecia (partial)
Skin changes (erythema, rash, pruritus)
Fluid and electrolyte imbalances (hypocalcemia, hypomagnesemia)
Bone marrow suppression (pancytopenia)

---

areas that are affected include the bone marrow, hair follicles, and gastrointestinal tract. Table 5-4 lists major side effects of common drugs used in CNS tumors.[6,18]

Biotherapy

Side effects of biotherapy are related to dose and combined modality (see box above).[26]

Surgery

The box, top right, lists postoperative surgical complications. Size and location of tumor and the overall preop-

erative state of the patient enhance the potential for complications.[10,25]

Steroidal Therapy

Use of steroids preoperatively and postoperatively can also produce a variety of treatment side effects that can produce local and systemic effects (see box above).[6] Steroids are administered to produce an antiinflammatory response and reduce cerebral swelling. Steroidal therapy may begin after an initial dose of mannitol, which may be used before, during, or after surgery to reduce immediate cerebral edema. Postoperative management with titration is performed with steroids such as dexamethasone.

POSTOPERATIVE CARE

Surgery for CNS tumors may be done by standard craniotomy or use of laser surgery. Use of laser surgery is limited but has several advantages: (1) it decreases the

PATIENT TEACHING PRIORITIES
Radiation Therapy

Knowledge of treatment schedule
Knowledge of skin care routine
    Marks are not to be washed off
    No creams or lotions to treatment site
Knowledge of radiation complications

PATIENT TEACHING PRIORITIES
Chemotherapy and Biotherapy

Knowledge of drug administration route and schedule
Knowledge of side effects and supportive measures:
    Weight changes and loss of appetite
    Nausea
    Bruising and bleeding episodes
    Temperature changes
    Oral hygiene routine

amount of dissection to surrounding tissue, and (2) it has the ability to reach tumors that were formerly inaccessible. Spinal tumors can also be removed by laser surgery or standard decompression laminectomy. Surgery is always indicated to assist with histologic typing and debulking of tumor mass. Inoperable tumors may respond by the relief of general symptoms of compression and intracranial pressure.

Radiation Therapy

If the tumor excision has been incomplete and the histologic report reveals a radiosensitive tumor, a patient may receive radiation therapy treatments after postoperative healing has taken place. Patient and family will need information on the length of treatment and expected side effects (see box above).

Spinal cord tumors are also treated with radiation, although the dose and treatment time may vary. The most serious consequence of spinal cord radiation is radiation myelopathy, which results in paraplegia and loss of bowel and bladder control. This is usually a late occurrence (6 to 15 months posttherapy). Family and patients need to be instructed to notify their physician if any symptoms occur. Symptoms of therapy complication may also manifest tumor recurrence. Constant anxiety exists even for those patients with better prognostic factors. Assessment of the emotional stability of the family and patient is ongoing and a critical nursing factor.

Chemotherapy and Biotherapy

Nursing management of those patients receiving chemotherapy and biotherapy treatments includes providing knowledge about drugs and their expected side effects (see box top right). Monitoring side effects and appropriate treatment can ensure patient comfort and safety.[6]

GERIATRIC CONSIDERATIONS

The normal age-related changes in the geriatric population may lead to a delay or misdiagnosis of CNS tumors. Altered ambulation patterns, sensory impairment, de-

GERIATRIC CONSIDERATIONS
CNS Tumors

Diagnostic difficulties
Increased assessment (preoperatively and postoperatively)
Treatment modality complications
Rehabilitation
Home care referral

creased visual and hearing acuity, and changes in cognition are similar to CNS tumor changes. Once diagnosed, these normal physiologic changes will also interfere with adequate postoperative assessment and the speed of recovery. Response to extensive surgery and treatment modalities may also produce increased side effects in elderly persons. Rehabilitation needs and expanded home care referrals are required to assist the expansion needs of the geriatric population. The box above summarizes these specific concerns.

PROGNOSIS

The ultimate prognosis of CNS tumors is determined by the following factors: histologic type, tumor grade, size and extent of tumor, patient's age, performance status, and residual tumor.[11] Survival rates range from complete cure to rapid deterioration and death. Glioblastoma multiforme (grade IV) has the poorest prognosis and a life expectancy of 9 to 12 months. Younger individuals who are neurologically intact survive longer than the geriatric (elderly) patient.

Metastatic lesions present a different prognosis and vary depending on whether the tumor is a single lesion or disseminated, size and cell type of primary tumor, other metastatic lesions, patient age, performance status, and the time from the treatment of the primary lesions until the start of the metastasis.[11]

Text continued on p. 79.

NURSING MANAGEMENT

The diagnosis of cancer produces high levels of anxiety and fear in most patients and families; of particular concern are those patients diagnosed with CNS tumors. Emotional distress is brought on by the rapid onset of debilitation, physical and emotional changes, and the ultimate poor prognostic factors. Preparation time from the onset of symptoms to diagnosis and surgery is limited and often allows little time for emotional support and education. Most information on the treatment course will be provided after surgery and is based on tumor size, type, and location and ability to remove tumor mass.

Lack of past experience with hospitalization and surgery further increases the anxiety and fear patterns. Paralysis, coma, and neurologic defects may all be a postoperative reality. For patients with metastatic disease who have already undergone treatment, the knowledge of cancer recurrences can be devastating.

NURSING DIAGNOSES

• *Fear and anxiety related to diagnosis and postoperative outcomes*
• *Knowledge deficit related to limited experience with diagnostic preoperative and postoperative routines*

OUTCOME GOALS

Patient will be able to:
• Verbalize expression of concerns (fears and anxiety) related to diagnoses and postoperative outcomes.
• State knowledge of preoperative and postoperative routines.

INTERVENTIONS

Interventions are based on providing emotional support through information and teaching on expected outcomes. Assessment of past coping mechanisms and support systems within the family structure are needed. Education should be based on teaching learning principles and include visual information. A basic review of the anatomy and physiology of the CNS system will assist in the understanding of tumor locations and causes of present symptoms. Discussion should include an explanation of tests and procedures, their diagnostic indications, postoperative routines, monitoring devices, potential postoperative complications, and expected body image alterations. Patients with altered cognition from extensive CNS involvement may not be able to participate. These families will need additional support systems of family, clergy, or other hospital supports that may be available. The inclusion of a clinical nurse specialist in neurology is helpful and can provide additional information on postoperative concerns. The box below summarizes patient/family education needs related to surgery.

PATIENT TEACHING PRIORITIES
CNS Tumor Surgery

Explanation of surgical diagnostic procedures
Basic review of anatomy and physiology of CNS system
   Tumor location
   Expected signs/symptoms
Postoperative monitoring
   Equipment
Postoperative nursing care routines
Postoperative complications
Body image concerns

NURSING MANAGEMENT

The postoperative course requires extensive monitoring for complications. Further treatment is based on operative results, tumor histology, and patient complications. Families continue to need intense emotional support during the postoperative course. For those patients with inoperable tumors, a referral for home care or hospice is appropriate.

NURSING DIAGNOSES

• *Self-care deficit related to postoperative procedure*
• *Body image disturbance related to altered physical status*
• *Sensory/perceptual alterations related to neurologic deficits*
• *Injury, risk for, related to altered cognition and side effect of medications*
• *Pain related to surgical procedure*
• *Coping, ineffective family: compromised, and coping, ineffective individual, related to prognostic factors*

OUTCOME GOALS

Patient will be able to:
• Demonstrate ability to increase self-care deficits.
• Express concerns related to altered body image.
• Maintain sensory and perceptual abilities during postoperative period.
• Demonstrate effective coping skills during postoperative period.

INTERVENTIONS

Postoperative care of the patient with a craniotomy includes frequent neurologic examinations, measurement of vital signs, supportive nursing care of positioning, and administration of medications, including pain, steroids, and anticonvulsant therapy. Observation of increased ICP and brain herniation is a critical factor in the postoperative course.[10,21] Common postoperative complications are included in the box, p. 73.

Neurologic examinations should include measurement of the level of consciousness, orientation, emotional response to surgery, and motor and sensory perception. Pupils are observed for inequality. Vital signs should be observed for decreased respirations and pulse and widened pulse pressure. The patient should be placed in a quiet, nonstimulating environment and positioned according to physician protocol. The most common position is with the head of the bed at a 30-degree angle to reduce cerebral edema and stress on the suture line. Dressings and drains are monitored for the type and amount of drainage. Coughing, deep breathing techniques, and suctioning are done in a nonaggressive manner to reduce increased ICP.

The patient will experience a self-care deficit for several days and require skin and mouth care as well as maintenance of bowel and urinary function. Assessment of the patient's comfort level is done during administration of care. Restlessness and moaning or increased head movement may indicate pain. Positioning, maintenance of a quiet environment, and low doses of mild pain medication are provided. Safety measures for those patients with potential seizure activity may include seizure pads and the administration of anticonvulsant therapy.

Management of increased ICP is through administration of mannitol and corticosteroids such as dexamethasone.[6,21] Long-term use of steroids to reduce edema can cause serious side effects (see box, p. 73) and therefore requires a titration schedule to reduce the amount and frequency of the drug.

After the immediate postoperative care the patient and family need further evaluation and continued support. Postoperative changes such as hair loss, edema, and generalized weight loss can cause extreme depression because of altered body image. Patients left with residual neurologic deficits may require nutritional supplements, tube feedings, or hyperalimentation depending on the ultimate prognosis. Rehabilitation and supportive equipment may also assist in caring for the patient at home.

Patients with primary spinal cord tumors experience a similar but a less aggressive postoperative course. Nursing observations include observation of neurologic function and level of motor and sensory function. Bowel and bladder control may be altered depending on the location of the tumor. Paralysis or motor deficits require additional rehabilitative consults. Prognostic factors and the amount of deficit will determine the amount of aggressive rehabilitative therapy. Support and follow-up are needed to assist patients and families during this critical period.

Metastatic spinal cord tumors represent an oncology emergency that requires immediate medical intervention. Early signs include neck and back pain, motor weakness, and loss of sensation. Treatment includes radiation therapy followed by surgery if the tumor does not respond to radiation and use of steroids.

NURSING MANAGEMENT

NURSING DIAGNOSES

• *Knowledge deficit related to lack of experience with chemotherapy routine and side effects*
• *Nutrition, altered: less than body requirements related to chemotherapy-induced nausea*
• *Oral mucous membrane, altered, related to chemotherapy administration*
• *Infection, risk for, related to altered immune status*
• *Self-esteem disturbance related to chemotherapy-induced side effects*

OUTCOME GOALS

Patient will be able to:
• Express knowledge of chemotherapy routine and side effects.
• Maintain nutritional status and maintain body weight within 10% of prechemotherapy state.
• Maintain oral mucous membranes through chemotherapy regimen.
• Demonstrate no evidence of signs or symptoms of infection throughout chemotherapy regimen.

INTERVENTIONS

Knowledge of the limited use and experimental nature of chemotherapy and biotherapy is important for patients and family. Because of the blood-brain barrier, a limited number of drugs are considered effective therapy for CNS tumors. Patients need to understand drug treatment schedules, follow-up blood work, and expected side effects.[20,24]

Potential side effects of biotherapy are listed in the box, p. 73. Nursing interventions include assessment of the patient's nutritional status, administration of antiemetics, small frequent bland feedings, monitoring intake and output, weight checks, and providing nutritional consultations.

Blood counts assist with monitoring the hematologic and immune status alterations produced by chemotherapy treatments. Limiting visitors with colds, vigilant handwashing, monitoring changes in temperature, and observation of signs and symptoms of infection all are critical for those patients with lowered WBC counts. Reduction of hemoglobin and platelets may produce cellular damage. Patients should be observed for shortness of breath, weakness, fatigue, bruises, petechiae, and signs of active bleeding. Applying pressure to injection sites and limited use of rectal medications are also methods of controlling increased trauma and induction of bleeding.

Oral hygiene is essential to reduce risk of infection and to promote cleanliness and comfort. Oral assessment for evidence of yeast infections or lesions should be done daily. Specific mouth care protocols should follow physician's routine.

The administration of steroids is a common occurrence for many chemotherapy protocols, particularly CNS tumors. Common side effects from steroidal therapy can be found in the box, p. 73.[21] The nurse monitors the patient's response to steroid therapy by continued observation of vital signs, blood sugars, changes in emotional state, and potential gastrointestinal bleeding. Administration of antacids or gastric antagonists assists with potential gastric complications. Body image changes from steroidal therapy, hair loss, or residual neurologic deficits may cause increased depression and withdrawal. Supportive care is required for both patients and family.

Biotherapy treatment requires constant observation for side effects. Treatment with biotherapy may be part of an experimental or research protocol. The box, p. 73, includes common side effects of biotherapy. Patients who experience increased symptoms may require removal from treatment because of an effort to keep data collection complete. Patients and families may experience anger and frustration over removal from the last hope of treatment.

NURSING MANAGEMENT

NURSING DIAGNOSES

- *Knowledge deficit related to lack of experience with radiation routine and side effects*
- *Skin integrity, impaired, related to radiation treatment modality*
- *Self-esteem disturbance related to change in physical appearance/therapy markings, skin changes, and hair loss*
- *Sensory/perceptual alterations related to postradiation damage*

OUTCOME GOALS

Patient will be able to:
- Verbalize knowledge of radiation routine and side effects.
- Maintain skin integrity.
- Verbalize alterations in self-esteem related to body image change.

INTERVENTIONS

Patients and family should be informed of the number of treatments that will be required. Normal treatments are daily for 4 to 8 weeks. Transportation arrangements may be indicated if mobility limitations are present. A brief introduction to the radiation department and an explanation of the use of radiation therapy helps to eliminate additional anxieties.

Included in teaching of side effects is knowledge of skin markings, hair loss, and skin changes near the radiation site. Instructions on skin care include not washing marks off and no application of creams near treatment sites. If treatments are given near the ear or in a visual field, hearing and vision may become impaired. Radiation treatments may also cause an increase in ICP and may require additional steroid therapy. Reporting signs and symptoms of headache or changes in personality is an important consideration. Emotional support is needed to deal with additional self-esteem concerns.

CONCLUSION

Despite the low incidence of CNS tumors, they continue to produce rapid deterioration, debilitation, and higher mortality than most primary cancers. Metastatic CNS tumors represent a continued challenge to the medical community. New clinical trials and surgical modalities are under investigation in the hopes of providing relief of symptoms and increased survival rates.

■ CHAPTER QUESTIONS

1. Possible causes of CNS tumors include all *except* which of the following?
   a. Neurofibromatosis
   b. Chemical exposures to petrochemicals
   c. Epstein-Barr virus
   d. Head injuries
2. Common diagnostic assessments used to diagnose CNS tumors include all *except* which of the following?
   a. Computed tomography
   b. Magnetic resonance imaging
   c. Lumbar puncture
   d. Positron emission tomography
3. The most common clinical feature of a CNS tumor is:
   a. Personality change
   b. Sensory and motor defects
   c. Headache
   d. Seizures
4. The treatment of choice for CNS tumors is:
   a. Dexamethasone therapy
   b. Surgery
   c. Radiation therapy
   d. Chemotherapy
5. Lowered drug response in CNS tumor management is a result of which of the following?
   a. Late diagnosis
   b. Existence of multiple metastatic lesions
   c. Poor patient tolerance for chemotherapy-related side effects
   d. Blood-brain barrier mechanism
6. Signs of intracranial pressure include all *except* which of the following?
   a. Headache
   b. Nausea and vomiting
   c. Narrow pulse pressure
   d. Irregular respirations
7. A possible radiation side effect is:
   a. Radiation myelopathy
   b. Pain
   c. Hypersensitivity reaction
   d. Personality change
8. All *except* which of the following are possible chemotherapy drugs used to treat CNS tumors?
   a. BCNU
   b. Cisplatin
   c. Methotrexate
   d. Adriamycin
9. Steroid therapy includes all *except* which of the following complications?
   a. Relocation of fat deposits
   b. Fluid retention
   c. Hyperkalemia
   d. Hyperglycemia
10. The least appropriate reference for a patient with a CNS tumor include all *except* which of the following?
    a. Hospice
    b. Physical therapy
    c. Occupational therapy
    d. Sex therapy

BIBLIOGRAPHY

1. Abner B, Collins J: *Cancer chemotherapy and practice,* Philadelphia, 1990, Lippincott.
2. Alvarez F and others: Malignant and atypical meningiomas: a reappraisal of clinical, histological, and computer tomographic features, *Neurosurgery* 20:688, 1987.
3. Amato CA: Malignant glioma: coping with a devastating illness, *J Neurosci Nurs* 23:20, 1991.
4. American Cancer Society: *Cancer facts and figures—1996,* Atlanta, 1996, The Society.
5. American Joint Committee on Cancer: *Manual of staging of cancer,* ed 3, Philadelphia, 1992, Lippincott.
6. American Brain Tumor Association: *A primer of brain tumors,* ed 5, Chicago, 1991, The Association.
7. Baird SB and others: *A cancer source book for nurses,* Atlanta, 1991, American Cancer Society.
8. Bernstein M and others: Interstitial brachytherapy for malignant brain tumors: preliminary results, *Neurosurgery* 26:371, 1990.
9. Blaney SM, Balis FM, Poplack DC: Pharmacologic approaches to the treatment of meningeal malignancy, *Oncology* 5:107, 1991.
10. Boss BJ, Heath J, Sunderland PM: Alteration of neurologic function. In McCance KL, Heuther SE, editors: *Pathophysiology: the biologic basis for disease in adults and children,* St Louis, 1990, Mosby.
11. Cammermeyer M, Appledome C, editors: *Core curriculum for oncology nursing,* ed 3, Park Ridge, Ill, 1990, American Association of Neuroscience Nurses.
12. *Chemotherapy and you: a guide to self help during treatment,* No 91-1136, Bethesda, Md, 1990, National Cancer Institute.
13. DeAngelis LM and others: Primary CNS lymphoma: managing patients with spontaneous and AIDS-related disease, *Oncology* 1:52, 1987.
14. Doenges ME, Moorhowe MF, Geissler AC, editors: *Nursing care plans,* ed 2, Philadelphia, 1993, Davis.
15. Drummond BC: Preventing increased intracranial pressure: nursing can make a difference, *Focus Crit Care* 17:116, 1990.
16. Edwards DK, Stupperick TK, Welsh DM: Hyperthermia treatment for malignant tumors: nursing management during therapy, *J Neurosci Nurs* 23:34, 1991.
17. Edwards MS and others: Hyperfractioned radiation therapy for

brain-stem glioma: a phase I-II trial, *J Neurosurg* 70:691, 1989.

18. Gullatte MM, Graves T: Advances in antineoplastic therapy, *Oncol Nurs Forum* 17:867, 1990.

19. Hart S: Neurological care. In Shaw M and others, editors: *Illustrated manual of nursing practice,* Springhouse, Pa, 1991, Springhouse.

20. Hickey JV: *The clinical practice of neurological and neurosurgical nursing,* ed 2, Philadelphia, 1986, Lippincott.

21. Kornblith P, Walker M, Cassady JR: *Neurologic oncology,* Philadelphia, 1987, Lippincott.

22. Leibel SA and others: Survival and quality of life after interstitial implantation of removable high-activity iodine-125 sources for treatment of patients with recurrent malignant gliomas, *Int J Radiat Oncol Biol Phys* 17:1129, 1989.

23. Levin VA, Sheline GE, Gutin PH: Neoplasms of the central nervous system. In DeVita VT, Hellman S, Rosenberg SP, editors: *Cancer: principles and practice of oncology,* ed 4, Philadelphia, 1993, Lippincott.

24. Levin VA and others: Superiority of post-radiotherapy adjuvant chemotherapy with CCNU, procardazine, vincristine (PCV) over BCNU for anaplastic gliomas: (NCOG final report), *Int J Radiat Oncol Biol Phys* 18:321, 1990.

25. Loeffler JA and others: Radiosurgery for brain metastases, *PPO Updates* 5:1, 1991.

26. Owens B: Neurological cancer. In Clark J, McGee R, editors: *Core curriculum for oncology nursing,* ed 2, Philadelphia, 1992, Saunders.

27. *Radiation therapy and you: a guide to self help during treatment,* No 91-2227, 1990, National Cancer Institute.

28. Ransohoff R, Koslow M, Cooper P: Cancer of the central nervous system and pituitary. In Lawrence W, Jr, Lenhard RE, Jr, Murphy GP, editors: *ACS textbook of clinical oncology,* ed 2, Atlanta, 1995, American Cancer Society.

29. Robinson C, Roy C, Seager M: Central nervous system cancers. In Baird S, McCorkle R, Grant M, editors: *Cancer nursing: a comprehensive textbook,* Philadelphia, 1991, Saunders.

30. Rodriquez L, Levin V: Does chemotherapy benefit the patient with a central nervous system glioma? *Oncology (Huntingt)* 1:29, 1987.

31. Rowland LP: *Merritt's textbook of neurology,* ed 8, Philadelphia, 1989, Lea & Febiger.

32. Saba MT, Magolan JM: Understanding cerebral edema: implications for oncology nurses, *Oncol Nurs Forum* 18:499, 1991.

33. Saleman M, Kaplan RS: Intracranial tumors in adults. In Haskell CM, editor: *Cancer treatment,* ed 3, Philadelphia, 1990, Saunders.

34. Schein PS: *Decision making in oncology,* Philadelphia, 1989, Decker.

35. Schenk E: Management of persons with neurologic problems. In Phipps WJ and others, editors: *Medical-surgical nursing: concepts and clinical practice,* ed 5, St Louis, 1994, Mosby.

36. Shalter M, Mariebe EN: *The nurse, pharmacology and drug therapy,* Redwood City, Calif, 1989, Addison-Wesley.

37. Shaw EG and others: Radiation therapy in the management of low grade supratentorial astrocytomas, *J Neurosurg* 70:853, 1989.

38. Speea WG, McArthur JC: Headache. In Harvey AM and others, editors: *The principles and practice of medicine,* East Norwalk, Conn, 1988, Appleton & Lange.

39. Sunderson N, Suite ND: Optimal use of the Ommaya reservoir in clinical oncology, *Oncol Nurs Forum* 3:15, 1989.

40. Tennebaum L: *Cancer chemotherapy: a reference guide,* Philadelphia, 1989, Saunders.

41. Walleck C: Intracranial problems. In Lewis SM, Collier IC, editors: *Medical-surgical nursing: assessment and management of clinical problems,* ed 4, St Louis, 1996, Mosby.

42. Wegmann JA, Hakius P: Central nervous system cancers. In Groenwald SL and others, editors: *Cancer nursing: principles and practice,* ed 2, Boston, 1990, Jones & Bartlett.

43. Yasko S: *Care of the client receiving external radiation therapy,* Reston, Va, 1982, Reston-Hall.

44. Zulch KJ: Histological typing of tumors of the central nervous system, *Int Histol Classification Tumors* 21:19, 1979.

CHAPTER 6
Breast Cancers

REBECCA CRANE

Breast cancer is a major public health concern throughout the world. In almost all parts of Europe and in North America, Australia, and New Zealand, breast cancer is the most frequent cancer in women as well as the leading cause of death for 35- to 54-year-old women.[169,189] The incidence of breast cancer is increasing throughout the world for reasons not fully understood. It is predicted that by the year 2000, female breast cancer will be seen as often in developing countries as in developed countries.[131]

In the United States, public awareness of breast cancer has grown considerably in recent years. Women in the public eye have spoken out about their experiences with breast cancer; media coverage has expanded to include breast health as well as breast cancer care information; legislative efforts have made screening mammography more available under insurance coverage; and grass-roots movements have placed women's health care issues into the forefront in the competition for research dollars.[219]

It has been only in the past 20 years that the Halsted radical mastectomy has been replaced with more conservative surgery.[201,237] The "one-step" procedure (biopsy with frozen-section diagnosis and immediate surgery) has been replaced with the two-step procedure. Women are expected to be involved in their treatment planning. The knowledge that breast cancer needed to be considered a systemic disease at the time of diagnosis led to increasing justification for the use of chemotherapy and hormonal manipulation as adjuncts to surgery to improve survival. Several questions regarding such adjuvant therapy continue to be addressed in ongoing national clinical trials:

1. Which women with negative nodes and smaller tumors should receive systemic treatment?
2. What is the optimal timing for initiation of treatment?
3. What is the optimal combination of drugs, the dose size, and intensity to be used?
4. What is the optimal duration of treatment?

Randomized clinical trials continue to assess the value of autologous bone marrow transplant in the treatment of women with breast cancer at high risk for recurrence and with advanced disease. New technologies in molecular genetics have led to the localization of two breast cancer susceptibility genes, BRCA1 and BRCA2.[168,247] Researchers continue to study tumor suppressor genes and oncogenes to understand better their effects on breast cancer initiation and development and their role as prognostic variables. Each of these endeavors lends hope that new and better methods for the treatment of breast cancer will lead to reductions in mortality. In addition, a major randomized multicenter clinical trial was begun in 1992 to assess the effects of tamoxifen for breast cancer prevention in 16,000 women at high risk for breast cancer. More than 11,000 women have been recruited to participate in the Breast Cancer Prevention Trial to date.[200] Two other clinical trials are in progress to address the question of the effects of a reduced fat diet on breast cancer: the Women's Health Initiative and the Women's Intervention Nutrition Study (WINS).[33,167] The future in breast cancer prevention and treatment, as in all health care, is charged with clinical, social, and economic challenges.[74]

Early detection remains the key to breast cancer control. Breast cancer screening guidelines continue to come under discussion, with efforts by major organizations to achieve widespread acceptance.[7,52,130,166] Mammography remains the mainstay for finding breast cancer before it has become clinically detectable. Coupled with regular and thorough breast self-examination (BSE) and regular periodic examination of the breasts by a professional, breast cancer can be found early, when it is more likely to be cured, often with conservative surgical management. Studies of socioeconomic and ethnic differences in the practice of breast cancer control activities as well as stage at diagnosis and survival have pointed out the need for more attention to these factors in all phases of the breast care continuum.[12,60,73,76,115] As the population of women in the United States ages, more consideration must also be given to the needs of an elderly population of women at risk for, diagnosed with, or followed after treatment for breast cancer.

The psychosocial impact of breast cancer screening, diagnosis, and treatment on the individual or family remains a major clinical and research responsibility for nursing, particularly in such challenging arenas as socioeconomic and ethnic diversity, the aging female population, and pregnancy after breast cancer. Because research results are at times confusing, conflicting, and controversial, women need help in integrating the information they are given, whether regarding risk of developing breast cancer or treatment options after the diagnosis. Nurses have a key role in advocating for women, whether in the political arena or at the bedside. Nurses need to be knowledgeable about current trends in breast cancer management so they can assist women throughout their treatment process. Nurses are also vital to public education efforts directed at breast cancer screening, teaching BSE and guidelines for mammography and professional breast examinations, and portraying the hope of breast cancer cure with early detection.

EPIDEMIOLOGY

The average American woman's risk for ever developing invasive breast cancer is one in eight.[189] This translates into 184,300 newly diagnosed female cases in the United States during 1996. Men rarely develop breast cancer by comparison, accounting for only 1400 new cases during the same year. It is predicted that 44,300 women and 260 men will die from the disease in 1996—fewer than in prior years.[189] These numbers reflect cases of invasive breast cancer. Carcinoma in situ (CIS) (discussed later in this chapter) accounted for about 30,000 additional new cases of breast cancer in women in 1996, increased from 5000 cases in 1988, 10,000 in 1989, 15,000 in 1990, 20,000 in 1992, and 25,000 in 1993.[189]

Overall, breast cancer incidence rates in women have continued to increase by about 2% per year since 1980.[7] This may result partly from increased use of screening programs and therefore earlier detection, as well as from an aging population. However, other reasons for the increase remain unknown. Mortality rates have remained essentially unchanged for 50 years, despite improvements in treatment and earlier detection. However, it appears that mortality rates may be declining worldwide, primarily for younger and white women.[7,99,233] In contrast, lung cancer death rates in women increased by 451% between 1959-1961 and 1989-1991.[7] Since 1987, more American women have died from lung cancer than breast cancer.[7] Breast cancer remains the most common site of cancer in American women.

The highest incidence rates of breast cancer in the world are in the United States (by country), and specifically by population group, Hawaiians in Hawaii, white women in Hawaii, and white women in Alameda County in Northern California.[169] Although black women generally have a lower incidence rate of breast cancer than white women in the United States, incidence rates have been increasing at a greater rate for black women.[8] Mortality rates for white women in the United States remain relatively stable, but rates for black women have increased by 19.4% over the same time.[8] Black women in the United States are more likely to be diagnosed with breast cancer at a later stage and subsequently have a 5-year relative survival rate that is nearly 15% lower than that for white women.[60,189] A disproportionate number of blacks in the United States are at lower socioeconomic levels; associated with an inadequate social and physical environment, inadequate information and education, a risk-promoting life-style, and impaired access to health care, this most likely accounts for more of the differences in cancer survival than race.[3,14,73]

ETIOLOGY AND RISK FACTORS

Research has shown that there is no known single cause of breast cancer. It is a heterogeneous disease, most likely developing as a result of many different factors that are not the same from woman to woman and most of which are yet unknown. Several characteristics appear to increase the probability of a woman developing breast cancer.[53,99] These characteristics, or *risk factors,* when present, have been shown to be associated with a greater incidence of breast cancer than when such factors are absent.[173] Women diagnosed with breast cancer may or may not have any of the risk factors. In fact, in one large prospective study by the American Cancer Society (ACS), 75% of the breast cancers detected occurred in women who had none of the most widely recognized higher risk factors.[216] It is therefore understandable that the concept of risk in breast cancer is often confusing and frequently fear inducing. Many women overestimate their risk of developing breast cancer.[122] This can lead to extremes of reaction from that of avoidance of health care to that of the opposite—worry and seeking of unnecessary repeated evaluations. Health care providers who do not understand risk may reinforce such fears. It is important for women and their nurses to understand the concept of risk and current knowledge of risk factors to develop individualized breast health plans of care.

Understanding Breast Cancer Risk

Breast cancer risk can be expressed as risk of development or risk of death from the disease. This chapter emphasizes risk as it relates to the development of breast cancer. *Absolute risk* is the number of breast cancer cases in a given population divided by the number of women in the population, expressed as an *average risk* for every woman in that population.[79] For white women in the United States today, this comes out to be about a 12.6% chance of developing breast cancer, most commonly expressed as the often-quoted "1 in 8" statistic.[189] This can be deceiving. This percentage is a cumulative lifetime risk based on the sum of risks at different ages *(age-specific risks)* for all women from birth to 110 years of age.[79,122] This does not take into account an individual woman's situation (her estimated life span, her current age, or the presence of other potentially high-risk factors). Absolute risk is sometimes expressed as age-specific risk for women in different age brackets. For example, American women ages 40 to 59 have a risk of developing breast cancer of approximately 4% (1 in 26), whereas at ages 60 to 79 they have a 7% (1 in 14) age-specific risk of developing breast cancer.[189] The risk is higher for older women because breast cancer occurs more frequently as age increases. The cumulative lifetime risk for white women 35 years of age (to the age of 110) is 10%, whereas at age 65 there is a 6.3% risk of developing breast cancer by the age of 110.[99] The cumulative lifetime risk is lower for the 65-year-old woman because she has fewer years left to be at risk (even if she did live to be 110, because it is still a comparison based on years of life remaining). This risk for developing breast cancer is also lower for nonwhite women in both age groups because their overall incidence is lower.[122,146] Because absolute risk can be presented in different ways and does not take into account individual situations, it may be difficult to derive personal meaning from such numbers. Absolute risk may underestimate the risk to some women (e.g., those with a family history of breast cancer) and overestimate the risk for others (e.g., nonwhite women).[79] However, absolute risk is a very meaningful statistic when addressing the magnitude of the breast cancer problem in the United States or for a very specific population.[79,122]

Relative risk is the incidence rate of breast cancer in a population of women with a known or suspected risk factor divided by the incidence rate of breast cancer in a population of women without that risk factor.[79,122] It is most often stated in studies addressing the epidemiology of breast cancer.[79] A woman with no risk factors would have a relative risk of 1.0; a relative risk greater than 1.0 indicates a greater likelihood of developing breast cancer than individuals without the risk factors.[146,226] For example, if the relative risk for a woman is 2.0, she is two times more likely than the population to develop breast cancer.[123] Relative risk expresses the excess risk of cancer that can be attributed to the risk factor.[79] The relative risk will increase as the number of risk factors increases.[216] To determine individual risk, one cannot multiply the cumulative lifetime risk (absolute risk) by the relative risk and obtain a meaningful number. However, *multiplying the age-specific risk by the relative risk* will give a percent risk, for example, for the next 10 years of life; that is, the woman age 40 with an age-specific risk of 4% between the ages of 40 and 59 and a relative risk of 2.0 would have about an 8% chance of developing breast cancer over the next 19 years.[79,122,146,189]

Attributable risk is the number of cancer cases in a population that are associated with given risk factors and that could potentially be prevented by alteration or removal of those factors.[146,216] It is most useful in public health policy and planning for cancer prevention and control. Unlike lung cancer, where there is a clear causal link with smoking, there are no such factors in breast cancer. Attributable risk does not account for the majority of breast cancer cases.[216] Where a known associated risk exists for some women, the factors involved (e.g., family history, nulliparity or late age at first birth) are ones over which they generally have little or no control.[123,165,216]

Risk Factors

The following information covers those risk factors most widely acknowledged or suspected to increase the probability of a woman developing breast cancer.

Gender. Women are more likely than men to develop breast cancer. Breast cancer accounts for 31% of all invasive cancers in women and less than 1% of the cancers in men.[189]

Age. The incidence of breast cancer increases with age. Most breast cancer cases are diagnosed in women 40 years of age and older.[6,122] Eighty percent of cases occur in women over age 50.[146] Most women who develop breast cancer will have no known risk factors other than being female and over 40 years of age.

Personal history of cancer. A previous diagnosis of breast cancer increases a woman's lifetime risk for developing a second breast cancer in the opposite (contralateral) breast. Estimates are that this lifetime risk is approximately 15%,[79] or a relative risk in the range of 3.0 to 4.0.[123] The risk has been shown to be even higher in women who also have a family history of breast cancer.[79,123] In addition, a previous history of primary ovarian or endometrial cancer has been associated with an increased risk of breast cancer (relative risk under 1.5).[79,123,165]

Family history of cancer and genetics. Women with a family history of breast cancer in a first-degree relative (mother, sister, or daughter) have a relative risk of 2.0 to 3.0.[79,123] This is a risk two to three times that of the general population. Risk increases further if both the mother and sister have had breast cancer (relative risk greater than 5.0).[99,123] Risk is greatest when the occurrence of breast cancer was premenopausal and bilateral.[99] A paternal history of breast cancer also has been shown to increase an individual's risk of developing breast cancer.[122] In some families this clustering of breast cancer may be accounted for only by chance or possibly from interactions among shared environmental, cultural, or socioeconomic factors that are less well understood.[240]

In other families, *genetics* may be a critical factor. Clinical features of possible hereditary breast cancer include a younger age at diagnosis, bilateral occurrence, multiple family members affected over three or more generations, and the occurrence of cancers in other sites (e.g., colon, ovary, uterus).[99,150,240] The presence of these features warrants further exploration for the implications of genetic testing and risk counseling. Recent advances in molecular technology have enabled scientists to study in great detail the genetic structure of individual chromosomes and thus some of the mechanisms by which tumor suppressor genes and growth factors work to produce cancer. In 1990 the discovery was made of the tumor suppressor gene (oncogene) p53 on the short arm of chromosome 17.[154] Mutations of this tumor suppressor gene are found in patients with Li-Fraumeni familial syndrome, a rare syndrome associated with a high incidence of familial cancers, including breast cancer.[154,240] Mutations of p53 may account for only 1% of all breast cancers in women under age 40.[18]

In 1994 the BRCA1 tumor suppressor gene was isolated on the long arm of chromosome 17.[168] Female carriers of a mutation of this gene are at great risk of developing breast cancer or ovarian cancer. Also in 1994 the second tumor suppressor gene, BRCA2, was localized on the long arm of chromosome 13.[246,247] It appears that BRCA2 mutations confer a high risk of breast cancer but not the same high risk of ovarian cancer as BRCA1.[247] Such inherited genetic mutations are estimated to account for only 5% to 10% of breast cancer cases.[8,99,240] However, in women who are carriers of either mutation, the lifetime risk of breast cancer to age 80 can reach 87%.[240] It is possible that the presence of mutations in BRCA1 or BRCA2 may also occur in noninherited or sporadic breast cancer cases.[134]

This is perhaps the most exciting area of research, with the hope of improved understanding of breast cancer inheritance and development, associated risk factors, and potentially prevention.[123] Testing has only recently become available on a limited basis for some families, to look for the presence of mutations in the BRCA1 or BRCA2 genes. However, such testing will not be a definite predictor of the likelihood of developing or not developing breast cancer. Other mutations may exist and have yet to be discovered. Most women at risk do not have the inherited gene mutation but a series of genetically determined factors that interact with life-style and environmental factors to predispose them to the development of breast cancer.[46] In families with a high incidence of cancer, risk counseling should include a thorough family cancer history, a review of environmental and life-style risk factors, personal medical history, and an individualized plan of screening and follow-up.[46,122,146] Because most women do not have inherited mutations of this gene, widespread genetic testing in the absence of a family history is not indicated at this time.[99]

Early menarche and late menopause. The exact role of hormones in the etiology of breast cancer has not been precisely determined. *Early onset of menarche* (before age 12) and *late menopause* (after age 50) are each associated with increased risk of breast cancer.[98,123] Studies have shown that risk also increases as the time interval lengthens between menarche and menopause.[98] Regular ovulatory cycles with cumulative exposure to estrogen therefore appears to be the major determinant of this risk.[98] The greater the number of years of menstrual activity (e.g., 40), the greater is the risk of developing breast cancer.[79,98] The lifetime exposure of the breast to estrogen appears to be the most convincing factor,[98] although of great significance is the role of other circulating hormones and metabolites, such as estradiol, progesterone, and prolactin.[123] Factors that have contributed to trends toward a lowering of the age at menarche in countries such as the United States include better nutrition and infectious disease control.[98] Surgically induced or radiation-induced menopause (e.g., bilateral oophorectomy, pelvic irradiation) reduces breast cancer risk, perhaps slightly greater than with natural menopause.[98]

Reproductive history. Having no children (*nulliparity*) or the *first full-term pregnancy after age 30* places a woman at an increased risk.[99,123] The relative risk is higher for the woman who delays childbirth than for the nulliparous woman.[122,123] Childbirth at an early age (before age 20) has been shown to have a protective effect.[98,122,123] The mechanism behind this reduction in risk remains unknown but most likely results from changes in the actual breast tissue or the hormones that make the breast tissue less susceptible to cancer formation.[123] The trend for more American women to delay pregnancy until a later age, thus increasing the exposure of breast tissue to estrogen, has potentially contributed to the increasing incidence of breast cancer.[165] Some authors[122,123] suggest that more studies of such women are needed, since most current studies reflect benefits to women who became pregnant many years ago or who were diagnosed with breast cancer after age 50.

Some studies have shown that as the number of months of breastfeeding increases, an associated reduction occurs in the risk of developing breast cancer, particularly for premenopausal women.[123,165] Such findings are not without question, although it would appear that if the number of ovulatory cycles and exposure to estrogens is related to breast cancer risk, this risk would also be reduced if lactation led to a reduction in the exposure to estrogen.[98]

Benign breast disease. The term *benign breast disease* is frequently misunderstood in discussions of risk.[122] The term encompasses a broad array of histopathologic diagnoses that are typically experienced by women clinically at some time in their lives but that are never biopsied. Some question why such a common condition should be termed a "disease." Many of these so-called diseases are not associated with any increased risk of breast cancer. "Fibrocystic disease" is a catchall phrase to describe clinical symptoms and findings of local or generalized lumpiness, pain, or cystic changes. *Fibrocystic changes* may be a more appropriate term to describe these often normal breast changes.

Benign breast lesions, when pathologic diagnosis is made, are classified into three groups. *Nonproliferative lesions,* when found alone, are not associated with any increased risk of breast cancer. These include histologically diagnosed cysts, apocrine metaplasia, papillary apocrine change, epithelial-related calcifications, fibroadenomas, and mild hyperplasia.[211] The presence of gross cysts in women with a family history of breast cancer has been shown to be associated with increased risk.[211]

Proliferative lesions without atypia include moderate or florid hyperplasias of the usual type, sclerosing adenosis, and intraductal papillomas. Some evidence indicates that multiple as opposed to single papillomas, occurring peripherally rather than centrally, are susceptible to breast cancer development.[211] Occurring in the ductal or glandular tissue of the breast, proliferative lesions without atypia have been associated with only a slightly increased risk (1.5 to 2.0) of breast cancer during the 10 to 20 years after biopsy.[56,186,187,211]

Proliferative lesions with atypia, or *atypical hyperplasia,* constitute the third category of benign breast disease and are most associated with increased breast cancer risk.[186,187] Only 3% to 5% of benign breast disease biopsies are found to have atypical cells.[122,186] Atypical hyperplasia can be found in either ductal or lobular tissue. It is a proliferation of abnormal-looking cells within the duct or lobule.[122,165,186,187,196] The diagnosis by biopsy of atypical ductal or lobular hyperplasia is associated with a relative risk of 4.0 to 5.0 during the 10 to 20 years after biopsy.[123,186,187]

If these cells continue to proliferate and take on the appearance of cancer cells, the lesion then becomes *carcinoma in situ,* or cancer confined to the site of origin, and further increases the risk of developing invasive breast cancer.[122,146,186,187] Treatment of women with this diagnosis is discussed later in this chapter.

Obesity and dietary fat. *Obesity* has been shown to be associated with increased risk of developing breast cancer in postmenopausal women.[123,165] Excess adipose tissue is rich in the necessary enzyme to convert estrone and estradiol from their precursors.[112] Consequently, obese women may have increased levels of circulating estrogens, which can affect hormone-dependent breast cancer cells.[112] Another observation has been that obesity is associated with decreased levels of sex hormone–binding globulin (SHBG), which normally binds estradiol and would prevent stimulation of breast cancer cells.[112,123] Seidman and others[216] used the measure of "relative weight index 110 or more" in their study of high-risk categories, defined as 10% or more above the average weight for a given woman's height and age.

Kelsey and Gammon[123] described being "heavy" as associated with a relative risk of 1.1 to 1.9. Others have described being 40% above ideal body weight as increasing one's risk of developing breast cancer.[6]

Incidence of breast cancer is increased in industrialized countries with a high socioeconomic status and an increased consumption of *dietary fat,* suggesting a relationship. Migrant studies evaluating the daughters of immigrants from Japan (where incidence of breast cancer is low and dietary fat consumption is low) to California have shown rates of breast cancer similar to those for American white women.[169,225] Dietary factors said to be associated with these variations in breast cancer incidence also are different for premenopausal and postmenopausal women.[122,225] However, the studies to date are difficult to interpret.[80,225] Dietary fat consumption in these studies has ranged from 25% to 49% or more of total calories from fat; the U.S. per capita fat intake was about 36.5% of total calories in 1985.[225] A reduction in fat intake to 20% to 30% of total calories and the addition of high-fiber foods have been suggested as healthy dietary habits because of the potential for cancer risk reduction as well as risk reduction in other illnesses such as heart disease.[6,99,146] Further studies are in progress to address the relationship between dietary factors and estrogen or other hormones and breast cancer risk and clarify the association with breast cancer.[33,167]

Radiation exposure. A greater than expected incidence of breast cancer has been seen in women exposed to ionizing radiation for the treatment of tuberculosis or postpartum mastitis or in survivors of the atomic bombs at Hiroshima and Nagasaki.[21,159,169] Sensitivity to the effects of radiation is greatest in childhood (ages 10 to 14) and decreased to almost negligible by age 40.[169] This susceptibility to radiation is important when considering potential risk from radiation with such procedures as mammography.[169] The current availability of low-dose mammography coupled with regular use in women *over 40* years of age makes the risk from radiation exposure almost negligible.[170]

Exogenous hormones. Because breast cancers are thought to be hormone related, numerous studies have been done to evaluate the risk associated with the use of *oral contraceptives* (OCs) and *estrogen replacement therapy* (ERT). Research results have been contradictory and inconclusive. The majority of these studies have shown no increased risk for most women.[98,122,123,165,194]

OC use became widespread in the early 1960s. Adequate follow-up data are only recently becoming available to identify possible latent effects associated with OC use and to estimate the resulting breast cancer risk. Some studies have suggested an increased risk associated with early onset of use and long-term use (more than 6 years).[98,99] Important considerations in future studies include the differences in OC composition over time (earlier OCs had higher estrogen content than many available today), age at onset of use, duration of use, and use by women with existing known other high-risk factors.[79,98] Others suggest, after reviewing the data, that cautious use of OCs might be prudent in very young or perimenopausal women.[79]

In January 1989 the Fertility and Maternal Health Drugs Advisory Committee of the U.S. Food and Drug Administration (FDA) concluded no relationship exists between OC use and breast cancer and recommended further studies. In fall 1989 the Committee on the Relationship Between Oral Contraceptives and Breast Cancer within the Institute of Medicine[113] was assembled to examine the etiology of breast cancer as related to OCs. Its report recommended that no fundamental change in clinical practice with respect to the use of OCs is supported by the knowledge to date about OCs and risk of breast cancer.[113] It also recommended that women seeking contraception be given adequate information and counseling as to the current ambiguities in the knowledge to date of the relationship between OCs and breast cancer.[113]

ERT in postmenopausal women has been available in the United States since 1942, with widespread use since the 1960s.[122] With new concern about endometrial cancer risk in the late 1970s, progesterone was added for a cyclic regimen.[98] In postmenopausal women, such ERT has been used to manage the menopausal symptoms of hot flashes and dyspareunia secondary to atrophic vaginitis. In recent years, ERT has also been employed to prevent osteoporosis and reduce the risk of cardiovascular disease. Studies to date of the relationship between ERT and breast cancer remain controversial, with some suggestion of slight increased risk when use is prolonged (more than 15 years), when estradiol is used rather than conjugated estrogens, and perhaps when progesterone is added.[79,98,99,123,194] No data exist for women who have taken estrogen for 20 years or more.[194] Women who take unopposed estrogens have an increased risk for endometrial cancer.[194] Until further studies address these issues, women should be advised of current knowledge and should weigh the potential benefits and risks before undertaking ERT.[79,98,122,146]

Alcohol consumption. Several studies have shown a slightly increased risk associated with alcohol consumption.[123] Unfortunately, the studies have been inconsistent with respect to the amount and type of alcohol use correlated with an increased risk. The age at which drinking begins (under 30 years of age), volume, and duration of use appear to be important variables in understanding risk with alcohol consumption.[122,123] The association with younger age at onset of alcohol consumption may be related to the developing and potentially susceptible breast tissue.[225] Heavy alcohol consumption may also be associated with poor nutrition.[122] Further study is needed of each of these variables.

Other factors. Associations between mammographic parenchymal (tissue) patterns and breast cancer risk remain unclear.[79,123] Higher socioeconomic status is associated with a higher risk of developing breast cancer, but lower socioeconomic status is associated with a greater risk of dying from the disease.[22,73] Ethnicity also is associated with risk, with nonwhite women being less at risk of developing breast cancer but at greater risk of dying from the disease.[22,73] No clear associations with increased risk of breast cancer have been found for cigarette smoking, stress, personality type, cerumen (ear wax), exposure to electromagnetic fields, caffeine, or hair dyes.[79,122,123]

For the woman who appears to have an increased risk based on family history or other factors, a detailed assessment should be conducted to determine actual individual risk. *Risk analysis* services are available in many breast centers throughout the United States.[46,122,226] This risk assessment should thoroughly explore a woman's perceptions of risk, her attitudes toward and beliefs about early detection methods (BSE, clinical breast examination [CBE], mammography) as well as her participation in each, and her need for information. An important message for women and their family members is that risk relates to developing breast cancer and not to dying from it.[226] Screening guidelines should be vigorously followed; some suggest an earlier age for beginning mammography and more frequent CBE.[46,79,226] There is no clear preventive intervention. Reduction in alcohol and dietary fat intake and weight loss if postmenopausal and obese are some measures that the individual can take, but none has a clear association with breast cancer prevention. Prophylactic mastectomy is quite controversial.[18,79,226] The Society of Surgical Oncology developed a statement that indications for this procedure are a clearly increased risk of breast cancer or clinical conditions that make evaluation extremely difficult.[221] This would include a family history of premenopausal bilateral breast cancer, a history of biopsy-proven atypical hyperplasia or lobular carcinoma in situ (LCIS), and dense, nodular breasts with or without diffuse microcalcifications.[221]

There remains much to learn about risk factors for breast cancer and the effects of combinations of risk factors now known or suspected. New risk factors need to be identified, risk quantified, and control measures studied. Most women who will be diagnosed with breast cancer have no known risk factors. Current knowledge about risk factors in breast cancer will help the nurse guide the patient in obtaining personally meaningful information. In most cases, interventions will need to be focused less on risk factor reduction and more on developing a plan of care for the early detection of breast cancer when it occurs.

PREVENTION, SCREENING, AND DETECTION

It is not known what causes breast cancer or how to prevent the disease. Breast cancer is a *heterogeneous disease;* in other words, it is a disease of many characteristics, varying from woman to woman in its potential for development, growth, and metastasis. The epidemiology of the disease indicates that it is hormonally influenced, with the duration of exposure to elevated levels of circulating estrogens being a primary factor in the promotion of cancer cell development over several years. This period of cell promotion is characterized by reversibility. If this exposure could be reduced or if the adverse effects of the exposure could be prevented, breast cancer might be prevented.

The Breast Cancer Prevention Trial described at the beginning of this chapter is one study to evaluate the role of tamoxifen for breast cancer prevention in a group of women at higher risk for breast cancer development. This is a placebo-controlled trial, meaning that women who consent to participate in the study are randomized to either the tamoxifen or a placebo. Because no known means exist to prevent breast cancer, the placebo is necessary to control for any bias that might result. To participate in the study, women must be 60 years of age or older or 35 years of age or older with a risk profile that meets preestablished criteria. Women who participate will be taking the medication (tamoxifen or placebo) for 5 years and followed regularly thereafter as well. Because estrogens are known to have an important role in reducing rates of coronary heart disease and osteoporosis in postmenopausal women, these will be closely monitored as part of the study. The purpose of the trial is to test the effectiveness of long-term tamoxifen in preventing the occurrence of invasive breast cancer as well as in reducing mortality from the disease. It will be some time before the results of this or other studies evaluating prevention will translate into interventions that clearly have a major impact on the female population.

Early detection is therefore the most important means for control of breast cancer. Research has shown that survival is directly related to the stage of the disease at diagnosis. The ACS has developed *screening guidelines* for asymptomatic women that incorporate the following three methods of early detection[8,52]:

1. *Breast self-examination (BSE)* should be performed monthly by all women beginning at age 20.
2. *Clinical breast examination (CBE)* by a health professional should be done every 3 years for women ages 20 to 40 and annually after age 40.
3. *Mammography* should begin by age 40. Routine screening mammography should be performed every 1 to 2 years for women ages 40 to 49 and then every year beginning at age 50.

A woman with known risk factors (e.g., family history) or chronic symptomatology should be advised to consult with her physician regarding the frequency and specificity of CBEs and mammography for her situation. Nurses have a major role in teaching these potentially lifesaving guidelines to all women. For greatest effectiveness, frequency (regular and periodic) and proficiency (skill and thoroughness) are key concepts to consider in each screening method.

Mammography

Mammography is the only proven means of detecting breast cancer before it can be detected by CBE or BSE. Screening mammography is used to detect cancer in *asymptomatic* women. By the time a lesion is 1 cm in diameter and detectable by palpation, it has been estimated that it may have been present for 8 or more years.[95] Figure 6-1 depicts the average-size lump detected with BSE and mammography. Since the Health Insurance Plan of New York (HIP) study in the early 1960s and the Breast Cancer Detection Demonstration Project (BCDDP) in the 1970s, screening mammography has repeatedly been shown to be effective in reducing the num-

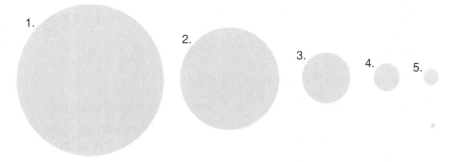

Figure 6-1   **1**, Average-size lump found by women untrained in breast self-examination (BSE). **2**, Average-size lump found by women practicing occasional BSE. **3**, Average-size lump found by women practicing regular BSE. **4**, Average-size lump found by first mammogram. **5**, Average-size lump found by regular mammograms. (From Spence W: *Breast care: the good news,* Waco, Texas, 1986, Health Edco.)

ber of deaths associated with breast cancer through the detection of clinically occult lesions less than 1 mm in size.[16,65,107,215] Mammography is also useful in evaluating high-risk women and women with breasts difficult to palpate (e.g., breasts that are large and pendulous or with severe fibrocystic changes). Ultrasound is helpful in conjunction with mammography for diagnostic purposes to help differentiate a fluid-filled cyst from a solid mass. Other methods for imaging the breasts, such as thermography, diaphonography (transillumination), and magnetic resonance imaging (MRI), have been evaluated but have not been shown to be effective in screening for breast cancer.[99] MRI may be useful in evaluating the augmented breast.[228] When properly performed, mammography can effectively detect 85% to 90% of breast cancers. It is possible for 10% to 15% of malignant lesions to be undetected.[16] Therefore, in women with clinical symptoms, a negative mammogram does not rule out the need for a biopsy. Dense breast tissue is the major reason for false-negative readings, but faulty equipment, skill of the technologist, or errors in interpretation can also be the cause.[16] *Scintimammography* is an investigational procedure and adjunct to mammography that involves injection of a radioisotope (technetium-99m sestamibi) followed by a nuclear medicine scan of the breasts. Preliminary reports reveal high specificity for differentiating benign from malignant lesions found initially on mammogram.[228]

Screening mammography generally consists of two views of each breast: one from side to side (mediolateral oblique) and one from top to bottom (craniocaudal).[231] For each view the breast is compressed to decrease the thickness of the breast and enable better visualization of the structures of the tissue, also reducing the amount of radiation.[16] It may be uncomfortable, but an explanation that proper breast compression is one of the most important factors in a quality mammogram may help women understand the importance of that momentary discomfort.[231] It is also helpful if premenstrual women do not have the screening mammogram immediately before their menses for the similar concern about comfort. *Xeromammography* was popular for several years beginning in the early 1970s. However, refinements in technology have made film-screen mammography the preferred breast imaging method because of its higher image contrast, lower radiation dose, and less equipment downtime.[16,231]

Concern has been expressed regarding the risks related to the radiation exposure from mammograms. The radiation dose delivered has been significantly lowered since the 1960s, and with equipment dedicated solely to mammography, the risk is negligible. The benefits must always be weighed against the potential risk of having breast cancer undiagnosed. Because of this and other concerns about mammography, the Mammography Qual-

ity Standards Act (MQSA), passed by Congress in 1992 and effective Oct. 1, 1994, established federal quality standards for equipment, personnel, and recordkeeping at all mammography facilities and required each to be accredited by the FDA.[231] These quality standards include the presence of the following[231]:

- Dedicated mammographic equipment with regular monitoring to ensure that the minimum necessary radiation dose is administered and that the quality of films processed is maintained
- Radiologic technologists who are specially trained and experienced in mammography
- Radiologists with demonstrated experience and competence in mammography
- Records of mammography that include comparisons with prior films, findings, and recommendations

Cost can prohibit some women from obtaining screening mammograms. The cost for a screening mammogram can range from $10 to $225, with a national average of about $89 in 1994.[105] Through efforts of the ACS, National Cancer Institute (NCI), and other organizations, costs for screening mammography have been declining in many parts of the United States and insurance coverage has increased.

Despite its value, mammography is still underutilized. One reason has been physician disagreement with following the ACS guidelines for mammography. A 1989 survey of more than 1000 U.S. physicians revealed that although physicians reported a greater inclination (since 5 years previously) to order screening mammography in asymptomatic women, reasons given for not ordering a mammogram included concerns about affordability and cost, reliability of the test, availability of a qualified radiologist or equipment, doubt of need if no symptoms or family history, and radiation risk.[5] In studies of women's attitudes about mammography, most have heard of the test but fewer (who are eligible) have had a mammogram.[6,16,231] One of the major reasons has been the lack of a referral or recommendation from their physician.[6,16,72,170] Fear of radiation, discomfort, or cancer; the cost; belief one is not at risk; and sometimes the belief that other tests (e.g., CBE) are adequate have also been reported as barriers.[5,16,72,153,231] Physician and public education efforts are important to overcome such barriers.

Breast Self-Examination

BSE is a free, private, and relatively simple examination. The majority of palpable breast lumps are discovered by the woman herself. Many physicians advocate BSE as a useful health care practice, and the technique essentially has no adverse effects.[6,99,131] In areas of the world where mammography or health care is not readily available, BSE may have important applicability.[170] Increasing evidence in the research literature indicates that women who perform BSE sometimes or regularly are more likely to discover smaller tumors and to have a smaller number of positive lymph nodes at diagnosis compared with women whose cancer is discovered accidentally.[13,38,71,109,220] Estimates are that regular practice of BSE could reduce the overall breast cancer mortality by approximately 19%.[88] The first prospective randomized controlled trial to evaluate the effectiveness of BSE was begun in 1985 in Leningrad and Moscow with the World Health Organization (WHO).[131] More than 120,000 women ages 40 to 64 years have participated in the study. Preliminary results indicate that women taught BSE were more likely to seek care for breast problems but were no different from the women not taught BSE in terms of breast cancer incidence or stage at diagnosis.[217] Ongoing follow-up of study participants will continue to the year 1999.

Most women in the United States know about BSE, but only 19% to 40% of them report practicing BSE on a regular basis.[38] Many women who practice BSE do not do it thoroughly (proficiently).[1] Compliance may be poor for a variety of reasons,* such as inadequate knowledge of how to do BSE, lack of confidence in ability to perform BSE and to detect abnormalities, fear of finding something, discomfort with touching breasts, lack of confidence in BSE as a means of detecting changes, forgetfulness, and lack of motivation. How effective will a woman be if she performs BSE monthly but poorly or thoroughly but less often?

Through one-on-one education that is repeated at intervals, monthly reminders, and encouragement by health professionals, compliance rates may improve. Studies have shown that education needs to include factual information about normal breast changes, breast cancer, and early detection and should promote positive attitudes or values.[38] Pamphlets and video instruction are passive teaching methods that have not been shown to be effective when used alone.[11] They also may not be ethnically sensitive, in the language of the woman being taught, or at a reading level that is appropriate.[163] BSE is a motor skill that entails coordination of palpation, movement, and sensation.[121] Opportunities for women to practice on silicone breast models and on themselves with feedback during the practice are crucial and may also enhance self-confidence in BSE performance.†

Women should be advised to perform BSE monthly. Premenopausal women should examine their breasts 5 to 7 days after their menstrual period begins. At this time their breasts may be less engorged and tender, thus allowing a more thorough and less distorted examination. Nonmenstruating or postmenopausal women should select the same day each month to do BSE. Selecting an anniversary or birth date is one suggestion to encourage women to remember. Women who are pregnant or breast-feeding should still examine themselves monthly, but the breastfeeding mother should do so soon after her breasts have been emptied. Women who have had breast cancer surgery should still perform BSE, with special attention to any surgical scar area and to the chest wall (postmastectomy).

BSE includes inspection and palpation of the breasts in both standing and lying positions. Attention is focused on evaluating for change. It is best done in an atmosphere that is unhurried and most comfortable for the individual woman. A thorough BSE will usually take 20 to 30 minutes. The ACS and NCI are two sources of patient and professional educational materials on BSE. The MammaCare Learning System is perhaps the most comprehensive and researched program, emphasizing proficiency through individualized instruction, the use of specially designed breast palpation models, an instruction manual, and a video program for self-learning.[155] Use of this system as well as other reviews of BSE proficiency are in the literature.* The components of BSE for proficiency in practice include *inspection* of the breasts in front of a mirror, *palpation* of the entire area of the breast using the flat *pads of the fingers* at different levels of *pressure,* in a specific *pattern* and *motion* within that pattern (i.e., small dime-sized circles in a vertical strip, wedge, or circular pattern), most easily done when in a flat or partial side-lying (upper body turned at 45-degree angle) *position* (Figure 6-2).[6,39,206]

Inspection of the breasts is best conducted standing in front of a mirror, with the arms at the sides and both breasts exposed for complete visualization of the skin surface, nipple/areola complex, and breast contour. Turning slightly side to side, the breasts are inspected for any evidence of skin retraction, puckering, dimpling, erythema, vein prominence, and presence of other characteristics such as nevi. The nipples should be noted as everted or inverted. Women with pendulous breasts should lift the breast on either side to inspect the skin on the lower side of the breasts and the chest area. It is normal that one breast may be slightly larger than the other. With hands on the hips pressing in and down, the same observation is repeated. This is further repeated with the arms over the head and with the arms in front while leaning forward.

Palpation is then performed lying down as previously described. Lotion can be applied to the flat pads of the fingers to smooth the skin. With respect to areas of the breast that may warrant additional attention, the upper outer quadrant of the breast is the most common location of most types of breast cancer, followed by the central area of the breast around the nipple.[197] Common er-

---

*References 11, 31, 32, 39, 54, 68, 206.
†References 11, 38, 39, 54, 151, 206.

*References 6, 39, 68, 182, 191, 206.

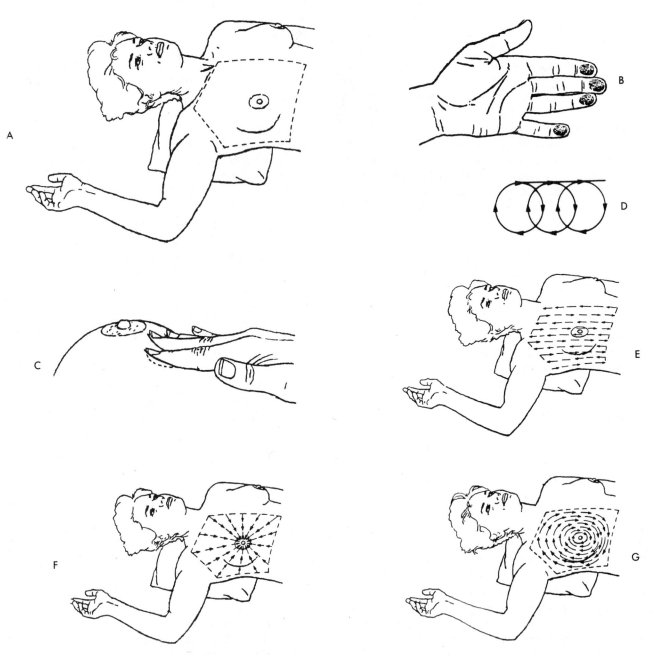

Figure 6-2   Breast self-examination (BSE). **A,** Perimeter of area to be examined should include all breast tissue. This area is bounded by a line that extends vertically from middle of axilla (armpit) to rib just beneath breast and continues horizontally along underside of breast to midsternum (middle of breastbone). It continues up midsternum to clavicle (collarbone) and along lower border of clavicle to shoulder and back to midaxilla. **B,** Palpation is performed with pads of fingers. **C** and **D,** Move your fingers (three or four) in small circles about the size of a dime. Varying levels of pressure (light, medium, and firm) should be applied to each spot palpated. Moderate pressure is illustrated. The following patterns can be used for the examination: **E,** vertical strip; **F,** wedge; and **G,** circle. (Courtesy American Cancer Society, California Division.)

rors in technique include *not palpating at different levels of pressure, not palpating the entire breast tissue area including behind the nipple,* and *using the fingertips for palpation rather than the flat pads of the three middle fingers.* Palpation needs to be done at three levels of pressure: light, medium, and firm. The light pressure will detect any changes in the skin that too-firm pressure might push away. Medium pressure will enable a woman to feel the glandular and fatty tissue of the breast. Firm pressure allows examination of the breast tissue close to the underlying ribs and muscle. The fingertips should be avoided because they are less sensitive than the finger pads. Women should be reminded not to do the examination too hurriedly. Beginning at the axilla or in the upper outer quadrant, the entire breast, axilla, and supraclavicular areas need to be examined. This area extends from the axilla to the bra line, over to the sternum, up to the supraclavicular notch, along the clavicle to the shoulder, and back to the axilla.[206] This completed pattern is followed by a gentle pressure, or milking action, on the breast and nipple to check for nipple discharge, and additional palpation in the axilla. Some women may also want to repeat the entire BSE in the shower.

It is crucial to emphasize that when first performing BSE, a woman is learning her normal breast characteristics so that any future variations or changes can be recognized and evaluated. If she notices a change on one breast, she may want to check the other breast for symmetry. She should be encouraged to have a plan of action should she detect a change that needs evaluation. This might be to call her health care provider for an appointment. Prompt medical attention should be sought if any of the clinical features or common symptoms of breast cancer are present (see box, p. 93). Although fear is a common feeling experienced when a new change or symptom is discovered, women can be encouraged when told that most breast lumps discovered are benign.[6,7]

Clinical Breast Examination

CBE is the most commonly employed screening technique for breast cancer today.[5,67] In the HIP study previously described, CBE contributed significantly to reductions in mortality for women in the 40- to 49-year-old group who were diagnosed with breast cancer.[170]

The importance of the BCDDP findings was that each of the screening measures (mammography, CBE, BSE) detected breast cancer cases not initially found by the other.[6] Studies have estimated that a lump of 0.3 cm can be detected by palpation in silicone breast models.[67] For CBE to be as effective as possible, the professional performing the examination needs to be proficient. Research suggests, however, that health professionals vary considerably in their confidence in and ability to perform CBE.[67,170] One study of registered nurses found an association between high confidence in their own BSE and

use of CBE in elderly women.[149] Unfortunately, many women relegate the examination of their breasts solely to their health care providers. A physician or other health professional does not have the advantage of being familiar with a woman's normal monthly breast irregularities when examinations are performed only yearly. The California Division of the ACS developed a program to help health professionals become more proficient in their performance of CBE, outlined in a publication describing seven areas of proficiency, modeled after those for BSE (see Figure 6-2).[4]

During CBE the health professional can demonstrate BSE technique, explain the rationale for each step, and encourage women to be partners in their care by continuing monthly BSE at home. In addition, a woman's particular normal anatomic variations can be pointed out. Signs and symptoms of breast abnormalities can be discussed and risk factors for breast cancer reviewed, with particular attention to what that means to the individual woman. The establishment of a relationship of trust between the health professional and the patient may lead to improved participation in breast cancer screening activities.

In the United States the goal for breast cancer screening by the year 2000 is that 80% of women ages 50 to 70 will be receiving annual CBE and mammography. This is increased from 45% for CBE alone and 15% for mammography.[89] Particular attention needs to be paid to special populations for all aspects of breast cancer screening. Problems in access, knowledge, and priorities are evident in socioeconomically disadvantaged women, with resultant higher mortality.[3,73,245] Reports of cancer screening availability for women in public health clinics[242] or rural settings[87] and studies of mammography utilization[26,117] and BSE practice by nonwhite women,[84,115,179,243] elderly persons,[40,43,151] or high-risk women[106,119] graphically demonstrate the need to find improved ways of reaching these populations with breast cancer screening.

Regular mammograms for eligible women, regular physical examinations, and monthly BSE can detect early breast cancers. All three components must be included in breast cancer screening. None of them is as effective individually as when combined. Early detection provides the opportunity for women and their physicians to select treatment options for managing small breast cancers and results in improved survival. These breast cancer detection recommendations are to be taught to all women, and women should be encouraged to incorporate these behaviors into their individual life-styles.

CLASSIFICATION

Knowledge of the anatomy of the breast helps in understanding the classification of breast cancer. The breast is

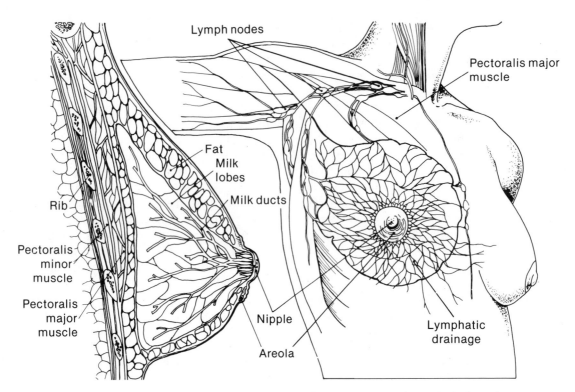

Figure 6-3 Anatomy of the female breast. (From DiSaia PJ: *Clinical gynecological oncology,* ed 3, St Louis, 1989, Mosby.)

a gland located on the chest wall (Figure 6-3). The overlying skin contains hair follicles and sweat and sebaceous glands. The pigmented area surrounding the nipple is known as the *areola,* and this has sebaceous glands that secrete a lubricant during breastfeeding. Fibrous strands called *Cooper's ligaments* pass through the glandular and fatty tissues from the skin to the underlying muscle, giving the breast support. The glandular tissue is made up of 15 to 20 lobes arranged in a radial pattern, capable of producing milk and connecting with ducts that drain into the nipple. An extensive lymphatic and vascular supply is present. Breast tissue extends to the clavicle, sternum, latissimus dorsi muscles, and up into the axilla. The axillary lymph nodes drain approximately 60% of the lymph from the breast. They are distributed from low in the armpit, at the lateral border of the pectoralis minor muscle (level I), to midway behind the pectoralis minor muscle (level II), and above at the medial border of the pectoralis minor (level III). Lymph nodes located between the pectoralis major and minor muscles are known as *Rotter's nodes.* The remainder of the lymph is drained from the internal mammary nodes.[128,184,202]

Primary breast cancers are grouped as invasive or noninvasive. A malignancy confined to the ducts or lobules is classified as noninvasive, or *carcinoma in situ.* If it arose in the ductal system, it is referred to as *ductal carcinoma in situ* (DCIS); in the lobule system it is called *lobular carcinoma in situ* (LCIS). Once the malignant cells penetrate the tissue outside the ducts or lobules, the cancer is described as infiltrating or invasive. Most breast malignancies are carcinomas and classified as ductal or lobular, with a small number of sarcomas and metastatic tumors reported. *Infiltrating ductal carcinoma* accounts for approximately 80% of all breast carcinomas and *infiltrating lobular carcinomas* about 10%.[99] *Paget's disease* of the nipple occurs infrequently (2% of all cases) and is most often associated with invasive carcinoma.[197] Also uncommon is *inflammatory carcinoma,* which is characterized by swelling, erythema, and invasion of the dermal lymphatics (giving the classic peau d'orange, or orange peel, appearance). When noninvasive cancer is found with invasive cancer, the staging and treatment planning are based on the characteristics of the invasive carcinoma.

CLINICAL FEATURES

In asymptomatic women, mammography serves to detect microscopic changes indicative of cancer, such as a small, irregular mass, microcalcifications, skin thickening, distortion of the ductal or ligament structures, or asymmetric density.[15] Palpable breast masses may also have these characteristics, often with peripheral spiculations, as well as nipple or skin retraction when underly-

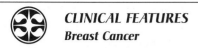

CLINICAL FEATURES
Breast Cancer

Most common symptoms at presentation

Mass (particularly if hard, irregular, nontender) or
thickening in breast or axilla

Spontaneous, persistent, unilateral nipple discharge that is
serosanguineous, bloody, or watery in character

Nipple retraction or inversion

Change in size, shape, or texture of breast (asymmetry)

Dimpling or puckering of skin

Scaly skin around nipple

Symptoms of local or regional spread

Redness, ulceration, edema, or dilated veins

Peau d'orange skin changes

Enlargement of lymph nodes in axilla

Evidence of metastatic disease

Enlargement of lymph nodes in supraclavicular
(collarbone) cervical area

Abnormal chest x-ray film with or without pleural
effusion

Elevated alkaline phosphatase, elevated calcium, positive
bone scan, and/or bone pain related to bone
involvement

Abnormal liver function tests

---

ing structures are involved.[15] The box above lists additional clinical signs and symptoms of breast cancer at presentation.

DIAGNOSIS AND STAGING
Tissue Diagnosis

Breast cancer can be diagnosed after cytologic (cells) or histologic (tissue) evaluation. Examination of tissue will give a definitive diagnosis. *Fine-needle aspiration (FNA) biopsy* for cytology is the preferred technique when dominant masses are palpable. It is a relatively simple procedure involving the aspiration of material from the mass using a syringe and 21- to 23-gauge needle.[188] The content of the aspiration is mounted on slides and processed for review. In skilled hands it is highly accurate; false-negative and false-positive results are rare. A negative result in the presence of a suspicious mass warrants further evaluation. Although FNA can lead to the diagnosis of carcinoma, it cannot distinguish whether it is invasive or noninvasive.[99] Some advantages of the FNA are the ease with which it can be done in the office setting, using minimal local anesthesia, and the low incidence of damage to surrounding tissue. When the results are cancer, it also prevents the necessity of surgical biopsy before treatment planning for definitive surgery.[188]

Core needle biopsy provides a core of tissue from a dominant mass. Insertion of a specially designed 14-gauge needle into the palpable mass is accomplished either manually or with the aid of an automated device.[188] This procedure requires some local anesthesia and has been associated with more bleeding and pain than the FNA, especially when deeper lesions are involved. False-positive results may be a greater problem than with FNA, although they are still low in incidence. A core needle biopsy may be helpful after a nondiagnostic or suspicious FNA. Because it provides a larger sample of tissue, core needle biopsy can differentiate in situ from invasive cancer.[188] *Incisional biopsy* is performed when the mass is large; it involves removal of only a portion of the mass. *Excisional biopsy* involves removal of the entire mass and a margin of normal tissue around it. It is used for palpable and nonpalpable lesions.

Nonpalpable abnormalities detected only on mammogram need to be evaluated under radiographic guidance. The *needle localization biopsy* involves a radiologist localizing the suspicious area under mammography guidance by directing a small wire with a hook on the end into the lesion. The wire is then taped to the patient's skin, the patient is transferred to the operating room, and the abnormality and needle are excised by the surgeon. The tissue removed is radiographed to verify removal of the suspicious area (or to direct further excision). The tissue is then examined microscopically in permanent sections. Although this is not a difficult procedure, it is not an exact procedure and more tissue than necessary may be removed.[210]

Stereotactic FNA or core needle biopsy is intended to improve on the needle localization biopsy procedure both in accuracy and in patient comfort. It is now available in many breast centers. For this procedure, patients are positioned prone on an examination table, with their affected breast suspended through an opening in the table. The breast is compressed as for mammography, films are taken, the skin anesthetized, and the biopsy needle mechanically and precisely aligned by radiograph to the area of abnormality.[210] Two major advantages of the stereotactic needle biopsy are the precision of the technique and the possible elimination of some unnecessary excisional biopsies for benign lesions.[210] *Ultrasound-guided biopsy* is also used in some settings. In this case the woman is positioned supine, the lesion localized with ultrasound, and the biopsy needle guided manually by the physician.

It is rare today that any woman would have a definitive surgical procedure for breast cancer without first learning she has cancer through some preliminary diagnostic test such as an FNA or some type of tissue biopsy.[99] For women who have already had an FNA or core needle biopsy diagnosis of carcinoma, a biopsy is usually performed intraoperatively to reconfirm the diagnosis just before the definitive surgical procedure. These procedures enable the determination of a definitive diagnosis of cancer and the opportunity for a woman to be involved in her treatment plan. Women need to be assured that the interval between diagnosis and definitive treatment, to obtain recommendations regarding management options, does not adversely affect survival.

Staging

Breast cancer is most frequently staged according to the *TNM classification* system, which evaluates the tumor size *(T)*, involvement of regional lymph nodes *(N)*, and distant spread of the disease or metastases *(M)* (discussed in detail in Chapter 4). The stages may be simply classified as follows[9]:

Stage 0	Carcinoma in situ (Tis-N0-M0)
Stage I	Tumor under 2 cm with negative nodes (T1-N0-M0)
Stage IIA	Tumor 0 to 2 cm with positive nodes or 2 to 5 cm with negative nodes (T0-N1, T1-N1, T2-N0, all M0)
Stage IIB	Tumor 2 to 5 cm with positive nodes or greater than 5 cm with negative nodes (T2-N1, T3-N0, all M0)
Stage IIIA	Tumor less than 5 cm with positive movable or nonmovable nodes (T0-N2, T1-N2, T2-N2, T3-N1, T3-N2, all M0)
Stage IIIB	Tumor of any size with direct extension to chest wall or skin, positive nodes, with or without positive internal mammary lymph nodes (T4-any N, any T-N3, all M0)
Stage IV	Any distant metastasis (includes ipsilateral supraclavicular nodes)

The historical classification of stage, still seen in national statistical reports, classifies stage as *local* (no lymph nodes involved), *regional,* and *distant.* Of breast cancer patients diagnosed between 1986 and 1991 in the United States, 58% had local disease, 32% regional disease, and 6% distant (metastatic) disease at diagnosis.[189] Black women (43%) were less likely than white women (52%) to have their breast cancer diagnosed at a local stage from 1981 to 1987.[22]

Evaluating the extent of disease allows appropriate therapy to be planned, determines the overall prognosis, and permits comparison of research results related to treatment.[99] The clinical staging process routinely begins preoperatively with a thorough history and physical examination, bilateral mammography, complete blood count, liver function tests, alkaline phosphatase, and calcium. Pathologic staging is based on the histologic review of the primary tumor from surgical specimens (type, size, and margins) and, when invasive carcinoma is present, the lymph nodes. Evaluation of a patient's bony structure, liver, and head is individualized according to the patient's specific symptoms, laboratory test results, and clinical evidence of enlarged axillary nodes. For example, elevated liver enzymes with or without hepatomegaly would warrant a computed tomography (CT) scan of the abdomen or liver scan to rule out liver metastases. Specific complaints of bone pain or an elevated alkaline phosphatase or calcium level would be evaluated with a bone scan or bone survey. Extensive local surgery might be contraindicated if distant metastases are discovered at the initial diagnosis.

A variety of substances known to be secreted by some tumors are being evaluated for their applicability in breast cancer. Presently they are not considered part of the staging process. The potential value is in monitoring response to therapy and detecting early recurrence. Serial levels that show a pattern of continued increase over time are evidence of metastasis.[97] Two of these *tumor markers* with some value in breast cancer are *carcinoembryonic antigen* (CEA) and *CA-15-3.* CEA has been the most widely studied marker.[97] A normal value preoperatively provides a baseline by which to follow the patient with serial levels. This marker, however, is limited in its value because it can be elevated with other conditions, such as benign breast disease or smoking. Also, less than half of all patients with known breast cancer metastases show an elevation in the CEA (greater than 10 ng/ml).[97]

CA-15-3 may also be elevated in benign breast conditions but is not elevated in smokers. From studies to date, it appears to be a more sensitive marker for breast cancer metastases than CEA, with elevated levels (greater than 22 U/ml) in 70% to 85% of such patients.[97] In patients with *primary* early-stage breast cancer, CA-15-3 levels are elevated in 20% to 50% of patients, compared with only 10% to 30% of patients who will have an elevated CEA.[97] Neither test is specific enough to be routinely used for staging and follow-up.

PROGNOSTIC FACTORS

Tumor size and lymph node status, incorporated into the staging system, have long been recognized as pathologic characteristics that alone have value in predicting survival. The staging system, however, although it has provided direction for treatment, has not provided the means by which to predict which women in a particular stage group will have disease recurrence and which will not. It is now recognized that 20% to 30% of women with negative lymph nodes at the time of breast cancer diagnosis will develop distant metastases within 10 years. Adjuvant therapy would be most appropriately directed to those women if one could somehow identify them by additional pathologic studies of the tumor.[95] Several pathologic characteristics have been studied for their ability to determine risk of local recurrence, metastasis, response to therapy, and overall prognosis. These are known as *prognostic factors,* shown in the box, p. 95.

Tumor Size

Small tumor size at diagnosis is associated with (1) a decreased incidence of axillary nodal metastasis at diagnosis, (2) potential eligibility for breast-preserving surgery,

---

PROGNOSTIC FACTORS IN BREAST CANCER

Tumor size
Lymph node status
Histologic and nuclear grade
Estrogen and progesterone receptors
DNA content analysis
   Ploidy
   S-phase fraction (SPF)
Vascular and lymphatic invasion
Oncogenes (e.g., HER-2/*neu*)
Tumor suppressor genes
Epidermal growth factor (EGF)
Cathepsin D
Heat shock stress response proteins
Necrosis
Margins of resection
Inflammatory response
Multicentricity
Extensive intraductal component *(EIC)*
Demographic characteristics

   Under investigation for many of these factors is their interaction with each other and the influence of each on tumor growth, local recurrence, metastasis, or response to therapy.

Table 6-1   Ten-Year Survival According to the Number of Nodes Involved

Number of nodes	10-year survival (%)
0	65-70
1-3	48-63
4-9	28
≥10	18

From Henderson IC: Breast cancer. In Murphy GP and others: *American Cancer Society textbook of clinical oncology,* ed 2, Atlanta, 1995, American Cancer Society.

---

and (3) less chance of tumor recurrence within the breast or axilla.[248] The 5-year survival rate is 99% when tumor size is less than 0.5 cm, 80% for tumors less than 2 to 5 cm, and 50% to 60% for tumors greater than 5 cm.[95,248]

Axillary Lymph Node Status

The larger the tumor, the greater is the likelihood that lymph nodes will be involved. The most important predictor of disease recurrence and survival is the presence of axillary lymph node metastasis. When the lymph nodes are involved, a greater probability exists that distant micrometastases are present. Survival is influenced by the number of lymph nodes involved (Table 6-1). Women with negative lymph nodes have a higher rate of survival than women with involved lymph nodes. Similarly, women with one to three involved lymph nodes do better than women with four or more involved lymph nodes.[95,248] Involvement of the level I nodes has a better prognosis than involvement of the level III nodes.[95,120,248] Surgical evaluation of the nodes is important because clinically negative nodes will be pathologically involved in 30% of patients.[95,128]

Estrogen and Progesterone Receptors

Since 1971 a biochemical assay has been available to analyze breast cancer cells, removed at the time of diagnosis, for the presence of estrogen and progesterone re-

ceptors (ERs/PRs). These receptors are located in the nucleus or on the surface of the cell and bind to circulating steroid hormones. The receptor-hormone complex then works within the cell nucleus to promote cellular growth and division.[183] Patients are said to be positive or negative for ERs and PRs based on the level of binding receptors present. If the primary lesion is too small, an inadequate amount of tissue may be available to submit for this analysis. Newer assays that estimate ER and PR levels on smaller tissue specimens have been developed and are being evaluated.[183] Care should be taken at the time of biopsy and definitive surgery to ensure that tissue that is malignant is sent for ER and PR measurement. Approximately 60% to 70% of breast cancers are ER positive, and 40% to 50% are PR positive.[183]

The presence of ERs and PRs in breast cancer tissue has been used widely in planning treatment based on predicted responsiveness to hormonal therapy. The greatest likelihood of response to hormonal therapy is related to high levels of both ERs and PRs. Tumors that are ER negative and PR positive have shown more responsiveness than ER-negative and PR-negative tumors.[183] In addition, receptor status correlates with a variety of clinical and biologic parameters, some of which are also noted as prognostic factors (Table 6-2). Only recently have ERs and PRs been considered for their role in predicting prognosis.[183] PRs may be a better determinant of prognosis and ERs a better predictor of endocrine response.[120] Receptor-positive tumors are seen more frequently in postmenopausal women, are associated with a lower recurrence rate, and generally have a better overall prognosis.[183]

Histologic and Nuclear Grade

Pathologists also report the *histologic grade* (cellular arrangement) of the tumor, which includes *mitotic index,* defined as whether the cellular structure is well differentiated (grade I), moderately well differentiated (grade II), or poorly differentiated (grade III).[120,248] Poorly differentiated tumors (with high mitotic rate) are generally considered to be associated with a poorer prognosis. *Nuclear grade* refers to the differentiation of the tumor

Table 6-2 Clinical and Biologic Differences between ER-Positive and ER-Negative Tumors

Biologic parameter	ER positive	ER negative
Tumor differentiation	Well differentiated (low grade)	Poorly differentiated (high grade)
DNA content	Normal (diploid)	Abnormal (aneuploid)
Nuclear grade	Cell nuclei well differentiated	Poorly differentiated cell nuclei
S-phase fraction	Low percentage of cells in S phase (DNA synthesis)	High percentage of cells in S phase
Age/menopausal status	≥50 postmenopausal	<50 premenopausal
Clinical course of disease	Prolonged disease-free survival and overall survival	Shorter time to recurrence and shorter overall survival
Type of metastases	Bone and soft tissue	Visceral involvement (lung, liver, brain)
Response to endocrine therapy	Responsive	Unresponsive

Data from Osborne CK: Receptors. In Harris JR and others, editors: *Breast diseases,* ed 2, Philadelphia, 1991, Lippincott.

cell nuclei. In the Scarf-Bloom-Richardson grading system, a low number refers to a well-differentiated tumor (and better prognosis), whereas a score of 9 at the other end of the scale reflects a poorly differentiated tumor (and poorer prognosis).[99] Nuclear grade is considered to be more important than histologic grade as a prognostic factor. Both have been criticized because of the subjective means by which they are determined.[99,248] Computer technology that allows objective measurement has been evaluated and may enable more consistent reporting. Also, developing a standardized means for measuring the amount, for example, of ductoglandular differentiation or mitotic rate, would enhance objectivity.[248]

Lymphatic and Blood Vessel Invasion

The presence of lymphatic and blood vessel invasion by tumor cells is generally associated with a greater incidence of disease recurrence and a worse prognosis.[111,156] No specific, completely objective laboratory method is available to identify lymphatic or blood vessel invasion.[111,248]

DNA Content

Recent advances have been made in understanding the proliferative potential of breast cancer cells. *Flow cytometry* evaluates the aggressiveness of a neoplasm by analyzing the cellular deoxyribonucleic acid (DNA) content *(ploidy)* and the percentage of cells in the S phase of cellular division *(S-phase fraction,* or SPF). Tumors are classified as *diploid* (normal DNA content) or *aneuploid* (abnormal DNA content) and with high or low SPF.[41,99,101] Cutoff values for high versus low SPF have varied in studies to date.[41,101] No widely accepted values distinguish between a good prognosis and a poor prognosis tumor, although results above the median values often are viewed as being worse.[99,156] A greater risk of recurrence and worse prognosis are associated with aneuploid tumors and cells with a high percentage of

cells in the S phase. The combination of ploidy and SPF has greater prognostic value than ploidy alone.[111] Type I DNA histograms refer to diploid and low-SPF tumors, type II are diploid and high SPF, and type III are aneuploid and high SPF, the latter being associated with poor differentiation and poorer prognosis.[41,85,111,156] Studies are currently in progress to evaluate the clinical applicability of these tests in determining prognosis.[156] This information may be most useful in defining subsets of node-negative breast cancer patients who are not cured by surgery alone and therefore need systemic adjuvant therapy. The *thymidine labeling index* (TLI) is another method of measuring cell proliferation, expressed as a percentage of cells taking up labeled thymidine. This method of evaluating proliferation has largely been replaced by flow cytometry.[101]

Oncogenes

Proto-oncogenes are normally involved in regulating cell growth and differentiation. When altered, they become known as *oncogenes,* the genes responsible for cancer.[175] Abnormalities of amplification (multiple copies) or overexpression (multiple quantities) of the proto-oncogene HER-2/*neu* (or c-*erb*B-2) in the DNA of some breast cancers has been associated with tumor growth, more aggressive cancers, local or distant recurrence, and poorer overall survival.[156,175] Other proto-oncogenes under investigation are c-*myc* and Ha-*ras*. *Tumor suppressor genes,* or *antioncogenes,* may be absent or not functional. Normally inhibiting cancer growth, their absence has significance in cancer cell growth. Currently under study are p53, Rb-1, and nm23.[28] As discussed earlier in this chapter, the inheritance of either the BRCA1 or BRCA2 damaged gene significantly increases a woman's risk of developing breast cancer. The study of oncogenes has promise for adding prognostic factors that will differentiate higher-risk women with negative lymph nodes who will benefit from adjuvant therapy. In addition, therapies may be developed that are able to target the genetic aberrations.[28,101,156]

Epidermal Growth Factor

Epidermal growth factor (EGF) influences breast cancer growth by binding with receptors. The presence of increased numbers of receptors for EGF (EGF-R) has been associated with more aggressive tumors, metastases occurrence and location, and poorer prognosis.[101,156]

Cathepsin D

Cathepsin D is a glycoprotein that can be induced by estrogen and/or growth factors in breast cancer cells, resulting in effects on the extracellular matrix and basement membrane that in turn may mediate tumor proliferation, invasion, and metastasis.[101] High values of cathepsin D may be associated with greater recurrence and decreased survival.[156] Although the assay for measuring cathepsin D is commercially available in the United States, further study is needed to determine cutoff values for identifying good or poor prognosis in node-negative versus node-positive women.[101,156]

Other Factors

Several other prognostic factors, such as heat shock or stress response proteins, are currently under study to determine their value in predicting disease response and survival.[99] The relationships among microscopic tumor necrosis, inflammatory response, and margins of resection have been inconclusively associated with prognosis.[248]

Tumor type and size, lymph node status, estrogen and progesterone receptor status, histologic and nuclear grade, and DNA content (ploidy, SPF) are the most frequently considered evaluations in use today for determining prognosis and treatment plans.[160] The heterogeneity of breast cancer complicates precise determination of prognosis and treatment given the present understanding of the prognostic factors described and the technology available.[101,175] Further study will refine laboratory methods of measurement, consistency in reporting, and measures of interactions among prognostic factors.

Mortality rates have not changed significantly during the past 50 years.[7] However, the number of women diagnosed at an earlier stage has increased. Fewer women are being diagnosed with large tumors (greater than 5 cm in diameter).[177] Most of the increase has been in women diagnosed with tumors less than 2 cm in diameter with negative lymph nodes.[177] Approximately two thirds of all cases of invasive breast cancer diagnosed today will not involve axillary nodes,[160,177] and approximately 70% of those patients will be cured without adjuvant therapy.[160] The use of prognostic factors will be most helpful in identifying high-risk groups of women in need of adjuvant therapy.[101,120,160]

METASTASIS

Adjuvant systemic therapy has been shown to improve overall survival and prevent or delay the development of metastatic disease. Once metastatic disease develops, the goal of treatment is palliation. Breast cancer spreads by direct invasion of surrounding tissues, along mammary ducts, or by way of lymphatic vessels. The major site of regional spread is the axillary lymph nodes. These nodes are positive in approximately 50% of patients who have palpable tumors at diagnosis.[95] Systemic or distant spread of the disease can occur in a variety of organs and tissues. The most frequent sites are bone, lung, pleura, liver, and adrenals. Other less common sites are the brain, thyroid, leptomeninges, eye, pericardium, and ovary.[95,102] Symptoms described by patients that should be considered potentially associated with the existence of metastasis include bone pain, shortness of breath, nausea and/or vomiting not associated with chemotherapy, loss of appetite, loss of weight, or neurologic changes.[102] Elevations of the serum alkaline phosphatase, calcium, and liver function tests may be indicative of site-specific metastases, when seen in combination with clinical and radiographic findings (see box, p. 93).

Two serious complications of metastatic disease, considered oncologic emergencies, are *spinal cord compression* and *hypercalcemia*. Metastatic tumor compressing the spinal cord results in motor weakness and progresses to autonomic or sensory deficits and paralysis. Preservation of neurologic function depends on early diagnosis and prompt treatment. Therapeutic options include radiotherapy alone or in combination with surgical decompression. Further palliative systemic treatment may be added. Hypercalcemia is generally a reversible metabolic problem. The symptoms are nonspecific: nausea, constipation, weakness, confusion, and lethargy. This problem may be the result of progressive bone metastases or compromised renal function or part of a "flare reaction." Another complication associated with breast cancer metastasis is *malignant pleural effusion*. Gradual to acute onset of increasing respiratory distress, particularly dyspnea on exertion, is the most common sign. (See Chapter 19 for further information on oncologic complications.)

The median survival from the appearance of metastases is longer than 2 years, although some patients (25% to 35%) may live for 5 years and others (10%) for more than 10 years.[99,102] Patients who were diagnosed with metastases a longer time after their initial breast cancer diagnosis and who have metastases to the bone or soft tissue areas have a better prognosis.[102] Metastatic breast cancer is not considered curable, but therapies are usually available that will control or perhaps alleviate the symptoms altogether and prolong life.

TREATMENT MODALITIES

Surgery

Surgical management of breast cancer is centuries old, before anesthesia and before antisepsis, but it has been only within the past century that surgical intervention has shown survival benefits.[128] The primary goal of surgery has always been to achieve local and regional control of the disease. The halstedian view that breast cancer spreads in an orderly fashion from the breast to the lymph nodes prompted the extensive resection characteristic of the radical mastectomy. Newer views of the nature of breast cancer as a systemic disease at diagnosis and the lack of support for the view that lymph nodes serve as a barrier to metastasis prompted further investigation into less extensive surgery and the role of adjuvant systemic therapy.[95] Early diagnosis and local/regional treatment may also be adequate for some patients. Modified radical mastectomy has replaced the radical mastectomy in the past 20 years, and currently, breast-conserving surgical procedures with axillary node dissection are the preferred treatment for many small invasive breast cancers. Removal of regional lymph nodes at levels I and II is suggested as the best method for determining nodal status in patients with invasive breast cancer and clinically negative nodes, with full dissection to level III in patients with clinically positive nodes.[128,171,202] Axillary node sampling is not recommended.[128,171] The box at right describes surgical procedures in the treatment of breast cancer.

Primary therapy. The type of surgery selected is based on clinical stage of the disease (tumor size, fixation, histology, nodes, metastases), mammographic findings (including evidence of cancer cells in other areas of the breast separate from the primary), the tumor location, patient history, available surgical and radiotherapeutic expertise, breast size and shape, and patient preference.

Some research has suggested timing of breast cancer surgery during the menstrual cycle may influence recurrence and survival.[108] The hypothesis that surgery is associated with the highest curability when performed in midcycle is based on animal studies demonstrating the greatest function of natural killer cells and interleukin-2 production occurs during this time.[108] The clinical studies have been retrospective, and problems controlling for other variables might influence outcome, such as irregular cycles, individual variability in tumor characteristics or immune function, and the incidence of other procedures before surgery (e.g., an excisional biopsy within a few days before a mastectomy). Although the timing of breast cancer surgery during the menstrual cycle may

---

SURGICAL PROCEDURES IN TREATMENT OF BREAST CANCER[128]

Modified radical mastectomy (also referred to as *total mastectomy with axillary node dissection*). The entire breast is removed along with axillary lymph nodes and the lining over the pectoralis major muscle. The pectoralis major muscle is not removed. The pectoralis minor muscle may or may not be removed.

Total mastectomy (also referred to as *simple mastectomy*). All the breast tissue, including the nipple-areolar complex and the lining over the pectoralis major muscle, is removed. There is no axillary node dissection. Chest wall muscles are not removed.

Lumpectomy (or *excision; tumorectomy*). The tumor is removed and the major portion of the breast is left. A *tylectomy* refers to a wide excision with at least 3 cm of normal breast tissue around the tumor.

Wide excision (limited resection, partial mastectomy). Excision of the tumor with grossly clean margins of normal breast tissue.[177]

Quadrantectomy (also referred to as *partial mastectomy*). The entire quadrant of the breast containing the tumor is removed along with the overlying skin and the lining over the pectoralis major muscle.

NOTE: In each of the breast-conserving surgical procedures (lumpectomy, wide excision, and quadrantectomy) axillary node dissection is usually performed through a separate incision, and surgical intervention is followed by radiation therapy to the remaining breast tissue to treat any undetected cancer and achieve local control.[177]

---

have some clinical application in the future, further study is needed. Patients who desire scheduling of surgery in accord with their menstrual cycle should be encouraged to discuss this option with their physician.

Nearly all patients with operable breast cancer are candidates for the *modified radical mastectomy*. In large tumors this procedure allows for local control and pathologic staging. For most women with smaller tumors (stages I and II disease), *breast-conserving treatment* is now recognized as appropriate therapy with proven equivalence to modified radical mastectomy in terms of overall and relapse-free survival rates.[36,66,99,177,244] Adequate time should be allowed in all cases for full discussion with the patient as to her options, advantages, and disadvantages.[207] Critical to the success of breast-conserving surgery is appropriate patient selection and a multidisciplinary approach. Patients are selected for breast-conserving treatment based on the factors noted in the box, p. 99.[99,128,244]

Studies of utilization patterns of breast-conserving surgery in women with stage I or II disease have been undertaken to assess implementation of the NIH Consensus Development Conference recommendations released in 1990.[139,177,185] Some studies indicate that in certain

CONSIDERATIONS IN PATIENT SELECTION FOR BREAST-CONSERVING TREATMENT[66,99,128,177,244]

1. *Tumor size.* Local control is best with relatively small tumors. Most published experience in treating patients has been with tumors a maximum of 4 to 5 cm in diameter. *Contraindications* are the existence of stage III or IV disease.
2. *Tumor location.* Peripheral tumors are best, with clinically negative axillary lymph nodes. *Contraindications* include two or more gross malignancies in other quadrants of the breast or mammographic indications of suspicious diffuse calcifications (multifocal or multicentric disease). Lesions located centrally in the breast, such as beneath the nipple area, usually necessitate removal of the entire nipple-areolar complex; cosmesis then is a consideration.
3. *Breast size.* The tumor/breast size ratio influences the cosmetic results. If lumpectomy will result in a large surgical defect, a mastectomy followed by breast reconstruction may be more appropriate. A *contraindication* may be large pendulous breasts because of difficulties encountered with radiation therapy: reproducing the positioning of the patient and availability of equipment to provide dose homogeneity.
4. *Patient preference and attitude.* A woman's desire to save her breast and a willingness to undergo 5 to 6 weeks of daily outpatient radiation therapy are important factors. A short hospital stay may also be required if radiation implants are used. Some women might consider this extended treatment an unacceptable cost and inconvenience, or they may achieve greater peace of mind with the physical certainty of surgical removal. Nurses can be supportive of patients in this decision-making process by facilitating communications, providing information, and helping them explore their personal values and relationships.[30,232,238,239] Many studies to date have shown no significant differences for general measures of emotional distress in women undergoing mastectomy or breast-conserving surgery.[136,137,244] However, studies have shown that women undergoing breast-conserving surgery may have a more positive sexual and body image and fewer problems with clothing but may need additional psychosocial support during radiation therapy.[78,124,136,137,213]
5. Other *contraindications* are prior irradiation to the breast region that would limit therapeutic dosing for breast cancer treatment; a history of collagen vascular disorder, which has been associated with poor tolerance of radiation; and pregnancy. Women in first- or second-trimester pregnancies would be unable to undergo radiation therapy; women in their third trimester could feasibly receive breast irradiation after delivery.

areas of the United States, breast-conserving treatment is not being applied appropriately.[91,139,177,185] Availability of radiation facilities and of surgeons and radiation oncologists who specialize in the management of breast cancer is important for optimal results. Lack of such expertise may be one factor of underutilization of breast-conserving surgery. Public and professional education and costs may be other reasons. The finding in one study that young and elderly women were more likely to receive breast-conserving surgery but that elderly women were less likely to receive radiation therapy when indicated raises further questions for investigation.[139]

To prevent breast cancer in certain high-risk women, *prophylactic mastectomies* (unilateral or bilateral), with or without reconstruction, may be considered after careful discussion of potential risks and benefits. Women for whom this procedure may be appropriate include those with the following[18]:

1. Strong family history of breast cancer (e.g., premenopausal bilateral breast cancer)
2. Biopsy-proven ductal or lobular carcinoma in situ or proliferative benign breast disease (atypical hyperplasia)
3. Personal history of contralateral multicentric carcinoma in situ or invasive breast cancer

When accompanied by any of these risk factors, the presence of extremely nodular or dense breasts that make clinical or mammographic examination difficult might be the strongest indication for prophylactic mastectomy.[18] Fear of cancer alone is not an indication for prophylactic mastectomy.

Subcutaneous mastectomy, consisting of removal of breast tissue through an inframammary incision, removes 90% to 95% of the tissue, retaining the skin and nipple-areolar complex. Because of the difficulty removing all the breast tissue and problems with cosmesis, it is not recommended, for primary surgical treatment of invasive breast cancer.[132,135,157]

Ductal and lobular carcinoma in situ (DCIS and LCIS), referred to earlier in this chapter, are noninvasive. In the past these were rarely seen. Because of mammography screenings, DCIS is seen much more frequently. Estimates currently suggest 15% to 20% of all breast cancers found on mammography are in situ.[69] LCIS is found *incidentally* in biopsies of suspicious lesions or masses. DCIS is associated with a high risk of development of invasive ductal carcinoma at or near the biopsy site, whereas LCIS appears to be an indicator of the possible future development of invasive cancer anywhere in either breast. The management of each is different and controversial.*

DCIS is primarily discovered on mammography, read out by the radiologist as suspicious clustered microcal-

---

*References 75, 92, 99, 125, 127, 212.

cifications.[92] As described previously, these lesions could be biopsied via the needle localization technique. It is not known whether all DCIS will progress to an invasive cancer or when. DCIS and occult invasive cancer may also be found incidentally near an invasive cancer. When found outside the area of the primary tumor, DCIS is referred to as *multicentric foci* (sites outside the quadrant of the breast where the primary tumor was found) or *multifocal* (sites within the same quadrant as the primary tumor).[75] It is not known whether these are actually separate sites of disease or continuous disease along the ducts. It is much more common as the size of the primary invasive tumor increases.[92]

Mastectomy has been the primary treatment for DCIS, with a cure rate of nearly 100%.[99] Axillary node dissection is not usually done, although this remains controversial for large areas of DCIS involvement. Studies of breast-conserving surgery and radiation therapy for these women have a short duration of follow-up. In progress are studies by the National Surgical Adjuvant Breast and Bowel Project (NSABP) to evaluate the role of breast-conserving surgery with or without radiation therapy and/or tamoxifen in the management of DCIS, which should lead to a better understanding of DCIS and its treatment.

LCIS, when found incidentally on a biopsy specimen, presents different management problems. It is not truly a precancerous lesion but an indicator of the risk of future invasive cancer, most often invasive ductal carcinoma.[127] It occurs primarily in premenopausal women and may be found diffusely in both breasts.[99] Treatment decisions for LCIS include no further surgery and close lifetime observation, bilateral total mastectomies, or total mastectomy on the side where LCIS was found with a biopsy of the opposite breast in the same location, with subsequent mastectomy if LCIS is found there as well.[99,127] Neither axillary node dissection nor radiation therapy would be necessary if only LCIS was present.[127]

Metastatic disease. Surgery also has a role in the management of metastatic disease. Examples include procedures to excise local recurrences, drain pleural effusions, debulk and decompress spinal cord metastasis, and remove ovaries to eliminate that source of endogenous estrogen.

Breast reconstruction. The disfigurement and loss associated with a mastectomy can be devastating for many women and their sexual partners. A woman's breasts are equated with femininity, sexual attractiveness, and nurturing behavior.[204] Physicians and patients now increasingly recognize the psychosexual consequences related to breast cancer surgery.* Consequently, reconstruction has become an important element in a woman's rehabilitation after breast cancer surgery. Improved

reconstructive techniques offer women hope for a more unaltered body image. A coordinated treatment approach by the surgeon, radiologist, and medical oncologist with the plastic surgeon will increase the likelihood of achieving the desired results.[132]

Some debate still surrounds the timing of breast reconstruction—whether it can be immediate (at the time of the mastectomy) or delayed to some future date after other treatment is completed. There are pros and cons with either approach. In the past there has been concern about reconstruction interfering with detection of local recurrence of breast cancer or with wound healing. If cancer does recur locally, it usually involves only the chest wall or the overlying skin, and recurrences in the pectoralis major muscle are rare.[199] Wound complications were found to be less in the immediate reconstruction group in one study.[235] Breast reconstruction has not been shown to hide or delay diagnosis of local recurrence.[132,135,199] Other reasons for delaying reconstruction have been beliefs that women needed first to adjust to the mastectomy and diagnosis before making a decision about reconstruction, as if this might somehow enable them to make a better decision and thus better appreciate the reconstructed breast.[132] It appears that such beliefs have been unfounded.[18,132] Patients undergoing immediate reconstruction have been found to experience less overall trauma with their mastectomy and recalled less intensely the pain of their initial surgery.[208,209] Another advantage of immediate reconstruction is the elimination of one other hospitalization and anesthesia for the first stage of reconstruction.[132] Immediate breast reconstruction is probably most appropriate in stage I or II disease and delayed reconstruction most appropriate for stage III locally advanced disease, when initiation of adjuvant therapy soon after surgery is critical.[18]

Initially, some women express a desire to have reconstructive surgery, but their enthusiasm may diminish with the passage of time. Some reasons for not pursuing reconstruction include fear of additional surgery, fear of recurrence of cancer, adjustment to their physical change, guilt feelings related to the desire to restore their breast, and reluctance to separate from their prosthesis.[208] Cost may be another variable. Costs for reconstruction vary based on the type of procedure and geographic area. Many insurance companies will cover reconstruction after mastectomy for breast cancer, although many will not cover reconstructive or cosmetic surgery on the opposite side to adjust for symmetry.[132] Women need to inquire whether their individual insurance policies will cover these procedures. Some cost savings may occur when hospitalization for mastectomy and reconstruction are combined.

Treatment of the breast cancer must remain the priority; thus treatment planning within the team will help clarify timing of reconstruction and/or adjuvant thera-

---

*References 63, 64, 78, 124, 132, 136, 137, 142.

pies. Scheduling of surgery should not be delayed unnecessarily because of coordination between the oncologic and plastic surgeons.[161] Unexpected complications can occur after mastectomy when combined with immediate reconstruction and thus can delay the onset of adjuvant chemotherapy or radiation therapy.[23,135] Such concern in itself may warrant a medical recommendation to delay reconstruction. When chemotherapy is given postoperatively, reconstruction is usually delayed for 3 to 6 months after completion of this therapy so that the white blood cell count, tissue response, and metabolism can stabilize.[23,135]

A thoughtful discussion of the options for reconstruction ideally should be incorporated within the initial treatment planning period. The amount of information about the diagnosis and treatment options, potential for adjuvant therapy, and clinical trial participation and the discussion of reconstruction can be overwhelming for the patient as she sifts through the details while experiencing distress over the diagnosis and potential losses. Whether or not she chooses to undergo reconstruction, having that information can inspire hope and show support that she does have options.

Most women with breast cancer preparing to have a mastectomy, particularly those with stage I or II disease, are candidates for reconstruction.[23] The patient's motivation and desire for a restored breast is one of the most important indicators for reconstruction.[23] The reasons women seek breast reconstruction are varied and may include a desire to feel whole again, to maintain a sense of femininity and positive body image, to eliminate an external prosthesis, or to reestablish physical symmetry and a sense of balance.[132] Some women will choose mastectomy with reconstruction over breast-conserving surgery because of a desire not to worry about remaining breast tissue or having to undergo radiation therapy.

Advanced age is not a contraindication for reconstruction as long as the woman is in sufficient health to tolerate the effects of surgery. Patients with unrealistic expectations that reconstruction will eliminate the physical and psychologic effects of mastectomy for a breast cancer diagnosis or will result in a perfect replication of the lost breast are more likely to be dissatisfied with the results. Women who are obese, are smokers, or have a history of diabetes or debilitating disease have the highest rates of complications.[161]

The goals of reconstructive surgery are to (1) construct a breast mound, (2) achieve symmetry with the opposite side, and (3) build a nipple-areolar complex.[132,135] Considerations for type of surgery include the quality and amount of skin, the size and shape of the opposite breast, the initial surgical procedure for cancer, and the patient's goals and general health.[135] Table 6-3 lists breast reconstructive surgery procedures.

The first breast *implants* were developed in the early 1960s and were silicone gel filled. Polyurethane foam–

Table 6-3   Breast Reconstructive Surgery Procedures in Breast Cancer[23,81,132,135]

Procedure	Method

Implant (with or without tissue expander)
  Silicone gel filled (use is limited to controlled clinical trials)
  Saline-filled silicone shells
	Surgically placed under skin and muscle of chest

Saline-filled tissue expanders	Valve under skin allows adjustments in saline until ideal size reached
Permanent	Valve must be removed
Postoperative adjustable	Valve does not need to be removed
Temporary	Implant is surgically replaced with permanent saline-filled implant
Myocutaneous flaps	Transfer of skin and underlying muscle with its intact blood supply to breast area
Latissimus dorsi Transverse rectus abdominis (TRAM)	

Free flap transfer
  Gluteus maximus
  Transverse rectus abdominis (TRAM)
	Transfer of skin, muscle, and blood vessels to breast area, with microsurgical reconnection of blood vessels to those in chest and axilla

Nipple-areolar complex	Areola: transfer of skin from lateral chest, inner thigh, or opposite areola and/or intradermal tattoo for color symmetry Nipple: skin flap raised from skin of breast mound, or graft used from opposite nipple
Symmetry	Augmentation Mastopexy (breast lift) Reduction

covered silicone gel prostheses were introduced in the early 1970s. Problems with deterioration of the polyurethane and concerns about safety resulted in those prostheses being withdrawn from the market. Silicone gel implants with a mechanically textured surface were also developed. Saline-filled silicone shells and *tissue expanders* have been more widely used in recent years. Tissue expanders consist of an elastomer or silicone shell liner and a valve or port through which the shell is inflated with saline gradually over several weeks. The shell-type expanders must be removed and replaced with a permanent prosthesis, whereas the gel-inflatable liner has a filling port that can usually be removed and thus leaves the implant as a permanent prosthesis.[23,135] The majority of the more than 2 million women with implants have undergone elective breast augmentation and not reconstruction for breast cancer.

The most common complication of implants is *capsular contracture,* or hardening of the scar tissue, resulting in firmness of the breast tissue and sometimes distortion of shape. Mechanical problems with inflation or deflation can occur with the tissue expanders but are uncommon. The potential also exists for a missed cancer on mammography, although an informed and skilled mammography technician will help reduce this risk. A controversy in recent years has been the possible risk of autoimmune diseases linked to rupture or leakage of silicone gel into the body tissues. These concerns have not been substantiated.[23] In 1991 the FDA asked manufacturers to stop selling any implants for which safety and effectiveness data had not been submitted. Thus, in 1992, gel-filled implants were restricted to use only in prospective controlled clinical studies for women who have a medically related need for the implant (e.g., breast cancer, rupture of old implant). This excludes women wanting the implants for breast augmentation. At present the saline-filled implants or expanders are available for any woman seeking reconstruction. A review of prospective studies of these implants is due in 1998 by the FDA.[23] Until further information is available, reconstruction with implants for women with breast cancer should continue to be preceded by a full discussion of the available options, risks, and benefits.

The *latissimus dorsi myocutaneous flap* from the upper back often is supplemented with an implant for full symmetry. It effectively fills the defect beneath the clavicle present because of removal of the pectoralis major muscle in women who have had a radical mastectomy.[132] The *transverse rectus abdominis myocutaneous flap* (TRAM) from the lower abdomen accomplishes a simultaneous abdominoplasty (similar to a "tummy tuck") and does not require the use of an implant. Complications with either of these procedures include flap loss from damage to the blood supply, skin necrosis, infection, hematoma, delayed wound healing, and fat necrosis or fibrosis, all being greater with the TRAM procedure.[23,132,135] Hernias at the donor site have occurred with the TRAM flap as well. In either procedure an additional scar is left, but the scar from the TRAM procedure is usually hidden within an acceptable "bikini" line. The TRAM flap can also be performed bilaterally. The TRAM procedure carries greater risk for the woman who has a history of smoking or obesity or is in otherwise compromised health.[23,135] *Free flap transfers* are rarely used because of the complexity of the surgical dissection and prolonged surgical time and a higher rate of failure than with the myocutaneous flaps.[132,135]

Augmentation, mastopexy (breast lift), or *reduction* of the remaining breast is sometimes necessary to achieve *symmetry.* This and any further refinements in the reconstructed breast should be completed before the nipple-areolar complex reconstruction.[135] Saving the nipple-areolar complex at the time of mastectomy for later reconstruction is not recommended. *Skin transfers* (see Table 6-3) have been the primary means of nipple and areola reconstruction. However, newer and more satisfactory techniques involve the raising of a flap of skin from the reconstructed breast mound and folding back sections of the flap to create the projecting nipple.[23,81,132,135] In all patients, *tattooing* of the nipple-areolar complex usually follows to achieve color symmetry.[23] Figure 6-4 illustrates optimal reconstructive results.

Radiation Therapy

Radiation therapy has localized effects on breast cancer and as such has a role in local/regional control of disease as adjuvant therapy and in combination therapy for local/regional advanced or metastatic disease. In the past, radiotherapy was routinely used after a modified radical mastectomy to decrease the risk of local/regional disease recurrence. The area irradiated included the chest wall, supraclavicular fossa, and axilla. This practice is now less common, reserved for patients who have a high risk for local recurrence of the disease (most often when the deep surgical margins of resection are involved). Other patients in whom benefit has been shown include those with tumors greater than 5 cm in size with four or more positive nodes.[93]

Radiation therapy in conjunction with breast-conserving surgery is administered to achieve local control of disease in women with early-stage (I or II) breast cancer. Multiple randomized clinical trials comparing mastectomy with breast-conserving surgery followed by radiation to the whole breast have demonstrated equivalence in terms of overall survival.[57,66,177] Radiation has also been shown to reduce the risk of subsequent invasive tumor growth in patients with a history of DCIS.[83] External beam radiotherapy begins 2 to 4 weeks after the wide excision and/or axillary node dissection, when ad-

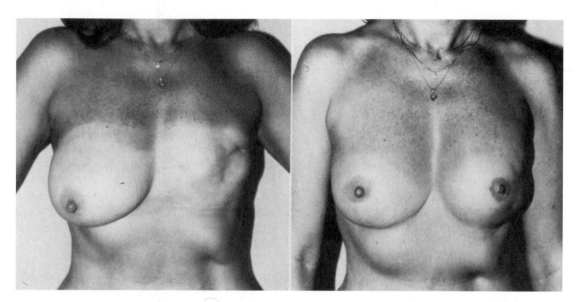

Figure 6-4 Breast reconstruction results. (From Bostwick J: *Aesthetic and reconstructive breast surgery*, St Louis, 1983, Mosby.)

equate healing has been achieved. Treatment planning is done to ensure homogeneity of dose through consistent reproducible positioning of the patient and the use of supervoltage equipment.[244] Each field is treated daily, Monday through Friday, to a total whole-breast dose of 4500 to 5000 centigrays (cGy), or rads, at 180 to 200 cGy per fraction. This therefore generally takes 4 to 5 weeks. A radiation boost to the original tumor site should always be given when surgical margins are involved or close, and it is usually given to all patients despite some controversy about the necessity.[177,218] It can be delivered by two methods: electron beam (external boost) or iridium-192 implanted temporarily in the tumor site. The latter requires a short hospital stay. The external boost is generally preferred because of cost, convenience, and cosmesis. The boost increases the total dose to the primary tumor site to 6000 to 6500 cGy.[177] Radiation to the axilla is generally not given when axillary node dissection has been completed at levels I and II, although controversy exists as to the possible benefits of such treatment when lymph nodes are involved or local invasion of the cancer has occurred beyond the lymph nodes.[177,218] Systemic adjuvant therapy also may be recommended. Future questions to be addressed include the optimal timing of adjuvant chemotherapy and radiation therapy postoperatively, with support for early initiation of each but not concurrently.[218]

Radiation therapy in combination with chemotherapy can be used to shrink inoperable breast lesions enough to allow surgical removal. For patients unable to undergo a surgical procedure, radiotherapy may be used as the primary therapy. In metastatic cancer, radiation therapy is palliative for painful bony metastases, shrinks meta-static brain lesions or tumors compressing the spinal cord, and relieves the symptoms of superior vena cava syndrome.

The toxicities associated with radiation therapy are generally mild and reversible. They include local skin changes, generalized fatigue, pain related to temporary inflammation of the nerves or the pectoral muscles in the radiation field, and occasionally sore throat. Extended axillary irradiation can aggravate lymphedema and range-of-motion difficulties. (For a more detailed discussion of the radiation-associated toxicities and specific nursing interventions, see Chapter 21 and the box, p. 110).

Systemic Therapy

Systemic treatment of breast cancer involves the use of chemotherapy or endocrine manipulation to treat patients with (1) axillary node involvement, (2) poor-prognosis node-negative disease, (3) advanced local/regional disease, or (4) distant metastases. The specific therapy recommended is influenced by the prognostic factors discussed earlier and the patient's general medical condition. Dosages used and the duration of therapy vary. Table 6-4 lists some common chemotherapy regimens used in adjuvant therapy, as well as individual drugs active in metastatic disease.

Adjuvant chemotherapy. Breast cancer can spread not only to axillary nodes but also to distant sites through the bloodstream. A percentage of women will therefore have micrometastases at diagnosis. Since 1972 adjuvant chemotherapy or hormone therapy has been given to prevent or delay the development of metastatic disease. It is given after the definitive surgical treatment while the tumor burden is small (micrometastases) and the cells are

Table 6-4 Major Chemotherapy Regimens for Breast Cancer[29,83,99,102]

Acronym	Drugs
ADJUVANT THERAPY	
CMF (6 months)	Cyclophosphamide (Cytoxan)
	Methotrexate
	5-Fluorouracil (5-FU)
AC (4 months)	Doxorubicin (Adriamycin)
	Cyclophosphamide (Cytoxan)
CAF or FAC (4-6 months)	Cyclophosphamide (Cytoxan)
	Doxorubicin (Adriamycin)
	5-Fluorouracil (5-FU)
RECURRENT OR METASTATIC DISEASE	
CMF, AC, CAF, or FAC	As noted for adjuvant therapy
OTHER ACTIVE AGENTS	Carboplatin
These have proven activity in breast cancer and are used and/or under investigation in combination chemotherapy for recurrent or metastatic disease, as well as in high-dose adjuvant therapy with peripheral blood stem cell transplant.	Carmustine
	Cisplatin
	Epirubicin
	Etoposide
	Ifosfamide
	Mitomycin C
	Mitoxantrone
	Paclitaxel (Taxol)
	Thiotepa
	Vinblastine
	Vinorelbine tartrate (Navelbine)

NOTE: Concurrent or sequential tamoxifen may also be recommended.

least likely to become drug resistant. Clinical trials have clearly demonstrated that adjuvant chemotherapy delays recurrence and improves overall survival, particularly in premenopausal, node-positive women.[58,83,99] This is also probably true for many women who are node negative, particularly if they are premenopausal or if their tumors are greater than 2 cm in size, high grade, and ER negative.[58,83]

There is no one optimal drug combination, treatment schedule, or duration of therapy for all patients, although some general guidelines have been established. Since 1985 the NIH has gathered panels of experts to evaluate the results of adjuvant clinical trials and to make treatment recommendations. For example, clinical trials to date have resulted in a gradual decrease in the total length of time recommended for adjuvant chemotherapy, to the current duration of 4 to 6 months as suitable for most patients.[83,99] The regimens most often used in adjuvant therapy contain a combination of *cyclophosphamide* (C), *methotrexate* (M), and *5-fluorouracil* (F). Because *doxorubicin* is one of the most active single agents for the treatment of metastatic breast cancer, it is often used in the adjuvant setting in combination regimens.[99] Dose in-

tensity and scheduling remain under investigation. In general, panel recommendations are made for treatment of patients not enrolled in a clinical trial. Consensus panel reports for treatment of early-stage breast cancer in 1990 and 1995 have addressed adjuvant therapy for subsets of women.[82,83,177] Table 6-5 summarizes standard practice recommendations at this time for women not registered in a clinical trial. These recommendations primarily consider menopausal status, lymph nodes, and ER status. It has been suggested that whenever possible, other prognostic factors (e.g., nuclear grade, DNA content) may be considered in estimating an individual woman's risk of recurrence.[177] However, much remains to be learned about the significance of these other prognostic factors.

In the past, node-negative patients were considered to have a good prognosis and no additional therapy after surgery was recommended. However, evidence suggests that 20% to 30% of these patients will develop recurrent disease.[83,95,99] The International Consensus Panel on the Treatment of Primary Breast Cancer concluded that women who have a greater than 10% mortality rate at 10 years benefit from adjuvant systemic therapy.[83] The difficulty lies in determining who those women are, the long-term toxicities, and risk/benefit ratio for these women.[45,99,177] The report of the 1990 NIH Consensus Conference, in summarizing the knowledge to date, recommended that outside of participation in a clinical trial, women with negative lymph nodes should be made aware of the risks and benefits of adjuvant chemotherapy based on current knowledge so as to be able to make an informed decision about such treatment.[82,177]

In general, women who will most clearly benefit from systemic chemotherapy with or without endocrine therapy are those with positive lymph nodes regardless of age and premenopausal women with larger tumors regardless of lymph node status.[58,83,99] Women with tumors less than 1 cm in diameter and negative lymph nodes may not warrant adjuvant chemotherapy outside of a clinical trial. Further studies in progress will identify the specific subsets of patients who need adjuvant chemotherapy and the most appropriate regimen.[83,99,177]

The medical decision to recommend adjuvant therapy and the patient's decision to receive it can be complex and difficult. As with decisions about the type of surgical procedure, patients need help understanding the concept of adjuvant therapy and information about the benefits and risks.[140,195,203] Although increased numbers of women have been given the opportunity to participate in clinical trials through the Community Clinical Oncology Programs (CCOP), emphasis should still be placed on participation by women and their physicians in clinical trials. Clinical trials are in progress to determine the benefits of perioperative chemotherapy (begun within hours after surgery), neoadjuvant therapy (administered for a

Table 6-5   Summary of Recommendations for Adjuvant Breast Cancer Therapy For Patients Not Enrolled in Clinical Trials (Invasive Cancer)[58,82,83,99,177]

Menopausal status	Tumor size	Hormone receptor status	Treatment
NODE NEGATIVE (BASED ON 10 OR MORE NODES)			
Premenopausal	≤1 cm	Negative or positive	None vs. ?*
	1-2 cm	Negative or positive	Chemotherapy* vs. none
	>2 cm	Negative	Chemotherapy
	>2 cm	Positive	Chemotherapy ± tamoxifen*
Postmenopausal	≤1 cm	Negative or positive	None vs. ?*
	1-2 cm	Negative	Chemotherapy* vs. none
	1-2 cm	Positive	Tamoxifen* vs. none
	>2 cm	Negative	Chemotherapy* ± tamoxifen*
	>2 cm	Positive	Tamoxifen
NODE POSITIVE			
Premenopausal	Any	Negative	Chemotherapy
	Any	Positive	Chemotherapy ± tamoxifen*
Postmenopausal	Any	Negative	Chemotherapy* ± tamoxifen* or none
	Any	Positive	Tamoxifen ± chemotherapy*

*These are areas of controversy as noted in the text, and the above summary may be revised as more research data become available. Note that some physicians will determine treatment based on additional prognostic factors, such as DNA content (ploidy) and S phase (measure of cell division). "High risk" has been described as the presence of tumors greater than 2 cm, receptor negative, aneuploid, or diploid with high S phase; from 1 up to 2 cm size tumors that are receptor positive, diploid, and low S phase as "good risk"; and "low to minimal risk" as the presence of tumors 1 cm or smaller, receptor positive, diploid, and low S phase.[83,99,177] These will likely prove most useful, via clinical trials, in determining treatment options for women with negative lymph nodes. For those situations when treatment is not well defined, patients should carefully review the risks and benefits of any treatment plan with their physician.

period before surgery), short-course intensive chemotherapy, and high-dose chemotherapy with peripheral blood stem cell transplant (discussed later in this chapter).[29,83,99]

Adjuvant endocrine therapy. *Tamoxifen* delays recurrence in postmenopausal breast cancer patients.[99] In studies of node-negative patients, tamoxifen also reduces the incidence of cancers in the opposite breast.[177] In the presence of ER-positive tumors, regardless of lymph node status, all women may benefit from tamoxifen. In premenopausal patients, however, the long-term risks of tamoxifen therapy secondary to endocrine abnormalities are not fully known.[99,177] The optimal duration of therapy has yet to be established. Current studies indicate long-term treatment, closer to 5 years, is probably better than therapy of 2 years' duration.[58,83,99] Therapy in excess of 5 years is not currently recommended.[99] Benefit from the addition of tamoxifen to multidrug chemotherapy in premenopausal women needs further study, whereas in postmenopausal women, benefit from the addition of chemotherapy to tamoxifen needs further study. All patients receiving tamoxifen need to be monitored for side effects, which may be disruptive enough to cause a woman to discontinue therapy. These primarily are hot flashes and gynecologic problems such as vaginal discharge, irritation, or dryness.[99,145,222] There is a slight increased risk of endometrial cancer but potential improvement in bone density and lipid values (high-

density lipoproteins [HDLs] and low-density lipoproteins [LDLs]).[145,222]

Treatment of advanced disease. Certain patients with features of *locally advanced disease* may be considered inoperable at diagnosis. This includes tumors with direct extension to the chest wall or skin, fixed axillary nodes or metastases greater than 2.5 cm, skin ulceration, and inflammatory changes. Although potentially resectable with radical mastectomy, the local recurrence rate is greater than 50%, and in most patients, overall survival is zero at 5 years.[176] Some, but not all, of these patients will have distant metastases at the time of diagnosis. Patients with locally advanced disease benefit from combination chemotherapy with or without endocrine therapy, followed by radiation therapy and/or surgical intervention for local control. The presence of supraclavicular or infraclavicular nodes or large, nonmovable axillary nodes at the initial diagnosis, and response to chemotherapy will determine whether the subsequent treatment is high-dose radiation therapy, mastectomy, or both. Systemic therapy is then resumed after local therapy. The optimum therapy for locally advanced disease still has not been determined in spite of improved responses with this sequential therapy.[176]

The goal of therapy in metastatic disease is control of the disease and palliation of symptoms. Metastatic breast cancer is incurable with either chemotherapy or hormone manipulation. These modalities are able to achieve temporary regression of the disease in a majority of patients, but these responses rarely last a long time. Overall, the median survival after the development of metastatic disease is less than 3 years.[100,236] As noted previously, a small percentage of these patients will be alive at 5 years and a very few will live 10 or more years.[99,102,236]

Women with receptor-positive cancers have more potentially beneficial treatment options available to them than those with receptor-negative cancers. Local/regional, soft tissue, and bony recurrences that are not life threatening are generally treated with endocrine therapy first. Radiation therapy may be used for local or symptomatic control. For more aggressive disease (liver, lymphangitic lung disease, and widespread, painful bony metastases), frontline treatment is chemotherapy. The regimen selected may be one of those listed in Table 6-4; selection is based on prior adjuvant treatment, prior response, and current physical condition.[236]

Chemotherapy. Responses to combination drug therapy occur in approximately 50% to 80% of patients. These disease regressions generally last from 5 to 13 months.[100] Doxorubicin (Adriamycin) is the most effective single agent in the treatment of metastatic breast cancer. Other active single agents typically employed in combination regimens include cyclophosphamide, methotrexate, and 5-fluorouracil.[100] Once initial therapy for distant metastases fails, subsequent treatment regimens often use mitomycin C, epirubicin, mitoxantrone, vinblastine, or paclitexal. Etoposide, ifosfamide, cisplatin, and carboplatin are not effective in patients who have failed after cyclophosphamide or doxorubicin therapy.[99] Docetaxel is the most recent drug showing promise for treatment of breast cancer resistant to anthracyclines, such as doxorubicin, or to paclitaxel (Taxol).[198] Because there is no "standard" therapy for metastatic disease, new approaches are regularly being tested in phases II and III research. Examples include non-cross-resistant therapy, new phase II agents, standard versus intensified dose therapy, intensive chemotherapy and autologous bone marrow transplantation, chemoendocrine combinations, weekly low-dose chemotherapy, and continuous infusion regimens.

Autologous transplant. For women with locally advanced (10 or more positive lymph nodes) or metastatic breast cancer, chemotherapy options are less effective and potentially associated with more myelosuppressive toxicity. This may be improved if the patient's own bone marrow is removed before high-dose treatment and reinfused after treatment, as with *autologous bone marrow transplant* (ABMT) or when the patient's peripheral blood stem cells are harvested and later reinfused (*peripheral stem cell transplant,* or PSCT). The addition of *granulocyte* and *granulocyte/macrophage colony-stimulating factors* (G-CSF and GM-CSF) to the treatment regimen has enabled more rapid recovery and re-

duced toxicities associated with myelosuppression. For patients with metastatic disease, the risk of occult, undetected bone marrow metastases is high, and thus the recurrence rate with ABMT and cost, morbidity, mortality, and toxicities associated with the procedure have been high. However, the response rate has been encouraging. PSCT appears to have lower costs, morbidity, and mortality and thus may be preferred to ABMT for patients with locally advanced or metastatic disease. PSCT is also being studied as initial adjuvant therapy in women with stage II or III disease. For PSCT, most treatment is conducted on an outpatient basis, with the patient and family closely involved in the procedures. The patient and significant other(s) need to remain close to the treatment facility. An experienced multidisciplinary transplant team that can ensure 24-hour access for patients is critical for the success of PSCT.[25,27] After a prescreening evaluation, medical evaluation, and insurance approval, the treatment begins with an alkylating agent followed by a series of self-injections of G-CSF or GM-CSF. These serve to "mobilize" the stem cells from the bone marrow into the peripheral circulation. Cells are harvested from the patient peripherally in a procedure known as *apheresis.* Several aphereses are performed over a week to 10 days to achieve an adequate volume of cells.[25] Dose-intensive chemotherapy is then administered, followed by the infusion of the PSCT. White blood cell and platelet counts usually return within 2 weeks.[25] Patients are then monitored closely on an outpatient basis for possible complications in the 2 to 3 weeks after PSCT. Many patients will return to their primary care physician or oncologist for further follow-up. Current follow-up suggests an improved 2-year survival rate for locally advanced disease (compared with conventional adjuvant chemotherapy), as well as for metastatic breast cancer.[224] Until further research results are available, eligible patients should be informed about the availability of this treatment option in the context of a randomized clinical trial.[83]

Hormonal manipulation. The ability to quantify ERs and PRs in breast cancer cells has allowed oncologists to predict with greater accuracy which women might respond to hormone manipulation. Receptor-positive patients respond 50% to 60% of the time, whereas only 10% of receptor-negative patients will respond. A variety of endocrine approaches are available. Metastatic tumors responding to one form of hormone therapy are more likely to respond to subsequent hormone maneuvers.[99] This type of therapy requires several weeks to be effective. Therefore it is not recommended in women with life-threatening liver, lung, or brain metastases. The dosage and duration of these therapies vary.

Tamoxifen is the primary *antiestrogen* used either as adjuvant therapy or as treatment of metastatic disease. It is the first choice in the management of postmenopausal women who are ER positive. Tamoxifen binds to ER sites in breast cancer cells, thereby blocking the uptake of estrogen necessary for cell proliferation. The drug is taken orally and has few toxicities. For premenopausal women, *ovarian ablation,* to reduce the level of circulating estrogens available to stimulate breast cancer cells, is a treatment of choice.[99,126] This can be achieved with bilateral oophorectomy, radiation therapy, or luteinizing hormone–releasing hormone (LHRH) agonists or antagonists (buserelin, leuprolide, goserelin). Recent studies have shown that tamoxifen and oophorectomy are equally effective in treating premenopausal women with distant metastases, and tamoxifen is associated with less toxicities. Therefore tamoxifen will usually be selected as first-line therapy for metastatic disease in premenopausal patients as well.[99]

Progression after tamoxifen or ovarian ablation usually requires a sequential trial of other endocrine therapies. However, simply discontinuing a form of therapy may also result in a "withdrawal response," when tumor regressions may occur.[99] For the postmenopausal woman who has progressed on tamoxifen, subsequent treatment might progress from progestins to aminoglutethimide, estrogens, or finally androgens.[99,126] Progestins followed by aminoglutethimide might be the sequence for premenopausal women.[99,126] The *progestins* most often used are megestrol acetate (Megace) and medroxyprogesterone acetate (Depo-Provera). Recent studies have shown these drugs to be as effective as other forms of hormone manipulation. The mechanism of action of progestins has not been established. Relatively few side effects are associated with their use; weight gain is the most frequently experienced side effect.[126] *Estrogens* such as Premarin or diethylstilbestrol (DES) can also result in tumor regressions in postmenopausal women. High doses of estrogen act at the level of the hypothalamus to inhibit the release of luteinizing hormone (LH), which normally stimulates the ovaries to produce estrogen. These drugs are as effective as tamoxifen but are associated with significant side effects (nausea, vomiting, anorexia, vaginal bleeding, breast engorgement, edema).[99,126]

Androgens, or male hormones, are less effective than estrogens or tamoxifen.[99] Testosterone and fluoxymesterone (Halotestin) have been evaluated, but fluoxymesterone is preferred. The exact mechanism of action of androgens is unknown. Side effects are minimal, but the usefulness of these compounds is limited because of the unacceptability of masculinizing effects (facial and body hair, deepening of the voice, alopecia). The flare response and hypercalcemia have been associated more frequently with androgen therapy than with any other endocrine therapy.[126]

With any endocrine therapy, "flare reaction" may occur during the first few weeks of treatment. The most frequent symptom of a flare reaction is abrupt onset of diffuse musculoskeletal aching, increased pain at sites of known disease, erythema at sites of skin metastases, or hypercalcemia.[99] Hypercalcemia is the most serious manifestation of a flare reaction. This reaction should not be confused with progressive disease and is not an indication of therapeutic response. The endocrine therapy should be continued unless the calcium levels exceed 14 mg/dl. A transient elevation of tumor markers (e.g., CA-15-3) may also occur in response to endocrine therapy.[99] Women receiving all endocrine therapies as well as postablative therapies (e.g., adrenalectomy, hypophysectomy) must be monitored for this reaction and provided treatment for their symptoms.

Adrenalectomy and *hypophysectomy* (surgical removal of the adrenals and pituitary glands, respectively) are no longer therapies of first choice for postmenopausal women because of the associated surgical morbidity and mortality and long-term side effects. Medical adrenalectomy can be achieved with the use of *aminoglutethimide.* The effects on the tumor are a result of inhibition of the enzyme that converts androgens (produced by the adrenal glands) to estrogens.[236] Patients generally receive hydrocortisone (HCT) to prevent adrenal insufficiency while receiving aminoglutethimide. They are encouraged not to discontinue the HCT abruptly while receiving aminoglutethimide or after it is discontinued. A gradual tapering of the dose is done until the patient's adrenal function returns. The most frequently experienced side effect with aminoglutethimide is lethargy, with less frequent occurrences of dizziness, skin rash, nausea/vomiting, and cushingoid symptoms.[126] Aminoglutethimide is not effective in premenopausal women unless there has been prior response to tamoxifen or ovarian ablation.[99] The effect of removal of the pituitary glands has been demonstrated medically through the use of levodopa or bromocriptine, which suppresses levels of prolactin, normally secreted via the pituitary.

Current trials of endocrine therapy in patients with metastatic disease include different agents alone or in combination with other therapies such as chemotherapy or biologic response modifiers.[126]

CONCLUSION

Breast cancer presents nurses with many challenges along a continuum of prevention, early detection, and treatment. The nurse must be knowledgeable about breast cancer and its ever-changing management; honest, realistic, and creative when providing support and care; skilled at symptom management; attentive to the patient's concerns within the context of the family or significant others; and ready to involve oneself in the professional and lay communities to promote breast health for all. Breast health care for elderly women will be a

Text continued on pg. 117.

NURSING MANAGEMENT

This section discusses selected nursing diagnoses and interventions. Further nursing diagnoses and interventions are based on patient age, clinical history, specific problems and concerns, concomitant physical and psychosocial problems, visual or auditory deficits, educational level, cultural influences, language, coping strategies, prior experience with illness, social support, medical diagnoses, and specific treatment goals and options planned. The role of nursing along a continuum of health care experiences for the woman at risk for or diagnosed with breast cancer is described by Thomas[229] and is reflected partly here in the discussion of phases of care.

PREDIAGNOSTIC PHASE

Nurses who work in public health clinics or outpatient facilities have many opportunities to interact with women who are entering the health care system for routine screening procedures. A valuable role for nurses is to offer public education programs on breast health and to reinforce the positive health care maintenance behaviors of individual women. When a woman notices a change in her breast, when her health care provider finds a palpable mass, or when she receives a report of an abnormal mammogram, anxiety and fear are likely to follow. Taking further action to learn the nature of the abnormality requires participation by the woman with her health care provider. Thomas[229] describes many factors that might influence a woman's actions during this time, such as usual coping style, experience with the health care system, beliefs about cancer, and cultural background. Access to the health care system and the services necessary, a problem for elderly and socioeconomically disadvantaged persons, could result in a delay in diagnosis.[73,91,203] Denial of the symptom or finding may result in a delay as well.[203,229] High optimism and expectations for positive outcomes may enhance care seeking for a breast problem.[138] Prior experience with breast problems or knowledge of other women who have had breast problems requiring evaluation may positively or negatively impact a woman's response. Nurses can be advocates to support women in seeking this follow-up.

DIAGNOSTIC PHASE

When a procedure is indicated to evaluate an abnormality, a woman may experience anxiety, fear, and even anticipatory grieving over the threat of the diagnosis of cancer and loss of the breast. Diagnostic procedures and tests can be overwhelming and frightening. Simply waiting for test results may seem unbearable. The stress at this time is also experienced by significant others.[181] The main components of nursing care during this phase include (1)

preparation of the patient for the procedures/tests, both physically and emotionally; (2) creation of a positive and supportive environment; and (3) provision of adequate information and resources to address patient and family concerns.

NURSING DIAGNOSIS

• *Anxiety related to fear of diagnosis of breast cancer*

OUTCOME GOALS

• Anxiety will be manageable so that patient will complete the diagnostic work-up.
• Patients without a cancer diagnosis will have a plan of care that prepares them for early detection of cancer and reduces anxiety as much as possible.
• Patients with a diagnosis of cancer will be supported in adjusting to the next phase of care.

INTERVENTIONS

• Explain purpose, preparation, and steps of procedures required for diagnosis (mammography, ultrasound, FNA, stereotactic or needle localization biopsy, excisional biopsy).[214]
• Provide literature as appropriate.
• Allow patient to ventilate fears and concerns regarding possible malignant diagnosis.
• Explain postprocedural care.
• Encourage patient to bring spouse/significant other/friend when returning for test results.
• Be present, if possible, when patient is given test and biopsy results. Continuity of care and a relationship of trust established early in the treatment phase do much to allay anxieties about the health care system.
• Patients who do not have a diagnosis of cancer will need information about follow-up specific to their diagnosis. This may be an opportune time to reinforce instruction in BSE, provide guidelines for follow-up with mammography and CBE, and offer general information about a healthy life-style and cancer risk reduction.[17] Some may need an individualized plan for regular screening. Women with benign proliferative breast disease and/or a strong family history of breast cancer who have concerns about personal breast cancer risk should be referred to appropriate resources for counseling regarding risk.[122,226]

PREOPERATIVE PERIOD

Patients who have been diagnosed with breast cancer are faced with an onslaught of information that ranges from the basic fact of the diagnosis of cancer to the complexity of choosing a type of surgical procedure with or without a second treatment (radiation therapy), with or without chemotherapy or hormonal therapy, and possibly within the context of a clinical research study. The decision about what to recommend to a patient and how that is subsequently explained to the patient can be equally complex for health care providers. It is important that patients are given adequate information from which they can make informed decisions. Many states now mandate that patients be given information on surgical treatment options. Some states also require second surgical opinions before any elective surgery.[203] Repeated discussions are often necessary to clarify information previously given but forgotten or not heard because of the stress experienced during the discussions.

Rowland and Holland[203] describe four potential responses of patients during this period: (1) deferral to the physician to make the decision, (2) permitting physicians to do only a certain procedure, (3) temporarily indecisive or potentially unable to make any decision, and (4) decisive based on a thoughtful review of the options. Most women benefit from some time to think over the information provided, discuss that information with significant others in their support network, and review again with the physician and treatment team.[30,203,232,238,239] Continuity of care providers is important for the continuity of information provided. Potential nursing diagnoses during this time can include (1) anticipatory grieving related to threatened changes in body image, work, or personal role relationships; (2) powerlessness related to inability to control diagnosis and perceived inability to make decisions; and (3) ineffective individual coping. Most women find their coping mechanisms challenged during this time and respond appropriately.

NURSING DIAGNOSIS

- *Powerlessness related to decisional conflict and informational overload regarding breast cancer treatment options and plan of care*

OUTCOME GOAL

Patient will be able to:
- Have adequate information and support to make an informed decision about treatment, involving her significant other(s) as appropriate.

INTERVENTIONS

- Be present with medical team, if possible, when the treatment plan is initially discussed and at subsequent discussions.
- Provide appropriate literature to supplement verbal discussion.
- Clarify information as appropriate.
- Act as liaison between patient and medical team.
- Anticipate patient and family concerns and questions and involve significant others as indicated by patient and situation. Identification of the social support network of patient will be helpful throughout treatment.[24,63,64]

- Allow patient and family to verbalize concerns openly, and reinforce normalcy of responses.[195]
- Clarify misinformation that women may have or may receive through other sources about breast cancer and its treatment; as Rabinowitz[195] suggests, this is a time to "demythologize."
- Assist decision making by helping patient review the pros and cons of her options and think through how she has made decisions in the past.[195]
- Consider referral to recovered patients who have undergone a specific treatment, such as breast-conserving surgery with radiation. The Reach to Recovery program of the ACS is one resource.
- Consider referral to professional resources for additional support in coping and adjustment for patients who have unusual difficulty processing the information and who do not follow through with making a treatment decision.

OPERATIVE PHASE

When Thomas[229] described the periods of care in breast cancer in 1978, many women were still undergoing a one-step procedure, waking up after a biopsy only to discover that they had indeed undergone a mastectomy. Fortunately, today this is not the case and women admitted to the hospital for surgical treatment are better prepared. Hospitalization and surgery alone are associated with stressors, such as separation from family, disruption in sense of control, and general anesthesia. Feelings of sadness at the anticipated loss (whether part or all of the breast), a sense of readiness for the surgery, and relief (that the cancer will be removed) are often interspersed postoperatively with concern about the final pathology report and the involvement of lymph nodes.

Wound care and remobilization of the arm are physical tasks of this period.[24,162] Some controversy exists as to the best time to begin mobilization of the arm and shoulder postoperatively and differences between patients undergoing mastectomy or breast-conserving surgery.[48,90,116,144,192] Concerns about early mobilization (days 1 to 2 postoperatively) have been related to the potential for increased drain tube output, delay in drain removal, postdrain seroma formation, and potential for impaired wound healing and infection. Concerns about late mobilization are related to arm and shoulder motion difficulties that may occur when exercise is not begun sooner. Restricted mobility carries the potential risk of later development of a "frozen shoulder." Some postoperative exercise to include flexion and extension of the hand, wrist, and elbow and limited movement for simple activities (eating, brushing teeth) seem reasonable immediately after surgery, gradually increasing exercises beginning within 3 to 5 days after surgery designed to regain full range of motion (ROM) of the shoulder joint. Often such exercise programs are designed by a treatment team from nursing, surgery, occupational therapy,

Continued.

and physical therapy. Because surgical admissions are of much shorter duration, much preoperative preparation takes place in the clinic or office setting along with post-operative education. Nurses have an important role not only in educating but in promoting the expression and exploration of feelings by the patient and her spouse or significant other. It is important to include both individuals in the treatment planning and follow-up (see box below and box on p. 116).

Possible nursing diagnoses during this phase include (1) grieving related to changes in body and body image; (2) risk for infection related to surgical wound and axillary lymph node dissection; (3) impaired physical mobility related to imposed restriction, pain, or fatigue; (4) body image disturbance; and (5) anxiety regarding final pathology report.

NURSING DIAGNOSIS

- *Injury, risk for (infection, delayed wound healing, immobility), related to surgical wound and impaired lymph drainage secondary to breast cancer surgery, complicated by failure to view and care for wound/drains*

OUTCOME GOALS

Patient will be able to:
- Be free of infection in the postoperative period, without delayed drain removal, excess fluid reaccumulation,

or delayed wound healing, and care successfully for her wound at home.
- View her operative site and begin to integrate this into her body image and sense of self, involving her spouse and significant others as appropriate.
- Describe arm care and demonstrate beginning ROM exercises.

INTERVENTIONS

- Inform patient and family about hospital and surgical routines.
- Describe postoperative activity (positioning and care of the arm on the operative side, drains, intravenous lines, ambulation) before surgery so that patient will be prepared to participate appropriately.
- Position arm on operative side slightly elevated with flat pillow or folded towel behind upper arm until patient is fully awake and ambulatory. Maintain position when reclining.
- Reinforce importance of early ambulation, coughing, and deep breathing.
- All intravenous access sites or venipunctures should be managed on the nonoperative side.
- Monitor wound for inflammation, tenderness, swelling, or purulent drainage. Change dressing when ordered using aseptic technique.
- Monitor drains and instruct patient simultaneously: intact, secured to the skin or clothing so as not to dangle, color and amount of fluid output.[51]
- Assess patient and medicate for pain or discomfort as ordered.
- Provide information on normal sensory sensations patient will experience postoperatively, such as paresthesias of the inner aspect of the upper arm and increased skin sensitivity.[42,133] "Phantom breast" experiences have also been reported.[133,143]
- Assess readiness to look at incision, and offer support when patient decides to view the incision. Description of the wound appearance may be helpful to some patients before actual viewing. Discuss possible response of patient's spouse/significant other toward viewing the incision and patient's readiness for this.
- Instruct patient in arm care and postsurgical arm exercises.[42,80,103,129,162] This will usually require further follow-up instruction in the outpatient setting, since the exercises should continue for a minimum of 6 weeks after surgery but may need to be continued for up to 6 months for full recovery and flexibility.[24,103] Examples of recommended exercises include squeezing a ball, brushing the hair, shoulder shrugs and circles, and finger climbing up a wall when facing the wall (standing about 6 inches away) and turned perpendicular to the wall. All exercises should begin gently without the sensation of pain. Gentle stretching of muscles, but not strain, is encouraged. Reach to Recovery volunteers

---

COMPLICATIONS
Breast Cancer Disease and Treatment

Disease related	Treatment related
Local/regional recurrence	**Surgery**
Ulceration	Impaired wound healing/ seroma
Lymphedema	Nerve injury
Brachial plexopathy	Lymphedema
	Shoulder dysfunction
Distant recurrence	
Spinal cord compression	**Radiation therapy**
Brain/leptomeningeal me-	Skin reactions
tastases	Lymphedema
Hypercalcemia	Shoulder dysfunction
Pathologic fractures	Marrow suppression
Pleural effusion	Fatigue
Lymphangitic spread	
Pericardial effusion/	**Chemotherapy**
tamponade	Marrow suppression
Superior vena cava syn-	(bleeding/sepsis)
drome	Stomatitis
	Anorexia/nausea/vomiting
	Extravasation/skin necrosis
	Hemorrhagic cystitis

also provide exercise instruction. Referral to occupational therapy or physical therapy may be helpful if not initially involved in the exercise instruction.

- Instruct patient in avoidance of strenuous household tasks such as vacuuming, sweeping, moving or rearranging furniture, and lifting objects more than 10 pounds until full surgical wound healing has occurred and ROM is improved.
- Instruct patient in use of temporary prosthesis and wearing of bra and possible options for patient after mastectomy for a sense of symmetry and balance before being fitted for a weighted prosthesis or before reconstruction. (See box below for arm exercises after a lymph node dissection.)

Breast Reconstruction

Preoperative nursing care of the patient who is to undergo immediate or delayed reconstruction focuses on the woman's perceptions and expectations of the specific reconstructive approach chosen. Problems and dissatisfaction can be minimized if the woman has realistic expectations of the procedure. Important aspects to reinforce from the physician's discussions with the patient include the appearance of the reconstructed breast, the type of scar(s), the surgical dressing and wound suction, and the use of a bra. A preoperative or postoperative visit by a woman who has had a successful breast reconstruction can be beneficial. Postoperative care will be dictated by the type of reconstructive procedure performed. Patients receiving breast implants will need to be taught wound care and bandaging, often inclusive of some type of external pressure support, eventual massage of the implants, and a restricted exercise routine (no heavy lifting or stretching for 4 to 6 weeks). Patients undergoing myocutaneous flap reconstruction will have more wound and drain care needs (e.g., major abdominal surgery with the TRAM flap) in the hospital.[162] Attention to skin care is vital because mobility may be restricted in the immediate postoperative period. Further discharge teaching should include the specifics of exercise appropriate to the surgical procedure.

Lymphedema

Lymphedema after breast cancer surgery is the accumulation of lymph fluid in the tissues of the upper extremity, extending from the upper arm and potentially to the hand and fingers. It occurs in less than 6% to 7% of all patients undergoing modified radical mastectomy.[86] Risk of developing lymphedema is increased by complete lymph node dissection (levels I, II, and III), radiation therapy to the axilla, obesity, poor nutritional status, increased age, and wound infection.[24,86] It may occur at any time after surgery. It is caused by the interruption or removal of lymph channels and nodes after axillary node dissection or radiation therapy. These procedures result in less efficient filtration of lymph fluid and an impaired ability to fight infection. Prevention of cosmetic deformity, emotional distress,[230] functional impairment, infection, and discomfort are the goals. Nurses can teach the importance of reporting any swelling or red appearance of the affected arm. Intervention should be instituted as soon as lymphedema is noted so as to prevent or reduce the extent of further progression. This includes elevation of the arm, ROM exercises, not carrying heavy objects with the affected arm, and avoidance of skin breaks to the arm (e.g., venipunctures, harsh detergents).[24] Massage, or manual lymph drainage, and mechanical decompression with a pneumatic pump and arm sleeve are further interventions that may be indicated.[110] Once a reduction in the swelling has been achieved, the patient can be fitted for an elastic sleeve and gauntlet that provides gradient pressure to the upper extremity from the hand to the shoulder. With new onset of lymphedema, the medical assessment includes evaluation for infection and other obstructive problems (vein thrombosis or tumor recurrence).[86] The second box, p. 112, lists specific arm care precautions for all patients to prevent trauma and infection in the arm on the operative side.

ARM EXERCISES AFTER LYMPH NODE DISSECTION
(Goal: Return to Full Range of Motion)

REMEMBER: These exercises are to be done slowly, to stretch muscles *gently,* and to return you back to your normal movement. They are not intended to cause pain. However, your muscles in your arm and shoulder may be very tired, stiff, or achy. If you find that you have a lot of tightness or soreness after doing your exercises one day, take it a little easier the next day. Doing these regularly and faithfully is more important than pushing yourself too hard too fast. If you do not do your exercises, you may develop problems with movement that are very difficult to treat.

Do each *four times a day.*
Rest briefly between exercises. Take a slow, deep breath before starting again.
Don't forget to breathe while you are doing the exercises!
You can always use your other arm to assist your weaker arm.

1. Open and close the fingers of your hand on the side of your surgery (make a fist and then relax your fingers). Repeat as often as you like.

Continued.

ARM EXERCISES AFTER LYMPH NODE DISSECTION—cont'd
(Goal: Return to Full Range of Motion)

2. Sitting, crawl up and down your thigh with your fingers on the surgery side. This should be pretty easy. Repeat as often as you like.
3. Bend and extend your elbow with it down at your side. Repeat as often as you like.
4. With your arm extended down at your side, twist your hand/wrist/lower arm in and then out. Repeat three times.
5. Look in the mirror if you can, and shrug your shoulders. See if you are favoring the shoulder on the side of your surgery. Eventually you should be able to raise both shoulders together when you are fully recovered.
   Shrug your shoulders. Roll your shoulders forward. Relax your shoulders down. Stretch your shoulders back, like a soldier standing at attention. Repeat three times. You may try this in reverse (shoulders up, back, down, forward). You may try this in a rolling motion or circle up, back, down, forward.
6. On the side where you had your surgery, take that hand and put it on your shoulder, like you had a "wing." Draw small circles in the air with your elbow, forward or back. Repeat this three times.
7. Take the hand on the side of your surgery, and crawl up your opposite arm to your shoulder, over your head, and to your other shoulder. Go back the other way. If you get tired during this exercise, rest your hand on your head or shoulder. After a short pause you may be able to continue. If you feel discomfort or fatigue, use your "good" hand to help your weak arm down to your side.
8. Try to reach your hand on the surgery side behind your back at your waist. Bring it back around to the front.

After the drain tube(s) have been removed:

9. "Wall climbing": Always do a few warm-up exercises before you try these.
   a. *Facing the wall.* Face a wall and stand about a foot away from it. Using both hands for balance, crawl or slide with your fingers up the wall, going as far as you can without causing pain. Pause. Take a deep breath and notice how far you have climbed. Crawl or slide back down the wall. Rest a moment and repeat three times. *Caution:* If you get to the top of where you can go, DO NOT drop your arms down. Always remember to crawl or slide back down. Goal: To reach all the way up, flat against the wall. You should notice gradual improvement every day.
   b. *With your side facing the wall.* Stand about a foot away from a wall, and crawl or slide your fingers (on the surgery side) up the wall, going as far as you can without causing pain. Pause. Take a deep breath and notice how far you have climbed. Crawl or slide back down the wall. Rest a moment and repeat three times. *Caution:* If you get to the top of where you can go, DO NOT drop your arms down. Always remember to crawl or slide back down. Goal: To reach all the way up, flat against the wall. *This is the most difficult exercise and the most important.* You should notice gradual improvement every day.
10. With your hands behind your head, bring your elbows in toward your face, and then back. Repeat this three times.
11. Laying down on a flat surface, bring your arm on the surgery side straight up from your side, and reach over your head. Return your arm to your side.

Swimming is a very good exercise to help your recovery. However, you should be able to do this exercise without much difficulty before you get into a pool. Check with your doctor about when you can begin this exercise.

Lifting anything over 10 pounds or vigorous and repeated movement that exerts strain on your arm should not be done until you have fully recovered from your surgery (4-6 weeks). This includes weight training. Ask your doctor about your recovery and if you want to know about beginning or returning to weight training.

If you notice any new swelling or redness in your arm on the side of your surgery and it lasts more than 24 hours, please contact the nurse or doctor's office.

*NOTE: Confirm with your physician before initiaing these exercises.

Data from Harbour UCLA Medical Center, Los Angeles.

ARM CARE PRECAUTIONS AFTER AXILLARY LYMPH NODE DISSECTION

Avoid sunburns or heavy sun exposure (and wear sunscreen).

Avoid burns while cooking, baking, or smoking.

Wear protective gloves when gardening.

Use the *unaffected* arm for injections, blood samples, intravenous access, or blood pressure readings.

Use thimble when sewing.

Watches, jewelry, and clothing should fit loosely on the arm and hand.

Use creams and lotions to keep cuticles soft; do not pull cuticles.

Treat cuts promptly and monitor for signs of infection.

No chemotherapy is to be given in the affected arm.

NURSING MANAGEMENT

ADJUVANT TREATMENT PHASE

During this period, patients will need continued reinforcement of exercise routines so as to regain full shoulder function. Wound healing will be completed and final pathology reports discussed. Patients face new decisions about adjuvant chemotherapy and/or hormonal therapy, and additional information needs to be clarified. Making a decision about treatment that potentially has side effects when one feels well is not easy. The discussion earlier in this chapter regarding facilitating a patient in decision making is applicable here.[140,195,203] Patients undergoing breast-conserving surgery will generally be receiving radiation therapy. Others will be receiving chemotherapy or hormonal therapy with tamoxifen.

The transition to this therapy phase and its completion constitute another important intervention period for nurses.[34,162] Sociocultural and psychosocial factors continue to be important throughout a physical treatment phase.[2,203] The impact of the diagnosis and treatment may be felt more fully during this time not only by the patient but also by her spouse/significant other and family members. The patient and her family may face new challenges to work and role relationships and to functioning. Loveys and Klaich[147] described "demands of illness" in a study of women after the diagnosis of cancer. Treatment issues, social interaction or support, change in life context or perspective, and acceptance of the illness were the most frequently identified concerns, although reconstructing the self, physical changes, uncertainty, financial or occupational concerns, loss, making comparisons, acquiring new knowledge, making choices, mortality issues, and making a contribution were also expressed as concerns. Interventions during this time are directed toward reducing the psychologic and physiologic distress these women experience.

Possible nursing diagnoses during this period include (1) risk for injury, infection, stomatitis, or bleeding secondary to chemotherapy, or impaired skin integrity related to radiation therapy[59,129,162,203]; (2) fatigue related to radiation and/or chemotherapy treatments and limiting energy and usual exercise routine[20]; (3) pain, hot flashes, decreased/absent vaginal secretions related to chemotherapy-induced or hormone therapy–induced ovarian suppression; (4) body image disturbance related to altered body image secondary to surgery, alopecia, weight gain or loss; (5) altered role performance related to disruption in life and work patterns secondary to treatments; (6) knowledge deficit related to chemotherapy side effects; and (7) anxiety related to completion of adjuvant therapy and transition to regular follow-up period.

NURSING DIAGNOSIS

- *Anxiety related to fear of side effects of additional treatment with chemotherapy and/or radiation therapy and to impact on resumption of usual activities in social and family life*

OUTCOME GOAL

Patient will be able to:
- Complete adjuvant therapy as close to schedule as possible with successful management of side effects and changes in role or daily activities.

INTERVENTIONS

- Explain rationale for adjuvant systemic therapy.
- Promote participation in breast cancer treatment clinical trials as appropriate.
- Describe specific treatment regimen schedule, route(s) of administration, anticipated side effects, and prevention or management of side effects.
- For premenopausal women, discuss effects of chemotherapy on menstrual function: irregularities, amenorrhea, and potential for pregnancy, with options for birth control while undergoing treatment.
- Provide postmenopausal women or premenopausal women undergoing tamoxifen therapy with information about potential side effects such as hot flashes and vaginal discharge and dryness. Tell patients to report such symptoms and provide subsequent guidance on the management of these problems.
- Emphasize and monitor compliance with the proposed treatment regimen.
- Monitor for potential side effects of treatment and intervene appropriately.
- Monitor for potential shoulder dysfunction secondary to a decrease in exercises. Also, assess involvement in other exercise activities.[249] Weight gain is a common problem during standard adjuvant chemotherapy.[50]
- Assist patient and her significant other in identifying real or imagined barriers that may influence resumption of normal sexual relations.
- Assist patient in locating resources for support, such as specifically targeted breast cancer patient support groups,[35,62,205,223] resources for fitting for a breast prosthesis, or other programs in the community. The Women in Nature program described by Johnson and Kelly[118] incorporates outdoor activities in the wilderness, exercise, and keeping a journal for women diagnosed with cancer. The benefits of exercise alone have also been described.[249]
- Encourage discussion of other psychosocial concerns, such as role functions in the home, return to work, vocational retraining, and family and social relationships.

Continued.

Patients may need assistance in identifying their emotional strengths, sources of support, and positive qualities separate from their appearance at a time when they are feeling vulnerable, threatened, and undesirable. Facilitating open communication between the patient and her significant other can be very helpful in the couple's adjustment to the cancer diagnosis and treatment. Referral to appropriate resources may be indicated.[37,80]

- For other specific interventions for patients undergoing radiation therapy and chemotherapy, see Chapters 21 and 22, respectively.

RECOVERY, REHABILITATION, AND LONG-TERM FOLLOW-UP PHASE

During this period, the patient is adjusting to the completion of chemotherapy and/or radiation therapy and may still be receiving tamoxifen therapy. The patient often has feelings of loss and anxiety associated with stopping adjuvant therapy or the fear that stopping such therapy may somehow allow the cancer to return. The patient, now free from regular frequent medical visits and perhaps beginning to feel more physically well again, faces a potential return to more usual patterns of living. The majority of breast cancer survivors who were employed before the diagnosis of cancer return to work.[37] It is usually not without some difficulty, however, including concerns about how co-workers will respond to her and about her own ability to withstand work pressures or physically being able to work the same schedule or type of work.[37] Loss of a job and loss of insurance benefits are of even greater concern in the 1990s. Job discrimination is also a real fear for those seeking employment.[37,42] Although discrimination against disabled persons is prohibited by The Federal Rehabilitation Act of 1973 and the Americans with Disabilities Act of 1990, some courts have decided that recovered cancer patients are not disabled (see Chapter 31). The California state law regarding handicapped and disabled persons specifically includes cancer patients.[80] However, discrimination is not always so obvious. *Reintegration* describes the process of assisting women with a history of breast cancer to return to work through a program with their employers and organizations that is directed to understanding the needs of each and how to work together.[37] Women who find that new employment is necessary may find help in vocational rehabilitation, often available through state or private industry programs.

After standard adjuvant chemotherapy is completed, premenopausal women often will resume menstrual function. The question of pregnancy after breast cancer has been well noted in recent literature.[47,96] Most studies of women who became pregnant after successful treatment of breast cancer have found that pregnancy did not negatively influence survival. The greatest risk for recurrence of breast cancer is in the first 2 years, so one suggestion has been to delay pregnancy until after that time.[47] Issues related to quality of life for a woman and her partner considering this decision may include exploring the desire for children, discussing the risk of recurrence and implications of single parenthood for the surviving parent, determining the support available from the extended social network, and exploring sociodemographic factors.[55,96] The issue of pregnancy after breast cancer, with more women delaying childbirth, is likely to remain an integral aspect of the nursing care of premenopausal women with breast cancer.

NURSING DIAGNOSIS

- *Social interaction, impaired*

OUTCOME GOAL

Patient will be able to:
- Effectively resume, reestablish, or begin anew personal and social relationships that are meaningful and rewarding and integrate the concept of survivorship.

INTERVENTIONS

- Assist patient to verbalize fears and concerns.
- Provide supportive information regarding those concerns and to ease fears, as appropriate, such as plans for continued medical follow-up, positive appraisal of her strengths, and services for vocational rehabilitation.
- Encourage and facilitate discussion with appropriate medical resources for pregnancy planning.
- Encourage participation in survivorship activities or group support, if desired.
- Encourage patient and/or family to resume participation in activities previously enjoyed.

RECURRENCE, METASTASIS, AND TERMINAL PHASE[44,142,229]

Fortunately, many women diagnosed with breast cancer today will not die from their disease. For those who face a recurrence, however, the experience may be much more traumatic than the initial diagnosis.[152,158] Local recurrences are often managed with local treatments, such as surgical resection or radiation therapy. For the woman experiencing a local recurrence after breast-conserving surgery, mastectomy may be recommended. Nursing care in such circumstances has been addressed previously.

The patient with metastatic recurrence (or disease at diagnosis) may exhibit physical signs or symptoms such as bone pain, hypercalcemia, dyspnea, or fatigue, or the recurrence may be suspected before symptoms present (e.g., elevated liver function tests, abnormal bone scan). This is a time when there is recognition that the previous treatment failed to control the disease completely. Coping strategies that worked will in the past may be stressed during this time. There is much uncertainty and anticipation of loss. The sense of hope may be challenged. It is a time when information about the next plan of action can give hope and direction. Many agents have demonstrated effectiveness against breast cancer, and although cure is no longer possible, palliation of symptoms and prolonged control of the disease are reasonable and worthwhile goals.

NURSING DIAGNOSIS

- *Grieving, anticipatory related to possible losses, including death*

OUTCOME GOALS

Patient will be able to:
- Effectively grieve the loss of the concept of cure and feel supported in resuming therapy, if indicated.
- Experience satisfactory control of side effects and complications of treatment.
- Come to some degree of acceptance of death in the terminal phase (see Chapter 31).

INTERVENTIONS

- Provide support when patient is informed of diagnosis and treatment plan.
- Explain rationale for treatments and side effects to anticipate and their management.
- Encourage patient and her significant other(s) to discuss openly their concerns. When conventional treatment fails or is difficult, unproven therapies often are sought; being able to discuss this with the health care team can help prevent complications (see Chapter 25).
- Assist patient and family to manage symptoms or complications of disease and/or treatment, such as pain and hypercalcemia.[10,164]
- Assess coping and support needs of patient and family. Assist patient and family in the terminal phase to verbalize feelings about the meaning of illness and death.
- Referrals to supportive resources may be indicated, such as home nursing care and hospice programs, support groups, pastoral care, and professional counselors for therapeutic intervention.

FOLLOW-UP

All patients with breast cancer require periodic follow-up evaluations for the remainder of their life. These evaluations are performed to monitor for recurrent disease and complications of treatment (see box, p. 110). Long-term effects of adjuvant chemotherapy, stem cell or bone marrow transplant, or other therapies are not fully known.[25,224] Regular evaluations also allow opportunity to assess the patient's level of coping and that of her husband/significant other and family.

Because the risk for recurrence is highest during the

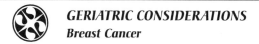

GERIATRIC CONSIDERATIONS
Breast Cancer

Prevention and detection*

Health assessments need to incorporate cognitive function, physical limitations/sensory deficits, and support network.

Education efforts should address knowledge, skill, and confidence in BSE, mammography and CBE, and benefits of early detection.

Continuity and participation may be enhanced when health care is coordinated by one or few providers (e.g., advocate, case manager).

Community-based breast cancer screening is beneficial.

Effectiveness of rescreening after age 70 is controversial.

Education of health care providers should emphasize continuing need for scheduled screening of elderly women in light of current data.

Diagnosis and treatment[19,70,178,227]

Importance of patient involvement in decision-making needs to be considered regardless of age.

Age alone should not determine type or extent of surgery or subsequent therapy.

Care throughout the operative phase includes careful preoperative assessment and intraoperative and postoperative physiologic monitoring.

Early *comprehensive discharge planning* should involve patient and significant other.

Side effects with radiation and chemotherapy may be enhanced or prolonged.

Most trials of systemic therapy have excluded women over 70 years of age.

Rehabilitation[61,77]

Return to or maintenance of precancer level of functioning is a reasonable goal.

Care should be taken to incorporate psychosexual assessment and intervention as appropriate for all ages.

Physical illness can impair developmental task completion.

Depression in elderly women may be masked by physical symptoms.

Metastatic disease[61]

Differential diagnosis of symptoms must differentiate normal or pathologic changes of aging from signs of metastatic disease.

Chronic pain may be indirectly expressed through other physical changes (e.g., anorexia, irritability, aching, insomnia).

Recurrent disease may exacerbate other felt losses of elderly women.

---

*References 40, 43, 49, 72, 148, 149, 151, 170, 190, 227, 241.

Continued.

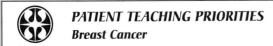

PATIENT TEACHING PRIORITIES
Breast Cancer

Prevention and early detection

Risk factors
Breast self-examination
Clinical breast examination
Mammography
Signs and symptoms to report to health care professional
(e.g., mass in breast or axilla; dimpling, puckering,
and/or scaly skin; spontaneous, persistent nipple
discharge)
Follow ACS guidelines for health care examination
Plan of action (appointments, who to call)

Treatment options

Biopsy procedures
Surgery
   Breast-conserving treatment
   Breast reconstruction
Radiation therapy
Chemotherapy
Hormonal therapy
Clinical trials

Disease-related and treatment-related complications

Disease recurrence, infection, impaired wound healing,
lymphedema, shoulder dysfunction, marrow
suppression, alopecia, stomatitis, hemorrhagic cystitis,
weight gain, "flare reaction," pain, anorexia

Other

Prosthesis options
Support groups
Recovery and long-term follow-up

first 2 years after diagnosis, physical assessments are recommended every 3 months for the first 2 to 3 years, biannually for the next 2 to 3 years, and then annually.[97] Serum chemistry tests are usually obtained at each evaluation, mammograms are done yearly, and chest x-ray films and bone scans may be done annually or as indicated.[97] Any signs or symptoms the patient has at the time of each evaluation will influence what additional tests or imaging studies are ordered or their frequency.

Northouse[180] reported that difficulties in psychosocial adjustment to breast cancer are not confined to the early phase of the illness but persist over time for both patients and husbands. Fear of disease recurrence, role adjustment problems, resource depletion, toxicities of therapy, and changes in body image, self-esteem, and patterns of sexuality are problems the patient and to some extent the husband/significant other may encounter. Cancer affects families, and children also may need support.[114] Emotional problems may require referrals to trained counselors or support groups available through the ACS, local hospitals, or community.

Husbands/significant others should be encouraged to come to the follow-up evaluations with the patients. This allows them to be included in the discussion regarding concerns and problems they are experiencing individually and as a couple. Special consideration also needs to be given to the elderly woman, who may have a limited social support network (see box, p. 115).

In addition to regular evaluations by a health professional, women must be encouraged to begin or continue monthly BSE and regular mammograms. It is also important to identify high-risk family members, to whom appropriate screening recommendations can be provided.

The box on left summarizes patient teaching priorities for the patient with breast cancer.

particular concern in the near future with the aging female population. Early detection outreach to socio-economically disadvantaged women will also be a focus of breast cancer control efforts, with potential for significant benefit in reducing the number of deaths from breast cancer. Nurses have a pivotal role in all these areas.

■ CHAPTER QUESTIONS

1. Which of the following statements about risk factors for breast cancer is *most* true?
   a. Dietary factors account for the greatest percentage of risk.
   b. Most cases of breast cancer can be attributed to family history and genetics.
   c. The primary risk factor for developing breast cancer is being female.
   d. A severe bump or blow to the breast can predispose someone to breast cancer.

2. *Relative risk* is a term that refers to which of the following?
   a. Average risk for every woman in a given population, such as in the United States (e.g., this is reported as one in eight)
   b. Risk to relatives of a woman who has been diagnosed with breast cancer
   c. Number of cancer cases in a population associated with given risk factors that could be prevented
   d. Incidence rate of breast cancer in a population of women with some risk factor, divided by the incidence rate of breast cancer in a population of women without that risk factor (e.g., this is reported in values of 1.0, 2.0, 3.0)

3. Which of the following environmental influences has *clearly* been associated with potentially increasing one's risk for breast cancer?
   a. Alcohol
   b. Obesity and dietary fat intake
   c. Electromagnetic fields
   d. Stress

4. A 51-year-old asymptomatic woman who is concerned about follow-up since she has breast implants would like to formulate a plan of breast health care. As a member of the health care team, besides teaching breast self-examination (BSE) technique, how would the nurse best advise her?
   a. Clinical breast examination (CBE) on a regular basis, annual mammography, and monthly BSE are her keys to early detection.
   b. CBE on an annual basis, mammography every 1 to 2 years, and monthly BSE would be recommended, but she should review this plan with her physician.
   c. Monthly BSE is difficult to perform and is not necessary if she has regular CBEs and annual mammography.
   d. Monthly BSE, annual CBE, and annual mammography by an accredited facility will help identify any changes promptly.

5. A 33-year-old patient recently diagnosed with invasive breast cancer has just met with the surgeon to learn about her surgical treatment options and wants to know more about breast-conserving surgery and radiation. How would the nurse best approach the patient?
   a. Determine the patient's specific questions before addressing aspects of the surgical routines, recovery, the treatments, and self-care management.
   b. Advise her about side effects of the radiation and self-care management strategies.
   c. Share experiences of other patients and ask if she has further questions.
   d. Arrange for an appointment with the radiation oncologist and a tour of the radiation therapy unit.

6. Which of the following *best* describes the purpose of giving standard adjuvant chemotherapy to women with invasive breast cancer?
   a. It is a systemic form of cancer treatment given to treat micrometastases after surgical removal of the primary site of cancer for certain high-risk women.
   b. It is a systemic form of cancer treatment given in conjunction with other treatments to enhance their effect.
   c. It is a systemic form of cancer treatment given to treat micrometastases after surgical removal of the primary site of cancer for certain high-risk women based on data from clinical trials.
   d. It is a systemic form of cancer treatment given to treat micrometastases before any other treatment.

7. A 63-year-old woman with metastatic breast cancer has recently started receiving tamoxifen. She calls the nurse at her physician's office with the complaint of aching all over and increased pain at her sites of bony metastases. What is the most likely explanation for her experience?
   a. Progressive disease
   b. "Flare reaction" to endocrine therapy
   c. An infection
   d. Fever

8. A patient who has just undergone a modified radical mastectomy returns to the clinic for a postoperative evaluation. She is dressed in oversized loose clothing and is accompanied by her husband. She expresses that he has taken very good care of her and emptied her drain tubes for her. In addition, she offers that neither he nor she has looked at her wound or the dressing covering it. After being escorted into an examination room, her husband seeks out the nurse to express concern about his wife's behavior, his desire to help her, and her refusal to let him see her wound. Which approach might the nurse use to *best* help the husband and patient?
   a. Offer to sit with them as a couple to talk over their concerns jointly.
   b. Suggest a referral to a counselor, therapist, or support group where other couples have received help.
   c. Explore the patient's experience of her surgery and recovery and whether she has viewed the mastectomy site over the dressing. Be present when the dressing is removed to assist her in viewing the site, and/or be present to have her husband do so with her.
   d. Explore the patient's experience of her surgery and re-

covery, offer to be present when the drain is removed, and place a referral to a support resource.

9. For the elderly woman, which of the following does *not* accurately reflect barriers to breast health care?
   a. Social isolation and low income may decrease participation in health care programs.
   b. Sensory changes of aging may delay identification of symptoms or decrease touch sensitivity in BSE.
   c. Physical symptoms may mask underlying depression and associated low motivation for self-care.
   d. Screening and breast cancer treatments are not effective after age 70.

10. A 41-year-old woman who was successfully treated for breast cancer a year ago reports to the nurse on her regular clinical follow-up that she is experiencing increasing stress at her work and frequently is in conflict with her husband and children. She has had new aches and pains that frighten her, but the physician said she was doing well. Her menstrual cycle has never returned after chemotherapy, but she has had no symptoms of menopause. The nurse could *best* help this patient by doing which of the following?
   a. Acknowledge her concerns and allow her to explore them further.
   b. Tell her this is a normal consequence of cancer treatment.
   c. Suggest she seek consultation with a gynecologist.
   d. Advise her to bring her husband and together talk further with her physician.

BIBLIOGRAPHY

1. Alagna SW, Reddy DM: Predictors of proficient technique in successful lesion detection in self breast examination, *Health Psychol* 3:113, 1984.
2. Ali NS, Khalil HZ: Identification of stressors, level of stress, coping strategies, and coping effectiveness among Egyptian mastectomy patients, *Cancer Nurs* 14:232, 1991.
3. American Cancer Society: *Special report on cancer in the economically disadvantaged,* New York, 1986, The Society.
4. American Cancer Society: *Clinical breast examination: proficiency criteria and guidelines,* Oakland, Calif, 1988, The Society, California Division.
5. American Cancer Society: 1989 survey of physicians' attitudes and practices in early cancer detection, *CA Cancer J Clin* 40:77, 1990.
6. American Cancer Society: *Special touch breast health trainer's guide,* ed 2, Oakland, Calif, 1990, The Society, California Division.
7. American Cancer Society: *Cancer facts and figures—1995,* Atlanta, 1995, The Society.
8. American Cancer Society: *Breast cancer facts and figures—1996,* Atlanta, 1996, The Society.
9. American Joint Committee on Cancer: *Manual for staging of cancer,* ed 4, Philadelphia, 1993, Lippincott.
10. Arathuzik D: Pain experience for metastatic breast cancer patients: unraveling the mystery, *Cancer Nurs* 14:41, 1991.
11. Assaf AR and others: Comparison of three methods of teaching women how to perform breast self-examination, *Health Educ Q* 12:259, 1985.
12. Ayanian JZ and others: The relation between health insurance coverage and clinical outcomes among women with breast cancer, *N Engl J Med* 329:326, 1993.
13. Baines CJ: Breast self-examination, *Cancer* 69:1942, 1992.
14. Baquet CR and others: Socioeconomic factors and cancer incidence among blacks and whites, *J Natl Cancer Inst* 83:551, 1991.
15. Bassett LW: Mammographic features of malignancy. In Mitchell GW, Bassett LW, editors: *The female breast and its disorders,* Baltimore, 1990, Williams & Wilkins.
16. Bassett LW, Gold RH: Introduction to mammography. In Mitchell GW, Bassett LW, editors: *The female breast and its disorders,* Baltimore, 1990, Williams & Wilkins.
17. Benedict S, Williams RD, Baron PL: The effect of benign breast biopsy on subsequent breast cancer detection practices, *Oncol Nurs Forum* 21:1467, 1994.
18. Bilimoria MM, Morrow M: The woman at increased risk for breast cancer: evaluation and management strategies, *CA Cancer J Clin* 45:263, 1995.
19. Blesch KS: The normal physiological changes of aging and their impact on the response to cancer treatment, *Semin Oncol Nurs* 4:178, 1988.
20. Blesch KS and others: Correlates of fatigue in people with breast or lung cancer, *Oncol Nurs Forum* 18:81, 1991.
21. Boice JD Jr, Monson RR: Breast cancer in women after repeated fluoroscopic examinations of the chest, *J Natl Cancer Inst* 59:823, 1977.
22. Boring CC: Cancer statistics for African Americans, *CA Cancer J Clin* 42:7, 1992.
23. Bostwick J III: Breast reconstruction following mastectomy, *CA Cancer J Clin* 45:289-304, 1995.
24. Brown M, Eyles H, Bland KI: Nursing care for the patient with breast cancer. In Bland KI, Copeland EM III, editors: *The breast: comprehensive management of benign and malignant diseases,* Philadelphia, 1991, Saunders.
25. Buchsel PC, Kapustay PM: Peripheral stem cell transplantation. In Hubbard SM, Goodman M, Knobf MT: *Oncology nursing: patient treatment and support,* Philadelphia, 1995, Lippincott.
26. Burack RC, Liang J: The acceptance and completion of mammography by older black women, *Am J Public Health* 79:721, 1989.
27. Burns JM and others: Critical pathway for administering high-dose chemotherapy followed by peripheral blood stem cell rescue in the outpatient setting, *Oncol Nurs Forum* 22:1219, 1995.
28. Callahan R and others: Somatic mutations and human breast cancer, *Cancer* 69:1582, 1992.
29. Castiglione-Gertsch M, Gelber RD, Goldhirsch A: Adjuvant systemic therapy: the issues of timing and sequence, *Recent Results Cancer Res* 140:201, 1996.
30. Cawley M, Kostic J, Cappello C: Informational and psychosocial needs of women choosing conservative surgery/primary radiation for early stage breast cancer, *Cancer Nurs* 13:90, 1990.
31. Champion VL: Attitudinal variables related to intention, frequency and proficiency of breast self-examination in women 35 and older, *Res Nurs Health* 11:283, 1988.
32. Champion VL: The relationship of selected variables to breast cancer detection behaviors in women 35 and older, *Oncol Nurs Forum* 18:733, 1991.

33. Chlebowski RT: Dietary fat intake reduction for patients with resected breast cancer, *Adv Exp Med Biol* 364:11, 1994.

34. Chou A: Breast health nursing. In Gross A, Itto D, editors: *Women talk about breast surgery,* New York, 1990, Clarkson Potter.

35. Christ GH and others: Educational and support programs for breast cancer patients and their families. In Harris JR and others, editors: *Breast diseases,* ed 2, Philadelphia, 1991, Lippincott.

36. Christian MC and others: The National Cancer Institute audit of the National Surgical Adjuvant Breast and Bowel Project protocol B-06, *N Engl J Med* 333:1469, 1995.

37. Clark JC, Landis LL: Reintegration and maintenance of employees with breast cancer in the workplace, *Am Assoc Occup Health Nurses* 37:186, 1989.

38. Coleman EA: Practice and effectiveness of breast self examination: a selective review of the literature (1977-1989), *J Cancer Educ* 6:83, 1991.

39. Coleman EA, Pennypacker H: Measuring breast self-examination proficiency, *Cancer Nurs* 14:211, 1991.

40. Coleman EA and others: Efficacy of breast self-examination teaching methods among older women, *Oncol Nurs Forum* 18:561, 1991.

41. Collins-Hattery AM, Blumberg BD: S phase index and ploidy prognostic markers in node negative breast cancer: information for nurses, *Oncol Nurs Forum* 18:59, 1991.

42. Cooley ME, Erikson B: Rehabilitation. In Fowble B and others, editors: *Breast cancer treatment: a comprehensive guide to management,* St Louis, 1991, Mosby.

43. Costanza ME: Breast cancer screening in older women: synopsis of a forum, *Cancer* 69:1925, 1992.

44. Coward DD: Self-transcendence and emotional well-being in women with advanced breast cancer, *Oncol Nurs Forum* 18:857, 1991.

45. Curtis RE and others: Risk of leukemia after chemotherapy and radiation treatment for breast cancer, *N Engl J Med* 326:1745, 1992.

46. Daly MB: New perspectives in breast cancer: the genetic revolution, *Oncol Nurs* 1:1, 1994.

47. Danforth DN: How subsequent pregnancy affects outcome in women with a prior breast cancer, *Oncology* 5:23, 1991.

48. Dawson I and others: Effect of shoulder immobilization on wound seroma and shoulder dysfunction following modified radical mastectomy: a randomized prospective clinical trial, *Br J Surg* 76:311, 1989.

49. Dellefield ME: Informational needs and approaches for early cancer detection in the elderly, *Semin Oncol Nurs* 4:156, 1988.

50. Demark-Wahnefried W, Winer EP, Rimer BK: Why women gain weight with adjuvant chemotherapy for breast cancer, *J Clin Oncol* 11:1418, 1993.

51. Dietrick-Gallagher M, Hyzinski MM: Teaching patients to care for drains after breast surgery for malignancy, *Oncol Nurs Forum* 16:263, 1989.

52. Dodd GD: American Cancer Society Guidelines on screening for breast cancer, *Cancer* 69(suppl):1885, 1992.

53. Donegan WL: Cancer of the breast in men, *CA Cancer J Clin* 41:339, 1991.

54. Dorsay RH and others: Breast self-examination: improving competence and frequency in a classroom setting, *Am J Public Health* 78:520, 1988.

55. Dow KH and others: Pregnancy after breast-conserving surgery and radiation therapy for breast cancer, *Monogr Natl Cancer Inst* 16:131, 1994.

56. Dupont WD, Page DL: Risk factors for breast cancer in women with proliferative breast disease, *N Engl J Med* 312:146, 1985.

57. Early Breast Cancer Trialists' Collaborative Group: Effects of radiotherapy and surgery in early breast cancer: an overview of the randomized trials, *N Engl J Med* 333:1444, 1995.

58. Early Breast Cancer Trialists' Collaborative Group: Systemic treatment of early breast cancer by hormonal, cytotoxic, or immune therapy, *Lancet* 339:1, 1995.

59. Ehlke G: Symptom distress in breast cancer patients receiving chemotherapy in the outpatient setting, *Oncol Nurs Forum* 15:343, 1988.

60. Eley JW and others: Racial differences in survival from breast cancer: results of the National Cancer Institute Black/White Cancer Survival Study, *JAMA* 272:947, 1994.

61. Engelking C: Comfort issues in geriatric oncology, *Semin Oncol Nurs* 4:198, 1988.

62. Fawzy FI, Fawzy NW: A structured psychoeducational intervention for cancer patients, *Gen Hosp Psychiatry* 16:149, 1994.

63. Feather BL, Wainstock JM: Perceptions of postmastectomy patients. Part I, *Cancer Nurs* 12:293, 1989.

64. Feather BL, Wainstock JM: Perceptions of postmastectomy patients. Part II, *Cancer Nurs* 12:301, 1989.

65. Feig SA: Decreased breast cancer mortality through mammography screening: results of clinical trials, *Radiology* 167:659, 1988.

66. Fisher B and others: Reanalysis and results after 12 years of follow-up in a randomized clinical trial comparing total mastectomy with lumpectomy with or without irradiation in the treatment of breast cancer, *N Engl J Med* 333:1456, 1995.

67. Fletcher SW, O'Malley MS, Bunce LA: Physician's abilities to detect lumps in silicone breast models, *JAMA* 253:2224, 1985.

68. Fletcher SW and others: How best to teach women breast self-examination: a randomized controlled trial, *Ann Intern Med* 112:772, 1990.

69. Forbes JF: Screening for breast cancer and treatment of early lesions (ductal carcinoma in situ): summary, *Recent Results Cancer Res* 140:155, 1996.

70. Forrest APM: Primary breast cancer in older women. In Balducci L, Lyman GH, Ershler WB, editors: *Geriatric oncology,* Philadelphia, 1992, Lippincott.

71. Foster RS and others: Breast self examination practices and breast cancer stage, *N Engl J Med* 299:265, 1978.

72. Fox SA, Murata PJ, Stein JA: The impact of physician compliance on screening mammography for older women, *Arch Intern Med* 151:50, 1991.

73. Freeman HP: Cancer in the socioeconomically disadvantaged, *CA Cancer J Clin* 39:266, 1989.

74. Friedell GH: The 'squeakywheel' and health care policy *JAMA* 265:3300, 1991 (commentary).

75. Frykberg ER, Ames FC, Bland KI: Current concepts for management of early (*in situ* and occult invasive) breast carcinoma. In Bland KI, Copeland EM III, editors: *The breast: comprehensive management of benign and malignant diseases,* Philadelphia, 1991, Saunders.

76. Fulton JP, Rakowski W, Jones AC: Determinants of breast cancer screening among inner-city Hispanic women in comparison with other inner-city women, *Public Health Rep* 110:476.

77. Ganz PA: Breast cancer in older women: quality-of-life considerations, *Cancer Control J Moffitt Cancer Ctr* 1:372, 1994.

78. Ganz PA and others: Breast conservation *versus* mastectomy, *Cancer* 69:1729, 1992.

79. Garber JE and others: Management of high-risk groups. In Harris JR and others, editors: *Breast diseases,* ed 2, Philadelphia, 1991, Lippincott.

80. Gaskin TA and others: Rehabilitation. In Bland KI, Copeland EM III, editors: *The breast: comprehensive management of benign and malignant diseases,* Philadelphia, 1991, Saunders.

81. Giomuso CB, Suster V: Free flap breast reconstruction, *Medsurg Nurs* 3:9, 1994.

82. Glick JH: Meeting highlights: adjuvant therapy for primary breast cancer, *J Natl Cancer Inst* 84:1476, 1992.

83. Goldhirsch A and others: Meeting highlights: International Consensus Panel on the Treatment of Primary Breast Cancer, *J Natl Cancer Inst* 87:1441, 1995.

84. Gonzalez JT: Factors relating to frequency of breast self-examination among low-income Mexican American women: implications for nursing practice, *Cancer Nurs* 13:134, 1990.

85. Goodman M: Adjuvant systemic therapy of stage I and II breast cancer, *Semin Oncol Nurs* 7:175, 1991.

86. Gottlieb LJ, Patel P-KK: Lymphedema following axillary surgery: elephantiasis chirurgica. In Harris JR and others, editors: *Breast diseases,* ed 2, Philadelphia, 1991, Lippincott.

87. Gray ME: Factors related to practice of breast self-examination in rural women, *Cancer Nurs* 13:100, 1990.

88. Greenwald P and others: Estimated effect of breast self-examination and routine physician examination on breast cancer mortality, *N Engl J Med* 299:271, 1978.

89. Greenwald P, Sondik EJ: Cancer control objectives for the nation 1985-2000, *Natl Cancer Inst Monogr* 2, 1986.

90. Gutman H and others: Achievements of physical therapy in patients after modified radical mastectomy compared with quadrantectomy, axillary dissection, and radiation for carcinoma of the breast, *Arch Surg* 125:389, 1990.

91. Hand R and others: Hospital variables associated with quality of care for breast cancer patients, *JAMA* 266:3429, 1991.

92. Harris JR: Clinical management of ductal carcinoma in situ. In Harris JR and others, editors: *Breast diseases,* ed 2, Philadelphia, 1991, Lippincott.

93. Harris JR: Postmastectomy radiotherapy. In Harris JR and others, editors: *Breast diseases,* ed 2, Philadelphia, 1991, Lippincott.

94. Harris JR: Staging of breast carcinoma. In Harris JR and others, editors: *Breast diseases,* ed 2, Philadelphia, 1991, Lippincott.

95. Harris JR, Hellman S: Natural history of breast cancer. In Harris JR and others, editors: *Breast diseases,* ed 2, Philadelphia, 1991, Lippincott.

96. Hassey KM: Pregnancy and parenthood after treatment for breast cancer, *Oncol Nurs Forum* 15:439, 1988.

97. Hayes DF: Serum (circulating) tumor markers for breast cancer, *Recent Results Cancer Res* 140:101, 1996.

98. Henderson BE, Bernstein L: The role of endogenous and exogenous hormones in the etiology of breast cancer. In Harris JR and others, editors: *Breast diseases,* ed 2, Philadelphia, 1991, Lippincott.

99. Henderson IC: Breast cancer. In Murphy GP and others: *American Cancer Society textbook of clinical oncology,* ed 2, Atlanta, 1995, American Cancer Society.

100. Henderson IC: Chemotherapy for metastatic disease. In Harris JR and others, editors: *Breast diseases,* ed 2, Philadelphia, 1991, Lippincott.

101. Henderson IC: Prognostic factors. In Harris JR and others, editors: *Breast diseases,* ed 2, Philadelphia, 1991, Lippincott.

102. Henderson IC, Harris JR: Integration of local and systemic therapies. In Harris JR and others, editors: *Breast diseases,* ed 2, Philadelphia, 1991, Lippincott.

103. Hicks JE: Exercise for cancer patients. In Basmajian JV, Wolf SL, editors: *Therapeutic exercise,* ed 5, Baltimore, 1990, Williams & Wilkins.

104. Hladiuk M and others: Arm function after axillary dissection for breast cancer: a pilot study to provide parameter estimates, *J Surg Oncol* 50:47, 1992.

105. Houn F, Brown ML: Current practice of screening mammography in the United States: data from the National Survey of Mammography Facilities, *Radiology* 190:209, 1994.

106. Houts PS and others: Using a state cancer registry to increase screening behaviors of sisters and daughters of breast cancer patients, *Am J Public Health* 81:386, 1991.

107. Howard J: Using mammography for cancer control: an unrealized potential, *CA Cancer J Clin* 37:33, 1987.

108. Hrushesky WJM: Menstrual cycle timing of breast cancer resection, *Recent Results Cancer Res* 140:27, 1996.

109. Huguley CM Jr and others: Breast self-examination and survival from breast cancer, *Cancer* 62:1389, 1988.

110. Humble CA: Lymphedema: incidence, pathophysiology, management, and nursing care, *Oncol Nurs Forum* 22:1503, 1995.

111. Hutter RVP: The role of the pathologist in the management of breast cancer, *CA Cancer J Clin* 41:283, 1991.

112. Ingram D and others: Obesity and breast disease: the role of the female sex hormones, *Cancer* 64:1049, 1989.

113. Institute of Medicine, Committee on the Relationship Between Oral Contraceptives and Breast Cancer, Division of Health Promotion and Disease Prevention: *Oral contraceptives and breast cancer,* Washington, DC, 1991, National Academy Press.

114. Issel LM, Ersek M, Lewis FM: How children cope with mother's breast cancer, *Oncol Nurs Forum* 17(S):5, 1990.

115. Jacob TC, Penn NE, Brown M: Breast self-examination: knowledge, attitudes, and performance among black women, *J Natl Med Assoc* 81:769, 1989.

116. Jansen RFM and others: Immediate versus delayed shoulder exercises after axillary lymph node dissection, *Am J Surg* 160:481, 1990.

117. Jepson C and others: Black-white differences in cancer prevention knowledge and behavior, *Am J Public Health* 81:501, 1991.

118. Johnson JB, Kelly AW: A multifaceted rehabilitation program for women with cancer, *Oncol Nurs Forum* 17:691, 1990.

119. Kaplan KM and others: Breast cancer screening among relatives of women with breast cancer, *Am J Public Health* 81:1174, 1991.
120. Kaufmann M: Review of known prognostic variables, *Recent Results Cancer Res* 140:77, 1996.
121. Kegeles SS: Education for breast self-examination: why, who, what, and how? *Prev Med* 14:702, 1985.
122. Kelly PT: *Understanding breast cancer risk,* Philadelphia, 1991, Temple University Press.
123. Kelsey JL, Gammon MD: The epidemiology of breast cancer, *CA Cancer J Clin* 41:146, 1991.
124. Kemeny MM, Wellisch DK, Schain WS: Psychosocial outcome in a randomized surgical trial for treatment of primary breast cancer, *Cancer* 62:1231, 1988.
125. Ketcham AS, Moffat FL: Vexed surgeons, perplexed patients, and breast cancer which may not be cancer, *Cancer* 65:387, 1990.
126. Kimmick G, Muss HB: Current status of endocrine therapy for metastatic breast cancer, *Oncology* 9:877, 1995.
127. Kinne DW: Clinical management of lobular carcinoma in situ. In Harris JR and others, editors: *Breast diseases,* ed 2, Philadelphia, 1991, Lippincott.
128. Kinne DW: Surgery. In Harris JR and others, editors: *Breast diseases,* ed 2, Philadelphia, 1991, Lippincott.
129. Knobf MT: Symptoms and rehabilitation needs of patients with early stage breast cancer during primary therapy, *Cancer* 66:1392, 1990.
130. Kopans DB: Mammography screening and the controversy concerning women aged 40 to 49, *Radiol Clin North Am* 33:1273, 1995.
131. Koroltchouk V, Stanley K, Stjernsward J: The control of breast cancer: a World Health Organization perspective, *Cancer* 65:2803, 1990.
132. Krizek TJ: Breast reconstruction after mastectomy. In Harris JR and others, editors: *Breast diseases,* ed 2, Philadelphia, 1991, Lippincott.
133. Kwekkeboom K: Postmastectomy pain syndromes, *Cancer Nurs* 19:37, 1996.
134. Langston AA and others: BRCA1 mutations in a population-based sample of young women with breast cancer, *N Engl J Med* 334:137.
135. LaRossa D: Reconstructive surgery. In Fowble B and others, editors: *Breast cancer treatment: a comprehensive guide to management,* St Louis, 1991, Mosby.
136. Lasry J-CM: Women's sexuality following breast cancer. In Osoba D, editor: *Effect of cancer on quality of life,* Boca Raton, Fla, 1991, CRC.
137. Lasry J-CM, Margolese RG: Fear of recurrence, breast-conserving surgery, and the trade-off hypothesis, *Cancer* 69:2111, 1992.
138. Lauver D, Tak Y: Optimism and coping with a breast cancer symptom, *Nurs Res* 44:202, 1995.
139. Lazovich D and others: Underutilization of breast-conserving surgery and radiation therapy among women with stage I or II breast cancer, *JAMA* 266:3433, 1991.
140. Levine MN and others: A bedside decision instrument to elicit a patient's preference concerning adjuvant chemotherapy for breast cancer, *Ann Intern Med* 1117:53, 1992.
141. Levy S and others: Mastectomy versus breast conservation surgery: mental health effects at long-term follow-up, *Health Psychol* 11:349, 1992.
142. Lewis FM, Deal LW: Balancing our lives: a study of the married couple's experience with breast cancer recurrence, *Oncol Nurs Forum* 22:943, 1995.
143. Lierman LM: Phantom breast experiences after mastectomy, *Oncol Nurs Forum* 15:41, 1988.
144. Lotze MT and others: Early versus delayed shoulder motion following axillary dissection, *Ann Surg* 193:288, 1981.
145. Love RR and others: Symptoms associated with tamoxifen treatment in postmenopausal women, *Arch Intern Med* 151:1842, 1991.
146. Love SM: Dr. *Susan Love's breast book,* ed 2, Reading, Mass, 1995, Addison-Wesley.
147. Loveys BJ, Klaich K: Breast cancer: demands of illness, *Oncol Nurs Forum* 18:75, 1991.
148. Ludwick R: Breast examination in the older adult, *Cancer Nurs* 11:99, 1988.
149. Ludwick R: Registered nurses' knowledge and practices of teaching and performing breast exams among elderly women, *Cancer Nurs* 15:61, 1992.
150. Lynch HT and others: Natural history and age at onset of hereditary breast cancer, *Cancer* 69:1404, 1992.
151. Maddox MA: The practice of breast self-examination among older women, *Oncol Nurs Forum* 18:1367, 1991.
152. Mahon SM: Managing the psychosocial consequences of cancer recurrence: implications for nurses, *Oncol Nurs Forum* 18:577, 1991.
153. Mahon SM, Casperson D: Teaching women about mammography through use of a brochure, *Oncol Nurs Forum* 18:1375, 1991.
154. Malkin D and others: Germ line p53 mutations in a familial syndrome of breast cancer, sarcomas, and other neoplasms, *Science* 250:1233.
155. MammaTech Corporation: *MammaCare learning system for breast self-examination,* Gainesville, Fla, 1990, MammaTech.
156. Mansour EG, Ravdin PM, Dressler L: Prognostic factors in early breast carcinoma, *Cancer* 74(1 suppl):381, 1994.
157. Marchant D: Surgery for breast cancer. In Mitchell GW Jr, Bassett LW, editors: *The female breast and its disorders,* Baltimore, 1990, Williams & Wilkins.
158. McEvoy MD, McCorkle R: Quality of life issues in patients with disseminated breast cancer, *Cancer* 66(S):1416, 1990.
159. McGregor D and others: Breast cancer incidence among atomic bomb survivors, Hiroshima and Nagasaki, 1950-1969, *J Natl Cancer Inst* 59:799, 1977.
160. McGuire WL, Clark GM: Prognostic factors and treatment decisions in axillary-node-negative breast cancer, *N Engl J Med* 326:1756, 1992.
161. McInnis WD: Plastic surgery of the breast. In Mitchell GW Jr, Bassett LW, editors: *The female breast and its disorders,* Baltimore, 1990, Williams & Wilkins.
162. McKenney S, Dow KMH: Patient rehabilitation and support: nursing. In Harris JR and others, editors: *Breast diseases,* ed 2, Philadelphia, 1991, Lippincott.
163. Meade CD, Diekmann J, Thornhill DG: Readability of American Cancer Society patient education literature, *Oncol Nurs Forum* 19:51, 1992.

164. Meriney DK: Application of Orem's conceptual framework to patients with hypercalcemia related to breast cancer, *Cancer Nurs* 13:316, 1990.

165. Mettlin C: Breast cancer risk factors, *Cancer* 69(suppl):1904, 1992.

166. Mettlin C, Smart CR: Breast cancer detection guidelines for women aged 40 to 49 years: rationale for the American Cancer Society reaffirmation of recommendations, *CA Cancer J Clin* 44:248, 1994.

167. Michels KB, Willett WC: The Women's Health Initiative: will it resolve the issues? *Recent Results Cancer Res* 140:295, 1996.

168. Miki Y and others: A strong candidate for the breast and ovarian cancer susceptibility gene BRCA1, *Science* 266:66, 1994.

169. Miller AB: Causes of breast cancer and high-risk groups. In Harris JR and others, editors: *Breast diseases,* ed 2, Philadelphia, 1991, Lippincott.

170. Miller AB: Early detection of breast cancer. In Harris JR and others, editors: *Breast diseases,* ed 2, Philadelphia, 1991, Lippincott.

171. Mitchell GW Jr: Ambulatory surgery for diagnosis and treatment. In Mitchell GW Jr, Bassett LW, editors: *The female breast and its disorders,* Baltimore, 1990, Williams & Wilkins.

172. Mitchell GW Jr: History and physical examination. In Mitchell GW Jr, Bassett LW, editors: *The female breast and its disorders,* Baltimore, 1990, Williams & Wilkins.

173. Morra ME, Blumberg BD: Women's perceptions of early detection in breast cancer: how are we doing? *Semin Oncol Nurs* 7:151, 1991.

174. Morris T: Psychosocial aspects of breast cancer: a review, *Eur J Cancer Clin Oncol* 19:1725, 1983.

175. Morrison BW: Oncogenes and breast cancer. In Harris JR and others, editors: *Breast diseases,* ed 2, Philadelphia, 1991, Lippincott.

176. Morrow M, Hoffman PC, Weichselbaum RR: Locally advanced breast cancer. In Harris JR and others, editors: *Breast diseases,* ed 2, Philadelphia, 1991, Lippincott.

177. National Institutes of Health Consensus Development Panel: Consensus statement: treatment of early-stage breast cancer. In Consensus Development Conference on the Treatment of Early-Stage Breast Cancer, *J Natl Cancer Inst Monogr* 11:1, NIH Publication No 90-3187, Washington, DC, 1992, US Government Printing Office.

178. Nattinger AB, Goodwin JS: Geographic and hospital variation in the management of older women with breast cancer, *Cancer Control J Moffitt Cancer Ctr* 1:334, 1994.

179. Nemcek MA: Factors influencing black women's breast self-examination practice, *Cancer Nurs* 12:339, 1989.

180. Northouse L: A longitudinal study of the adjustment of patients and husbands to breast cancer, *Oncol Nurs Forum* 17(S):39, 1990.

181. Northouse LL and others: Emotional distress reported by women and husbands prior to a breast biopsy, *Nurs Res* 44:196, 1995.

182. O'Malley MS: Cost-effectiveness of two nurse-led programs to teach breast self-examination, *Am J Prev Med* 9:139, 1993.

183. Osborne CK: Receptors. In Harris JR and others, editors: *Breast diseases,* ed 2, Philadelphia, 1991, Lippincott.

184. Osborne MP: Breast development and anatomy. In Harris JR and others, editors: *Breast diseases,* ed 2, Philadelphia, 1991, Lippincott.

185. Osteen RT and others: Regional differences in surgical management of breast cancer, *CA Cancer J Clin* 42:39, 1992.

186. Page DL, Dupont WD: Anatomic markers of human premalignancy and risk of breast cancer, *Cancer* 66:1326, 1990.

187. Page DL, Simpson JF: Benign, high-risk, and premalignant lesions of the mamma. In Bland KI, Copeland EM, editors: *The breast: comprehensive management of benign and malignant diseases,* Philadelphia, 1991, Saunders.

188. Parker SH: Needle selection. In Parker SH, Jobe WE: *Percutaneous breast biopsy,* New York, 1993, Raven.

189. Parker SL and others: Cancer statistics, 1996, *CA Cancer J Clin* 65:5, 1996.

190. Paul PB: The older woman: implications for care. In *Proceedings of the Sixth National Conference on Cancer Nursing: Cancer prevention, early detection and screening,* Atlanta, 1992, American Cancer Society.

191. Pennypacker HS and others: Toward an effective technology of instruction in breast self-examination, *Int J Ment Health* 11:98, 1982.

192. Petrek JA and others: Axillary lymphadenectomy: a prospective, randomized trial of 13 factors influencing drainage, including early or delayed arm mobilization, *Arch Surg* 125:378, 1990.

193. Phillips JM, Wilbur J: Adherence to breast cancer screening guidelines among African-American women of differing employment status, *Cancer Nurs* 18:258, 1995.

194. Pritchard KI, Roy J-A, Sawka CA: Sex hormones and breast cancer: the issue of hormone replacement, *Recent Results Cancer Res* 140:285, 1996.

195. Rabinowitz B: Guidelines for facilitating patient decision making, *Innov Oncol Nurs* 5:4, 1989.

196. Ramzy I: Pathology of benign breast disease. In Mitchell GW, Bassett LW, editors: *The female breast and its disorders,* Baltimore, 1990, Williams & Wilkins.

197. Ramzy I: Pathology of malignant neoplasms. In Mitchell GW, Bassett LW, editors: *The female breast and its disorders,* Baltimore, 1990, Williams & Wilkins.

198. Ravdin PM, Valero V: Review of docetaxel (Taxotere), a highly active new agent for the treatment of metastatic breast cancer, *Semin Oncol* 22(suppl 4):17, 1995.

199. Recht A, Hayes DF: Local recurrence following mastectomy. In Harris JR and others, editors: *Breast diseases,* ed 2, Philadelphia, 1991, Lippincott.

200. Redmond CK, Costantino JP: Design and current status of the NSABP Breast Cancer Prevention Trial, *Recent Results Cancer Res* 140:309, 1996.

201. Robinson JO: Treatment of breast cancer through the ages, *Am J Surg* 151:317, 1986.

202. Rosato EF, Curcillo PG II: Surgical considerations in the management of breast cancer. In Fowble B and others: editors: *Breast cancer treatment: a comprehensive guide to management,* St Louis, 1991, Mosby.

203. Rowland JH, Holland JC: Psychological reactions to breast cancer and its treatment. In Harris JR and others, editors: *Breast diseases,* ed 2, Philadelphia, 1991, Lippincott.

204. Sachs BC: Breasts: sex symbols and releasers, *Dis Breast* 4:26, 1978.

205. Samarel N, Fawcett J: Enhancing adaptation to breast cancer: the addition of coaching to support groups, *Oncol Nurs Forum* 19:591, 1992.

206. Saunders KJ, Pilgrim CA, Pennypacker HS: Increased proficiency of search in breast self-examination, *Cancer* 58:2531, 1986.

207. Schain WS: Physician-patient communication about breast cancer: a challenge for the 1990s, *Surg Clin North Am* 70:917, 1990.

208. Schain WS, Jacobs E, Wellisch DK: Psychosocial issues in breast reconstruction: intrapsychic, interpersonal and practical concerns. In Scheflan MB, editor: *Clinics in plastic surgery,* Philadelphia, 1984, Saunders.

209. Schain WS and others: The sooner the better: a study of psychological factors in women undergoing immediate versus delayed breast reconstruction, *Am J Psychiatry* 142:40, 1985.

210. Schmidt RA: Stereotactic breast biopsy, *CA Cancer J Clin* 44:172, 1994.

211. Schnitt SJ, Connolly JL: Benign breast disorders. In Harris JR and others, editors: *Breast diseases,* ed 2, Philadelphia, 1991, Lippincott.

212. Schnitt SJ, Harris JR: Ductal carcinoma in situ (intraductal carcinoma) of the breast, *PPO Updates* 2:1, 1988.

213. Schover LR: The impact of breast cancer on sexuality, body image, and intimate relationships, *CA Cancer J Clin* 41:112, 1991.

214. Sciartelli CH: Using a clinical pathway approach to document patient teaching for breast cancer surgical procedures, *Oncol Nurs Forum* 22:131, 1995.

215. Seidman H and others: Survival experience in the Breast Cancer Detection Demonstration Project, *CA Cancer J Clin* 37:258, 1987.

216. Seidman H, Stellman SD, Mushinski MH: A different perspective on breast cancer risk factors: some implications of the nonattributable risk, *CA Cancer J Clin* 32:301, 1982.

217. Semiglazov VF and others: The role of breast self-examination in early breast cancer detection (results of the 5-years USSR/WHO randomized study in Leningrad), *Eur J Epidemiol* 8:498, 1992.

218. Shank B: Controversies regarding irradiation after preservative surgery for breast cancer. In Wise L, Johnson H Jr: *Breast cancer: controversies in management,* Armonk, NY, 1994, Futura.

219. Sharp N: The politics of breast cancer, *Nurs Management* 22:24, 1991.

220. Shugg D and others: Practice of breast self-examination and the treatment of primary breast cancer, *Aust NZ J Surg* 60:455, 1990.

221. Society of Surgical Oncology: SSO develops position statement on prophylactic mastectomies, *SSO News,* Summer 1993, p 1.

222. Speroff L: Tamoxifen: special considerations for gynecologists, *Contemp Obstet Gynecol* 37:50, 1992.

223. Spiegel D: Facilitating emotional coping during treatment, *Cancer* 66:1422, 1990.

224. Stadtmauer EA: Peripheral blood stem cell transplantation in breast cancer, *Hematol Oncol Annu* 2:61, 1994.

225. Stampfer MJ, Bechtel SD, Hunter DJ: Fat, alcohol, selenium, and breast cancer risk, *Contemp Obstet Gynecol* 37:42, 1992.

226. Stefanek ME: Counseling women at high risk for breast cancer, *Oncology* 4:27, 1990.

227. Stewart JA, Foster RS Jr: Breast cancer and aging, *Semin Oncol* 16:41, 1989.

228. Stuntz ME and others: Breast imaging techniques and their application in breast disease, *Breast J* 1:284.

229. Thomas SG: Breast cancer: the psychosocial issues, *Cancer Nurs* 1:53, 1978.

230. Tobin MB and others: The psychological morbidity of breast cancer—related arm swelling, *Cancer* 72:3248, 1993.

231. US Dept of Health and Human Services: *Quality determinants of mammography,* Pub No 95-0632, Rockville, Md, 1994, Agency for Health Care Policy and Research.

232. Valanis BG, Rumpler CH: Helping women to choose breast cancer treatment alternatives, *Cancer Nurs* 8:167, 1985.

233. Veronesi U: The control of breast cancer: a look into the future, *Recent Results Cancer Res* 140:1, 1996.

234. Vinokur AD and others: Physical and psychosocial functioning and adjustment to breast cancer, *Cancer* 63:394, 1989.

235. Vinton AL, Traverso LW, Zehring RD: Immediate breast reconstruction following mastectomy is as safe as mastectomy alone, *Arch Surg* 125:1303, 1990.

236. Vogel CL: Treatment of metastatic breast cancer, *Semin Oncol Nurs* 7:194, 1991.

237. Wagner FB: History of breast disease and its treatment. In Bland KI, Copeland EM, editors: *The breast: comprehensive management of benign and malignant diseases,* Philadelphia, 1991, Saunders.

238. Ward S, Griffin J: Developing a test of knowledge of surgical options for breast cancer, *Cancer Nurs* 13:191, 1990.

239. Ward S, Heidrich S, Wolberg W: Factors women take into account when deciding upon type of surgery for breast cancer, *Cancer Nurs* 12:344, 1989.

240. Weber BL: Familial breast cancer, *Recent Results Cancer Res* 140:5, 1996.

241. Weisman CS and others: Cancer screening services for the elderly, *Public Health Rep* 104:209-214, 1989.

242. Whitman S and others: Patterns of breast and cervical cancer screening at three public health centers in an inner-city urban area, *Am J Public Health* 81:1651, 1991.

243. Willis MA and others: Inter-agency collaboration: teaching breast self-examination to black women, *Oncol Nurs Forum* 16:171, 1989.

244. Winchester DP, Cox JD: Standards for breast-conserving treatment, *CA Cancer J Clin* 42:134, 1992.

245. Woolhandler S, Himmelstein DU: Reverse targeting of preventive care due to lack of health insurance, *JAMA* 259:2872, 1988.

246. Wooster R and others: Identification of the breast cancer susceptibility gene BRCA2, *Nature* 378:789, 1995.

247. Wooster R and others: Localization of a breast cancer susceptibility gene, BRCA2, to chromosome 13q12-13, *Science* 265:2088, 1994.

248. Yeh IT and others: Pathologic assessment and pathologic prognostic factors in operable breast cancer. In Fowble B and others, editors: *Breast cancer treatment: a comprehensive guide to management,* St Louis, 1991, Mosby.

249. Young-McCaughan S, Sexton DL: A retrospective investigation of the relationship between aerobic exercise and quality of life in women with breast cancer, *Oncol Nurs Forum* 18:751, 1991.

CHAPTER 7
Colorectal Cancers

MARY E. MURPHY

Colorectal cancer is the fourth most common malignant tumor in the United States, second only to lung cancer in its incidence and mortality. An estimated 94,500 new cases develop each year, with an annual death rate of 46,400.[1,29] Continued research to investigate the cause and treatment of this disease are under investigation and remain a medical priority.

EPIDEMIOLOGY

Colorectal cancer affects both genders equally, with the incidence increasing significantly in persons over age 50. The mean age at the time of diagnosis is 62.[1,47] The disease occurs most frequently in Western industrialized countries of Northern America, Northern Europe, and New Zealand. Individuals from low-incidence countries who move to Western countries develop colorectal cancer at the same rate as in Western countries.[6,40] The incidence among the black population continues to increase.

ETIOLOGY AND RISK FACTORS

The cause of colorectal cancer is unknown, but recent research indicates that diet, genetics, and other predisposing factors such as bowel disorders may play an important role in its development.

Diet

The relationship between diet and colorectal cancer remains under investigation, but evidence shows that individuals with diets low in animal fats and high in fiber demonstrate a significantly lower incidence of disease.[20,46] Research indicates that fats and meat products may alter the concentration of normal body products such as cholesterol and fecal bile salts and also may change the normal intestinal flora of the bowel. This process may serve as a cancer promoter by damaging the colonic mucosa and increasing the proliferational activity of the colonic epithelium.

Reduced dietary fiber may also serve as a promoter of the carcinogenic process by increasing the amount of contact time that the carcinogenic substance has with colonic mucosa, therefore increasing the potential for mutagenic changes in the bowel wall.

Other dietary factors that serve as promoters of the carcinogenic process include genotoxic carcinogens such as charbroiled meats, fish, and fried foods. Dietary deficiencies of vitamins A, C, and E; selenium; and calcium have also been investigated and may result in future dietary recommendations.[13,14,22,32,46]

Genetic Factors

Genetic abnormalities and traits represent a new area of scientific technology that may help identify individuals at risk. Progressive genetic changes trigger a multistep process in which chromosomal and oncogenic changes occur and result in colorectal epithelium mutations forming malignant tumors in the colon.

Areas of investigation include the K-PAS proto-oncogene, APC gene, DCC antioncogene, and HNPCC gene, all of which demonstrate the relationship between genetic changes and colorectal carcinogenesis.

Genetics plays a role in the predisposition to colorectal cancer. Persons with first-degree relatives who have colorectal cancer have a threefold risk of having the disease themselves. Polyposis syndromes such as Gardner's, Turcot, and Peutz-Jeghers are linked to increased risks for the development of colorectal cancers. These autosomal dominant diseases are manifested by thousands of colonic adenomas that have a high malignant potential. As these adenomas grow and increase in size, cellular changes occur that result in a malignant transformation.[17,18,22,23,41]

Other Predisposing Factors

Other predisposing factors include ulcerative colitis and Crohn's disease. These inflammatory bowel disorders are associated with dysplasia and associated malignant lesions. Potential for the malignant process is correlated to the disease's duration. In addition to inflammatory bowel disease, polyposis adenomas are the most common bowel polyps and account for 80% of all types of bowel polyps.[8,40] These polyps increase their malignant potential as they grow larger and demonstrate cellular changes. This process takes 10 to 15 years from the time of diagnosis. Villous adenomas are another type of polyp that has been associated with increased malignancy and high fatality. These polyps produce excessive mucus and result in severe fluid and electrolyte disorders.

PREVENTION, SCREENING, AND DETECTION

The American Cancer Society (ACS) recommends specific protocols for the screening and prevention of colorectal cancers, especially diet and diagnostic examinations.

Dietary considerations focus on a low-fat, high-fiber diet, including whole-grain cereals, fruits, and vegetables. Cruciferous vegetables, such as Brussels sprouts, cauliflower, cabbage, kohlrabi, and broccoli, have been recommended to reduce colon cancer risk.[5,12,14,19] The relationship between diet and colon cancer continues to be investigated, and additional research is needed to provide more definitive information. The box below lists current dietary recommendations.

The ACS recommendations for colon cancer screening for an asymptomatic person include an annual digital rectal examination for persons over age 40 and an annual stool guaiac test for persons over age 50. Proctosigmoidoscopy should be done every 3 to 5 years after age 50 after two negative annual examinations (Table 7-1).[21,26,36,39] Persons at high risk may need screening at an earlier age and more frequently than the general population.[21]

DIETARY RECOMMENDATIONS FOR COLORECTAL CANCER PREVENTION

1. Reduce the amount of saturated and unsaturated fats in the diet from 40% to 30% of total daily caloric intake.
2. Increase the amount of fiber in the diet by eating fresh fruits, vegetables (including cruciferous vegetables: cabbage, broccoli, Brussels sprouts, kohlrabi, cauliflower), and whole-grain breads and cereals.
3. Eat foods rich in vitamin C: citrus fruits, strawberries, currants, cabbage, tomatoes, walnuts, and rosehips.
4. Eat foods rich in vitamin A: peaches, cantaloupe, apricots, and the dark-green and yellow vegetables (carrots, spinach, squash, asparagus, sweet potatoes).
5. Eat foods rich in vitamin E: vegetable oils (soybean, corn, cottonseed, sunflower seed), alfalfa, and lettuce leaves.

Because many tumors are found in the lower rectum, abdominal and rectal examinations should be performed at the time of a routine physical examination.

The *stool guaiac slide test* is an effective and inexpensive screening tool but does have limitations. False-negative and false-positive results may occur for a variety of reasons. The primary cause may be inadequate instruction on sample collection or poor compliance with specific directions. Instructions should include various dietary, medication, and collection procedures.

All individuals should be on a meat-free, high-residue diet for 2 days before specimen collection. Red meats may contain nonhuman hemoglobin, which yields false-positive tests. Foods with peroxidase activity, such as tomatoes, turnips, beets, radishes, and cherries, should be eliminated because their consumption will yield a false-positive test. High-residue diets are recommended to encourage bleeding from small colonic lesions.[36,49]

Medication ingestion may also yield false-negative or false-positive tests. Vitamin C and antacids produce false-negative results even in the presence of active bleeding. Iron, aspirin, cimetidine, cytochromes, and halogens are known for false-positive results and should be avoided during the testing period. Diseases such as diverticulosis, hemorrhoids, and other gastrointestinal pathology have yielded false-positive tests because of an alternate bleeding source.

Sample collection also has a direct impact on test results. Diluted specimens obtained from toilet water may result in fecal blood loss from the sample or may be affected by the halogens, such as chlorine, that may be present in the water. Stool samples either too dry or wet may also alter results. Two separate samples from each stool should be collected in designated containers for 3 consecutive days for a total of six samples. Testing should be done within 5 days of sample collection.

Further methods of screening include a fecal blood test, the Hemo-Quant (Smith-Kline Bio-Science Laboratories). The advantages of Hemo-Quant are that it can detect hemoglobin in smaller amounts of stool and that it is unaffected by other factors that interfere with a guaiac test. Immunochemical stool screening is also be-

Table 7-1 Summary of American Cancer Society Recommendations for the Early Detection of Colorectal Cancer in Asymptomatic Men and Women

Test or procedure	Age	Frequency
Proctosigmoidoscopy	50 and over	Every 3 to 5 years based on advice of physician
Stool guaiac slide test	Over 50	Every year
Digital rectal examination	Over 40	Every year

ing evaluated as a suitable method for colorectal screening and may show future benefits.[36]

Proctosigmoidoscopy is also an appropriate method of screening for cancerous lesions of the colon and rectum. Approximately 50% to 65% of all colorectal cancers can be found within the range of this particular instrument (25 cm, or 10 inches). A flexible fiberoptic sigmoidoscope is available that can reach to the splenic flexure (60 cm, or 24 inches). This instrument provides for increased visibility and patient comfort but requires additional time and cost for the procedure.[9,20]

CLASSIFICATION

The site of presentation is primarily the sigmoidorectal area. The majority (40% to 50%) of lesions occur in the rectum, and 20% to 35% occur in the descending and sigmoid colon. Only 8% occur in the transverse colon and 16% in the cecum and ascending colon. A small percentage (4% to 8%) may occur as a second primary site.[37,40,41]

Most bowel cancers are *adenocarcinomas* and are moderately differentiated to well-differentiated cancers. Other forms of colorectal cancers consist of epithelioma, squamous cell carcinoma, sarcoma, lymphoma, leiomyosarcoma, and melanoma. Cancer of the anus occurs rarely, but recent research has shown an increase in males with a history of homosexual and bisexual activity or a history of anal condylomata acuminata. Other anal cancers include squamous cell, basal cell, and melanomas.

CLINICAL FEATURES

General signs and symptoms exist for all colorectal cancers and may include a change in bowel habits, blood in the stool, abdominal pain, anorexia, flatulence, and indigestion. Later symptoms include loss of energy, weight loss, and a decline in general health. Symptoms may vary greatly according to size, location, tumor type, and the individual patient (Figure 7-1). Specific variances are seen between the right and left colon and the rectum. Patients with right-sided lesions do not display changes in bowel habits because of the liquid nature of the stool. Specific symptoms include a dull, vague abdominal pain radiating from abdomen to back. These tumors present as palpable masses in the right lower quadrant. Dark or mahogany-red blood may be present in the stool. Anemia leads to weakness and malaise, and indigestion and weight loss often occur.

In contrast, patients with left-sided lesions usually display a change in bowel habits because the area affected is the sigmoid colon and the rectum. Symptoms include cramps, gas pains, a decrease in the caliber of stool, bright-red bleeding, constipation, and a feeling of rectal pressure or incomplete evacuation of stool. Obstruction

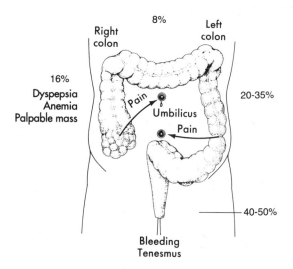

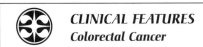

Figure 7-1 Signs and symptoms related to colon cancer. (From Beare P, Myers J: *Principles and practice of adult health nursing,* ed 2, St Louis, 1994, Mosby.)

CLINICAL FEATURES
Colorectal Cancer

- *General:* Change in bowel habits, blood in stool, abdominal pain, anorexia, flatulence, indigestion
- *Late symptoms:* Weight loss, fatigue, decline in general health
- *Right-sided lesions:* Dull vague abdominal pain radiating to back, dark/mahogany-red blood in stool, weakness, anemia, malaise, indigestion, weight loss, liquid stool
- *Left-sided lesions:* Change in bowel habits—cramps, gas pains, decrease in caliber of stool, bright-red bleeding, constipation, rectal pressure, incomplete evacuation of stool
- *Transverse colon:* Palpable masses, obstruction, changes in bowel habits, bloody stools
- *Rectal:* Changes in bowel habits, bright-red bleeding, tenesmus, severe pain in groin, labia, scrotum, legs, or penis

---

may occur and result in emergency surgery. Patients with transverse colon tumors have palpable masses, obstruction, a change in bowel habits, and bloody stools. Those with rectal cancers may display similar symptoms, such as changes in bowel habits, bright-red bleeding, tenesmus, and a late symptom of severe pain in the groin, labia, scrotum, legs, or penis (see box above). Unfortu-

---

DIAGNOSTIC WORK-UP FOR COLORECTAL CANCER

Barium enema
Colonoscopy
Chest x-ray film
Liver scan
Bone scan
CBC, AST (SGOT), LDH, ALP, BUN*
Carcinoembryonic antigen (CEA)

---

*See text for abbreviations.

nately, colorectal cancer may be advanced before symptoms occur. Pain may only be the last symptom, and metastasis may be present before treatment is sought.

DIAGNOSIS

Persons at high risk for disease or who have symptoms and are guaiac positive require additional diagnostic testing (see box above). A *barium enema* provides a clear picture of the large intestine and is useful for detecting smaller tumors. *Colonoscopy* may be performed at this time, especially if surgery is indicated. This examination provides increased visualization and the ability to biopsy lesions. Potential metastatic lesions are evaluated using chest x-ray films and liver, bone, and other scans. Laboratory work includes a complete blood count (CBC), serum aspartate aminotransferase (AST, glutamic-oxaloacetic transaminase), lactate dehydrogenase (LDH), alkaline phosphatase (ALP), and blood urea nitrogen (BUN). A *carcinoembryonic antigen* (CEA) test may be used. This biologic marker is elevated in later stages of colorectal cancer and may have prognostic value at diagnosis or disease recurrence. Other tests are currently being evaluated for their usefulness as diagnostic tools and involve antigens, such as *colon-specific antigens* (CSAs) and *colon-specific antigen protein* (CSAP).[43] Diagnosis is confirmed by tissue biopsy from the suspected site. Additional diagnostic evaluation includes a variety of procedures.

STAGING

The most widely used method for colorectal surgery is the *Duke's classification* or some modification of the original form, which was developed in 1932. The Duke's system classifies tumor into four major categories based on the degree and depth of tumor involvement and presence of lymph nodes. Subcategories were developed by Astler and Collier in 1954 in an attempt to delineate the importance of tumor wall penetration, as follows:

Table 7-2 Comparison of Staging Systems

TMN system	Duke's system
Tis-N0-M0	
Tis: carcinoma in situ	
T1 or T2-N0-M0	A
T1: tumor invading submucosa	
T2: invading muscle layer	
T3 or T4-N0-M0	B
T3: tumor invades through muscle layer, into subserosa	
T4: tumor directly invades other organs or perforates visceral peritoneum	
Any T-N1, N2, or N3-M0	C
N1: one to three pericolic or perirectal lymph node metastases	
N2: four pericolic or perirectal lymph node metastases	
N3: any nodal metastasis along vascular trunk or apical node	
Any T-any N-M1	D
M1: distant metastasis	

Duke's classification

Stage A	Carcinoma limited to the mucosa
Stage B1	Carcinoma invades the muscle but is confined to the bowel wall
Stage B2	Carcinoma penetrates through the muscularis propria into the serosa and connective tissue
Stage B3	Same as B2 with adherence or invasion into adjacent organs, but with negative nodes
Stage C1	Lymph nodes positive for metastatic disease, but main tumor confined to bowel wall
Stage C2	Lymph nodes positive for metastatic disease, and tumor completely penetrates bowel wall
Stage C3	Same as B3, with positive nodes
Stage D	Distant metastasis

The variances and minor modifications of various systems of colorectal staging resulted in the promotion of the *TNM system* by the Committee of the International Union Against Cancer (UICC). In this system, *T* refers to tumor, *N* to node involvement, and *M* to distant metastasis. Additional numbers are added to each letter to specify the extent of tumor growth. No uniform or widely accepted staging is used for anal cancers. Table 7-2 compares the Duke's system and TNM system.[25]

METASTASIS

Most colorectal cancers spread by direct extension and penetration into layers of the bowel. Local invasion occurs to surrounding organs. Lymph node involvement and invasion into the vascular bed allow for disseminated disease. Lymphatic disease is present in 50% of all diagnosed cases. Nodal chains follow the pathway of the superior and mesenteric arteries. Colon cancer and cancer of the upper one half of the rectum spread by direct

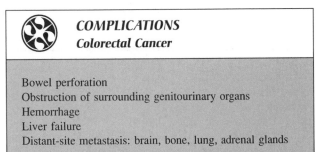

COMPLICATIONS
Colorectal Cancer

Bowel perforation
Obstruction of surrounding genitourinary organs
Hemorrhage
Liver failure
Distant-site metastasis: brain, bone, lung, adrenal glands

Table 7-3   Major Surgeries for Colorectal Cancer

Location	Tumor site	Procedure
Right colon	Cecum, ascending colon, proximal and midtransverse colon	Right colectomy or colostomy
Left colon	Splenic flexure and descending colon	Colectomy or colostomy
Sigmoid colon	Sigmoid portion of bowel	Sigmoid resection
Upper rectum	12 cm from anal verge	Anterior colon resection
Middle rectum	7-11 cm from anal verge	Pull-through procedure
Lower rectum	7 cm from anal verge	Abdominal perineal resection and colostomy

extension to the liver. Cancer of the lower half of the rectum spreads to portal veins and the inferior vena cava. Venous invasion permits distant metastasis, with the liver and lung as the most common sites. Additional sites include the brain, bone, and adrenal glands. Anal cancers spread directly into local muscles and to genitourinary organs. Metastatic spread at diagnosis significantly alters prognosis and treatment modalities. The box above summarizes disease-related complications of colorectal cancer.

Liver Metastasis

Of all patients diagnosed with colorectal cancer, 25% will have liver metastasis at the time of their diagnosis. As many as 70% will display metastatic disease as the disease progresses. Methods to treat metastatic liver cancer include surgical resection, cryosurgery, regional infusion therapy, and vascular interruption with hepatic artery ligation. Each procedure has specific eligibility criteria based on the extensiveness of the metastatic disease. Risks and benefits vary. To date, no one specific treatment has been documented to be successful to manage liver metastasis.[3,11,44] (For specific instructions on the use of the Infusaid, Medtronic, and other pumps as treatment approaches, see Chapters 20 and 26.)

TREATMENT MODALITIES
Surgery

Colon resection with disease-free margins remains the surgical goal. Tumor and associated blood vessels are resected en bloc with the vascular and lymphatic structures to prevent seeding of malignant cells. A biopsy of the liver and regional lymph nodes is taken at the time of surgery to evaluate the extent of disease. Extensive procedures may be needed to attain the goal of reanastomosis and return to normal bowel function. Tumor size, tumor location, and additional metastases determine the type and the extent of surgery. Three major surgeries performed for colorectal cancer are *colon resection with reanastomosis, colostomy* (temporary or permanent), and *abdominal perineal resection*[6,37,40] (Figure 7-2). Table

7-3 outlines site-specific surgeries that may be done for various portions of the colon and rectum.

The most questionable procedure is surgery of the middle rectal tumors, which requires judgment, surgical skill, and intense evaluation of the potential for cure over a sphincter-sparing procedure (Figure 7-3). The use of the end-to-end stapler has permitted increased success with these lesions. This instrument facilitates an anastomosis from the low rectal area to the colon. Procedures such as this spare patients from the bladder dysfunction and sexual dysfunction that result from radical abdominal perineal resection. Research continues to evaluate the success of these procedures versus the likelihood of disease recurrence.

In addition to surgical guidelines for general tumor site, each case must be evaluated individually to meet specific patient needs. Age, nutritional status, metastases, and such complications as perforation and obstruction may alter the surgical course. Additional surgical modalities may be required for palliation even when cure is not possible. Relief of pain, odor, or bleeding may be the ultimate goal. Extensive metastases may also require more radical surgeries such as *pelvic exenteration,* in which the entire bladder and rectum and other structures are removed and an ileal conduit and sigmoid colostomy are created. Figure 7-4 illustrates the best sites for ostomies.

Chemotherapy

Chemotherapy alone has not been proved to be effective against colorectal cancer. Chemotherapy continues to be considered an adjunct to the initial surgical intervention. Various forms of combination drug therapy have been evaluated, including 5-fluorouracil (5-FU) alone and in combination with methyl lomustine (MeCCNU, semustine), mitomycin-C, vincristine, cisplatin, methotrexate, and biotherapy such as bacille Calmette-Guérin (BCG),

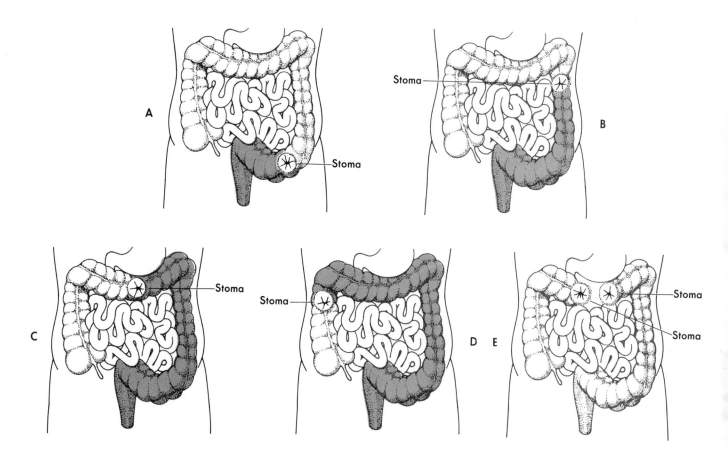

Figure 7-2 **A,** Sigmoid colostomy. **B,** Descending colostomy. **C,** Transverse colostomy. **D,** Ascending colostomy. **E,** Double-barrel colostomy. (From Beare P, Myers J: *Principles and practice of adult health nursing,* ed 1, St Louis, 1990, Mosby.)

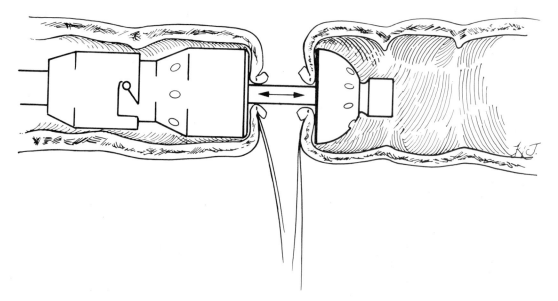

Figure 7-3 Sphincter-sparing procedure. (From Broadwell D, Jackson B: *Principles of ostomy care,* St Louis, 1982, Mosby.)

methanol-extractable residue (MER), and interferon. Leucovorin has been combined with 5-FU to enhance the effectiveness of 5-FU. Levamisole plus 5-FU given after surgery to reduce disease recurrence has shown a significant benefit to improve survival in patients with stage C disease. 5-FU continues to remain the drug of choice for treatment of colorectal cancer.[2,24,27,35]

Chemotherapy has also been used in attempts to prevent unresectable tumors confined to the liver from metastasizing. 5-FU has been administered by intraarterial catheter into the hepatic artery, and floxuridine (FUDR), an analogue of 5-FU, has been administered by an implanted pump known as an Infusaid or Medtronic. The role of regional hepatic perfusion remains controversial in the treatment of metastatic disease. Additional studies with 5-FU, leucovorin, and methotrexate are under investigation (see box and Table 7-4).

Radiation Therapy

The role of radiation therapy in the management of colon tumors remain under investigation, but it is often used for patients with extensive microscopic tumor penetration, lymph node involvement, and direct tumor extension into the viscera or perineum. Various combination approaches have been attempted, including preoperative radiation, postoperative radiation, and a combination of both known as the "sandwich technique." *Preoperative* radiation therapy may damage malignant cells that could disseminate during surgery and may help shrink unresectable lesions. *Intraoperative* therapy is a modality that allows delivery of radiation to a large treatment area after the tumor is resected. Normal organs are moved from the pathway of radiation, and a large, single fraction beam is directed onto the tumor site. Technical and financial difficulties arise in the ability to place expensive equipment with protective devices in an operating room. Ongoing research is necessary to predict outcomes and complications.[42] *Postoperative* radiation has proved effective in prevention of disease recurrence in high-risk persons. Palliation may result from radiation treatment through reduction of tumor size, thereby relieving pain, bleeding, and pressure.[16,30,42]

PROGNOSIS

Persons diagnosed with colorectal cancer must receive follow-up treatment after initial surgery, including peri-

Table 7-4 Chemotherapy Drugs and Related Side Effects

Drug	Side effects
5-FU (5-fluorouracil)	Anorexia, nausea, vomiting, stomatitis, diarrhea, bone marrow suppression, alopecia, dermatitis, skin hyperpigmentation
MeCCNU (semustine)	Bone marrow suppression, nausea, alopecia, pulmonary fibrosis
Cisplatin	Anorexia, nausea, vomiting, stomatitis, bone marrow suppression, renal insufficiency, ototoxicity
Mitomycin-C	Nausea, vomiting, anorexia, stomatitis, bone marrow suppression, alopecia, necrosis
Methotrexate	Bone marrow suppression, renal tubular necrosis, stomatitis, diarrhea, hepatic dysfunction
Vincristine	Extravasation, peripheral neuropathy, intestinal obstruction

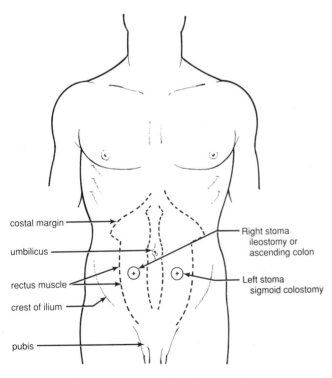

Figure 7-4 Best sites for ostomies.

costal margin

umbilicus

rectus muscle

crest of ilium

pubis

Right stoma ileostomy or ascending colon

Left stoma sigmoid colostomy

COMMON CHEMOTHERAPY DRUGS USED IN TREATMENT OF COLORECTAL CANCER

5-Fluorouracil (5-FU)
Methyl lomustine (MeCCNU, semustine)
Mitomycin-C
Vincristine
Cisplatin
Methotrexate
5-FU and levamisole
Advanced cancer:
    Floxuridine (FUDR) (via pump)
    5-FU and leucovorin
    Methotrexate, 5-FU, and leucovorin

odic physical examinations, colonoscopy, CEA levels, and traditional x-ray films as needed. Symptoms of weight loss and pain should be evaluated immediately. Disease recurrence may be observed locally or regionally in distant organs. Local recurrence at the original tumor site is a possibility and may cause obstruction and hemorrhage. Penetration beyond the bowel wall may result in fistula formation. Further surgery or combined adjunctive therapy may be indicated.

Spread to distant organs has a direct impact on the prognosis and the patient's ultimate survival. Survival time for persons with metastasis usually is less than 1 year. Age is an additional factor that affects the survival rate; persons under age 30 have a poorer prognosis, and patients over age 70 have a higher surgical morbidity rate. High CEA titers before surgery, the presence of obstruction at diagnosis, and poorly differentiated cancers also decrease the survival rate. Rectal tumors continue to be associated with poor prognosis, especially those located near the lower one third of the rectum. The overall survival rate of all stages is 40%. Survival rates continue to change as new treatment modalities and early detection methods are developed.[6,19,29,37] Table 7-5 lists specific prognosis rates.

CONCLUSION

Colorectal cancer provides an exciting challenge to the medical profession. Knowledge of the impact of dietary and environmental factors on colorectal statistics is a critical goal of research. Promotion of the American Cancer Society guidelines and large-scale, cost-effective screening may improve statistics and survival rates. Clinical trial research also provides hope for new treatment modalities with drug protocols and combined radiation therapy. Nursing will play an important role in health care teaching and promotion of future health care practices.

Text continued on p. 138.

Table 7-5 Prognosis Rates for Colorectal Cancer

Duke's classification	Survival rate
A	80%-90%
B	60%
C	25%-45%
D	5%
Anal cancer	48%-66%

NURSING MANAGEMENT

SURGERY
Preoperative Teaching

Patient teaching and preoperative counseling are essential elements of nursing care for the patient preparing for colorectal surgery. Many patients will have already had several diagnostic and laboratory tests in an outpatient setting before they reach the hospital. Often they are aware of their diagnosis but may be in the stage of denial or disbelief. Patients and their families may be anxious or even angry at the diagnosis and will require additional attention and reinforcement of teaching preoperatively and postoperatively.

Teaching may begin with preparation of the colon for surgery. Most protocols involve a regimen of 2 or 3 days of liquid diets, a combination of laxatives and/or enemas, and the use of oral antibiotics to sterilize the bowel before surgery.[31,33] Antibiotics suppress both anaerobic and aerobic colonic organisms and reduce septic complications after surgery. Patients with bowel obstructions do not receive the usual bowel preparation.

NURSING DIAGNOSES

- *Knowledge deficit related to lack of experience in surgical routine and procedure*
- *Fear related to the diagnosis of cancer and outcomes of surgical procedure*
- *Knowledge deficit related to ostomy*

OUTCOME GOALS

Patient will be able to:
- Verbalize understanding of surgical procedure and postoperative routine.
- Express fears and use effective coping mechanisms.
- Demonstrate care of ostomy, including stoma, peristomal skin, application of appliance, dietary concerns, and changes in life-style patterns.

INTERVENTIONS

The nurse must provide support to an already anxious patient by explaining the rationale for the bowel preparation regimen. Close observation of the patient's tolerance of laxatives and enemas must be reported, including the side effects of nausea, vomiting, abdominal discomfort, and excessive diarrhea and the symptoms of electrolyte imbalance. Elderly and debilitated patients are at the greatest risk for discomfort and complications.

Preoperative Care

Preoperative teaching may begin at this time and should include a review of the patient's past experience with surgery. Basic teaching should include a review of the preoperative routine: preoperative medications, intravenous lines, recovery room procedures, and placement of a

Continued.

Foley catheter, nasogastric tube, and abdominal dressings. Postoperative exercises, such as coughing and deep breathing, wound splinting, and leg exercises, should be reviewed and practiced. Concerns about pain medication and diet restrictions may be discussed preoperatively. A basic review of anatomy is necessary for the person to understand the surgical procedure and colostomy placement.

Psychosocial issues and concerns must be addressed and support systems identified. A review of past coping mechanisms allows the individual to evaluate strengths and weaknesses. Ample time to discuss fears and concerns must be permitted to evaluate the dynamics of interpersonal relationships between patients and their support systems. Quality preoperative assessment allows for more effective intervention postoperatively.

If a colostomy is performed, a referral to an enterostomal therapist or other appropriate resource should be made as soon as possible. Preoperative teaching should review the type of surgery, a description of an ostomy, various pouching methods available, and marking of the stoma site. Marking the stoma site is important to eliminate the possibility of future skin problems and difficult pouch applications. One of the basic rules for stoma marking is that the stoma should be away from the waistline, folds, scars, or where the abdominal incision will be placed (see Figure 7-4). The stoma should be placed so that the patient will be able to see and reach the pouch easily. The stoma site will be placed through the rectus abdominis muscle, which runs vertically through the abdomen. Approximately 3 inches (7.5 cm) of skin will be necessary to provide adequate pouch placement. Various positions should be attempted before marking the stoma. The stoma should be visualized in sitting, standing, and lying positions. The site is usually below the umbilicus and at the infraumbilical bulge. The stoma site is then marked with a dye such as methylene blue or gentian violet.[15] Marking the stoma validates the reality of the ostomy. Documentation of the patient's and family's reaction is important to meet future emotional needs.

Postoperative Care
NURSING DIAGNOSES

- *Pain related to incisional discomfort*
- *Infection, risk for, related to improper wound healing*
- *Bowel incontinence (or other elimination problem) related to loss of normal bowel function*
- *Skin integrity, impaired, related to abdominal incision and stoma drainage*

OUTCOME GOALS

Patient will be able to:
- Verbalize level of comfort at pain-rating score of 0 to 3.

- Be free of signs and symptoms of infection, as demonstrated by adequate wound healing.
- Have adequate bowel function, as evidenced by evacuation of stool in 1 to 3 days.
- Maintain intact skin at incision and peristomal site.

INTERVENTIONS

Care during the postoperative period focuses on meeting the patient's physical and metabolic needs. Observing the patient for initial complications includes assessment of vital signs and lung and bowel sounds. The incision is inspected for drainage or bleeding and approximation. The nasogastric tube and Foley catheter, if present, are monitored for the amount and color of drainage and patency. Accurate recording of intake and output is necessary to provide proper electrolyte balance. The stoma site is observed at each shift initially for color and size. A postoperative pouch usually covers the stoma, allowing for easy visibility. The stoma should appear pink and moist. Signs of necrosis and ischemia are present if the stoma appears blue or black or has a dusky appearance. This observation should be reported at once because this indicates stoma death. Drainage from the stoma should be scant and blood tinged. A strict postoperative routine of coughing, deep breathing exercises, early ambulation, and adequate pain control assists the patient toward early recovery and limits potential complications (see box below).

Despite good nursing care, postoperative complications may occur, including infection, paralytic ileus, pulmonary complications, anastomotic leak, urinary problems, stoma retraction, and prolapse.[5,8,15,40] Fevers may result from infection, respiratory difficulty, urinary infections, or thrombophlebitis. Elderly patients with preexisting medical illness such as diabetes and lung disease are at greatest risk.

Anastomotic leaks are more common in lower resections and often result in fistula formation. Skin care and adequate nutrition are essential components of proper wound healing. Paralytic ileus, a common complication after bowel surgery, results from the surgical manipula-

COMPLICATIONS
Bowel Surgery

Infection (wound, urinary, lung)
Thrombophlebitis
Paralytic ileus
Pulmonary embolus
Hemorrhage
Anastomotic leaks

tion of the bowels in surgery and can last up to 14 days or more. Increased abdominal girth, distention, nausea, and vomiting are classic signs of an ileus. Decompression of the bowel with a nasogastric tube, maintenance of the NPO (nothing by mouth) status, and increased activity usually result in a return to normal bowel function.

Postoperative wound infection is not usually a major concern because of prophylactic antibiotics and reduction of wound contamination with postoperative stoma pouching. Those patients with abdominoperineal resections are at greater risk for wound complications and infections. Sitz baths, dressing changes, and topical ointments assist in the healing process. Healing may be very slow, and meticulous skin care remains essential.

Postoperative Teaching
NURSING DIAGNOSES

- *Sexual dysfunction related to body function alteration and body changes*
- *Self-esteem disturbance related to altered body image*
- *Family processes, altered, related to diagnosis of cancer and ostomy placement*
- *Health maintenance, altered, related to knowledge deficit regarding diet modifications and ostomy care*

OUTCOME GOALS

- Patient will express concerns related to sexual dysfunction and identify alternatives to cope with modification.
- Patient will verbalize concerns related to self-concept and express positive self-esteem.
- Patient and family will verbalize changes in family patterns and identify methods to incorporate new changes into life-style.
- Patient will verbalize understanding of dietary restrictions and ostomy care.

INTERVENTIONS

Postoperative teaching addresses the patient's emotional and physical changes resulting from the ostomy and involves appropriate referral to resources as needed. Postoperative pouch application and stoma care should be a step-by-step process, moving from the simple to the complex components. Ostomy care includes pouch applications, emptying of the pouch, and use of skin products.

Pouch selection is based on the site of the stoma, manual dexterity, cost, and patient preference; all pouches should be well fitted and odor proof and should provide skin protection.[15] Special skin barriers may also be necessary, depending on the type of effluent discharged. Ileostomy drainage is particularly wet and contains enzymes that can cause skin irritation. Sigmoid colostomy effluent is solid but may also cause skin problems. Odor is managed with pouching, and ostomy deodorant sprays must be discussed. The enterostomal

Table 7-6 Ostomy Supplies*

Product	Use
Skin barriers	Paste, wafers, rings, or powders used to protect skin
Skin sealants	Plasticizing agents that produce a thin, protective film around skin
Skin cleaners	Foams, wipes, sprays, or liquids used to clean or remove residue from skin
Skin adhesives	Sprays or liquids used to increase adhesion of ostomy equipment
Pouches	Wafers cut to fit and presized: one piece or two piece, disposable or reusable
Belts and binders	Provide support and keep equipment in place
Convex inserts	Provide support and convexity
Pouch covers	Protect skin from moisture and provide concealment
Tail closures	Close end of pouches to prevent leakage
Tapes	Help pouches stay in place; prevent leakage; provide waterproofing
Stoma guide strips	Assist with centering pouches over stoma
Solvents	Assist with removal of residual tape or water residue

*Patient should be referred to appropriate resources, including the enterostomal therapy nurse, American Cancer Society, and United Ostomy Association.

therapist is invaluable in selecting the appropriate product for the patient (Table 7-6).

Colostomy irrigations may be an option for patients with a sigmoid colostomy. Patients should be told the advantages of both systems, that irrigation control takes patience, and that a daily schedule can be established over time. Other types of ostomies cannot be regulated by irrigation because the effluent is constant and liquid.

The special dietary needs and restrictions of the ostomy patient are discussed, including adequate fluid intake and the avoidance of certain foods that may cause blockage, odor, or gas. A list of medications that are not absorbed in the intestine and may be expelled through the colostomy is also provided. Foods that contain seeds, nuts, or excessive bulk should be avoided because blockage is likely. Gas- and odor-producing foods are frequently the same foods that caused problems before surgery and usually are related to beans, cabbage, and brussel sprouts.

Trial and error and the use of commercial deodorant products assist with this problem. Discharge teaching includes specific problems that may be encountered, such as diarrhea or blockage. A dietary consultant can assist the patient in appropriate diet selection. A physician or

Continued.

enterostomal therapist should be notified if these problems arise. Stoma prolapse and stoma retraction also may occur if there is undue pressure on the stoma from an appliance or from edema or scar formation. Specific skin problems and use of products are discussed with the patient at this time. Discharge teaching may be an overwhelming task for a patient who is emotionally and physically drained from the events of surgery. Scheduling short visits with repetition is the most reliable method of teaching. Readiness to learn has the greatest impact on ostomy teaching.

Body image and sexuality concerns are discussed preoperatively and postoperatively. Signs of difficulty in dealing with the new ostomy may include failure to look at the stoma, making remarks about the stoma, or not permitting the significant other to assist with care of the appliance. Common concerns are fear of rejection, shame, a sense of disfigurement, and concerns of others' reactions. Continued feelings of low self-esteem lead to depression, withdrawal, and sexual dysfunction.[10,34,38] An ostomy visitor with a similar background may provide the additional support and encouragement needed at this time. Meeting a person who is able to work and continue with outside activities provides the patient with a positive outlook and encouragement.

Sexual counseling begins while the patient is in the hospital. A discussion about sexuality concerns ultimately includes the spouse or significant other.[10] Suggestions to assist couples to deal with sexuality issues should begin with open communication and gradual introduction of sexual activity. Body image concerns may be dealt with by the use of pouch covers, nightgowns and shirts, or other methods to conceal the ostomy until the patient is comfortable with the issue. Altered sexual positions that are more comfortable and less traumatic on the stoma should also be discussed. Patients with abdominoperineal resections require referrals for further counseling, since 30% to 100% of all men with this surgery experience erectile impotence. Damage to the parasympathetic nerve and loss of sensation have a severe impact on sexual performance. Referral to a urologist for a semirigid or inflatable penile implant is necessary if the patient finds he is unable to perform sexually and desires further medical intervention. Research on females with abdominoperineal resections is not conclusive, but reports include changes in sensation that alter the orgasmic process.[10]

Rehabilitation

Rehabilitation of the patient with colorectal cancer requires the combined efforts of several professionals. Physical, emotional, and spiritual concerns must be met to return the patient to the preoperative state of functioning. The ultimate goal of rehabilitation is to provide patients with the knowledge and support to reach their maximum capabilities within the limits of their condition. The United Ostomy Association and ACS can provide additional support and information for the patient and family. Additional referrals for counseling to deal with emotional and sexual concerns may also be necessary for long-term support. The availability of an enterostomal therapist and adequate access to ostomy supplies are additional supports for those patients who have had ostomy surgery.

RADIATION THERAPY
NURSING DIAGNOSES
- *Skin integrity, impaired, risk for, related to effects of radiation treatment*
- *Diarrhea related to treatment side effects*
- *Fluid volume deficit, risk for, related to nausea and vomiting*
- *Health maintenance, altered, related to knowledge deficit regarding radiation side effects*

OUTCOME GOALS

Patient will be able to:
- Maintain skin integrity without complications.
- Have normal bowel evacuation in 1 to 3 days.
- Control nausea and vomiting without evidence of fluid and electrolyte loss.
- Verbalize knowledge of side effects of radiation therapy.

INTERVENTIONS

Patients receiving radiation therapy to the abdominal cavity require emotional and physical support throughout their treatment. Preradiation instruction reviews the frequency and length of treatments, skin markings and their care, and potential side effects and their management. Patients who have an ostomy may need additional information about skin care to their stomas. Side effects experienced by patients receiving abdominal radiation include nausea, vomiting, diarrhea, cystitis, sexual dysfunction, bone marrow suppression, local skin reaction, and fatigue (see box below).[48]

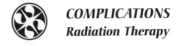

COMPLICATIONS
Radiation Therapy

Skin irritation
Proctitis
Nausea/vomiting
Cystitis
Sexual dysfunction
Bone marrow suppression
Fatigue

Nausea and vomiting are of particular concern to patients receiving radiation therapy over the abdominal area. This is primarily related to the destruction of the epithelial lining of the bowel wall. The toxic waste production from cellular destruction produces increased stimuli to the nausea receptors in the medulla. Prolonged nausea and vomiting may produce weight loss and dehydration. Appropriate nursing measures include use of antiemetics 1 to 2 hours before radiation therapy and up to 12 hours after each treatment. Small, frequent meals are encouraged, with high protein and liquid supplements if needed. Weight, dietary intake, and hydration status should be monitored weekly. For patients with an ostomy, significant weight loss causes stoma shrinkage. Measurement of the stoma and pouch sizes may be needed.[15]

Diarrhea is another common symptom. It begins about 1 or 2 weeks after the start of radiation treatment and is caused by the rapid proliferation of the epithelial cells in the intestinal wall. Patients experiencing diarrhea should be instructed to eat low-residue, high-protein, high-carbohydrate diets. Fluids high in potassium are encouraged; milk products are discouraged. Antidiarrheal products are effective in controlling diarrhea. Patients are instructed to record the number and consistency of bowel movements. Rectal irritation from bowel movements or from radiation therapy to the rectum requires sitz baths, topical creams, and assessment by the radiologist and enterostomal therapist. Ostomy patients require increased pouch changes, assessment of peristomal skin, and use of a skin barrier to protect their skin. Severe excoriation of the peristomal skin requires a referral to the enterostomal therapist or the discontinuation of treatments until symptoms subside.[15]

Abdominal radiation causes inflammation of the bladder, resulting in symptoms of cystitis, burning, back pain, hematuria, and foul-smelling urine. Instructions should be given on increasing fluid intake to 2 to 3 quarts of liquids per day and limiting caffeine products. Urine cultures, sensitivity specimens, and monitoring intake and output may be necessary.

Sexual dysfunction occurs for a variety of emotional and physical reasons. Changes in self-concept, decreased libido, impotence, fertility concerns, and vaginal lining changes may all occur as a result of radiation therapy. Instructions include alternative forms of sexual contact, use of a water-based lubricant, and appropriate referrals for severe sexual concerns and fertility issues.

Bone marrow suppression may also occur because of the proximity of the radiation dose to the treatment site and the pelvic bones. The significance of suppression depends on the length of treatment cycles, number of treatments, and total dose delivered. Patients are monitored for fatigue, infection, bleeding, and fever. Weekly laboratory studies should be obtained. Patient instructions include prudent handwashing to minimize the potential for infection.

Local skin reactions may occur at any time, resulting from the destruction of epithelial tissue. Reactions include itchy, dry skin, darkened areas near the radiation site, and mild excoriation. Patients are instructed to avoid excessive heat or cold and not to use creams or lotions near the treatment site. Only skin products applied by the radiologist should be used because an increased skin reaction occurs with nonprescribed creams.

Patients with ostomies experience increased radiation dermatitis near the peristomal skin site because of the direct exposure of mucous membrane to treatment field. Pouches are often removed before treatments and cause the patient increased concern about skin exposure. Assessment of the peristomal skin is done at this time. Careful skin cleansing and skin barriers assist with adequate protection. Severely excoriated areas require additional creams or powders near the stoma site. A referral to the enterostomal therapist should always be made if the skin condition worsens. Treatments are often delayed if symptoms progress.

CHEMOTHERAPY
NURSING DIAGNOSES

- *Knowledge deficit related to potential chemotherapy side effects*
- *Oral mucous membrane, altered, related to side effects of chemotherapy drugs*
- *Nutrition, altered: less than body requirements, related to nausea and vomiting*
- *Infection, risk for, related to altered immune status*
- *Injury, risk for, related to change in clotting factor*
- *Diarrhea related to chemotherapy side effects*
- *Self-esteem disturbance related to hair loss and body changes*

OUTCOME GOALS

Patient will be able to:
- Verbalize knowledge of chemotherapy side effects.
- Maintain normal mucous membranes.
- Maintain body weight within 10% of pretherapy state.
- Be free of infection and have temperature within normal limits.
- Maintain normal platelet count.
- Maintain normal bowel evacuation pattern of 1 to 3 days.
- Verbalize changes in body image and methods to promote self-esteem.

INTERVENTIONS

Patients receiving chemotherapy for colorectal cancer may be treated with a single or multidrug protocol as well as a combination of chemotherapy, radiation, and biotherapy. Side effects are usually dose, drug, and patient

Continued.

specific. General side effects include nausea, vomiting, diarrhea, and myelosuppression. (See Table 7-4 for specific drugs and their side effects.)

Nursing measures include adequate instructions on potential drug side effects. Diarrhea is of particular concern to the ostomy patient because skin breakdown may easily occur. Use of a protective barrier and additional paste or powder may be necessary. Recording the number and consistency of stools is of vital importance to assess hydration status. Small, frequent, high-protein meals rich in potassium are encouraged. Antidiarrheal agents may become necessary if bowel movements are too frequent.[15]

Constipation is treated with fluids, stool softeners, laxatives, and irrigations of the stoma if necessary. Mucositis is also found around the peristomal skin and the stoma itself. Bowel drainage from infused chemotherapy agents requires the use of protective skin barriers, careful pouch changes, and proper skin cleansing. Fungal infections near the stoma site may also result from prolonged myelosuppression. Antifungal powders near the peristomal skin assist in wound healing. Local trauma

from low platelet counts may also be experienced near the stoma. Careful pouch removal is necessary to avoid trauma.[15]

Nausea and vomiting cause excessive weight loss that changes stoma size. This often requires a pouch change or size variance. Consultation for the appropriate pouch should be done before any significant changes.

Body image and self-esteem disturbances require emotional support to deal with the additional body changes of hair loss and ostomy formation. Support groups and counseling should be provided for these individuals.

Specialized treatment of metastatic liver cancer may be accomplished with an infusion pump. The Medtronics Infusion Pump allows patients increased freedom from hospitalization but requires extensive patient teaching concerning the pump's placement and management. Its placement is a surgical procedure; a disk-shaped pump is placed into a subcutaneous pocket, allowing access to the hepatic artery. The pump contains an access port, a chamber for the fluid to be infused, and a chamber filled with fluorocarbon. The vapor pressure of fluorocarbon at normal body temperature results in expan-

---

 PATIENT TEACHING PRIORITIES
Colorectal Cancer

SURGERY (PREOPERATIVE CARE)

Turning, coughing, deep breathing
Wound splinting
Ambulation
Pain management
Pouch application
Bowel preparation
Postoperative complications

CHEMOTHERAPY

Drug name/regimen
Side effects
Complications
Follow-up schedule

CULTURE

Relationships
Communication
Values
Sexual concerns
Food habits
Health care beliefs
Teaching/learning process
Religious concerns
Body image
Pain
Death/dying beliefs

SURGERY (POSTOPERATIVE CARE)

Ostomy and skin care
Pouch application
Diet modifications
Complications
Sexuality issues
Rehabilitation
Community support

RADIATION

Treatment schedule
Side effects
Skin care
Dietary constraints

COMMUNITY

Availability of enterostomal therapist services, hospital, clinics, ostomy supplier
Support groups
Home care agencies
Housing (privacy/bathroom facilities)
Acceptance of differences
Family resources (financial/emotional/physical availability)
Transportation resources
Rehabilitation resources
Community screening programs

sion of the pump and release of the chemotherapeutic drug (see Figure 20-9).[3] Postoperative complications include development of a seroma, an accumulation of sterile fluid in the pump pocket. Seromas may require draining. Infections may also occur within the pocket site and may require surgical removal of the pump. Percutaneous access is employed to fill the pump on a 2- to 4-week schedule. Each patient's schedule will vary. FUDR and a heparin solution are infused every 2 weeks. Between the doses of FUDR, a solution of normal saline and heparin is used to keep the pump open. Access to the pump for filling is done by a perfusion scan and injection of radioactive material to assist with proper placement.

NURSING DIAGNOSIS

• *Knowledge deficit related to care of infusion pump and management of side effects from pump*

OUTCOME GOALS

Patient will be able to:
• Explain correct use and care of infusion pump.
• Verbalize knowledge of the management of side effects from infusion pump placement and use.

Specific teaching concerning the pump includes understanding its use and particular filling schedule. Side effects of FUDR must also be discussed and managed. Common side effects include nausea, vomiting, abdominal pain, diarrhea, fatigue, and chemical hepatitis. Symptoms are treated systemically except for hepatitis, which requires the removal of the drug from the pump. Patients must also be instructed to avoid blunt trauma to the pump site and to limit exposure to extremes of temperature and altitude, which may interfere with drug administration. The effect of intraarterial chemotherapy and its effectiveness in hepatic metastasis are still under evaluation.

Continued patient teaching is needed to support the patient with colorectal cancer through the postoperative course and through various treatment modalities. The box, p. 136, summarizes teaching implications for these patients.

GERIATRIC CONSIDERATIONS

Special considerations should be given to the elderly population, who may demonstrate a lack of awareness of increased risk factors, signs and symptoms, and recommended screening for colorectal cancer. Awareness of the ACS guidelines and the availability of community screening programs are imperative to early diagnosis. Once a diagnosis is made and treatment indicated, the elderly patient may experience increased side effects from preexisting medical conditions and lack of physical stamina to tolerate aggressive therapy.

Postoperatively, elderly patients are at increased risk for pulmonary, circulatory, and bowel complications. Additional treatment modalities of radiation and chemotherapy impose further complications of fluid and electrolyte imbalance, infection, and skin concerns. Monitoring the immune and nutritional status of this population is essential.

Postoperative teaching of elderly patients may also require added time to allow for any vision and hearing impairment as well as dexterity with pouch applications. Community resources and referrals should be made to assist with physical and financial support. The box below summarizes geriatric considerations.[45]

GERIATRIC CONSIDERATIONS
Colorectal Cancer

Education needs
Awareness of screening recommendations
Knowledge of signs and symptoms
Understanding of risk factors

Treatment complications
Surgery
  Pulmonary
  Circulatory
  Bowel

Chemotherapy and radiation
  Fluid and electrolyte imbalance
  Infection
  Skin impairment

Teaching concerns
  Vision/hearing impairment
  Dexterity for pouch applications

Community resources
  Financial/home care referral

■ CHAPTER QUESTIONS

1. Risk factors for colorectal cancer include:
   a. High alcohol intake
   b. History of constipation
   c. Abnormal bowel habits
   d. Combination of factors, including diet, genetics, and predisposing factors such as bowel disorders
2. Reduced dietary fiber promotes carcinogenic changes by:
   a. Increasing the contact time of carcinogenic substances with the colonic mucosa
   b. Promoting growth of polyps
   c. Promoting constipation concerns
   d. Reabsorbing fluids
3. The American Cancer Society recommendations for colon cancer screening include:
   a. Digital rectal examination every year
   b. Proctosigmoidoscopy every year for patients over age 50
   c. Need for persons at high risk to increase screening at an earlier age than the normal population
   d. Colonoscopy examinations for every rectal bleeding episode
4. The primary location for presentation of colorectal cancer is the:
   a. Rectum
   b. Descending colon
   c. Transverse colon
   d. Ascending colon
5. Late symptoms of colorectal cancer include:
   a. Change in bowel habits
   b. Blood in the stool
   c. Weight loss
   d. Anorexia
6. Treatment modalities for colon and metastatic liver cancer include all *except* which of the following?
   a. Intraarterial infusion of FUDR
   b. Local infusion of FUDR
   c. Radiation therapy, including intraoperative therapy
   d. Surgical dissection
7. Appropriate immediate postoperative nursing diagnoses for a patient with colon cancer and a bowel resection include all *except* which of the following?
   a. Pain
   b. Impaired skin integrity
   c. Sexual dysfunction
   d. Risk for infection
8. Home care teaching for surgical interventions includes all *except* which of the following?
   a. Dietary modifications
   b. Alterations in sexual functioning
   c. Management of skin integrity concerns
   d. Management of chemotherapy-related side effects
9. Complications of abdominal radiation include:
   a. Constipation
   b. Urinary retention
   c. Cystitis
   d. Appetite increase
10. Considerations for patient teaching include all *except* which of the following:
    a. Cultural variations
    b. Community resources
    c. Age differences
    d. Genetic variances

BIBLIOGRAPHY

1. American Cancer Society: *Cancer facts and figures—1995,* Atlanta, 1996, The Society.
2. Baltzer L, Berkery R: *Oncology pocket guide to chemotherapy,* St Louis, 1995, Mosby.
3. Buchwald H: Implantable pump: recent progress and anticipated future advances, *ASAIO J* 38(4):772, 1992.
4. Clark JC, Gwin RR: An overview of cancers in bowel and bladder diversion, *Progressions* 4:15, 1992.
5. Cohen A, Minsky B, Schilsky R. Colon cancer. In DeVita VT, Hellman S, Rosenberg SA, editors, *Cancer: principles and practice of oncology,* ed 4, Philadelphia, 1993, Lippincott.
6. Cohen A, Winaner S: *Cancer of the colon and rectum and anus,* St Louis, 1995, McGraw-Hill.
7. Corman M: *Colon and rectal surgery,* Philadelphia, 1993, Lippincott.
8. Decrosse J, Tsioulias G, Jacobson J: Colorectal cancer detection, treatment, and rehabilitation, *CA Cancer J Clin* 44:1, 1994.
9. Fazio VW: Surgery of colonic carcinoma techniques, *Semin Colon Rectal Surg* 2:36, 1991.
10. Fogel CL, Lauber D: *Sexual health promotion,* Philadelphia, 1990, Saunders.
11. Fong Y, Blumgart L, Cohen A: Surgical treatment of colorectal cancer and metastasis to the liver, *CA Cancer J Clin* 45:1, 1995.
12. Garland CF, Garland FC, Gorham ED: Can colorectal incidence and death rates be reduced with calcium and vitamin D? *Am J Clin Nutr* 54:1935, 1994.
13. Greenwald P, Witkin KM: Large bowel cancer: policy prevention research and treatment. In Rozen P, Reich CB, Winaner SJ, editors: *Frontiers of gastrointestinal research,* New York, 1991, Karger.
14. Hampton B: Gastrointestinal cancer, colon, rectum, anus. In Baird S, McCorkle R, Grant M, editors: *Cancer nursing,* ed 3, Philadelphia, 1991, Saunders.
15. Hampton B, Bryant R: *Ostomies and continent diversions: nursing management,* St Louis, 1992, Mosby.
16. Harrison LB, Enker WE, Anderson LL: High-dose-rate intraoperative radiation therapy for colorectal cancer. Parts I and II, *Oncology* 9:679, 1995.
17. Jagelman DG: Choice of operation and familial adenomatous polyposis, *World J Surg* 15:47, 1991.
18. Kemp C: *Terminal illness: a guide to nursing care,* Philadelphia, 1995, Lippincott.
19. Kritechvsky D: Diet and nutrition, *CA Cancer J Clin* 41:328, 1991.
20. Kurtz R, Lightdall C, Ginsber R: Specialized techniques of cancer management and diagnosis. In DeVita VT, Hellman S,

Rosenberg SA, editors: *Cancer: principles and practice of oncology,* ed 4, Philadelphia, 1993, Lippincott.

21. Levin B, Murphy CP: Revision in American Cancer Society recommendations for early detection of colorectal cancer, *CA Cancer J Clin* 42, 1992.

22. Loescheneril L: Genetics in cancer prediction, screening and counseling. Part I, *Oncol Nurs Forum* 22:2, 1995.

23. Lydon J: Metastasis. Part I. Biology and prevention. In *Oncology nursing: patient treatment and support,* Philadelphia, 1995, Lippincott-Raven.

24. MacDonald JS, Schnall SF: The role of 5-FU plus levamisole in therapy of colon cancer, *PPO Updates* 5, 1991.

25. *Manual of staging cancer,* Philadelphia, 1992, Lippincott.

26. Mahon S: Using brochures to educate the public about early detection of prostate and colorectal cancer, *Oncol Nurs Forum* 22:9, 1995.

27. Moertel CG: Chemotherapy for colorectal cancer, *N Engl J Med* 330, 1994.

28. Neiderhuber T, Ensminger W: Treatment of metastatic disease. In DeVita VT, Hellman S, Rosenberg SA, editors: *Cancer: principles and practice of oncology,* ed 4, Philadelphia, 1993, Lippincott.

29. Parker S and others: Cancer statistics, 1996, *CA Cancer J Clin* 46:1, 1996.

30. *Radiation therapy and your guide to self help during treatment,* No 91:10, Bethesda, Md, 1990, National Cancer Institute.

31. Rhedune A, Gooding BA: Social support, coping strategies, and long-term adaptation to ostomy among self-help members, *J Enterostom Ther* 18:11, 1991.

32. Roncucci LR and others: Antioxidant vitamins or lactulose for prevention of the recurrence of colorectal adenomas, *Dis Colon Rectum* 36(3):227, 1993.

33. Salvadalena GB: An enterostomal therapy nursing data base for use with ostomy surgery patients, *J Enterostom Ther* 18:100, 1991.

34. Schalz J: Cultural expressions affecting patients' care, *Dimens Oncol Nurs* 4:16, 1990.

35. Schilsky RL, Brachman DG: Adjuvant chemotherapy and radiation therapy in colorectal cancer care, *PPO Updates* 6:1, 1992.

36. Selby JV: How should we screen for colorectal cancer? *JAMA* 274(14):1294, 1996.

37. Shank A, Minsky B, Freidman M: Rectal cancer. In DeVita VT, Hellman S, Rosenberg SA, editors: *Cancer: principles and practice of oncology,* ed 4, Philadelphia, 1993, Lippincott.

38. Shell JA: The psychosexual impact of ostomy surgery, *Progressions* 4:4, 1992.

39. Soloman MS, McLeod RS: Screen strategies for colorectal cancer, *Surg Clin North Am* 73(1):31, 1993.

40. Steele W and others: Adenocarcinoma of the colon and rectum. In Holland J and others: *Cancer medicine,* Philadelphia, ed 3, 1993, Lea & Febiger.

41. Strohl RA: Colorectal cancer. In Clark JC, McGee RF, editors: *Core curriculum for oncology nursing,* ed 2, Philadelphia, 1992, Saunders.

42. Tepper J: Intraoperative radiation strategies. In Cohen A, Winaner S, editors: *Cancer of the colon and rectum and anus,* St Louis, 1995, McGraw-Hill.

43. Torosian MH, Daley JM: An evaluation of the clinical usefulness of CEA in colorectal cancer, *Oncology* 5:41, 1991.

44. Wadler S: The treatment of advanced colorectal carcinoma, *Oncoline* 6:1, 1991.

45. Weinrich SP and others: Knowledge of colorectal cancer among older adults, *Cancer Nurs* 15(5):332, 1992.

46. Weisburger JH and others: Dietary fat intake and cancer, *Hematol Oncol Clin North Am* 5(1):7, 1991.

47. Wingo P, Tong T, Bolden S: Cancer statistics, 1995, *CA Cancer J Clin* 45(1):8, 1995.

48. Yasko J: *Care of the client receiving radiation therapy,* Reston, Va, 1982, Reston-Hall.

49. Zanca JA: If people understood what to do, they'll do it, *Cancer Nurs* 10:1, 1992.

CHAPTER 8

Gastrointestinal Cancers

BETTY THOMAS DANIEL

Gastrointestinal (GI) cancers accounted for 21% of the new cases of cancer diagnosed in the United States in 1996 and 23% of the cancer deaths in the same period. This represents a total of 222,500 new cases and 125,410 cancer deaths.[46] Progress has been made in treating some of the GI cancers, but others remain difficult to control. Symptoms of many of these cancers are vague and nonspecific until advanced disease develops, which makes treatment difficult and long-term survival rates low. However, prevention and early detection can reduce the impact of the disease and prolong survival.

Nurses have an important role to play in the prevention, early detection, diagnosis, and treatment of GI cancers. In some instances, prevention and early detection are not possible, but knowledge of the course of disease may improve the patient's quality of life.

CANCER OF THE ESOPHAGUS

EPIDEMIOLOGY

Cancer of the esophagus is a fairly uncommon cancer in the United States, but its incidence varies greatly throughout the world. It is considered endemic in the Lin Xian region of central China and along the east coast of southern Africa, where its incidence is reported to be as high as 50 cases per 100,000 men.[20] In the United States the estimated number of new cases in 1996 was 12,300, and 11,200 of these patients will die of their disease.[46] Esophageal cancer is most common in elderly males, and the male-to-female ratio is approximately 3:1.[23] The incidence and mortality rates are more than three times higher among blacks than whites.[7]

ETIOLOGY AND RISK FACTORS

Although the etiology of esophageal cancer is not well defined, some identified risk factors are associated with chronic irritation of the esophagus. In the United States and Western Europe, smoking and alcohol ingestion are the most prominent factors.[26] In some Asian countries and South America, the consumption of hot tea and a hot beverage called *mate* have been identified as risk factors. Other factors that are implicated include a previous history of squamous cell carcinoma of the head and neck, a diet high in nitrosamines, the presence of Barrett's esophagus, a history of lye ingestion, esophageal achalasia, Plummer-Vinson syndrome, tylosis, and a variety of nutritional deficiencies.[20,23,26,37]

PREVENTION, SCREENING, AND DETECTION

Prevention of the disease focuses on counseling regarding alcohol and tobacco use and instructing patients with risk factors to report any problems with *dysphagia* (difficulty in swallowing) or *odynophagia* (pain on swallowing). These patients must be evaluated immediately so that any cancer present may be diagnosed as early as possible.[37] In areas where esophageal cancer is endemic, mass screening by brushing techniques is feasible, but in the United States the incidence of the disease does not justify this approach.

CLASSIFICATION

The most common types of esophageal carcinomas are squamous cell carcinoma (60%) and adenocarcinoma (35%).[35] *Squamous cell carcinomas* arise from the surface epithelium and are found most often in the middle and lower esophagus. *Adenocarcinomas* most often occur in the lower third of the esophagus and probably arise from the gastric fundus. They are rarely found in the upper and middle esophagus. Fewer than 1% of all esophageal tumors are sarcomas.[23]

CLINICAL FEATURES

Dysphagia and weight loss are the most common presenting symptoms of this disease, occurring in 90% of patients.[49] Many of the patients do not seek medical at-

CLINICAL FEATURES
Advanced Carcinoma of Esophagus

Pain radiating to back on swallowing
Dysphonia (laryngeal paralysis)
Diaphragmatic paralysis (involvement of phrenic nerve)
Coughing when swallowing (tracheoesophageal fistula)
Superior vena cava syndrome
Palpable supraclavicular or cervical nodes
Malignant pleural effusion
Malignant ascites
Bone pain

From DeVita V and others, editors: *Cancer: principles and practice of oncology,* ed 4, Philadelphia, 1993, Lippincott.

TNM SYSTEM FOR CLASSIFICATION AND STAGING OF ESOPHAGEAL CANCER

PRIMARY TUMOR (T)

T1: tumor invading lamina propria or submucosa
T2: tumor invading muscularis propria
T3: tumor invading adventitia
T4: tumor invading adjacent structures

REGIONAL LYMPH NODES (N)

N0: no regional lymph node metastasis
N1: regional lymph node metastasis

DISTANT METASTASIS (M)

M0: no distant metastasis
M1: distant metastasis

STAGE GROUPING

Stage I: T1-N0-M0
Stage IIA: T2-N0-M0
         T3-N0-M0
Stage IIB: T1-N1-M0
         T2-N1-M0
Stage III: T3-N1-M0
         T4-any N-M0
Stage IV: any T-any N-M1

tention at first, but instead adjust their diets to soft and then to liquid foods. Odynophagia is present in about 50% of patients.[49] A 40- to 50-pound (18 to 22 kg) weight loss over 2 to 3 months may occur before the patient is seen by a physician. Because of this delay, most patients present with advanced disease. The symptoms of advanced disease usually result from the invasion or involvement of surrounding organs and structures (see box above).

DIAGNOSIS AND STAGING

All patients complaining of dysphagia should be tested by a barium swallow and an upper GI endoscopy.[37] Esophageal tumors have a characteristic irregular, ragged mucosal pattern with narrowing of the lumen.[23] Endoscopy is required to confirm the presence of a malignant tumor. Biopsies and brushings can be obtained through the endoscope to confirm the diagnosis. Endoscopic ultrasonography may be used to identify invasion of the tumor into the tissue layers and involvement of lymph nodes to aid in staging of disease. The use of chromoscopy, a staining technique, is helpful in identifying areas for biopsy during endoscopic procedures. Computed tomography (CT) provides information about the enlargement of lymph nodes and involvement of neighboring organs.[37]

The American Joint Committee on Cancer's tumor, node, metastasis (TNM) staging system is used for staging both cervical and thoracic esophageal carcinomas (see box above, right).

METASTASIS

Esophageal cancer can spread to almost any part of the body, but distant metastases usually are not present on initial diagnosis. However, they are almost always found

during autopsy. Primary sites of metastasis include the liver, lung, stomach, peritoneum, kidney, adrenal gland, brain, and bone.[49] Cancer of the esophagus is characterized by extensive invasion of local or adjacent tissue and organs. The aorta and trachea are threatened by this invasion, exacerbating the poor prognosis of these patients.

TREATMENT MODALITIES

The most effective approach to the treatment of esophageal cancer is a combined-modality therapy. Chemotherapy with surgery or radiation therapy appears to be the most promising approach. Frequently, the patient's weakened cardiopulmonary status makes him or her a poor surgical risk.[49] Metastasis to the liver, peritoneum, or neck glands is often considered a contraindication to radical surgery.[30]

Surgery

The choice of surgical approach to an *esophagogastrectomy* and *esophagogastrostomy* depends on the tumor's extent and location. Lesions involving the esophagogastric junction or lower thoracic esophagus are approached by a left thoracotomy (Figure 8-1). For lesions of the upper esophagus, a total esophagectomy using an upper midline incision and right thoracotomy (Ivor Lewis) or a transhiatal approach may be used (Figures 8-2 and 8-3).

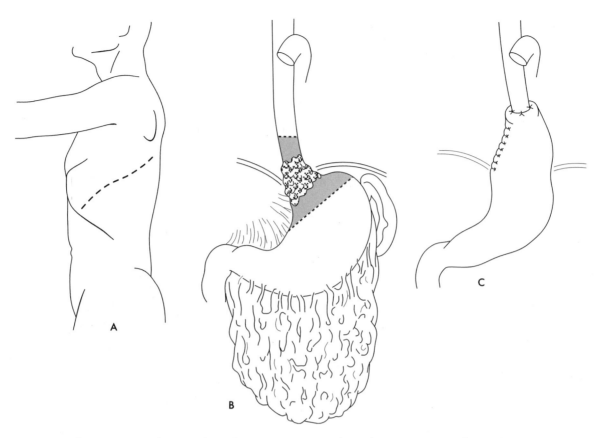

Figure 8-1   Technique of esophagogastrectomy and esophagogastrostomy for carcinoma of cardia. **A,** Site of incision; **B,** extent of resection *(shaded area)*; **C,** completed esophagogastrostomy. (From Ellis HF Jr, Shahlan DM: Tumors of the esophagus. In Glenn WWL and others, editors: *Thoracic and cardiovascular surgery,* ed 4, East Norwalk, Conn, 1983, Appleton & Lange.)

The *transhiatal approach* has been used for lesions at every level of the esophagus. If the patient has had a surgical procedure involving the stomach, or if the tumor extends so far as to require a total esophagectomy, the esophagus must be reconstructed using a portion of the small or large intestine. The left colon is most commonly used (Figure 8-4).

Radiation Therapy

Both squamous cell carcinoma and adenocarcinoma of the esophagus are sensitive to radiation therapy, which is used most often as palliation for obstruction and for pain control for patients who are not candidates for surgical procedures.[39] Unfortunately, this relief is short term for more than 50% of the patients.[49] Radiation therapy is seldom used as a primary therapy, since a course of treatment usually lasts 6 to 8 weeks and median survival for these patients is only a few months. Patients offered radiation therapy alone are those with widespread metastasis, advanced and obstructing tumors, or a poor functional status that does not permit combined-modality therapy.[37]

Both preoperative and postoperative radiation therapy are typically used. Preoperative radiation therapy is used to reduce large tumors to a resectable size and to decrease the risk of dissemination of viable cancer cells during surgical manipulation.[42] Postoperative radiation therapy is used to eliminate microscopic disease and reduce local tumor. Results of clinical trials show that relapse occurs in at least 80% of patients treated with combined therapy, again making palliation an important application of radiation therapy.[28]

Chemotherapy

Single-agent chemotherapy has shown some effectiveness in treating squamous cell carcinoma but not in adenocarcinoma of the esophagus and cardia.[37] Both patients with local disease and patients with advanced disease respond to single-agent or combination chemotherapy, but the response duration is measured only in

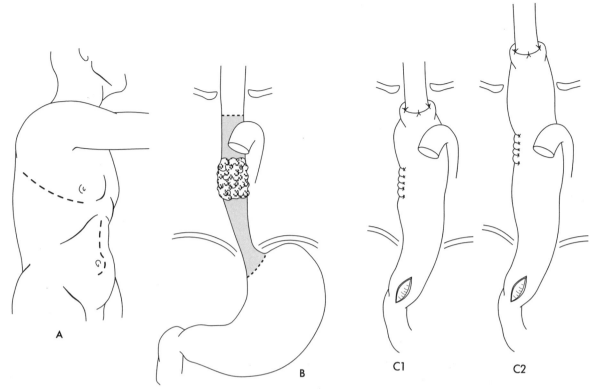

Figure 8-2   Esophagogastrectomy with thoracoabdominal approach. **A,** Combined abdominal incision and right thoracotomy for lesions of the upper thoracic esophagus; **B,** extent of resection *(shaded area);* **C1,** esophagogastrostomy in the chest; **C2,** if submucosal spread is great, cervical anastomosis can be performed through a third incision. (From Ellis FH Jr: Esophagogastrectomy for carcinoma: technical considerations based on anatomic location of lesion, *Surg Clin North Am* 60:273, 1980.)

months.[34] *Cisplatin* appears to be the most effective agent, and many of the combination protocols are based on this drug. Other frequently used agents, both as single agents and in combination, include bleomycin, mitomycin, doxorubicin, methotrexate, and 5-fluorouracil (5-FU).[49]

The chemotherapy may be given before surgery or radiation therapy. Preoperative *(neoadjuvant)* chemotherapy may provide the advantages of enhancing surgical outcome by reducing the tumor burden, minimizing the probability of developing drug resistance, and allowing in vivo evaluation of the effectiveness of the agents given.[48] Adverse side effects depend on the agents used and may include nausea, vomiting, myelosuppression, nephrotoxicity, and peripheral neuropathy.

A number of studies have used concurrent neoadjuvant chemotherapy and radiation therapy. The purpose of preoperative radiation therapy is to control local recurrence while improving the resectability of the primary tumor. The purpose of chemotherapy is to eliminate metastatic disease. A large percentage of

esophageal cancer patients die of metastatic disease, but most have local/regional recurrence as well, which explains the increase in the number of clinical trials of preoperative chemoradiotherapy.[2] Researchers have learned that not only does thoracic radiation therapy control local recurrence, but a number of the chemotherapeutic agents used to treat esophageal cancer, such as 5-FU and cisplatin, act to potentiate the effect of radiation as well. However, patterns of failure in the reported trials show that the majority of patients had only distant disease. This leads researchers to believe that a more intensive chemotherapy component in multimodality therapies is needed.[2]

The box, p. 144, summarizes potential treatment-related complications of esophageal cancer.

PROGNOSIS

The prognosis for persons with esophageal cancer is very poor. From 1986 to 1991, the 5-year survival rate reported was 11% for whites and 7% for blacks.[46] Therefore 90% to 95% of patients are in need of palliative care

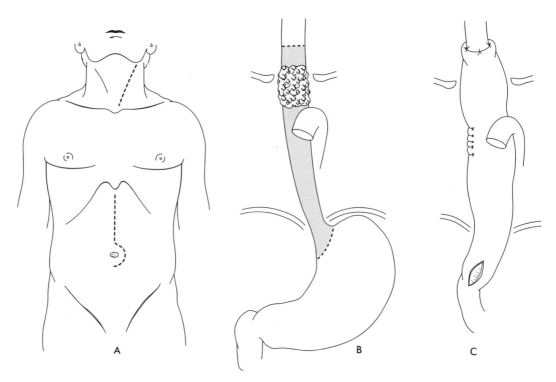

Figure 8-3 Transhiatal approach (esophagectomy without thoracotomy). **A,** Upper midline and left cervical incision; **B,** extent of resection; **C,** completed anastomosis. (From Ellis FH Jr: Esophagogastrectomy for carcinoma: technical considerations based on anatomic location of lesion, *Surg Clin North Am* 60:276, 1980.)

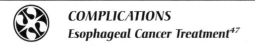

COMPLICATIONS
Esophageal Cancer Treatment[47]

After esophageal resection

Respiratory insufficiency
Congestive heart failure
Pulmonary embolism
Wound infection or dehiscence
Obstruction at esophageal hiatus
Ruptured spleen
Phlebitis
Subphrenic abscess
Torsion, gangrene, or rupture of GI replacement
Hemorrhage
Anastomotic leak and strictures

Related to radiation therapy

Radiation pneumonitis
Pericarditis
Myocarditis
Spinal cord damage
Stricture
Fistula formation
Hemorrhage

at diagnosis or shortly thereafter. The major problems experienced by patients with advanced disease include dysphagia, chest pain, and malnutrition.[11] Palliative surgery is not always an option; alternatives include peroral dilation, peroral esophageal prosthesis, and laser ablation of obstructing lesions. An investigational treatment for obstructive lesions is *photodynamic therapy* (PDT), in which patients are given a photosensitizer such as dihematoporphyrin ether (DHE), then are treated with light delivered from an argon pump dye laser. This treatment has shown promise as an alternate.[32] These procedures usually allow the patient to continue oral feedings of liquids and possibly soft foods. If the patient develops anorexia or is unable to continue oral feedings, enteral feedings may be used. Percutaneous endoscopic gastrostomy is a low-risk method of placing a feeding tube. It avoids the need for a laparotomy and general anesthesia in severely ill patients.[11] Total parenteral nutrition is usually not used in these patients if another route is possible. Chronic severe mediastinal and posterior chest pain is indicative of regional spread of cancer and is very incapacitating. If the patient is unable to take oral sustained-release analgesics, he or she may require a patient-controlled analgesia (PCA) pump for maximum comfort.

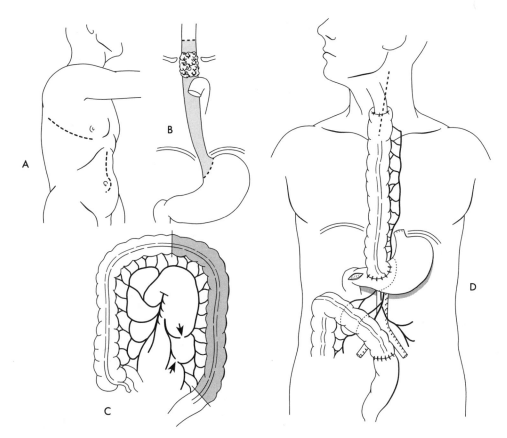

Figure 8-4   Esophagectomy with colon interposition. **A**, Right thoracotomy and midline incision; **B**, extent of resection; **C**, segment of left colon used; **D**, completed resection. (From Ellis FH Jr: Esophagogastrectomy for carcinoma: technical considerations based on anatomic location of lesion, *Surg Clin North Am* 60:277, 1980.)

CANCER OF THE STOMACH

Although cancer of the stomach has shown a significant decline in incidence, about 60% from the 1930s to the 1970s, it remains the eighth most common cause of cancer deaths in the United States.[39] The reason for the decline in incidence in some parts of the world but not in others remains an enigma. It is postulated that the increased consumption of refrigerated foods rather than spiced, smoked, and pickled foods may be a factor.[19] Although the United States reports an incidence of 10 per 100,000 population, Japan's incidence is 90 per 100,000. Iceland and certain parts of Central and South America report incidences similar to that in Japan.[39]

EPIDEMIOLOGY

In the United States an estimated 22,800 new cases of stomach cancer were diagnosed in 1996, and a total of 14,000 deaths were attributed to the disease.[46] Gastric cancer is more common in men than women; the ratio reported is 1.7:1.[35] It is found more often in people between 50 and 70 years of age[35] and is three times more common in semiskilled and unskilled labor groups than in executive and professional groups.[19]

ETIOLOGY AND RISK FACTORS

Several dietary factors have been associated with the development of cancer of the stomach. Immigrant studies show that the second generation of families emigrating from countries of high incidence to low incidence have fewer cases of gastric cancer. This decrease may be attributed to changes in dietary habits. High consumption of smoked or salted foods or foods contaminated with aflatoxin has been associated with increased incidence of stomach cancer.[6]

Occupational risk factors have also been associated with higher incidence of stomach cancer. Workers in coal mining, farming (in Japan), nickel refining (in Russia), rubber processing, timber processing, and asbestos processing have all been shown to have higher than normal

NURSING MANAGEMENT

The nurse can assume a significant role in identifying persons at risk for esophageal cancer and in providing counseling on the signs and symptoms of esophageal cancer, life-style modifications to eliminate or reduce risk factors, and importance of annual health examinations by a health care professional. Because there are few or no early signs of esophageal cancer, other than vague GI symptoms of pressure, indigestion, or heartburn (pyrosis), nurses should be aware of persons who are chronic users of home remedies or over-the-counter medications for GI distress. Nurses should urge these persons to seek medical attention immediately.

NURSING DIAGNOSIS

• *Knowledge deficit regarding prevention and early detection of esophageal cancer related to unfamiliar information*

OUTCOME GOALS

Patient will be able to:
• Identify risk factors associated with development of esophageal cancer.
• Identify measures to minimize risks.
• Identify signs and symptoms to be reported to health care professionals related to early detection of esophageal cancer.

INTERVENTIONS

• Assess for high-risk factors such as heavy alcohol and cigarette use or history of reflux esophagitis, hiatal hernia, or Barrett's esophagus.
• Provide instructions on healthy life-style behaviors:
  —Have annual health examination by a health care professional.
  —Stop use of cigarettes through a smoking cessation program.
  —Eliminate or reduce consumption of alcoholic beverages.
  —Eat balanced diet with adequate portions of recommended food groups.
• Provide instructions to report these signs and symptoms: persistent GI distress (regurgitation, reflux, heartburn, epigastric pain) requiring use of antacids, difficulty swallowing requiring changes in diet, or weight loss.

Many persons with esophageal cancer have had a significant weight loss just before they are diagnosed. They usually are experiencing dysphagia and have had to make some dietary adjustments. Depending on the severity of the dysphagia, they will need to change their oral intake and receive enteral feeding, or even total parenteral nutrition (TPN).

NURSING DIAGNOSIS

• *Nutrition, altered: less than body requirements, related to dysphagia*

OUTCOME GOALS

Patient will be able to:
• Identify signs and symptoms to report to health care professionals.
• Identify measures to obtain adequate nutrition.
• Demonstrate a stable nutritional status.[27]

INTERVENTIONS: *Mild Dysphagia*

• Assess patient for choking or regurgitation during and after meals.
• Obtain dietary consultation for calorie count and dietary modification as needed.
• Weigh patient every other day.
• Instruct patient to sit upright for meals and 30 minutes after meals. If in bed, raise head to at least 45-degree angle.
• Offer six to eight small feedings per day of high-protein, high-calorie liquified foods and nutritional supplements.
• Avoid feedings within 2 hours of bedtime.
• Teach patient to use oral suction if he or she is anxious about aspiration.
• Provide oral and written instructions of measures to maintain stable nutritional status and prevent aspiration.

INTERVENTIONS: *Severe Dysphagia (in Addition to Mild Dysphagia)*

• Monitor food and fluid intake daily.
• Weigh patient daily.
• Assess for fatigue, altered mental status, weight loss of 2 pounds (1 kg) or more, and decreased serum albumin.
• Obtain dietary consultation for alternate routes of nutrition (enteral feedings via nasogastric or gastrostomy tubes or TPN).
• Administer feedings per physician's orders.
• Instruct patient/caregiver to administer feedings.
• Instruct patient/caregiver to provide oral hygiene frequently.
• Instruct patient/caregiver about signs and symptoms to report to health care professionals.

incidence.[6] However, this may be associated with social class rather than the actual occupational hazard.

Familial occurrence of gastric cancer is rare, but a small increase in incidence has been noted in direct relatives of some people who have had gastric cancer. The most notable family with this disease is that of Napolean Bonaparte.[35] It has been reported that diffuse gastric cancer is significantly more common in patients with blood group A, in relatives of patients with diffuse gastric cancer, and in cases of familial hypogammaglobulinemia.[19]

Pathologies or past medical history associated with the development of gastric cancer include gastric polyps, especially the villous adenoma; pernicious anemia; chronic reflux esophagitis; *Helicobacter pylori* infection; and gastric resection for benign peptic ulcer disease.[6] It is suggested that the presence of atrophic gastritis and achlorhydria in persons with pernicious anemia may contribute to the development of gastric cancer.[38]

PREVENTION, SCREENING, AND EARLY DETECTION

The key to prevention of cancer of the stomach lies in dietary intake. As previously indicated, people of geographic areas and socioeconomic groups associated with the lowest incidence consume a diet different from those of highest incidence. Nutrition counseling to prevent gastric cancer should stress the importance of consuming a balanced diet high in fresh fruits and vegetables and moderate in amount of animal protein and fats. Salted, smoked, and pickled foods should be consumed in low quantities.

Screening and early detection programs have been very successful in Japan. Upper GI endoscopic examinations and upper GI series are the techniques used most. The diagnosis of early gastric cancer in Japan increased from 1.3% in 1941 through 1945 to 36% in 1965.[24]

In Western countries, where the incidence of gastric cancer is low, widespread screening programs are not considered useful because of the low yield. It is important, however, to identify persons at high risk and follow them with annual endoscopic examinations. The high-risk group includes those with atrophic gastritis, pernicious anemia, intestinal metaplasia, gastric polyps, familial hypogammaglobulinemia, previous gastric surgery, or dysplasia.[19]

CLASSIFICATION

Adenocarcinomas represent almost 95% of the malignant tumors of the stomach.[6] *Lymphoma* accounts for up to 8%, and *leiomyosarcoma* makes up from 1% to 3%. Other, rarer types of malignant gastric tumors include carcinoids, plasmacytomas, and metastatic cancers.[35]

Several classification systems are used for stomach cancer. One developed by Borrmann identifies five different types of stomach cancer: *type 1* includes polypoid or fungating cancers; *type 2* includes ulcerating lesions with elevated borders; *type 3* includes ulcerating lesions infiltrating the gastric wall; *type 4* includes diffusely infiltrating carcinomas; and *type 5* includes unclassifiable cancers.[6,35,39] Lauren developed the *DIO system,* which identifies two main groups of gastric cancers: diffuse gastric cancer *(D)* and intestinal gastric cancer *(I).* These two groups account for 90% of all stomach cancers; the remainder are referred to as *other (O). Intestinal gastric cancers* are characterized by polypoid or fungating lesions that may ulcerate centrally. *Diffuse gastric cancers* infiltrate the gastric wall without forming large discrete masses and are associated with a very poor prognosis. They are frequently seen in patients with pernicious anemia and familial hypogammaglobulinemia. A classic example is linitis plastica.[19] Broder's classification system is based on degree of histologic differentiation. Tumor cells are graded from *1 (well differentiated)* to *4 (anaplastic).* An example of grade 4 is linitis plastica, typically a poorly differentiated cell type. Polypoid tumors are most likely to have well-differentiated grade 1 tumor cells.[6]

CLINICAL FEATURES

One of gastric cancer's most frustrating aspects is that it has no early symptoms. Most patients present with locally advanced or metastatic disease.[39] The symptoms are vague and may have been present for several months. They include indigestion and epigastric discomfort (which the patient may have been treating with antacids), malaise, early satiety, postprandial fullness, and loss of appetite.[19] Back pain may indicate that the cancer has spread to the pancreas. Dysphagia is associated with lesions in the cardia. Vomiting after meals is seen in obstructing tumors of the middle third and pyloric regions of the stomach.[19] Hematemesis occurs infrequently with gastric carcinoma but may indicate leiomyosarcoma of the stomach.[39]

DIAGNOSIS AND STAGING

Physical examination of the patient suspected of having gastric cancer should include palpation of the abdomen for masses and nodules around the umbilicus. Attention should also be paid to whether the supraclavicular and axillary nodes are enlarged. A digital rectal examination should be performed to assess for the presence of a shelf of metastatic deposits.

The two most useful diagnostic procedures for gastric cancer are the *upper GI endoscopy* and the *double-contrast upper GI series.*[6,19,39] The latter is able to identify the site of the lesion and, with special compression

TNM CLASSIFICATION AND STAGING FOR STOMACH CANCER

PRIMARY TUMOR (T)

T1: tumor invading lamina propria or submucosa

T2: tumor invading muscularis propria or subserosa

T3: tumor penetrating serosa (visceral peritoneum) without invasion of adjacent structures

T4: tumor invading adjacent structures

REGIONAL LYMPH NODES (N)

N0: no regional lymph node metastasis

N1: metastasis in perigastric lymph node(s) within 3 cm of edge of primary tumor

N2: metastasis in perigastric lymph node(s) more than 3 cm from edge of primary tumor or in lymph nodes along left gastric, common hepatic, splenic, or celiac arteries

DISTANT METASTASIS (M)

M0: no distant metastasis

M1: distant metastasis

STAGE GROUPING FOR CANCER OF STOMACH

Stage IA:	T1-N0-M0
Stage IB:	T1-N1-M0
	T2-N0-M0
Stage II:	T1-N2-M0
	T2-N1-M0
	T3-N0-M0
Stage IIIA:	T2-N2-M0
	T3-N1-M0
	T4-N0-M0
Stage IIIB:	T3-N2-M0
	T4-N1-M0
Stage IV:	T4-N2-M0
	any T-any N-M1

techniques, detect depressions and elevations of the gastric mucosa. The fiberoptic gastroscope permits the skilled endoscopist to obtain multiple biopsies of all suspicious lesions and brush cytologic specimens. In patients with a stiffened stomach that insufflates poorly, an exploratory laparotomy is usually indicated to make a diagnosis.[39] CT scans and ultrasonography are helpful in defining sites of metastatic spread, but not the primary tumor. Endoscopic ultrasonography is used to stage gastric cancer and identify the presence of adenopathy.[39]

The box above outlines the American Joint Commission on Cancer's TNM criteria for classification and staging of cancer of the stomach.[9]

METASTASIS

In addition to local extension to nearby organs and tissue, cancer of the stomach metastasizes most frequently to the liver, lungs, bone, and brain. Stomach cancer also spreads to local lymph nodes, Virchow's node in the left supraclavicular area, and the left axillary node (Irish's node). Peritoneal metastasis is also known to occur, and *Krukenburg's tumor* (metastasis to the ovary) is one indication of metastasis to the peritoneum. Another is the identification of periumbilical nodules (Sister Joseph nodes). *Blumer's rectal shelf* is another form of peritoneal metastasis that may be identified by rectal examination. It is described as a stony-hard indurated area of prerectal tumor that feels like a shelf.[39]

COMPLICATIONS
Gastric Cancer Disease and Treatment

DISEASE-RELATED COMPLICATIONS

Pain
Obstruction
Bleeding
Dysphagia

TREATMENT-RELATED COMPLICATIONS

Postoperative Complications[57]

Early	Late
Infection	Dumping syndrome
Hemorrhage	Reflux esophagitis
Acute pancreatitis	Chronic weight loss
Ileus, jaundice	Anemia
Anastomotic leak	Hypoproteinemia

Radiation Therapy Complications

During treatment[14]	Late
Anorexia	Radiation nephritis
Nausea	Hypertension
Vomiting	GI bleeding
Weight loss	Duodenal ulcers

Chemotherapy Complications

Myelosuppression	Alopecia
Stomatitis	Extravasation
Nausea/vomiting	Fatigue
Diarrhea	Nephrotoxic

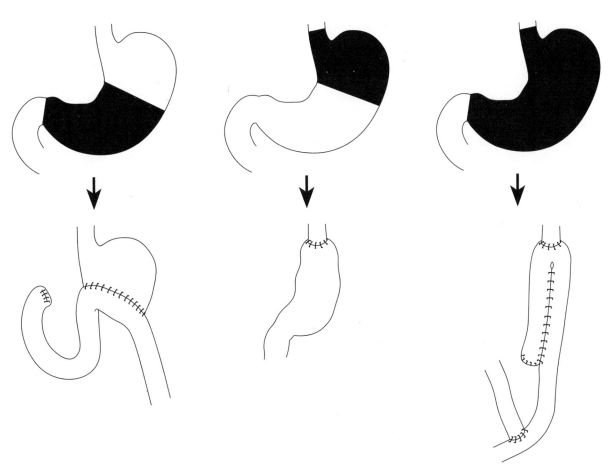

Figure 8-5 Surgical resections and reconstruction for the three locations of gastric cancer. (From Lawrence W Jr: Gastric neoplasms. In Lawrence W Jr, Lenhard RE Jr, Murphy GP, editors: *American Cancer Society textbook of clinical oncology*, ed 2, Atlanta, 1995, American Cancer Society.)

TREATMENT MODALITIES

Surgery, chemotherapy, and radiation therapy are used to treat cancer of the stomach and have potential complications (see box, p. 148).

Surgery

Surgery is the major treatment modality and is used for both cure and palliation. It is recommended that any patient with biopsy-proven gastric cancer and no evidence of distant metastasis should undergo an exploratory laparotomy or celiotomy to determine whether the patient should undergo a curative procedure or a palliative one. Fewer than 40% of patients who have a laparotomy are determined to be curable.[35]

The operative procedure chosen depends on the anatomic location of the tumor and knowledge of the pattern of spread from that particular location.[51] For selection of procedure, the stomach may be divided into thirds. The proximal third includes the gastroesophageal junction and the fundus; the middle third includes the fundus to midsection of the lesser curvature; and the distal third includes the remaining portion to the pylorus.[51] For tumors in the proximal third, choice of surgical procedure remains controversial, but usually either a *radical subtotal gastrectomy*[51] or a *total gastrectomy* is used.[57] Tumors in the middle section usually require a total gastrectomy to obtain tumor-free margins.[51] Tumors located in the distal third are usually treated with a radical subtotal gastrectomy.[51,57] Figure 8-5 illustrates the surgical resections and reconstruction for each procedure.[35]

Chemotherapy

Gastric cancer does seem more responsive to chemotherapy than some of the other malignancies.[29,58] Chemotherapy is now being studied as adjuvant therapy for fully resected tumors, for advanced gastric cancer, and in combination with radiation therapy. One of the older regimens that has been widely studied is *FAM* (5-FU, doxorubicin [Adriamycin], mitomycin-C). It shows a consistent response rate of approximately 35% but has a minimal impact on survival.[29] A newer regimen is *EAP* (etoposide, doxorubicin [Adriamycin], cisplatin [Platinol]). Although this regimen is associated with significant dose-limiting myelosuppression, it has been associated with a significant improvement in survival compared with FAM.[13] A third regimen that is currently showing good responses is *FAMTX* (5-FU, doxorubicin [Adriamycin], high-dose methotrexate, leukovorin rescue). EAP and FAMTX are also being used preoperatively, but it remains unclear whether they significantly affect surgical results.[13]

Radiation Therapy

Radiation therapy is important in the treatment of locally advanced or recurrent gastric cancer. Although radiation therapy has been used alone with some response, it has greatest benefit when combined with chemotherapy.[6] Controversy exists regarding the preferred method of combining radiation with surgery; preoperative, intraoperative, and postoperative schedules have all been proposed. A tolerable dose is 45 to 50 Gy delivered in 1.8 Gy fractions per day.[14] *Intraoperative radiation therapy* (IORT) has been useful in the control of microscopic disease with a maximum tolerated dose of 15 to 20 Gy.[14] The advantage of IORT is that radiosensitive normal tissue can be removed from the field. Combining IORT and postoperative radiation has been studied and may increase the long-term survival of patients with stage II, III, or IV disease.[1] Another method that increases the effectiveness of radiation therapy is administering 5-FU as a radiosensitizer over the first 3 days of the radiation schedule.[40]

PROGNOSIS

The prognosis for patients with gastric cancer depends on the extent of the disease and on the treatment. The 5-year survival rate reported for the period of 1986 to 1991 was 11%.[46] Therefore the prognosis for these patients remains poor. It has been reported that two thirds of patients are not candidates for curative surgery at diagnosis.[35] The only option for these patients is palliative resection of the tumor, which may alleviate the symptoms of obstruction, bleeding, and pain.[51] Patients experiencing dysphagia with tumors of the proximal stomach unable to undergo a resection may benefit temporarily from dilations, laser ablation of tumor, PDT, or placement of an endoprosthesis.[57]

CANCER OF THE LIVER

Hepatocellular carcinoma (HCC) is relatively uncommon in the United States but is one of the most common malignancies in some parts of the world, especially parts of Africa and Asia. There are no effective controls against this disease, and it continues to be rapidly fatal in areas of high incidence.

EPIDEMIOLOGY

For reporting purposes in the United States, HCC is combined with biliary tract cancers (gallbladder carcinoma, cholangiocarcinoma, and periampullary carcinoma). Therefore the incidence data are not completely reliable for primary liver cancer (HCC) alone. The estimated number of new cases of liver and biliary tract cancers in 1996 was 19,900, which resulted in 15,200 deaths.[46] It has been estimated that the number of deaths from HCC is about 4000 annually in the United States; black men have a three times higher risk of getting the disease than women or white men.[4]

This situation is quite different in Asia and Africa. In Mozambique the incidence is 500 times that in the United States. In Japan, HCC is the third leading cause of cancer deaths among men and fifth among women.[4]

ETIOLOGY AND RISK FACTORS

Because of the widespread geographic variations in incidence, researchers have been particularly interested in studying the environmental factors implicated in the development of HCC. The box below summarizes the etiologic and risk factors known to be associated with primary liver cancers. Hepatitis B virus (HBV) and hepatitis C virus (HCV) infections are probably the most important cause worldwide. A positive correlation exists between the presence of hepatitis B surface antigen (HBsAG) in the serum of patients and HCC. HCV is also associated with an increased risk of developing HCC. Hepatitis A virus (HAV), however, does not appear to be related to the development of HCC.[4]

Cirrhosis and alcohol consumption have been associated with the development of HCC. Cirrhosis associated with chronic HBV infection and hemachromatosis is a

---

SUMMARY OF CONDITIONS ASSOCIATED WITH HEPATOCELLULAR CARCINOMA (HCC)

Hepatitis B virus	Aflatoxins
Hepatitis C virus	Alcoholism
Hemochromatosis	Occupational exposure to
Cirrhosis	pesticides and herbicides
Anabolic steroid use	
Immunosuppressive agents	

NURSING MANAGEMENT

As with patients with cancer of the esophagus, patients with cancer of the stomach experience profound weight loss caused by the disease process and the treatment modalities, particularly radical subtotal or total gastrectomy. The preoperative patient assessment should include a nutritional evaluation encompassing a diet and weight loss history (especially the type and consistency of diet consumed), laboratory values (serum albumin, leukocyte count, total iron-binding capacity, ferritin, electrolytes), and calorie intake.[50]

NURSING DIAGNOSIS

• *Nutrition, altered: less than body requirements, related to gastrectomy*

OUTCOME GOALS

Patient will be able to:
• Explain rationale for altered nutrition and factors that contribute to malnourishment.
• Demonstrate measures to manage nutritional status.
• List signs and symptoms to report to the health care team.
• Demonstrate a stable nutritional status consistent with stage of disease.

INTERVENTIONS[15]

• Weigh patient daily.
• Take accurate intake and output readings every 24 hours.
• Monitor laboratory values, including electrolytes and leukocyte count.
• Provide patient/caregiver dietary instructions:
—Eat six small feedings per day.
—Limit fluids at mealtime, and drink fluids between meals.
—Progress slowly from liquid to soft diet.
—Choose high-protein and moderate-carbohydrate foods.
—Avoid greasy foods.
—Eat slowly.
• Provide instructions on signs and symptoms to report to health care team:
—Diarrhea
—Clay-colored stools
—Fatty stools
—Abdominal cramps
—Weakness
—Faintness
—Rapid heartbeat
• Provide instructions for diet if diarrhea occurs:
—Choose low-residue, bulk-forming foods (refined breads and cereals, pasta, rice, cheese, fish, chicken, bananas, applesauce, cooked vegetables).
—Avoid foods such as whole-grain breads or cereals, fresh fruits and vegetables, gas-forming foods, citrus fruits, and juices.
—Eat slowly.
—Notify health care team of need for antidiarrheal and/or antispasmodic agents.
• Provide instructions for diet if dumping syndrome occurs:
—Choose foods high in protein and fat and low in carbohydrates.
—Avoid concentrated sweets.
—Drink liquids between meals.
—Rest after meals for at least 30 minutes.
—Notify health care team if symptoms continue.
• Obtain dietary consult for assistance, evaluation, and diet planning.
• Administer enteral/parenteral feedings if ordered and provide instructions to patient/caregiver if necessary before discharge.

---

major risk factor in Asia and Africa. In the Western world, however, alcoholic cirrhosis is more common and therefore may be a more important risk factor. Once cirrhosis has developed, the risk of developing cancer does not diminish, even if alcohol consumption is stopped.[4]

Aflatoxin is a carcinogen produced by fungus growing in contaminated grain and other foods improperly stored in warm, moist places. This is a widespread problem in humid regions of Africa and Asia, where HCC is most common.[4]

A number of chemical agents have been implicated in the development of primary liver cancer. These include 16 different pesticides and herbicides, along with industrial chemicals such as cycasin and nitrosamines that are known to produce liver cancer in laboratory animals.[4] Thorotrast, a contrast medium used until the 1950s, is associated with the development of angiosarcoma of the liver.[38] The use of oral contraceptives has also been reported to lead to HCC, but this is very rare; benign liver adenomas and focal nodular hyperplasia are more common in users of oral contraceptives.[4]

PREVENTION, SCREENING, AND DETECTION

Technologic advances in the agricultural field and in storage of grains have reduced contamination of food by aflatoxin in developed countries, but these advances have not yet been made in the developing countries. The advent of the vaccine against HBV may significantly reduce morbidity and mortality from HCC in high-risk areas.[44] High-risk patients with chronic HBV or cirrhosis may be screened for the tumor marker alpha(α-)-fetoprotein (AFP) and by abdominal ultrasonography.[38]

CLASSIFICATION

The histopathologic types of primary cancers of the liver include hepatomas or hepatocellular carcinomas, intrahepatic bile duct carcinomas or cholangiocarcinomas, and mixed types.[9] Almost 95% of all primary liver tumors are malignant. The benign liver tumors include adenomas, focal nodular hyperplasia, hamartomas, and hemangiomas.[8] In the United States, almost 90% of the primary liver cancers are HCC, and intrahepatic cholangiocarcinomas represent about 7%; the remainder are angiosarcomas, hepatoblastomas, and primary lymphomas.[4]

CLINICAL FEATURES

The most common presenting symptoms of HCC are a right upper quadrant abdominal mass, pain, and epigastric fullness.[21] The pain is usually located in the right upper quadrant of the abdomen and may be described as dull or aching and may radiate to the right shoulder.[4,38] The box at right lists other signs and symptoms.[4] HCC is also associated with several paraneoplastic syndromes, including hyperglycemia, hypoglycemia, Cushing's syndrome, precocious puberty, hyperlipidemia, polycythemia, microangiopathic hemolytic anemia, leukocytosis, and disseminated intravascular coagulation.[44]

DIAGNOSIS AND STAGING

Diagnosis of liver cancer can be challenging. Patients presenting with a right upper quadrant abdominal mass should have a diagnostic work-up at once. The initial studies should include blood tests, x-ray films, and ultrasound.

Blood tests should include AFP and hepatitis surface antigens. AFP is the principal tumor marker associated with HCC and is elevated in more than 70% of patients with the disease.[38] The normal value for AFP is 40 ng/ml, and elevations to greater than 400 ng/ml are almost always diagnostic for HCC. It is important to note, however, that a significant number of patients with HCC will have normal AFP.[4]

Radiologic studies should specifically include an ultrasound and CT. The ultrasound is inexpensive, noninvasive, and nontoxic[38]; it will detect lesions less than 3

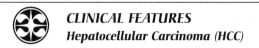

CLINICAL FEATURES
Hepatocellular Carcinoma (HCC)

Symptoms
  Abdominal pain
  Weight loss
  Anorexia
  Nausea/vomiting
  Abdominal mass
  Weakness, fatigue, malaise
  GI bleeding
  Diarrhea

Clinical Signs
  Abdominal mass/hepatomegaly
  Jaundice
  Ascites
  Fever

cm in size. CT is able to detect and demonstrate the extent of the liver tumors and is helpful in identifying any metastatic disease.[4,38] For any tumor that appears to be resectable, an arteriogram is necessary to provide information regarding arterial and venous involvement. This information is also invaluable if the patient requires hepatic artery infusions.

A biopsy is ultimately necessary to make a definitive diagnosis. If the tumor appears resectable, a surgical approach is best for obtaining a tissue specimen. Resection should be attempted only for local lesions limited to one lobe or segment that is without extrahepatic spread.[38] For unresectable tumors the percutaneous route is preferred and may be done with either sonographic or CT guidance. Hemorrhage is a risk for vascular lesions but is usually self-limiting. Peritoneoscopy is another approach for obtaining a specimen that allows direct visualization of the liver and decreases the risk of hemorrhage.[38]

In 1988 the American Joint Commission on Cancer adopted a staging system based on degree of liver involvement, extent of vascular invasion, nodal involvement, and the presence or absence of distant metastasis (TNM).[9] The box, p. 153, summarizes this system.

METASTASIS

The usual sites for HCC metastasis are the regional nodes, lung, bone, adrenal gland, and brain. Approximately 40% of the HCC patients have tumor cells in the regional nodes, but other metastatic sites are rare. At surgery, few patients have metastasis, but more than 50% have metastasis at the time of autopsy.[38] Spread also occurs by direct invasion of adjacent structures such as the stomach and diaphragm.[50]

TNM CLASSIFICATION AND STAGING FOR LIVER CANCER

PRIMARY TUMOR (T)

T1: solitary tumor 2 cm or less in greatest dimension without vascular invasion

T2: solitary tumor 2 cm or less in greatest dimension with vascular invasion, or multiple tumors limited to one lobe, none more than 2 cm in greatest dimension, without vascular invasion, or a solitary tumor more than 2 cm in greatest dimension without vascular invasion

T3: solitary tumor more than 2 cm in greatest dimension with vascular invasion, or multiple tumors limited to one lobe, none more than 2 cm in greatest dimension, with vascular invasion, or multiple tumors limited to one lobe, any more than 2 cm in greatest dimension, with or without vascular invasion

T4: multiple tumors in more than one lobe, or tumor(s) involve(s) a major branch of portal or hepatic vein(s)

LYMPH NODE (N)

N0: no regional lymph node metastasis
N1: regional lymph node metastasis

DISTANT METASTASIS (M)

M0: no distant metastasis
M1: distant metastasis

STAGE GROUPING

Stage I:	T1-N0-M0
Stage II:	T2-N0-M0
Stage III:	T1-N1-M0
	T2-N1-M0
	T3-N0-M0
	T3-N1-M0
Stage IVA:	T4-any N-M0
Stage IVB:	any T-any N-M1

TREATMENT MODALITIES

Surgery

Surgery is the only potentially curative treatment modality for patients with HCC. Unfortunately, less than 25% of the patients meet the criteria for liver resection. Patients with extrahepatic involvement of major vessels or structure are ineligible, as are those with poor hepatic reserve or severe coagulopathy.[4,36] Patients with cirrhosis are not usually candidates for resection because of the risk of intraoperative hemorrhage and postoperative hepatic failure.[51] Although liver resections have become much safer, operative mortality is still 3% to 15%.

Hepatic resection involves either a bilateral subcostal or thoracoabdominal incision. After the incision there are four recognized resection techniques: right lobectomy, left lobectomy, trisegmentectomy, and lateral segmentectomy. The lateral segmentectomy involves the removal of the outer portion of the left lobe. The trisegmentectomy is the removal of the right lobe and the inner portion of the left lobe.[4] Figure 8-6 illustrates the four approaches to liver resection.

Liver transplantation is an option for very few primary liver cancer patients. Because of high cancer recurrence rates and limited donor organs, it remains controversial. Patients with HCC, cholangiocarcinoma, some bile duct cancers, and some liver metastasis are considered candidates for transplantation. Unfortunately, results depend on the stage of the disease. Five-year survival rates reported range from 75% for stage I to only 10% for stage IVA.

Chemotherapy

No single-system chemotherapeutic agent has shown high activity against HCC. Doxorubicin has been the most active, but the true response rate is substantially less than 20%. A number of combinations of agents have been studied, but none has been recognized as a standard therapy and none has demonstrated a survival advantage over any other.[4]

Because a large number of HCC patients have significant unresectable liver tumors without extrahepatic spread, regional chemotherapy has been investigated. *Regional chemotherapy* involves infusion of agents that are highly metabolized by the liver via the hepatic artery. This greatly increases the dose of drug delivered to the tumor but minimizes the systemic side effects.[4] *Intraarterial chemotherapy* can be administered through temporary catheters placed into the axillary or femoral arteries. This method requires that the patient remain in bed for the duration of the infusion, which may be up to 5 days. Complications of this method include thrombosis of the hepatic and other intraabdominal arteries, catheter displacement, sepsis, and hemorrhage. Drugs may also be administered via an *implantable pump,* which offers the advantages of allowing the patient to remain ambulatory and reducing catheter-related complications. The most common problems associated with the implantable pump have been gastroduodenal ulceration and inflammation.[35] The agents used most frequently for intraarterial chemotherapy are floxuridine (FUDR) and 5-FU. Other drugs used include cisplatin, doxorubicin, mitomycin-C, and dichloromethotrexate.[4] Combination therapy via the hepatic artery is currently being investigated.

Embolization and Chemoembolization

Embolization is the selective occlusion of hepatic vessels by injecting nondegradable particles, typically Gelfoam and Ivalon. Embolizations usually need to be repeated because of the formation of collateral circulation. *Chemoembolization* involves occlusion by particles into which chemotherapeutic agents have been ad-

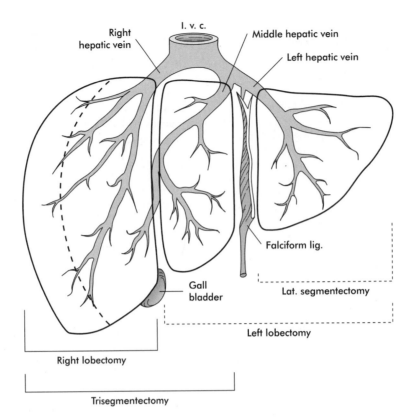

Figure 8-6   Four approaches to liver resection. *I.V.C.,* Inferior vena cava; *Lat.,* lateral; *lig.,* ligament. (From Starzl TE and others: Hepatic trisegmentectomy and other liver resections, *Surg Gynecol Obstet* 141:729, 1975.)

sorbed. Drugs used in this application include doxorubicin, cisplatin, mitomycin-C, aclarubicin, and carmustine (BCNU).[4,38]

Radiation Therapy

Even though HCC is considered a radiosensitive tumor, the use of radiation therapy is restricted by the relative intolerance of the normal liver parenchyma. The whole liver will tolerate 3000 cGy. At this dose the incidence of radiation hepatitis is 5% to 10%. A cure or long-term remission of HCC requires significantly higher doses. To improve results, radiolabeled antibodies have been used with some success. The high concentration of ferritin in HCC has led to the use of antiferritin antibodies labeled with iodine-131; this technique allows tolerance of high doses. The dose-limiting toxicity is thrombocytopenia, since the bone marrow has a significant uptake of the antiferritin antibodies.[4] The box, p. 156, summarizes typical treatment-related complications.

PROGNOSIS

Overall prognosis for the patient with primary liver cancer is poor. The relative 5-year survival rate for cancer of the liver is 5%.[46] For those with resectable disease this rate increases to 10%.[45]

CANCER OF THE GALLBLADDER

Gallbladder cancer is an uncommon malignancy, representing about 75% of the extrahepatic biliary tract cancers. Patients are usually asymptomatic until the disease is advanced; therefore most present with extensive disease. The overall 5-year survival rate for gallbladder cancer is less than 5%. The most common signs and symptoms include abdominal pain, nausea and vomiting, weight loss, jaundice, abdominal mass, and hepatomegaly. It is more common in females, and the median age of patients is 70 years.

The most common tumor type is *adenocarcinoma,* accounting for 85% of cases. Overall survival of patients with gallbladder cancer is poor, with a 5-year survival of 5%. The treatment of choice is *surgical resection.* A small number of patients are diagnosed during a cholecystectomy for chronic cholecystitis, when surgery alone is usually adequate. Patients with more extensive disease require more radical procedures.

The role of *radiation therapy* is controversial. Local recurrence is a common cause of death in patients who relapse after cholecystectomy. Thus adjuvant radiation therapy is often used. Intraoperative radiation therapy also has been used to prevent local recurrence. However, little data support using radiation therapy as a part of standard therapy.

NURSING MANAGEMENT

The nursing care of the patient with primary liver cancer is very challenging. Because most patients with HCC are not candidates for liver resection, many will be treated by hepatic artery infusion therapy via an implanted infusion pump. The nurse's primary responsibility is educating the patient and family to manage this form of therapy.[18]

NURSING DIAGNOSIS

• *Knowledge deficit regarding management of hepatic artery infusion therapy related to lack of exposure*

OUTCOME GOALS

Patient will be able to:
• State rationale for use of hepatic artery infusion.
• Demonstrate measures for care of implanted pump and management of side effects of chemotherapy.
• Identify signs and symptoms to report to health care team.

INTERVENTIONS

• Assess patient's understanding of treatment, goals, patient's ability to manage care postoperatively, and availability of support from family and friends.

• Provide both verbal and written instructions regarding the implanted pump and chemotherapy:
  —Purpose of pump and where catheter is placed anatomically in liver
  —Management of pocket site: keep incision clean and dry until healed; resume usual activities when healed; avoid activities that may lead to blunt trauma to pump pocket or that may cause increased temperature, pressure, or altitude
  —What to report to health care team: temperature greater than 101° F (38.3° C) for more than 24 hours, air travel, or change in residence requiring a change in altitude
  —Side effects of chemotherapy drug(s) being infused and other medications
• Provide written list of phone numbers of health care team members and schedule of treatment cycles.

The role of *chemotherapy* has not been well defined. The common agents that have been used include 5-FU, doxorubicin, methotrexate, lomustine, etoposide, and cisplatin. These are used alone or in combination. Although patients who receive chemotherapy have better survival rates, studies are not conclusive because of the low incidence of this cancer.

CANCER OF THE PANCREAS

Pancreatic cancer is the second most common GI cancer and the fourth leading cause of cancer death in the United States.[10] Cancers of the pancreas fall into three different categories: those in the exocrine pancreas, those around the ampulla of Vater, and those in the islets of Langerhans. The pathologic and etiologic characteristics of the three types differ. The term *pancreatic cancer* usually refers to cancer of the exocrine pancreas.

EPIDEMIOLOGY

The estimated number of new cases of cancer of the pancreas reported in 1996 is 26,300, which resulted in 25,800 deaths. This represents 3% of the cancers diagnosed and 5% of the cancer deaths in women, and 2% of the cancers diagnosed and 4% of deaths in men. Over the past 60 years the incidence of cancer of the pancreas has been slowly but steadily increasing.[46] The median age of patients with pancreatic cancer is about 70. The incidence is about 35% higher in the black population than in the white population; the American black male is the person at highest risk worldwide.[3]

ETIOLOGY AND RISK FACTORS

Cigarette smoke is the most clearly identified carcinogen in pancreatic cancer. Cigarette smoke contains carcinogens, including nitrosamines, that have induced pancreatic cancer in laboratory animals.[12] Several dietary carcinogens have been implicated, but no conclusive data have been reported. High-risk dietary components include excessive consumption of meat, coffee, and alcohol. Occupational exposure to solvents and petroleum compounds is associated with increased risk of pancreatic cancer, as is history of chronic pancreatitis and diabetes mellitus.[12]

PREVENTION, SCREENING, AND DETECTION

Because no specific risk factors have been conclusively identified for pancreatic cancer, it is impossible to determine how to prevent the disease. Avoiding cigarette

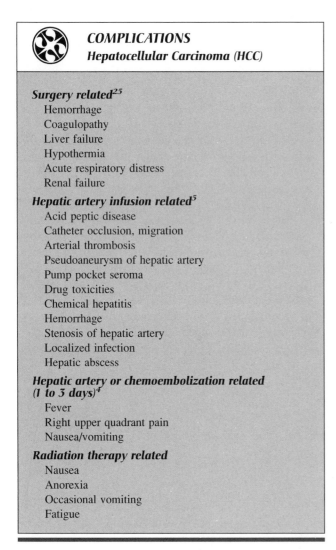

COMPLICATIONS
Hepatocellular Carcinoma (HCC)

Surgery related[25]
Hemorrhage
Coagulopathy
Liver failure
Hypothermia
Acute respiratory distress
Renal failure

Hepatic artery infusion related[5]
Acid peptic disease
Catheter occlusion, migration
Arterial thrombosis
Pseudoaneurysm of hepatic artery
Pump pocket seroma
Drug toxicities
Chemical hepatitis
Hemorrhage
Stenosis of hepatic artery
Localized infection
Hepatic abscess

Hepatic artery or chemoembolization related (1 to 3 days)[4]
Fever
Right upper quadrant pain
Nausea/vomiting

Radiation therapy related
Nausea
Anorexia
Occasional vomiting
Fatigue

Table 8-1 Clinical Features of Pancreatic Cancer According to Site of Lesion

| | Percent of patients | |
Sign or symptom	Head	Body and tail
SYMPTOMS		
Weight loss	92	100
Pain	72	87
Anorexia	64	33
Nausea	45	43
Vomiting	37	37
Diarrhea	18	
CLINICAL SIGNS		
Jaundice	87	23
Palpable liver	83	33
Palpable gallbladder	29	
Abdominal tenderness		27
Abdominal mass	13	23
Ascites	14	20

Modified from Ahlgren JD, Hill MC, Roberts IM: Pancreatic cancer: patterns, diagnosis, and approaches to treatment. In Ahlgren J, MacDonald J, editors: *Gastrointestinal oncology,* Philadelphia, 1992, Lippincott.

smoke and eating a healthy balanced diet would probably reduce risk. The occupational exposure is decreased if safety precautions are employed when working with known carcinogens. No cost-effective test has been found that could be used to screen the asymptomatic population and identify patients for more invasive procedures.[41]

CLASSIFICATION

Ninety-five percent of cancers involving the pancreas arise from the exocrine gland.[3,13] *Ductal adenocarcinoma* accounts for 80% of all pancreatic cancers. Other less common types include squamous cell carcinomas, giant cell carcinomas, and carcinosarcomas.[12] Primary lymphomas and plasmacytomas occur rarely.[3] The majority of the carcinomas occur in the proximal gland, which includes the head, neck, and uncinate process of the pancreas. Twenty percent occur in the body of the pancreas, and 5% to 10% occur in the tail.[12]

CLINICAL FEATURES

Pain is the most common symptom in patients with pancreatic cancer and is often the reason the patient seeks medical attention. The pain is generally described as gnawing and is located in the epigastrium. Occasionally the pain may be relieved with meals, mimicking the pain associated with peptic ulcer disease. Severe pain is usually indicative of invasion of the splanchic plexus and is a sign of unresectability.[12]

Two other common symptoms are *anorexia* and *weight loss*. A typical patient has lost more than 10% of his body weight at diagnosis. The exact cause of the weight loss is unknown, but it may be related to malabsorption. Table 8-1 summarizes signs and symptoms according to the location of the tumor.[3]

DIAGNOSIS AND STAGING

Ultrasonography is an effective and relatively inexpensive means of demonstrating a mass in the pancreas, but CT may be necessary for the diagnosis of pancreatic cancer. CT can show a mass in the pancreas, involvement of the liver or bile ducts, ascites, and the presence of metastases.[12] It is also used for staging.[3] Endoscopic retrograde cholangiopancreatography (ERCP) is used to identify tumors of the ampulla or obstructed stenotic or sclerosed ducts. Angiography is helpful in determining any abnormal vasculature and whether the tumor is resectable. To confirm the diagnosis of pancreatic cancer, a biopsy is needed. If the patient is not a candidate for a laparotomy, a percutaneous biopsy may be obtained using ultrasound or CT guidance.[3]

The American Joint Commission for Cancer has accepted a staging system for pancreatic cancer based on local, regional nodal, and distant metastatic involvement using the TNM system. The box at right lists the established staging criteria.[9]

METASTASIS

Because of the location of the pancreas, early invasion of adjacent organs by pancreatic tumors is common. These adjacent organs include the major vessels, duodenum, stomach, bile duct, retroperitoneum, spleen, kidney, and colon. Widespread carcinomatosis and ascites are common because of intraperitoneal seeding.[3] Distant metastasis occurs most often to the liver, but other sites are the lung, bone, and brain.[12]

TREATMENT MODALITIES

Even with the advances in treatment in recent years, pancreatic cancer continues to be the most difficult to treat of all GI cancers. Surgery is probably the only effective treatment. Unfortunately, the cancer is unsymptomatic until it invades adjacent organs or metastasizes. Only 15% of patients meet the criteria for curative surgery. Radiation therapy offers a chance for extended survival to patients with locally advanced disease, but the majority of patients are not candidates for curative surgery or radiation therapy. These patients require palliative therapy to relieve pain and maintain quality of life.[3]

Surgery

The majority of pancreatic cancers occur in the head of the pancreas. Patients who are amenable to curative resection will undergo either a pancreatoduodenectomy (or Whipple operation) or a total pancreatectomy. The *pancreatoduodenectomy* involves the removal of the distal stomach, the gallbladder, the common bile duct, the head of the pancreas, the duodenum, and the upper jejunum.[41] Figure 8-7 illustrates the pancreatoduodenectomy, or *Whipple resection* of the pancreas.[56] Reconstruction after the pancreatoduodenectomy involves three steps. As part of the choledochojejunostomy, the jejunum is anastomosed to the common hepatic duct. A pancreatojejunostomy attaches the remaining pancreas to the small bowel. The standard gastrojejunostomy is then performed.[31]

A *total pancreatectomy* is an extension of the pancreatoduodenectomy and in addition involves removal of the body and tail of the pancreas and the spleen and a more extensive regional lymphadenectomy. Controversy continues over the advantages and disadvantages of the two procedures.[41]

TNM CLASSIFICATION AND STAGING FOR PANCREATIC CANCER

PRIMARY TUMOR (T)

T1: tumor invading mucosa or muscle layer
T1a: tumor invading mucosa
T1b: tumor invading muscle layer
T2: tumor invading perimuscular connective tissue; no extension beyond serosa or into liver
T3: tumor invading beyond serosa or into one adjacent organ, or both (extension 2 cm or less into liver)
T4: tumor extending more than 2 cm into liver, and/or into two or more adjacent organs (stomach, duodenum, colon, pancreas, omentum, extrahepatic bile ducts, any involvement of liver)

REGIONAL LYMPH NODES (N)

N0: no regional lymph node metastasis
N1: regional lymph node metastasis
N1a: metastasis in cystic duct, pericholedochal, and/or hilar lymph nodes (i.e., in hepatoduodenal ligament)
N1b: metastasis in peripancreatic (head only), periduodenal, periportal, celiac, and/or superior mesenteric lymph nodes

DISTANT METASTASIS (M)

M0: no distant metastasis
M1: distant metastasis

STAGE GROUPING

Stage I: T1-N0-M0
Stage II: T2-N0-M0
Stage III: T1-N1-M0
T2-N1-M0
T3-any N-M0
Stage IV: T4-any N-M0
any T-any N-M1

Palliation for cancer of the head of the pancreas is the objective of surgery more often than is cure. Jaundice, gastric outlet obstruction, and pain are the problems most often relieved through surgical intervention. If the patient is a candidate for a surgical procedure, but not a curative resection, palliative surgery is warranted to relieve symptoms and improve quality of life. A laparotomy may be performed to establish tissue diagnosis. At this time the biliary tract is internally decompressed to relieve jaundice and pruritus and prevent ascending cholangitis, progressive liver failure, and coagulopathy.[41] A choledochojejunostomy or cholecystojejunostomy may be indicated to bypass distal obstruction of the biliary tree.[3] Duodenal obstruction is a late symptom of pancreatic cancer, but a gastrojejunostomy may be performed prophylactically or if compression or invasion of the duodenum is present. A chemical splanchnicectomy may also be indicated for relief of pain.[41]

If surgery is not an option for the patient, obstructive jaundice may be relieved by either the endoscopic placement of a stent, which will provide internal drainage of bile, or the placement of percutaneous transhepatic catheter, which will provide either external or internal-external drainage. The percutaneous transhepatic catheter may be used to internalize the drainage via a stent. Complications of these procedures include cholangitis, hemorrhage, bile leak, and catheter obstruction.[3]

Chemotherapy

For unknown reasons, pancreatic cancer cells are relatively chemoresistant.[12] Both single and multiple chemo-therapeutic agents have been tried with generally poor results. 5-FU, mitomycin-C, and gemcitabine are the most responsive single agents,[41] but combinations now in use that show improved responses include streptozotocin, mitomycin-C, and 5-FU (SMF); 5-FU, doxorubicin (Adriamycin), and mitomycin-C (FAM); and FAM with the addition of streptozotocin.[41] Studies are also in progress investigating the usefulness of biologic therapies in treating pancreatic cancer.[12]

Radiation Therapy

The use of radiation therapy in treating cancer of the pancreas is limited by the proximity of the pancreas to dose-limiting structures such as the kidneys, bowel, liver, and spinal cord. With the development of new techniques, however, radiation is now being used to improve local disease control and long-term survival.

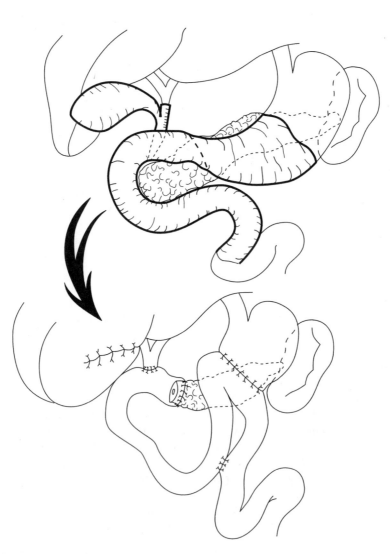

Figure 8-7   Extent of pancreatoduodenectomy or Whipple resection *(top)*, and technique of resection *(bottom)*. (From Trede M, Schwall G, Saeger H: Survival after pancreatoduodenectomy, *Ann Surg* 211:454, 1990.)

Adjuvant radiation therapy is being studied for resectable tumors. Researchers are using postoperative external beam radiation with or without 5-FU as a radiosensitizer. Intraoperative radiation therapy (IORT) is also being studied. IORT has the advantage of being able to deliver tumor-specific high-dose radiation therapy while avoiding adjacent normal tissue.[3] Radiation therapy is the primary treatment for patients with unresectable disease. External beam therapy, IORT, and combinations of these continue to have a 50% probability of local failure. The standard treatment remains 5-FU and external beam radiation therapy, since it consistently has extended median survival from the range of 6 months to 1 year.[3] The box below summarizes treatment-related complications.

PROGNOSIS

The prognosis for persons with cancer of the pancreas is relatively poor. The reported 5-year survival rate for pancreatic cancer is 3%.[17] This figure has increased only slightly from that reported in the early 1960s.[11] Improved surgical techniques and supportive care have not led to improved survival. Median survival in patients who have had a pancreatoduodenectomy ranges from 16 to 30 months.

CANCER OF THE SMALL INTESTINES

Neoplasms of the small intestines are rare. They comprise only 1% of GI malignancies. The estimated number of new cases for 1996 was 4600, which resulted in 1140 deaths.[46] Small bowel cancers have been reported in patients from 1 year to 84 years of age, but the average age is 57 years.[16] The types of neoplasms found in the small intestines include adenocarcinoma, lymphoma, leiomyosarcoma, liposarcoma, neurofibrosarcoma, malignant schwannoma, carcinoid, fibrosarcoma, hemangiosarcoma, and lymphangiosarcoma.[52] Risk factors that have been associated with small bowel cancers include inflammatory bowel disease, Crohn's disease, Peutz-Jeghers syndrome, familial polyposis, Gardner's syndrome, celiac disease, and neurofibromatosis.[16]

Symptoms of cancer of the small intestine are vague and not localizing,[52] occurring late in the disease course. There is usually a delay of months before a diagnosis is made. Symptoms may include pain, symptoms of small bowel obstruction, bleeding, and weight loss. Because

---

COMPLICATIONS
Pancreatic Cancer Treatment[31]

Hemorrhage, intraoperative and postoperative in first 24 to 48 hours

Fistula (pancreatic or biliary)

Cardiovascular problems (myocardial infarction, congestive heart failure, rhythm disturbances)

Vascular thrombosis, most often in portal vein

Infection (lung, urinary tract, incisional wound, peritoneal cavity)

Renal or hepatic failure

Pancreatitis

Gastric retention

Late complications (jaundice, gastrointestinal ulceration, diabetes mellitus, dumping syndrome)

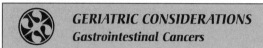

GERIATRIC CONSIDERATIONS
Gastrointestinal Cancers

Factors related to cancer prevention and early detection

Encourage low-fat, high-fiber diet within ethnic, social, and economic limitations.

Encourage smoking cessation and avoidance of exposure to other health hazards (e.g., sun, chemicals, petroleum products).

Be suspicious of symptoms such as malaise, fatigue, anorexia, weight loss, and altered bowel habits as possible indicators of cancer and not automatically attributed to nonmalignant illnesses associated with aging.

Factors related to modalities of therapy

Alterations in hepatic and renal function may necessitate adjustment of dosage and schedule of chemotherapy protocols.

Decreased bone marrow cellularity may place patient at risk for prolonged myelosuppression chemotherapy with toxic effects on bone marrow.

Decreased nutritional intake may be exacerbated because of nausea and taste changes associated with many chemotherapeutic agents typically used for GI malignancies.

Fatigue may be increasing problem after courses of therapy, requiring additional assistance with activities of daily living.

Comorbid disease (e.g., obesity, poor nutritional status, lung and cardiovascular disease, altered immune function) places older adult at greater risk for surgical morbidity and mortality.

Teaching should be tailored to take into account older adult's life experiences and cognitive and physical impairments (e.g., reading comprehension, decreased vision and hearing, altered tactile sense, misconceptions regarding cancer and cancer treatment, past experience with cancer and family members).

Modified from Boyle DM and others: Oncology nursing society position paper on cancer and aging: the mandate for oncology nursing, *Oncol Nurs Forum* 19:913, 1992.

NURSING MANAGEMENT

Patients who have had surgical intervention for pancreatic cancer have complex and challenging nursing needs. Preoperative assessment includes both psychologic and physical parameters, including nutritional history, elimination problems, pain, jaundice, pruritus, fatigue or weakness, depression, or anxiety; laboratory values must be monitored for anemia and coagulation abnormalities. Postoperatively, nurses should be aware of the extent of the surgical resection and the reconstruction the patient has undergone to anticipate potential problems and plan for the care of the patient.

NURSING DIAGNOSIS

• *Fluid volume deficit related to extensive abdominal surgery*

OUTCOME GOALS

Patient will be able to:
• State rationale for potential and actual fluid loss.
• Demonstrate measures to correct or maintain adequate fluid volume.
• Maintain fluid volume evidenced by normal laboratory parameters.

INTERVENTIONS: *Potential Fluid Loss*

• Check assessment parameters:
 —Monitor fluid intake and output, and note fluid preferences.
 —Examine mucous membranes for moistness and integrity.
 —Monitor weight and vital signs.
 —Monitor laboratory values: blood urea nitrogen (BUN), creatinine, electrolytes, serum osmolality, and hematocrit.
• Provide patient instructions:
 —List signs and symptoms to report to health care team: thirst, dry skin and mucous membranes, fatigue, constipation, nausea/vomiting, diarrhea, or fever.
 —Monitor appropriate fluid intake per day, as well as type and timing of fluid intake, to avoid possible problems such as dumping syndrome.
 —Administer medications to minimize fluid loss.

INTERVENTIONS: *Actual Fluid Loss*

• In addition to above assessment parameters, monitor type and amount of output (diarrhea, wound drainage, emesis), and weigh patient daily.
• Administer intravenous fluids per physician's orders.
• Offer small amount of fluids by mouth as appropriate.
• Administer replacement electrolytes per physician's orders.
• If tube feedings or TPN is ordered, administer and provide instructions to patient/caregiver as appropriate.
• When oral feedings are resumed, administer pancreatic enzymes per physician's orders, and provide instructions on same to the patient.

NURSING DIAGNOSIS

• *Injury, risk for, related to unstable blood glucose levels*

OUTCOME GOALS

Patient will be able to:
• State rationale for potential changes in blood sugar.
• Demonstrate self–blood glucose monitoring, urine testing, and insulin injection.
• Identify signs and symptoms of hypoglycemia and hyperglycemia and measures to prevent/treat.

INTERVENTIONS

• Assess patient for signs and symptoms of hypoglycemia and hyperglycemia; report to physician if occurs.
• Test urine for acetone every 4 to 6 hours or as ordered by physician.
• Monitor blood glucose levels every 6 hours, and administer sliding-scale insulin per physician's order.
• If patient is not receiving TPN, blood glucose may be monitored before breakfast and evening meal with a daily dose of neutral protamine Hagedorn (NPH) insulin in the morning and sliding scale regular insulin in the evening.
• Provide patient with written and verbal instructions regarding diabetic management.
• Evaluate for the need for home health referral.

PATIENT TEACHING PRIORITIES
Gastrointestinal Cancers

Prevention and early detection

Risk factors
Dietary habits
Avoidance of cigarette smoking
Moderate or no alcohol consumption
Signs and symptoms to report to health care
  professional (e.g., dysphagia, odynophagia, chronic
  indigestion, jaundice, weight loss not associated with
  dieting, change in bowel habits)
Annual physical examination and cancer checkup

Diagnostic procedures

Purpose of procedure
Preparation needed by patient
Procedure description
Postprocedural care by patient

Treatment modalities

Surgery—preoperative instructions include operative
  experience and immediate postoperative period;
  discharge instructions include self-care needs and
  any further treatment plans
Chemotherapy—name of agent, possible side effects
  and measures to control, route of administration,
  dose, schedule, and any directions needed for
  self-administration
Radiation therapy—description of procedure and
  schedule and duration of treatment, skin care
  measures, and management of any side effects

Supportive care

Community resources (e.g., home health care agencies,
  inpatient and outpatient hospice care)
Use of any medical equipment in the home
Referrals necessary for psychosocial support for patient
  and caregiver
Referrals for financial assistance if needed

the signs and symptoms are not specific, diagnosis may not be confirmed until surgery is performed. Treatment depends on the histologic type of tumor, but surgery is indicated in all symptomatic tumors. Radiation therapy and chemotherapy have little impact on primary small intestinal cancer, although adjuvant therapy is currently being investigated.

• • •

Nursing care guidelines for patients with GI cancer follow the practices recommended for the patient's particular therapy (see boxes, p. 159 and above). Refer to Chapter 31 for interventions related to death and dying.

CONCLUSION

Gastrointestinal cancers remain a nursing practice challenge. The overall prognosis ranges from 5% to 15%. Progress has been made in treatment modalities. However, prevention, early detection, and the seeking of health care early when initial symptoms occur can reduce the impact and prolong patient survival.

■ CHAPTER QUESTIONS

1. For an esophageal cancer patient receiving chemotherapy who is experiencing mild dysphagia, what would the nurse want to include in patient teaching?
   a. Instructions regarding alternate feeding routes
   b. Instructions for six to eight small feedings per day
   c. Instructions to lie down immediately after eating
   d. Instructions for clear-liquid diet
2. In interviewing a patient, the nurse learns that the patient is a chronic user of antacids for indigestion and epigastric pain. He is 62 years old and has come to the clinic because his wife is concerned that the symptoms are not relieved by the antacids as well as they had been. What advice should the nurse give them?
   a. Referral to a gastroenterologist for upper GI endoscopy is needed for further work-up of symptoms
   b. Change to a bland diet
   c. Change to a different antacid
   d. Eating six to eight small meals a day
3. A close association exists between which of these risk factors and hepatocellular cancer?
   a. Epstein-Barr virus
   b. *Helicobacter pylori* infection
   c. Hepatitis B infection
   d. Human immunodeficiency virus
4. The treatment of choice for cancer of the pancreas is:
   a. Bone marrow transplant
   b. Radiation therapy
   c. Chemotherapy
   d. Surgery
5. Which of the following statements is *true?*
   a. In the United States, almost 90% of all primary liver cancers are hepatocellular carcinomas.
   b. The most common type of esophageal cancer is adenocarcinoma.
   c. Lymphomas account for up to 50% of the gastric malignancies.
   d. The most common cancers in the pancreas are endocrine in origin.
6. Which of the following is the second most common GI malignancy?
   a. Esophageal
   b. Gastric
   c. Liver
   d. Pancreatic
7. If you were counseling a client regarding risk factors for pancreatic cancer, which of the following would you include?
   a. Avoid use of tobacco and alcohol.
   b. Avoid diets high in nitrosamines.

c. Avoid exposure to pesticides and herbicides.

d. Avoid tobacco, and drink alcohol and coffee in moderation only.

8. Your patient has been recently diagnosed with hepatocellular carcinoma. He tells you he read about a person who had a liver transplant, and he wonders if he might be able to have one. How would you respond?

   a. Liver transplants are not an option for persons with cancer.

   b. Liver transplants are an option for select patients with cancer, but donors are scarce and the outcome for many patients is no better than with surgery and chemotherapy.

   c. Liver transplants have become an acceptable treatment modality for primary liver cancer if the patient is able to find a donor.

   d. The use of liver transplants for cancer patients is still being investigated.

9. Cancer of the small intestines occurs in what age-group?

   a. Over 50 years

   b. 35 to 75 years

   c. 15 to 80 years

   d. 1 to 84 years

10. How would you describe cancer of the gallbladder?

   a. Rare form of GI malignancy with a poor prognosis

   b. Uncommon cancer that has one of the better prognoses in relation to other GI cancers

   c. Slow-growing cancer that affects middle-age adults

   d. Form of cancer that does not require any treatment until it becomes symptomatic

BIBLIOGRAPHY

1. Abe M and others: Japan trials in intraoperative radiotherapy, *Int J Radiat Oncol Biol Phys* 5:1431, 1979.

2. Ahlgren JD: Esophageal cancer: chemotherapy and combined modalities. In Ahlgren JD, McDonald JS, editors: *Gastrointestinal oncology,* Philadelphia, 1992, Lippincott.

3. Ahlgren JD, Hill MD, Roberts IM: Pancreatic cancer: patterns, diagnosis and approaches to treatment. In Ahlgren JD, McDonald JS, editors: *Gastrointestinal oncology,* Philadelphia, 1992, Lippincott.

4. Ahlgren JD, Wanebo HF, Hill MC: Hepatocellular carcinoma. In Ahlgren JD, McDonald JS, editors: *Gastrointestinal oncology,* Philadelphia, 1992, Lippincott.

5. Ahmed T, Friedland ML: Chemotherapy of primary and metastatic hepatic neoplasms. In Hodgson WJB, editor: *Liver tumors: multidisciplinary management,* St Louis, 1988, Green.

6. Alexander HR, Kelsen DP, Tepper JE: Cancer of the stomach. In Devita VT Jr, Hellman S, Rosenberg SA, editors: *Cancer: principles and practice of oncology,* ed 4, Philadelphia, 1993, Lippincott.

7. American Cancer Society: *Cancer facts and figures—1996,* Atlanta, 1996, The Society.

8. Anderson BB and others: Primary tumors of the liver, *J Natl Med Assoc* 84:129, 1992.

9. Beahrs OH and others: *Manual for staging of cancer,* ed 4, Philadelphia, 1992, Lippincott.

10. Beazley RM, Cohn I Jr: Tumors of the pancreas, gallbladder, and extrahepatic ducts. In Murphy GP, Lawrence W Jr, Lenhard RE Jr, editors: *American Cancer Society textbook of clinical oncology,* Atlanta, 1995, American Cancer Society.

11. Boyce HW: Palliation of advanced esophageal cancer, *Semin Oncol* 11:186, 1984.

12. Brennan MF, Kinsella T, Casper ES: Cancer of the pancreas. In DeVita VT Jr, Hellman S, Rosenberg SA, editors: *Cancer: principles and practice of oncology,* ed 4, Philadelphia, 1993, Lippincott.

13. Brown TD, McDonald JS: Gastric, biliary, and pancreatic cancer: combined modality therapy and chemotherapy. In Brain MC, Carbone PP, editors: *Current therapy in hematology-oncology,* ed 5, St Louis, 1995, Mosby.

14. Caudry M: Gastric cancer: radiotherapy and approaches to locally unresectable or recurrent disease. In Ahlgren JD, McDonald JS, editors: *Gastrointestinal oncology,* Philadelphia, 1992, Lippincott.

15. Cimprich B: Esophagogastrectomy. In Brown MH and others, editors: *Standards of oncology nursing practice,* New York, 1986, Wiley & Sons.

16. Coit DG: Cancer of the small intestine. In Devita VT Jr, Hellman S, Rosenberg SA, editors: *Cancer: principles and practice of oncology,* ed 4, Philadelphia, 1993, Lippincott.

17. Connolly MM and others: Survival in 1001 patients with carcinoma of the pancreas, *Ann Surg* 206:366, 1987.

18. Cozzi E and others: Nursing management of patients receiving hepatic artery chemotherapy through an implanted infusion pump, *Cancer Nurs* 7:229, 1984.

19. Cuschieri A: Tumors of the stomach. In Moossa AR, Schimpff SC, Robson MC, editors: *Comprehensive textbook of oncology,* ed 2, Baltimore, 1991, Williams & Wilkins.

20. Douglas HO Jr: Overview of gastrointestinal cancer: two decades of progress. In Moossa AR, Schimpff SC, Robson MC, editors: *Comprehensive textbook of oncology,* ed 2, Baltimore, 1991, Williams & Wilkins.

21. Edmondson HA, Craig JR: Neoplasms of the liver. In Schiff L, Schiff ER, editors: *Diseases of the liver,* ed 6, Philadelphia, 1987, Lippincott.

22. Ellis FH Jr: Esophagogastrectomy for carcinoma: technical considerations based on anatomic location of lesion, *Surg Clin North Am* 60:265, 1980.

23. Ellis FH, Huberman M, Busse P: Cancer of the esophagus. In Murphy GP, Lawrence W Jr, Lenhard RE Jr, editors: *American Cancer Society textbook of clinical oncology,* Atlanta, 1995, American Cancer Society.

24. Farley DR, Donohue JH: Early gastric cancer, *Surg Clin North Am* 72:401, 1992.

25. Foster JH Jr: Liver resection techniques, *Surg Clin North Am* 69:235, 1989.

26. Frank-Stromberg M: The epidemiology and primary prevention of gastric and esophageal cancer: a worldwide perspective, *Cancer Nurs* 12:53, 1989.

27. Grady R, Farnen J, Ascheman P: Nutrition, alteration in: less than body requirements related to dysphagia. In McNally JC and others, editors: *Guidelines for oncology nursing practice,* ed 2, Philadelphia, 1991, Saunders.

28. Hancock SL, Glatstein E: Radiation therapy of esophageal cancer, *Semin Oncol* 11:144, 1984.
29. Havlin KA, McDonald JS: Gastric cancer: chemotherapy of advanced disease. In Ahlgren JD, McDonald JS, editors: *Gastrointestinal oncology,* Philadelphia, 1992, Lippincott.
30. Jackson JW: Operations for carcinomas of the thoracic and oesophagus and cardia. In Jackson JW, Cooper DKC, editors: *Rob & Smith's operative surgery,* ed 4, London, 1986, Butterworths.
31. Jordan GL Jr: Pancreatic resection for pancreatic cancer, *Surg Clin North Am* 69:569, 1989.
32. Kadish SL, Kochman ML: Endoscopic diagnosis and management of gastrointestinal malignancies, *Oncology* 9:967, 1995.
33. Kellum JM, Clark J, Miller HH: Pancreaticoduodenectomy for resectable malignant periampullary tumors, *Surg Gynecol Obstet* 157:362, 1983.
34. Kelsen DP: Chemotherapy of esophageal cancer. In Roth JA, Ruckdeschel JC, Weisenburger TH, editors: *Thoracic surgery,* Philadelphia, 1989, Saunders.
35. Lawrence W Jr, Zfuss, A: Gastric neoplasms. In Murphy GP, Lawrence W Jr, Lenhard RE Jr, editors: *American Cancer Society textbook of clinical oncology,* Atlanta, 1995, American Cancer Society.
36. Lightdale CJ, Daly J: Management of primary and metastatic cancer of the liver. In Schiff L, Schiff ER, editors: *Diseases of the liver,* ed 6, Philadelphia, 1987, Lippincott.
37. Little AG, McGregor BD: Tumors of the esophagus. In Moossa AR, Schimpff SC, Robson MC, editors: *Comprehensive textbook of oncology,* ed 2, Baltimore, 1991, Williams & Wilkins.
38. Lotze MT, Flickinger JC, Carr BI: Hepatobiliary neoplasms. In Devita VT Jr, Hellman S, Rosenberg SA, editors: *Cancer: principles and practice of oncology,* ed 4, Philadelphia, 1993, Lippincott.
39. McDonald JS, Hill MC, Roberts JM: Gastric cancer: epidemiology, pathology, detection, and staging. In Ahlgren JD, McDonald JS, editors: *Gastrointestinal oncology,* Philadelphia, 1992, Lippincott.
40. Moertel CG and others: Combined 5-FU and radiation therapy as a surgical adjuvant for poor prognosis gastric carcinoma, *J Clin Oncol* 2:1249, 1984.
41. Moossa AR: Tumors of the pancreas. In Moossa AR, Schimpff SC, Robson MC, editors: *Comprehensive textbook of oncology,* ed 2, Baltimore, 1991, Williams & Wilkins.
42. Naden G, Phillips TL: Radiation therapy for cancer of the esophagus. In Roth JA, Ruckdeschel JC, Weisenburger TH, editors: *Thoracic oncology,* Philadelphia, 1989, Saunders.
43. Nerenstone SR, Friedman MA, Ihde DC: Primary liver cancer. In Moossa AR, Schimpff SC, Robson MC, editors: *Comprehensive textbook of oncology,* ed 2, Baltimore, 1991, Williams & Wilkins.
44. Niederhuber JE: Tumors of the liver. In Murphy GP, Lawrence W Jr, Lenhard RE Jr, editors: *American Cancer Society textbook of clinical oncology,* ed 2, Atlanta, 1995, American Cancer Society.
45. Niederhuber JE, Ensminger WD: Surgical considerations in the management of hepatic neoplasia, *Semin Oncol* 10:135, 1983.
46. Parker SL and others: Cancer statistics, 1996, *CA Cancer J Clin* 46:5, 1996.
47. Rosenberg JC, Lichter AS, Leichman LP: Cancer of the esophagus. In DeVita VT Jr, Hellman S, Rosenberg SA, editors: *Cancer: principles and practice of oncology,* ed 3, Philadelphia, 1989, Lippincott.
48. Roth JA, Kelsen DP: Surgery and adjuvant chemotherapy for carcinoma of the esophagus. In Roth JA, Ruckdeschel JC, Weisenburger TA, editors: *Thoracic oncology,* Philadelphia, 1989, Saunders.
49. Roth JA and others: Cancer of the esophagus. In DeVita VT Jr, Hellman S, Rosenberg SA, editors: *Cancer: principles and practice of oncology,* ed 4, Philadelphia, 1993, Lippincott.
50. Sandor C: Nutrition, alteration in: less than body requirements related to disease process and treatment. In McNally JC and others, editors: *Guidelines for oncology nursing practice,* ed 2, Philadelphia, 1991, Saunders.
51. Smith JW, Brennan MF: Surgical treatment of gastric cancer, *Surg Clin North Am* 72:381, 1992.
52. Smith LE, Hill MC: Cancer and other tumors of the small bowel. In Ahlgren JD, McDonald JS, editors: *Gastrointestinal oncology,* Philadelphia, 1992, Lippincott.
53. Smith SL, Ciferni M: Liver transplantation. In Smith SL, editor: *AACN tissue and organ transplantation: implications for professional nursing practice,* St Louis, 1990, Mosby.
54. Starzl TE and others: Hepatic trisegmentectomy and other liver resections, *Surg Gynecol Obstet* 141:729, 1975.
55. Stone MD, Benotti PN: Liver resection: preoperative and postoperative care, *Surg Clin North Am* 69:383, 1989.
56. Trede M, Schwall G, Saeger H: Survival after pancreatoduodenectomy, *Ann Surg* 211:447, 1990.
57. Vezeridis MP, Wanebo HJ: Gastric cancer: surgical approach. In Ahlgren JD, McDonald JS, editors: *Gastrointestinal oncology,* Philadelphia, 1992, Lippincott.
58. Wooley PV, Treat J: Nonsurgical treatment of gastric cancer. In Moossa AR, Schimpff SC, Robson MC, editors: *Comprehensive textbook of oncology,* ed 2, Baltimore, 1991, Williams & Wilkins.

CHAPTER 9
Genitourinary Cancers

JEANNE PARZUCHOWSKI
MICHELLE WALLACE

Genitourinary (GU) malignancies include cancers of the urinary and genital organs in males and urinary organs in females. As a group, in 1996, GU tumors in the United States represent 401,000 cases of all cancer in males and 72,190 cases of male deaths, 53,400 cases of cancer in females and 17,200 cases of deaths in females.[119] Transrectal ultrasonography, computed tomography (CT) scan, and magnetic resonance imaging (MRI) are now routinely used to establish diagnoses. Recent developments in GU pathology include whole-mount techniques for prostate gland visualizations and elucidation of a range of biologic markers, including alpha(α-)-fetoprotein (AFP), human chorionic gonadotropin (HCG), and prostate-specific antigen (PSA).[118,119]

Refinements in the traditional therapeutic modalities and sophistication in newer treatment modalities, including laser therapy, three-dimensional imaging, and biologic response modifiers, have resulted in enormous progress in the management of GU cancers.

This chapter reviews principles and practices in the diagnosis and management of GU malignancies, including prostate, testis, bladder, kidney, and penis cancer, with special emphasis on issues related to prevention, early detection, and continuing care.

PROSTATE CANCER
EPIDEMIOLOGY

Prostate cancer represents the most common malignancy in the United States, accounting for 41% of all newly diagnosed cancer in men. The median age at diagnosis is 72, with the incidence rate increasing with each decade after age 50. For black men the incidence rate is nearly twice that of the general population, and the death

rate is as much as three times greater.[119] The global distribution of prostate cancer reveals a predominance in the United States and Northern European countries, most notably Sweden, with the lowest incidence being in Eastern Europe and Asia. However, Asians living in the United States are beginning to experience a rate of prostate cancer approaching that of the white population. This is supported by the observation that immigrants who move from low-risk areas to the United States gradually assume the higher risk of the U.S. population.[118]

Prostate cancer is associated with the aging process. After age 50 years, both incidence and mortality rates from prostate cancer increase at nearly exponential rates. It remains unclear why this cancer increases with age so much more than other cancers. Autopsy study data from many countries demonstrate that 15% to 30% of men older than 50 years have histologic evidence of prostate cancer.[118,119]

ETIOLOGY AND RISK FACTORS

The exact etiology of prostate cancer is unknown, although it appears that prostate cancer results from an interplay between endogenous hormones and environmental influences, most prominently dietary fat.[90,125]

Several studies have suggested that the incidence of prostate cancer is higher in men whose male relatives were affected with prostate cancer. Black men living in the United States have a higher incidence of prostate cancer at all ages.[123] The relative risk for prostate cancer increases over time after vasectomy. Vasectomy appears to confer an increased risk for the development of prostate cancer.[52,102] Epidemiologic research and migrant studies have associated a high-fat diet with prostate cancer, but how dietary fat is related to prostate cancer is unclear. The effect of dietary fat may be mediated through endogenous hormones. A low-fat, high-fiber diet has been shown to affect male sex hormone metabolism by decreasing circulating testosterone. Testosterone is necessary for normal prostate epithelium to grow. Early

The authors would like to express their appreciation to Jeffrey Forman, MD, Kimberly B. Hart, MD, Bruce Redman, DO, Ms. Joan Richardson, and Jason Parzuchowski for their support in writing the manuscript and providing the illustrations in this chapter.

prostate cancer has been shown to be estrogen dependent. The absence of prostate cancer in androgen-deficient males and the reduction of prostate cancer in experimental animals by prolonged administration of male sex hormones suggest that altered hormone metabolism may play a role in the progression of prostate cancer.[5]

ANATOMY

The prostate gland is a small, walnut-size, firm organ weighing about 20 g and shaped like an inverted pyramid. The superior surface referred, to as the *base*, lies at the neck of the urinary bladder; the *inferior apex* rests on the urogenital diaphragm (Figure 9-1). The portion of the urethra passing centrally from the superior base to the inferior apex is referred to as the *prostatic urethra*. Dense, fibrous tissue surrounds the gland. The ejaculatory ducts penetrate the gland posteriorly and superiorly. There are no true lobar divisions in the gland.

Visualizing the prostate gland as having a central area or zone, a submucosal or transitional zone, and a horseshoe-shaped peripheral area may help with understanding disease distribution and the area accessible to digital rectal examination (DRE). Palpable areas include posterior or posterolateral region of the peripheral zone with a median furrow, which is felt as a shallow midline depression, and the two superiorly positioned seminal vesicles are identifiable landmarks on rectal palpation. The prostate serves as a sex accessory gland, with the seminal vesicles contributing viscous secretions to semen.

PREVENTION, SCREENING, AND DETECTION

Prostate cancer screening and early detection remain controversial,[55,82,83] since no randomized, controlled study has ever demonstrated disease-specific mortality reduction from any test or procedure, including a DRE.[9] Therefore the major challenge in prostate cancer is the

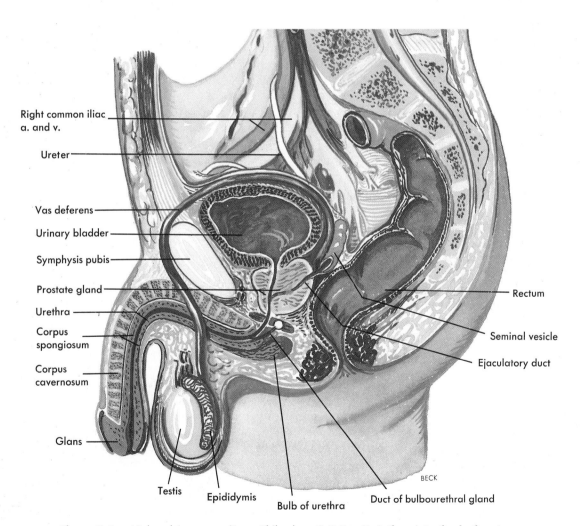

Figure 9-1   Male pelvic organs. (From Thibodeau G, Patton K: *Anthony's textbook of anatomy and physiology*, ed 14, St Louis, 1994, Mosby.)

promotion of early detection when the cancer is confined to the prostate gland and is curable. The American Cancer Society (ACS) recommended annual DRE of the prostate gland beginning at age 40. Recent guidelines issued by ACS recommend PSA level quantification annually for men 50 years of age and older for white men and 40 years of age and older for black men or men with a family history.[3,5,11,25,34]

To perform a DRE, wearing a lubricated glove, the examiner inserts the index finger approximately 2 to 3 cm (about 1 inch) into the anal orifice and gently presses against the lower wall of the rectum, systematically palpating the accessible surface of the prostate gland. This examination is facilitated when the subject is leaning forward with arms resting on the examination table, toes pointed inward, and the knees slightly flexed. Any change in size, consistency, or contour detected in the gland may represent an inflammatory process, infarction, or calculus, in addition to tumor. When a suspicious area is identified in the prostate, a biopsy is indicated. Prostatic needle biopsy for a core of tissue is accomplished easily with good yield and low morbidity by rectal approach. Since the introduction of a spring-loaded biopsy device, a relatively painless collection of multiple prostate tissue specimens can provide excellent material for pathology review and such ancillary studies as flow cytometry to assess deoxyribonucleic acid (DNA) content and morphometry to assess nuclear configuration.

High-frequency transducers in transrectal ultrasonography have enabled the visualization of internal prostatic anatomy, an opportunity previously available only to pathologists studying radical prostatectomy or autopsy specimens. Transrectal ultrasonography shows most prostatic lesions, both malignant and benign, as hypoechoic.* MRI, with its ability to illustrate glandular subtleties and determine capsular penetration and seminal vesicle involvement, may be helpful in the staging of prostate cancer.[148,149] CT continues to be the primary modality for evaluation of nodes, tissue, and organs; radionuclide scanning continues to be a primary modality for detecting or confirming metastatic bone involvement.

CLINICAL PREVENTION TRIALS

In response to recent developments in the diagnosis of prostate cancer and increasing disease prevalence, the Southwest Oncology Group (SWOG) is currently conducting an intergroup prostate cancer prevention trial, anticipated to register more than 12,000 men over a 2-year period. Eligible participants will include men ages 55 and older with normal prostates and PSA levels within nor-

mal range. At registration, participants are randomized to receive finasteride (Proscar), a 5-α-reductase inhibitor that prevents conversion of testosterone to dihydrotestosterone, or a placebo. Annual DRE and PSA level measurements will be done. Biopsy will be performed if PSA level reaches 4.0 ng/ml or greater in the placebo group. An equal percentage of men in the finasteride group will also be biopsied.

CLASSIFICATION

Ninety-five percent of prostate cancers are *adenocarcinomas. Ductal carcinomas,* including transitional and squamous cell carcinomas, endometrioid carcinomas, and sarcomas, account for the remainder. The classically employed *Gleason system* ascertains a degree of glandular differentiation and tumor growth pattern in relation to prostate stroma. A score is assigned both to the predominant pattern of differentiation, ranging from well-formed to undifferentiated tumors, and to any secondary pattern of differentiation observed microscopically. The histologic grading systems assign grade based on the most undifferentiated portion or on the predominant pattern observed. Scores range from 2 to 10 and have been shown to be predictive of associated lymph node metastases.* In general, degree of tumor differentiation and abnormality of histologic growth pattern directly correlate with likelihood of metastases and with death.[34,113,114,120] Prognosis is worse in patients with pelvic lymph node involvement. Recently, ductal-acinar dysplasia, identified by nuclear and cytoplasmic abnormalities, has been characterized as *prostatic intraepithelial neoplasia* (PIN). Early studies suggest that PIN meets the criteria for premalignant lesions, defined as those with the ability to progress to invasive cancer.

DIAGNOSIS, STAGING, AND CLINICAL FEATURES

The first clinical staging system was introduced by Whitmore and Jewett.[72] The American urologic system consists of ABCD stages that have been translated into tumor-node-metastasis (TNM) categories by the American Joint Commission on Cancer (AJCC)[14,72,130] and the Committee of the International Union Against Cancer (UICC).[9,130] Table 9-1 outlines the TNM classification for prostate cancer. Stage A, or T1, disease is asymptomatic, suspected on DRE, and found incidentally on pathologic examination of resected prostate tissue for management of prostatic hypertrophy. Stage A is further subdivided into A$_1$, or T1a, which is a pathologically graded, well-differentiated tumor or tumor foci representing 5% or less of resected tissue; and A$_2$, or T1b, which is a mod-

---

Table 9-1 Prostate Cancer Staging Systems

Whitmore-Jewett	Description	AJCC
A	*Incidental finding of carcinoma on examination of prostate tissue after prostatectomy or trans-urethral resection*	T1
A_1	Histologically well- or moderately well-differentiated tumor or tumor consisting of <5% of resected specimen	T1a
A_2	Histologically poorly differentiated or anaplastic tumor or tumor consisting of >5% of resected specimen	T1b
B	*Clinically palpable tumor confined to prostate*	T2
B_1	Focal ≤1.5 cm	T2a
B_2	Diffuse >1.5 cm ≥two foci	T2b
C	*Extension beyond prostate capsule to seminal vesicles or contiguous tissue*	T3
D	*Metastatic tumor*	N-M
D_1	Regional nodal involvement	M1 to M3
D_2	Metastasis to any of the following: Bone Lymph nodes above aortic bifurcation Other organ(s)	M

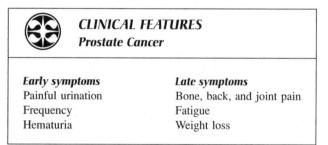

CLINICAL FEATURES
Prostate Cancer

Early symptoms	**Late symptoms**
Painful urination	Bone, back, and joint pain
Frequency	Fatigue
Hematuria	Weight loss

erately or poorly differentiated tumor involving greater than 5% of the resection. Stage B, or T2, disease is a palpable tumor confined to the prostate. B_1, or T2a, disease is a focal lesion 1.5 cm or less in diameter; B_2, or T2b, is diffuse disease greater than 1.5 cm in diameter or two or more foci of tumor foci at a time. Stage B_1, or T2, prostate cancer may also be asymptomatic. Clinically determined involvement of seminal vesicles or adjacent structures is staged as C, or T3, disease. At this stage, local irritative symptoms include painful urination, frequency, and hematuria. Stage D, or N-M, represents metastatic disease with D_1, or M, indicative of tumor metastatic to bone, other organs, or nodes above the aortic bifurcation.[103]

Symptoms associated with advanced disease may include painful urination; urinary frequency; hematuria; bone, back, or joint pain; weight loss; and fatigue (see box above). Prostate cancer spreads by direct extension to the seminal vesicles and contiguous structures, bladder, membranous urethra, and pelvic side walls. The rectum is essentially spared because it is offered a degree of protection by Denonvilliers' fascia. Lymphatic spread to pelvic nodes or hematogeneous deposition to bone is frequently encountered.

BIOLOGIC MARKERS

Laboratory quantification of PSA provides a marker for monitoring response to therapy.* PSA, a glycoprotein produced by normal and neoplastic ductal epithelium, serves to lyse the seminal coagulum. First purified from normal prostate tissue in 1979, PSA has since been found in seminal fluids, in benign hypertrophied prostate tissue, and in cancerous tissue. Monoclonal and polyclonal antibodies that react with PSA have been developed to provide laboratory determination of the level of PSA present. The ability of PSA to predict localized disease reliably is being evaluated. Because PSA is specific for prostatic cellular activity, it offers the clinician an additional marker to assess the likelihood of disease recurrence after definitive therapy.[3,47,85,140] For example, a rising PSA after radical prostatectomy suggests clinical recurrence[47,189] in men without prostatic disease; the normal range with the Tandem-R assay is 0 to 4 ng/ml.[170]

TREATMENT MODALITIES

Therapeutic maneuvers viewed with optimism in all stages of prostate cancer are also surrounded by controversy.[5,168,178,181]

In disease confined to the prostate gland, complete response to therapy and attainment of a normal life span are reasonable goals.[1,5,20,25,125] More extensive disease involvement can be managed effectively, with results varying from a complete response to partial remission.[3,25,33] In contrast to many other tumors, the therapy of advanced disease can be accompanied by partial re-

---

*References 38, 69, 85, 113, 114, 164.

mission or stable disease for a gratifying period.[90] The optimal management of men with localized prostate carcinoma remains controversial. No treatment with close observation is a viable option in select patients such as those with stage A_1 disease, very advanced age, or poor medical health.[43] Treatment options include a radical prostatectomy, external beam or interstitial radiotherapy, and hormonal therapy.[179] Selection of treatment is based on projected survival, as well as patient and physician preferences. Even when the cancer appears clinically localized to the prostate gland, a substantial percentage of patients will develop disseminated tumor after local therapy with surgery or irradiation.[179] This is caused by the high incidence of clinical understaging even with current diagnostic techniques. Metastatic tumor is currently not curable.

Surgery

Surgery has historically been the primary therapy for prostate cancer in the form of *radical prostatectomy* for localized cancer,[20,97,191] *transurethral resection* for tumor causing bladder outlet obstruction, or *bilateral orchiectomy* for management of metastatic disease. Stages A, B_1, B_2, T1, and T2 lesions may be treated surgically by radical prostatectomy.[1,180,191] Surgery is usually reserved for patients in good health who are under age 70 and require selective surgical intervention. These patients should have tumors confined to the prostate (stages A and B) and a negative bone scan. Patients appear to have a better prognosis than those with significant lymph node involvement. The technique of radical prostatectomy by perineal approach, introduced in this country by Hugh Hampton Young in 1903, demonstrated the feasibility of removal of the prostate and seminal vesicles in the management of prostatic malignancy. This is still used, particularly in patients with early-stage clinical disease. It offers advantageous exposure and a shorter operating time, a consideration in many elderly men. The retropubic approach is employed most often because it provides access to regional lymph nodes in the pelvis. Regional node sampling permits assessment of the presence or absence of tumor in adjacent nodes. If tumor is present in nodes, radical prostatectomy may be deferred. For patients with prostate cancer confined to the gland, radical prostatectomy is one of the most effective methods for definitively eradicating the tumor.[7,20,179,180,191] Postoperative complications of incontinence and urethral stricture are seen in fewer than 5% of patients. Previously, impotence was a major complication of radical prostatectomy. Postoperatively, 85% to 90% of men were incapable of sustaining an erection adequate for vaginal penetration. However, new surgical techniques popularized by Walsh and Lepor[180] spare the cavernous nerves and retain the physiologic responses required to maintain po-

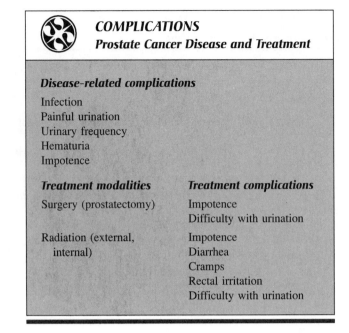

COMPLICATIONS
Prostate Cancer Disease and Treatment

Disease-related complications

Infection
Painful urination
Urinary frequency
Hematuria
Impotence

Treatment modalities	*Treatment complications*
Surgery (prostatectomy)	Impotence
	Difficulty with urination
Radiation (external, internal)	Impotence
	Diarrhea
	Cramps
	Rectal irritation
	Difficulty with urination

tency.[17,18,74,94] Pharmacologic erection or surgical implantation of a penile prosthesis may manage disease-related or treatment-related impotence. After radical prostatectomy, whole-mount techniques add a new dimension to pathologic assessment of the prostate capsule and seminal vesicles because the pathologist can reconstruct the gland, allowing for accurate measurement of tumor volume, visualization of foci of tumor, and analysis of surgical margins. The box above summarizes potential disease-related and treatment-related complications.

Postoperative radiotherapy may be considered in patients who are found to have capsular penetration or seminal vesicle invasion by tumor at the time of prostatectomy or a detectable PSA level more than 3 weeks after surgery.[190]

Radiation Therapy

External beam radiotherapy, with or without interstitial radiation implantation, can result in long-term remissions paralleling those achieved with radical prostatectomy.[17,48,141,166]

Local control is more difficult to achieve in patients with advanced disease.[19,40,156] More aggressive treatment strategies, such as radiation dose escalation studies, supplemental interstitial boosts,[128,166] hyperthermia, neutron irradiation,[88,90,128,154] or neoadjuvant hormonal therapy, are being evaluated to improve local control in these patients.[48,80,142]

Radiation therapy is delivered daily over 7 weeks. The radiation field includes the prostate and seminal vesicles, with a margin to allow for patient motion. With the advent of systems based on three-dimensional CT scans, radiation can be delivered *conformally*.[141,142] This technique allows an increased dose to be given to the tumor volume while limiting toxicity to normal tissues.[16] The risk of treatment-related side effects is influenced by the dose to normal tissue and volume of tissue treated. Acute toxicity, occurring within 6 months of treatment, is usually reversible and occurs within rapidly dividing cells. Chronic reactions occur in more slowly dividing cells and may be permanent. Many patients report fatigue during and immediately after treatment. Frequent rest periods should be encouraged. Symptoms relating to bladder toxicity include cystitis, urethral stricture, urinary frequency, dysuria, and nocturia. The rate of urinary incontinence is 2% to 3%. Tenesmus, diarrhea, and mucosal bleeding may result from gastrointestinal (GI) irritation. Surgical management is rarely indicated. Pharmacologic management of these symptoms is achieved with the use of antispasmodics and antidiarrheal agents. Patients should be instructed to maintain adequate elimination patterns and to monitor for signs and symptoms of urinary or rectal irritation.[16] Treated areas should not be exposed to sunlight because local skin reactions have been reported.

Potency is affected by radiation. Age and concomitant conditions, such as diabetes and hypertension, also play an additive role in impotency. Patients with good erectile function before treatment tend to remain potent, in contrast to those with poor initial function. Patients should be directed to urologists specializing in sexual dysfunction if they want to improve their potency. Radiation also plays a role in palliation for prostate cancer. External beam irradiation to selected sites or hemibody radiation therapy provides significant pain relief. Strontium-89, a systemic radioisotope, targets specific sites of metastatic disease when administered intravenously.[129,136] Response rates of 70% to 80% have been reported.[136]

Brachytherapy, the interstitial implantation of radioisotopes, offers another treatment option of prostate cancer management. Radioactive sources may be permanently implanted or may be temporarily implanted in the tumor volume for a short time.[80] Temporary implants are often used in combination with external beam radiotherapy.[128] Extensive planning with CT imaging and transrectal ultrasound facilitates needle and seed placement. Only patients with negative seminal vesicle biopsies and no evidence of metastatic disease are eligible for implantation.[80] Reported side effects include nocturia, frequency, dysuria, and urgency.

Nursing considerations, regardless of treatment options, include obtaining a comprehensive medical history with emphasis on baseline urologic and erectile function. Pretreatment cystograms offer objective data evaluating

bladder capacity and sphincter competency. Baseline erectile function can be obtained by Doppler studies. Patient education should encompass expectations of the entire treatment process.

Hormonal Therapy

Hormonal therapy may offer effective disease management in conjunction with a good quality of life for patients with metastatic carcinoma.[41]

Because prostatic epithelial cells depend on dihydrotestosterone for growth and differentiation, an understanding of the hypothalamic-pituitary-gonadal axis that regulates the physiologic balance of circulating testosterone is essential (Figure 9-2). Removal of the testes, the source of 95% of the major circulating androgen, testosterone, through bilateral orchiectomy, as introduced by Huggins and Hedges in 1941, is a cost-effective, well-tolerated intervention that interrupts the gonadal portion of the axis.

In 1971 a decapeptide, *luteinizing hormone–releasing hormone* (LHRH), was described by Schally. *Luteinizing hormone* (LH), released from the anterior pituitary in response to pulsatile release of LHRH, which is synthesized in the supraoptic nucleus of the hypothalamus, results in the testicular secretion of a physiologic level of testosterone with corresponding spermatogenesis (production of spermatozoa). Administration of exogenous estrogens such as *diethylstilbestrol* (DES) profoundly inhibit pituitary LH secretion, thereby reducing circulating testosterone to castrate level while increasing sex steroid–binding globulin and promoting prolactin secretion. This mechanism led to widespread application of DES in varying daily doses in the treatment of metastatic prostate cancer. The use of DES with cardiovascular morbidity led to a decline in DES use.[183]

Subsequently, a synthetic LHRH analogue was produced with a potency of up to 100 times that of naturally occurring LHRH. Initially, it was thought that the synthetic LHRH would stimulate pituitary release of follicle-stimulating hormone (FSH) and LH. However, it was discovered that in hypophysiologic concentration, LHRH analogues actually demonstrated a paradoxic effect. After an initial stimulation of gonadotropin release, long-term administration of LHRH analogues results in an enduring inhibition with corresponding gonadal down-regulation, including inhibition of prostatic growth. This may be the result of pituitary desensitization to the overabundance of LHRH. After an initial rise, serum testosterone falls to castrate levels with chronic LHRH therapy. LHRH agonists (e.g., leuprolide acetate, goserelin acetate)[122,178] have been established as effective options in the treatment of advanced prostate cancer.

Peripheral tissue and adrenal androgens account for

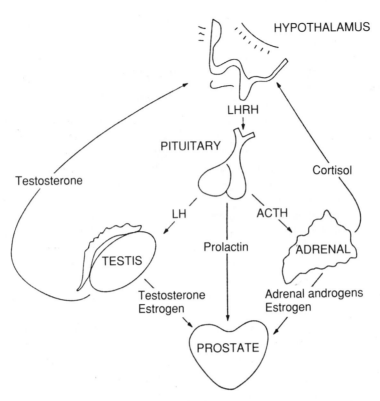

Figure 9-2 Hypothalamic-pituitary-testicular-adrenal axis. *LHRH,* Luteinizing hormone–releasing hormone; *LH,* luteinizing hormone; *ACTH,* adrenocorticotropic hormone. (Modified from Crawford ED: Combined androgen blockade, *Urology* 34[suppl]:24, 1989.)

the remaining 5% of circulating testosterone. *Anti-androgens,* both steroidal and nonsteroidal agents, such as flutamide (Eulexin, Casodex), compete with dihydrotestosterone for binding sites on prostatic cells.[10,32,78,144] Through this action, antiandrogens do not alter the level of circulating male hormone but rather block the hormone from reaching the target tissue, the prostate gland. The antiandrogens do not interfere with sexual potency because they do not alter testosterone levels.

High-dose *ketoconazole* (1200 mg daily), an anti-fungal agent, affects both gonadal and adrenal androgens, rapidly lowering unbound testosterone to castrate levels within 1 to 2 days. However, the GI intolerance and potential for hepatotoxicity associated with it limit its clinical use. *Aminoglutethimide* effectively blocks adrenal steroidogenesis and synthesis of mineralocorticoids, glucocorticoids, and sex steroids but must be coupled with hydrocortisone to circumvent moderate to fatal adrenal insufficiency.[128,144] Surgical *adrenalectomy* and surgical *hypophysectomy* are not cost-effective or therapeutically advantageous options. Table 9-2 summarizes potential treatment complications associated with surgical and hormonal therapy for prostate cancer.

Cryotherapy

Cryotherapy is another modality under investigation for both primary treatment and disease recurrence. Lower impotency rates have been reported for cryotherapy. The results with this modality are preliminary, and long-term follow-up is necessary to determine the role of cryotherapy in the treatment of prostate cancer.

Chemotherapy

In prostate cancer, recurrent or persistent disease is challenging.[10,99] Selection of further treatment depends on multiple factors, including prior treatment, site of recurrence, comorbid conditions, and individual patient considerations. Prolonged disease control is often possible with hormone therapy,[10,33,120] with median cancer-specific survival of 6 years after local failure.[98,178] Chemotherapy has limited value in the treatment of patients with refractory disease after hormonal therapy. Many drugs have been used as second-line hormonal therapy. Response rates usually approximate 20%, and duration of response is usually less than 6 months. Phases I and II clinical trials of chemotherapy consisting of combinations of VP-16–Emcyt (etoposide-extramustine) and biologic agents in hormone-refractory patients are ongoing.[67,106,125]

Table 9-2 Hormone Therapy for Prostate Cancer: Potential Treatment Complications

Treatment	Cardiovascular	Impotence	Gastrointestinal	Hot flashes	Testosterone flare	Permanent	Cost
Bilateral orchiectomy	—	↑↑↑	—	↑↑	—	↑↑↑	$
Estrogens	↑	↑↑↑	↑	↑	—	—	$ to $$$*
LHRH analogues	—	↑↑↑	—	↑↑	↑↑	—	$$$
Antiandrogens	—	↑	↑↑↑	↑	—	—	$$$
Progestational agents	—	↑↑↑	↑	↑	↑	—	$$
Ketoconazole	—	↑↑↑	↑↑↑	↑	—	—	$$$
Aminoglutethimide	—	↑↑↑	↑↑	—	—	—	$$

From Davis MA, Crawford ED: Unpublished data, 1991.
*Thromboembolic management.

TESTICULAR CANCER

EPIDEMIOLOGY

Testicular cancer is a relatively uncommon disease, with an estimated 3000 cases per year. Testicular cancer represents the most common malignancy in men from ages 15 to 35 and the second most common malignancy from ages 35 to 39. Occurring during the prime of life for most patients, testicular cancer has a major emotional impact. Testicular tumors occur more often in white males than black males in the United States.[118] The disease represents one of the most curable solid tumors and serves as a paradigm for the multimodal treatment of solid malignancies. Dramatic increases in survival are a result of a combination of effective diagnostic techniques, improvement in tumor markers, effective multidrug chemotherapeutic regimens, and modification of surgical techniques. All these advances have led to a significant decline in the morbidity and mortality from this disease.[81,153]

Better understanding of serum tumor markers has allowed for early diagnosis and follow-up, with intervention earlier in the course of the disease, when widespread metastases on presentation, including brain metastases, may be curable.[131,163]

ETIOLOGY AND RISK FACTORS

The etiology of testicular cancer is unknown, but certain conditions are associated with an increased incidence of this malignancy. Specifically, testicular tumors are more likely to occur in an atrophic testis or a cryptorchid (undescended) testis; the likelihood of subsequent development of cancer in an undescended testis is 40 times greater than in a normal testis. *Orchiopexy,* surgical descent of the cryptorchid testis, before a boy is 2 years old may reduce the probability of subsequent development of a testicular tumor.[32,37]

Testicular tumors have certain characteristics that favor successful treatment. Men who have had an undescended testicle are at a higher risk of developing cancer than other men whose testicles have moved down into the scrotum. The relative risk of testicular cancer in patients with cryptorchidism is thought to be 3 to 14 times the normal expected incidence.[37] Patients may have an antecedent history of scrotal trauma. However, no evidence implicates trauma as a causative factor. A history of mumps or orchitis has been reported as well.[32]

PREVENTION, SCREENING, AND DETECTION

Prevention of testicular cancer is not a reasonable expectation because etiologic factors are unknown. However, early detection is accomplished best by *testicular self-examination* (TSE) and is recommended for patients with a prior history of testicular malignancy. As recommended by the ACS, young men from puberty through age 40 need to be instructed and encouraged to perform monthly TSE (Figure 9-3). Patients who have been cured of testicular cancer have approximately a 5% cumulative risk of developing a cancer in the opposite testicle over 31 years after the initial diagnosis.[112] These patients should be instructed to do TSE and should have periodic examinations aimed at early detection.[112,171]

TSE is facilitated by the heat of a warm bath or shower. Each testicle is examined with both hands. The index and middle fingers are placed on one side of the testicle. The thumbs are placed on the other side. A gentle rolling motion allows for complete palpation of each testicle. One testicle may be larger than the other. Any lump, new finding, or worrisome area needs to be reported. The normal testis is homogeneous in consistency, freely movable, and separable from the epididymis.

The classic presentation of a testicular tumor is a nontender, enlarged testis noted incidentally by the patient or his sexual partner. This is described as a lump or hardness of the testis, with occasional heaviness or a dull, aching sensation in the lower abdomen or scrotum. Acute pain is the presenting symptom in about 10% of patients. On rare occasions, infertility is the presenting complaint.

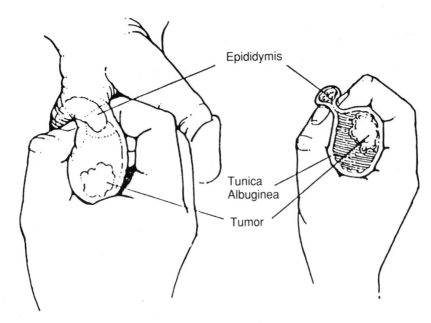

Figure 9-3 Testicular self-examination (TSE). Care is taken with digital separation of testis from posterior elements, including epididymis and cord, for thorough palpation of intrascrotal contents. (Modified from Donohue JP: The testis. In Paulson DF, editor: *Genitourinary surgery*, 1984, Churchill Livingstone.)

Typically, there are no early symptoms. However, a scrotal mass may represent a variety of conditions, including epididymitis, spermatocele, hydrocele, torsion, testicular trauma, or infarction. In many instances, diagnosis of a testicular tumor is delayed because of a man's reluctance to seek medical attention for a troublesome testis condition or the clinician's assumption that a scrotal mass represents an infectious or inflammatory process.

A history of trauma, mumps, orchitis, episodic testicular pain, low back pain, groin pain, or abdominal aching or gynecomastia with or without tenderness is often reported. More than half the testicular tumors are initially considered to represent epididymitis. If symptoms persist after completion of antibiotics prescribed for suspected epididymitis, testicular cancer must be considered. Ultrasound of the scrotum is usually not performed if a solid tumor is thought to originate from the testicle on physician examination but may be helpful in equivocal cases.[161]

The physician should palpate the testes and surrounding structures for a scrotal mass, examine the breasts for gynecomastia, transilluminate intrascrotal lesions, and perform abdominal examination for a palpable mass, as well as evaluate the supraclavicular region, axillae, and inguinal area for adenopathy. Proper examination of a scrotal mass, including separation of the anterior testis within the tunica albuginea from the posterior adnexal elements, including the epididymis and cord, must be performed so that the intrascrotal contents may be palpated (Figure 9-3). The tunica albuginea functions as a natural barrier to expansive local growth. Once a palpable nodule exists within the testicle, local involvement or metastases may occur via either the lymphatic (in an orderly manner) or the hematogeneous route. Lymphatic metastasis generally tends to follow the spermatic vessels to primary landing sites in the retroperitoneum. Involvement of the epididymis or spermatic cord may lead to pelvic and inguinal lymph node metastases. Common sites of distant metastases include the lungs, bone, or liver and may occur as a direct tumor invasion.[81]

Lymphatic metastasis is common to all forms of germinal testicular tumors. Distant metastases occur most frequently to the pulmonary region. Subsequent spread may occur in the liver, viscera, brain, or bone. Bony metastases are encountered late in the course of the disease. Central nervous system metastases may occur.[163] Posteroanterior and lateral chest x-ray films provide an initial assessment of the lung parenchyma and mediastinal structures. Chest CT may be ordered to detect pulmonary metastases. Abdominal and pelvic CT scans (or MRI) remain the most effective way to identify retroperitoneal lymph node involvement.[27] CT scanning can generally identify lymph nodes less than 2.0 cm in diameter in the upper paraaortic regions and provide three-dimensional estimates of tumor size as well as involvement of soft tissue structures. CT scanning, however, has limitations when evaluating thin patients or differences between fibrous or other malignancies. Many of the early

NURSING MANAGEMENT

Nurses and physicians must promote compliance with screening recommendations, especially in men with a family history of prostate cancer. Black men especially need to be aware of their increased risk for disease and disease-associated mortality.

Because prostate cancer has become a major tumor afflicting the American male, a corresponding awareness of the disease and its potential for morbidity needs to be emphasized. Clinical support services of a multidisciplinary professional team with expertise in diagnosis and management of prostate cancer must address the issues of pain control, nutritional support, financial impact, sexuality, and emotional support. See box below for geriatric considerations and pp. 187-189 for detailed nursing interventions.

 GERIATRIC CONSIDERATIONS

Since approximately 87% of prostate cancer patients are 65 years of age or older, awareness of the concerns of this population is appropriate. With the transition to older adulthood and accommodation to the gradual shift in family responsibilities, retirement, and declining economic opportunities, the aging adult is challenged to achieve ego integrity. Along with the acceptance of age-related limitations, the senior adult is adjusting to physiologic aging, retirement, reduced income, and deaths of relatives, friends, and conceivably spouse while maintaining a safe and solvent environment, often in a relocation setting. The older person is customarily concerned about finances, loss of independence, and placing a burden on family or society. Frequently the senior adult approaches the health care system and care providers from a docile perspective and may not aggressively pursue or report symptoms, thus resulting in delay of diagnosis or lack of symptom resolution. The older adult with Medicare has acute care coverage but may not have comprehensive coverage for preventive or supportive care, including oral and subcutaneous medications. Intellectual function is usually maintained in older adulthood, although short-term memory may gradually decline, underscoring the need for application of recall and repetitive techniques. Special attention to establishing a framework for open communication and identifying components of the individual's dilemma, such as reimbursement, are suggested for facilitating compliance and rehabilitation for the older adult. And last, the older adult may accommodate the disease-related symptoms, interpreting them as age-related rather than disease-related, thus delay in seeking prudent medical intervention.

---

and late symptoms are a result of lymphatic enlargement and pressure on adjacent structures. The box at right outlines clinical features associated with testicular cancer.

CLASSIFICATION

Approximately 97% of all testicular tumors are germ cell tumors originating in the primordial germ cells essential for spermatogenesis. Testicular tumors are classically categorized according to the histologic types.

Testicular cancer is broadly divided into two groups: a pure form or a mixture of cell types. Most clinicians distinguish primarily between *pure seminoma* and *nonseminoma*. Seminomas are more sensitive to radiation therapy. For patients with seminoma (all stages combined) the cure rate exceeds 80%. For patients with early-stage disease the cure rate approaches 100%. Tumors that have a mixture of seminomatous and nonseminomatous components are treated as nonseminoma. Tumors that ap-

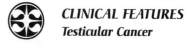 **CLINICAL FEATURES**
Testicular Cancer

Classic presentation
Nontender, enlarged testis
History
Trauma
Mumps, orchitis
Episodic testicular pain or heaviness
Symptoms
Abdominal aching
Low back pain
Gynecomastia
Breast tenderness

pear to have a seminomatous histology in patients with elevated serum levels of AFP are treated as nonseminomas. Elevation of the β-subunit of HCG alone is found in approximately 10% of patients with pure seminoma. Nonseminoma includes embryonal carcinoma, teratoma, yolk sac carcinoma, and choriocarcinoma, or various combinations of these cell types. Risk for metastases is highest with choriocarcinoma and lowest with teratoma.

CLINICAL STAGING

Clinical examination and radical orchiectomy are required for clinical staging. Histopathologic cell types are divided into two groups, seminomatous and nonseminomatous testicular tumors unlike other tumor types. The extent of the primary tumor (T) is classified after radical orchiectomy.[173] In testicular cancer the most important aspect in the pathology is whether there has been invasion of the cord, epididymis, tunica albuginea, rete testis, scrotum, lymphatic system, or blood vessels; patients having tumors with such histologic features typically are excluded from surveillance and undergo staging *retroperitoneal lymph node dissection* (RPLND). The extent of staging in part determines treatment decisions but also dictates prognosis.[173]

The pathologic confirmation of testicular cancer is made after high ligation of the cord is performed followed by *orchiectomy,* when the testis is surgically removed. An inguinal incision rather than a transscrotal incision is made to approach the mass. Violation of the scrotal lymphatic vessels and open biopsy are avoided to prevent lymphatic spread.[27] Transscrotal biopsy is always contraindicated with diagnostic evaluation because of the risk of local dissemination of tumor.[91]

BIOLOGIC MARKERS

Testicular cancer is one of the few malignancies for which specific serologic tumor markers are available.[6,13] Germinal testicular tumors produce marker proteins that are relatively specific and measurable in minute quantities. Tumor markers may be capable of detecting small tumor burdens that cannot be detected by imaging techniques. Two markers are clinically useful in diagnosis, staging, and monitoring of treatment responses in patients with germ cell neoplasms. AFP and the β-subunit of HCG as serum markers provide valuable information for assessment. Any elevation in AFP or HCG raises the clinical index of suspicion. Serum tumor marker proteins should be obtained before an orchiectomy so that the efficacy of the removal of the primary testicular malignancy may be assessed. The half-life of AFP is approximately 5 days, and the half-life of HCG is approximately 24 to 36 hours. Elevation in serum tumor markers after appropriate treatment may indicate persistent or metastatic disease.

Not all patients have elevated serum marker proteins. Therefore these serum marker proteins are useful only when they are initially abnormal or when one or both illustrate a rising pattern after normalization, indicating disease recurrence. Elevated HCG is possible with pure seminoma. An elevated AFP is never observed in pure seminoma. If the AFP is elevated, the tumor is not pure seminoma but rather a mixed cell type. High levels of HCG are suspicious in the patient considered to have pure seminoma.

FERTILITY AND PRETREATMENT PLANNING

The ability to preserve or "bank" human sperm by cryogenic methods has been developed and successfully applied in reproductive biology.[153] A major application of a sperm bank is to preserve the sperm from men who face permanent injury to spermatogenesis through surgery, chemotherapy, or radiation. Exclusion criteria for sperm banking at most centers include those individuals with health histories outlined in the box, p. 175.

Many of the patients successfully treated for testicular tumors need pretreatment counseling to discuss options for planned parenthood and the effects of therapy on fertility. In one prospective study of 41 patients before therapy, 77% were oligospermic (sperm deficient), 17% were azoospermic (completely lacked sperm), and only 66% could meet the requirements for sperm banking. In this same group of patients, 96% were azoospermic after 2 months of therapy. A retrospective review of a group of 28 patients with solitary lesions indicated sperm counts in 46% of patients after chemotherapy.[29,55,58,111,165]

Although reviews indicate that combination chemotherapy does affect spermatic function, a high degree of recovery of spermatogenesis is experienced 2 to 3 years after initiation of treatment. Subsequent successful pregnancies with no increased incidence of fetal abnormalities or tumors in offspring have been reported.[42] It is important to emphasize in the pretreatment phase and throughout that radiotherapeutic and chemotherapeutic treatments should not be considered as substitutes for standard methods of birth control. Men should be instructed that conception can occur during therapy.

TREATMENT MODALITIES
Seminoma Therapy

Seminomas, which account for 40% of germ cell tumors of the testis, tend to be homogeneous neoplasms on gross examination, often pale gray to yellow, with a slightly lobulated consistency.[70] Pure seminomas exhibit dramatic radiosensitivity. Tumors possessing both seminomatous and nonseminomatous properties or seminoma in patients with elevated AFP levels should be managed as nonseminomas. Pure seminoma may exhibit elevated

---

CRITERIA FOR SPERM BANKING: INITIAL VISIT

HISTORICAL SCREENING (FOR EXCLUSION PURPOSES)

Identification of at-risk groups for acquired immunodeficiency syndrome (AIDS):

    Men with any homosexual contact since 1978

    Intravenous drug users

    Sexual partners of persons in AIDS risk groups

    Donor from geographic areas where sex ratio of AIDS patients is close to 1:1

    More than one sexual partner within 6 months

    Evidence of sexually transmitted disease (STD) within past 6 months:

        Dysuria

        Urethral discharge

        Genital ulcer

        Positive syphilis test (VDRL or RPR)

        Sexual partner with frequent episodes of *Trichomonas* infection

    Any history of:

        Genital herpes

        Genital wart

        Chronic hepatitis

        Previous exclusion from blood donation unless for noninfectious reason

PHYSICAL EXAMINATION

Ensure none of the following is present:

    Urethral discharge

    Genital wart

    Genital ulcer

Perform urethral cultures:

    Neisseria gonorrhoeae

    Chlamydia trachomatis

    Mycoplasma hominis

    Trichomonas vaginalis

SEROLOGY

Hepatitis B surface antigen and core antibody

Human immunodeficiency virus (HIV)

Cytomegalovirus (CMV)

VDRL or RPR

VDRL, Venereal Disease Research Laboratories; *RPR,* rapid plasma reagin.

---

levels of β-HCG. Removal of the affected testicle, or radical inguinal orchiectomy, is the initial treatment for all stages of seminomas.

For stage I seminoma, after orchiectomy, radiation is delivered to the pelvic and ipsilateral lymph nodes to an approximate cumulative dose of 25 to 30 cGy. Retroperitoneal nodes are prophylactically irradiated even with a negative lymphangiogram or CT scan because approximately 15% will have occult nodal spread that can be cured with irradiation.[70,168] The contralateral testis is shielded from the radiation beam. Cure rates with this approach are 95%. Nonbulky stage I seminomas, tumors measuring less than 3.0 cm on CT scan, have a cure rate of 90%. The abdominal and pelvic lymph nodes are irradiated in bulky tumors not exceeding 5.0 cm. Although earlier studies reported that bulky stage II seminomas had a cure rate of 70% with radiation alone, studies using improved treatment planning and equipment as well as careful selection of patients (including use of tumor markers) have reported an improvement in the results of radiation in the treatment of bulky stage II seminoma.[7] Elective irradiation of the mediastinum is no longer recommended. Combination chemotherapy with a cisplatin, etoposide, and bleomycin regimen is effective in treating bulky tumors. Recurrence rate is higher for bulky stage II tumors rather than radiation for nonbulky tumors, leading some to recommend primary chemotherapy for patients with bulky disease.[98] Platinum-based chemotherapy is the treatment of choice for stage III disease, advanced supradiaphragmatic adenopathy, or widespread metastatic disease. The role of radiotherapy in advanced seminoma is reserved for salvage of chemotherapy failures or palliation[12] in patients who do not achieve remission with high-dose chemotherapy with autologous bone marrow transplantation.[15]

Nursing considerations are directed at decreasing the treatment-induced symptomatology in the management of seminoma. After orchiectomy, measures are taken to promote comfort and to minimize postoperative morbidity. Discussions regarding concerns about body image and sexuality should be encouraged. Reassurance is needed that potency is not permanently impaired. Radiotherapy to the retroperitoneal area is generally well tolerated. Mild nausea and vomiting, diarrhea, myelosuppression, and azoospermia may occur as a result of the radiation or chemotherapy. Antiemetics may be employed during treatment. Patients should be instructed to increase fluid intake and begin a low-residue diet that is high in protein and carbohydrates. Foods or beverages that increase GI motility should be eliminated. Measures should be taken to prevent infection and bleeding from chemotherapy-induced myelosuppression. Fertility-related issues are discussed earlier in this chapter.

Nonseminoma Therapy

The majority of nonseminomas have more than one cell type. The cell type is important for deciding chemotherapy and risk of metastases.

Stage I nonseminoma. Stage I nonseminoma is highly curable, with more than 95% of patients treated successfully. Standard treatment includes removal of the testicle through the groin followed by retroperitoneal lymph node dissection. If preservation of fertility is an important aspect of the treatment and rehabilitation, a nerve-sparing *retroperitoneal lymphadenectomy* (RPL) that preserves ejaculation can be performed.[42] In patients

---

CHEMOTHERAPY REGIMENS FOR
STAGE II NONSEMINOMA

BEP: bleomycin + etoposide + cisplatin (Platinol)
EP: etoposide + cisplatin (Platinol)

---

with pathologic stage I disease after RPL, the presence of lymphatic or venous invasion from the primary tumor appears to predict relapse.[153] AFP cannot be used as a predictable indicator of presence or absence of disease, since marker-negative patients may be marker positive at relapse and marker-positive patients may be marker negative at relapse.[15,37,81]

Stage II nonseminoma. Stage II nonseminoma is also highly curable, with success rates greater than 95%. Radical inguinal orchiectomy followed by RPLND with or without fertility-preserving technique, along with follow-up, remains a standard of care. Patients whose markers do not return to normal after RPLND are treated with chemotherapy.[169] The option of surgery and careful follow-up, reserving chemotherapy for relapse, may be considered as a treatment alternative in patients who have less than six positive nodes in the RPLND, none of which is greater than 2.0 cm in diameter or has invaded outside the lymph node capsule. Most patients are curable even with relapse.[169] The third approach for stage II nonseminoma includes radical inguinal orchiectomy followed by chemotherapy with delayed surgery for removal of any residual tumor (if present), then monthly checkups. The box above outlines chemotherapy regimens. Surgery usually is performed after completion of three or four courses of chemotherapy and normalization of markers. Clinical trials are currently evaluating the role of combined chemotherapy with patients who have small-volume retroperitoneal disease in an effort to avoid RPLND.[45,169]

Stage III nonseminoma. The cure rate for stage III nonseminoma with standard chemotherapy is about 70%. Patients who are not cured with standard chemotherapy usually have large, bulky disease. Patients with brain metastases should be treated with chemotherapy and simultaneous whole-brain irradiation and consideration of surgical excision.

Chemotherapy

Considerable excitement has been generated with the success of chemotherapy for testicular tumors. *Cisplatin* was discovered to have a profound inhibitory effect on bacteria replication by Rosenberg in 1965. Before that, a number of single agents had demonstrated activity in disseminated testicular cancer, most notably actinomy-

---

 COMPLICATIONS
Testicular Cancer Disease and Treatment

Potential organ system, body image, and reproductive capacity complications associated with testicular cancer and treatment are serious and significant. Compliance is paramount to achievement of optimal success in the management of testicular tumors. With cure a likely expectation, the individual with a testicular tumor, his support network, and his clinicians are encouraged to maintain an outcome-focused approach while mandating compliance with proven therapeutic regimens with their acceptable and generally reversible profile of complications. Key elements in potential complications are highlighted below.

Treatment modality	*Treatment complications*
Orchiectomy	Body image concern
Retroperitoneal lymph node dissection (RPLND)	Body image concern
	Spermatogenesis deficiency
Chemotherapy	Body image concern
	Bone marrow suppression
	Organ function impairment:
	Renal
	Neurologic
	Otologic
	Pulmonary
	Alopecia
	Fatigue
	Spermatogenesis impairment
Radiation therapy	Body image concern
	Spermatogenesis impairment
	Skin integrity compromise

---

cin D, methotrexate, chlorambucil, vinblastine, mithramycin, and bleomycin. However, enduring complete remissions occurred in less than 20% of patients. With the introduction of cisplatin-based chemotherapy, this percentage dramatically increased to 80% to 90%. The coupling of cisplatin with vinblastine and bleomycin rendered a substantial number of patients disease free.[7,65,92,96,107] Etoposide and ifosfamide have demonstrated notable activity in germ cell tumors. No other tumor type appears to have so many viable chemotherapeutic agents for induction and, if necessary, for salvage therapy.[7] Meticulous attention needs to be paid to the selection of appropriate combinations of drugs with proven efficacy, employing dosages and schedules as determined in clinical trials. Patients need to comply with their therapeutic regimens, and clinicians need to encourage these patients in their compliance efforts.

The box, p. 176, summarizes testicular cancer treatment modalities and potential complications.

PROGNOSIS

With the cure rates seen in both seminomatous and non-seminomatous disease, testicular tumors are truly a model of success for combination-agent chemotherapy and multimodality therapy. At this time, clinicians have the luxury of striving for achieving a higher percentage of early-stage diagnoses through promoting TSE and motivating males to seek clinical evaluation on discovery of the primary tumor, evaluation for metastatic disease status, and proper coordination of the appropriate therapeutic interventions of surgery, chemotherapy, and radiotherapy to guarantee dramatic successes. With current economic constraints and quality of life issues, persons with cancer are being treated in their local communities outside the referral and university-based centers. However, a slight but troubling decline is being seen in the percentage of complete and enduring cures for testicular tumors. The tendency to consider a milder dose of chemotherapy, adhering to the patient's work and social schedules, needs to be tempered with the realization that any reduction in dosages or disruption in timing may compromise the patient's chance for a complete remission and a cure.

RENAL CELL CANCER

EPIDEMIOLOGY

Approximately 3% of all tumors diagnosed in the United States each year are tumors of the kidney.[118] *Wilms' tumors* are usually diagnosed in children under age 5 years and account for approximately 4% of all kidney cancers.[57] In adults, kidney cancer occurs more often in men than women (2:1 ratio). Renal cancer is most frequently encountered in adults over age 40, with a median age at diagnosis of 64.3 years for whites and 58.2 years for blacks.

ETIOLOGY AND RISK FACTORS

The etiology of renal cancer is unknown. Renal cell carcinoma arises from the proximal convoluted tubule. Associated abnormalities include deviations of the short arm of chromosome 3 and abnormalities of the p53 gene.[134]

Although no specific agent has been definitely identified as the cause of renal carcinoma, many epidemiologic studies imply that tobacco may pay a significant role in this disease. Studies report an increased risk of 1.5:2.2 for tobacco users. Patients with von Hippel-Lindau disease have a higher incidence of renal cell cancer, as do

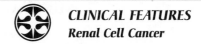

CLINICAL FEATURES
Renal Cell Cancer

Pain
Hematuria
   Intermittent
   Uncontrolled
Anemia
Fever
Fatigue

patients with acquired cystic disease. Familial renal cell carcinoma has been reported.

CLASSIFICATION AND STAGING

Renal cell carcinomas are historically characterized by a mixture of clear, granular, or spindlelike sarcomatoid cells arranged in solid, cystic, tubular, or papillary patterns. More than 95% of parenchymal tumors are adenocarcinomas and are referred to as *hypernephroma, renal cell carcinoma, clear cell cancer,* or *Grawitz's tumor.* Squamous cell carcinoma and nephroblastoma are also identified.[24] Renal carcinomas locally invade the capsule, are highly angioinvasive and often spread to the renal vein and vena cava, and result in widespread hematogeneous and lymphatic metastases. The most common sites for nonlymphatic metastases are lung, bone, liver, and brain. Renal cell carcinoma can metastasize to unusual sites, such as the testes and skin. Another unique and rare aspect related to this carcinoma is the tumor's ability to regress spontaneously.[115]

The staging system for renal cell cancer is based on the degree of tumor spread beyond the kidney.[24] Blood vessel involvement may not always signify a poor prognostic indicator. The TNM system defined by the AJCC can be abbreviated into a tumor stage grouping as follows: T1, tumor confined to the kidney and capsule; T2, tumor larger than 2.5 cm and limited to the kidney; T3, tumor extending into major veins or exhibiting perinephric invasion; and T4, tumor invading beyond Gerota's fascia.

CLINICAL FEATURES

The classic triad of hematuria, palpable flank mass, and flank pain is associated with advanced tumors (see box above). Analgesics generally relieve the pain. Pain unresponsive to additional treatments may indicate invasion of adjacent muscle and nerve routes. Early-stage renal cell cancer is usually "silent" and is coincidentally detected when the patient is undergoing work-up for a non-

Diagnostic and therapeutic maneuvers for the management of testicular tumors are difficult for patients. However, the results are so dramatic and exciting that encouraging persons to comply is not just suggested but mandated. Compliance with treatment regimens of appropriate drugs, dosages, and sequencing of timing will result in enduring disease-free remissions in an extraordinarily high percentage of patients. Although the group at risk for developing testicular tumors is at an age when body image concerns are paramount, temporary body image distortions, although deeply troubling, are a small price to pay for what appears to be the promise of a normal life span once appropriate therapy, with subsequent resolution of tumor, has been completed. See pp. 187-189 for detailed nursing interventions.

SYNDROMES ASSOCIATED WITH RENAL CARCINOMAS

SYNDROMES

Hypercalcemia
Nonmetastatic hepatopathy
Hypertension
Erythrocytosis
Pyrexia
Galactorrhea
Cushing's syndrome
Gynecomastia
Serum glucose abnormalities

SEROLOGIC FACTORS AND OTHER SYNDROMES

Prostaglandins
Alkaline phosphatase
Neuromyopathy
Amyloidosis
Coagulation factors
Iron metabolism
γ-Enolase
α-Fetoprotein
Vasculitis
Fibroblast growth factor

From Sufrin G and others: Paraneoplastic and serologic syndromes of renal adenocarcinoma, *Semin Urol* 7(3):159, 1989.

cancer-related procedure such as cardiac angiography or gallbladder ultrasound. Renal cell carcinomas are known to secrete hormones, including parathyroid hormone and erythropoietin, which cause hypercalcemia and erythrocytosis. Hypertension is typically encountered and may be mediated by tumor secretion of renin. Stauffer's syndrome, a reversible hepatorenal condition that results in abnormal liver function, may also be observed.

Unfortunately, approximately 34% of patients have metastases at diagnosis.[24] The box at left lists paraneoplastic syndromes associated with renal malignancies.

DIAGNOSIS

The distinction between well-differentiated renal carcinomas and renal adenomas can be difficult. The diagnosis is usually made arbitrarily on the basis of size of the mass, but size alone should not influence the treatment approach, since metastases can occur in lesions as small as 0.5 cm. A renal mass can be detected on intravenous pyelography (IVP) or ultrasound. Ultrasound differentiates cystic from solid lesions. With the increased improvements in the quality of ultrasound, abdominal CT, and other imaging modalities, early detection and staging of clinically asymptomatic patients are possible.

Tumor size, its density, extent of local invasion, renal vein or vena cava involvement, lymph node metastasis, and liver and lung involvement should be identified. CT scan with contrast or MRI with gadolinium injection may be used to delineate tumors. MRI is used to identify thrombus that may have formed in the renal vein or renal vena cava. X-ray films of the chest are important to rule out lung involvement. Laboratory tests that include a complete blood count with an SMA-12 and liver chemistries should be obtained. Selective renal arteriography is generally performed only when renal-sparing procedures are planned.

TREATMENT MODALITIES

Currently, state-of-the-art treatment using surgery cures more than half the patients with early-stage renal cell cancer. Poor prognosis is associated with a patient with stage IV disease as a result of the tumor's lack of sensitivity to existing chemotherapy and radiotherapy. Patients with advanced-stage disease should be considered for clinical experimental protocols.[149,185]

Surgery

For more than two decades, *radical nephrectomy* has proved to be an efficient treatment modality for localized renal carcinomas. The first description of renal carcinoma was made in 1613 when Sennent described "a hard tumor" that he believed to be "incurable."

Surgical resection is the standard curative therapy for stage I or II renal cell carcinoma. Resection may be simple or radical. In a radical nephrectomy the kidney, perinephric fat, Gerota's capsule, and regional nodes are removed.[119,124,152] In advanced stages of disease, palliative nephrectomy may be performed for control of intractable bleeding and pain control. Arterial embolization may be considered as a palliative measure for controlling bleeding in patients with inoperable disease. For bilateral tumors, which occur in 1% of patients, treatment consists of nephrectomy for the larger lesion and partial nephrectomy or a bilateral partial nephrectomy. If the patient has contralateral disease and undergoes bilateral nephrectomy, the patient and family require education regarding the need for long-term hemodialysis or peritoneal dialysis.

A surgical resection remains the standard of care in stage III renal disease. The resection should include a radical procedure, as outlined earlier, with or without lymph node dissection.[124] The surgery is extended to remove the renal vein and caval thrombus with a portion of the vena cava as necessary. The value of preoperative or postoperative radiotherapy affecting survival remains inconclusive but may serve as a source of palliation. Clinical trials that incorporate the use of adjuvant α-interferon are currently under investigation.[4,50,105,137]

Advanced stage IV renal cell cancers present a major challenge to the clinician because almost all these patients are incurable. Palliation of symptoms caused by the primary tumor can include external beam irradiation, embolization, or nephrectomy.

Responses to cytotoxic chemotherapy with any regimen or with progestational agents have remained low. Biologic therapies are under evaluation.[50,132,138] α-Interferons have been used in select patient populations with a reported 15% objective response rate. More promising treatments currently under evaluation in clinical trials incorporate the administration of interleukin-2 (IL-2) with or without lymphokine-activated killer (LAK) lymphocytes.[185]

PROGNOSIS

Unfortunately, the prognosis for any patient with treated renal cell cancer who has relapsing, recurring, or progressing disease, regardless of stage or cell type, is poor. Survival is equated with early diagnosis of incident carcinoma. Local recurrence occurs infrequently, and failure is related to metastatic disease through nodal or hematogeneous spread.

BLADDER CANCER

EPIDEMIOLOGY

Bladder carcinoma is the most common malignant tumor of the urinary tract, with approximately 52,900 new cases reported in 1996.[118,119] Most bladder tumors are found on the lateral and posterior walls of the bladder as well as the trigone.

ETIOLOGY AND RISK FACTORS

Numerous studies have identified a variety of agents associated with the development of bladder cancer, such as aniline dye, used in textile, rubber and cable, paint, and printing industries; β-naphthamine; 4-aminodiphenyl; and tobacco tar. In humans, cigarette smoking is associated with a sixfold higher incidence. Bladder irritants (e.g., schistosomiasis, bladder calculi, urinary tract infections) in the presence of nitrosamines may act as cocarcinogens. Adenocarcinoma may occur in exstrophy of the bladder or in a urachal remnant.[132,176]

CLASSIFICATION

Transitional cell carcinoma derived from the uroepithelium is the most common carcinoma of the bladder in the United States, accounting for 90% of cases. The remainder of the cancers are squamous cell carcinoma (5%) and adenocarcinoma (less than 1%). Egypt has a much higher incidence of squamous cell carcinoma secondary to irritants such as parasitic infections and schistosomiasis. Pathologic grade, which is based on cell atypia, nuclear abnormalities, and number of mitotic features, is of great prognostic importance.

CLINICAL FEATURES

About 75% of patients with bladder cancer have gross hematuria. This hematuria is often described as "painless," and bladder irritability (urgency, dysuria, or strangury) is likely to be present. Intermittent bleeding is characteristic, and patients report one or more episodes of hematuria over 6 months to a year. Late diagnosis may occur because the patient or physician may delay work-up if the urine clears. Because urinary tract infections (UTIs) are often seen, many patients with cancer of the bladder are treated with antibiotics for what is thought to be hemorrhagic cystitis, a common phenomenon in females. Another large group of patients have vesical irritability, including frequency, spasms, and pain

NURSING MANAGEMENT

With the identification of certain etiologic factors, lifestyle or environmental modification to decrease the risk of developing kidney cancer is a reasonable goal. Specifically, encouraging cessation or moderation of tobacco use, promoting avoidance of developing a tobacco habit in youth, and stressing dietary modification to decrease or limit high-fat content are positive steps in decreasing cancer risk. Minimizing occupational or life-style exposure to petrochemicals is also suggested. See pp. 187-189 for detailed nursing interventions.

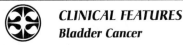

CLINICAL FEATURES
Bladder Cancer

Classic presentation
Hematuria
   Solitary
   Recurrent
Infection
   Absent
   Present
History
Exogenous exposure
   Present
   Absent
Tobacco habit
   Present
   Absent
Symptoms
Vesical irritability
   Frequency
   Spasms
   Pain

(see box above). The presence of unexplained gross or microscopic hematuria should always be evaluated.

DIAGNOSIS AND STAGING

The clinical staging of bladder carcinoma is based on determining the depth of invasion of the bladder wall by the tumor.[171,172,174,176] The diagnostic steps indicated in a patient with hematuria include urinalysis, IVP, cystoscopy, and urine cytology. IVP allows for visualization of the upper tracts to help exclude a nonvesical source of hematuria and to determine if there is any evidence of obstruction or a persistent bladder-filling defect.

Cystoscopy is used to verify the presence of a bladder tumor and to characterize its gross appearance. Areas of erythema (especially with a "velvety" appearance) may represent carcinoma in situ (CIS). Cystoscopy with random bladder biopsies are performed with the patient un-

der local anesthesia using an intraurethral topical anesthetic with or without intravenous sedation. Associated procedures, such as transurethral resection, bimanual examination, or retrograde studies of the upper tracts, are more readily performed with the patient sedated. A bimanual pelvic examination helps to determine the presence of a palpable or fixed mass. In addition to tissue biopsies, cells may be captured from bladder mucosa through bladder washings or voided urine, since malignant cells from urinary epithelial surfaces exhibit characteristic morphologic changes. *Urine cytology* is relatively reliable, inexpensive, and safe and facilitates follow-up in treatment of bladder tumors. It complements but does not replace endoscopic and radiographic studies.

If the tumor is invasive, additional studies may be indicated, including abdominal and pelvic CT scans, chest x-ray films, and bone scans (only if bone metastasis is clinically suspected). Urine cytology may be of screening value in industrial settings and can be used to detect lesions at early-stage follow-up. DNA flow cytometry of urine may be used as a diagnostic and screening mechanism in high-risk patients. Clinical staging, even with CT or MRI, often underestimates the extent of tumor, particularly in less-differentiated and more deeply invasive cancers.[176]

The management and prognosis of bladder cancer are determined by many factors. Recurrence and progression depend on the initial anatomic and histologic classification, multiplicity, location of tumor,[2,174] associated GU problems (e.g., UTI, ureteral obstruction, compromised renal function), and the patient's general health and ability to tolerate and care for a urinary diversion if required.

Treatment planning is based on the depth and degree to which the cancer has penetrated into the bladder wall. Before treatment it is essential to determine if the tumor has seeded downward from the renal pelvis or has originated as a ureteral primary. Metastasis occurs by lymphatic and hematogeneous routes and usually spreads to the lymph nodes, liver, lung, and bones.

The bladder is also a common site for contiguous spread from anaplastic lesions of neighboring viscera, most notably the uterine cervix and prostate. The bladder may be invaded by carcinoma of the sigmoid colon, rectum, or uterine body. Secondary tumors can promote urinary irritative symptoms or obstruction.

BIOLOGIC MARKERS

Flow cytometry assigns an automated semiquantitative value to qualitative cellular and nuclear abnormalities observed under the microscope. Epithelial cells are stained and passed through the light produced by the argon laser. The stained DNA emits a pulse of green fluorescence, and stained ribonucleic acid (RNA) emits a pulse of red fluorescence. The flow cytometer can then profile the DNA and RNA content and size of each cell. The cells can be analyzed in sequence. Presence of tumor should be suspected when greater than 15% of cells with DNA fluorescence are encountered above the *diploid* (normal) level of chromosomes or when there is a clearly *aneuploid* (abnormal) tumor cell line with fewer or more than half the number of chromosomes characteristically found.[93] Specimens obtained by bladder washing are preferred for flow cytometry because of the higher total cell yield. Flow cytometry appears to be somewhat more sensitive than conventional urinary cytology in diagnosing low-grade tumors of the bladder, but its application in urologic oncology is still being defined. The pathologist has a major role in identifying the grade of the bladder cancer tumor and determining whether invasion has occurred.[132]

Research investigations into the development of reliable tumor markers are ongoing. Nonspecific substances in urine, including polyamines, cholesterol, and fibrin degradation products, or carcinoembryonic antigen (CEA) may be increased when bladder tumors are present. Studies are being conducted to determine the diagnostic value of the presence or absence of blood group antigens in transitional cell carcinomas.

TREATMENT MODALITIES
Noninvasive Therapy

Historically, most patients with noninvasive stage I bladder cancer (T1-N0-M0, stage A) have been managed with *transurethral resection* (TUR) and *fulguration* with or without intravesical therapy.[162] Treatment of multiple papillary transitional cell lesions with TUR depends on the tumor's location and size. Most surgeons begin removing lesions at the dome of the bladder. Therefore, if bleeding occurs, it goes to the bladder base, not obscuring the surgeon's vision. In patients with tumors that cannot be removed by standard TUR, cystectomy must be considered.[2] Sessile lesions are usually associated with higher-grade, infiltrating bladder cancers rather than the papillary type. TUR of superficially invasive or sessile lesions is rarely performed.

Agents such as thiotepa may be instilled postopera-

tively. Unless the resection is small, an indwelling catheter may be left in place. The catheter may be connected to gravity drainage or a continuous irrigation system. The catheter is left in place for 2 to 3 days or until the urine is clear. It is important to monitor the patient for any signs of clot retention and urinary outlet obstruction. Patients should be informed that they may experience some bleeding on urination as the postoperative site heals.

Patients are followed postoperatively with periodic cystoscopies and bladder washings for cytology, usually every 3 months for the first year and at 6-month intervals for the next 2 years. If cystoscopies and cytologies are negative, the patient is then cystoscoped annually. Electrofulguration may be performed on patients who have been previously diagnosed with appropriate biopsies and histologic variables. This procedure is used on small lesions 2 to 3 mm in size or when lesions are located near the bladder neck and are not accessible to resection. The major problem with fulguration is that it destroys cellular morphology and does not provide adequate information on the depth of invasion. The depth of penetration through the bladder wall with this technique is approximately 2 mm.

On lesions that are smaller than 1 cm, argon or neodymium : yttrium-aluminum-garnet (Nd : YAG) lasers may be used. The depth of penetration is about 1 mm. Nd:YAG lasers create transmural thermal coagulation of the bladder wall, which allows for the treatment of larger tumors. Laser procedures are thought to prevent local spread and recurrence and are done with the patient under local anesthesia. Although these bloodless procedures offer a new dimension in future treatment, they remain costly and require special training and equipment.

Intravesical therapy with thiotepa, mitomycin, doxorubicin, or bacille Calmette-Guérin (BCG) may be administered to patients with multiple tumors or recurrent tumors or to high-risk patients after TUR. Treatment with BCG has proved to be efficacious in delaying progression to muscle invasion or metastatic disease and has resulted in improved bladder preservation and decreased death rates related to bladder cancer. Patients with T1 tumors who have persistent CIS after a second 6-week BCG course are high risk for developing muscle invasion and need to be evaluated for cystectomy.[11,61,86] To date, BCG appears to provide a complete response rate in about 70% of patients and delays tumor recurrence and progression. Future use of maintenance doses of BCG may prolong a patient's disease-free interval after a 6-week induction course has been given.[86]

Clinical evaluation of photodynamic therapy after intravenous administration of *hematoporphyrin derivatives* (HPDs) of tumor cells sensitized to light is under investigation.[131] HPDs are selectively concentrated in dysplastic and neoplastic transitional cells, including CIS, and emit a red fluorescence on exposure to deep-blue light to allow location of the tumor. After HPD therapy, patients may experience significant photosensitivity, which may persist up to a month after therapy. Patients should be instructed to keep all exposed areas of the body shielded from the sunlight for at least 6 to 8 weeks after treatment. Irritative bladder symptoms are also an expected side effect of this treatment.[131] This treatment modality is considered experimental.

Intravesical interferon alfa-2a has shown activity against papillary tumors and in situ as a primary treatment or as a secondary treatment after failure of intravesical agents.[11]

Invasive Therapy

Stage II bladder cancer (T2-N0-M0, stage B) with invasion into superficial muscle may be controlled by TUR, but often more aggressive treatment is required related to the multiplicity, size, and undifferentiated grade of the neoplasms. Segmental cystectomy may be performed only in select patients.

The role of radiation therapy in the management of bladder cancer has many uses. Its effect on urinary patterns varies, depending on radiation dose delivered and the chemotherapeutic and surgical approaches used.[66] Radiation delivered after surgery or with chemotherapy may intensify the effects and delay tissue healing. Therefore treatment is withheld for 4 to 6 weeks postoperatively. Cumulative doses of 6500 to 7000 cGy delivered over 6 to 7 weeks can be tolerated by the whole bladder.

Early reactions to radiation usually occur during the first 3 or 4 weeks of therapy and tend to resolve within 4 weeks of completion. Urinary frequency, urgency, and dysuria may occur as bladder capacity is reduced. Hematuria may result from mucosal inflammation. Patients occasionally require a respite from treatment as symptoms intensify or as skin integrity becomes compromised. Pharmacologic treatments provide relief and are used to prevent infection. Antispasmodics or parasympathetic blockers provide relief of symptoms and promote analgesia. Patients are instructed to empty the bladder frequently and increase intake of fluids, such as water and cranberry juice. Caffeine, alcohol, tobacco, and spices tend to irritate the bladder mucosa and should be avoided.

Late effects of radiation occur 1 or more years after treatment. Internal fibrosis, telangiectasia, chronic urinary frequency, and permanent diminished bladder capacity may occur. Combined modalities of surgery and radiotherapy may lead to fistula formation, but this complication occurs infrequently, affecting less than 5% of patients.[145,150,162,168] Development of a fistula after treatment may indicate tumor recurrence.

Although radical cystectomy remains a definitive form of treatment, bladder preservation treatment modalities (initial TUR, with chemotherapy and concomitant radio-

therapy)[150,172] are options in certain patients. Some reports indicate that radiation therapy with salvage cystectomy allows preservation of bladder and sexual function.[71] In patients who are not candidates for surgery, choice of appropriate treatment is always affected by the patient's overall health status and ability to tolerate the side effects of the therapy (see box below). Although TUR and fulguration are the most common conservative forms of management for early-stage disease, radical cystectomy is used in the management of bladder cancers that have penetrated the muscularis of the bladder wall.

Radical cystectomy implies the en bloc removal of the anterior pelvic organs: the prostate, seminal vesicles, and bladder with its visceral peritoneum and perivesical fat in men; and the urethra, bladder, cervix, vaginal cuff, uterus, ovaries, and anterior pelvic peritoneum in women. Pelvic iliac lymph node dissection may or may not be performed. The *ileal conduit* is constructed from a small piece of bowel. The ureters are anchored into the ileal conduit, which protrudes through the skin as a bud stoma in the right lower quadrant for application of an external ileostomy drainage device (Figure 9-4). *Continent diversion* has been used successfully in selected male and female populations. In a Kock pouch procedure a midportion of isolated ileum is folded and opened onto itself, creating a continent pouch with a nipple-valve stoma.[158] The stoma is generally below the undergarment

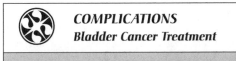

COMPLICATIONS
Bladder Cancer Treatment

Treatment modality	Treatment complications
Intravesical therapy	Body image concern
Thiotepa	Myelosuppression
Bacille Calmette-Guérin (BCG)	Irritative symptoms
	Constitutional "tuberculosis-like" granulomatosis
Radical cystectomy	Body image concern
Diffuse, recurrent carcinoma in situ or muscle-invasive transitional cell carcinoma	Loss of body function
	Sexuality/sensuality disturbance
Systemic chemotherapy	Body image concern
	Bone marrow suppression
	Organ function impairment:
	Renal
	Cardiac
	Neurologic
	Alopecia
	Fatigue

line. A small gauze pad may cover the stoma, which provides access for intermittent catheterization by the individual approximately every 6 hours.

Preoperative consultation and education with an enterostomal therapist (ET) is essential to treatment and rehabilitation. Pretreatment management of the ileal stoma site should be done jointly with the surgeon and the ET while the patient is in the supine, sitting, and standing positions. Optimal stomal placement is crucial for postoperative management. The standard of care for urinary diversion focuses on patient adjustment to body image and quality of life. The surgeon positions the ileostomy location below the belt line and close to the pubis for concealment, since these patients do not wear external appliances.[100] If cosmetic concealment is of little concern to the patient, placement higher on the abdominal wall may make intermittent catheterization easier.

The first attempt to create a continent diversion was done in 1852, when Simon attempted to divert urinary drainage in his patient by creating a communication between the ureters and the rectum. Bricker established the ileal conduit diversion in 1950. Since then, great milestones have been achieved in the area of continent diversions. Urinary diversions of the lower urinary tract should ideally fulfill the criteria outlined in the box, p. 184.

It is imperative to remember that there is no panacea in surgical reconstructions of bladders. However, with

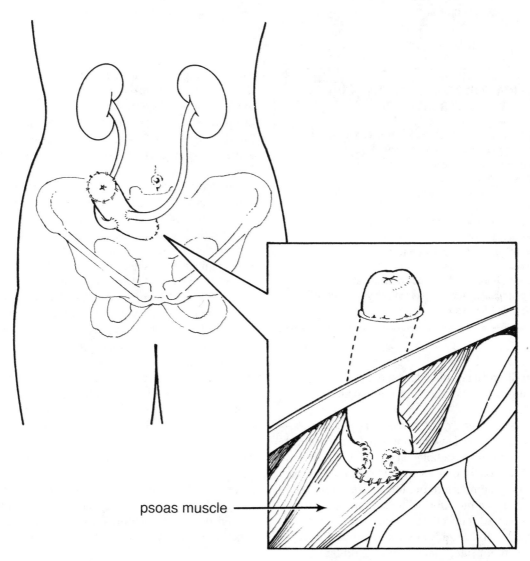

psoas muscle

Figure 9-4 Completed ileal loop. Ileal conduit has been anchored to psoas muscle, and ureters lie without tension or angulation. A protruding bud stoma has been created. (Modified from Richie JP: Techniques of ureterointestinal anastomoses and conduit construction. In Crawford ED, Borden TA, editors: *Genitourinary cancer surgery*, Philadelphia, 1982, Lea & Febiger.)

Reduction of risk factors associated with development and promotion of bladder neoplasms is necessary. Nurses should encourage individual and collective efforts to moderate or stop the use of tobacco products or to avoid development of tobacco habits. This intervention could significantly decrease the morbidity and mortality associated with bladder cancer. A solitary episode of hematuria in the absence or presence of other symptomatology requires further investigation.

Approximately 80% of bladder cancers are superficial when first diagnosed. These superficial presentations have a demonstrated pattern of recurrence. Patients must view the disease as a chronic process requiring a life-time pattern of serial cystoscopies, cytology, surgical resection for pathologic evaluation of suspicious lesions, and intravesical chemotherapy as indicated. Postponement of potentially curative therapy (i.e., radical cystectomy) in the event of bladder cancer locally confined to the muscularis may render salvage therapy useless. The development of measures to promote patient compliance to established regimens of surveillance in superficial bladder cancer for early detection and initiation of effective therapy with recurrences is suggested as an area for nursing research. This need is underscored by the high mortality associated with bladder cancer. See pp. 187-189 for detailed nursing interventions.

CRITERIA FOR CONTINENT URINARY DIVERSIONS

1. The reservoir substitute for the lower tract should collect and store urine under low pressure.
2. The diversion must prevent reflux into the upper urinary tracts.
3. The diversion should not cause recurrent infections from stasis or reflux.
4. The diversion should not cause fluid and electrolyte or acid-base imbalances.
5. Malabsorption nutritional disorders should be minimized.
6. Continence should be maintained so that patients can control emptying of the reservoir at socially acceptable and convenient intervals.

---

the inception of artificial sphincters and new surgical approaches, the impact on improving the patient's quality of life can be significant.[44,158]

Treatment with concurrent chemotherapy and radiotherapy has been associated with improved rates of local control compared with radiotherapy alone. Currently, multiple trials are under investigation to evaluate the role of chemotherapy administered before cystectomy, after cystectomy, or in conjunction with radiotherapy to improve local disease, prevent distant metastases, or preserve the bladder. Recent advances in combination chemotherapy (methotrexate, vinblastine, doxorubicin, cisplatin) have produced pathologically complete responses in 20% of patients treated before definitive surgery.[95]

Stage III disease carries a high risk for extramural tumor and lymph node involvement. Preoperative radiotherapy followed by radical cystectomy has been widely used for stage III cancer. Because the frequency of distant metastases is becoming apparent with improved surgical techniques, systemic preoperative or postoperative chemotherapy is now being evaluated in clinical trials. To date, improved rates of local control have been achieved using a combination of cisplatin and external beam radiotherapy.

Currently, a small percentage of patients with advanced stage IV bladder cancer can be cured. The prognosis of patients with T4 tumors is generally poor with either radical cystectomy or radiotherapy. The focus of care for many stage IV patients should be on symptom management and supportive care. Urinary diversions generally are ineffective with either radical cystectomy or radiotherapy. The focus of care for many stage IV patients should be on symptom management and supportive care. Urinary diversion may be indicated not only for palliation of symptoms related to bladder tumors, bleeding, and pain, but also for preservation of renal function in patients who are candidates for chemotherapy. Because of the overall poor results with drug treatment, patients with metastatic renal cell cancer should be provided with the opportunity to participate in clinical research trials. Recent combination chemotherapy regimens that include cisplatin, methotrexate, and vinblastine with or without doxorubicin have demonstrated some complete responses. As mentioned, these trials are designed to evaluate the impact of chemotherapy administered before cystectomy, after cystectomy, or in conjunction with radiotherapy.[150]

PENILE CANCER

The most common presentation for penile cancer is a mass, persistent sore, or ulcer on the glans or foreskin. A few patients have inguinal lymphadenopathy. More than half of patients fail to seek medical attention for longer than 1 year.[36,123]

TREATMENT

Wide excision or *partial penectomy* is the treatment for small and well-localized tumors.[123] Adequate margins must be obtained to prevent recurrence. From 35% to 60% of patients with penile cancer present with palpable inguinal lymph nodes.[114] However, 40% of palpable lymph nodes are false positive because of inflammation and infection; therefore clinical assessment of lymph nodes should be delayed until the patient has a 4- to 6-week course of antibiotics. Current treatment recommendations for lymph node dissection include (1) observation for patients with noninvasive tumor and clinically negative nodes and (2) bilateral groin dissection for patients with clinically positive nodes. Radiation therapy may be used as an organ preservation strategy. Methods used include interstitial implantation and external beam radiation. The whole shaft of the penis is treated with 40 cGy, with a boost of 20 cGy to the tumor. This approach has a 70% to 80% local control rate. Inguinal and pelvic nodal irradiation to 50 cGy should be administered in patients unable to have lymph node dissection.[64,101]

Common radiation side effects include meatal/urethral stricture, mucosal changes, and telangiectasias. Palliation is the focus in the treatment of stage IV penile cancer. Surgery may be considered for control of local lesions to prevent necrosis, infection, or hemorrhage. Laser treatments offer a noninvasive alternative to surgery.[139] Chemotherapy has been used in several small series; common regimens include bleomycin, methotrexate, or cisplatin. The experience thus far has been limited, and results have been difficult to document.

SEXUAL REHABILITATION

Impotence is a topic that can arouse fear and anxiety in men and women. The lack of knowledge about the sexual process compounds the problem. An initial consultation with the patient should include evaluation of a potential or existing functional disability to identify the potential etiology involved. The initial consultation is critical in establishing the patient-professional relationship and setting realistic goals before and after genitourinary surgery. One of the major goals of the initial consultation is to restore the individual and partner to a healthy physical and emotional state, and then focus on improving whatever success may result from the ultimate treatment of sexual dysfunction.

A sexual history before definitive treatment can often provide an accurate assessment of the patient's social situation and marital status. Determining the presence of erectile dysfunction, decreased libido, ejaculatory dys-

function, and orgasmic difficulties before treatment is critical for the development of an appropriate rehabilitation plan. It is important to assess the patient's level of sexual functioning. Baseline questions should address frequency of sexual intercourse, quality of erections, and ability to maintain erections (the first sign of organic dysfunction is the inability to maintain an erection). It is also important to document if the patient states that he is impotent or reports that sexual functioning is not important; the direction of counseling then can focus on other aspects of treatment and rehabilitation.

In the preoperative evaluation, if a patient has never experienced erectile dysfunction, he must be prepared for the potential physiologic changes if a nerve-sparing procedure cannot be accomplished or in case a radical prostatectomy is planned. This is extremely important if a man has a sexually insecure partner; the onset of impotence can create serious problems in their relationship. The partner may feel unattractive, sexually undesirable, or rejected. Couples who experience sexual dysfunction before or after a surgical procedure often blame one another, become angry, and withdraw sexually. It is important in the pretreatment phase to determine how the couple dealt with conflict or pressure in times of stress. The couple's ability to speak openly about sexual issues should be evaluated. Once erectile dysfunction occurs, couples with good, open sexual communication are much better at adapting to the situation than couples who have inhibited sexual communication skills. These couples will continue to relate sexually, employing a repertoire of pleasurable activities that do not depend on an erection. Inhibited couples generally stop all sexual activity when erections dissipate. Once a man has experienced erectile dysfunction, he tends to worry about whether his next sexual experience will be a failure. The more he worries, the greater the anxiety. This can evolve into a cycle of performance anxiety that causes him to become a spectator, disrupting his quality of life.

Recent research advances in the neuroanatomy, physiology, hemodynamics, and pharmacology of penile erection have provided clinicians with the ability to plan for erectile rehabilitation in the pretreatment phase before radical prostatectomy. The introduction of intracorporeal injection of vasoactive drugs has provided a mechanism to induce penile erection and evaluate impotence.

EMPHASIS ON QUALITY OF LIFE

Just as clinicians stage and plan primary cancer treatments based on baseline data (e.g., scans, radiographs, laboratory tests), diagnostic testing to evaluate erectile function should be performed.

The *nocturnal penile tumescence test* allows one to assess penile tumescence and the degree of rigidity the patient experiences. A device called a RigiScan with a

Table 9-3 Semirigid Penile Prostheses

Type	Advantages	Disadvantages
Simple	Least expensive	Difficulty with outward erectile appearance
Hinged	Has softer zone for positioning for micturition	Cost
	No dressing	Postoperative complications
	Fewer sizes necessary	
Malleable	Central metal core so penis can be bent down and up for coitus	Postoperative complications
		Cost
	Best rigidity	
Positionable	Central cable that runs through a series of polyfone segments	Postoperative complications
		Cost
	Superior cosmetic results	
Mechanically activated	Only nonhydraulic device available	Most expensive

strain gauge at the base of the penis tip has the ability to record tumescence and rigidity during erections. If normal tumescence and rigidity are demonstrated during sleep, vascular impotence is less likely. Doppler pulse wave form analysis initially was used to evaluate penile arterial vasculature. This procedure has now been replaced with high-resolution ultrasonography and pulsed Doppler spectrum analysis. This test evaluates the function of the arterial system during vasodilator-induced secretions (penile injections). High-resolution imaging and identification of the arteries can be done, and the whole penis can be scanned to assess the internal corporeal tissue. The inner diameter of the cavernous arteries and blood flow velocity are assessed before and after injection of a vasodilator. The ultrasound and pulsed Doppler evaluations are done in a flaccid state. After this, the patient assumes a supine position, a rubber band is placed on the base of the penis, and a vasodilator is injected into the corpora cavernosa. Arterial dilation and flow are evaluated, as well as cavernosa venous emptying capacity (CVOD). Baseline organic erectile functioning results from failure to initiate (neurogenic), failure to fill (arteriogenic), or failure to store (CVOD).

Options for treatment after a radical prostatectomy or radical cystoprostatectomy can involve *intracorporeal pharmacotherapy, penile implants,* or *external devices.* External devices are generally recommended for individuals who are receiving anticoagulant therapy or who have blood dyscrasias. Because no single penile prosthesis is ideal for every patient, a man who is a candidate for a penile implant should be offered a choice between a semirigid rod device and an inflatable implant. Compared with inflatable protheses, *semirigid devices* are not as expensive, are easier to implant, and have lower long-term mechanical failure rates. Men who have penile fibrosis as a result of other diseases or infection may not be candidates for implants. Table 9-3 outlines the different types of implants available.

Common complications related to implant procedures include perforations during dilation of the corpora, erosion, infection, or mechanical complications related to the implant.

Impotence after a TUR of the prostate and its etiology depend on the physiologic and psychologic factors discussed earlier. Recently, nerve-sparing procedures have been considered in select patients. It is critical to note that nerve-sparing procedures should never compromise a curative approach. Adequate resection of the tumor is the primary concern, and preservation of sexual function should be of secondary importance. Size, extent of disease, and intraoperative findings in clinically localized prostate cancer may require wide resection of tissue, including the neurovascular bundle. Inadvertent injury to these nerves can affect sexual functioning postoperatively. Assessment of the patient's baseline erection functioning before treatment can assist the clinician in planning a sexual recovery program. Erectile function may return spontaneously up to 2 years after a radical prostatectomy. Support and appropriate management of the impotent patient are essential to maintaining the patient's sexual quality of life during this period.

CONCLUSION

Effective multimodality therapeutic maneuvers are instituted for a wide array of genitourinary malignancies. Because these tumors as a group may involve physiologic systems associated with comfort, as measured by kidney and bladder integrity, erectile function, and fertility in males as well as body image considerations in both males and females, quality of life issues are being investigated. Surgical refinements, including nerve-sparing radical prostatectomy and investigations into the degree of vascular damage precipitated by radiotherapy and its effects on erectile function, are addressing critical components of libido and potency. Data about alterations in sexual

NURSING MANAGEMENT

This section highlights nursing assessment and strategy development, implementation, and evaluation for genitourinary (GU) malignancies. Nursing interventions are predicated on continuous acknowledgment of the individuality of each patient, maintenance of a patient-centered focus rather than a disease-centered approach, and awareness of predictable points in the cancer continuum that may precipitate or exacerbate stress. These focus points include the diagnostic phase, initiation and completion of therapy, evaluation of response to therapy, introduction of a treatment modality new to the patient, discovery of metastatic or recurrent disease, and finally the exhaustion of all viable treatment options.[9,31]

The selected nursing diagnoses include anxiety, health-seeking behaviors, altered urinary elimination, and altered sexuality patterns. Interventions follow each diagnostic grouping as a guide for creation of evaluative and therapeutic nursing strategies. The box at right lists teaching priorities for prevention, early detection, and risk modification tactics.

NURSING DIAGNOSES

- *Anxiety related to:*
  - *—GU cancer incidence and mortality rates*
  - *—Screening (digital rectal examination [DRE], testicular self-examination [TSE], physical examination)*
  - *—Diagnostic procedures: biopsies for histologic and cytologic review*
  - *—Staging extent of disease: imaging modalities*
  - *—Localized disease: surgery, radiation therapy, laser therapy, bladder instillation of chemotherapy and biologic response modifier (BRM) therapy*
  - *—Locally, regionally advanced, or metastatic disease: radical surgery, radiation therapy, chemotherapy, BRM therapy, hormonal therapy*
  - *—Continuing care: encounters with health care professionals and systems, outcome or response to therapy, finances*
  - *—Supportive care: pain control, maintenance of independence, nutrition, mobility, quality-of-life issues*

OUTCOME GOAL

Patient will be able to:
- Demonstrate decreased anxiety and be knowledgeable of planned treatment.

INTERVENTIONS

- Review purpose of surgery, radiation therapy, chemotherapy, hormonal therapy, and BRM therapy treatments and rationale for treatment.
- Explain common terms and procedures, provide written literature, and show actual equipment.

PATIENT TEACHING PRIORITIES
Genitourinary Cancers

Prevention

Avoid or limit exposure to exogenous carcinogens.
Discourage development of tobacco habits.
Maintain low-fat diet.

Early detection

Encourage early investigation of GU findings, such as mass, pain, hematuria, and altered urinary patterns.

American Cancer Society (ACS) screening guidelines

Perform monthly TSE.
Have annual DRE (males 40 years and older).
Have annual prostate-specific antigen (PSA) test (males 50 years and older).

Risk modification

Encourage cessation or moderation of tobacco habits.
Avoid obesity.
Limit exposure to petrochemicals.

- Familiarize patient with terminology, equipment, simulation, dosimetry port films, linear accelerator, and implants.
- Discuss potential sequelae of radiation, surgery, and chemotherapy, such as alteration in skin integrity and change in elimination patterns.
- Explain role of various medical personnel patient with whom patient will interact.
- Allow time for discussions, write down key words or expressions, and provide diagrams or models reviewing anatomic and physiologic functions for clarification.
- Encourage patient to write down questions as they arise, and discuss concerns about cancer and the treatment as a strategy for eliciting individual concerns.
- Elicit degree of comprehension and comfort using a technique for recall of information previously presented.

NURSING DIAGNOSES

- *Health-seeking behaviors related to:*
  - *—Prevention or risk reduction in development of GU cancers, specifically bladder and kidney cancer*
  - *—Promotion of early detection:*
    Monthly TSE
    Annual DRE for males 40 years and older

Continued.

Annual PSA test for males 50 years and older
Evaluation by health care professional of any epi-
*   sode of hematuria*

OUTCOME GOALS

Patient will be able to:
- Effectively communicate feelings, demonstrate ability to perform self-care, and seek assistance as necessary.
- State name, type, and treatment and description of surgery, reason for therapy, expected outcomes and potential side effects, and professionals involved.

INTERVENTIONS

- Encourage cessation or moderation of tobacco habits.
- Discourage development of tobacco habits.
- Promote low-fat diet.
- Avoid or minimize exposure to exogenous chemicals or agents known to be associated with initiation or promotion of malignancies.
- Encourage early investigation of any GU findings, including a mass, pain, hematuria, or alteration of urinary patterns.
- Provide current and accurate information on diagnostic and therapeutic modalities.
- Encourage positive outlook with a view of the positive statistics on disease remission or disease stabilization.

NURSING DIAGNOSES

- *Urinary elimination, altered, related to:*
—*Decreased bladder capacity secondary to partial cystectomy, instillation of intravesical agents, radiation therapy*
—*Urinary diversion: radical cystectomy with ileal conduit or continence techniques*
—*Obstruction: cancerous tissue growth or edematous or fibrous tissue reaction to therapy*
—*Retention: possible chronic or intermittent catheterization after prostatectomy or drug therapy related (e.g., antihistamines, epidural analgesics)*
—*Incontinence from urethral instrumentation or after prostatectomy*
—*Increased gastrointestinal motility secondary to radiation therapy*

OUTCOME GOALS

Patient will be able to:
- Monitor changes in patterns of elimination and report to health care provider.
- Adhere to diet as recommended.
- Report rectal bleeding, diarrhea, tenesmus, abdominal discomfort, urinary frequency, nocturia, urinary urgency, dysuria, hematuria, or lower back pain.
- Communicate feelings about body image changes.

INTERVENTIONS

- Promote acceptance of change in body image secondary to disease or treatment process.
- Provide information and ensure continuing care for the individual with a urinary diversion.
- Provide resource and referral information for patients on a bladder catheterization program and those experiencing any degree of incontinence.
- Instruct patient about signs and symptoms of cystitis and avoidance of foods that irritate the bladder lining.
- Assess and document ongoing patterns of bowel elimination.
- Teach patient signs and symptoms of proctitis.
- Monitor weight and nutritional status weekly, and observe for evidence of fluid volume depletion. Provide patient with low-residue, high-protein, and high-carbohydrate diet.

NURSING DIAGNOSES

- *Sexuality patterns, altered, related to:*
—*Pathophysiologic changes associated with cancer or treatment:*
  Diagnostic procedures: urethral stricture, scarring from instrumentation, erosion and scarring from bladder biopsies
  Surgery: unilateral or bilateral orchiectomy, transurethral resection, modified or extensive node dissection, interruption of neural pathways essential for potency preservation
  Radiation therapy: interstitial prostatic implants or external beam therapy
  Hormonal manipulation
  Chemotherapy
  BRM therapy
—*Self-image and self-esteem disturbances:*
  Diagnosis
  Loss of body part or function
  Potential loss of autonomy and independence
  Financial concern
  Temporary or permanent role changes
  Decreased libido
—*Physiologic function:*
  Males
  Potential for fertility impairment related to disease, chemotherapy, radiation therapy, surgical interventions
  Potential for impotence: hormonal, systemic, or surgical ablative therapy; arteriosclerotic changes promoted by radiation therapy; cavernous nerve removal (radical prostatectomy)
  Dry orgasms after removal of prostate and seminal vesicles
  Females
  Inadequate vaginal lubrication and infertility secondary to surgical procedure

Radical cystectomy with removal of ovaries, fallopian tubes, uterus, cervix, and anterior portion of vagina

INTERVENTIONS

- Assess patterns of sexuality expression before diagnosis as a guide to predicting or planning for similar pattern of maintenance or attainment during and after treatment.
- Consider technique of permission granting general discussion regarding disease and treatment followed by specific individual questions.
- Review anticipated physiologic impact of disease and treatment on libido and potency.
- Consider general themes associated with age, gender, disease, and treatment modalities while focusing on the person's perception of cancer and potential impact on life-style.
- Maintain an awareness of personal biases and values, and allow for possibility of nontraditional partner or expressions of sexuality.
- Encourage enhancement of satisfaction and pleasure from everyday encounters.
- Review options for management of impotence, including injectable drugs (prostaglandins, papaverine), oral drugs (yohimbine), vascular reconstruction, surgery, vacuum devices, and surgically implanted semirigid or inflatable penile prostheses.
- Ensure that patient/partner can identify aspects of sexuality and sexual function that may be threatened by the surgical procedure (e.g., prostatectomy, cystectomy, ileal conduit).
- State factors that influence sexual identity, and identify behaviors that facilitate acceptance of surgery.
- Maintain satisfying social and sexual role concept.
- Verbalize importance of seeking professional assistance if normal life-style, socialization, or sexual function is impaired.
- Provide patient/partner with factual information; give assurance that it is okay to share feelings and concerns; assist with coping and adjustment to illness.
- See box on geriatric considerations, p. 173.
- Refer to Chapters 31 and 32 for further psychosocial and sexuality interventions.

function are being extrapolated retrospectively from males and females after radical cystectomy. Degree of recovery of spermatogenesis is being assessed in males with testicular tumors after multimodality therapy. Additional areas for research in epidemiology, etiology, and morbidity and mortality from disease and therapy are being identified and pursued. Traditional and newer diagnostic and therapeutic interventions offer promise and support the goals of prevention and early detection of genitourinary malignancies while suggesting strategies to enhance quality of life in the continuing care of persons living with advanced disease.

■ CHAPTER QUESTIONS

1. Which of the following biologic markers are useful for diagnosis and follow-up care of patients with testicular cancer?
   (1) PSA and testosterone
   (2) HCG
   (3) AFP
   (4) CEA
   (5) CA-19-9
   (6) CA-125
   a. (1) and (2)
   b. (2) and (3)
   c. (3) and (6)
   d. (2) and (5)

2. Which of the following statements is false regarding the management of seminoma?
   (1) Cure rates are less than 50%.
   (2) Seminoma is an extremely radiosensitive tumor.
   (3) Radical inguinal orchiectomy is the initial treatment for all stages of seminoma.
   (4) Pure seminoma may exhibit elevated levels of β-HCG.
   a. (1) and (2)
   b. (2) and (3)
   c. (2) and (4)
   d. (1) and (3)

3. The site of action of leuprolide (Lupron) is:
   a. Pituitary-hypothalamic axis
   b. Adrenal gland
   c. Testes
   d. Liver

4. Which of these items is *not* a risk factor for bladder cancer?
   a. Aniline dyes
   b. Smoking
   c. High dietary fat
   d. Schistosomiasis

5. Impotency can result from all the following *except:*
   a. Radiation therapy
   b. Radical prostatectomy
   c. Diabetes
   d. Mumps

6. Prostate cancer continues to play a prominent role in cancer statistics for men. In 1996, prostate cancer was:
   a. Number 1 in incidence and number 1 in mortality
   b. Number 1 in incidence and number 2 in mortality

c. Number 2 in incidence and number 1 in mortality
d. Number 2 in incidence and number 3 in mortality

7. The purpose of the Prostate Cancer Prevention Trial (PCPT) is to determine whether the drug finasteride will:
   a. Delay onset of prostate cancer
   b. Determine efficacy of the drug in treatment of prostate cancer
   c. Prevent development of prostate cancer
   d. Reduce incidence of prostate cancer in high-risk men

8. All men receiving treatment for testicular cancer are candidates for sperm banking.
   a. True
   b. False

9. Approximately 90% of cancers of the bladder are:
   a. Adenocarcinoma
   b. Ductal carcinoma
   c. Squamous cell carcinoma
   d. Transitional cell carcinoma

10. The clinical features of renal cell carcinoma include:
    a. Pain, hematuria, fever, anemia
    b. Hematuria, low back pain, gynecomastia, infection
    c. Bladder spasms, infection, hematuria, low back pain
    d. Frequent urination, hematuria, bone pain, weight loss

BIBLIOGRAPHY

1. Adolfsson J, Steineck G, Whitemore WF: Recent results of management of palpable clinically localized prostate cancer, *CA Cancer J Clin* 72(2):310-322, 1993.

2. Amling CL and others: Radical cystectomy for stages TA, TIS and T1 transitional cell carcinoma of the bladder, *J Urol* 151(1):31, 1994.

3. Andriole GL: Serum prostate-specific antigen: the most useful tumor marker, *J Clin Oncol* 10(8):1205, 1992.

4. Atkins MB and others: Randomized phase II trial of high-dose interleukin-2 either alone or in combination with interferon alpha-2b in advanced renal cell carcinoma, *J Clin Oncol* 11(4):661, 1993.

5. Austenfeld MS and others: Meta-analysis of the literature: guideline development for prostate cancer treatment, *J Urol* 152(5):1866, 1994.

6. Bajorin DF, Bosl GJ: The use of serum tumor markers in the prognosis and treatment of germ cell tumors, *Cancer Principles Pract Oncol Updates* 6(1):1, 1992.

7. Bajorin DF and others: Randomized trial of etoposide and cisplatin versus etoposide and carboplatin in patients with good-risk germ cell tumors: a multi-institutional study, *J Clin Oncol* 11(4):598, 1993.

8. Baniel J and others: Late relapse of testicular cancer, *J Clin Oncol* 13(5):1170, 1995.

9. Beahrs OH and others: *American Joint Committee on Cancer manual for staging of cancer,* ed 4, Philadelphia, 1992, Lippincott.

10. Bertgna C and others: Efficacy of the combination of flutamide plus orchidectomy in patients with metastatic prostatic cancer: a meta-analysis of seven randomized double-blind trials (1056 patients), *Br J Urol* 73(4):396, 1994.

11. Boccardo F and others: Prophylaxis of superficial bladder cancer with mitomycin or interferon alfa-2b: results of a multicentric Italian study, *J Clin Oncol* 12(1):7, 1994.

12. Boring CC, Squires TC, Jong T: Cancer statistics, 1994, *CA Cancer J Clin* 44:19, 1994.

13. Bosel GJ and others: Serum tumor markers in patients with metastatic germ cell tumors of the testis: a 10 year experience, *Am J Med* 75:29, 1983.

14. Bostwick DG and others: Staging of prostate cancer, *Semin Surg Oncol* 10(1):60, 1994.

15. Broun ER and others: Long-term outcome of patients with relapsed and refractor germ cell tumors treated with high-dose chemotherapy and autologous bone marrow rescue, *Ann Intern Med* 117(2):124, 1992.

16. Bucholtz JD: Implications of radiation therapy for nursing. In *Oncology Nursing Society core curriculum for oncology nursing,* ed 2, Philadelphia, 1992, Saunders.

17. Catalona WJ: Management of cancer of the prostate, *N Engl J Med* 331(15):996, 1994.

18. Catalona WJ, Basler JW: Return of erections and urinary continence following nerve-sparing radical retropubic prostatectomy, *J Urol* 150(3):905, 1993.

19. Catalona WJ, Bigg SW: Nerve-sparing radical prostatectomy: evaluation of results after 250 patients, *J Urol* 143(3):538, 1990.

20. Chodak GW and others: Results of conservative management of clinically localized prostate cancer, *N Engl J Med* 330(4):242, 1994.

21. Cooper MA, Einhorn LH: Maintenance chemotherapy with daily oral etoposide following salvage therapy in patients with germ cell tumors, *J Clin Oncol* 13(5):1167, 1995.

22. Coopin C and others: Improved local control of invasive bladder cancer by concurrent cisplatin and preoperative radical radiation, *Proc Am Soc Clin Oncol* 11:A-67, 198, 1992.

23. Daniels GF, McNeal JE, Stamey TA: Predictive value of contralateral biopsies in unilaterally palpable prostate cancer, *J Urol* 147(3, pt 2):870, 1992.

24. deKernion JB, Berry D: The diagnosis and treatment of renal cell carcinoma, *Cancer* 45(7 suppl):1947, 1980.

25. del Regato JA, Trailins AH, Pittman DD: Twenty years follow-up of patients with inoperable cancer of the prostate (stage C) treated by radiotherapy: report of a national cooperative study, *Int J Radiat Oncol Biol Phys* 26(2):197, 1993.

26. Desmond PM and others: Morbidity with contemporary prostate biopsy, *J Urol* 150(5, pt 1):1425, 1993.

27. Donohue JP and others: The role of the retroperitoneal lymphadenectomy in clinical stage B testis cancer: the Indiana University experience (1965-1989), *J Urol* 153(1):85, 1995.

28. Dowsett M and others: The effects of aminoglutethimide and hydrocortisone, alone and combined, on androgen levels in postorchiectomy prostate patients, *Br J Cancer* 57:190, 1988.

29. Drasga RE and others: Fertility after chemotherapy for testicular cancer, *J Clin Oncol* 1(3):179, 1983.

30. Duchesne GM and others: Orchiectomy alone for stage I seminoma of the testis, *Cancer* 65(5):1115, 1990.

31. Einhorn LH, Donohue JP: Cisdiamine dichloroplatinum, vinblastine, and bleomycin combination chemotherapy in disseminated testicular cancer, *Ann Intern Med* 87:293, 1977.

32. Einhorn LN, Richie JP, Shipley WU: Cancer of the testis. In Devita VT, Hellman S, Rosenberg SA, editors: *Cancer: principles and practice of oncology,* ed 4, Philadelphia, 1993, Lippincott.

33. Eisenberger MA, Southwest Oncology Group (SWOG): Phase III comparison of flutamide vs placebo following bilateral orchiectomy in patients with stage D2 adenocarcinoma of the prostate (summary last modified 12/92), SWOG-8894, clinical trial closed, San Antonio, Tex, Sept 15, 1994, SWOG.

34. Epstein JI, Carmichael M, Walsh PC: Adenocarcinoma of the prostate invading the seminal vesicle: definition and relation of tumor volume, grade and margins of resection to prognosis, *J Urol* 149(5):1040, 1993.

35. Esriq D and others: Accumulation of nuclear and tumor progression in bladder cancer, *N Engl J Med* 331(19):1259, 1993.

36. Fair RW, Fuks ZY, Scher HI: Cancer of the urethra and penis. In DeVita VT, Hellman S, Rosenberg SA, editors: *Cancer: principles and practice of oncology,* ed 4, Philadelphia, 1993, Lippincott.

37. Farrer JH, Walker AH, Rajfer J: Management of postpubertal crytorcchio testes: a statistical review, *J Urol* 134:1071, 1985.

38. Fijuth J and others: Serum prostate-specific antigen in monitoring the response of carcinoma of the prostate to radiation therapy, *Radiother Oncol* 23(4):236, 1992.

39. Fisher RI and others: Metastatic renal cancer treated with interleukin-2 and lymphokine-activated killer cells: a phase II clinical trial, *Ann Intern Med* 108(4):518, 1988.

40. Forman JD: The management of localized and locally advanced prostate cancer, *Radiation Oncology Investigation* 4:1996.

41. Fossa SD and others: Prognostic factors in hormone-resistant progressing cancer of the prostate, *Ann Oncol* 3(5):361, 1992.

42. Foster RS and others: The fertility of patients with clinical stage I testis cancer managed by nerve-sparing retroperitoneal lymph node dissection, *J Urol* 152(4):1139, 1994.

43. Fowler FJ and others: Patient-reported complications and follow-up treatment after radical prostatectomy—the National Medicare experience: 1988-1990 (updated June 1993), *Urology* 42(6):622, 1993.

44. Fowler JE: Continent urinary reservoirs and bladder substitutes in the adult. Parts I and II, *Monogr Urol* 8(2), 1987.

45. Fox EP and others: Outcome analysis for patients with persistent nonteratomatous lymph node dissections, *J Clin Oncol* 11(7):1294, 1993.

46. Fraley EE and others: The role of ilioinguinal lymphadenectomy and significance of histological differentiation in treatment of carcinoma of the penis, *J Urol* 142(6):1478, 1989.

47. Frazier HA and others: Is prostate specific antigen of clinical importance in evaluating outcome after radical prostatectomy? *J Urol* 149(3):516, 1993.

48. Freeman JA and others: Radical retropubic prostatectomy and postoperative adjuvant radiation for pathological stage C (PCNO) prostate cancer from 1976 to 1989: intermediate findings, *J Urol* 149(5):1029, 1993.

49. Friedman EL and others: Therapeutic guidelines and results in advanced seminars, *J Clin Oncol* 3(10):1325, 1985.

50. Fyfe G and others: Results of treatment of 255 patients with metastatic renal cell carcinoma who received high-dose recombinant interleukin-2 therapy, *J Clin Oncol* 13(3):688, 1995.

51. Gerber GS, Goldberg R, Chodak GW: Local staging of prostate cancer by tumor volume, prostate-specific antigen, and transrectal ultrasound, *Urology* 40(4):311, 1992.

52. Giovannucci E and others: A prospective cohort study of vasectomy and prostate cancer in U.S. men, *JAMA* 269:873, 1992.

53. Gleason DF: Histologic grading and clinical staging of prostatic carcinoma. In Tannenbaum M: *Urologic pathology: the prostate,* Philadelphia, 1977, Lea & Febiger.

54. Gleason DF, Mellinger GT: Prediction of prognosis for prostatic adenocarcinoma by combined histological grading and clinical staging, *J Urol* 111(1):58, 1974.

55. Gohagan JK: Early Detection Branch, Early Detection and Community Oncology Program, DCPC, National Cancer Institute, National Institutes of Health: A 16-year randomized screening trial for prostate, lung, colorectal, and ovarian cancer—PLCO trial (summary last modified 5/95), PLCO-1, clinical trial active, Bethesda, Md, Nov 16, 1993.

56. Golimbu M and others: Renal cell carcinoma: survival and prognostic factors, *Urology* 27(4):291, 1986.

57. Green DM and others: Wilms tumor, *CA Cancer J Clin* 46(1):996, 1996.

58. Hansen PV and others: Testicular function patients with testicular cancer treated with orchiectomy alone or orchiectomy plus cisplatin-based chemotherapy, *J Natl Cancer Inst* 81(6):1246, 1989.

59. Hautmann RE and others: The ileal neobladder: 6 years of experience with more than 200 patients, *J Urol* 150(1):40, 1993.

60. Herr HW and others: Bacillus Calmette-Guérin therapy for superficial bladder cancer: a 10-year follow-up, *J Urol* 147(4):1020, 1992.

61. Herr HW and others: Intravesical Bacillus Calmette-Guérin therapy prevents tumor progression and death from superficial bladder cancer: ten-year follow-up of a prospective randomized trial, *J Clin Oncol* 13(6):1404, 1995.

62. Hofstetter A, Frank F: Laser use in urology. In Dixon JA, editor: *Surgical application of lasers,* Chicago, 1983, Year Book.

63. Holmang S and others: The relationship among multiple recurrences, progression and prognosis of patients with stages TA and T1 transitional cell cancer of the bladder followed for at least 20 years, *J Urol* 153(6):1823, 1995.

64. Horenblas S and others: Squamous cell carcinoma of the penis. II. Treatment of primary tumor, *J Urol* 147(6):1533, 1992.

65. Horwich A and others: Effectiveness of carboplatin, etoposide, and bleomycin combination chemotherapy in good-prognosis metastatic testicular nonseminomatous germ cell tumors, *J Clin Oncol* 9(1):62, 1991.

66. Housset M and others: Combined radiation and chemotherapy for invasive transitional-cell carcinoma of the bladder: a prospective study, *J Clin Oncol* 11(11):2150, 1993.

67. Hudes GR and others: Phase II study of estramustine and vinblastine, two microtubule inhibitors, in hormone-refractory prostate cancer, *J Clin Oncol* 10(11):1754, 1992.

68. Hudson MA, Herr HW: Carcinoma in situ of the bladder, *J Urol* 153 (3, pt 1):564, 1995.

69. Huncharek M, Muscat J: Serum prostate-specific antigen as a predictor of radiographic staging studies in newly diagnosed prostate cancer, *Cancer Invest* 13(1):31, 1995.

70. Hussay DH: The testicle. In Cox JD: *Moss' radiation oncology: rationale, technique, results,* ed 7, St Louis, 1994, Mosby.

71. Jahnson S, Pedersen J, Westman G: Bladder carcinoma—a 20-year review of radical irradiation therapy, *Radiother Oncol* 22(2):111, 1991.

72. Jewett HJ: The present status of radical prostatectomy for stages A and B prostatic cancer, *Urol Clin North Am* 2(1):105, 1975.

73. Johansson JE: Expectant management of early stage prostate cancer: Swedish experience, *J Urol* 152(5):1753, 1994.

74. Jonler M and others: Sequelae of radical prostatectomy, *Br J Urol* 74(3):352, 1994.

75. Karling P, Hammar M, Varenhorst E: Prevalence and duration of hot flushes after surgical or medical castration in men with prostatic carcinoma, *J Urol* 152(4):1170, 1994.

76. Kaufman DS and others: Selective bladder preservation by combination treatment of invasive bladder cancer, *NJ Med* 3929(19):1377, 1993.

77. Kelly WK and others: Prostate-specific antigen as a measure of disease outcome in metastatic hormone-refractory prostate cancer, *J Clin Oncol* 11(4):607, 1993.

78. Kennealey GT, Furr BJ: Use of the nonsteroidal anti-androgen Casodex in advanced prostatic carcinoma, *Urol Clin North Am* 18(1):99, 1991.

79. Kidney. In Beahrs OH and others: *American Joint Commission on Cancer manual for staging of cancer,* Philadelphia, ed 4, Philadelphia, 1992, Lippincott.

80. Kleinberg L and others: Treatment-related symptoms during the first year following transperineal ^{125}I prostate implantation, *Int Radiat Oncol Biol Phys* 4(2):985, 1994.

81. Klepp O and others: Prognostic factors in clinical state I non-seminomatous germ cell tumors of the testis: multivariate analysis of a prospective multicenter study, *J Clin Oncol* 8(3):509, 1990.

82. Kramer BS and others: Prostate cancer screening: what we know and we need to know, *Ann Intern Med* 119(9):914, 1993.

83. Krahn MD and others: Screening for prostate cancer: a decision analytic view, *JAMA* 272(10):773, 1994.

84. Krown SE: Interferon treatment of renal cell carcinoma: current status and future prospects, *Cancer* 59(3 suppl):647, 1987.

85. Kuban DA, El-Mahdi AM, Schellhammer PF: Prostate-specific antigen for pretreatment prediction and post treatment evaluation of outcome after definitive irradiation for prostate cancer, *Int J Radiat Oncol Biol Phys* 32:307, 1995.

86. Lamm DL, Griffith JG: Intravesical therapy: does it affect the natural history of superficial bladder cancer? *Semin Urol* 10(1):39, 1992.

87. Lamm DL and others: Maintenance BCG immunotherapy of superficial bladder cancer: a randomized prospective Southwest Oncology Group study, *Proc Am Soc Clin Oncol* 11:A-627, 203, 1992.

88. Laramore GE and others: Fast neutron radiotherapy for locally advanced prostate cancer: final report of a Radiation Therapy Oncology Group randomized clinical trial, *Am J Clin Oncol* 16(2):164, 1993.

89. LaVecchia C: Cancers associated with high fat diets, *Monogr Natl Cancer Inst* 12:79, 1992.

90. Lawton CA and others: Is long-term survival possible with external beam irradiation for Stage D1 adenocarcinoma of the prostate? *Cancer* 69(11):2761, 1992.

91. Leibovitch I and others: The clinical implications of procedural deviations during orchiectomy for nonseminomatous germ testes cancer, *J Urol* 151a(93):939, 1995.

92. Levi JA and others: The importance of bleomycin in combination chemotherapy for good-prognosis germ cell carcinoma, *J Clin Oncol* 11(7):1300, 1993.

93. Lipponen PK: Over expression of p53 nuclear oncoprotein in transitional-cell bladder cancer and its prognostic value, *Int J Cancer* 53:365, 1993.

94. Litwin MS and others: Quality-of-life outcomes in men treated for localized prostate cancer, *JAMA* 273(2):129, 1995.

95. Loehrer PJ and others: A randomized comparison of cisplatin alone or in combination with methotrexate, vinblastine, and doxorubicin in patients with metastatic urothelial carcinoma: a cooperative group study, *J Clin Oncol* 10(7):1066, 1992.

96. Loehrer PJ and others: Importance of bleomycin in favorable-prognosis disseminated germ cell tumors: an Eastern Cooperative Oncology Group trial, *J Clin Oncol* 13(2):470, 1995.

97. Lu-Yao GL and others: An assessment of radical prostatectomy: time trends, geographic variation, and outcomes, *JAMA* 269(20):2633, 1993.

98. Mason BR, Kearsley JH: Radiotherapy for stage II testicular seminoma: the prognostic influence of tumor bulk, *J Clin Oncol* (12):1856, 1988.

99. Matzkin H and others: Prognostic significance of changes in prostate-specific markers after endocrine treatment of stage D2 prostatic cancer, *Cancer* 70(9):2302, 1992.

100. McCarthy CP: Altered patterns of elimination. In *Nursing care in radiation oncology,* Philadelphia, 1992, Saunders.

101. McLean M and others: The results of primary radiation therapy in the management of squamous cell carcinoma of the penis, *Int J Radiat Oncol Biol Phys* 25(4):623, 1993.

102. Mettlin C, Natarujau H, Habum R: Vasectomy and prostate cancer risk, *Am J Epidemiol* 132:1056, 1990.

103. Montie JE: Staging of prostate cancer: current TNM classification and future prospects for prognostic factors, *CA Cancer J Clin* 5(7, suppl):1814, 1995.

104. Morse MJ, Whitmore WF: Neoplasm of the testis. In Walsh PC, Gittes RF and others, editors: *Campbell's urology,* ed 5, Philadelphia, 1986, Saunders.

105. Muss HB: The role to biological response modifiers in metastatic renal cell carcinoma, *Semin Oncol* 15(5, suppl 5):30, 1988.

106. Myers C and others: Suramin: a novel growth factor antagonist with activity in hormone-refractory metastatic prostate cancer, *J Clin Oncol* 10(6):881, 1992.

107. Narayan P and others: Is adjuvant chemotherapy necessary following retroperitoneal lymph node dissection for nonseminomatous testicular cancer? *Urol Clin North Am* 7(3):747, 1980.

108. National Institute of Health: National Institute of Health Consensus Development Conference: magnetic resonance imaging, *JAMA* 259(14):2132, 1988.

109. Novick AC and others: Conservative surgery for renal cell carcinoma: a single-center experience with 100 patients, *J Urol* 141(4):835, 1989.

110. Neves RJ, Zincke H, Taylor WF: Metastatic renal cell carcinoma and radical nephrectomy: identification of prognostic factors and patient survival, *J Urol* 139(6):1173, 1988.

111. Nijman JM and others: Gonadal function after surgery and chemotherapy in men with stage II and III nonseminomatous testicular tumors, *J Clin Oncol* 5(4):651, 1987.

112. Oesterling A and others: Risk of bilateral testicular germ cell cancer in Denmark: 1960-1983, *J Anat Can Inst* 83(10):1391, 1991.

113. Oesterling JE and others: Correlation of clinical stage, serum prostatic acid phosphatase and preoperative Gleason grade with final pathological stage in 275 patients with clinically localized adenocarcinoma of the prostate, *J Urol* 138(1):92, 1987.

114. Oesterling JE and others: The use of prostate-specific antigen in staging patients with newly diagnosed prostate cancer, *JAMA* 269(1):57, 1993.

115. Oliver RT, Nethersell AB, Bottomley JM: Unexplained spontaneous regression and alpha-interferon as treatment for metastatic renal carcinoma, *Br J Urol* 62(2):128, 1989.

116. Olsson CA: Management of invasive carcinoma of the bladder. In deKernion JB, Paulson DF, editors: *Genitourinary cancer management,* Philadelphia, 1987, Lea & Febiger.

117. Ornellas AA and others: Surgical treatment of invasive squamous cell carcinoma of the penis: retrospective analysis of 350 cases, *J Urol* 151(5):1244, 1994.

118. Parker SL and others: Cancer statistics, 1995, *CA Cancer J Clin* 45(1):8, 1995.

119. Parker SL and others: Cancer statistics, 1996, *CA Cancer J Clin* 46(1):5, 1995.

120. Partin AW and others: Use of nuclear morphometry, Gleason histologic scoring, clinical stage, and age to predict disease-free survival among patients with prostate cancer, *CA Cancer J Clin* 42(1):161, 1992.

121. Pearse DH: The urinary bladder. In Cox JD: *Moss' radiation oncology: rationale, technique, results,* ed 7, St Louis, 1994, Mosby.

122. Peeling WB: Phase III studies to compare goserelin (Zoladex) with orchiectomy and with diethylstilbestrol in treatment of prostatic carcinoma, *Urology* 33(5, suppl):45, 1989.

123. Penis. In Beahrs OH and others: *American Joint Commission on Cancer manual for staging of cancer,* ed 4, Philadelphia, 1992, Lippincott.

124. Phillips E, Messing EM: Role of lymphadenectomy in the treatment of renal cell carcinoma, *Urology* 41(1):9, 1993.

125. Pienta K, Esper PS: Risk factors for prostate cancer, *Ann Intern Med* 118(10):793, 1993.

126. Pienta KJ and others: Phase II evaluation of oral estramustine and oral etoposide in hormone-refractory adenocarcinoma of the prostate, *J Clin Oncol* 12(10):2005, 1994.

127. Pisansky TM and others: Prostate-specific antigen as a pretherapy prognostic factor in patients treated with radiation therapy for clinically localized prostate cancer, *J Clin Oncol* 11(11):2158, 1993.

128. Porter AT, Forman JD: Prostate brachytherapy—an overview, Department of Radiation Oncology, UHC and DMC, *Cancer* 71(3):950, 1993.

129. Porter AT and others: Results of a randomized Phase-III trial to evaluate the efficacy of strontium-89 adjuvant to local external beam irradiation in the management of endocrine resistant metastatic prostate cancer, *Int J Radiat Oncol Biol Phys* 25:805, 1993.

130. Prostate. In Beahrs OH and others: *American Joint Commission on Cancer manual for staging of cancer,* ed 4, Philadelphia, 1992 Lippincott.

131. Prout GR and others: Photodynamic therapy with hematoporphyrin derivative in the treatment of superficial transitional-cell carcinoma of the bladder, *N Engl J Med* 317(20):1251, 1987.

132. Raghavan D, Huben R: Management of bladder cancer, *Curr Probl Cancer* 19(1):1, 1995.

133. Richie JP: Surgery for invasive bladder cancer, *Hematol Oncol Clin North Am* 5(1):129, 1992.

134. Richie JP, Garnick MB: Primary renal and ureteral cancer. In Rieselback RE, Garnick MG: *Cancer and the kidney,* Philadelphia, 1982, Lea & Febiger.

135. Ritter MA and others: Prostate-specific antigen as a predictor of radiotherapy response and patterns of failure in localized prostate cancer, *J Clin Oncol* 10(8):1208, 1992.

136. Robinson RG: Strontium-89: precursor targeted therapy for pain relief of blastic metastatic disease, *Cancer* 72(11, suppl):3433, 1993.

137. Rosenberg SA and others: A progress report on the treatment of 157 patients with advanced cancer using lymphokine-activated killer cells and interleukin-2 or high-dose interleukin-2 alone, *N Engl J Med* 316(15):889, 1987.

138. Rosenberg SA and others: Treatment of 283 consecutive patients with metastatic melanoma or renal cell cancer using high-dose bolus interleukin 2, *JAMA* 271(12):907, 1994.

139. Rosenberg SK, Fuller TA: Carbon dioxide rapid superpulsed laser treatment of erythroplasia of Queyrat, *Urology* 16(2):181, 1980.

140. Ruckle HC, Klee GG, Oesterling JE: Prostate-specific antigen: concepts for staging prostate cancer and monitoring response to therapy, *Mayo Clin Proc* 69(1):69, 1994.

141. Russell KJ, Boileau MA: Current status of prostate-specific antigen in the radiotherapeutic management of prostatic cancer, *Semin Radiat Oncol* 3(3):154, 1993.

142. Saffer EM and others: Conformal static field radiation therapy treatments of early prostate cancer versus nonconformal techniques: a reduction in acute morbidity, *Int J Radiat Oncol Biol Phys* 3(24):485, 1992.

143. Sarkis AS and others: Prognostic value of p53 nuclear over expression in patients with invasive bladder cancer treated with neoadjuvant MVAC, *J Clin Oncol* 13(6):1384, 1995.

144. Sartor O and others: Surprising activity of flutamide withdrawal, when combined with aminoglutethimide, in treatment of "hormone-refractory" prostate cancer, *J Natl Cancer Inst* 86(3):222, 1994.

145. Sauer R and others: Preliminary results of treatment of invasive bladder carcinoma with radiotherapy and cisplatin, *Int J Radiat Oncol Biol Phys* 15:871, 1988.

146. Schellhammer PF, Kuban DA, El-Mahdi AM: Treatment of clinical local failure after radiation therapy for prostate carcinoma, *J Urol* 150(6):1851, 1993.

147. Schellhammer PF and others: Morbidity and mortality of local failure after definitive therapy for prostate cancer, *J Urol* 141(3):567, 1989.

148. Schiebler ML and others: MR imaging in adenocarcinoma of the prostate: interobserver variation and efficacy for determining stage C disease, *J Radiol* 158(3):559, 1992.

149. Schiebler ML and others: Current role of MR imaging in the staging of adenocarcinoma of the prostate, *Radiology* 189(2):339, 1993.

150. Sell A and others: Treatment of advanced bladder cancer category T2, T3 and T4a: a randomized multicenter study of preoperative irradiation and cystectomy versus radical irradiation and early salvage cystectomy for residual tumor: DAVECA protocol 8201, *Scand J Urol Nephrol* 138(suppl):193, 1991.

151. Selli C and others: Stratification of risk factors in renal cell carcinoma, *Cancer* 52(5):899, 1983.

152. Sene AP and others: Renal carcinoma in patients undergoing nephrectomy: analysis of survival and prognostic factors, *Br J Urol* 70(2):125, 1992.

153. Sesterhenn IA and others: Prognosis and other clinical correlates of pathologic review in stage I and II testicular carcinoma: a report from the Testicular Cancer Intergroup Study, *J Clin Oncol* 10(1):69, 1992.

154. Sherman JK: Semen cryopreservation, *American Association of Tissue Banks/Reproductive Council* 11(1):1, 1988.

155. Shinohara K and others: Comparison of prostate-specific antigen with prostate-specific antigen density for 8 clinical applications, *J Urol* 152(1):120, 1994.

156. Shipley WU and others: Advanced prostate cancer: the results of a randomized comparative trial of high dose irradiation boosting with conformal protons compared with conventional dose irradiation using photons alone, *Int J Radiat Oncol Biol Phys* 32(1):3, 1995.

157. Shipley WU and others: Treatment of invasive bladder cancer by cisplatin and radiation in patients unsuited for surgery, *JAMA* 258:931, 1987.

158. Skinner DG, Boyd SD, Lieskovsky G: Clinical experience with the Kock continent ileal reservoir for urinary diversion, *J Urol* 132(6):1101, 1984.

159. Skinner DG and others: The role of adjuvant chemotherapy following cystectomy for invasive bladder cancer: a prospective comparative trial, *J Urol* 145(3):459, 1991.

160. Smiley SR and others: Radiotherapy as initial treatment for bulky stage II testicular seminomas, *J Clin Oncol* 3(10):1333, 1985.

161. Socinski MA, Stomper PC: Radiologic evaluation of nonseminomatous germ cell tumor of the testis, *Semin Urol* 6(3):205, 1988.

162. Soloway MS: The management of superficial bladder cancer. In Javadpour N, editor: *Principles and management of urologic cancer,* ed 2, Baltimore, 1983, Williams & Wilkins.

163. Spears and others: Brain metastases and testicular tumors: long-term survival, *Int J Radiat Oncol Biol Phys* 22(1):17, 1992.

164. Stamey TA, Ferrari MK, Schmid HP: The value of serial prostate-specific antigen determinations 5 years after radiotherapy: steeply increasing values characterize 80% of patients, *J Urol* 130(6):1856, 1993.

165. Stephenson WT and others: Evaluation of reproductive capacity in germ cell tumor patients following treatment with cisplatin, etoposide, and bleomycin, *J Clin Oncol* 13(9):2278, 1995.

166. Stock RG and others: A modified technique allowing interactive ultrasound-guided three-dimensional transperineal prostate implantations, *Int J Radiat Oncol Biol Phys* 32(1):219, 1995.

167. Stomper PC and others: CT and pathologic predictive features of residual mass histologic findings after chemotherapy for nonseminomatous germ cell tumors: can residual malignancy or teratoma be excluded? *Radiology* 180:711, 1991.

168. Stuzman RE, McLeod DG: Radiation therapy: a primary treatment modality for seminoma, *Urol Clin North Am* 7(3):757, 1980.

169. Sujka SK, Huben RP: Clinical stage I nonseminomatous germ cell tumors of testis: observation vs retroperitoneal lymph node dissection, *Urology* 38(1):29, 1991.

170. Takayama TK, Vessella RL, Lange PH: Newer applications of serum prostate-specific antigen in the management of prostate cancer, *Semin Oncol* 21(5):542, 1994.

171. Terris MK and others: Efficacy of transrectal ultrasound-guided seminal vesicle biopsies in the detection of seminal vesicle invasion by prostate cancer, *J Urol* 149(5):1035, 1993.

172. Tester W and others: Combined modality program with possible organ preservation for invasive bladder cancer: results of RTOG Protocol 85-12, *Int J Radiat Oncol Biol Phys* 25(5):78, 1993.

173. Testis. In Beahrs OH and others: *American Joint Committee on Cancer manual for staging of cancer,* ed 4, Philadelphia, 1992, Lippincott.

174. Thrasher JB, Crawford ED: Current management of invasive and metastatic transitional cell carcinoma of the bladder, *J Urol* 149(5):957, 1993.

175. Toner GC and others: Adjunctive surgery after chemotherapy for nonseminomatous germ cell tumors: recommendations for patient selection, *J Clin Oncol* 8(10):1683, 1990.

176. Urinary bladder. In Beahrs OH and others: *American Joint Committee on Cancer manual for staging of cancer,* ed 4, Philadelphia, 1992, Lippincott.

177. van Leeuwen FE and others: Second cancer risk following testicular cancer: a follow-up study of 1,909 patients, *J Clin Oncol* 11(2):415, 1993.

178. Vogelzang NJ and others: Goserelin versus orchiectomy in the treatment of advanced prostate cancer: final results of a randomized trial, *Urology* 46(2):220, 1995.

179. Waaler G, Stenwig AE: Prognosis of localized prostatic cancer managed by "watch and wait" policy, *Br J Urol* 72(2):214, 1993.

180. Walsh PC, Lepor H: The role of radical prostatectomy in the management of prostate cancer, *CA Cancer J Clin* 60:562, 1987.

181. Warde P and others: Stage I testicular seminoma: results of adjuvant irradiation and surveillance, *J Clin Oncol* 13(9):2255, 1995.

182. Wasson JH and others: A structured literature review of treatment for localized prostate cancer, *Arch Fam Med* 2:487, 1993.

183. Waymont B and others: Phase III randomized study of Zoladex versus stilbestrol in the treatment of advanced prostate cancer, *Br J Urol* 69(6):614, 1992.

184. Webb JA, Shanmuganathan K, McLean A: Complications of ultrasound-guided transperineal prostate biopsy: a prospective study, *Br J Urol* 72(5):775, 1993.

185. Weiss GR and others: A randomized phase II trial of continuous infusion interleukin-2 or bolus injection interleukin-2 plus lymphokine-activated killer cells for advanced renal cell carcinoma, *J Clin Oncol* 10(2):275, 1992.

186. Whitmore WF: Expectant management of clinically localized prostatic cancer, *Semin Oncol* 21(5):560, 1994.

187. Wolfe JS and others: Combined role of transrectal ultrasonography, Gleason score, and prostate-specific antigen in predicting organ-confined prostate cancer, *Urology* 42(2):131, 1993.

188. Wozniak AJ and others: A randomized trial of cisplatin, vinblastine, and bleomycin versus vinblastine, cisplatin, and etoposide in the treatment of advanced germ cell tumors of the testis: a Southwest Oncology Group Study, *J Clin Oncol* 9(1):70, 1991.

189. Zenter PG and others: Prostate-specific antigen density: a new prognostic indicator for prostate cancer, *Int J Radiat Oncol Biol Phys* 27(21):47, 1993.

190. Zietman AL and others: Radical radiation therapy in the management of prostatic adenocarcinoma: the initial prostate-specific antigen value as a predictor of treatment outcome, *J Urol* 151(3):640, 1994.

191. Zincke H and others: Radical prostatectomy for clinically localized prostate cancer: long-term results of 1,143 patients from a single institution, *J Clin Oncol* 12(11):2254, 1994.

CHAPTER 10

Gynecologic Cancers

JANE C. CLARK

The American Cancer Society (ACS) estimates that 82,100 women were diagnosed with a malignancy of the female genital tract in 1996. Although dramatic improvements in the prevention, diagnosis, and treatment of women with gynecologic cancers have occurred during the past decade, an estimated 26,900 women died from gynecologic malignancies in 1996.[1]

This chapter reviews the epidemiology, etiology, risk factors, routes and sites of metastasis, and treatment strategies for gynecologic cancer. The nurse's role in the education of the public about preventive health behaviors, self-examination skills, and recommended screening activities is discussed. In addition, critical elements of nursing care for the patient diagnosed with specific gynecologic cancers are described.

CERVICAL CANCER

EPIDEMIOLOGY

Although the incidence rates of invasive cervical cancer have steadily declined since the 1940s, the ACS estimates that 15,700 women were diagnosed with the disease in 1996.[1] Patterns of occurrence have been described based on age and socioeconomic status. Invasive cervical cancer occurs most often among women between ages 35 and 50 years. Recent trends indicate an increasing incidence of cervical cancer in younger women and women of low socioeconomic status (SES).*

Cervical cancer develops primarily at the *squamocolumnar junction,* the area on the cervix where squamous cells that line the vagina and cover the outer portion of the cervix and where columnar cells that line the endocervical canal meet. The squamocolumnar junction occurs on the outer portion of the cervix *(exocervix)* in younger women. As women age, changes in the vaginal pH trigger a process of squamous metaplasia in which the squamous cells begin to cover the columnar cells, re-

---

*References 1, 3, 8, 11, 13, 18, 19, 24.

sulting in an area called the *transformation zone.* Over time, the squamocolumnar junction moves from the exocervix into the endocervical canal.[8]

Invasive cervical cancer is usually preceded by a 10- to 20-year history of preinvasive cellular changes ranging from mild dysplasia to carcinoma in situ (CIS) (Figure 10-1). If untreated, a small proportion of women with mild dysplasia will eventually develop invasive cancer. In prospective studies, however, 40% to 71% of women with CIS developed invasive cancer over a 10- to 12-year follow-up period.[4,8,13,17] Even with the widespread use of the Papanicolaou (Pap) smear for early detection of preinvasive and invasive cervical disease, an estimated 4900 women died of cervical cancer in 1996.[1,4,8,13]

ETIOLOGY AND RISK FACTORS

The etiology of cervical cancer is unknown. Data have suggested a strong association between sexual history and practices and the incidence of cervical cancer. In addition, diet and life-style have been identified as cofactors for development of the disease.

Sexual practices associated with an increased risk for cervical cancer include onset of sexual intercourse before 18 years of age and multiple sexual partners. Increasingly, data have indicated that the number of sexual partners of the male partner(s) also may play a significant role in the development of cervical cancer. A history of infection with sexually transmitted viruses, such as herpes simplex virus type 2 (HSV-2) and the human papillomavirus (HPV, specifically types HPV-16 and HPV-18), initial pregnancy before 18 years of age, and multiple pregnancies place an individual woman at increased risk for cervical intraepithelial neoplasia (CIN) and invasive cervical cancers.[3,8,11,13,19]

Cofactors associated with an increased risk include decreased levels of vitamins A and C and folic acid in the diet, tobacco use, and alcohol abuse. The role of genital hygiene also is being explored as a possible cofactor in the development of cervical cancer.[13]

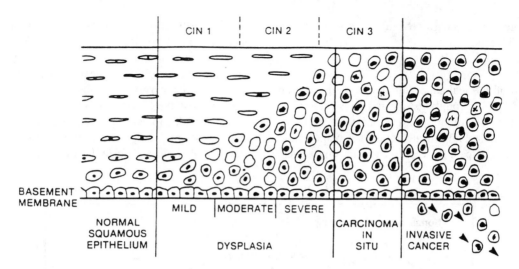

Figure 10-1   Progression of cervical intraepithelial neoplasia *(CIN)*. (From Jones HW, Wentz AC, Burnett LS: *Novak's textbook of gynecology,* ed 11, Baltimore, 1988, Williams & Wilkins.)

In the late 1960s an increase in the incidence of clear cell adenocarcinoma of the cervix was noted in women younger than 30 years. On review of medical histories for these women, a commonality was noted. Most of the women had been exposed in utero to *diethylstilbestrol* (DES), a synthetic estrogen given to women with high-risk pregnancies. Although the use of DES during pregnancy was discontinued in the early 1960s, a study of the incidence of cervical and vaginal carcinomas among DES-exposed women continues.[8]

PREVENTION, SCREENING, AND DETECTION
Prevention

Prevention is the key strategy for eradication of cervical cancer. Based on available knowledge about factors that place women at high risk for cervical cancer, the nurse can develop cervical cancer prevention programs for the public. Programs for teenagers may include strategies such as avoidance of penile-vaginal intercourse and use of barrier contraceptives to prevent pregnancy and sexually transmitted diseases (STDs). For women of all ages, limitation of the number of sexual partners and use of barrier contraceptives, such as condoms and diaphragms, are recommended to reduce the risk of cervical cancer. Dietary modifications that may reduce the risk of cervical cancer include increased ingestion of foods high in vitamins A and C and folic acid. In addition, strategies to prevent initiation or to encourage discontinuation of tobacco and alcohol use could be included.[4,7,10] Since invasive cervical cancer is preceded by a preinvasive stage in most patients, the ACS guidelines for screening should be taught as a cancer prevention strategy.

The target population for teaching prevention of cervical cancer is teenagers. Points to be stressed include an overview of normal physiologic changes that occur on the cervix during puberty and adolescence, the importance of using barrier contraception, and initiation of routine Pap smears and pelvic examinations whenever the teenager becomes sexually active. Emphasis on the ability to diagnose preinvasive lesions of the cervix and on the effectiveness of conservative treatment in eradicating preinvasive disease may lessen the fear of cancer and enhance compliance.

Screening

The primary screening test for cervical cancer is the *Papanicolaou smear.* The specimen is obtained by collecting a sample of cells from the squamocolumnar junction with a cotton swab, wooden spatula, or a cytobrush. The lowest false-negative rate and the highest predictability are achieved by sampling cells from the exocervix and the endocervical canal.[13] A *pelvic examination* is also recommended to evaluate the shape and consistency of the cervix and adjacent tissues.

The ACS recommendations for screening of asymptomatic women for cervical cancer include an annual Pap smear and pelvic examination for all women who are or have been sexually active or who are 18 years of age. After three or more normal, consecutive, annual Pap smears, the Pap smear and pelvic examination can be performed less frequently at the physician's discretion.[1] Although debate continues about the cost-effectiveness of the Pap smear for women older than 65 years, data indicate that the incidence of invasive cervical cancer increases with age in general and particularly among older, lower socioeconomic women who have never had a Pap smear. Therefore women should not be denied the opportunity to have a Pap smear and pelvic examination based on age alone.

Recent changes in medicare coverage allow for a Pap smear every 3 years.

Detection

The detection of cervical cancer in symptomatic women is determined by a thorough history and physical examination. A clinical examination is performed to visualize the cervix, obtain a Pap smear, conduct a colposcopic examination, and palpate the cervix and adjacent tissues.

The majority of invasive cervical carcinomas may be visualized on inspection. Cervical carcinoma presents in two primary patterns. The most common presentation is an *exophytic lesion*. These lesions occur primarily on the portio of the cervix, resemble polyps, spread superficially across the cervix, and bleed easily. *Endophytic lesions* invade toward the endocervical canal. These tumors often go undetected as they expand within the endocervical canal and form a barrel-shaped lesion.[3,8,13]

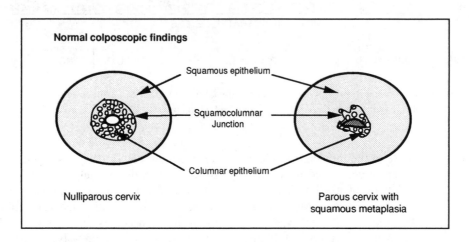

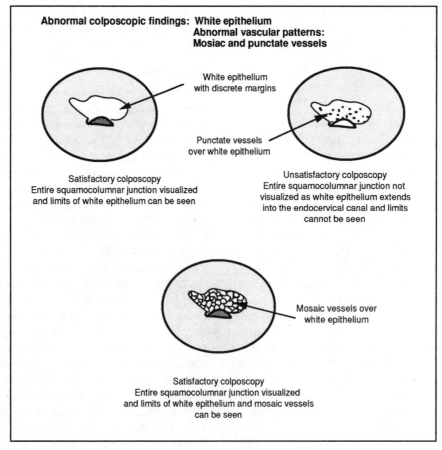

Figure 10-2   Graphic representation of cervical findings using the colposcope.

A colposcopic examination may be performed in women with significant symptoms or grossly suspicious lesions on the cervix. The *colposcope* is a binocular optical device used to magnify and illuminate the cervical tissues. After application of a 3% to 5% acetic acid solution, the clinician evaluates the transformation zone and the squamocolumnar junction, if visible, for abnormalities in color and contour of tissues and vascular patterns (Figure 10-2). The clinician obtains a colposcopically directed biopsy from the most abnormal areas for evaluation.

The rectovaginal, bimanual examination allows the clinician to evaluate the size, contour, and consistency of the cervix, corpus, ovaries, and vaginal and rectal tissues. Gross extension of the tumor to adjacent structures such as the rectum, vagina, and paracervical tissues also can be evaluated.

CLASSIFICATION

Cervical carcinomas are classified histologically by the tissue of origin. Historically, more than 90% of cervical cancers are *squamous cell carcinomas.* Squamous cell carcinomas have been divided further into *keratinizing, nonkeratinizing,* and *small cell* types based on histologic descriptors. *Adenocarcinomas* and *adenosquamous carcinomas* account for an increasingly greater proportion of cervical cancers (11% to 16%), particularly in women

under 35 years of age. The increase in cervical cancers with adenomatous features is important because of the poorer prognosis associated with the disease.[4,8,13]

CLINICAL FEATURES

The most common presenting symptom of women with cervical cancer is *abnormal vaginal bleeding,* which may present as a decrease in the interval between the menstrual periods, an increase in the length or amount of menstrual flow, or intermenstrual bleeding. The woman also may describe episodes of "contact" bleeding after intercourse or douching. Less often the woman may complain of a persistent, thin, watery, blood-tinged, odoriferous vaginal discharge.* Symptoms of more advanced disease include urinary complaints such as difficulty starting the stream of urine, urinary urgency, hematuria, or pain with urination. Advanced disease resulting in pressure or invasion of the rectum may result in constipation, rectal tenesmus, or rectal bleeding. Involvement of regional lymph nodes may result in edema of the lower extremities. Pain of the lower back, groins, and lower extremities also may be present with advanced disease.*

The boxes below list clinical features and complications of gynecologic cancers.

---

*References 3, 8, 11, 13, 18, 19.

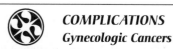

CLINICAL FEATURES
Gynecologic Cancers

Cervical: abnormal vaginal bleeding—increase in the amount, frequency, and/or length; contact bleeding related to intercourse; urinary urgency; dysuria; hematuria

Endometrial: bleeding—may be prolonged, irregular, and/or excessive; pain in the hypogastric, pelvis, and/or lumbosacral area

Ovarian: dyspepsia, indigestion, anorexia, and/or early satiety; urinary frequency; constipation; pelvic pressure; pain

Vulvar: pain, pruritus, bleeding, discharge, dysuria, presence of lump or mass in vulvar area

Vaginal: Vaginal bleeding—perimenopausal and postmenopausal; foul-smelling vaginal discharge; pain; dyspareunia

Fallopian: vaginal bleeding; intermittent, colicky, dull, aching pain; profuse, watery vaginal discharge

Gestational trophoblastic disease: first-trimester vaginal bleeding, hyperemesis, abnormal enlargement of uterus, absence of fetal heart sounds and movement

COMPLICATIONS
Gynecologic Cancers

Disease related

Sexual dysfunction
Infertility
Sterility
Alteration in bowel and bladder function
Loss of pregnancy
Changes in self-concept

Treatment related

Infertility
Sterility (temporary/permanent)
Fistula formation
Infection
Bleeding
Wound dehiscence
Vaginal fibrosis/stenosis
Ureteral obstruction
Myelosuppression
Alopecia
Alteration in bowel and bladder function
Termination of pregnancy
Altered sexual function

DIAGNOSIS AND STAGING

Diagnosis and staging form the basis of treatment for cervical carcinomas. A tissue biopsy is required for the diagnosis of cervical cancer. The exocervix and the endocervical canal are easily accessible to punch biopsy and curettage, respectively. Since the treatment of preinvasive cervical disease is more conservative, the tissue biopsy is needed to rule out or confirm the presence of invasive cancer. If an adequate tissue sampling for making the determination is not obtained, a more extensive tissue sampling with conization of the cervix is required (Figure 10-3). Pathologic confirmation of preinvasive or invasive disease is mandatory before initiation of treatment.[8,13]

Staging for cervical cancer is done clinically. Data obtained from the clinical examination (inspection, palpation, colposcopy), radiographic examinations (chest, kidneys, sigmoid colon and rectum, skeleton), and pathologic evaluation of biopsy and curettage materials are used to determine the extent of disease and ultimately plan treatment. Table 10-1 presents staging systems for cervical cancer that have been developed by the American Joint Committee on Cancer (AJCC) and the International Federation of Gynecology and Obstetrics (FIGO).[8,11,13,18,19]

METASTASIS

Cervical carcinomas are slow-growing tumors that invade by direct extension to adjacent tissues of the uterus, vagina, rectum, bladder, and parametrial tissues. Lymphatic invasion also occurs in regional and distant lymphatic channels. Cervical cancer rarely spreads hematologically; however, metastatic disease can occur in the lungs or liver.[8,13,18,19]

TREATMENT MODALITIES

The treatment of preinvasive cervical disease is based on the extent of disease (Figure 10-4). Women with preinvasive disease may be treated conservatively with *cryosurgery, electrocautery,* or *laser vaporization*. Each of these techniques allows destruction of superficially abnormal cells with cold, heat, or light energy, respectively. Of the three methods, the laser vaporization allows for more control of the pattern and depth of tissue destruction.[8,13]

A *cold-knife conization* or *loop electrosurgical excision procedure* (LEEP) of the cervix may be used as treatment. With either procedure, the entire transformation zone and squamocolumnar junction are removed (see Figure 10-3). Conization of the cervix often is recommended as treatment for women who desire to maintain fertility. However, many physicians recommend hysterectomy after completion of childbearing. For women with preinvasive disease who do not desire to maintain

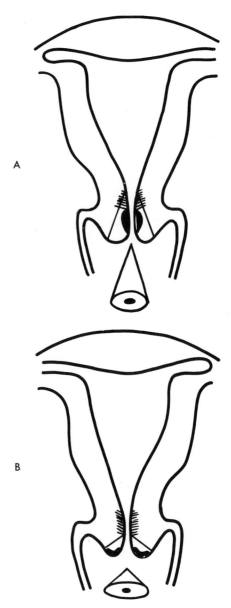

Figure 10-3 Cone biopsy for endocervical and exocervical disease. **A,** Endocervical disease: increased depth of cone biopsy to remove all abnormal areas. **B,** Exocervical disease: increased width of cone biopsy to remove all abnormal areas. (From DiSaia PJ, Creasman WT: *Clinical gynecologic oncology,* ed 4, St Louis, 1993, Mosby.)

fertility or who are high risk for noncompliance with follow-up examinations, hysterectomy may be considered as definitive treatment.[8,13]

Localized cervical carcinoma (stages I to IIA) may be treated with surgery alone, radiation therapy alone, or a combination of both. Comparable survival rates have been demonstrated among the three treatment plans. The choice of treatment is based on extent of disease and the patient's general health status, desire to maintain childbearing function, and indication of intent to comply with

Table 10-1 Staging Classification for Cervical Cancer

	Primary tumor (T)	
TNM	FIGO	Definition
TX		Primary tumor cannot be assessed
T0		No evidence of primary tumor
Tis	0	Carcinoma in situ
T1	I	Cervical carcinoma confined to uterus (extension to corpus should be disregarded)
T1a	Ia	Preclinical invasive carcinoma, diagnosed by microscopy only
T1a1	Ia1	Minimal microscopic stromal invasion
T1a2	Ia2	Tumor with invasive component 5 mm or less in depth taken from base of epithelium and 7 mm or less in horizontal spread
T1b	Ib	Tumor larger than T1a2
T2	II	Cervical carcinoma invades beyond uterus but not to pelvic wall or to lower third of vagina
T2a	IIa	Without parametrial invasion
T2b	IIb	With parametrial invasion
T3	III	Cervical carcinoma extends to pelvic wall and/or involves lower third of vagina and/or causes hydronephrosis or nonfunctioning kidney
T3a	IIIa	Tumor involves lower third of vagina, no extension to pelvic wall
T3b	IIIb	Tumor extends to pelvic wall and/or causes hydronephrosis or nonfunctioning kidney
T4	IVa	Tumor invades mucosa of bladder or rectum and/or extends beyond true pelvis
M1	IVb	Distant metastasis

Regional lymph nodes (N)

Regional lymph nodes include paracervical, parametrial, hypogastric (obturator), common, internal and external iliac, presacral, and sacral

TMN	Definition
NX	Regional lymph nodes cannot be assessed
N0	No regional lymph node metastasis
N1	Regional lymph node metastasis

Distant metastasis (M)

TMN	FIGO	Definition
MX		Presence of distant metastasis cannot be assessed
M0		No distant metastasis
M1	IVb	Distant metastasis

Stage grouping

Stage 0:	Tis-N0-M0
Stage IA:	T1a-N0-M0
Stage IB:	T1b-N0-M0
Stage IIA:	T2a-N0-M0
Stage IIB:	T2b-N0-M0
Stage IIIA:	T3a-N0-M0
Stage IIIB:	T1-N1-M0
	T2-N1-M0
	T3a-N1-M0
	T3b-any N-M0
Stage IVA:	T4-any N-M0
Stage IVB:	any T-any N-M1

From American Joint Committee on Cancer: *Manual for staging cancer,* ed 4, Philadelphia, 1992, Lippincott.

follow-up recommendations. Ideally the treatment decision should be made jointly by the woman, the gynecologic oncologist, and the radiation therapist after review of the risks and benefits of treatment alternatives.*

Surgical treatment of women with invasive cervical cancer most often includes a *radical hysterectomy* with *bilateral pelvic lymphadenectomy*. Advantages of a radical approach to treatment include the gathering of additional pathologic information about the spread of the disease to local and regional lymph nodes and the need for adjuvant radiation therapy and maintenance of ovarian function. Disadvantages of radical surgical treatment include the high costs of hospitalization, risks of intraoperative and postoperative complications, and the loss of childbearing function. For a select number of women with stage IA disease who desire to maintain fertility,

conization of the cervix may be used as definitive treatment. Follow-up with cervical cytology, colposcopy, and pelvic examination at 3-month intervals is recommended for early detection of recurrent invasive cervical cancer.[8,13]

Radiation with external beam *(teletherapy)* and internal or interstitial beam *(brachytherapy)* offers women with early-stage disease equally effective treatment. Advantages of radiation are that the treatment can be given on an outpatient basis, intraoperative and postoperative complications are avoided, and treatment time is shorter.[19] Disadvantages include long-term effects of radiation on normal tissues, such as radiation enteritis, bladder damage, fistula formation, vaginal stenosis, and ureteral obstruction.[8,19]

Advanced cervical carcinoma (stages IIB to IV) is treated primarily with radiation therapy alone, although recent clinical trials include antineoplastic agents, radio-

*References 3, 8, 13, 18, 19, 24.

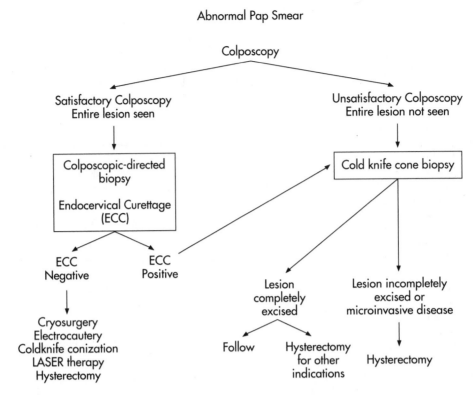

Figure 10-4 Decision tree for management of cervical intraepithelial neoplasia (CIN). (From Flannery M: Reproductive cancers. In Clark JC, McGee RF, editors: *Core curriculum for oncology nursing,* Philadelphia, 1992, Saunders.)

sensitizing agents, hyperbaric oxygen, and hyperthermia administered in conjunction with radiation. Coordination between the medical oncologist and the radiation oncologist is mandatory to maximize therapeutic benefit while carefully monitoring immediate and long-term consequences of combined therapy.

The incidence of persistent or recurrent cervical cancer is approximately 35%. Women with advanced-stage disease at diagnosis are in the highest-risk group. For locally recurrent or persistent disease, treatment options include pelvic exenteration, radiation therapy to previously nonradiated areas, and antineoplastic therapy.

Pelvic exenteration is considered for curative treatment of women with recurrent disease if no evidence of extrapelvic disease, tumor fixed to the pelvic wall, or ureteral obstruction from the tumor is present preoperatively. The procedure consists of removal of the uterus, cervix, vagina, rectum, bladder, urethra, and lateral supporting tissues and carries significant morbidity.[8,13] In women whose disease has not spread to the bladder or rectum, variations on the procedure may be performed: a posterior pelvic exenteration or anterior pelvic exenteration, respectively (Figure 10-5). Patients must be monitored carefully after the surgery for potential complications of the procedure, such as infection, bleeding,

wound dehiscence, and fistula formation.[8,13,18] In addition, the patient is faced with learning new self-care skills (ostomy care), evaluating components of self-image and body image, and learning new sexual expression behaviors and attitudes.

Radiation therapy is used to treat some women with recurrent disease. Women with a central recurrence who have not received prior radiation therapy to the area are candidates for this form of treatment.

Antineoplastic agents, as single agents or in combination, have been used to treat women with recurrent cervical cancer; however, responses to treatment have been modest, ranging from 10% to 40%. Researchers and clinicians postulate that the low response rates are caused by three primary factors:

1. Previous radiation therapy to the pelvis may result in fibrosis of the bone marrow and a decreased tolerance of the agents' hematologic effects.
2. Decreased vascularization of recurrent tumors may limit the agents' ability to reach the target tissues.
3. Fibrosis from previous radiation therapy can also damage and obstruct the ureters.

The combination of ureteral obstruction and nephrotoxicity of many antineoplastic agents may result in the kidneys being unable to clear the drug metabolites from the

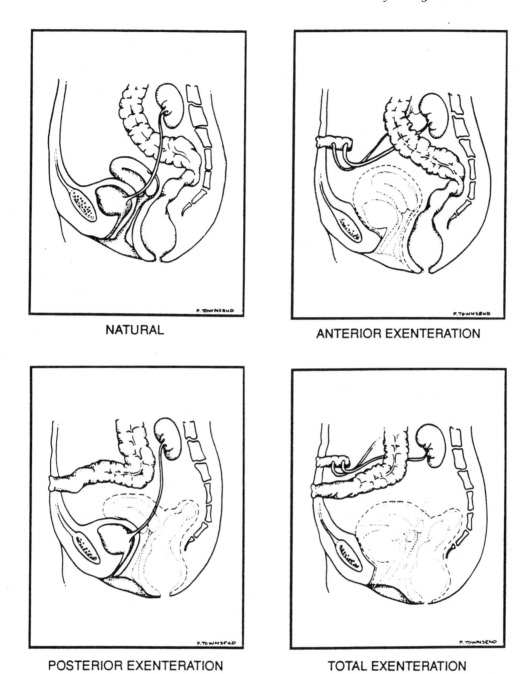

NATURAL

ANTERIOR EXENTERATION

POSTERIOR EXENTERATION

TOTAL EXENTERATION

Figure 10-5   Pelvic exenteration for treatment of cervical cancer. (From Martin LK, Braly PS: Gynecologic cancers. In Baird SB, McCorkle R, Grant M, editors: *Cancer nursing: a comprehensive textbook*, Philadelphia, 1991, Saunders.)

body. The goal of current treatment with antineoplastic agents for recurrent cervical cancer is palliation.[3,8,13,19]

TREATMENT DURING PREGNANCY

As the incidence of preinvasive and invasive cancer is increasing in younger women of childbearing age, the issue of treatment for the woman who is pregnant has be-

come more common. Careful discussion among the woman, partner, gynecologic oncologist, and obstetrician about potential risks of the disease, evaluation procedures, and treatment is recommended at each step of the evaluation and treatment process.[8,13]

Pregnant women with an abnormal Pap smear are evaluated with colposcopy and biopsies. If the squamocolumnar junction can be visualized entirely with colposcopy and if directed biopsies are sufficient to rule out the presence of invasive cancer, the clinician can follow the woman to term with interval Pap smears and colposcopy examinations. Appropriate treatment is deferred until after delivery. If, however, the limits of the colposcopically abnormal area are not visualized or if biopsies cannot rule out invasive cancer, a conization of the cervix is recommended. Profuse bleeding and spontaneous abortion of the fetus are potential complications of the procedure.[8,13]

Invasive cancer of the cervix occurs in 1 of 2205 pregnancies. Women with stage IA disease usually can be followed with Pap smears, colposcopy, and biopsies to term. In the presence of invasive cancer, immediate treatment is recommended. For women at less than 24 weeks' gestation, the pregnancy is terminated. Radical hysterectomy or radiation therapy can be used as primary treatment. Treatment of women between 24 and 28 weeks' gestation is more complicated. The risk of delaying treatment to allow for fetal development must be weighed carefully against the risk of progressive disease. After 28 weeks' gestation, the fetus is considered viable and is delivered by cesarean section to decrease the risk of maternal bleeding and spread of the disease. Radical hysterectomy is performed for definitive treatment after delivery.[13]

PROGNOSIS

Prognosis in cervical cancer is determined primarily by stage of disease. The 5-year survival rate for patients diagnosed with CIS approaches 100%; with local disease, 91%; regional disease, 50%; and distant metastasis, 9%. Overall survival trends have improved since the 1940s.[1]

ENDOMETRIAL CANCER

EPIDEMIOLOGY

Endometrial cancer is the most common gynecologic malignancy among women older than 50 years. Of the estimated 34,000 women diagnosed with endometrial cancer in 1996, approximately 70% were older than 50 years.[1,8,13] For reasons that are not clear, the incidence of the disease is increasing, particularly among women younger than 50 years.

ETIOLOGY AND RISK FACTORS

Although the etiology of endometrial cancer is unknown, abnormal balance of endogenous and exogenous *estrogen* is thought to play a role in development of the disease. With advancing age the amount of estrogen produced by the body decreases. However, researchers have suggested that as estrogen production is lowered, the

body increases the production of estrogen precursors. These estrogen precursors are known to have carcinogenic potential and may play a role in the development of *adenomatous hyperplasia,* a premalignant condition.[13,18,19]

Additional evidence of the association of estrogen to the development of endometrial cancer is found clinically in situations where the endometrium is exposed to unopposed estrogen stimulation. Women who have Stein-Leventhal syndrome or who have an intact uterus and are receiving hormone replacement therapy with estrogen alone, as opposed to estrogen and progesterone combination therapy, are at higher risk of developing endometrial cancer. Risk factors for cancer of the endometrium include advancing age, early onset of menstruation, late menopause, and concurrent conditions. Women who have a history of postmenopausal bleeding and have never been pregnant are at higher risk for cancer of the endometrium. Concurrent conditions, such as obesity, diabetes, hypertension, endometrial hyperplasia, use of tamoxifen, or previous history of breast, colon, or ovarian cancer, also increase the risk for endometrial cancer.[3,8,13,18,19]

PREVENTION, SCREENING, AND DETECTION
Prevention

As knowledge of the etiology of endometrial cancer evolves, the primary focus of prevention is targeted toward high-risk women. Maintenance of ideal body weight is recommended to avoid obesity and to decrease the risk of hypertension and diabetes. Treatment of premalignant changes of the endometrium such as endometrial hyperplasia with progesterone is suggested as a prevention strategy. To control the symptoms of menopause in women with an intact uterus, the addition of cyclic progesterone to the estrogen replacement regimen is recommended to reduce the risk of development of endometrial cancer.[8,13]

Screening

No reliable, valid, and cost-effective tests are recommended for periodic screening of asymptomatic women for endometrial cancer. However, the ACS recommends that asymptomatic, high-risk women have an endometrial tissue sampling done at menopause.[1]

Detection

The detection of endometrial cancer in symptomatic women is guided by a complete history, physical examination, and diagnostic evaluation. The history includes a review of risk factors and the presence of clinical signs and symptoms for endometrial cancer. The physical examination includes evaluation of the size, consistency, and shape of the uterus, which are determined by palpation on the rectovaginal, bimanual examination. The depth of the uterine cavity is determined by inserting a uterine sound. An endometrial biopsy is obtained for histologic confirmation of the disease.

CLASSIFICATION

Five primary types of endometrial cancer are seen: adenocarcinoma, mixed müllerian tumors, sarcomas, clear cell carcinoma, and epidermoid carcinoma.[13] More than 90% of endometrial cancers are *adenocarcinomas.* These exophytic or polypoid lesions tend to invade the uterine muscle. Variants of adenocarcinoma include *adenocanthoma* (contains benign squamous elements) and *adenosquamous carcinoma* (contains malignant squamous elements). The aggressive nature of these lesions results in a higher incidence of invasion of the myometrium and lymph nodes, distant metastases, and a lower survival rate compared with adenocarcinomas. Mixed müllerian tumors, sarcomas, clear cell carcinomas, and epidermoid carcinomas are rare and are associated with higher incidences of local and distant metastases and lower survival rates than adenocarcinomas.[3,8,13]

CLINICAL FEATURES

The most common presenting symptom in women with endometrial cancer is prolonged, excessive, or irregular *premenopausal or postmenopausal bleeding.* Additional symptoms may include a yellow, watery vaginal discharge, *pyometria* (accumulation of pus in the uterus), *hematometria* (accumulation of blood in the uterus), or pain in the hypogastric or lumbosacral areas or the pelvis. Women with advanced disease may present with intestinal obstruction, ascites, jaundice, respiratory distress, or hemorrhage.[8,10,13,18,19]

On physical examination, the uterus may be enlarged or have an irregular contour. In advanced stages, extension of tumor into the vagina, bladder, or bowel may be palpated on bimanual, rectovaginal examination. Enlarged inguinal lymph nodes also may be palpated. (See box, p. 199.)

DIAGNOSIS AND STAGING

The diagnostic evaluation includes physical examination, tissue sampling, and laboratory and radiographic studies to determine the histologic type, degree of differentiation, and extent of disease. Ideally the gynecologic oncologist and radiation oncologist collaborate on the physical examination and a thorough evaluation of potential sites of metastatic disease: cervix, vagina, tissues surrounding the urethral meatus, parametria, and regional lymph nodes. Cervical biopsies, endocervical curettage, endometrial biopsy, and/or a fractional dilation and cu-

rettage (D&C) are done to rule out the presence of a cervical malignancy and to obtain a tissue sample for diagnosis. Cervical biopsies and endocervical curettage are collected first to minimize the risk of contamination of the cervical specimen with endometrial tissue that may be dislodged by the uterine sound or dilator.[8,13] Although obtaining the necessary specimens can be uncomfortable for the patient, the diagnostic evaluation usually can be performed in the outpatient setting.

Laboratory studies routinely include a complete blood count (CBC), blood chemistry profile (SMA), and liver and renal chemistries. Additional radiographic studies to determine the presence of metastatic disease may include a chest x-ray film, magnetic resonance imaging (MRI), and computed tomography (CT). If involvement of the bladder or rectum is suspected, intravenous pyelography (IVP), barium enema, proctosigmoidoscopy, and cystoscopy may be done.

Endometrial cancer is staged surgically. Staging is based on the depth of myometrial invasion, degree of cellular differentiation, and the extent of metastatic disease. Table 10-2 presents the schema for staging cancer of the endometrium.

METASTASIS

Most endometrial cancers originate in the fundus of the uterus and spread by direct extension to the entire endometrium, through the layers of the uterine wall (myometrium and serosa), or through the endocervical canal to the cervix. The disease may also spread outside the uterus to the structures of the parametria and abdominal cavity, such as the ovaries, fallopian tubes, vagina, bladder, rectum, omentum, or bowel. Lymphatic metastases occur primarily to the pelvic and paraaortic lymph nodes. The endometrium is highly vascular; therefore hematogeneous spread, particularly with sarcomas, is common. Lung, liver, bone, and brain metastases may occur.[3,8,13,18,19]

TREATMENT MODALITIES

Development of a plan for treatment of endometrial cancer is a collaborative effort between the gynecologic oncologist and radiation oncologist. Factors that influence the treatment plan selected include the type of tumor, degree of differentiation, stage of disease, and the woman's general health status.

Surgery

Since abnormal bleeding brings most women to the health care system with early-stage disease, localized treatment is typically chosen. Surgery, usually a *total abdominal hysterectomy* and *bilateral salpingo-oophorectomy* (TAH-BSO), is the most common primary

Table 10-2   Corpus Uteri (Endometrium)

Data Form for Cancer Staging		
Patient identification	Institution identification	Grade (G) _____
Name _____	Hospital or clinic _____	Date of classification _____
Address _____	Address _____	Chronology of classification
Hospital or clinic number _____	**Oncology Record**	[ ] Clinical (use all data prior to first treatment)
Age ____ Sex ____ Race _____	Anatomic site of cancer _____	[ ] Pathologic (if definitively resected specimen
	Histologic type _____	available)

Clin	Path	TNM category	FICO* stage	DEFINITIONS
				Primary Tumor (T)
[ ]	[ ]	TX		Primary tumor cannot be assessed
[ ]	[ ]	T0		No evidence of primary tumor
[ ]	[ ]	Tis		Carcinoma in situ
[ ]	[ ]	T1	I	Tumor confined to corpus uteri
[ ]	[ ]	T1a	IA	Tumor limited to endometrium
[ ]	[ ]	T1b	IB	Tumor invades up to or less than one half of the myometrium
[ ]	[ ]	T1c	IC	Tumor invades more than one half of the myometrium
[ ]	[ ]	T2	II	Tumor invades cervic but does not extend beyond uterus
[ ]	[ ]	T2a	IIA	Endocervical glandular involvement only
[ ]	[ ]	T2b	IIB	Cervical stromal invasion
[ ]	[ ]	T3 &/or N1	III	Local and/or regional spread as specified in T3a, b, N1 and FIGO IIIA, B, and C below
[ ]	[ ]	T3a	IIIA	Tumor involves serosa and/or adnexae (direct extension or metastasis) and/or cancer cells in ascites or peritoneal washings
[ ]	[ ]	T3b	IIIB	Vaginal involvement (direct extension or metastasis)
[ ]	[ ]	N1	IIIC	Metastasis to the pelvic and /or paraaortic lymph nodes
[ ]	[ ]	T4†	IVA	Tumor invades bladder mucosa and/or bowel mucosa
[ ]	[ ]	M1	IVB	Distant metastasis. (*Excluding* metastasis to vagina, pelvic serosa or adnexae. *Including* metastasis to intraabdominal lymph nodes other than paraaortic, and/or inguinal lymph nodes.)
				Lymph Node (N)
[ ]	[ ]	NX		Regional lymph nodes cannot be assessed
[ ]	[ ]	N0		No regional lymph node metastasis
[ ]	[ ]	N1		Regional lymph node metastasis
				Distant Metastasis (M)
[ ]	[ ]	MX		Presence of distant metastasis cannot be assessed
[ ]	[ ]	M0		No distant metastasis
[ ]	[ ]	M1	IVB	Distant metastasis

Clin	Path	Stage AJCC/UICC				FIGO
[ ]	[ ]	0	Tis	N0	M0	
[ ]	[ ]	IA	T1a	N0	M0	Stage IA
		IB	T1b	N0	M0	Stage IB
		IC	T1c	N0	M0	Stage IC
[ ]	[ ]	IIA	T2a	N0	M0	Stage IIA
		IIB	T2b	N0	M0	Stage IIB
[ ]	[ ]	IIIA	T3a	N0	M0	Stage IIIA
[ ]	[ ]	IIIB	T3b	N0	M0	Stage IIIB
[ ]	[ ]	IIIC	T1	N1	M0	Stage IIIC
			T2	N1	M0	
			T3a	N1	M0	
			T3b	N1	M0	
[ ]	[ ]	IVA	T4	any N	M0	Stage IVA
[ ]	[ ]	IVB	any T	any N	M1	Stage IVB

Staged by _____ M.D.

_____ Registrar

Date _____

Data from American Joint Committee on Cancer: *Manual for staging cancer,* ed 4, Philadelphia, 1992, Lippincott.
*FIGO: Federation Internationale de Gynecologie et d'Obstetrique
†Note: The presence of bullous edema is not sufficient evidence to classify a tumor T4.

treatment for women with early-stage disease. More extensive surgery, radical abdominal hysterectomy and bilateral pelvic lymphadenectomy, has been used for treatment, but surgical risks are higher and no significant improvement in survival rates has been reported.[3,8,13]

Radiation Therapy

Radiation therapy is used as primary treatment for women with other health problems that increase the risks of surgical complications. However, survival rates for women treated with radiation therapy alone, even with early-stage disease, are not as high as those observed when surgery alone is used as the primary treatment. In women with bulky disease, poorly differentiated tumors, or greater depth of myometrial invasion, the addition of preoperative or postoperative radiation therapy may be recommended. Radiation may consist of brachytherapy, teletherapy, or a combination of both. Advantages of preoperative and postoperative radiation therapy are detailed in the literature.[3,8,13]

Hormonal Therapy

Endometrial cancer is a hormone-dependent tumor. Increased levels of progesterone and estrogen receptors

have been identified in more well-differentiated tumors. Therefore clinicians are using estrogen and progesterone receptor analyses as one factor to determine those women who may benefit from hormone manipulation either as an adjuvant therapy or as treatment for recurrent disease. Depo-Provera, Provera, Delalutin, and Megace are the most common progestational agents currently used for women who are estrogen and progesterone receptor positive. Response rates with hormonal manipulation range from 30% to 70%, with the highest response rate occurring in women with well-differentiated tumors.[3,8,13]

Chemotherapy

Antineoplastic agents are reserved for women who have estrogen/progesterone-negative tumors, who have failed hormone therapy, or who have disseminated disease. However, antineoplastic agents, used either as single agents or in combination, have resulted in no significant improvement in survival rates from endometrial cancer. Agents typically used include doxorubicin, 5-fluorouracil (5-FU), vincristine, cisplatin, and cyclophosphamide. Evaluation of the effectiveness of combined hormonal and antineoplastic agents in women with endometrial cancer is ongoing.

PROGNOSIS

Relative 5-year survival rates associated with a diagnosis of endometrial cancer have improved significantly between 1960-1962 and 1990-1992.[1] The 5-year survival rate for women diagnosed with early-stage endometrial cancer is 83%; if diagnosed at a regional stage, 65%; and with distant metastasis, 26%.[1]

OVARIAN CANCER

EPIDEMIOLOGY

The 26,700 new cases of ovarian cancer account for only 25% of all gynecologic cancers diagnosed in the United States in 1996.[1] However, the disease is the leading cause of death (14,800 deaths in 1996) in women diagnosed with gynecologic cancers.[1] The highest incidence of ovarian cancer is reported in highly industrialized countries. The disease occurs less frequently in women from Asia and Latin America.[3,8,25]

The ACS estimates that 1 of every 70 women will develop ovarian cancer during her lifetime.[1] This statistic is particularly alarming, since early disease is asymptomatic and no cost-effective, reliable, and valid screening tests are available.

ETIOLOGY AND RISK FACTORS

The etiology of ovarian cancer is unknown. However, age, genetics, history of other cancers, and menstrual history have been associated with an increased incidence of the disease. Most ovarian cancers are diagnosed in the 50- to 59-year-old age-group. Families with a history of ovarian cancer across multiple generations have been identified but are uncommon. A familial or personal history of other cancers, including breast, colon, and uterine, increases the risk of ovarian cancer. The incidence of ovarian cancer is greater among women who are single, nulliparous, and infertile; the incidence is lower among women who use oral contraceptives. Researchers are currently evaluating the role of uninterrupted ovulation in the pathogenesis of ovarian cancer.[3,8,25]

PREVENTION, SCREENING, AND DETECTION
Prevention and Screening

Because the etiology of ovarian cancer remains a mystery, no recommendations exist for prevention of the disease. Women in higher-risk categories, as described previously, are encouraged to seek routine gynecologic care, including an annual pelvic examination. Palpation of a normal-size ovary in postmenopausal women is cause for a further diagnostic evaluation. However, the overall yield of 1 case of ovarian cancer in 10,000 pelvic examinations is low. Furthermore, the occurrence of widely disseminated metastatic disease in women with palpable disease is high, and survival rates in this group are low.[3,8,19,25]

Recently the cost-effectiveness of the use of tumor markers and vaginal ultrasound to screen high-risk women for ovarian cancer has been studied. Researchers have noted variable specificity and sensitivity outcomes with tumor markers, such as alpha(α-)-fetoprotein (AFP) for rare endodermal sinus tumors, carcinoembryonic antigen (CEA), and CA-125 for epithelial ovarian tumors. Because of the variability in results, none of the tests is recommended for screening asymptomatic populations. However, serial CA-125 levels have been used to monitor selected high-risk women with a strong familial history of ovarian cancer. A third method of screening women at high risk for ovarian cancer has been serial vaginal ultrasounds. No long-term, large, prospective studies have been done to date that demonstrate cost-effectiveness of this procedure in detecting ovarian carcinoma in asymptomatic women.[3,8,18,25]

In summary, ovarian cancer is "silent" in the early stages. No effective methods of screening have been identified. Therefore most women continue to be diagnosed with ovarian cancer after the disease has spread throughout the abdominal cavity, lymphatic channels, and vascular system.

Detection

Most women with early-stage ovarian cancer are asymptomatic. Therefore the clinician must maintain an index of suspicion for ovarian cancer. A careful personal and family history is important to identify women at high risk for the disease. Attention to generalized, vague complaints among women during their middle-age years often will alert the clinician to the possibility of ovarian cancer. Finally, a pelvic examination and palpation of an adnexal mass or a postmenopausal ovary raise suspicion for ovarian cancer.

CLASSIFICATION

Ovarian carcinomas are classified as epithelial, sex cord–stromal, or lipid cell tumors. *Epithelial tumors,* most frequently found in women 40 to 65 years of age, account for 85% of all ovarian malignancies diagnosed in the United States. *Sex cord–stromal tumors* occur much less frequently than the epithelial tumors. These tumors often are associated with femininizing or masculinizing effects. Women with sex cord–stromal tumors have a better prognosis than women with epithelial malignancies. *Lipid cell tumors* account for less than 5% of all ovarian malignancies. These tumors, particularly dysgerminoma, endodermal sinus tumors, and embryonal carcinoma, occur most frequently in younger women.[25] Since most ovarian malignancies are epithelial tumors, the remainder of this section focuses on this specific ovarian neoplasm.

CLINICAL FEATURES

Vague gastrointestinal symptoms such as dyspepsia, indigestion, anorexia, and early satiety may be some of the first symptoms of ovarian cancer. Pressure of the tumor on the rectum and bladder may result in symptoms of urinary frequency, constipation, or pelvic pressure and discomfort. Progressive disease is marked by an increase in abdominal girth, pain, shortness of breath, intestinal or ureteral obstruction, and muscle wasting.* (See box, p. 199.)

---

*References 1, 3, 8, 11, 18, 19, 24, 25.

DIAGNOSIS AND STAGING

Diagnosis and staging (Table 10-3) of women with ovarian cancer are achieved by tissue sampling and inspection of the abdominal cavity at the time of exploratory laparotomy. The initial approach and exploration of the abdomen are well defined and methodic to allow careful evaluation of the extent of disease and to remove (debulk) as much of the tumor burden as possible. Before surgical exploration, however, a series of laboratory and radiographic tests is recommended. A CBC, biochemical profile, and CA-125 level are obtained. In addition, a chest x-ray film, cystoscopy, proctoscopy,

Table 10-3   Staging Classification for Ovarian Cancer

Primary tumor (T)		
TNM	**FIGO**	**Definition**
TX		Primary tumor cannot be assessed
T0		No evidence of primary tumor
T1	I	Tumor limited to ovaries
T1a	Ia	Tumor limited to one ovary; capsule intact, no tumor on ovarian surface
T1b	Ib	Tumor limited to both ovaries; capsules intact, no tumor on ovarian surface
T1c	Ic	Tumor limited to one or both ovaries with any of the following: capsule ruptured, tumor on ovarian surface, malignant cells in ascites, peritoneal washing
T2	II	Tumor involves one or both ovaries with pelvic extension
T2a	IIa	Extension and/or implants on uterus and/or tube(s)
T2b	IIb	Extension to other pelvic tissues
T2c	IIc	Pelvic extension (2a or 2b) with malignant cells in ascites or peritoneal washing
T3 and/or N1	III	Tumor involves one or both ovaries with microscopically confirmed peritoneal metastasis outside pelvis and/or regional lymph node metastasis
T3a	IIIa	Microscopic peritoneal metastasis beyond pelvis
T3b	IIIb	Macroscopic peritoneal metastasis beyond pelvis 2 cm or less in greatest dimension
T3c and/or N1	IIIc	Peritoneal metastasis beyond pelvis more than 2 cm in greatest dimension and/or regional lymph node metastasis
M1	IV	Distant metastasis (excludes peritoneal metastasis)

Regional lymph nodes (N)

Regional lymph nodes include hypogastric (obturator), common iliac, external iliac, internal iliac, lateral sacral, paraaortic, and inguinal

TMN	Definition
NX	Regional lymph nodes cannot be assessed
N0	No regional lymph node metastasis
N1	Regional lymph node metastasis

Distant metastasis (M)

TMN	FIGO	Definition
MX		Presence of distant metastasis cannot be assessed
M0		No distant metastasis
M1	IV	Distant metastasis (excludes peritoneal metastasis)

Stage grouping

Stage IA:	T1a-N0-M0
Stage IB:	T1b-N0-M0
Stage IC:	T1c-N0-M0
Stage IIA:	T2a-N0-M0
Stage IIB:	T2b-N0-M0
Stage IIC:	T2c-N0-M0
Stage IIIA:	T3a-N0-M0
Stage IIIB:	T3b-N0-M0
Stage IIIC:	T3c-N0-M0
	any T-N1-M0
Stage IV:	any T-any N-M1

Data from American Joint Committee on Cancer: *Manual for staging cancer,* ed 4, Philadelphia, 1992, Lippincott.

IVP, barium enema, CT, MRI, or ultrasound may be ordered.[3,8,13,25]

METASTASIS

Ovarian carcinoma spreads by direct extension to adjacent pelvic organs such as the opposite ovary, uterus, fallopian tubes, bladder, rectum, and peritoneum, seeding of the peritoneal cavity, and lymphatic and vascular channels (Figure 10-6). Spread occurs primarily by shedding of malignant cells that float within and form micrometastases throughout the peritoneal cavity. Common sites of metastatic disease include the omentum and surfaces of the bowel, uterus, bladder, and peritoneum. Free-floating malignant cells are washed beneath the diaphragm and removed through lymphatic channels located in the diaphragm. This pattern of flow of peritoneal fluid accounts for the high incidence of metastatic ovarian disease found on the undersurfaces of the diaphragm.[25]

Lymphatic invasion can occur in the pelvic, paraaortic, and aortic nodes even in early-stage disease. Partial or complete obstruction of lymphatic channels in the diaphragm result in the accumulation of malignant ascitic fluid.

Although rare, metastasis can occur through vascular invasion to distant sites. The most common sites of hematogenous spread include the liver, lung, and pleura.[3,8,11,19,25]

TREATMENT MODALITIES

Treatment of ovarian cancer is based on surgical staging of the disease, malignant potential of the tumor, and the bulk of remaining disease. Surgery, radiation therapy, and chemotherapy may be used as single or combined modalities.

Surgery

Surgery plays a role in the diagnosis, primary treatment, evaluation of response to therapy, and palliative care for women with ovarian cancer (see box, p. 210). In addition to the exploratory laparotomy required for staging, surgery is used as primary treatment for women with borderline and malignant tumors of the ovary. For younger women with tumors of borderline malignant potential, conservative treatment with unilateral oophorectomy may be considered definitive treatment. However, in women beyond childbearing years, every attempt is made to remove the uterus, cervix, fallopian tubes, and ovaries if the disease is considered surgically resectable. Beyond a TAH-BSO, surgical resection of the bulk of remaining tumor is attempted. Resection of the bladder, colon, or omentum may be indicated. The extent of the debulking procedure is based on evaluation of potential risks of more extensive resection and potential benefits in terms of survival and quality of life.[3,8,25]

The use of surgical exploration (second-look procedure) to evaluate the response to primary therapy for

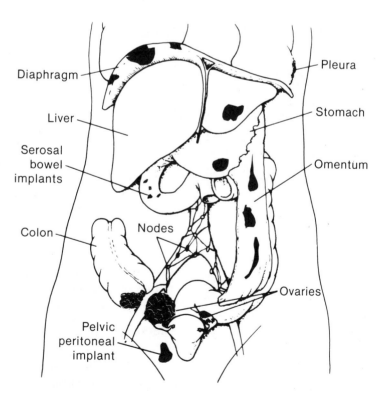

Figure 10-6 Patterns of metastasis for ovarian cancer. (From DiSaia PJ: *Hosp Pract* 22(4):235, 1987.)

STEPS IN SURGICALLY STAGING OVARIAN CANCER

Step 1. If ascites is present, remove as much as possible for cytology. If no ascites is present, obtain cell washings from the pelvis, both abdominal gutters, and both subdiaphragmatic areas.

Step 2. Determine whether the mass is malignant; if malignant, perform appropriate pelvic procedure (total abdominal hysterectomy and bilateral salpingo-oophorectomy unless patient desires further childbearing and there is no evidence of spread beyond the ovary).

Step 3. Carefully examine pelvic peritoneum; if lesions are present, remove as much as possible and biopsy any lesion that cannot be removed. If no lesions are seen, sample at a minimum the peritoneum of lateral pelvic side walls, bladder, rectosigmoid, and cul-de-sac.

Step 4. Examine the paracolic gutters, and remove any lesions seen. If no lesions are seen, obtain a 1 × 3 cm strip of peritoneum on either side.

Step 5. Examine the omentum, and remove any that contains visible tumor (including the supracolic omentum if involved by tumor). If no lesions are seen, remove the infracolic omentum.

Step 6. Examine and palpate both diaphragms and surface of the spleen and liver. If lesions are present, remove as much as possible; biopsy if they cannot be removed. If no lesions are seen, a 1 × 2 cm strip of peritoneum should be carefully excised from the right hemidiaphragm. (NOTE: Only peritoneum is needed, and care should be taken not to create a pneumothorax.)

Step 7. Beginning at either the rectum or cecum, carefully inspect the entire large colon and remove and/or biopsy any suspicious lesion of the intestine or mesentery.*

Step 8. Beginning at either the ileocecal valve or ligament of Treitz, carefully inspect the entire small bowel and mesentery and remove and/or biopsy any lesions.*

Step 9. If, after all the above procedures, no gross disease larger than 1 or 2 cm is left, the pelvic and paraaortic lymph nodes should be sampled.

From Hoskins WJ, Perez CA, Young RC: Cancer of the ovary. In DeVita VT Jr, Hellman S, Rosenberg SA, editors: *Cancer: principles and practice of oncology,* ed 4, Philadelphia, 1993, Lippincott.

*If resection of intestine is necessary to cytoreduce the tumor optimally or to relieve obstruction, this should be performed.

ovarian cancer is controversial. Advocates of second-look procedures indicate that the procedure allows for direct inspection of the abdominal cavity, sampling of ascitic fluid, and sampling of abdominal tissues at risk for persistent microscopic disease. If persistent disease is found, the surgeon is able to debulk the tumor burden before retreatment. If no disease is documented, therapy is usually discontinued and the woman enters a clinical follow-up scheme. Opponents of the second-look procedure argue that the procedure requires hospitalization, a major abdominal surgery, and disruption of the patient's normal activities. In addition, the ultimate benefit of the procedure is questioned given the high incidence of recurrent disease (15% to 20%) among women who have had negative findings at second-look procedure.[3,8,19,25]

Surgery has also been used in providing palliative care to women with advanced ovarian cancer. Bowel resection and bowel or urinary diversion may be done to relieve obstructive symptoms in selected patients. The relative risks and benefits of such procedures are weighed carefully before surgical intervention.

Radiation Therapy

Teletherapy to the pelvis and abdomen and the instillation of radioactive isotopes in the peritoneal cavity have been used in the treatment of women with early stages (I and II) of ovarian cancer. Although adequate doses of radiation can be delivered to the pelvis and abdomen to eradicate the disease, the tolerance of normal tissues within the treatment field to the tumoricidal doses is limited. To overcome this barrier, shielding techniques for vital organs such as the kidneys and liver, multifield techniques, and various fractionation techniques have been used to limit damage to normal tissues and organs.

The response to radiation therapy is determined by the extent of residual disease and the differentiation of the tumor. Women with well-differentiated tumors that are less than 2 cm in size have the best response rates.[8,19,25]

Radioactive isotopes (e.g., ^{32}P) have been used to treat residual disease in the peritoneal cavity. Women who have limited residual disease, less than 2 cm, are the most likely candidates for ^{32}P therapy. Disadvantages of the treatment include potential inability of the entire peritoneal cavity to be exposed to the isotope because of adhesions or loculation and the occurrence of small bowel obstruction or stenosis.[3,8,25]

Chemotherapy

For women with high-risk, early-stage, epithelial ovarian tumors and for women with disseminated disease, antineoplastic therapy has resulted in improved length of survival. Historically, alkylating agents have been used most often as either single agents or in combination regimens for treatment of women with ovarian cancer. Systemic melphalan, 5-FU, thiotepa, and cyclophosphamide have shown tumoricidal activity. Altretamine, cisplatin, carboplatin, doxorubicin, ifosfamide, etoposide, docetaxel, and paclitaxel also have been used, with response rates ranging from 27% to 78%.[8,19,25] In general, systemic combination therapy with cisplatin and cyclophosphamide has resulted in improved response rates, increased disease-free survival, and increased survival when compared with other multiagent regimens with significantly more severe toxicities.[25] The use of dose-intensive, combination chemotherapy with autologus bone marrow rescue is being evaluated for efficacy in the patient with ovarian cancer.

Because metastasis in ovarian cancer occurs primarily through exfoliation of malignant cells within the peritoneal cavity, researchers have explored the use of antineoplastic agents intraperitoneally to treat the disease. For individuals with no residual disease but who are at high risk for recurrence, intraperitoneal chemotherapy has been used as adjuvant therapy. In women with minimal residual disease, the intraperitoneal route of administration has been used to provide high concentrations of antineoplastic drug(s) to disease within the peritoneal cavity while limiting the concentrations of the agent(s) in the circulation and thus limiting systemic toxic effects. However, controversy still exists about the use and benefits of intraperitoneal chemotherapy in the treatment of ovarian cancer.[3,19,25]

PROGNOSIS

Although the relative 5-year survival rates improved significantly from the mid-1970s to the mid-1990s, the rates remain dismally low (44%). Prognosis improves (91%) when the disease is diagnosed at an early stage and treated aggressively. Since early ovarian cancer is typically asymptomatic, only 23% of patients are diagnosed with localized disease. Patients with distant metastasis at the time of diagnosis have a 23% 5-year survival rate.[1]

VULVAR CANCER

EPIDEMIOLOGY

Vulvar carcinoma accounts for approximately 5% of all gynecologic malignancies. Although the incidence of invasive vulvar cancer is small, the incidence rates of *vulvar intraepithelial neoplasia* (VIN) and CIS are increasing. VIN occurs most often in women in their 40s, CIS in women in their 50s, and invasive disease in women in their 60s. No ethnic or geographic variations have

GERIATRIC CONSIDERATIONS
Gynecologic Cancers

Vulvar and vaginal cancer disease onset occurs in the late fifth decade to the sixth decade of life.

Patients should be taught the need for annual health examinations, including bimanual pelvic examination with a thorough inspection and palpation of the perineal and vaginal areas.

Other chronic diseases (e.g., hypertension, diabetes, arthritis) may exacerbate with the onset or progression of the disease and the side effects of the multiple therapies.

Age-related modifications may require a reduction in drug regimens and other therapies.

Elderly women may live alone and have limited financial, social, and health care resources. Nurses should assess needs and intervention strategies and consult with multiple referral systems (e.g., American Cancer Society, social services, Meals on Wheels, home health care agencies).

been noted in the incidence rates. The most frequent sites for vulvar carcinoma include the labia majora, labia minora, and clitoris.*

ETIOLOGY AND RISK FACTORS

The etiology of vulvar carcinoma is unknown. However, several factors have been associated with an increased incidence of the disease. These include concurrent diseases such as hypertension, diabetes, cardiovascular disease, obesity, cervical cancer, early menopause, and chronic vulvar irritation.[3,13,16,18,24]

PREVENTION, SCREENING, AND DETECTION
Prevention and Screening

No specific measures are recommended for the prevention of vulvar cancer. In recent years, emphasis has been placed on teaching women vulvar self-examination as a strategy for screening in asymptomatic women.[13]

Detection

Many women with vulvar cancer are asymptomatic. Therefore a thorough history and physical examination are required to identify women with existing risk factors and to inspect and palpate vulvar tissue for abnormalities. Physical examination of the vulva, groins, and pelvis is mandatory.[8,13] (See box above.)

---

*References 3, 8, 13, 18, 19, 24.

CLASSIFICATION

Invasive cancers of the vulva are classified as squamous cell, basal cell, adenocarcinoma, and malignant melanoma. Ninety percent of all malignancies of the vulva are squamous cell carcinomas.[13]

CLINICAL FEATURES

Symptomatic women with vulvar cancer most often have a vulvar lump or mass, pain, or pruritus of several months' duration. Vulvar tissues may be reddened, white, warty, or abnormally pigmented. Vulvar bleeding, discharge, and dysuria may be present. (See box, p. 199.)

DIAGNOSIS AND STAGING

Diagnosis of vulvar cancer is made by biopsy of abnormal areas noted on inspection, palpation, or colposcopic examination. Once a diagnosis of invasive disease is made, the woman undergoes a metastatic work-up that may consist of cystoscopy, proctoscopy, barium enema, IVP, lymphangiography, CT, and MRI.[3,8,13]

Staging for vulvar carcinoma is done clinically. Table 10-4 presents the classification system for staging.

METASTASIS

Carcinomas of the vulva follow a predictable, slow pattern of spread by direct extension to local tissues and by lymphatic spread to inguinal and pelvic lymph nodes. With the exception of melanomas of the vulva, hematogenous spread rarely occurs. Approximately one third of women with disease confined to the vulva will have nodal metastasis.[8,13,19]

Table 10-4 Vulva

Data Form for Cancer Staging	Institution identification	Grade (G) _____
Patient identification	Hospital or clinic _____	Date of classification _____
Name _____	Address _____	Chronology of classification
Address _____	**Oncology Record**	[ ] Clinical (use all data prior to first treatment)
Hospital or clinic number _____	Anatomic site of cancer _____	[ ] Pathologic (if definitively resected specimen
Age _____ Sex _____ Race _____	Histologic type _____	available)

Clin	Path			DEFINITIONS
				Primary Tumor (T)
[ ]	[ ]		TX	Primary tumor cannot be assessed
[ ]	[ ]		T0	No evidence of primary tumor
[ ]	[ ]		Tis	Preinvasive carcinoma (carcinoma *in situ*)
[ ]	[ ]		T1	Tumor confined to the vulva or to the vulva and perineum, 2 cm or less in greatest dimension
[ ]	[ ]		T2	Tumor confined to the vulva or to the vulva and perineum, more than 2 cm in greatest dimension
[ ]	[ ]		T3	Tumor involves any of the following: lower urethra, vagina, or anus
[ ]	[ ]		T4	Tumor involves any of the following: bladder mucosa, upper part of urethral mucosa, rectal mucosa or tumor fixed to the bone
				Lymph Node (N)
				Regional lymph nodes are the femoral and inguinal nodes
[ ]	[ ]		NX	Regional lymph nodes cannot be assessed
[ ]	[ ]		N0	No regional lymph node metastasis
[ ]	[ ]		N1	Unilateral regional lymph node metastasis
[ ]	[ ]		N2	Bilateral regional lymph node metastasis
				Distant Metastasis (M)
[ ]	[ ]		MX	Presence of distant metastasis cannot be assessed
[ ]	[ ]		M0	No distant metastasis
[ ]	[ ]		M1	Distant metastasis (Pelvic lymph node metastasis is M1)

Clin	Path	Stage Grouping AJCC/IUCC				
[ ]	[ ]	0	Tis	N0	M0	
[ ]	[ ]	I	T1	N0	M0	I
[ ]	[ ]	II	T2	N0	M0	II
[ ]	[ ]	III	T1	N1	M0	III
			T2	N1	M0	
			T3	N0	M0	
			T3	N1	M0	
[ ]	[ ]	IVA	T1	N2	M0	IVA
			T2	N2	M0	
			T3	N2	M0	
			T4	any N	M0	
[ ]	[ ]	IVB	any T	any N	M1	IVB

Staged by _____ M.D.

_____ Registrar

Date _____

Data from American Joint Committee on Cancer: *Manual for staging cancer,* ed 4, Philadelphia, 1992, Lippincott.

TREATMENT MODALITIES

Treatment of women with vulvar cancer is based on the size and extent of the lesion as well as depth of invasion. The clinician also considers functional and cosmetic results when planning treatment. For women with preinvasive disease, VIN, or CIS, in a limited area, a conservative approach with topical 5-FU, cryotherapy, laser therapy, wide local excision, skinning vulvectomy, or simple vulvectomy can be used for primary treatment. With each treatment the chance for control of disease with minimal disruption of function or cosmesis in carefully selected women is good. Women undergoing conservative treatment must be followed at 3- to 6-month intervals.

In women with invasive disease less than 2 cm in diameter, less than 5 mm of invasion, and negative inguinal lymph nodes on frozen section, wide local excision alone may be done. If the inguinal lymph nodes are positive, a radical vulvectomy with complete, bilateral groin dissection is done.[8,25] For women who are not candidates for surgical intervention, radiation therapy for early-stage disease has been used successfully.

Historically, clinicians have used a surgical approach to the treatment of vulvar carcinoma, although the risks of wound breakdown, lymphedema, and sexual dysfunction were high. Radiation therapy was not used because of the high incidence of short-term side effects (moist desquamation, maceration) on the skin over the vulvar, perineal, and groin areas. Given the advanced age of women usually diagnosed with the disease, concurrent health problems that increase surgical risks, and improved techniques of delivering high doses of radiation therapy while sparing the skin, clinicians again are evaluating the role of radiation therapy in the treatment of women with vulvar cancer.

The treatment plan for women with locally advanced disease can consist of a combination of surgery, radical surgery (vulvectomy, anterior exenteration, posterior exenteration), and preoperative or postoperative radiation therapy. For women with distant metastasis, a combination of radiation therapy to control central disease and chemotherapy for systemic disease is typically used as palliative treatment.

Chemotherapy has been used to treat limited numbers of women with vulvar cancer. Other than the use of topical agents to treat preinvasive disease, results have been disappointing. Clinical trials are currently in progress to evaluate the effectiveness of mitomycin-C, 5-FU, and cisplatin in combination with radiation therapy in the treatment of women with advanced disease.[3,13,19,24]

PROGNOSIS

Survival of patients with vulvar cancer is associated with the stage of disease at diagnosis and more specifically the status of pelvic lymph nodes. Survival for patients with stages I and II ranges from 90% to 98%. If nodes are negative, regardless of stage, survival rates range from 69% to 100%. A marked decrease in survival (21% to 53%) is noted for patients with positive nodes.[8]

VAGINAL CANCER

EPIDEMIOLOGY

Carcinoma of the vagina accounts for approximately 2% of all gynecologic cancers. The disease, preinvasive and invasive, occurs primarily in the fifth and sixth decades of life, respectively. Incidence rates have been declining with the use of screening cytology for cervical disease and development of more rigid diagnostic criteria for vagina carcinoma.[3,8,13] However, 300 deaths related to vaginal cancer were estimated for 1996.[1]

ETIOLOGY AND RISK FACTORS

The etiology of vaginal cancer is unknown. However, prior radiation to a field including the vagina; DES exposure in utero; and increasing age place a woman at higher risk for the disease.[8,13,19]

PREVENTION, SCREENING, AND DETECTION
Prevention and Screening

No recommendations for the prevention and screening of women for vaginal cancers exist. However, a thorough physical examination including inspection and palpation of the vaginal tissues, cervical cytology, and bimanual examination should be done routinely as part of a gynecologic examination for women who are sexually active or 18 years of age or older.

Detection

Many women with vaginal carcinoma are asymptomatic. Detection of preinvasive and invasive lesions is accomplished by thorough inspection of the vaginal tissues, colposcopic examination, and palpation of the tissues along the length of the vaginal wall. Preinvasive lesions of the vagina may only be visualized by colposcopic examination that reveals areas of whitened tissues or atypical vascular patterns. Lesions occur most often on the posterior wall and the upper third of the vagina.[3,8,13,19,24]

CLASSIFICATION

Most carcinomas of the vagina are squamous cell cancers (93% to 97%). Other cell types include clear cell carcinomas associated with exposure to DES in utero, malignant melanomas, and sarcomas.[13]

CLINICAL FEATURES

Symptomatic women with vaginal cancer have one or more of the following symptoms: abnormal perimenopausal, postmenopausal, or postcoital vaginal bleeding; dyspareunia; and foul-smelling vaginal discharge. With advanced disease, changes in patterns of urination and pelvic pain may occur. (See box, p. 199.)

DIAGNOSIS AND STAGING

Diagnosis of preinvasive and invasive carcinoma of the vagina is made by biopsy. Usually the biopsy can be obtained in the outpatient setting.

Staging is done clinically based on inspection of the vagina and palpation of pelvic structures on rectovaginal, bimanual examination. The clinician pays special attention to the location and size of the primary lesion. Metastatic disease is assessed by review of findings from laboratory and radiographic studies, including biochemical profile, chest x-ray film, IVP, barium enema, cystoscopy, and proctoscopy. MRI, CT, and lymphangiography may be used to rule out metastatic disease.[3,8,13] Table 10-5 presents staging system for carcinoma of the vagina.

METASTASIS

Squamous cell carcinoma of the vagina spreads primarily by direct extension to adjacent tissues, including the urethra, bladder, rectum, parametria, and pelvic side wall. In addition, spread can occur through extensive lymphatic channels surrounding the vagina and can extend to the rectal, pelvic, paraaortic, and femoral lymph nodes.

Other types of vaginal cancer have a greater tendency to spread through the lymphatic and hematogenous routes. Frequent sites of metastasis include the supraclavicular nodes and lungs.[3,8,13]

TREATMENT MODALITIES

Treatment of vaginal neoplasia is based on the stage of disease and general health status of the woman. For women with premalignant lesions of the vagina, local excision, carbon dioxide laser, or topical chemotherapy (5-FU) may be used for primary treatment. Partial or total vaginectomy may be done for treatment of women with multifocal disease involving more than a single portion or the full length of the vagina. Radiation therapy for treatment of preinvasive vaginal neoplasia is reserved for women who are poor surgical candidates.[3,8,13]

Surgery

Surgery is recommended as treatment for women with early-stage disease (stage I). Based on the location, size, and extent of the lesion, a total hysterectomy, radical hysterectomy, partial vaginectomy and pelvic lymphadenectomy, or in very selected cases anterior or posterior exenteration (see Figure 10-5) may be recommended. Surgery may also be recommended for women who have locally recurrent disease after primary treatment with radiation therapy.

Radiation Therapy

Because of the proximity of the bladder and rectum as well as the potential for local and regional lymph node metastasis, radiation therapy alone or in combination with surgery is recommended as treatment for women with stage II and higher carcinoma of the vagina. Teletherapy with or without brachytherapy may be used.[8,13]

Chemotherapy

The results of chemotherapy in treating women with advanced or recurrent vaginal carcinomas, including clear cell and melanoma, have been disappointing. Cisplatin, 5-FU, vincristine, cyclophosphamide, and doxorubicin have been used as single agents and in combined protocols with minimal response rates. More promising results have occurred with chemotherapy used to treat women with vaginal sarcomas and endodermal sinus tract tumors.[8]

PROGNOSIS

A marked improvement in the survival rates in patients with vaginal cancer has occurred in the past three decades. Survival at 5 years after diagnosis for all stages ranges from 42% to 56%. The most promising results occur in women who have been diagnosed with stage I (65% to 100%) and stage II (42% to 75%) disease.[8]

FALLOPIAN TUBE CANCER

EPIDEMIOLOGY

Cancer of the fallopian tubes accounts for only 0.1% of all cancers of the female reproductive system. The disease occurs in women 19 to 80 years of age, with most women diagnosed between 40 and 65 years of age. Fallopian tube carcinoma occurs in both tubes in 5% to 31% of women diagnosed with the disease.[8,13]

ETIOLOGY AND RISK FACTORS

The etiology of cancer of the fallopian tubes is unknown. Researchers have hypothesized that chronic inflammation of the tubes and tubal tuberculosis may contribute to the development of the disease. However, since the number of cases of fallopian tube cancer is so small, meaningful data with respect to etiology and risk factors are limited.[8,13]

Table 10-5   Staging Classification for Vaginal Cancer

Primary tumor (T)		
TNM	**FIGO**	**Definition**
TX		Primary tumor cannot be assessed
T0		No evidence of primary tumor
Tis	0	Carcinoma in situ
T1	I	Tumor confined to vagina
T2	II	Tumor invades paravaginal tissues but not to pelvic wall
T3	III	Tumor extends to pelvic wall
T4	IVa	Tumor invades mucosa of bladder or rectum and/or extends beyond true pelvis
M1	IVb	Distant metastasis

Regional lymph nodes (N)	
TMN	**Definition**
NX	Regional lymph nodes cannot be assessed
N0	No regional lymph node metastasis
Upper two thirds of vagina:	
N1	Pelvic lymph node metastasis
Lower one third of vagina:	
N1	Unilateral inguinal lymph node metastasis
N2	Bilateral inguinal lymph node metastasis

Distant metastasis (M)		
TNM	**FIGO**	**Definition**
MX		Presence of distant metastasis cannot be assessed
M0		No distant metastasis
M1	IVb	Distant metastasis

Stage grouping		
Stage 0:	Tis-N0-M0	
Stage I:	T1-N0-M0	
Stage II:	T2-N0-M0	
Stage III:	T1-N1-M0	
	T2-N1-M0	
	T3-N0, N1-M0	
Stage IVA:	T1-N2-M0	
	T2-N2-M0	
	T3-N2-M0	
	T4-any N-M0	
Stage IVB:	any T-any N-M1	

Data from American Joint Committee on Cancer: *Manual for staging cancer,* ed 4, Philadelphia, 1992, Lippincott.

PREVENTION, SCREENING, AND DETECTION
Prevention and Screening

Currently, no recommendations are made specifically for the prevention and screening of women for cancer of the fallopian tubes. However, as the pelvic examination is done for screening for other gynecologic malignancies, the clinician must always be alert to the possibility of a pelvic mass being cancer of the fallopian tube. The presence of persistent positive cervical cytology in a woman without evidence of cervical, endometrial, or vaginal cancers should alert the clinician to possible cancer of the fallopian tube.[3,8,13]

Detection

Clinical examination is done to detect the presence of ascites and a pelvic mass. A pelvic mass is palpable in more than 50% of women with fallopian tube cancer.[3,8,13] Since fallopian tube carcinoma is rare and symptoms and clinical findings are similar to those in ovarian carcinoma, the diagnosis is rarely made before surgery.

CLASSIFICATION

Adenocarcinoma is the most common histologic type of cancer of the fallopian tube. Sarcomas, mixed mesoder-mal tumors, lymphomas, hydatidiform moles, and choriocarcinoma have also been reported. Since the number of cases of carcinoma of the fallopian tube is so small, the clinical significance of both histology and grade of the tumor is unknown.[8,13]

CLINICAL FEATURES

The postmenopausal women may present with symptoms of vaginal bleeding; intermittent, colicky, dull, aching pain; and profuse, watery, vaginal discharge. If the tumor is large, pressure or a sense of heaviness on the bladder or rectum may be reported. In women with metastatic disease, ascites may be present and the woman may complain of abdominal fullness and pressure. (See box, p. 199.)

DIAGNOSIS AND STAGING

Diagnosis of fallopian tube carcinoma is made at the time of surgery for definitive treatment of a pelvic mass. Since the disease has a pattern of spread similar to that of ovarian cancer, a similar surgical approach is recommended. Although many clinicians use the FIGO system for ovarian cancer, no official staging system for cancer of the fallopian tube exists.

METASTASIS

Carcinoma of the fallopian tube metastasizes primarily by direct extension to adjacent tissues and organs, seeding of the abdominal cavity, and lymphatic spread to local and regional nodes. The pattern of metastasis is thought to be related to the site of the primary lesion. For women with lesions in the proximal portion of the tube, metastasis is more likely to occur in the myometrium and endometrium. For women with lesions in the lateral position of the tube, metastasis is more likely to occur to the ovaries and aortic nodes.

TREATMENT MODALITIES

Surgery with TAH-BSO and omentectomy is the treatment of choice for fallopian tube carcinoma. Debulking of the tumor burden is the primary goal. For women with residual disease, treatment with interperitoneal radioactive isotopes (^{32}P or ^{198}Au), pelvic and/or abdominal teletherapy, or systemic single agent or combination chemotherapy with cyclophosphamide, doxorubicin, progestins, cisplatin, or chlorambucil, is recommended.[3,8,13]

PROGNOSIS

The prognosis for patients with cancer of the fallopian tube is similar to that of patients with ovarian cancer and is related to stage of disease in general and specifically to depth of penetration of the tubal wall. The survival rate for all stages has been reported as 38%, with the rate as high as 88% in patients with stage I disease. Survival data are not as reliable for fallopian tube cancer as for other gynecologic malignancies because the number of cases is low and treatment varies considerably across published reports.[8]

GESTATIONAL TROPHOBLASTIC DISEASE

EPIDEMIOLOGY

Gestational trophoblastic disease (GTD) can occur with a molar pregnancy or after an abortion, ectopic pregnancy, or normal-term delivery. Although the disease accounts for only 1% of all cancers of the female reproductive system in the United States, incidence rates in Asia and South America have been reported as high as 1:120 pregnancies.[8,13]

ETIOLOGY AND RISK FACTORS

GTD includes a variety of tumors that originate in the trophoblastic layer of the chorionic villae during pregnancy. The tumors may range from benign hydatidiform moles to locally invasive moles to choriocarcinomas. Although the etiology is unknown, empiric data indicate that low-protein diets, poverty, and increasing age may contribute to development of the disease.[8,13]

PREVENTION, SCREENING, AND DETECTION
Prevention and Screening

No recommendations for prevention or screening of asymptomatic women for GTD are available.

Detection

The detection of GTD is based on careful review of findings on history, clinical examination, and laboratory studies. Disparities in gestational dates, uterine size, and human chorionic gonadotropin (HCG) levels are keys to the early detection of GTD.

CLASSIFICATION

GTD is classified morphologically as either hydatidiform moles, invasive moles, or choriocarcinoma. Invasive moles and choriocarcinoma have a higher incidence of metastasis to surrounding tissues and thus carry a poor prognosis.[8,13]

CLINICAL FEATURES

The most common symptom of GTD is vaginal bleeding, particularly during the first trimester. A history of hyperemesis may be reported. Clinical examination reveals enlargement of the uterus in excess of the estimated length of gestation. Fetal heart sounds are absent, and fetal parts cannot be palpated. Finally, elevations of the HCG titers that exceed those found during the course of a normal pregnancy and postpartum period should alert the clinician to the possibility of the disease.[8,13] (See box, p. 199.)

DIAGNOSIS AND STAGING

Diagnosis of GTD is confirmed by tissue examination from expulsion of grapelike villi, vaginal bleeding, or evacuation of tissues from the uterus. Clinical examination of the uterus, pelvis, and vagina before and during surgery for evidence of metastasis is recommended. The lungs, brain, and liver are evaluated by laboratory and radiographic studies to rule out the presence of metastatic disease.

No uniform system of staging for GTD exists. However, clinicians typically use a system developed by the New England Trophoblastic Disease Center (Table 10-6).

Table 10-6 Staging Classification for Gestational Trophoblastic Disease (GTD)

Stage	Definition
0	Molar pregnancy
	A. Low risk
	B. High risk
I	Confined to uterine corpus
II	Metastases to pelvis and vagina
III	Metastasis to lung
IV	Distant metastasis

Modified from Goldstein DP, Berkowitz RS: The management of gestational trophoblastic neoplasms, *Curr Probl Obstet Gynecol* 4(1), 1980.

METASTASIS

Metastasis from GTD occurs primarily by local extension to surrounding tissues of the pelvis or through hematogenous spread. The most common sites of distant metastasis include the lungs, brain, and liver.[8,13]

TREATMENT MODALITIES

Treatment of GTD is based on the staging. For women with local disease, surgery is the primary treatment. For women at high risk for or with invasive disease and metastasis, a combination of surgery, chemotherapy, and radiation therapy may be used.

Surgery

Surgery, including evacuation of the uterus and D&C, is the primary treatment for women with hydatidiform moles. Surgery, including hysterectomy, also plays a role in the treatment of women with other types of GTD. Radical surgery has not been shown to be beneficial in terms of increasing survival rates.

Chemotherapy

Treatment with antineoplastic agents is used for women with hydatidiform moles who have plateau or elevated weekly β-HCG titers after evacuation or develop metastatic disease and for women with invasive moles or choriocarcinoma who have metastatic disease. The most effective agents include methotrexate, with or without leucovorin rescue; actinomycin-D; and chlorambucil. Salvage treatment with combination drug regimens, including methotrexate, cisplatin, vincristine or vinblastine, bleomycin, and etoposide, has been recommended.[3,8,13]

Radiation Therapy

Radiation therapy also plays a role in the treatment of women with metastatic disease. Women with metastasis to the brain or elevated levels of HCG in the spinal fluid receive whole-brain radiation. Metastatic lesions to the liver may be treated with radiation therapy.[8,13]

Response to Therapy

Response to treatment is based on serial β-HCG levels. After evacuation of hydatidiform moles, β-HCG levels are monitored weekly. For approximately 80% of women diagnosed, the levels return to normal and no additional treatment is needed.

For women with metastatic disease, β-HCG levels are evaluated before each course of treatment. Once the β-HCG levels have returned to normal and have remained within normal levels for 3 weeks, monitoring at monthly intervals is begun and continued for 1 year. Current recommendations include measures to prevent pregnancy during the 1-year follow-up period.

PROGNOSIS

Prognosis for patients with GTD is reported based on the percentage of patients that achieve remission with treatment. For patients with nonmetastatic disease, remission (HCG levels within normal range for 3 consecutive weeks) rates with single-agent chemotherapy range from 90% to 100%. Remission rates for patients with metastatic disease are related to the site(s) of metastasis. With combined chemotherapy and radiation therapy, patients with metastatic disease to the lungs or vagina had higher remission rates (74%) than those with metastatic disease at other sites.[8]

CONCLUSION

The specialty of gynecologic oncology has experienced some of the most impressive successes in the use of screening, early diagnosis, and treatment techniques to modify the natural history and incidence of selected gynecologic cancers. These successes have resulted in a significant decrease in mortality. Throughout the phases of care, prevention, screening, diagnosis, treatment, and rehabilitation, nurses play a critical role in improving the quantity and quality of survival. Challenges remain, but the rewards are seen in the daily lives of the many survivors of gynecologic cancers. Patients are often faced with adjusting to significant structural, functional, and cosmetic changes as a result of the disease and treatment. The nurse assumes a key role in addressing rehabilitation concerns. In collaboration with others on the health care team, identification of rehabilitation needs for both the woman and her significant others and referral to appropriate rehabilitation personnel and services may be necessary. The nurse also plays an important role in the long-term evaluation of the success of rehabilitative efforts.

Text continued on p. 224.

NURSING MANAGEMENT

Women at risk or with a diagnosis of gynecologic malignancy present a range of challenges to the nurse. Prevention, screening, and early detection activities are nursing interventions that have the potential to improve both survival and quality of survival for these women.

Counseling on healthy life-style choices that can reduce cancer risks; teaching and valuing the importance of routine gynecologic surveillance and care, including self-examination skills, Pap smear, and bimanual pelvic examination; and educating women about the early signs and symptoms of gynecologic cancers are critical elements of the role the nurse plays in prevention and early detection. The box at right presents specific content for a teaching plan for women at risk for selected gynecologic malignancies.

Throughout the diagnostic phase the nurse becomes an advocate and resource for the woman and her significant others. The nurse is responsible for instruction on the rationale for, procedures involved in, and sensations experienced during diagnostic tests and pretest and posttest care. The nurse also assumes a role in listening to concerns that the woman and her significant others may have about the requirements and results of the diagnostic evaluation.

During the treatment phase the nurse assists the woman in meeting the physical and psychosocial demands imposed by the disease and treatment. In collaboration with the patient, significant others, physician, social worker, physical, respiratory, and occupational therapists, nutritionist, and chaplain, the nurse develops and coordinates implementation of a plan of care designed to provide a safe environment, minimize the incidence of complications from disease and treatment, monitor for signs and symptoms of complications of the disease and treatment, promote independence in self-care, include significant others in the plan of care, and promote coping strategies that foster self-worth and a positive self-concept.* Elements common to the nursing care of patients receiving surgery, radiation therapy, chemotherapy, biotherapy, and bone marrow transplantation are included in Chapters 20, 21, 22, 23, and 24, respectively.

Women facing gynecologic cancers have the potential to experience many common responses to the disease and treatment. Structural changes in anatomy resulting from surgery and radiation therapy for gynecologic cancers may result in altered sexuality patterns.

Aggressive treatment and progressive disease place the patient at risk for complications. Common complications associated with progressive disease include altered bowel elimination related to obstruction; fluid volume excess: ascites related to intraabdominal metas-

*References 2, 5, 6, 9, 12, 14, 15, 20-23.

PATIENT TEACHING PRIORITIES
Gynecologic Cancers

Patient teaching reflects cultural sensitivity and use of multiple reinforcers: written, audio, visual, and verbal. Teaching includes content that represents the identified needs of patients across the care continuum, including the following:

Prevention, screening, and detection practices for all the gynecologic cancers

Disease symptomology (cervical, endometrial, ovarian, vaginal, vulvar, fallopian cancers; gestational trophoblastic disease)

Treatment modalities with pertinent side effects and purpose, rationale, and potential schedule

Monitoring of blood counts

Wound management

Bowel and bladder elimination

Self-care management

Signs of infection (fever, chills, erythema, bleeding, drainage with odor)

Sexual dysfunction issues (infertility, sterility, libido, intercourse)

---

tasis; and fluid volume excess: lymphedema related to blocked lymphatic channels. Nursing care for patients experiencing these problems focuses on maintaining safety, comfort, and mobility.

Aggressive treatment for gynecologic cancers carries increased risks of complications. Since the bladder and bowel lie in proximity to the female reproductive system, altered bowel and urinary elimination related to treatment may result. Problems experienced include decreased sensation to defecate or void, enteritis, cystitis, and fistula formation. Radical surgery and radiation therapy, particularly involving the vulva, may result in impaired skin integrity.

Women with gynecologic cancers are often faced with adjusting to significant structural, functional, and cosmetic changes as a result of the disease and treatment. The nurse assumes a key role in addressing rehabilitation concerns, which may range from care of ostomies resulting from pelvic exenteration, sexual counseling (Chapter 32), health maintenance issues, and psychologic concerns (Chapter 31). In collaboration with others on the health care team, identification of rehabilitation needs for both the woman and her significant others and referral to appropriate rehabilitation services and agencies may be necessary. Potential agencies include the United Ostomy Association, National Coalition for Cancer Survivorship,

American Cancer Society, and the National Lymphedema Network. Women can be encouraged to participate in support programs or groups such as Can-Surmount. The nurse also plays an important continuous role in long-term evaluation of the success of rehabilitative efforts.

NURSING DIAGNOSIS

• *Knowledge deficit related to prevention and early detection of gynecologic malignancies*

CERVIX

ASSESSMENTS

• Assess baseline knowledge of personal risk factors for cervical cancer.
• Identify personal risk factors for cervical cancer: age at onset of sexual activity, number of sexual partners, sexual history of partners, number of pregnancies, history of sexually transmitted diseases (STDs), history of cervical dysplasia, method of contraception, genital hygiene measures, and history of alcohol or tobacco abuse. Identify any concerns the woman may have related to personal risks for cervical cancer.

OUTCOME GOAL

Patient will be able to:
• Describe personal risk factors for cervical malignancies.

INTERVENTIONS

• Teach advantages of barrier contraception use.
• Teach methods to discontinue smoking: "cold" turkey, nicotine patch or gum, I Quit, and hypnosis.
• Educate woman about the benefits and schedule of routine Pap smears and pelvic examinations.
• Review signs and symptoms of cervical cancer: abnormal menstrual, intramenstrual, or postcoital bleeding; vaginal discharge; and pain.
• Provide age-appropriate and culturally sensitive written materials about cervical cancer.
• Provide a list of community resources for information and services available to women at risk or with a diagnosis of cervical cancer.

VULVA

ASSESSMENTS

• Assess knowledge of personal risk factors for vulvar cancer.
• Identify personal risk factors for vulvar cancer: age; chronic vulvar irritation; concurrent diseases such as hypertension, diabetes, cardiovascular disease, and obesity; and history of cervical cancer.
• Identify any concerns the woman may have related to personal risks for vulvar cancer.

OUTCOME GOAL

Patient will be able to:
• Participate in life-style choices that modify the risk of vulvar malignancies.

INTERVENTIONS

• Teach steps of vulvar self-examination: inspection and palpation.
• Encourage woman to report significant changes in the texture, color, or sensations of the vulva to a physician: a lump, pruritus, bleeding, or discharge.
• Educate women about the benefits of an annual health examination, including evaluation of the vulva and groins.
• Provide age-appropriate and culturally sensitive written materials on vulvar cancer.
• Provide a list of community resources for information and services available to women at risk or with a diagnosis of vulvar cancer.

ENDOMETRIUM

ASSESSMENTS

• Assess baseline knowledge of personal risk factors for endometrial cancer.
• Identify personal risk factors for endometrial cancer: young age at onset of menstruation; menopause after 52 years of age; nulliparity; obesity; history of Stein-Leventhal syndrome, diabetes, or hypertension; family history of breast, colon, or endometrial cancer; and use of exogenous estrogens.
• Identify concerns that the woman may have related to personal risks for endometrial cancer.

OUTCOME GOAL

Patient will be able to:
• Demonstrate compliance with recommended screening behaviors to detect endometrial malignancies in asymptomatic women.

INTERVENTIONS

• Discuss life-style choices that can reduce endometrial cancer risks: maintenance of ideal body weight and reduction of fat intake to 30% of total caloric intake.
• Describe health promotion activities to screen for endometrial cancer: annual Pap smear and bimanual pelvic examination and endometrial biopsy in women at high risk for endometrial cancer.
• Review signs and symptoms of endometrial cancer: prolonged, excessive, or intramenstrual bleeding in premenopausal women; postmenopausal spotting or bleeding; or yellow, watery, vaginal discharge.
• Provide age-appropriate and culturally sensitive written materials about endometrial cancer.

Continued.

• Provide a list of community resources for information and services available to women at risk or with a diagnosis of endometrial cancer.

OVARY

ASSESSMENTS

• Assess baseline knowledge of personal risk factors for ovarian cancer.
• Identify personal risk factors for ovarian cancer: history of infertility, nulliparity, and personal or family history of breast, ovarian, colon, or uterine cancer.
• Identify concerns that women may have related to personal risks for ovarian cancer.

OUTCOME GOAL

Patient will be able to:
• Report signs and symptoms of ovarian malignancies to a member of the health care team.

INTERVENTIONS

• Discuss life-style choices that can reduce ovarian cancer risks: use of oral contraceptives, serial CA-125 levels, and vaginal ultrasounds for high-risk women.
• Describe health promotion activities to screen for ovarian cancer: annual bimanual pelvic examination.
• Review signs and symptoms of ovarian cancer: dyspepsia, indigestion, loss of appetite, early satiety, pelvic pressure or discomfort, urinary frequency, increasing abdominal girth, and weight loss.
• Provide age-appropriate and culturally sensitive written materials about ovarian cancer.
• Provide a list of community resources for information and services available to women at risk or with a diagnosis of ovarian cancer.

NURSING DIAGNOSIS

• *Sexuality patterns, altered, related to impact of structural, functional, and psychologic changes associated with treatment for gynecologic cancers*

ASSESSMENTS

• Assess woman's and significant other's perception of patient as a sexual being.
• Evaluate factors that contribute to woman's self-concept and expression of sexuality.
• Identify perceived threats to sexuality imposed by disease and treatment.
• Assess factors that may facilitate or hinder adaptation to the structural, functional, and psychologic changes resulting from treatment.

OUTCOME GOALS

Patient will be able to:
• Identify potential threats to sexual expression of patient

and partner resulting from diagnosis and treatment of gynecologic cancers.
• Discuss effects of surgery, radiation therapy, chemotherapy, biologic therapy, and bone marrow transplantation on sexuality.
• Participate in self-care activities to minimize impact of disease and treatment for gynecologic cancers on sexuality and patterns of sexual behavior.
• Report nonacceptable changes in sexual expression and behaviors related to disease and treatment to member of health care team.

INTERVENTIONS

• Review normal anatomy and physiology of the reproductive system with woman and significant other.
• Describe strategies recommended for minimizing effects of treatment that can influence sexuality patterns.
• Discuss the potential structural, functional, or psychologic effects of treatment: surgery, radiation therapy, and/or chemotherapy.

INTERVENTIONS: SURGERY

• Inform woman that only a small portion of vagina is resected as a component of either a simple or radical hysterectomy. Edges of vagina are sutured to form a closed tube. Vagina has ability to stretch during intercourse.
• Discuss that removal of ovaries results in lack of estrogen. Vaginal tissues may become dry and loose elasticity. Oral estrogen replacement therapy or vaginal estrogen creams may be ordered by physician unless contraindicated by presence of a hormone-dependent tumor (i.e., endometrial or breast cancer).

INTERVENTIONS: RADIATION THERAPY

• Inform woman that radiation also can affect vaginal tissues, making them thinner, drier, and less elastic over time. If woman is not sexually active, vaginal stenosis may occur after radiation therapy.
• Teach use of vaginal dilators to prevent vaginal stenosis:
  —Lubricate dilator with water-based lubricant or estrogen cream.
  —Insert dilator gradually to full length of vagina.
  —Leave dilator inserted in vagina for 10 minutes each day.
  —Remove and wash dilator thoroughly with soap and water.

INTERVENTIONS: CHEMOTHERAPY

• Inform woman that common side effects of chemotherapy, including hair loss, stomatitis, nausea, vomiting, and fatigue, can influence both perceptions of body image and self-concept and desire for sexual intimacy.

—Encourage open discussions about perceptions of body image and self-concept with health care team and significant others.

—Encourage patient to assume an active role in decision making about care.

—Recognize incremental achievements in progress toward patient outcome goals.

—Recommend participation in American Cancer Society's Look Good, Feel Better program.

• Encourage open discussions with patient and partner about potential effects of treatment on sexuality patterns.

• Teach patient and partner strategies to reexplore pleasurable experiences during intimacy.

• Suggest increasing the length of time for foreplay to allow for adequate vaginal lubrication.

• Suggest use of vaginal water-based lubricant or vaginal estrogen cream.

• Describe sexual positions that provide woman with more control over depth of penetration.

• Discuss benefits of engaging in sexual behaviors that require minimal energy (hugging, kissing, closeness) and that are initiated when well rested.

• Recommend a schedule for resuming sexual activity.

• Review signs and symptoms of altered sexuality patterns to be reported to the health care team: feelings of decreased self-worth, negative feelings about body image or self-concept, and any changes in expression of sexuality that are not satisfying or pleasurable to self or partner.

• Evaluate impact of disease, treatment, and effectiveness of suggestions in maintaining a satisfactory sexuality pattern.

• Refer for sexual counseling if problems persist.

NURSING DIAGNOSIS

• *Fluid volume excess: ascites related to intraabdominal metastasis*

ASSESSMENTS

• Assess weight and abdominal girth daily.

• Assess condition of skin over abdomen, buttocks, bony prominences, and back for changes in color, temperature, or texture.

• Evaluate effect of ascites on level of comfort, mobility, respiratory effort, and activities of daily living (ADLs).

OUTCOME GOALS

Patient will be able to:

• Report effects of ascites on ADLs and comfort to member of health care team.

• Participate in strategies to minimize untoward effects of ascites.

• List signs and symptoms that require immediate medical intervention.

INTERVENTIONS

• Position patient with head elevated 30 to 90 degrees to allow for maximum respiratory expansion with minimal effort.

• Monitor intake and output ratio each day.

• Assist patient with ADLs as needed.

• Encourage wearing loose clothing around the trunk and abdomen: larger-size bra, bikini-cut panties, and pantyhose made for pregnant women.

• Encourage compliance with low-salt diet.

• Monitor for signs and symptoms of respiratory or gastrointestinal distress that require medical intervention: marked shortness of breath, protracted nausea or vomiting, and acute changes in pattern of pain.

• Provide supportive care as physician performs palliative paracentesis:

—Instruct patient in terms of what will be involved in procedure, what sensations may be experienced during and after procedure, and elements of postprocedural care.

—Position patient in comfortable position.

—Administer any premedications ordered for anxiety.

—Measure amount of ascitic fluid removed and prepare specimen for laboratory as ordered.

—Monitor subjective (pain, relief of shortness of breath) and objective responses (blood pressure, pulse, respirations) of patient to procedure.

—Observe site after procedure for continued drainage, discharge, redness, pain, or warmth.

NURSING DIAGNOSIS

• *Fluid volume excess: lymphedema related to blocked lymphatic channels*

ASSESSMENTS

• Assess for predisposing factors that could contribute to occurrence of lymphedema of lower extremities: concurrent cardiac, renal, or liver disease; previous lymphadenectomy or radiation therapy of pelvic nodes; and diet.

• Assess pattern of lymphedema: onset, location, and aggravating and alleviating factors.

• Evaluate impact of lymphedema on life-style, comfort, skin integrity, and ADLs.

• Evaluate serial measurements, presence on peripheral pulses, and range of motion of affected extremities.

OUTCOME GOALS

Patient will be able to:

• List personal risk factors for lymphedema.

• Describe pattern of lymphedema to member of health care team.

• Discuss impact of lymphedema on ADLs and comfort.

• Participate in strategies to minimize risk of complications of lymphedema.

• Report significant changes in lymphedema to member of health care team.

Continued.

INTERVENTIONS

- Protect affected extremity: wear loose, protective clothing and avoid restrictive jewelry, irritants, and temperature extremes.
- Avoid invasive procedures to affected extremity.
- Elevate extremity as much as possible.
- Monitor for and report changes in color, temperature, intactness of skin over the affected extremity, and quality of peripheral pulses to physician.
- Consult physical therapy to evaluate use of compression equipment and to develop program of exercise to maintain range of motion in extremity.

NURSING DIAGNOSIS

- *Bowel elimination, altered (e.g., bowel incontinence; diarrhea; constipation), related to disease or treatment for gynecologic cancers*

ASSESSMENTS

- Assess characteristics of stool: amount, consistency, odor, and color.
- Assess bowel elimination patterns: frequency, presence of constipation, diarrhea, pain with defecation, or incontinence.
- Identify factors that contribute to bowel elimination patterns: dietary intake, fluid intake, activity level, and medication history.

OUTCOME GOALS

Patient will be able to:

- Discuss personal risk factors for changes in bowel or bladder elimination.
- Perform self-care activities related to management of altered bowel or bladder elimination.
- Participate in activities to minimize risk of complications of altered bowel or bladder elimination.
- List community resources available related to management of changes in bowel or bladder elimination.
- List signs and symptoms of complications of altered bowel and bladder elimination that require immediate professional intervention.

INTERVENTION

- Discuss changes that may occur in bowel elimination patterns after surgery or radiation therapy: adhesions with bowel obstruction, decreased sensation of need to defecate, radiation enteritis, and rectovaginal fistula.

INTERVENTIONS: SURGERY

- Discuss that women treated with hysterectomy or radical hysterectomy will note decreased bowel function postoperatively because of manipulation of bowel during surgery. Bowel is kept at rest postoperatively by avoiding oral fluid and food intake until bowel sounds return. Flatulence is common and may be uncomfort-

able. Attention to pattern of bowel elimination is necessary in first weeks after surgery to minimize risk of constipation associated with use of pain medication, changes in fluid and food intake, and inactivity.
  - —Ensure that woman institutes bowel regimen as ordered by physician before surgery to cleanse bowel of stool.
  - —Encourage strategies to stimulate bowel function: walking, heating pads, and bowel stimulants.
  - —Monitor bowel sounds every 8 hours.
  - —Instruct patient to notify team of presence of flatulence or passage of stool.
- Discuss that for women undergoing a total or posterior pelvic exenteration, a bowel diversion will be constructed.
  - —Instruct patient in skills to evaluate condition of stoma, application of collection devices, care of peristomal skin, and irrigation techniques.
  - —Teach critical changes in character of stool, condition of stoma or peristomal skin, or functioning of diversion to report to health care team.

INTERVENTIONS: RADIATION THERAPY

- Inform woman that the most common immediate side effect of radiation therapy to bowel is diarrhea.
  - —Observe for signs and symptoms of dehydration.
  - —Assess condition of the perianal and perineal skin.
  - —Teach women elements of good perineal hygiene after each bowel movement: cleanse the area with water, pat area dry thoroughly, and apply barrier cream as needed to maintain skin integrity.
  - —Instruct in dietary changes to increase bulk of stool: avoid fresh fruits and vegetables.
  - —Administer antidiarrheals as ordered by physician.
- Discuss that long-term effects of radiation therapy on bowel include radiation enteritis and rectovaginal fistula formation.
  - —Place bowel at rest.
  - —Instruct in dietary changes to increase bulk of stool: avoid fresh fruits and vegetables.
  - —Administer antidiarrheals as ordered by physician.
  - —Administer antiinflammatory agents to decrease inflammation in bowel.
  - —Teach significant changes to be reported to health care team: blood in stool, marked increase in the volume of diarrhea, symptoms of dehydration, and passage of stool from vagina.

INTERVENTIONS: PROGRESSIVE DISEASE

- Inform woman that bowel obstruction is a common symptom of progressive disease.
  - —Monitor for signs of bowel obstruction: colicky, cramping, lower abdominal pain; alternating diarrhea and constipation; abdominal distention; vomiting; and hyperactive, high-pitched bowel sounds above

obstruction and absent bowel sounds below obstruction.
—Prepare patient for nasogastric tube as ordered by physician.
—Report significant changes in character of symptoms that indicate need for immediate medical attention: increase in severity of pain, decrease in abdominal girth, rebound tenderness, and acute absence of bowel sounds.

NURSING DIAGNOSIS

• *Urinary elimination, altered, related to disease or treatment for gynecologic cancers*

ASSESSMENTS

• Assess urinary elimination patterns before initiation of treatment: frequency, nocturia, and incontinence.
• Identify factors that contribute to urinary elimination patterns: volume and timing of fluid intake, concurrent diseases such as diabetes, and medications.

INTERVENTION

• Discuss changes that may occur as a result of surgery or radiation therapy: decreased sensation to void, incomplete emptying of bladder, cystitis, and vesicovaginal fistula formation.

INTERVENTIONS: SURGERY

• Inform woman that after hysterectomy or radical hysterectomy, innervation to bladder may be damaged. Decreased sensation of need to void and incontinence are common effects. A suprapubic catheter is usually placed after surgery. Bladder retraining occurs with catheter in place until residual urines of less than 50 ml are achieved after voiding.
—Encourage to drink as much fluid as possible.
—Limit fluid intake after 7 PM.
—Establish regular schedule for voiding.
• Discuss that for women undergoing a total or anterior pelvic exenteration, a urinary diversion will be constructed.
—Teach skills to evaluate condition of stoma, application of collection devices, and care of peristomal skin.
—Discuss critical changes in character of urine, condition of stoma or peristomal skin, and functioning of diversion to report to health care team.

INTERVENTIONS: RADIATION THERAPY

• Inform woman that the primary short-term effect of radiation on bladder tissues is radiation cystitis. Frequency, dysuria, and bleeding are common symptoms.
—Encourage a daily fluid intake of 3000 ml.
—Consult physician to order medications to minimize discomfort.

—Reassure patient that symptoms will improve with time.
• Discuss that the primary long-term effect of radiation therapy is weakening of tissues between vagina and bladder and formation of a fistula. Depending on size of fistula, urine may leak or flow through vagina. Approaches to treatment range from catheter placement to surgical repair.
—Institute care strategies to keep patient dry: pouching, indwelling catheter, and protective clothing.
—Teach perineal care measures: rinse perineum thoroughly with warm water after each voiding, pat area dry, and apply skin barrier as ordered.
—Monitor condition of perineal skin daily.
• Review signs and symptoms of alteration in urinary elimination to report to health care team: frequency, pain, changes in the amount or character of the urine, inability to void, and passage of urine through vagina.

NURSING DIAGNOSIS

• *Skin integrity, impaired, related to surgery or radiation therapy for treatment of vulvar cancer*

ASSESSMENTS

• Assess skin over vulva, perineum, gluteal folds, and groin areas before initiation of treatment.
• Evaluate for factors that predispose woman to impaired skin integrity: presence of diabetes, obesity, and age.
• Assess steps in routine perineal hygiene measures.
• Evaluate perceived and actual ability (skill and range of motion) of patient to provide self-care during treatment.

OUTCOME GOALS

Patient will be able to:
• Discuss personal risk factors for impaired skin integrity.
• Perform self-care activities to minimize risk of impaired skin integrity.
• List signs and symptoms of complications of impaired skin integrity that require immediate professional intervention.

INTERVENTIONS

• Discuss potential structural and functional effects of treatment of vulvar cancer with surgery (wound breakdown) and radiation therapy (erythema, dry to moist desquamation).
• Develop a plan of care to minimize risks of side effects of treatment.

INTERVENTIONS: SURGERY

• Discuss that wounds from a radical vulvectomy are difficult to heal, particularly if preoperative radiation therapy has been given. Key elements of wound care for these patients are keeping wound clean and dry.
—Irrigate surgical wounds with half-strength hydrogen peroxide.

Continued.

—Pack wounds with gauze.

—Dry perineum with a hair dryer on coolest setting.

—Use bed cradles and positioning to increase circulation of air to wound.

INTERVENTIONS: RADIATION THERAPY

• Discuss that tissues of vulva, perineum, and groin areas are extremely radiosensitive. Erythema often occurs early in course of therapy and is associated with edema, warmth, and tenderness of tissues. Moist desquamation occurs later in course of treatment and is accompanied by marked redness of tissues, serous drainage, and pain. Radiation is usually stopped until changes subside.

—Suggest comfort measures such as wearing loose cotton panties or no panties, avoiding pantyhose, using cool compresses to the perineum, and taking pain medications as ordered by physician.

—Recommend measures to keep tissues clean and dry.

—Discourage use of any topical agents other than those recommended by radiation oncologist.

• Review signs and symptoms of infection and skin breakdown that should be reported to health care team: redness, increased pain, purulent drainage, foul-smelling discharge, fever, swelling, and ulceration.

NURSING DIAGNOSIS

• *Health maintenance, altered, related to lack of endogenous estrogen in presence of estrogen/progesterone-dependent malignancy*

ASSESSMENTS

• Assess life-style factors that contribute to health maintenance: diet, activity, and stress reduction techniques.

• Assess woman's perception of physical and psychologic changes experienced attributed to lack of estrogen.

• Evaluate extent to which changes have a negative impact on quality of life.

• Evaluate personal and family history for presence of osteoporosis, cardiac disease, and psychiatric problems.

OUTCOME GOALS

Patient will be able to:

• Discuss relative risks and benefits of estrogen replacement.

• Participate in alternative strategies to minimize postmenopausal symptoms and decrease risks of osteoporosis and heart disease.

INTERVENTIONS

• Discuss rationale for avoiding estrogen replacement therapy in presence of estrogen/progesterone-dependent cancer.

• Describe potential risks to health maintenance from lack of estrogen: increased risks of osteoporosis, cardiovascular disease, psychiatric disease, and vasomotor changes.

• Instruct in strategies to maintain bone integrity: diet rich in calcium-containing foods, calcium supplements, regular exercise program, modifications in home environment to decrease risk of falls, and periodic evaluation of bone density in high-risk women.

• Teach strategies to minimize risk of cardiovascular disease: low-fat diet, regular exercise program, and periodic evaluation of serum cholesterol and triglyceride levels.

• Discuss alternate methods to minimize postmenopausal symptoms: diet, exercise, and medications such as Bellergal-S.

• Suggest use of water-based lubricants for vaginal dryness.

• Encourage expression of psychologic responses to disease and treatment. If depressive symptoms persist or if woman has suicidal ideations, refer to psychologist or psychiatrist for medical management.

■ CHAPTER QUESTIONS

1. In counseling women about cancer prevention, which of the following behaviors would be most important to include to reduce the incidence of cervical cancer?
   a. Obtain a Pap smear at least every 3 years after three consecutive annual Pap smears.
   b. Include foods high in vitamins A and C in the diet.
   c. Use a barrier form of contraception.
   d. Abstain from alcohol consumption.

2. The nurse is assessing a 65-year-old female who underwent natural menopause more than 10 years ago. Which of the following statements by the patient would mandate that the nurse obtain additional information from the patient?
   a. "I am satisfied with my sexual activity at this time."
   b. "I have not had any hot flashes since I started taking Premarin."

   c. "I read that if you take estrogen, you reduce your risks of heart disease."
   d. "I hope I don't get osteoporosis like my father's sisters."

3. The most common presenting complaint of a woman with cervical cancer is:
   a. Thin, watery vaginal discharge
   b. Urinary urgency
   c. Pain with defecation
   d. Abnormal vaginal bleeding

4. The nurse is teaching a 58-year-old patient with vaginal cancer who has completed a course of radiation therapy as primary treatment for the disease. The patient is not currently sexually active. Which of the following instructions is most important for the nurse to include?
   a. Use of a vaginal dilator
   b. Compliance with hormone replacement therapy

c. Importance of reporting presence of a clear vaginal discharge

d. Use of condoms if patient resumes intercourse

5. A 35-year-old woman has had a radical hysterectomy and right oophorectomy as primary treatment for a stage IB carcinoma of the cervix. The nurse is evaluating the effectiveness of discharge teaching. Which of the following statements made by the patient indicates a need for additional instruction?

a. "I will not have to take any hormone replacement therapy."

b. "I can resume intercourse in about 6 weeks."

c. "I will probably notice a decrease in the strength of my orgasm."

d. "I will probably notice no change in my sexual drive."

6. Which of the following tests is most frequently used in screening asymptomatic women for ovarian cancer?

a. Pelvic examination

b. CA-125

c. Pap smear

d. Vaginal ultrasound

7. The nurse is caring for a patient with ascites secondary to intraabdominal metastatic ovarian carcinoma. Which of the following suggestions made by the nurse would be most helpful to increase the comfort of the patient?

a. Elevate the head of the bed no more than 20 degrees.

b. Wear supportive undergarments.

c. Eat several small meals during the day.

d. Wash the abdominal skin with an antibacterial soap.

8. The nurse is providing care to a patient who had a right groin lymphadenectomy as part of primary therapy for cancer of the right labium. The patient has a concurrent diagnosis of diabetes. Which of the following self-care strategies would be most important for the nurse to teach the patient to decrease the risk of complications from lymphedema of the right leg?

a. Avoid insulin injections in the right leg.

b. Avoid testing the temperature of the bath water with the left leg.

c. Wear clothing that protects the legs from the effects of the sun.

d. Report any changes in the color of the skin over the right leg to the health care team.

9. A 28-year-old woman who had a radical hysterectomy 7 days ago is returning to the office for follow-up care. The patient has a suprapubic catheter in place. Which of the following assessments would be most important for the nurse to make in determining whether the catheter can be removed?

a. Total urinary output over 24 hours

b. Ratio of oral intake to urinary output

c. Volume of postvoiding residuals

d. Presence of urinary incontinence

10. A woman is completing the fourth of 6 weeks of pelvic irradiation for endometrial carcinoma. The patient had experienced an increase in the frequency and amount of diarrhea. Which of the following interventions would be most appropriate for the nurse to suggest to minimize complications of diarrhea?

a. Clean the perineum with an antibacterial soap after each bowel movement.

b. Apply a skin barrier after briskly drying the perineal skin.

c. Increase the number of fresh fruits in the diet.

d. Drink at least 3000 ml of cool or iced fluid each day.

BIBLIOGRAPHY

1. American Cancer Society: *Cancer facts and figures—1996,* Atlanta, 1996, The Society.

2. Anderson BL: Psychosexual adjustment following pelvic exenteration, *Obstet Gynecol* 61(3):331, 1983.

3. Barber HRK: *Manual of gynecologic oncology,* ed 2, Philadelphia, 1989, Lippincott.

4. Cashavelly BJ: Cervical dysplasia: an overview of current concepts in epidemiology, diagnosis, and treatment, *Cancer Nurs* 10(4):199, 1987.

5. Clark J: Mucous membrane integrity, impairment of: related to vaginal changes. In McNally JC and others, editors: *Guidelines for oncology nursing practice,* ed 2, Philadelphia, 1991, Saunders.

6. Clark JC, McGee RF, Preston R: Nursing management of responses to the cancer experience. In Clark JC, McGee RF, editors: *Core curriculum for oncology nursing,* Philadelphia, 1992, Saunders.

7. Davis M: Secondary prevention in oncology nursing practice. In Clark JC, McGee RF, editors: *Core curriculum for oncology nursing,* Philadelphia, 1992, Saunders.

8. DiSaia PJ, Creasman WT: *Clinical gynecologic oncology,* ed 4, St Louis, 1993, Mosby.

9. Donovan MI, Girton SE: *Cancer care nursing,* ed 2, Norwalk, Conn, 1984, Appleton-Century-Crofts.

10. Fanslow J: Knowledge deficit related to prevention and early detection of cervical and uterine (endometrial) cancer. In McNally JC and others, editors: *Guidelines for oncology nursing practice,* ed 2, Philadelphia, 1991, Saunders.

11. Flannery M: Reproductive cancers. In Clark JC, McGee RF, editors: *Core curriculum for oncology nursing,* Philadelphia, 1992, Saunders.

12. Fleming C, Scanlon C, D'Agostino NS: A study of the comfort needs of patients with advanced cancer, *Cancer Nurs* 10(5):237, 1987.

13. Hoskins WJ, Perez C, Young RC: Gynecologic tumors. In DeVita VT Jr, Hellman S, Rosenberg SA, editors: *Cancer: principles and practice of oncology,* ed 4, Philadelphia, 1993, Lippincott.

14. Jenkins B: Patients' report of sexual changes after treatment for gynecological cancer, *Oncol Nurs Forum* 15(3):349, 1988.

15. Krouse HG: A psychological model of adjustment in gynecologic cancer patients, *Oncol Nurs Forum* 12(6):45, 1985.

16. Lamb M: Vulvar cancer: patient information booklet, *Oncol Nurs Forum* 13(6):79, 1986.

17. Lovejoy NC: Precancerous lesions of the cervix, *Cancer Nurs* 10(1):2, 1987.

18. Martin LK, Braly PS: Gynecologic cancers. In Baird SB, McCorkle R, Grant M, editors: *Cancer nursing: a comprehensive textbook,* Philadelphia, 1991, Saunders.

19. Otte DM: Gynecologic cancers. In Groenwald SL and others, editors: *Cancer nursing: principles and practice,* ed 2, Boston, 1990, Jones and Bartlett.

20. Richards S, Hiratzka S: Vaginal dilatation post pelvic irradiation: a patient education tool, *Oncol Nurs Forum* 13(4):89, 1986.

21. Spencer MM: Bowel elimination, alteration in: diversional methods. In McNally JC and others, editors: *Guidelines for oncology nursing practice,* ed 2, Philadelphia, 1991, Saunders.

22. Spencer MM: Urinary elimination, alteration in: diversional methods. In McNally JC and others, editors: *Guidelines for oncology nursing practice,* ed 2, Philadelphia, 1991, Saunders.

23. Swihart J: Bowel elimination, alteration in: bowel obstruction. In McNally JC and others, editors: *Guidelines for oncology nursing practice,* ed 2, Philadelphia, 1991, Saunders.

24. Tombes MB: Gynecologic malignancies. In Baird SB and others, editors: *A cancer source book for nurses,* Atlanta, 1991, American Cancer Society.

25. Young RC, Fuks A, Hoskins WJ: Cancer of the ovary. In DeVita VT Jr, Hellman S, Rosenberg SA, editors: *Cancer: principles and practice of oncology,* ed 4, Philadelphia, 1993, Lippincott.

CHAPTER 11
Head and Neck Cancers

ANDREA SAMPSON HAGGOOD

The old adage "a picture is worth a thousand words" conceptually underlies the degree of psychologic trauma that can be associated with the diagnosis, treatment, and rehabilitation of persons with head and neck cancer. It is one's face, even more so than one's voice, spoken words, emotions (verbalized and withheld), or mannerisms (involuntary and intentional), that presents each individual to the world. Although not among the five leading causes of death from cancer in the United States, the significance of head and neck cancers lies in what they represent to the patient, family, and professional as an acutely visible and disabling threat to future function and well-being. Left untreated, cancers in this area can result in disabilities and lead to fatalities. Even if treated, patients and their significant others will have to face the potential for disfigurement, physiologic dysfunction, sensory loss, changes in body image, altered social interaction, altered sexuality, spiritual distress, and cancer-related death.

Providing care and education for these patients and their significant others can present a significant challenge for the nurse. However, nurses are uniquely skilled and positioned to support and guide the patient and family through their adjustment to illness, treatment, and rehabilitation, ultimately impacting future quality of life. Given the intricacies involved in patient care and disease management for the person with head and neck cancer, nursing care is presented in great detail in this chapter. Nursing care guidelines are included throughout for surgery, cosmesis, radiation therapy, and self-care management.

EPIDEMIOLOGY AND ETIOLOGY

In the United States, carcinomas of the aerodigestive tract account for approximately 4% of all malignancies, and approximately 56,600 new head and neck malignancies and 13,720 deaths occurred in 1996.[11,108,129] The worldwide incidence consists of more than 500,000 cases of head and neck neoplasms.[120,129] In other parts of the world (e.g., India, Southeast Asia, other developing countries), where oral cancers account for as many as 35% of all malignancies, head and neck cancer is much more prevalent.[128] From 90% to 95% of head and neck cancers are of *squamous cell* histology.[74,120,128,129,155] Other cell types include various salivary gland tumors (e.g., adenocarcinoma, adenoid cystic tumor, mucoepidermoid cancer), thyroid tumors, verrucous carcinomas, lymphoepitheliomas, and rare lymphomas and soft tissue sarcomas.[21,113]

The most common site of head and neck cancer is the oral cavity, followed by the larynx and then the pharynx. At diagnosis, more than two thirds of patients have locally advanced (stages III and IV) disease.[128] Although in the past 10 years more patients have been seen in their third and fourth decade of life, especially with oral cavity malignancies,[128] the incidence of head and neck malignancies is highest after age 40,[101,128] with more than 50% occurring in persons over age 65.[113] There continues to be a higher incidence of head and neck cancers among males, except for thyroid cancers, which have a higher incidence in females. In the 5 to 10 years before 1995 the male/female incidence ratio in the United States decreased from 4 to 5:1 to approximately 3:1, with an estimated ratio of 2:1 in 1996.[11,107,128] This trend is attributed to the increasing consumption of tobacco and alcohol by females. In blacks the incidence and mortality rates of laryngeal cancer are significantly higher than for whites.[11] There has also been a trend of increasing incidence of pharyngeal cancers over the past 20 years.[128] Whereas in white men an increasing trend in survival rates has been seen in cases of oral and pharyngeal can-

The author would like to express her appreciation to J. Parzuchowski for the years of mentoring and support in ENT and head and neck surgery and oncology. The author also gives special thanks to P.B. Haggood, J. Andersen, MD, and L. Littsey for their support in the writing of this chapter.

227

cers diagnosed between 1970-1973 (43%) and 1974-1976 (55%) (remaining stable at 55% between 1974-1976 and 1980-1982 and between 1980-1982 and 1986-1991), a decreasing survival rate has been seen when comparing rates between 1974-1976 (36%) and 1980-1982 (31%) for black men, with a slight increase in survival between 1980-1982 and 1986-1991 (33%).[11] In one study the most important explanatory factor for ethnic differences in oral and pharyngeal cancer incidence was alcohol consumption. After controlling for smoking, heavy drinking (more than 30 drinks per week) resulted in a ninefold increase risk of oral and pharyngeal cancers among whites, in contrast to a seventeenfold increase in blacks.[121] The American Cancer Society (ACS) suggests that survival differences can largely be attributed to the more advanced stage of disease at diagnosis among blacks.[11]

The aerodigestive tract serves as a conduit for air, fluid, and food. Therefore the body is constantly exposed to a broad range of potential carcinogenic agents. Lifestyle choices and occupational exposures have been studied and correlate positively to head and neck cancer. Although extensive evidence exists regarding risk of tobacco and alcohol consumption and the associated development of head and neck cancer, the degree of risk associated with other etiologic factors is not as well documented. Further investigation is clearly indicated, particularly in areas such as molecular genetics, where much of the research is fragmented and preliminary.[25] Table 11-1 summarizes various etiologic factors implicated in the incidence of head and neck cancer.

PREVENTION, SCREENING, AND DETECTION

The primary risk factor for developing cancer of the oral cavity, pharynx, and larynx is *tobacco use* (smoked and smokeless).[24,120,121] It acts as an initiator, promoter, and cocarcinogen, having a linear dose-effect response on the tissues with which it has contact, with smokers having a relative risk 6 to 25 times that of nonsmokers.[121] The level of risk depends on the type of tobacco, daily amount consumed, the duration of the habit, the types of tobacco, the manner in which it is used, and depth of inhalation.[121,137] "Tar" (polycyclic aromatic hydrocarbons) is the primary source of tumorigenic activity in tobacco smoke. Benzo(a)pyrene, vinyl chloride, polonium-210, nickel, and cadmium are some other carcinogenic agents identified in tobacco smoke.[121] The primary constituent responsible for oral cancers is thought to be N^1-nitrosonor nicotine, which has tumor-promoting properties in animals and is present in cigarette smoke condensate, chewing tobacco, and snuff. Relative risk decreases significantly with each year of smoking cessation, but the risk for head and neck neoplasia never returns to that of a nonsmoker.[120]

In combination with *alcohol,* tobacco has been associated with 80% to more than 95% of squamous cell cancers of the head and neck.[128,129] The risk factors of alcohol and tobacco have a maximum effect in the oral cavity and oropharynx in the horseshoe-shaped area that includes the anterior floor of the mouth, the ventrolateral tongue, and the lingual aspect of the retromolar trigone (where saliva pools), as well as the soft palate.[121] Some studies suggest that alcohol, which is both a solvent and an irritant, has an independent carcinogenic action on the oral cavity, pharynx, and larynx, in addition to its synergistic effects with tobacco, when consumed in large amounts.[121,129] Marijuana smoke, which contains a higher concentration of "tar" than tobacco smoke, has been implicated in the development of head and neck cancer.[28,137] Precancerous lesions (erythroplakia more so than leukoplakia) are associated with cancers of the oral cavity, alveolar ridge, gums, and floor of the mouth in people who have dipped or chewed tobacco.[94,133]

Up to 15% of malignancies of the aerodigestive tract may have viral etiologies.[128] The *Epstein-Barr virus* (EBV) related to nasopharyngeal cancer is the virus best described as a risk factor for head and neck cancer. Now mounting evidence exists that the human papillomaviruses (HPVs) and herpes simplex virus type 1 (HSV-1) may be involved in the development of cancers in the aerodigestive tract.[90,120,155] Cancers of the thyroid have been found to occur more frequently in persons who received small doses of radiation therapy 20 previously for acne, chronic tonsillitis, enlarged thymus, or middle ear disease. Nutritional deficiencies (e.g., Plummer-Vinson syndrome), poor oral hygiene, mechanical irritation, occupational exposures, and immunosuppression have also been linked with cancer development in specific sites within the aerodigestive tract.

Risk for second primary tumors in patients with head and neck cancer ranges from 10% to 40%; they may be *synchronous* primaries (simultaneous lesions or those presenting within 6 months of initial diagnosis) or *metachronous* second primaries (appearing 6 months or more after initial diagnosis).* Second and sometimes third primaries, usually occurring in the lung, head, and neck region and esophagus, are explained by the concept of a diffuse mucosal atypia called "field cancerization."[120] This concept poses that once mucosal surfaces of the upper aerodigestive tract have undergone changes (initiation, promotion, and proliferation), changes occur in surrounding tissues.[134] Genetic alterations resulting in the inactivation of oncogenes, inactivation or mutation of tumor-suppressor genes, and amplification of growth factors and their receptors have been linked with the development of head and neck neoplasms.[120] Since these malignancies occur in a small percentage of patients who

---

*References 24, 35, 70, 89, 120, 133.

Table 11-1   Etiology of Head and Neck Cancer: Specific Sites

Site	Carcinogens/occupations	Other factors
Skin	Inorganic arsenics in drugs, water, or occupational environment Ultraviolet rays of sun, ionizing radiation Polycyclic aromatic hydrocarbons, coke ovens, gas workers Chloroprene (neoprene) in synthetic rubber	Burns Riboflavin deficiency Syphilis: lip
Nose and sinuses	Wood dust (furniture industry) Shoe industry (leather manufacturing) Textile workers Radiochemical (Thorotrast) Radium dial painters and chemists (osteogenic sarcomas) Mustard gas Nickel refining Isoprophyl oil BCME: bis(chloromethyl)ether—alkylating agent (produces esthesioneuroepithelioma in animals)	?Chronic sinusitis ?Cigarette smoke
Nasopharynx	Nitrosamines (*N*-nitrosodimethylamine)	Epstein-Barr virus Genetics: Chinese from Kwantung province 25 times more susceptible Vitamin C deficiency Salted fish
Oral cavity	Cigarettes, reverse smoking Ethyl alcohol Snuff, chewing tobacco, betel nut Textile industries Coke ovens Leather manufacturing	Syphilis: tongue Nutrition: vitamin B (riboflavin) deficiencies
Hypopharynx-larynx	Cigarettes Asbestos (ship builders) Mustard gas Polycyclic aromatic hydrocarbons (coke ovens) Ethyl alcohol Wood exposure	Nutrition: riboflavin deficiency
Esophagus	Ethyl alcohol Cigarettes	Nutrition: riboflavin, nitrosamines Race and nationality: Eskimos, Iranians, blacks
Thyroid	Radiation exposure	Iodine deficiencies Genetics
Salivary glands	Radiation	Genetics: Eskimos

Modified from Jesse TC: Etiology of head and neck cancer. In Suen JW, Myers EN, editors: *Cancer of head and neck,* New York, 1981, Churchill Livingstone.

neither smoke nor drink, they may have a genetic predisposition to developing head and neck cancer.[129]

CLASSIFICATION

Carcinomas arising in the head and neck region are classified according to *anatomic regions* rather than cell type. These regions include the (1) oral cavity, (2) oropharynx, (3) nasal cavity, (4) nasopharynx, (5) paranasal sinuses, (6) hypopharynx, (7) larynx, (8) salivary glands, and (9) thyroid gland. Each of these regions is subdivided into specific sites (Figure 11-1 and Table 11-2).

The tumor characteristics of each area, therapeutic management, and prognosis may differ depending on the disease's natural history, the sites of metastases, and the disease's biologic behavior.

DIAGNOSIS

Optimal treatment and patient survival require accurate identification of the primary tumor, local/regional spread and invasiveness, distant metastasis, and synchronous second primaries. All patients should undergo a thorough head and neck examination with the use of a mirror

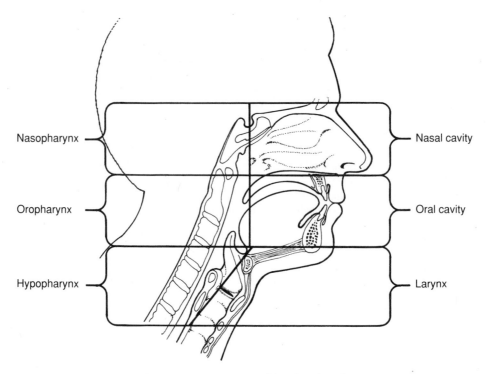

Figure 11-1   Regions of head and neck.

and/or a fiberoptic nasopharyngolaryngoscope. Radiologic examinations should be completed before obtaining a biopsy. A biopsy can alter the mucosa and bone detail and can cause the radiologist to misinterpret the film. Direct triple endoscopy or *panendoscopy* (laryngoscopy, bronchoscopy, laryngoscopy, and selectively employed nasopharyngoscopy) with multiple biopsies performed under general anesthesia is the definitive diagnostic and staging procedure.[120,128] Fine-needle aspiration (FNA) of a suspicious cervical node is performed if no obvious primary is identified. Since open biopsy may jeopardize curative therapy, it is a last resort if panendoscopy and FNA fail to identify a primary site or histopathology.[120] An essential element in head and neck staging is the physician's documentation, including a precise diagram and written description of the extent of disease, to provide all consulting disciplines with accurate data.

STAGING

Head and neck tumors are classified by the American Joint Committee for Cancer Staging and End Results Reporting. Patient information that affects clinical staging of head and neck tumors is listed in the box at right. Head and neck *T classifications* are a general indication of the extent of the primary tumor. These T classifications can be subclassified according to how the tumor affects other anatomic sites. Tumors of the oral cavity and lip are clas-

---

PATIENT INFORMATION NEEDED FOR STAGING HEAD AND NECK TUMORS

FACTS ABOUT TUMOR

Exact location
Histologic type
Estimated degree of local invasion
Local behavior (e.g., exophytic or invasive)
Cytologic grade
Involvement of other structures

LOCAL LYMPH NODE INVOLVEMENT

Location of all suspicious nodes (unilateral/bilateral)
Size
Firmness
Presence of extracapsular spread

DISTANT METASTASIS

Organ system involved
Degree of tumor replacement

PRESENCE OR ABSENCE OF SECOND CANCER

---

sified primarily by the T stage of the lesion. Cancer staging of tumors of the pharynx (nasopharynx, oropharynx, hypopharynx), larynx, and paranasal sinuses is determined by the extent of the primary tumor, depth of tumor invasion, and the number of sites involved. The

Table 11-2 Major Subdivisions of Aerodigestive Tract

Site	Function	Anatomic relationship	Clinical features
Oral cavity	Maintain oral competency for swallowing, articulation	Sensory motor innervation of tongue is bilateral; central chamber of salivary system; sensory innervation mediated by lingual nerve (V); motor innervation to muscles by hypoglossal nerve (XII) Lymphatic drainage to submaxillary and upper cervical lymph nodes and retropharyngeal lymph nodes	Early symptoms: painless "white spot," persistent ulcerations, difficulty with denture fit, difficulty swallowing, blood-tinged sputum
Oropharynx	Mouth and pharynx perform together in alimentary functions of swallowing, emesis, and respiratory functions of crying, speaking, coughing, and yawning	Boundaries include soft palate, tonsils, tonsillar fossa, and base of tongue; glossopharyngeal nerve (IX) mediates motor and sensory innervation to pharynx and posterior one third of tongue; soft palate and pharynx innervated by vagus nerve (X) Lymphatic drainage to jugulodigastric (tonsillar) node and retropharyngeal lymph nodes	Irregular ulcerations of mucosal surfaces, painless growth, dysphagia, pain on swallowing, otalgia, persistent sore throat Late symptoms: speech difficulties, palatal resultant incompetence with nasal regurgitation, dysphagia with or without aspiration, trismus
Nasal cavity	Conditions affecting inspired air before entrance: olfaction humidification, temperature control, cleansing, antibacterial and antiviral protection	First cranial nerve (olfactory) innervates mucous membranes to mediate sense of smell Drainage into submandibular nodes	Similar to chronic sinusitis
Nasopharynx	Anatomic boundary that lies behind nasal cavities and above soft palate	Open space situated just below base of skull behind nasal cavity; inferior wall bordered by soft palate, pharyngeal orifice of eustachian tube, abducens nerve (VI), oculomotor nerve (III), trochlear nerve (IV), and optic nerve (II) Behind eustachian tube lies internal carotid artery, internal jugular vein, and glossopharyngeal (IX), vagus (X), spinal accessory (X), and hypoglossal (XII) nerves Lymph node chain that drains these areas: posterior cervical triangles, supraclavicular nodes, and jugular chain	Persistent poorly localized frontal headaches; temporal, parietal, and orificial pain; decreased hearing, tinnitus; multiple nerve palsies, sensory losses Blood in postnasal drip very significant Profuse epistaxis an infrequent presenting symptom
Paranasal sinuses	Air-filled cavities within bones of skull lined by mucous membranes that drain into nasal cavities	Four pair of maxillary, ethmoid, and frontal sphenoid tumors drain into submaxillary, retropharyngeal, and jugular lymph nodes	Chronic sinusitis, bump on hard palate, swelling, numbness and/or pain of cheek, swelling gums, toothache, increased lacrimation, visual changes: diplopia exophthalmos Persistent unilateral rhinorrhea: epistaxis

Continued.

Table 11-2 Major Subdivisions of Aerodigestive Tract—cont'd

Site	Function	Anatomic relationship	Clinical features
Hypopharynx	Anatomic boundary extending from tip of epiglottis to lower border of cricoid cartilage Structures important for swallowing and airway protection	Lower subdivision of oropharynx, also called laryngopharynx, divided into pyriform sinuses and posterior cricoid area; posterior and lateral pharyngeal walls Pharyngeal constrictions innervated by glossopharyngeal (IX) and vagus (X) nerves Lymphatic drainage: primary along internal jugular vein and retropharyngeal and paratracheal nodes	Painless, enlarged cervical lymph nodes; odynophagia accompanied with progressive dysphagia and rapid weight loss Otalgia on same side of tumor Hoarseness, dysphagia
Larynx	Serves for speech production, maintenance of airway, and airway protection	Located directly below hypopharynx; sensory innervation supplied from internal laryngeal branch of superior laryngeal nerve of vagus and recurrent laryngeal nerve Divided into three anatomic sites: (1) supraglottic, (2) glottic, and (3) subglottic Lymph drainage to anterior jugular nodes	Persistent hoarseness; change in quality, pitch, voice; pain; hemoptysis; dysphagia; cough; aspiration
Salivary glands	Production of saliva	Divided into major glands: paired parotid, submandibular, sublingual, and minor salivary glands Lymphatic drainage usually to deep jugular or intraglandular or paraglandular lymph nodes; innervation of this area includes mandibular branch of seventh cranial, lingual, and hypoglossal (XII) nerves	Painless, rapidly growing mass with or without associated nerve paralysis
Thyroid gland	Endocrine gland	Highly vascular gland located in anterior and lower part of neck; composed of small central part, isthmus, and two lobes; isthmus covers second, third, and fourth tracheal rings; thyroid related medially to esophagus and recurrent laryngeal nerve and laterally to carotid sheath, containing carotid artery; internal jugular vein and vagus nerve Lymphatic drainage of thyroid gland mainly through lymphatic vessels that accompany arterial blood supply	Neck pain, tightness or fullness in neck, hoarseness, dysphagia, dyspnea

depth of invasion can significantly affect normal function and mobility of involved and neighboring structures, such as in the hypopharyngeal/laryngeal region, where the tumor may invade bone or affect cranial nerves (e.g., nasopharyngeal cancer). The *N classifications* indicate location (unilateral or bilateral), number, and size of cervical lymph node metastasis and are uniform for all sites. *M classifications,* which indicate distant spread of disease, are determined by clinical and radiographic findings.[19,129] Using the concept of the greater the T size, the greater the stage, increased extension or invasion results in a higher stage; increased stage of disease is directly related to a poorer prognosis. Staging of head and neck disease is as follows: stage I—Tis or T1-N0-M0; stage II—T2-N0-M0; stage III—T3-N0-M0/T1, T2, or T3-N1-M0/T3-N2-M0; and stage IV—T4-N0 or N1-M0/any T-N2 or N3-M0/any T-any N-M1.[19]

PRETREATMENT EVALUATION
Rationale for Treatment Options

The therapeutic measures available for the management of head and neck cancer include surgery, radiation therapy, and chemotherapy. Treatment modalities may be used alone or in combination. Surgery or radiation therapy is used as standard treatment for patients with very early limited or advanced resectable head and neck cancers. The ultimate goal of all head and neck therapy is patient survival and quality of life. Treatments may be given in an attempt to achieve cure, control, or palliation. If the goal is cure, treatment focuses on local control of the disease and prolonged relapse-free survival. When cure is no longer possible, palliation and control of symptoms become the focus of therapy. Table 11-3 outlines the advantages and disadvantages of the three therapeutic measures, which are briefly discussed next.

Surgery. Surgery is as effective as radiation in eliminating limited cancers of the head and neck region. Surgery may be done effectively without functional and cosmetic loss in small early cancers, which are easily accessible. Surgical failures are usually related to the surgeon's inability to remove the tumor en bloc. A disadvantage of surgery is the potential for structural, functional, or cosmetic loss.

Radiation therapy. Radiation therapy can control the disease in situ, avoids surgical sacrifice of anatomic parts, and preserves functions of speech, swallowing, smell, and cosmesis. Despite acute and long-term sequelae, radiation is classified as the best "tissue and organ sparing" treatment available. Radiation therapy has excellent cure rates for patients with limited disease (T1-N0-M0 and T2-N0-M0).[12,24,31,136,138] Failed radiation therapy in head and neck cancers differs from failed surgery or chemotherapy. Cancer cells that are hypoxic are insensitive to radiation and do not respond well to treatment. Local failure also can occur when occult malignant cells outside the irradiated field are present, when distant metastases through lymphatic and hematogenous spread are present at treatment, or when tissue and organ tolerance to radiation is less than that of the tumor.

Chemotherapy. Chemotherapy is being used in the treatment of patients with advanced or recurrent disease. The curative role of chemotherapy is still undergoing evaluation; however, its adjuvant or palliative roles in the treatment of this disease have been recognized. Normal epithelial tissues depend on certain substances to maintain their integrity and to promote cellular renewal. The role of chemotherapy is now being evaluated for its preventive potential in premalignant lesions (e.g., leukoplakia or erythroplasia of the oral cavity). Vitamin A and its natural analogues, retinoids, are necessary for the normal development and differentiation of epithelial tissues.

Table 11-3 Advantages and Disadvantages of Treatments for Head and Neck Cancers

Modality	Advantages	Disadvantages
Surgery	Ability to remove central-resistant hypoxic tumor cells Immediate reconstruction Provides most accurate estimate of disease extent No carcinogenic effect No biologic resistance by tumor	Potential for structural, functional, or cosmetic loss Only provides local/regional treatment May leave behind viable malignant tissue Must sacrifice some healthy tissue to excise malignancy effectively
Radiation therapy	Curative if disease is small and localized Acute side effects generally disappear after treatment Limited residual deformity or functional loss (in most patients) Focused delivery of tumoricidal dose	Time consuming Not effective as single treatment for large tumors Potential long-term sequelae: soft tissue damage May have carcinogenic effects Some tumors radioresistant
Chemotherapy/biologic therapy	Potential chemopreventive systemic treatment for killing lymphatic and hematogenous metastasis Minimal residual deformity or loss of function	Limiting factors: normal tissue tolerance and tumor responsiveness

(See Chapters 22 and 23 for discussions of drug side effects, specific chemotherapy and biotherapy agents, and treatment combinations.)

Combined research. The ultimate goal of clinical head and neck research is to provide optimal therapies for each patient. Historically, treatment recommendations may have been based on limited experience and knowledge. The Southwest Oncology Group, Radiation Oncology Group, Veterans Administration Head and Neck Study Group, and other intergroup study groups have attempted to answer questions about the natural history and treatment of head and neck cancers as well as patient rehabilitation. These diversified groups are evaluating new therapies, including drugs, surgical techniques, radiation delivery systems, and biologic approaches. The strength of the cooperative group studies is that larger populations are evaluable, which can support statistically significant findings that will direct diagnosis and treatment of patients diagnosed with head and neck cancer.*

Factors Affecting Treatment Decisions

Treatment decisions are always affected by factors related to the tumor, patient, and the health care provider. In choosing a treatment option, especially in head and neck cancer, the treatment team must put in perspective what is to be achieved. Clearly, survival is important and easily measured, but the quality of life during that survival is even more important.[1,20,30,55] The choice of treatment modalities depends on many factors: (1) tumor site and size, (2) extent of lesion and disease, (3) histology and aggressiveness, (4) need for reconstruction, (5) previous treatment, (6) patient's physical and emotional condition, (7) availability of health care providers and resources to provide comprehensive treatment and rehabilitation programs, and (8) quality of life. *Quality of life* is especially relevant because the patient's adjustment to illness can be significantly affected by symptoms and side effects of the disease and treatment. Quality of life issues emphasize the impact of these symptoms on the patient's physical function, physiologic and emotional status, social function and well-being, and financial status, in contrast to the standard performance scales currently used (e.g., Karnofsky and Zubrod).[1,31] Since the potential for disease recurrence still remains high, quality of life is of significant value when making treatment decisions.

Tumor-related factors. Appropriate therapy requires an accurate assessment of the tumor. The size and extent of the primary tumor are equally as important as type and site in determining the treatment. A guide to size and extent of primary head and neck tumors may be found in the American Joint Commission on Cancer Staging and End Results Reporting studies.[19,75] In general,

smaller cancers without metastases (T1 or T2-N0) do not require multimodality treatment. For larger primary tumors (T3 or T4), combined modalities offer a greater chance for quality survival. Patients with regional metastasis classified as N1 or with extension into soft tissues of the neck have benefited from the addition of radiation, which has been shown to prevent recurrence within the neck. Primary lesions that present with regional metastases or distant disease may be best approached by combination therapy incorporating surgery, radiation, and systemic or regional chemotherapy.*

Patient-related factors. Patient-related factors that affect treatment decisions include general health, previous therapy, dental health, social habits, motivation, economic resources, individual needs, and cultural beliefs and values. Many patients have other health conditions (e.g., chronic lung, cardiovascular, hepatic, or renal disease) that limit the clinician's ability to perform surgery or give maximum doses of chemotherapy. The patient brings a unique set of psychosocial experiences to the treatment milieu. An evaluation of the psychosocial status of the patient and significant others may be more important and more difficult to obtain than an evaluation of the patient's physical status.† Many patients with head and neck cancer are chemical (alcohol/tobacco) abusers and may have associated personality disorders. An evaluation of the patient's smoking and drinking habits is essential in forming the treatment plan. History of previous psychiatric difficulties (e.g., clinical depression) can be a "red flag" indicating those at risk for ineffective coping during or after treatment.[138] The nurse must assess the patient for orientation to current medical status, appropriateness of responses to questions and health care directions, and interactions with family or significant others. Often the choice of therapy is influenced by myths and misconceptions the patient or family hold based on previous health-related experiences. With the initial assessment the nurse should attempt to determine how motivated the patient is to comply with the demands of illness and treatment and to survive. Insight into motivation may be gained by obtaining information related to previous ability to work and work habits; life-style; economic status; social networks; perceived resources; health-seeking behaviors and history; culturally related attitudes, values, and beliefs that affect the patient's perception of health and illness; compliance with treatment regimens; and self-care practices.‡ Finally, the nurse must remember that treatment cannot be administered if patients choose not to have therapy. The treatment team has the responsibility to educate patients who elect to take their "chances" about the natural course of their dis-

---

*References 5, 6-8, 51, 60, 78, 81, 111.

---

*References 3, 7-9, 12, 51, 53, 60, 73, 77, 84, 98, 111, 127.
†References 30, 57, 61, 68, 83, 96, 135.
‡References 33, 44, 67, 72, 96, 131, 132.

ease and the ultimate outcome. Regardless of the patient's decision, physical support and symptom control should be offered and continued. Offering educational materials and activating support systems early within the course of disease provide the patient with opportunities for control and self-care and facilitate the nurse-patient relationship.

Health care resources. Treatment of head and neck cancers is influenced by availability of specialists, facilities, equipment, resources, and health care reimbursement and the patient's ability to access care. The skills and experience of the head and neck surgeon, radiotherapist, and medical oncologist vary in each treatment center. Patients receiving treatment in centers that participate in clinical research trials are afforded opportunities to participate in treatment protocols otherwise unavailable. Patients ideally should receive treatment where a comprehensive rehabilitation team is readily available, including dentists, maxillofacial prosthodontists, speech pathologists, nurse specialists, social workers, physical and occupational therapists, and clinical dietitians. If these opportunities are limited, it may be efficacious for the physician to refer the patient to centers that provide such services.

Treatment and Rehabilitative Planning

Treatment and rehabilitative planning are always dictated by the anatomic location and extent of the primary tumor. Before initiation of treatment the patient should be evaluated by an interdisciplinary team.[44,67] Pretreatment assessment by the interdisciplinary groups can accomplish several goals: establish the diagnosis, stage the disease, plan treatment, and integrate prescriptive rehabilitative programs.* Nursing assessment in the pretreatment phase identifies any potential or actual nursing diagnoses that can minimize complications of therapy and promote adjustment of patient and family or significant others to the illness, treatment, and rehabilitation.†

Psychosocial assessment. In general, patients with head and neck cancer and their families respond to the diagnosis of cancer with shock, anxiety, fear, denial, and grief.[55,57,79,91] The patient is faced with a potential threat to body image and self-esteem. The patient may experience severe and permanent facial disfigurement and functional loss that closely resemble those experienced by the burn patient.[14] The face and neck left uncovered by clothing are subject to full view of others. Physical disfigurement or functional loss may pose a threat to the patient's coping, sexuality, and socialization patterns.[14] Patients may feel stigmatized and may become socially isolated. Depression related to the prognosis, altered

body image, or decreased self-esteem can become a major impediment to the rehabilitative process.[67] If surgery is planned, the patient may fear undergoing anesthesia or dying during the surgical procedure.

Potential altered body image or a patient's perception of distortion in body image often plays a significant role in the ability to cope with the illness and the treatment plan.[20,27,30,55,56] A person's body image is a picture or concept of the physical and emotional self, which is incorporated into the person's psychologic construct. Many head and neck cancer patients initially refuse surgery in an attempt to preserve or maintain the concepts of self and function.[57] Body image, self-esteem, and sexuality can be threatened by the results of the surgical procedure. The patient who faces loss of cosmesis, structure, or function (e.g., laryngectomy, tongue or jaw/neck dissection) experiences a major adjustment in body image and may have problems coping. The degree of disfigurement and the patient's perceptions associated with the surgery may intensify the emotional response. The nurse must remember that patients diagnosed with early-stage disease may not face the same issues as those with advanced or recurrent disease. A nursing diagnosis of potential altered patterns of sexuality can be related to changes in appearance, fear of the partner, change in oral and respiratory function, alcohol abuse, or nonacceptance of surgery. Salient questions that should be incorporated into a psychosocial nursing assessment and suggested interventions are listed later in this chapter. These nursing interventions support both patient and family and assist the patient to cope with and adjust to illness.*

Pulmonary assessment and health history. Patients with head and neck cancer may have other significant medical problems. The physician will evaluate the patient for a history of cardiopulmonary disease, diabetes, bleeding disorders, and renal disease. Careful review and documentation of preexisting medical disorders, along with routine paraclinical data, blood chemistries, cardiography, and chest x-ray films, should be evaluated. Disorders such as hypertension, end-stage cardiopulmonary disease, uncontrolled or labile diabetes, or bleeding disorders may preclude or significantly modify surgical interventions. Prognostic signs associated with cardiac disease that carry a high surgical risk for the patient include (1) history of poor exercise tolerance, (2) increasing angina, (3) chronic diabetes, (4) uncontrolled or acute congestive heart failure, (5) severe uncontrolled hypertension, (6) dysrhythmias, (7) acute electrocardiographic (ECG) changes indicating injury or ischemia, and (8) myocardial infarction within 6 months of surgery. Patients with respiratory insufficiency or a significant smoking history should undergo a respiratory evaluation. Patients with respiratory insufficiency or chronic ob-

---

*References 33, 44, 64, 67, 72, 85, 131, 154.
†References 14, 44, 57, 61, 64, 67, 91.

*References 14, 61, 81, 86, 91, 93, 96, 100.

structive lung disease cannot adequately meet the body's oxygenation needs during stress. An aggressive pulmonary hygiene and rehabilitation program can be implemented by the nurse or respiratory therapist.[109] To circumvent complications of atelectasis or aspiration pneumonia, the patient should be instructed on proper posture, lung expansion techniques, and breathing exercises.

Nicotine ingestion is clearly a source that contributes to poor wound healing and loss of reconstructive flaps. Some patients are more sensitive to the peripheral vasoconstrictive and ischemic effects of nicotine than others, and the harmful microcirculatory effects of nicotine may persist weeks after cessation of smoking. When cessation of smoking is critical to the survival of the flap, as with a free island flap, the physician may order preoperative urine nicotine levels. Treatment decisions may be significantly influenced by the patient's ability to quit smoking.[56,62,78,153] A lengthy discussion of smoking cessation programs is not within the scope of this text, but programs such as Fresh Start (American Cancer Society) and In Control (American Lung Association) are among the available resources. A thorough nursing assessment also should include documentation of the use of drugs or chemicals.

Alcoholism is common in this patient population; thus a large percentage of these patients will also have associated medical and psychologic problems related to acute and chronic abuse (e.g., chronic liver disease, peripheral neuropathies, damaged central nervous system [CNS]). Liver function tests and standard coagulation screening tests, including platelet count, partial thromboplastin time, and prothrombin time, should be evaluated. If chronic alcohol abuse is suspected, the nurse should monitor the patient for clinical problems and signs and symptoms related to withdrawal. The alcohol withdrawal syndrome, which includes symptoms ranging from mild tremulousness to delirium tremens, represents the body's defense reaction to withdrawal of the CNS depressant. Anxiety, tremulousness, increased visual imagery, and tachycardia are compensatory mechanisms that are no longer depressed by alcohol. Manifestations of symptoms may be quite variable from time of cessation of alcohol. Agitation, increased anxiety, and mild tremulousness usually occur within the first 24 to 36 hours. Seizures related to withdrawal most frequently occur within 24 to 48 hours, and delirium tremens is often preceded by tremulousness and agitation. In some patients, severe manifestations may be delayed for 3 to 5 days after cessation of drinking. The medical management of alcohol withdrawal syndrome should include (1) maintaining patient hydration, (2) providing adequate calories, (3) administering vitamin supplementation, (4) suppressing CNS hyperactivity with sedation, and (5) monitoring for electrolyte imbalance, metabolic imbalance, and acidosis.

Nutritional assessment. Each of the three major treatment modalities used singly or in combination may affect the patient's nutritional status. Limited caloric intake for extended periods can deplete protein stores.[54,64,115,123] A pretreatment nutritional assessment should be completed because weight loss is common among these patients before, during, and after treatment.[18,26,32,123,144] A recent loss of 10% or more of actual body weight unrelated to dieting or other concurrent medical conditions (e.g., diabetes, infection, alcoholism) is a critical indicator for continued nursing assessment and implementation of a nutritional plan.[40,45,63,72]

The aim of nutritional support in head and neck cancer patients is twofold: to rebuild or maintain protein and to maintain fat stores. Reduced nutritional intake places the patient at risk for a physiologic state of negative nitrogen balance with a resultant loss of protein stores. A reduction in total plasma volume places the patient at risk for blood loss and hypotension and poor wound healing. If the patient is unable to maintain adequate nutrition, the physician may prescribe oral high-calorie, high-protein supplemental feedings. Most physicians choose the oral or enteral route if the patient has a functional gastrointestinal tract. Patients may require placement of a nasogastric, gastrostomy, or jejunostomy feeding tube.[24,141] Jejunostomy tubes are placed when the patient is at high risk for aspiration. The nurse may need to prepare the patient psychologically and educationally if placement of a feeding tube is required. The psychologic and social impact of not being able to eat normally can be devastating to the patient and can result in ineffective coping or social isolation. Nursing education and interventions directed at assisting the patient to cope with these physical changes can help the patient circumvent feelings of not being "normal" or of being "socially unacceptable." Patients should be afforded the opportunity to continue experiencing all sensory input (e.g., smell, sight) and maintaining normal socialization patterns and life-style. The nurse and clinical dietitian may encourage the patient and family to puree normal high-calorie, high-protein meals in the blender before administration. Prepackaged supplements are also available if normal food preparation and blenderized meals are not a practical option. (See Chapter 28 for a complete review of nursing diagnoses, assessment, interventions, and care plans related to nutrition.)

Communication and cognitive motor skills. A thorough nursing assessment of the patient's reading, comprehension, and communication skills should be accomplished before the initiation of the definitive therapy. Education should be tailored to the patient's specific need and educational level. If patients have limited reading or writing skills, education may need to be accomplished by using simple explanations, pictures, or videos. Explanations without medical jargon facilitate effec-

Table 11-4   Functional Loss Associated with Laryngectomy

Procedure	Structures removed	Structures remaining	Functions
TOTAL LARYNGECTOMY Loss of laryngeal sphincter mechanism may lead to aspiration. Swallowing mechanism must be intact so that when food lands on vocal cords, patient coughs to remove it and swallows instantly.	Hyoid bone Entire larynx Epiglottis, false/true cords Cricoid cartilage Two/three rings of trachea	Tongue Pharyngeal walls Lower trachea	Loss of voice (resulting from tracheal laryngectomy) Normal swallowing
PARTIAL SUPRAGLOTTIC/ HORIZONTAL LARYNGECTOMY During supraglottic laryngectomy, muscles that elevate larynx are transected, thereby limiting elevation of larynx. This, along with loss of supraglottic structures, further downgrades swallowing. Because cough is necessary to clear larynx, patient's pulmonary functions must be adequate.	Hyoid bone Epiglottis False cords	True cords Cricoid cartilage Trachea	Normal voice Increased risk for aspiration Normal airway
HEMIVERTICAL LARYNGECTOMY Interferes very little with swallowing. Removal of arytenoid cartilage may cause aspiration in a small percentage of patients. Free or pedicled muscle or submucosal cartilage grafts may prevent aspiration. If surgical resection extends to base of tongue, swallowing may be affected related to inability to move bolus. Aspiration may occur.	One true cord, one false cord Arytenoid cartilage One-half thyroid cartilage	Epiglottis One true cord, one false cord Cricoid	Hoarse but serviceable voice Normal airway Normal swallowing
PARTIAL LARYNGECTOMY/ LARYNGOFISSURE Procedure may affect predominantly deglutition and phonation.	One vocal cord	All other structures	Hoarse but serviceable voice Normal airway Normal swallowing

tive communication. Alternative forms of communication will need to be established with the patient before undergoing definitive surgical procedures such as laryngectomy, glossectomy, or palatal resection. Also, a thorough hearing, speech, and visual examination should be accomplished in patients undergoing these procedures. Deficits in any of these functional areas need to be identified before surgery to facilitate appropriate rehabilitation. Table 11-4 outlines functional losses related to the four types of laryngectomies. Pretreatment consultation with a speech pathologist facilitates communication among the patient, family, and nurse; establishes a trusting relationship among professional, patient, and family;

and decreases anxiety. Meeting members of the rehabilitation team before treatment serves as a nonverbal statement to the patient that wellness and rehabilitation are the primary treatment foci. If the patient is scheduled for a laryngectomy, a presurgical visit by a trained laryngologist before hospital admission may allay the patient's fears and anxieties.

Dental Assessment

Dental care is important before, during, and after head and neck cancer treatment.[24,69,90,105,129] Assessing the dental history gives the nurse insight into the patient's knowledge, beliefs, and resources toward preventive care, as well as susceptibility to dental disease. Oral pathology may be present if the patient has not been evaluated or treated by a dentist. An accurate dental history is critical to prevention of oral complications during therapy. The following questions should be incorporated into a nursing dental history:

1. When was the patient's last dental visit, and what type of procedures were done?
2. How often does the patient see a dentist?
3. Does the patient have a relevant history of:
   a. Sore swollen gums, drainage, or boils?
   b. Toothaches or teeth sensitive to hot, cold, or chewing?
   c. Loose teeth?
4. Does the patient have loose, poorly fitting dentures or recurring problems with denture sores?
5. Does the patient have bad breath odor?
6. What kind of toothpaste or dental floss does the patient use?

Oral assessment by the dentist, hygienist, or nurse can facilitate identification of oral disease. The hard and soft oral tissue should be systematically and thoroughly examined. Equipment needed for an oral examination includes good light source, gloves, tongue blade, and unsterile 2 × 2 gauze square. Labial mucosa, vestibule, anterior dentition, and gingiva can be examined by retracting the lips. Buccal mucosa, vestibule, posterior dentition, and gingiva can be examined by retracting the cheeks. Dorsum and lateral surfaces of the tongue can be inspected by grasping the tip of the tongue using a 2 × 2 gauze. Wrapping tongue to palate allows for examination of the floor of the mouth and lingual frenulum. By tilting the patient's head back, with chin up and mouth wide open, the hard palate, maxillary dentition, and gingiva can be inspected. All patients with dentures should have them evaluated for proper fit. Instability and excessive movement of the dentures potentially cause irritation and may become a source of infection. The nurse should pay particular attention to all denture-bearing surfaces: floor of mouth, hard and soft palate, and lateral borders of the tongue. Demonstrated gingival recession, hypertrophy or decayed teeth, denture sores, or exposed roots should be documented, and the dentist should be consulted.

An individual dental treatment plan that reflects the patient's present and future dental needs should be developed. All corrective procedures should be completed before initiation of any treatment. The dentist or hygienist will take a full-mouth x-ray film (panorex), scale the teeth, and evaluate the roots. A pretreatment panorex identifies the presence of teeth in edentulate patients when radiation to this area is planned. Teeth should be extracted and restored, dental plaque and calculus removed, and periodontal disease corrected before initiation of treatment. If advanced periodontal disease ex-

ists on the teeth, it is best to extract the teeth in the involved area. Periodontal disease and poor oral care are major sources of infection during treatment. All these procedures should be completed 10 to 14 days before the initiation of therapy. This waiting period allows for adequate healing of extraction sites. The nurse should enlist the patient's active participation in his or her dental care and oral hygiene. Patient education should include (1) oral hygiene instructions emphasizing the importance of cessation of use of tobacco and alcohol products; (2) fluoride application and oral hygiene instructions taught initially and on an individual basis or as outlined on the radiation care plan; (3) nutritional counseling, especially limiting sucrose intake; and (4) avoiding commercially available mouthwashes that contain alcohol. The type of floss is not as important as compliance. The mechanical action of vertically moving the floss against the tooth disrupts bacterial colonization. Daily fluoride application should be encouraged as part of a preventive dental and oral care regimen. Fluoride is an anticarious agent with antibacterial properties that promotes remineralization of the enamel. Three types of fluoride are available for use: acidulated phosphate fluoride, neutral sodium fluoride, and stannous fluoride.[69] The fluoride of choice, as with oral rinses and toothpastes, should be nonirritating to the mucosa, readily available, and convenient. Patients undergoing radiation therapy with teeth included in the treatment field should have custom fluoride carrier trays, which will need to be prescribed by the dentist. These fluoride-filled trays are placed over dry teeth for at least 5 minutes to obtain a therapeutic effect (Figure 11-2). The patient should spit out the excess fluoride after removing the tray, but should not rinse, eat, or drink for

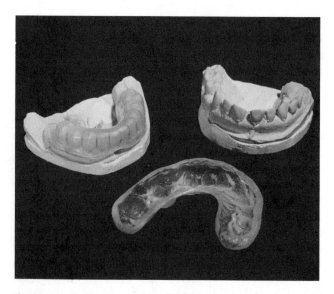

Figure 11-2 Oral cavity molds used to prepare individual carrier fluoride trays.

Table 11-5 Fluoride Sources

Type	Method of application
Sodium fluoride	Carrier technique
Stannous fluoride	Mixed with water and brushed on
Acidulated phosphate fluoride	Brushed on

30 minutes after application. When patients are experiencing episodes of severe mucositis or xerostomia, they may need to convert to a brush-on technique if placement of carrier trays is painful. Regardless of the fluoride delivery method employed, fluoride must be used daily and continuously when patients undergo radiation.

Most dentists will recommend a neutral sodium or stannous fluoride gel. It is important for the nurse to understand the differences in fluoride preparations and application techniques (Table 11-5). All patients with dentures should be instructed to keep the dentures and denture-soaking containers clean. Ideally, soaking containers should be disposable and the cleaning solution (any commercial brand) should be discarded and replaced daily.[41] Common soaking solutions that have been found to inhibit microbial growth include chlorhexidine gluconate (Stuart Pharmaceuticals, Wilmington, Del), Chloroseptic (Norwich Eaton Pharmaceuticals, Norwich, NY), or Efferdent (Warner-Lambert Company, Morris Plains, NJ). Chlorhexidine oral rinse is used as an anticarious agent. *Streptococcus mutans,* a component of caries-producing dental plaque, has proved to be sensitive to chlorhexidine rinse solutions.[41,148] Mouth rinses with 0.1% or 0.2% aqueous solution of chlorhexidine used twice a day have proved effective in inhibiting plaque formation. In addition to a meticulous oral care program, the nurse should educate the patient about the importance of a balanced diet that emphasizes limiting sucrose intake. Sugarless gum and mints are acceptable and should be encouraged.

TREATMENT MODALITIES

Marked improvements in the treatment of head and neck cancer have been made in the 1990s compared with therapies offered in the 1960s. New surgical techniques, radiotherapeutic approaches, and chemotherapy are now used earlier in patient management. However, only 30% of patients with resected cancers are alive after 5 years. Unfortunately, the incidence of local/regional failures is as high as 60%, with systemic metastases developing in more than 10% of this patient population. The sites of occurrence for second primary tumors vary from 10% in the larynx to 40% in the oropharynx, with the remainder in the esophagus, lung, and bladder. The second tumors usually prove to be the cause of death.

Surgery

The primary goal of surgery for head and neck cancer is removal of the primary disease and all metastatic lymph nodes in hope of controlling local disease and preventing recurrent disease. A secondary goal is to preserve structure and function as much as possible without compromising the treatment.[39] A final goal is to maximize the cosmetic and functional outcome.*

Surgery plays a major role in the diagnosis and staging of head and neck tumors. Surgical approaches to the treatment of these tumors depend greatly on the site and size of the primary lesion, the presence of cervical lymph nodes, and whether the patient has distant metastases.[24,75,129] Although surgical management of benign lesions usually involves local excision, malignant lesions require wide resections with or without regional lymphadenectomy and reconstruction at the time of definitive procedure. When cure is no longer within the scope of treatment, the physician can offer palliative surgical options (e.g., tracheostomy, gastrostomy, jejunostomy placement, venous access, implantable ports).

Presurgical assessment. Preoperative patient assessment, medical evaluation, and health team communication focused on rehabilitation can minimize postoperative complications and help the patient to cope with illness. Additional time spent in preoperative education and planning may actually decrease postoperative complications, decrease the period of inpatient convalescence, and improve the overall quality of postoperative survival. Guidelines for preoperative and postoperative nursing care are presented later in this section.

A presurgical nutritional evaluation is essential because patients with head and neck cancer often experience weight loss and interference with food and fluid intake. A reduction in nutritional intake, protein stores, and total plasma volume places the patient at risk for blood loss and hypotension. The nurse should monitor the patient for clinical signs and symptoms of hypovolemia, such as persistent tachycardia, dizziness, or syncope. The physician may order a volume replacement with red blood cells, albumin, or normal saline. The most efficient tissue oxygenation in microcirculation takes place in normal persons with a hemoglobin level greater than 10 g and a hematocrit level greater than 30%.† The nurse should be aware that if volume depletion has occurred rapidly, a false increase in the hemoglobin and hematocrit levels may be present for a short time. Preoperatively, the nurse should initiate a dietary consultation. It may be necessary to give the patient oral supplements, enteral feedings by tube, or short-term parenteral therapies before surgery. Follow-up nutritional support should be

---

*References 27, 34, 56, 65, 66, 71, 83, 92, 95, 103, 117, 118, 153, 156.
†References 18, 26, 45, 54, 62, 63, 78, 82, 115.

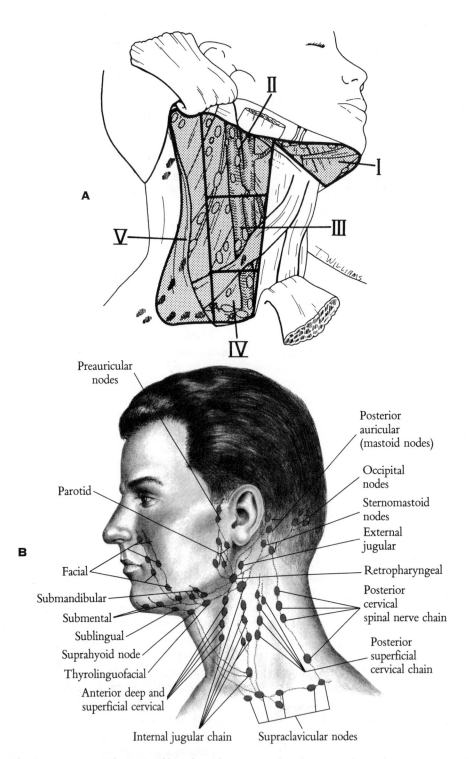

Figure 11-3 **A,** Schematic of lymph node regions of neck. **B,** Lymphatic drainage system of head and neck. (**A** from Cummings CW and others, editors: *Otolaryngology–head and neck surgery*, ed 2, St Louis, 1993, Mosby; **B** from Seidel HM and others: *Mosby's guide to physical examination*, ed 3, St Louis, 1995, Mosby.)

The following exercises have been developed to increase the movement and strength in your neck, arms, and shoulders.

Neck Range of Motion

1. Bring chin to chest in a relaxed way and then let it fall gently backwards so a stretch on the neck muscles is felt.
2. Slowly turn head as far as possible to one side as if attempting to look over that shoulder. Do the same to the other side.
3. Bend the head toward the shoulder on the unaffected side. A stretching will be felt on the operated side.

Shoulder Mobility

1. Standing with shoulders relaxed and head facing forward, let arm on the affected side hang freely. Make circles with the shoulder by moving it:
   a) forward
   b) upward
   c) backward
   d) downward
2. With a wand or cane in front of body and shoulders and arms relaxed, raise wand as high as possible keeping elbows extended. After you are able to raise it directly overhead, slowly lower it behind the neck. Raise wand overhead and return it to starting position.
3. Stand facing a wall with your feet a few inches from it. Slide the hand on your affected side up the wall as far as possible, using the wall for support. Perform the same exercise with your affected side facing the wall. Repeat the motion of sliding your hand up the wall but do not turn your body when doing this exercise.

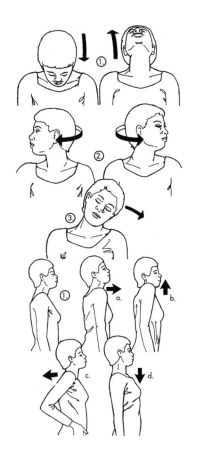

Figure 11-4   Exercises after neck dissection. (From Sigler BA, Schuring LT: *Ear, nose, and throat disorders*, St Louis, 1993, Mosby.)

evaluated on an ongoing basis by the nurse, dietitian, physician, and patient.

During the preoperative phase the nurse needs to assess the patient's cognitive skills, motor skills, and ability to communicate. Any potential sensory deficits (e.g., vision, hearing, fine motor writing skills) could affect the patient's ability to participate in the postoperative rehabilitative process.

Surgical procedures. Cosmesis, body image, and function can be affected significantly by the type of primary and reconstructive procedures.* In addition to the primary surgery, the patient may require a lymph node dissection. The head and neck have about 300 lymph nodes, about 30% of the total lymph nodes in the body. Approximately 75 nodes are present on each side of the neck, most of which are in the deep jugular and spinal accessory chains (Figure 11-3).

The nodes most frequently involved in metastatic carcinoma are those in the deep jugular chain, which extends from the base of the skull to the clavicle. The decision to perform a neck dissection is based on the presence of lymph nodes or, in a clinically negative neck, based on the probability of metastasis.[75,98,107] Table 11-6 lists the types of radical neck procedures, structures removed, and advantages and disadvantages of each procedure. *Modified neck dissection* is a term used to describe several different procedures that are modified from the classic, complete, or radical neck dissections.

Patients who have had a radical or modified procedure may benefit from a preoperative physical therapy evaluation. Functional parameters that are evaluated include head rotation and arm and shoulder mobility (Figure 11-4).

When the spinal accessory nerve has been sacrificed, the head and shoulder range of mobility is significantly affected and the patient faces the potential for permanent disability and chronic pain.[42,124]

Reconstruction. The primary goal of most head and neck surgery before 1981 was to remove the cancer, replace the anatomic structure, and restore cosmesis. With the advent of muscle, musculocutaneous, and free tissue transfer, more attention is dedicated to restoration of functional losses and rehabilitation. Surgeon and communication scientists are coordinating efforts to identify and improve reconstructions of the oral cavity that focus on functions of swallowing and speech. Videofluoro-

---

*References 4, 16, 17, 27, 34, 39, 66, 71, 92, 95, 103, 122, 124, 125, 143-147, 149, 153.

Table 11-6 Radical Neck Procedures

Procedure	Structures removed	Advantages	Disadvantages
Comprehensive (classic) neck dissection: bilateral or unilateral			
Radical neck dissection	En bloc removal of nodal regions I to VI and all lymph node–bearing tissues on one side of neck, superficial and deep fascia, sternocleidomastoid muscle, omohyoid muscle, submandibular gland, tail of parotid gland, internal and external jugular veins, connective tissue of carotid sheath, transverse cervical vessels, spinal accessory nerve, greater auricular nerve, cutaneous branches of the cervical plexus; excision may also include external carotid artery, portion of digastric muscle, branches of vagus nerve, and hypoglossal nerve	Low probability of leaving nodal disease behind	Trapezius muscle dysfunction with shoulder drop, resulting in pain and limitation in motion Mild to moderate neck deformity If bilateral procedure is performed, cerebral edema may persist Painful neuromas may occur Loss of carotid artery
Modified radical neck dissection	Unilateral removal of nodal regions I to V with preservation of spinal accessory nerve, internal jugular, and/or sternocleidomastoid muscle	Low incidence of shoulder drop and shoulder disability Carotid artery not sacrificed Cosmetic deformity not as severe as with comprehensive neck dissection If cervical plexus preserved, decreased incidence of sensory deficit and painful neuromas	Possible omission of occult positive nodes Increased risk of hematoma under sternocleidomastoid muscle Increased risk of surgeon cutting into positive nodes and seeding neck Increased difficulty in performing secondary procedure and if disease recurs
Type I	Spinal accessory nerve preserved		
Type II	Spinal accessory nerve and internal jugular preserved		
Type III (functional or Bocca) neck dissection	Spinal accessory nerve, internal jugular, and sternocleidomastoid preserved		
Selective neck dissection	Spinal accessory, internal jugular, and sternocleidomastoid muscles preserved	Same as for modified neck dissection, plus improved lymphatic drainage because selected lymph node groups retained	Increased possibility of cutting into or omitting occult positive nodes
Lateral neck dissection	En bloc removed of nodal regions II, III, and IV		
Anterolateral neck dissection	Supraomohoid neck dissection: en bloc removal of nodal regions II, III, and IV Expanded supraomohyoid neck dissection: en bloc removal of nodal regions I, II, III, and IV		
Posterolateral neck dissection	Removal of suboccipital and retroauricular lymph node groups and nodal regions II, III, IV, and V		
Extended neck dissection	Any neck dissection extended to include lymph node groups not usually removed or structures not routinely removed (e.g., carotid artery, levator scapular muscle)	Lower probability of leaving occult disease behind	Increased risk of cerebrovascular accident (stroke) if carotid is resected Increased risk of shoulder dysfunction if levator scapular muscle excised

Data from Medina JE, Rigual NM: Neck dissection. In Cummings CW and others, editors: *Otolaryngology–head and neck surgery,* ed 2, St Louis, 1993, Mosby.

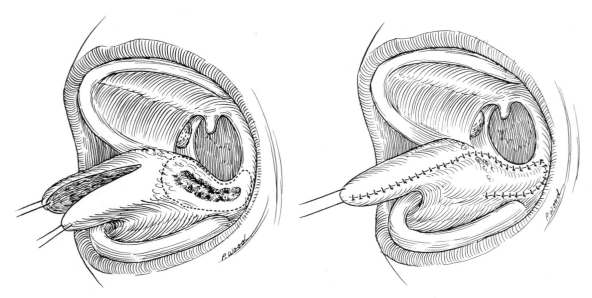

Figure 11-5 Tongue flap used for reconstruction of lateral oropharynx. (From Cummings CW and others, editors: *Otolaryngology–head and neck surgery*, ed 2, St Louis, 1993, Mosby.)

scopic studies are done to evaluate the patient's communicative ability, tongue strength, and range of motion. When done preoperatively and postoperatively, these studies can help measure the patient's progress in rehabilitation. Patient education is essential to a patient's adjustment to illness, empowerment, and rehabilitation when considering reconstructive surgery.

The goals of reconstructive surgery are better accepted if the patient understands the reasons for considering various surgical options, such as flap versus graft or secondary wound healing. Patients must understand that no restorative surgery can return them to complete normalcy and that function and imperfection in contour are an expected outcome. When immediate reconstruction is performed, it is important and reasonable to anticipate possible need for revisions or future procedures. Surgical removal of head and neck tumors can result in functional and socially unacceptable cosmetic deformities. Many patients undergo immediate reconstruction. Patients may be faced with more than one surgical procedure for reconstruction, including autogenous tissue and all-aplastic material.* Normal physiology is best achieved when the surgeon uses autogenous tissue. Soft tissue defects can be closed by direct approximation (suturing), free skin grafts, pediculed tissue (using local, regional, or distant flaps), or free flaps transferred by microvascular anastomoses. Skeletal tissue is best provided by living vascularized bone grafts or flaps.† Nonvascularized bone grafts or all-aplastic material can be used for bone re-

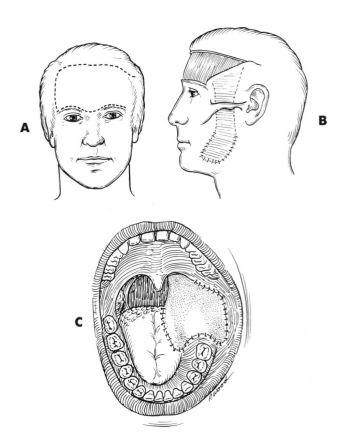

Figure 11-6 **A**, Forehead flap based on superficial temporal artery and portions of occipital artery. **B**, Rotation of forehead flap medial to zygomatic arch for reconstruction of oropharynx. Flap is pulled interiorly to fill resected area. **C**, Completion of forehead flap reconstruction. (From Cummings CW and others, editors: *Otolaryngology–head and neck surgery*, ed 2, St Louis, 1993, Mosby.)

---

*References 15, 17, 34, 43, 65, 66, 71, 82, 92, 103, 114, 117, 124, 125, 142, 146, 149, 156.
†References 15, 17, 114, 142, 145, 153.

placement.[128,129] Small defects can usually be covered by primary closure.

Moderate-size defects may require skin grafting or local skin flaps (Figures 11-5 and 11-6). Table 11-7 outlines factors that affect the surgeon's choice of flap. Several types of flaps are available for reconstruction: (1) tongue flaps are used to cover internal mucosal defects such as floor of mouth, pharyngeal wall, or cheek; (2) skin flaps consist of skin, the subcutaneous tissues, and the fascia of the underlying muscle; and (3) myocutaneous flaps incorporate an island of desired skin and underlying subcutaneous tissue, and fascia is severed from

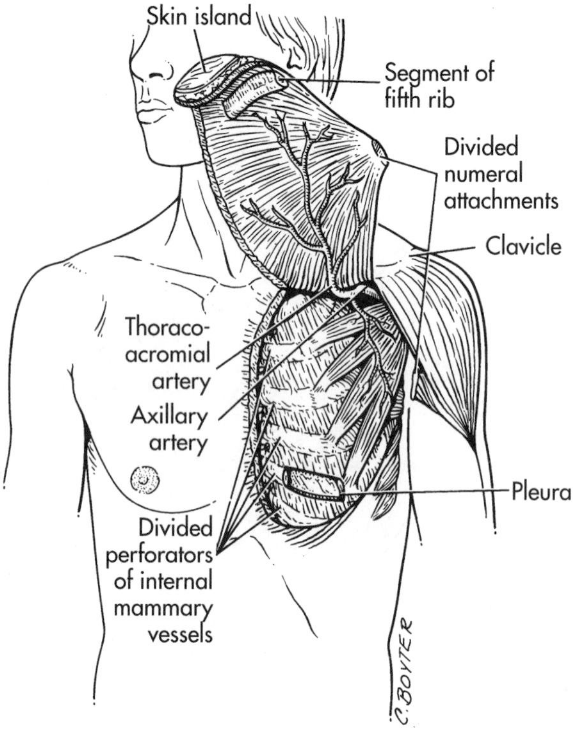

Figure 11-7   Diagrammatic representation of myocutaneous flap procedure. (From Mathes S, Nahai F: *Clinical applications for muscle and musculocutaneous flaps,* St Louis, 1982, Mosby.)

An opening (fistula) has been created between the tracheostoma (windpipe) and esophagus (food passage) in order to place a speech valve (prosthesis). Temporarily, a red rubber catheter will stent the fistula open. Once healing has taken place, a speech prosthesis will replace the catheter.

If the Prosthesis Comes Out

1. Insert a red rubber catheter (10, 12, 14 Fr) into fistula approximately 6-8 inches.
2. Tie a knot in the external end of the catheter to prevent passage of stomach contents.
3. Tape external end of catheter to skin of chest.
4. If catheter cannot be inserted, contact your physician or speech therapist immediately. This may indicate closure of the fistula.

Replacing the Prosthesis

1. Remove prosthesis.
2. Cleanse neck and stoma.

3. Using inserter that is supplied with prosthesis, reinsert clean prosthesis into fistula.
4. Tape in place.
5. Clean prosthesis with hydrogen peroxide and water. Rinse well.
6. The voice prosthesis will last from 2 weeks to several months between changes. The length of time a prosthesis remains in place is dependent upon you. If food or fluid leaks around the prosthesis, it should be changed. If leakage continues, contact your speech therapist for a new size or length of prosthesis.

To Use the Prosthesis

1. Cover your stoma with your thumb. This will allow air from your lungs to pass through the opening of the prosthesis into the esophagus. The walls of your throat and the structures in your mouth will form the words for speech.

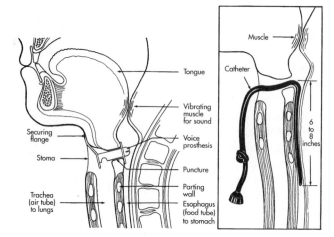

Figure 11-8   Care of tracheoesophageal puncture. (From Sigler BA, Schuring LT: *Ear, nose, and throat disorders,* St Louis, 1993, Mosby.)

Table 11-7 Factors that Affect Surgeon's Choice of Flaps

Tissue considerations	Physician considerations
Size of arc	Will the flap cover the defect?
Vascular supply	Will the flap survive?
Accessibility	How close to defect is the new tissue?
Donor site	Functional loss and contour of donor site
Sensation	Maintain nerve supply

all surrounding tissues (Figure 11-7). A full thickness of underlying muscle is lifted with its blood supply. When reconstruction is not technically feasible, the patient may require fitting with a prosthesis (e.g., externally for a total ear or nose; internally for a palate). Preoperative consultation with a maxillofacial prosthodontist is necessary. This preoperative consultation allows the patient and professional to evaluate all options for reconstruction. The surgeon and prosthodontist must work collaboratively. Appropriate planning for surgical resection and reconstruction allows for the anchoring and stabilization of a prosthesis (Figure 11-8).

Radiation Therapy

Radiation therapy for head and neck tumors can be divided into three treatment categories: curative, palliative, or adjunctive to surgery or chemotherapy.* Treatment planning is based on the nature, size, location, and growth of the tumor; volume of disease; organs to be spared; and purpose of treatment. Radiation energies of 1 million volts or greater and radioactive isotopes are usually the primary sources of treatment in head and neck cancers. These are termed *megavoltage radiation sources,* and they possess some very important physical advantages in the treatment of head and neck cancers, such as skin-sparing effects, increase in depth of dose, formation of a sharp beam (which minimizes unnecessary damage to adjacent tissues and organs), and a bone-sparing effect related to decreased absorption by soft tissue and bone.[59,150]

In treatment of head and neck cancers, radiotherapy may be given preoperatively to prevent marginal recurrences and to control subclinical disease at the primary site or in the nodes. It is also used to convert technically inoperable tumors to operable ones. The combination of preoperative irradiation and surgery is successful in decreasing both local and regional recurrence.† However,

the major disadvantages of preoperative radiation are (1) the normal tissue reaction to radiation may obscure the surgeon's ability to determine the exact extent of the tumor margin, and (2) the risk for postoperative complications are higher. Preoperative radiation is usually given for 1 month, followed by a 1-month rest period, which allows time for the acute tissue reaction to subside but stays within a time frame when radioactive cell kill is still occurring.[152]

Postoperative radiation therapy may also be given to treat residual disease at the surgical margins and subclinical disease in the lymph nodes or may be implanted in the wound. Radiation treatments are usually given about 3 or 4 weeks (preferably no more than 6 weeks) after surgery to allow wound healing. Treatment usually lasts 6 to 8 weeks.

In addition to external beam radiation, *radioactive isotopes* and *intracavitary implants* are sources of radiation that may be applied closely to tumors by hollow containers loaded with radioactive sources. These techniques are beneficial when treating tumors of the antrum, sinuses, and nasal cavity. These interstitial or intracavitary implants can be used for the treatment of the tongue, tonsils, nasopharynx, oral cavity, and metastatic neck nodes.[73,112] Interstitial irradiation is often used in the management of early localized T1 lesions of the nasal vestibule with no detectable lymph nodes. Larger and more infiltrating (T2) squamous cell carcinomas are treated by implants alone or with external beam radiation. This technique is termed *brachytherapy.* The advantage of brachytherapy is that it permits the delivery of irradiation at a high volume over a short period while delivering a relatively low dose to surrounding tissues.[99] Interest in protocols that examine "organ preservation" have been developed in the area of advanced laryngeal cancers.

Pretreatment assessment. Immobilization devices (e.g., head straps, bite blocks, light cast molds), portal planning films, and simulation, and dosimetry port films all must be prepared before initiation of radiation treatment. Pretreatment medical work-ups, including physical examinations, radiographs with or without contrast, computed tomography (CT), magnetic resonance imaging (MRI), nutritional evaluation, and paraclinical laboratory studies, should be completed before initiation of treatment. If anemia, weight loss, or electrolyte imbalance exists, every medical effort should be made to correct imbalances, since anemic patients do not tolerate radiation therapy well and tumors do not respond as well. Once the type and amount of radiotherapy are determined, a pretreatment psychosocial assessment should be completed by the nurse, including the following questions:

• How does the patient interpret his or her current physical status?

*References 60, 73, 76, 77, 84, 98.
†References 7-9, 13, 59, 110.

Text continued on p. 251.

NURSING MANAGEMENT

HEAD AND NECK SURGERY

NURSING DIAGNOSES

- *Knowledge deficit related to surgery, preoperative/postoperative procedures*
- *Self-care deficit related to postoperative treatments*
- *Anxiety related to the surgical experience and unpredictable outcome*

INTERVENTIONS: Preoperative

- Review purpose of surgery and rationale (e.g., temporary versus permanent tracheostomy).

- Explain common terms and procedures, provide written literature (show videos), and show actual equipment. Patient will need to be familiar with terminology/equipment.
- Discuss potential sequelae of surgery:
  —Change in body appearance
  —Change in body function (e.g., breathing, speaking, swallowing, coughing, mobility)
- Explain roles of various medical and nursing personnel and purpose of visits:
  —Medicine
  —Respiratory therapy
  —Nursing/clinical nurse specialist/nurse practitioner
  —Home care coordinator
- Determine means of nonverbal communication to be used in the postoperative period (as appropriate).
- Instruct and have patient give verbal return demonstration on all self-care (e.g., coughing, deep breathing, ambulation).
- Document (in nursing notes):
  —Patient's level of understanding
  —Patient's ability to perform self-care behavior
  —Patient education materials given

INTERVENTIONS: Postoperative

- Instruct patient on self-care behaviors:
  —Provide patient education materials.
  —Teach patient to report symptoms of discomfort.
  —Teach patient the importance of ambulation, coughing, deep breathing, and rehabilitation.
- Document:
  —Patient's response to surgery, functional level, self-care level, and ability to perform procedures
  —Patient's level of understanding
  —Patient's ability to perform self-care
  —Patient education materials given

OUTCOME GOALS: Preoperative

Patient will be able to:
- Demonstrate decreased anxiety.
- Demonstrate knowledge about planned surgical procedure.
- Effectively communicate feelings.
- Demonstrate ability to perform self-care, and seek assistance as necessary.
- Name surgery and describe it.

- State reason for surgery, physical changes, and expected outcomes.

- State expectations of intraoperative care and professionals involved.

- State immediate postoperative care, and perform self-care behaviors.

- State he or she is less anxious when questioned.
- Describe nonverbal means of communication for use in postoperative period (as appropriate).

OUTCOME GOALS/RATIONALE: Postoperative

Patient will be able to:
- Demonstrate decreased anxiety.
- Demonstrate knowledge about postoperative care and rehabilitation.
- Effectively communicate feelings.
- Demonstrate ability to perform self-care.
- Demonstrate realistic expectations for assistance needed for postoperative care.

INTERVENTIONS: *Postoperative–cont'd*

- Discharge patient with written instructions:
- Specific self-care behaviors (e.g., tracheostomy/ laryngectomy care exercise, wound management, oral/ dental hygiene, signs and symptoms to report to physician)
- Tips for tracheostomy care:
  —When performing tracheostomy care at home, patient may use clean technique.
  —Keep peristomal area clean and dry to protect it from erosive secretions and prevent infections. From 3 to 5 ml of sterile or disinfected (e.g., quart of water boiled for 15 minutes with a teaspoon of salt added) saline may be instilled in tracheostomy to lavage and irritate trachea and bronchi, thereby stimulating a cough to clear tenacious secretions.
  —Wear stoma cover/bib to protect stoma, filter out dust and other airborne particles, warm the air entering the trachea, and help retain some of expired humidity.
  —Avoid extremes of temperatures; exposure to dust, gas fumes, and aerosolized vapors; and submersion of stoma under water.
- Emergency procedures (list of appropriate nursing/ medical personnel to contact in case of emergency)
- Medic-Alert wallet card and necklace/bracelet should be carried/worn at all times to indicate that person is a neck breather.
- Home care referral

OUTCOME GOALS/RATIONALE: *Postoperative–cont'd*

- State emergency procedures and names of personnel to contact.

NOTE: These instructions ensure a safe homebound environment even if patient demonstrates independence in hospital setting. It is not unusual for patient to become overwhelmed with information and experience difficulty processing it on discharge.

NURSING DIAGNOSES

- *Breathing pattern, ineffective, related to diversional methods (tracheostomy, laryngectomy)*
- *Airway clearance, ineffective, related to tracheal edema, secretions*
- *Injury, risk for, related to hematoma formation between flap and underlying tissue*
- *Tissue perfusion, altered, related to arterial erosion rupture around/at surgical site*
- *Skin integrity, impaired, related to surgery flap reconstruction, flap failure*
- *Swallowing, impaired, related to superior laryngeal nerve injury, loss or weakness of tongue*
- *Communication, impaired verbal, related to airway diversion or loss/weakness of tongue*

Potential Clinical/Collaborative Problems

- Respiratory distress
- Hypoxia, airway obstruction, tracheal edema, aspiration
- Hemorrhage
- Hematoma
- Arterial rupture
- Failure of flap survival
- Nerve damage

INTERVENTIONS: *Postoperative*

- Monitor signs and symptoms of respiratory distress:
  —Restlessness, agitation, confusion
  —Complaint of air hunger, inability to breathe
  —Diminished or absent air exchange in breath sounds over tracheostomy, laryngectomy tube

OUTCOME GOALS/RATIONALE: *Postoperative*

- If tracheostomy is not placed during surgical procedure, tissue swelling (tracheal edema) may occur during the first 24 hours; patient should be observed for airway obstruction. Intrinsic laryngeal edema or hematoma and increased anxiety or apprehension can

Continued.

INTERVENTIONS: *Postoperative–cont'd*

- —Use of accessory muscle retractions of soft tissues around airway
- Monitor signs and symptoms of hemorrhage:
  - —Continuous oozing of blood or bleeding around surgical site, drains, tracheostomy, laryngectomy, unrelated to manipulation of auctioning, reconstruction
  - —Presence of unusual edema around wound, stoma, reconstructive site, drainage tubes

- Monitor signs and symptoms of hematoma:
  - —Check drains for patency.
  - —Notify physician immediately if presence of air, serum, or milky fluids.
  - —Normal, excessive, absent.
    Air indicates dead space; milky drainage may indicate fistula formation with thoracic duct.
    Leakage can lead to severe fluid/electrolyte loss.

- Monitor signs and symptoms of infection:
  - —Vital signs
  - —Drainage/odor
  - —Intake/output
- Monitor wound and surrounding tissue for signs and symptoms of arterial erosion/rupture:
  - —Evidence of arterial erosion
  - —Color (red, pallor, black)
  - —Vascularity (evidence of bleeding and/or bruising, pulsations, arterial exposure)
  - —Temperature changes (warm, cool, unilateral)
  - —Edema (presence or absence)
  - —Turgor (taut, mobile)

- Monitor signs and symptoms of thoracic duct leakage:
  - —Milky white drainage often mixed with serous fluid in drainage tubes
- Monitor signs and symptoms of fluid and electrolyte imbalance.

- Monitor signs and symptoms of nerve injury:
  - —Superior laryngeal nerve dysphagia

  - —Recurrent laryngeal nerve

OUTCOME GOALS/RATIONALE: *Postoperative–cont'd*

increase potential for obstruction. Elevating patient's head to facilitate lymphatic arterial flow reduces edema.

- Continuous oozing of blood after first 24 hours postoperatively is not normal; may require surgical intervention for control.

- Surgical incision should be assessed carefully the first 24 hours for bleeding drainage and patency of drainage tubes. Serious complications can lead to skin flap wound breakdown. If suction apparatus and tubes are not functioning, skin flaps may not adhere, and necrosis may occur.

- If drains' suction becomes plugged, malfunctions, or has excessive oozing or bleeding, vascular link-up occurs and fluid collects; sets site for compromised circulation and infection.
- Drains prevent development of dead space. Continuous bloody drainage may indicate formation of hematoma or fistula formation.
- Hematoma formation is prevented by placement of suction catheter draining superiorly and anteriorly or placement of flap to recipient site, eliminating dead space. Fluid or air collects between flap and underlying tissue. Gravity permits venous drainage through flap.
- Meticulous wound care as ordered by physician should be provided.
- Careful monitoring of intake and output avoids overhydration or underhydration.

- Exposure of adventitial layer of artery to atmosphere facilitates drying and destroys blood supply of layers. Once artery is exposed to the air, destruction of wall occurs in approximately 6 to 10 days.
- Contributing factors to arterial erosion include poor wound healing, exposure of artery at surgery, tumor growth invasion, previous radiation, fistula formation, or infection.
- Raising head of patient's bed facilitates venous drainage; raising it 30 to 45 degrees promotes lymphatic venous drainage.
- Major lymphatic leak from thoracic duct represents loss of fluid and protein and may require surgical closure or protein replacement.

- Branch of vagus that innervates base of tongue may cause swallowing impairment.
- Responsible for adduction/abduction of vocal cords.
- Bilateral pareses require immediate tracheostomy.

INTERVENTIONS: *Postoperative–cont'd*

- —Lingual nerve
- —Hypoglossal nerve

- —Glossopharyngeal nerve

- —Facial nerve

- —Phrenic nerve
- —Spinal accessory nerve

- Monitor signs and symptoms of flap reconstructive failure:
  - —Monitor wound, flap, surrounding tissue every 2 hours for 72 hours, then every 4 hours.
  - —Color (redness, pallor, cyanosis), tension, kinking, pressure, hematoma
  - —Vascularity (presence or absence of blanching)
  - —Temperature (warm, cool, unilateral)
  - —Edema (presence or absence)
  - —Turgor (taut, mobile, shiny, wrinkled)
  - —Odor (not malodorous)
  - —"Red flap": flap appears bright red and when tested for capillary filling feels tense or thick on digital palpation. This occurs when blood flow is excessive. A red flap occurs when there is partial venous obstruction.
  - —"White flap": one that has limited or no blood supply; related to tension, constriction, pressure, or occlusion; can stop blood flow. With dearterialization, flap has no capillary refill, is cool to touch, and becomes white.
  - —"Blue Flap": occurs when input of blood exceeds output. This imbalance occurs when arterial pressure remains the same and venous pressure increases (e.g., hematoma) or with constriction of vascular pedicle related to patient lying on flap, with a tight pressure dressing, or with formation of a clot at venous anastomotic site.

- Monitor signs and symptoms of infection:
  - —Tenderness
  - —Thickness (inspect level of tissue repair, presence or absence of tumor)
  - —Moisture (dry; drainage—amount, color, odor; fistula formation)
- Monitor pressure—external pressure of flap.

OUTCOME GOALS: *Postoperative–cont'd*

- Numbness on ipsilateral tongue can occur if severed.
- If severed, unilateral tongue paralysis results, which causes impairment of speech and mastication; innervates the genioglossus muscle and is responsible for tongue movement.
- Innervates posterior two thirds of tongue. Damage can result in altered taste sensation on ipsilateral side and difficulty in swallowing.
- Result of trauma, especially in the area of parotid, may result in droop or asymmetry of musculature around the mouth (drooping periostosis).
- If severed, paralysis of diaphragm can result.
- Innervates trapezius muscle, which stabilizes and supports shoulder; allows lateral abduction of arm.
- Often affected in neck dissections. Injury results in painful shoulder, droopy atrophy of trapezius muscle, and immobility of head and shoulder.
- Major surgery can create deficits that may not be approximated and closed by direct suture. Skin flaps with or without muscle provide tissue and bulk protection to vital structures (e.g., carotid artery). Purpose is to maintain vascular integrity. Maximum redness should occur first 8 to 12 hours and decrease after 2 to 3 days. If arterial or venous supply is hindered, flap may necrose or slough. Flap and recipient sites should survive if no unusual kinking, pressure, hematoma, or infection occurs. Tension compromises blood supply; kinking causes decreased blood supply to distal portion of flap and compromises venous outflow, resulting in increased capillary permeability and occlusion of lymphatics and arterioles. Pressure compromises blood supply. Position patient to permit gradual flow of lymph and blood. Elevate head of bed 30 to 45 degrees.
- Normal tissue and flaps are warm to the touch and recover color slowly after tested for blanching. Flaps have fine wrinkles, an indication of minimal edema.
- Abnormal findings (shiny, taut, reddish) indicate circulatory embarrassment and venous congestion. After testing for blanching, flap recovers color quickly.
- Foul purulent drainage is seen.
- Room temperatures that are extreme cold can be a contributing factor to flap loss; maintain room temperature.

- Flap necrosis can lead to formation of fistula, septicemia, arterial rupture, and prolonged hospitalization.

- External pressure on muscle flap compromises circulation, facilitates venous congestion, and leads to decreased permeability and occlusion of lymphatics.

Continued.

INTERVENTIONS: *Postoperative–cont'd*

Postoperative nursing care should focus on preventing and minimizing complications. Immediate postoperative care focuses on maintaining and monitoring the airway. Patient's head should be elevated to reduce edema. Nurse should make sure that drains are kept functional and clear to avoid accumulations of fluid under surgical site or reconstructed flap. Intake and output must be monitored to avoid overhydration or underhydration. If patient has a nasogastric tube, first postoperative day patient is kept NPO, and tube is placed on suction to avoid gastric contents, air, vomiting, or aspiration from occurring. Feedings usually are initiated on second or third postoperative day. Early ambulation is encouraged, and upper aerodigestive system may require frequent, gentle suction to prevent atelectasis, infection, and aspiration. If patient has undergone a mandible/tongue or palatal or larynx resection, nurse must provide patient with paper or magic slate or picture board to facilitate communication. Speech rehabilitation should be started as soon as patient's surgical condition is stable. Whether or not patient is to receive any additional therapy, he or she should be monitored for local or regional recurrence or new disease. Nurse should instruct patient on the importance of maintaining all scheduled appointments; most physicians will follow patient monthly for the first year. During this period, patient should be prepared to undergo additional tests to evaluate his or her response to treatment or identify any recurrences or new disease (e.g., chest x-ray film, blood chemistries).

It is generally recommended that patient be seen every month for the first year, every 2 months for the second year, every 3 months for the third year, every 6 months for the fourth and fifth year, and every 6 to 12 months thereafter. Early detection of local or regional recurrences or a new primary lesion provides patient with the best opportunity for cure or control of disease.

NURSING DIAGNOSES

- *Body image disturbance related to head/neck cancer surgery*
- *Sexual dysfunction related to altered self-esteem and change in appearance*
- *Self-esteem disturbance related to anatomic changes, role disturbance, disruption of life-style, uncertain future, altered sexuality patterns, body image changes*

INTERVENTIONS: *Preoperative*

- Review purpose of interview: obtaining information and a sexual history early in a relationship with a patient validates to patient/partner that sexuality is an important part of health and rehabilitation and therefore it is appropriate for concerns to be discussed.
- Progress from less sensitive questions. Ask patient/partner if they have any questions at conclusion of history.

OUTCOME GOALS: *Preoperative*

Patient/partner will be able to:
- Identify aspects of sexuality/sexual function that may be threatened by surgical procedure (e.g., tracheostomy; laryngectomy; tongue, jaw/neck dissection/reconstruction).
- State factors that influence sexual identity.
- Identify behaviors that facilitate acceptance of surgery.

INTERVENTIONS: *Preoperative–cont'd*

- Include following components of preoperative nursing assessment in interview:
  —Specific sexual needs of patient/partner
  —Sexual history (provide privacy, assure confidentiality)
  —Coping style and adjustment to previous illness or surgery
  —Attitudes about sex
  —Patient's attitudes about altered body image and perception of sexuality
  —Effects of illness on partner/patient. Does patient's present or postoperative physical condition limit partner's ability for sexual expression?
  —Demonstration of nurse's acceptance; facilitation of patient's comfort and adjustment to illness and surgery
  —Determination of involvement of partner in providing actual physical care and whether or not partner is fatigued
  —Assessment of whether partner feels guilty about initiating or making sexual demands
  —Patient's/partner's reactions to impending physical change
  —Existence of pain, fatigue, depression, limited mobility that would affect normal expressions of sexuality
  —Interference by illness on patient's roles. Has being ill interfered with (mother, father, wife, husband, etc.)?
  —Impact of surgery on patient's self-perception
  —Effect of illness/disability on patient's sexual function

INTERVENTIONS: *Postoperative*

- Assess that patient/partner wants to know about surgical procedure and changes in function that may be related to surgical procedure.
- Assess patient's attitude about altered body image and perception of sexuality.
- Do pain, fatigue, and limited mobility affect normal expressions of sexuality?
- What is patient's/partner's reaction to altered body image?

OUTCOME GOALS: *Preoperative–cont'd*

- Maintain satisfying social and sexual/role concept.
- Verbalize importance of seeking professional assistance if normal life-style, socialization, or sexual function is impaired.

OUTCOME GOALS: *Postoperative*

Patient/partner will be able to:
- Provide factual information.
- Give assurance that it is acceptable to share feelings and concerns.
- Assist with coping/adjustments to illness.

- Is there a previous history of effective versus ineffective individual family coping and powerlessness?
- What is the patient's knowledge deficit related to radiation therapy, pretreatment planning, and actual treatment delivery?
- Does the patient demonstrate any cognitive or learning disabilities, such as illiteracy, sensory limitations, and vision, speech, hearing, or motor disabilities?

Patient education is developed based on information obtained in the initial nursing assessment. Simple, nontechnical, concise explanations should be used rather than medical terminology. Pretreatment patient education should include the rationale for why radiation therapy was chosen over other treatments, actual length of treatment session, duration of treatment, and oral, nutritional, and skin care. This education will eliminate the myths and misconceptions that the patient and family may experience related to radiation therapy and its side effects.

Although radiation therapy holds some distinct advantages over other treatment modalities, the patient remains at risk for acute and chronic side effects. Acute complications include mucositis and oral ulcerations with resultant pain or discomfort, superficial infections, dermatitis, and hypogeusia. Chronic side effects may include chronic xerostomia, radiation caries, soft tissue necrosis, osteoradionecrosis, and trismus.* The type and extent of complications vary depending on the dose, type, fractionation, duration of radiation, and the volume of tissue radiated. Therefore it is important to consider these factors before counseling patients regarding self-care behaviors. Most complications can be prevented or minimized with collaborative efforts of the patient, family, physician, nurse, dentist, dental hygienist, physical therapist, speech therapist, and dietitian, thus enhancing the patient's overall quality of life.†

Complications

Mucositis. Radiation-induced mucositis is a frequently occurring acute problem. Radiation impairs mitosis nonspecifically. Mucositis, ulceration, and inflammation of the mucous membranes are expected and often painful side effects of high-dose radiotherapy to the head and neck. Mucosal erythema usually begins within 2 to 3 weeks of the initiation of therapy. The normal mucosa thins from direct killing of parietal replicating cells. The rate of mucosal breakdown and ulceration is directly related to the timing and total dosage of radiotherapy. The daily dosage of radiotherapy will determine the degree of erythema, mucositis, or xerostomia. During this time the radiation destroys the basal cell layer at a rate faster than proliferation of new cells. Mucosal ulcerations result spontaneously or can be caused by minor trauma from dentures, abrasive foods, or teeth. The ulcerations vary in site and severity, generally occurring along the buccal and labial mucosa, adjacent to teeth. Preradiation patient teaching on oral care can circumvent ulcerations related to trauma. All these changes can compromise the natural epithelial barrier that protects the oral cavity from pathogenic bacteria and fungus. Preexisting periodontal disease exacerbates the ulcerations. Mucositis can develop and persist to a degree that radiation treatments may be temporarily discontinued.

Pain. Pain related to oral mucositis, if not managed properly, can have a profound negative effect on hydration, nutrition, and sleep. Pain or discomfort related to mucositis should not automatically limit the patient from

maintaining adequate hydration and nutrition or from practicing oral hygiene procedures. Adequate pain control can be achieved by prescribing topical anesthetics alone or in conjunction with nonnarcotic and narcotic analgesics. In addition, an early nursing consultation with a dietitian is one of the simplest ways to circumvent complications. The dietitian can make recommendations for alternative food preparation and supplements.

Infection. Oral mucositis with ulcerations puts the patient at risk for developing oral infections.[36] Oral infections seen in patients undergoing radiation may be bacterial, fungal, or viral in origin. One of the most common acute infections seen in patients is *candidiasis,* or *moniliasis,* resulting from radiation-induced changes of the normal oral flora. The nurse should monitor the patient for the classic white patches that scrape off, leaving burning tissue.

For *fungal infections,* topical and systemic antifungal agents may be prescribed by the physician. Antifungal agents are usually mixed with sucrose to make the drug more palatable. A non-sucrose-containing antifungal agent should be used by head and neck patients to prevent caries formation. A patient who wears a dental prosthesis or uses fluoride carrier trays must be instructed that these are to be removed from the oral cavity and immersed in an antifungal agent for 8 hours to avoid reintroductions of fungal organisms into the oral cavity. Toothbrushes and denture-soaking containers should be changed frequently.

The nurse performs a weekly routine oral examination to detect new lesions early in their development, noting carefully size, shape, location, and appearance. Cultures or smears of new lesions may be ordered by the physician to document and facilitate treatment of any superimposed infection.

Palliative treatment of mucositis related to radiation includes oral rinses and application of topical anesthetics. Sodium bicarbonate oral rinse (1 tsp baking soda in 32 oz water or normal saline) should be used at least six times a day. Topical anesthetics can be used, progressing from the least potent and toxic to the more potent and toxic.

Dermatitis. Dermatitis, an acute condition characterized by a sunburned appearance, results from radiation inhibiting mitosis of epithelial cells. The patient may experience significant pain or discomfort and become reluctant to perform any self-care. Treatment of this condition is discussed in detail in Chapter 30.

Xerostomia. Xerostomia (dry mouth) occurs when radiation therapy causes sclerosis of the acini of the salivary gland. Saliva regulates the pH in the oral cavity, which controls bacterial flora, and lubricates and cleanses the teeth. When the amount of saliva and consistency (thick) are changed, generalized oral disease can occur, creating an environment conducive to caries for

*References 13, 22, 52, 102, 105, 140.
†References 1, 18, 20, 30, 44, 61, 67, 79.

Text continued on p. 257.

NURSING MANAGEMENT

HEAD AND NECK RADIATION THERAPY

NURSING DIAGNOSES

- *Knowledge deficit regarding radiation therapy to head and neck*
- *Oral mucous membrane, altered, related to radiation therapy to head and neck (mucositis, xerostomia, caries)*
- *Nutrition, altered: less than body requirements related to oral pain, difficulty swallowing (dysphagia), difficulty chewing, xerostomia-imposed fluid restrictions, change in tolerance to temperatures of food (cold, hot), change in tolerance to acidic or highly seasoned food, change in taste (hypogeusia), poorly fitted dentures or inability to wear dentures (Table 11-8)*
- *Pain, acute, related to mucositis, xerostomia, difficulty chewing, swallowing*
- *Pain, chronic, related to radiation caries, or osteoradionecrosis*
- *Injury, risk for, related to oral hygiene*
- *Health maintenance, altered, related to osteoradionecrosis*

Table 11-8   Supraglottic Swallow

Action	Effect
Take deep breath	To aerate lungs
Perform Valsalva maneuver (bear down)	To approximate vocal cords
Place food in mouth and swallow	Some food will enter airway and remain on top of closed vocal cords
Cough	To remove food from top of vocal cords
Swallow	To swallow food moved from top of vocal cords
Breathe	Restoring breathing before cough-swallow sequence would result in aspiration of food collected by vocal cords

From Sigler BA, Shuring LT: *Ear, nose, and throat disorders,* St Louis, 1993, Mosby.

INTERVENTIONS

- Review purpose of radiation therapy and rationale for treatment.

- Explain common terms and procedures, provide written literature, and show actual equipment (e.g., light cast molds, bite blocks). Patient will need to be familiar with terminology and equipment (e.g., simulation/dosimetry port films, cobalt/linear accelerator implants).
- Discuss potential sequelae of radiation:
  —Change in body appearance (e.g., skin)

  —Change in body function (e.g., mucositis, xerostomia, swallowing)
  —Potential for infection
  —Potential for radiation caries
  —Potential for soft tissue and osteoradionecrosis
  —Nutritional stomatitis and taste loss
  —Trismus
- Explain roles of various medical, nursing personnel, technicians, dosimetrists, and purpose of visits.
- Instruct and have patient give verbal/return demonstration on all self-care:
  —Oral hygiene (for dentulous and edentulous patients)

OUTCOME GOALS/RATIONALE

Patient will be able to:
- Demonstrate decreased anxiety and be knowledgeable of planned radiation therapy.
- Effectively communicate feelings, demonstrate ability to do self-care, and seek assistance as necessary.
- State name, type, length of treatment, and description of radiation.

- State reason for radiation therapy, expected outcome, and potential side effects.
- Patient will state expectations of radiation treatment and professionals involved.
- Oral care instructions should be determined by the patient's physician, radiation oncologist, and dentist.

- Patient will state expectations and reasons for all oral care.
- Patients at risk for infection and radiation caries must adhere to a strict oral hygiene program coupled with
Continued.

INTERVENTIONS–cont'd

OUTCOME GOALS/RATIONALE–cont'd

dental visits. Patients who remain at risk for radiation caries should assume an active role in this prevention.

• Provide instructions for edentulous patients:
—Brush teeth often, especially after eating and at bedtime.
—Use soft, nylon toothbrush with even bristles.
—Place bristles at an angle to where your gums and teeth meet.
—Use short back-and-forth strokes to clean front, back, and all chewing surfaces of teeth and tongue.
—Tongue can harbor bacterial plaque and should be gently brushed.
—Use toothpaste that contains fluoride.

• Patient will brush teeth at least four times daily, particularly after meals and at bedtime.

• Patient will use Bass Technique of brushing, in which toothbrush bristles are adapted to teeth and gingiva at 45-degree angle and vibrated in short back strokes. This method is effective in cleaning gingival sulcus.

• Toothpaste is not necessary to remove plaque from teeth. Fluorinated paste is recommended if used.

—Use dental floss at least once a day to clean sides of teeth where toothbrush does not reach. Ease the floss between teeth so that it is close to the tooth as you guide it up and down. Do not snap floss between teeth because it may damage your gums.
—Oral hygiene—cleanse inside of mouth gently with moist clean gauze or toothette. Massage gums gently with finger.
—Clean dentures or partials every day with denture brush and denture cleaner (e.g., soap and water or baking soda and water).
—Change dental soaking cup and brush frequently—every 2 weeks.
—Store dentures in container of water to keep shape when not in mouth.
—Remove dentures several hours daily as prescribed by dentist.
• Instruct dentulous and edentulous patients to rinse mouth often:
—Rinse mouth several times daily. This helps relieve dryness and promotes comfort, cleansing, and healing.
—Mix solution (1 tsp table salt, 1 tsp baking soda, and 1 qt warm water), swish in mouth, and expectorate.
—Instruct dentulous patient on fluoride application—daily application of topical fluoride.
—Instruct on rationale/application of daily fluoride application after brushing, flossing, and rinsing.
—Instruct patient not to eat or drink anything for 30 minutes after application.

• Patient will use dental floss to cleanse the interproximal tooth surfaces inaccessible to toothbrush.

• Edentulous patients with or without prostheses will cleanse soft tissues of oral cavity gently to stimulate circulation.

• Patient will frequently change denture storage container and brush to decrease potential for infection/colonization of bacteria.

• Patient will remove dentures from oral cavity to allow oral tissues to rest.
• Frequent oral irrigations with alkaline lavage will help buffer acidity of oral cavity and promote cleansing lubrication of oral mucosa. Variations or other rinses may be recommended by physician and/or dentist.

• Patient will state self-care behaviors and will perform application.
• Patient will obtain a fluoride prescription and fluoride carrier tray from dentist.
• Five-minute application daily decreases radiation caries and dental sensitivity.
• Fluoride is available in gel, rinses, and tablets. A 11.23% neutral sodium gel applied in custom carrier is most often used.
• Edentulous patients do not require fluoride application.

• Instruct patient to report to physician/nurse/dentist clinical problems early related to:
—Xerostomia
—Loss of taste

• Patient will state expectations and rationale for regular dental visits and early reporting of symptoms.
• Patient will state reason for maintaining nutritional intake and self-care behaviors.

INTERVENTIONS–cont'd

- —Inability to maintain nutritional intake
- —Inability to maintain hydration
- —Infection
- Instruct patient on stomatitis/taste loss, nutritional maintenance, and foods to be avoided.
  - —Consult dietitian.
  - —Encourage patient to substitute aroma of foods for taste to stimulate appetite; eat frequent smaller meals; avoid extreme temperatures.
  - —Apply soothing ointments to lips for dryness/cracking.
  - —Moisten foods with sauces, gravies, creams, and other liquids.
  - —Eat pureed food.
  - —Chew sugarless gum.
  - —Take vitamin B complex if prescribed.
  - —Restrict all sucrose intake (i.e., candies, cakes, pastries).

POTENTIAL COLLABORATIVE/CLINICAL PROBLEMS

- Mucositis
- Xerostomia
- Radiation caries
- Soft tissue necrosis and osteoradionecrosis

During course of radiation therapy and at follow-up visits:

INTERVENTIONS: Mucositis

- Monitor signs and symptoms of mucositis:
  - —Oral pain
  - —Burning
  - —Discomfort
  - —Difficulty chewing/swallowing/speaking
  - —Sensitivity to temperature extremes/highly seasoned foods
  - —Unable to tolerate wearing dentures

Medical Interventions

- Have patient take systemic analgesic as prescribed.
- Apply viscous lidocaine to produce topical anesthesia. NOTE: Viscous lidocaine application may adversely affect patient's taste sensation. Patients may be unable to detect temperature extremes and inadvertently bite themselves.

OUTCOME GOALS/RATIONALE–cont'd

Patient will be able to:
- Maintain weight/hydration.
- State reason for nutritional maintenance.
- State expected outcome and rationale for avoiding:
  - —All forms of tobacco
  - —All forms of alcohol, including mouthwashes
  - —Having teeth pulled after radiation therapy
- Damage to microvilli and outer-surface taste cells of tongue and their innervating nerve fibers decreases ability to taste. Taste loss, xerostomia, soreness, dryness, difficulty chewing, swallowing, and sucrose restrictions can result in weight loss and nutrition deficiency.
- Taste acuity will return following therapy. Vitamin B complex therapy is effective for patients that experience angular cheilosis and lingual manifestation related to malnutrition. Angular cheilosis may also be caused by a loss of vertical dimension between mandible and maxilla.
- Sucrose intake for dentulous patients has little nutritional value and promotes radiation caries.

- Mucosal erythema is usually expected within 2 to 3 weeks after initiation of treatment. Radiation destroys basal cell layer, thereby thinning mucosa. Ulcerations can occur spontaneously or as a result of trauma from brushing, dentures, food, or teeth. Swallowing can become difficult if pharyngeal mucosa is involved.

Continued.

Nursing Interventions

- Maintain patient comfort:
  —Use moist gauze, toothette, or water rinse to cleanse teeth and mouth if toothbrush causes discomfort.
  —Temporarily suspend fluoride application if discomfort occurs.
  —Avoid alcohol or mouthwashes containing alcohol (alcohol drys and irritates mucous membranes).
  —Suggest methods to assist patient with cessation of alcohol and tobacco consumption.
  —Avoid coarse, spicy, acidic foods and extreme temperatures. Consult with dietitian.
  —Maintain soft bland or liquid diet.
  —Remove dentures or prosthesis that rests within radiation field (exception: mealtime, if tolerated).

INTERVENTIONS: Xerostomia

- Monitor signs and symptoms of xerostomia:
  —Dry mouth
  —Burning sensation
  —Difficulty swallowing
  —Difficulty speaking
  —Decreased ability to tolerate wearing a prosthetic appliance

Medical Intervention

- Refer patient to physician/dentist.

Nursing Interventions

- Encourage use of prescribed synthetic salivas to lubricate mouth and buffer oral microflora.
- Carry out frequent oral irrigations as prescribed.
- Have patient drink water and sugar-free beverages throughout day as prescribed.
- Puree foods or use food processor.
- Moisten foods with gravies and sauces.
- Have patient use humidifier at home.
- Encourage use of sugarless gum and candy and ice chips.
- Have dentist instruct on wearing dentures.

INTERVENTIONS: Radiation Caries

- Monitor signs and symptoms of radiation caries:
  —Tooth sensitivity
  —Pain
  —Destruction of teeth

Medical Intervention

- Refer patient to physician/dentist.
  —Maintenance of oral hygiene program
  —Frequent alkaline lavage
  —Restriction of sucrose intake

Nursing Intervention

- Reinforce all prescriptions.

- Radiation to the major and minor salivary glands results in a significant decrease in salivary secretions and changes in pH, viscosity, volume, and inorganic constituents of saliva. Alterations in quality and quantity of saliva inhibit saliva to cleanse, lubricate, and buffer the oral cavity, predisposing patient to caries and periodontal disease. Salivary flow decreases, and saliva is thick, viscous, and stringy. Saliva contains microbial compounds important in mechanical removal of pathogens from mouth.

- Xerostomia and associated changes in salivary flow related to radiation can create environment for a highly acidic and cariogenic oral microflora. Total output of salivary production results in reduction of caries-protective electrolytes and immunoproteins. Reduced consumption of high-detergent foods (coarse, roughage) that cleanse teeth also contributes to caries formation. Carious lesions can occur up to 3 months after radiation therapy, appear on the cervical margin of teeth, and progress to complete destruction of the crown. Patients are at risk for caries for their entire lives.

INTERVENTIONS: *Tissue Necrosis*

- Monitor signs and symptoms of tissue necrosis and osteoradionecrosis:
  —Throbbing pain
  —Bleeding
  —Suppuration
  —Fetid odor in breath
  —Difficulty eating

INTERVENTIONS: *Infection*

- Monitor signs and symptoms of infection:
  —Complaints of pain, burning, tenderness
  —Bleeding (gingiva)
  —Tooth mobility
  —Elevated temperature

Medical Interventions

- Use topical nystatin mouth rinses daily.
- Ensure frequent physician/dental visits.
- Administer antibiotics if indicated.

Nursing Interventions

- Maintain meticulous oral hygiene.
- Carry out oral irrigations.
- Provide for consistent monitoring of oral cavity.
- Monitor vital signs, specifically temperature.

INTERVENTIONS: *Trismus*

- Monitor signs and symptoms of trismus:
  —Impaired ability to open mouth widely
  —Impaired ability to chew
  —Impaired ability to speak

Medical Intervention

- Use prosthetic appliances and elastics prepared by dentist/prosthodontist.

Nursing Interventions

- Refer patient to physician/dentist.
- Instruct patient to exercise masticatory muscles before, during, and after treatment: opening and closing mouth 20 times in row three times a day.
- Maintain meticulous oral hygiene.

OUTCOME GOALS/RATIONALE—cont'd

- Soft tissue necrosis is the progressive enlarging of mucosal ulcers that become necrotic and may develop in radiated soft tissue as a result of radiation-induced fibrosis and impaired blood supply. Osteoradionecrosis is a progressive condition as a result of radiation on the osteocytes, regional blood supply, and bone marrow. Bony exposure, infection, and necrosis can occur, resulting in bone sequestration and fracture. Osteoradionecrosis is common in the mandible, usually results from trauma, and usually occurs within a year of treatment. This process can progress to pathologic fracture, infection of surrounding soft tissues, and oral-cutaneous fistula formation.

- Infection can occur during or after radiation. Oral infections are most common (e.g., candidiasis [thrush], periodontal disease [pyorrhea]). Periodontal disease is manifested by hyperemic and edematous gingiva.

- Muscles of mastication undergo fibrosis related to radiation. This may indicate disease recurrence and occurs 3 to 6 months after completion of therapy. Fibrosis of the muscles of mastication and temporomandibular joint, although uncommon, may result in trismus.

mation. The oral pH becomes more acidic when salivary flow decreases and allows a major caries-forming organism, *Streptococcus*, to grow. Salivary flow can be accurately measured before and after radiation therapy by having the patient undergo *sialometric testing*. This allows the clinician to measure the patient's ability to produce saliva when stimulated, either by total stimulation or stimulation of paired major salivary glands.

Radiation therapy also affects taste bud function. Alteration in taste *(dysgeusia)* and decreased taste *(hypo-*

geusesthesia) can occur. The degree of taste alteration and impairment depends on the site and dose of radiation. Taste sensations are decreased because food must be in solution to be tasted. Taste buds, as with other normal cells, will regenerate after completion of radiation if adequate nutrition is maintained. Most patients experience a degree of return of function within 4 to 12 months, but some patients may have permanent taste alterations. Most patients undergoing radiation therapy state that the taste sensation of sweetness lasts the longest. This is related to more taste buds normally being devoted to detection of sweet tastes than sour or salty tastes. The nurse must remember that with this alteration in taste sensation, the patient may naturally increase sugar intake to obtain the same level of sweetness. Alternative sources for sugar should be identified to prevent radiation caries.

Palliation of xerostomia, hypogeusia, and impaired swallowing can be achieved by adequate hydration of the oral cavity with nonsucrose liquids. Most salivary substitutes consist of sodium carboxymethyl cellulose combined with fluoride and other agents. In 1992 a multiinstitution, randomized, double-blind study demonstrated that pilocarpine has a direct treatment benefit for hyposalivation in patients after radiation therapy. Pilocarpine is a cholinergic parasympathomimetic agent that acts as an agonist on the muscarinic receptors. When given orally, it stimulates salivary flow.[87,116]

If the patient prefers not to carry a thermos of water or some other liquid to sip on frequently, several artificial saliva products are commercially available, such as Moi-Stir (Kingswood Laboratory, Carmel, Ind), Orex (Young Dental, Maryland Heights, Md), Sahvart (Westport Pharmaceuticals, Westport, Conn), and Xerolube (Scherer Laboratories, Dallas, Texas). In addition, the patient should be instructed to moisten the lips with lanolin or cocoa butter. Rinses or creams containing synthetic steroids (e.g., Kenalog) should be avoided because they have the potential to facilitate fungal growth in preexisting conditions conducive to fungus. Patients may stimulate unaffected salivary glands by sucking or chewing on sucrose-free sour candies or gum. A dietary consultation will aid the patient in learning additional food preparation techniques to facilitate chewing and swallowing (e.g., addition of sauces and gravies to dry foods, stimulation of taste sensations by the aroma of warm foods).*

Radiation caries. Radiation caries can result from radiation-induced xerostomia, poor oral hygiene, and high sucrose intake. These lesions form within 2 to 3 months compared with several months in the normal patient. Classically, radiation caries occur in areas of the tooth that are normally self-cleaning, such as the incisional edges of the anterior teeth, near the gum line, and

the cuspids. The preventive treatment regimen for radiation caries should include five key segments: pretreatment evaluation, periodontal care, oral hygiene instructions, daily fluoride application, and limited sucrose intake.[69] Once radiation caries form, teeth are at a high risk for fractures, and actual extractions are not recommended.

Osteoradionecrosis. Osteoradionecrosis (infection into the bone) is by far the most devastating of all the chronic sequelae of radiation to the head and neck. Despite improved technology of shielding and treatment delivery, patients remain at risk for this long-term side effect.[13,23,52,77]

Radiation causes hypoxic, hypocellular hypovascularization, resulting in tissue breakdown, cellular breakdown, cellular death, and collagen lysis that exceeds synthesis. Rather than a primary infection of irradiated bone, this has been described as a complex metabolic and tissue hemostastic deficiency created by radiation-induced cellular injury and replication. This injury weakens the bone and tissue, decreasing the ability to respond to injury, and produces favorable conditions for trauma and infection to occur. The mandible, with its single-source blood supply, has a higher incidence of osteoradionecrosis than the maxilla, which has a broad-based blood supply.[23,52,105]

Monitoring the patient for osteoradionecrosis is extremely important. Nurses play a significant role in prevention of this phenomenon. Patient education, postradiation follow-up appointments, and the importance of regular examinations should be presented as *essential* and *nonoptional.* At these visits the nurse should perform a thorough oral examination, documenting the presence or absence of chronic oral ulcerations, defective teeth, caries, defective restorations, or poorly fitting dentures. If any of these are identified, the patient should be immediately referred to the dentist for an examination. Follow-up visits should include concurrent medical and dental evaluations. Although prevention is the best approach to managing this potential clinical problem, local irrigations, high-dose extended antibiotics, and surgical procedures to remove dead bone tissue may be indicated.

Trismus. Patients who receive radiation that directly affects the muscles of mastication or the temporomandibular joint (TMJ) may develop trismus. Trismus may occur during therapy or may become problematic up until 6 months after completion of radiotherapy. Patient education about mouth-opening exercises is extremely important. A simple exercise of opening the mouth as widely as possible 20 times, three to four times a day, should minimize muscle fibrosis and loss of mobility. If trismus is noted, the degree of opening must be recorded and monitored at the patient's regular follow-up appointments. The dentist or maxillofacial prosthodontist may prescribe special appliances similar to those prescribed

---

*References 32, 45, 123, 131, 136, 141.

by an orthodontist, such as wedges, or appliances with screws, springs, or elastic for the patient to wear. Most physicians use all possible conservative measures to treat this side effect, leaving surgical interventions as a last approach. Any surgical procedure on devitalized tissue and bone may result in poor healing and infection.

Chronic side effects. Chronic side effects of radiation include anorexia, dysgeusia, and generalized lethargy.[136] Ideally, every patient undergoing radiation for head and neck cancer should be seen by a nurse and registered dietitian before, during, and after radiation. Nutritional evaluation and support should be provided for at least 6 months after completion of radiation. Weight loss or potential for weight loss should be anticipated during radiation therapy. Weight loss will continue after radiation, being maximal at 3 months and remaining virtually unchanged for 6 months after treatment.[18,22,26,32,141]

Health care education for patients undergoing radiation therapy should include the following:
- Importance of returning for all appointments
- Maintaining individualized oral hygiene program— brushing, flossing, fluoride, and ongoing dental assessment
- Nutrition, weight maintenance, and monitoring weight gain
- Maintaining or returning to normal life-styles, work, recreation, family, and social life

A comprehensive nursing care plan and guidelines for monitoring for potential collaborative and clinical problems are listed on pp. 253-257.

Chemotherapy

The role of chemotherapy in the treatment of head and neck cancer has changed since more single active agents and combinations have been discovered.[5,8,78] In the past, systemic chemotherapy was used as a palliative treatment or for patients who had persistent, recurrent disease or disseminated metastases after standard therapy (surgery/radiation).[3,50,51,60] A brief discussion of agents under evaluation for the treatment of head and neck cancers is included in this chapter. Individual agents, classification, metabolism, toxicity, and indications are discussed in Chapter 22.

Medical oncologists are using chemotherapy in conjunction with standard therapy, surgery, and radiation. Clinical trials designed to answer questions related to efficacy, timing, and sequencing of treatment are currently underway in national cooperative and intergroup studies.* Chemotherapy sequencing and timing may be given in three ways and are listed in the box above.

These sequences and combinations seek to answer the following questions related to treating head and neck cancer:

*References 5, 7-9, 50, 51, 58, 76, 77, 80, 84, 111.

> ### CHEMOTHERAPY SEQUENCING AND TIMING
>
> *Induction chemotherapy:* used before standard treatment; also called neoadjuvant, prostandard, or prestandard therapy
> *Concurrent chemotherapy:* used as total treatment or postoperatively in patients with resectable tumors
> *Sandwich chemotherapy:* used after surgery or before radiotherapy
> *Maintenance chemotherapy:* used after standard therapies

- What is the best combination to use?
- When should chemotherapy be included in the treatment plan?
- When and in what sequence should chemotherapy be used (e.g., preoperatively, before radiation, or in conjunction with radiation)?
- Is there a benefit of using chemotherapy as part of multimodality therapy?
- Does giving chemotherapy first delay or lessen the need for extensive radiation or surgery?
- Does chemotherapy have an effect on disease-free survival, overall survival, and quality of life?
- What is the incidence of chronic or delayed side effects?
- Does chemotherapy cause a change in patterns of recurrence?

The physician monitors the patient's response to chemotherapy by clinical and physical examination, by x-ray films, and by validating absence of tumor by having the surgeon obtain multiple biopsies. Nurses are responsible for educating and monitoring the patient for clinical problems related to the chemotherapy, such as adjustment to illness, knowledge deficits, potential for effective individual/family coping, altered comforts, and potential for infection.

Chemotherapeutic drugs that have demonstrated significant activity in head and neck cancer include methotrexate, bleomycin, Oncovin, cisplatin, carboplatin, and 5-fluorouracil (5-FU). These first-line agents are currently being used singly or in combinations for the treatment of head and neck cancer. If the patient fails to respond clinically, the physician may prescribe second-line therapies such as WR 2721 with high-dose cisplatin and 5-FU, or weekly intravenous methotrexate.[6,9,58,81] The nurse and patient need to monitor for transient, acute, subacute, and chronic side effects related to these agents. One of the most important aspects of nursing care is educating and reinforcing to the patient the importance of maintaining scheduled appointments. Response to therapy and early detection of toxicities or new lesions can be determined only if the patient keeps the appointment. Patients may be tempted to delay or skip a treatment until they "get stronger," "feel better," "gain weight," or "conduct personal business." Early detection of side effects related to chemotherapy can facilitate patient comfort and safety. Documentation of toxicities and side effects is critical because subsequent therapies are determined and calculated by the patient's tolerance to treatment.[65]

Pretreatment assessment. The general clinical status of the head and neck cancer patient is one of the best predictors of the patient's ability to tolerate chemotherapy, respond well to it, and survive. A pretreatment assessment of the patient's clinical status must be thoroughly evaluated and should include age; nutritional status; disease staging (TNM); documentation of other disease processes (e.g., cardiac, pulmonary, TB); function and reserve of lung, liver, kidney, bone marrow; and prior therapies (e.g., chemotherapy, radiation, surgery). The treatment of squamous cell carcinoma of the head and neck has reached the stage where chemotherapy may be potentially curative. Successful development of chemotherapeutic regimens that are curative in patients with advanced stages of disease hold the potential for effectively treating many nonadvanced patients.

Two techniques, MRI and flow cytometry, hold the potential to identify head and neck tumors or cellular characteristics that may direct the course of therapy. The use of flow cytometry to detect and measure tumor parameters has doubled over the past four decades. This technique involves passing a beam of light through a head and neck cancer cell. In theory, any part of the cell that can be caused to fluoresce by interruption of a beam of light when it passes through all the deoxyribonucleic acid/ribonucleic acid structures can be measured and studied. These techniques have proved efficacious in hematologic malignancies and may be able to identify tumor characteristics that could predict how head and neck tumors will respond to chemotherapy, radiotherapy, or surgery.*

The patient's overall performance status is consistently associated with prognostic outcome, including determining the response to systemic chemotherapy and survival. The better the patient's performance status, the greater is the patient's ability to tolerate therapy and the greater is the likelihood that he or she will respond and survive longer.

Al-Sarraf and co-workers[5] identified and reported two groups of prognostic factors that play an important role in determining the overall survival of the patient with recurrent or systemic disease (see box at right).

As many as 30% of patients who are unwilling to alter their life-styles, particularly those who continue to smoke and drink, experience the occurrence of second cancers.

A complete nursing biopsychosocial evaluation should be included in the pretreatment evaluation. Emphasis should be placed on determining the patient's level of education, educational needs, literacy, and ability to learn and comprehend. Toxic effects related to chemotherapy can be life-threatening in patients who are unable to understand and monitor for these side effects.

REHABILITATION

As treatment protocols increase, more patients are being diagnosed with secondary primary lesions or distant metastasis. The patient who has been treated for head and neck cancer is at significant risk for recurrent disease at the primary site or the neck.[103,107] The patient should also be monitored for a metachronous primary in the head and neck area, lung, or esophagus. Ongoing assessment and evaluation of response to treatment are essential for early diagnosis of disease and validation of health. Routine follow-up of patients should include a thorough examination of the head and neck with indi-

---

PROGNOSTIC FACTORS IN RECURRENT AND SYSTEMIC HEAD AND NECK CANCER

GOOD PROGNOSTIC FACTORS

- Good performance status
- Minimal disease
- Local recurrence only
- No bony erosion
- Good response to induction (adjuvant) chemotherapy
- Good response to previous chemotherapy
- Long disease-free interval (DFT)
- First-line chemotherapy
- Good organ function
- Complete response (CR) to chemotherapy

POOR PROGNOSTIC FACTORS

- Poor performance status
- Bulky disease
- Systemic/visceral disease
- Bone metastasis and/or hypercalcemia (and local bone invasion)
- Lymphangitis spread (skin)
- Failure of radiotherapy (persistent disease)
- Failure of induction (adjuvant) chemotherapy
- Patients receiving first-line chemotherapy for recurrent and/or systemic cancer
- Organ impairment
- Less than CR to chemotherapy

---

*References 37, 38, 46, 47, 49, 50.

Modified from Al-Sarraf M: *Semin Oncol* 15(1):70, 1988.

Individualized nursing care plans addressing lack of knowledge related to chemotherapy and monitoring for potential side effects related to chemotherapy should be established. Family or significant others should always be incorporated into the teaching and care plan because they can assist in monitoring the patient's response to treatment and adjustment to illness.

Routine home care nursing referral for patients receiving chemotherapy is recommended after the initial treatment and for those persons who continue to demonstrate knowledge deficits related to chemotherapy. The home care nurses can monitor for side effects of chemotherapy, reinforce patient teaching, validate the patient's ability to perform self-care, and monitor for adequate hydration and nutrition.

DENTAL EVALUATION

The goal of dental therapy for patients undergoing chemotherapy is the same as with radiation therapy and surgery[1]: to reduce potential infections and morbidity and avoid unnecessary delays of chemotherapeutic treatments. Chemotherapeutic agents such as 5-FU, methotrexate, or bleomycin, alone or in combination with radiation therapy, affect tissues with high turnover rates, such as the oral mucosa. Mucosal tissues, in general, are subject to chronic physical trauma and infection. As discussed previously, when the patient experiences decreased host resistance, changes in normal bacteria—viral and fungal flora—have the potential to become pathogens and infect the patient.

Once chemotherapy has been initiated, the focus of dental therapy should be directed at maintaining oral hygiene and decreasing the potential for infection. Guidelines for oral hygiene and dental care are similar to those for the patient undergoing radiotherapy.

NUTRITIONAL ASSESSMENT

Common nutritional problems experienced by these patients relate not only to the treatment modality, but also to altered physiologic function related to tumor involvement. A pretreatment nursing nutritional assessment is important to identify any anticipated problems related to the patient's ability to maintain weight and hydration. The nutritional assessment should include a careful dietary history (including previous alcohol exposure) and daily intake, weight loss, and patient completion of a 3-day dietary recall. These data enable the health care professional and patient to develop a reasonable pretreatment nutritional plan. The nutritional plan ideally should be implemented before initiation of chemotherapy and monitored closely throughout the entire course of treatment. Having the patient complete the 3-day recall provides the nurse and clinical dietitian with an excellent tool for patient education. Patient education booklets such as *Eating Hints* and other dietary materials are available free from the National Institutes of Health and American Cancer Society.

Fluctuations of 2 to 3 lb between monthly visits is acceptable, but any rapid weight loss unrelated to infection or chemotherapy side effects may require the physician to place the patient on short-term or long-term enteral or parenteral nutrition. Head and neck cancer patients undergoing combinations of chemotherapy that incorporate platinum or platinum derivatives should be monitored for signs and symptoms of dehydration and fluid and electrolyte imbalances.[65] These agents are extremely nephrotoxic, and a key nursing intervention to circumvent toxicity is to maintain hydration and have the patient maintain a strict intake and output record. Likewise, patients should be provided with written guidelines for the monitoring of their hydration and should know when to notify the nurse or physician if they are unable to maintain hydration. Patients should be provided information on alternative sources of fluid, such as ice cream, jello, popsicles, and milkshakes. Symptom control (e.g., nausea and vomiting) and prescriptive therapies will depend on the chemotherapeutic agent given and the patient's response to treatment.

rect laryngoscopy once a month for the first year, every 2 months during the second year, and every 3 months the fifth year after treatment. Patients with new symptoms of significant weight loss, dysphagia, chronic soreness, or persistent hoarseness should have an endoscopic examination with biopsy when tumor is not visible by examination. Nurses share the responsibility to educate patients and reinforce the importance of maintaining scheduled appointments. Careful and meticulous follow-up is a significant link to long-term survival in this patient group. Nurses should emphasize the importance of maintaining a healthy life-style. The patient should be educated on the importance of cessation of alcohol and tobacco, notifying physician of early symptoms, and keeping appointments.

RECURRENT DISEASE

Treatment options of recurrent disease are limited. The clinical management and treatment of recurrent disease depend on accurate specific site and staging of the disease. Recurrent head and neck cancer is, by definition, a

COMPLICATIONS
Head and Neck Cancer Treatment

Surgery

Potential for structural, functional, or cosmetic loss, such as changes in body appearance and function (breathing, speaking, swallowing, coughing, mobility)

Respiratory distress; hypoxia, airway obstruction, tracheal edema, aspiration; hemorrhage; hematoma; arterial rupture; failure of flap survival; nerve damage

Radiation therapy

Mucositis	Xerostomia
Pain	Radiation caries
Infection	Osteoradionecrosis
Dermatitis	Fungal infections
Trismus	Dysgeusia

Chemotherapy

Mucositis	Dehydration
Infection	Electrolyte imbalance
Immunosuppression	Nausea and vomiting
Weight loss	Diarrhea

General considerations

Patients with head and neck cancers receiving multimodality therapy may experience severe and permanent facial disfigurement and functional loss that resembles what is experienced by the burn patient.

PATIENT TEACHING PRIORITIES
Head and Neck Cancers

Rationale for pretreatment evaluation:
   Psychosocial assessment—potential changes in body image (structural, functional, and cosmetic changes)
   Cardiopulmonary assessment and health history
Nutritional assessment; communication/cognitive motor skills; dental assessment
Rationale for treatment:
   Surgery—review purpose, rationale, and potential sequelae; explain common terms and procedures; discuss preoperative and postoperative nursing interventions.
   Radiation therapy—review purpose, rationale, and potential side effects of the therapy; explain the procedures, purpose of positioning the body, and scheduling of the radiation therapy treatments.
   Chemotherapy—review purpose, rationale, and potential side effects of the therapy; discuss chemotherapy treatment schedule and need for weekly blood tests to monitor the side effects of drugs.
   Rehabilitation—initiate referrals to social worker, speech pathologist, physical therapist, occupational therapist, clinical dietician, and nurse specialist.

---

failure to the standard definitive local therapy. Approximately 40% of these patients will recur overall, 20% locoregionally, 10% with distant metastasis, and another 10% with both local and distant disease. Many of these patients relapse within 6 to 24 months after treatment and have a median survival of 6 months from initial diagnosis to recurrence. In the past, reirradiation of recurrent tumors in the head and neck was performed with extreme caution. In select patient populations, reirradiation has been combined with surgery and/or chemotherapy in attempts to control the disease.[110] Managing the psychosocial consequences of cancer recurrence provides nursing with a unique opportunity to implement interventions that can fulfill the emotional and spiritual needs of both patient and family.[93]

In addition to recurrent disease, the physician is often challenged with other common clinical problems, which may significantly limit treatment options. The physician must identify the treatment regimen that holds the highest therapeutic value and lowest risk/benefit ratio.[3,7-9,60,81] Diseases related to life-styles, chronic obstructive pulmonary disease, and liver or renal disease substantially affect the physician's ability to deliver ad-

equate therapeutic doses of chemotherapy such as cisplatin, bleomycin, or methotrexate. Age-related diseases, such as underlying cardiac problems, hypertension, and diabetes, can limit tolerance to chemotherapy.

Common tumor-related factors can impact the timing and choice of such treatment as 5-FU and cisplatin. Malnutrition secondary to tumor or alcohol can have a major negative influence on treatment. Meningeal carcinomatoses and cranial nerve involvement may occur when the patient's tumor involves the base of the skull. These patients may require lumbar punctures and placement of an Ommaya reservoir for intrathecal instillation of methotrexate. Hypercalcemia related to bone or tumor involvement will require aggressive hydration and furosemide treatment before chemotherapy can be administered. Infection related to local wound cellulitis or recurring aspiration pneumonia may result in sepsis, requiring antibiotic therapy and delaying the administration of chemotherapy. In addition, bleeding from the carotid or small vessels can produce a significant obstacle. Chemotherapies that cause nausea and vomiting can precipitate bleeding. Many patients may require surgical intervention for fulguration, or occasional embolization of the artery to control bleeding.

Choice of treatment for recurrent head and neck cancer is also significantly influenced by the patient's previous exposure to radiotherapy or chemotherapy and

GERIATRIC CONSIDERATIONS
Head and Neck Cancers

Age-related losses such as vision, hearing, communication, fine motor skills (writing), and swallowing/eating functions will be further compromised by effects of surgery/radiation therapy and/or chemotherapy.

Nutritional and dental assessment with appropriate interventions will need to be adapted to age-related changes (diet history—likes/dislikes; dentures and/or lack of because of age or finances).

Pretreatment evaluation: psychosocial, cardiopulmonary, and health history factors will require age-related adjustments and appropriate interventions.

Treatment-related factors: surgery, radiation therapy, chemotherapy, and rehabilitation will require age-related adjustments and appropriate interventions. Patients with chronic diseases such as hypertension, cardiopulmonary insufficiency, diabetes, chronic obstructive pulmonary disease, arthritis, and chronic renal disease will require medical treatment adjustments.

   Surgery: potential exists for longer recovery and rehabilitation period.

   Radiation therapy: treatment schedule may require adjustment for recovery of side effects; fatigue/immunosuppression, weight loss, stomatitis, and infection.

   Chemotherapy: drug dosage, frequency of infusion, and monitoring of blood count will require adjustment (drug toxicities may increase related to previously mentioned chronic diseases).

Transportation, financial and family resources, and home care responsibilities will require assessment and intervention based on the deficits and/or availability.

ability to tolerate further bone marrow suppressive treatments.[81,84]

The boxes on p. 262 and above list complications, patient teaching priorities, and geriatric considerations.

CONCLUSION

Cancers of the head and neck are estimated to be the most prevalent cancers in the world. Whereas the physician's goals are improving treatment and patient survival, the nurse is challenged with assisting the patient to adjustments related to the disease, treatment, and rehabilitative living. The most important nursing challenge, however, is in the areas of early detection, prevention, patient education, and quality of life.[30,31,44,79] The incidence of head and neck cancers will never significantly decrease until patient use of the most common cocarcinogen (tobacco) ceases. Herein lies a challenge to all health care professionals.

■ CHAPTER QUESTIONS

1. Most head and neck cancers are which of the following cell types?
   a. Adenocarcinoma
   b. Lymphoepithelioma
   c. Squamous cell carcinoma
   d. Verrucous carcinoma

2. The most common site of head and neck cancer is the:
   a. Larynx
   b. Oral cavity
   c. Paranasal sinus
   d. Pharynx

3. The primary risk factor for head and neck cancer is:
   a. Alcohol abuse
   b. Nutritional deficiencies
   c. Occupational exposures
   d. Tobacco use

4. Surgery is as effective as radiation therapy in curing early-stage (stages I and II) cancers of the head and neck.
   a. True
   b. False

5. Quality of life as an outcome of cancer treatment is determined by which of the following patient variables?
   a. Emotional status
   b. Physical function
   c. Social well-being
   d. All the above

6. If postoperative drains do not function effectively, what may be the result?
   a. A dead space may develop.
   b. Flap necrosis may occur.
   c. Fluid may collect under the flap.
   d. Any of the above may occur.

7. If a head and neck cancer patient has an intact gastrointestinal tract but is at high risk for aspiration and requires long-term nutritional supplementation, which of the following tubes is preferred for feedings?
   a. Gastrostomy
   b. Jejunostomy
   c. Nasogastric
   d. Nasojejunostomy

8. Tracheostomy care performed at home by the patient should be completed using:
   a. Clean technique
   b. Sterile technique

9. All the following can aggravate radiation therapy related mucositis *except:*
   a. Alcohol
   b. Alkaline lavage
   c. Smoking
   d. Spicy foods

10. In the first year after treatment for head and neck cancer, physician follow-up should occur every:
   a. 1 month
   b. 3 months
   c. 6 months
   d. 12 months

BIBLIOGRAPHY

1. Aaronson NK, Beckman J: *The quality of life for cancer patients,* New York, 1987, Raven.
2. Albertson BE: Cancers of the head and neck. In Baird SB and others, editors: *A cancer source book for nurses,* ed 6, Atlanta, 1991, American Cancer Society.
3. Al-Kourainy K and others: Excellent response to cis-platinum based chemotherapy in patients with recurrent or previously untreated advanced nasopharyngeal carcinoma, *Am J Clin Oncol* 11:427, 1988.
4. Allison GR, Rappaport I, Salibian AH: Adaptive mechanisms of speech and swallowing after combined jaw and tongue reconstruction in long-term survivors, *Am Surg* 154:419, 1987.
5. Al-Sarraf M: Head and neck cancer: chemotherapy concepts, *Semin Oncol* 15(1):70, 1988.
6. Al-Sarraf M and others: Current progress in head and neck cancer: The Wayne State Experience. In Jacobs JR and others, editors: *Head and neck cancer: scientific perspectives in management and strategies for cure,* New York, 1987, Elsevier.
7. Al-Sarraf M and others: Concurrent radiotherapy and chemotherapy with cisplatin inoperable squamous cell carcinoma of the head and neck: RTOG study, *Cancer* 54:259, 1987.
8. Al-Sarraf M and others: Combined modality therapy (CMT) in patients with head and neck cancer (HN-CA): timing of chemotherapy (CT). In Salton JT, editor: *Radiation Therapy Oncology Group (RTOG) 6 study: adjunct therapy of cancer,* Philadelphia, 1990, Saunders.
9. Al-Sarraf M and others: Concurrent radiotherapy and chemotherapy with *cis*-platinum inoperable squamous cell carcinoma of the head and neck: an RTOG study, *Cancer* 59:259, 1990.
10. American Cancer Society: *Head and neck cancer,* Document 09440, Atlanta, 1995, The Society.
11. American Cancer Society: *Cancer facts and figures—1996,* Atlanta, 1996, The Society.
12. Amerin PC, Fingert H, Weitzman SA: Cisplatin-vincristine-bleomycin therapy in squamous cell carcinoma of the head and neck, *J Clin Oncol* 1:421, 1983.
13. Amour RJ and others: Postoperative irradiation for squamous cell carcinoma of the head and neck: an analysis of treatment results and complications, *Int J Radiat Oncol Biol Phys* 16:25, 1989.
14. Anderson BL: Sexual functioning morbidity among cancer survivors, *Cancer* 55(7):1835, 1985.
15. Ariyan S: The pectoralis myocutaneous flap, *Plast Reconstr Surg* 63:73, 1979.
16. Baker SR, editor: *Microsurgical reconstruction of the head and neck,* New York, 1989, Churchill Livingstone.
17. Barton FE, Spicer TE, Byrd HS: Head and neck reconstruction with the latissimus dorsi myocutaneous flap: anatomic observations and report of 60 cases, *Plast Reconstr Surg* 71:1999, 1983.
18. Basset MR, Dobie RA: Patterns of nutritional deficiency in head and neck cancer, *Otolaryngol Head Neck Surg* 91:119, 1983.
19. Beahrs OH and others: *American Joint Commission on Cancer manual for staging of cancer,* ed 4, Philadelphia, 1992, Lippincott.
20. Belcher AE: Nursing aspects of quality of life enhancement in cancer patients, *Oncology* 4(5):197, 1990.
21. Belcher AE: *Cancer nursing,* St Louis, 1992, Mosby.
22. Beumer J, Curtis TA, Morrish RB: Radiation complications in edentulous patients, *J Prosthet Dent* 36:193, 1976.
23. Beumer J and others: Osteonecrosis: predisposing factors and outcomes of therapy, *Head Neck Surg* 6:819, 1984.
24. Bildstein CY: Head and neck malignancies. In Groenwald SL and others, editors: *Cancer nursing: principles and practices,* ed 3, Boston, 1993, Jones and Bartlett.
25. Brachman DG: Molecular biology of head and neck cancer, *Semin Oncol* 21:320, 1994.
26. Brookes GBH: Nutritional status: a prognostic indicator in head and neck cancer, *Otolaryngol Head Neck Surg* 93:69, 1985.
27. Buchbinder D and others: Functional mandibular reconstruction of patients with oral cancer, *Oral Surg Oral Med Pathol* 68(4):499, 1989.
28. Caplan GA, Brigham BA: Marijuana smoking and carcinoma of the tongue: is there an association? *Cancer* 66:1005, 1990.
29. Carpenito LJ: *Nursing careplans and documentation: nursing diagnosis and collaborative problems,* ed 2, Philadelphia, 1995, Lippincott.
30. Cassileth BR and others: The satisfaction and psychosocial status of patients during treatment of cancer, *J Psychosoc Oncol* 7(4):47, 1989.
31. Cella DF: Quality of life as an outcome of cancer treatment. In Groenwald SL and others, editors: *Cancer nursing: principles and practices,* ed 3, Boston, 1993, Jones and Bartlett.
32. Chencharick JD, Mossman KL: Nutritional consequences of radiotherapy of the head and neck cancer, *Cancer* 51:811, 1983.
33. Conti J: Cancer rehabilitation: why can't we get out of first gear? *J Rehabil* 56(4):19, 1990.
34. Cook TA and others: Cervical rotation flaps for midface resurfacing, *Arch Otolaryngol Head Neck Surg* 117:77, 1991.
35. Cooper JS and others: Second malignancies in patients who have head and neck cancers: incidence, effect on survival and implications for chemoprevention based on the RTOG experience, *Int J Radiat Oncol Biol Phys* 17:449, 1989.
36. Crane L: Infections in patients with head and neck cancer. In Jacobs JR and others, editors: *Head and neck cancer: scientific perspectives in management and strategies for cure,* New York, 1987, Elsevier.
37. Crissman JD: Prognostic value of histopathologic parameters in squamous cell carcinoma of the oropharynx, *Cancer* 54:2995, 1984.
38. Crissman JD and others: Histopathologic diagnosis of early cancer, *Head Neck Cancer* 1:134, 1985.
39. David DJ and others: Mandibular reconstruction with vascularized crest: a 10 year experience, *Plast Reconstr Surg* 82:792, 1988.
40. Deitel M, To TB: Major intestinal complications of radiotherapy, *Arch Surg* 122:1421, 1987.
41. Depalo LG, Minah GE: Isolation of pathogenic microorganisms for dentures and denture soaking containers of the myelosuppressed cancer patients, *J Prosthet Dent* 49:20, 1983.

42. DeSanto L, Beahrs OH: The modified and radical neck dissection for squamous cell carcinoma of the upper aerodigestive system. In Jacobs JR and others, editors: *Head and neck cancer: scientific and clinical perspectives in management and strategies for cure,* New York, 1987, Elsevier.

43. Duchateau J, Decity A, Lejour M: Innervation of the rectus abdominous muscle: implications for rectus flaps, *Plast Reconstr Surg* 82:223, 1988.

44. Dudas S, Carlson CE: Cancer rehabilitation, *Oncol Nurs Forum* 15:183, 1988.

45. Elias EG, McCaslin DL: Nutrition in the patient with compromised oral function. In Peterson DE and others, editors: *Head and neck management of the cancer patient,* Boston, 1986, Martinus Nijhoff.

46. Ensley JF, Kish JA, Al-Sarraf M: The pretherapeutic identification of prognostically important parameters predictive of tumor response in squamous cell cancers of the head and neck. In Vog SE, editor: *Contemporary issues in clinical oncology: head and neck cancer,* vol 7, New York, 1988, Churchill Livingstone.

47. Ensley JF and others: Cellular DNA content parameters in untreated squamous cell cancers of the head and neck, *Cytometry* 10:334, 1980.

48. Ensley JF and others: The impact of conventional morphological analysis on response rates and survival in patients with squamous cell cancers of the head and neck, *Cancer* 57:711, 1986.

49. Ensley JF and others: The significance of pretreatment identification of prognostically important subgroups of squamous cell cancers of the head and neck. In Jacobs JR and others, editors: *Head and neck cancer: scientific and clinical perspectives in management and strategies for cure,* New York, 1987, Elsevier.

50. Ensley JF and others: The correlation of specific variables of tumor differentiation with response rate of survival in patients with advanced head and neck cancer treated with induction chemotherapy, *Cancer* 63:1487, 1989.

51. Ensley JF and others: Improved responses to radiation and concurrent cisplatin (CACP) in patients with advanced head and neck cancer (SCCHN) that fail induction chemotherapy. In *Proceedings of the Sixth International Conference on Adjuvant Therapy of Cancer,* March 1990, Tucson, Ariz.

52. Epstein JB and others: Osteonecrosis: study of relationship of dental extractions in patients receiving radiotherapy, *Head Neck Surg* 10:48, 1987.

53. Ervin TJ and others: An analysis of induction and adjuvant chemotherapy in the multidisciplinary treatment of squamous-cell carcinoma of the head and neck, *J Clin Oncol* 5:10, 1987.

54. Fearon KCH and others: Influence of whole body protein turnover rate on resting energy expenditure in patients with cancer, *Cancer Res* 48:2590, 1988.

55. Ferrans C: Quality of life: conceptual issues, *Semin Oncol Nurs* 6:248, 1990.

56. Fisher J, Jackson T: Microvascular surgery as an adjunct to craniomaxillofacial reconstruction, *Br J Plast Surg* 42:146, 1989.

57. Fisher S: The psychosexual effects of cancer and cancer treatment, *Oncol Nurs Forum* 10(2):6367, 1983.

58. Forastiere AA and others: Phase II trial of AZQ in head and neck cancer, *Cancer Treat Rep* 66:2097, 1982.

59. Fowler JF: Rationales for high linear energy transfer radiotherapy. In Steel GG, Adams GS, Peckman MJ, editors: *The biological basis of radiotherapy,* New York, 1983, Elsevier.

60. Fu KK and others: Combined radiotherapy and chemotherapy with bleomycin and methotrexate in advanced inoperable head and neck cancer: update of a Northern California oncology group randomized trial, *J Clin Oncol* 5:1410, 1987.

61. Germino B: Cancer and the family. In Baird SB, McCorkle R, Grant M, editors: *Cancer nursing: a comprehensive textbook,* Philadelphia, 1991, Saunders.

62. Goltrup F and others: The dynamic properties of tissue oxygenation in healing flaps, *Surgery* 95:527, 1984.

63. Goodwin WJ, Torres J: The value of the prognostic nutritional index in the management of patients with advanced carcinoma of the neck, *Head Neck Surg* 6:932, 1984.

64. Gotay C: Research in cancer rehabilitation. In McGarvey C, editor: *Physical therapy for the cancer patient,* New York, 1990, Churchill Livingstone.

65. Gralla RJ and others: The management of chemotherapy-induced nausea and vomiting, *Med Clin North Am* 71:289, 1987.

66. Grayden JE: Factors that predict patients' functioning following treatment for cancer, *Int J Nurs Stud* 25(2):117, 1988.

67. Guillamondequi OM, Larson DL: The lateral trapezium musculocutaneous flap: its use in head and neck reconstruction, *Plast Reconstr Surg* 67:143, 1981.

68. Gullane PJ, Arena S: Extended palatal island mucoperiosteal flap, *Arch Otolaryngol* 111:330, 1985.

69. Harriot JC and others: Dental preservation in patients irradiated for head and neck tumors: a 10 year experience with topical fluoride and a randomized trial between two fluoridation methods, *Radiother Oncol* 1:72, 1983.

70. Harris L, Smith S: Chemotherapy in head and neck cancer, *Semin Oncol Nurs* 5(3):174, 1989.

71. Hidlago D: Aesthetic improvements in free flap mandible reconstruction, *Plast Reconstr Surg* 88(4):574, 1991.

72. Hooper JA, Sigler BA: Nursing care of the head and neck cancer patient. In Myers EN, Suen JY, editors: *Cancer of the head and neck,* New York, 1988, Churchill Livingstone.

73. Housset M and others: A perspective study of three treatment techniques for T1-T2 base of tongue lesions: surgery plus post op radiation, external radiation plus interstitial implantation and external irradiation alone, *Int J Radiat Oncol Biol Phys* 13:511, 1987.

74. Jacobs CD: Head and neck cancers. In Witts RE, editor: *Manual of oncologic therapeutics,* Philadelphia, 1991, Lippincott.

75. Jacobs J, Spitznagel E, Sessions D: Staging parameters for cancer of the head and neck: a multifactorial analysis, *Laryngoscope* 95:1378, 1985.

76. Jacobs JR and others: Cisplatin and 5-fluorouracil infusion therapy before definitive treatments in advanced head and neck carcinoma: an RTOG study, *Arch Otolaryngol* 113:193, 1987.

77. Jacobs JR and others: Chemotherapy following definitive surgery for advanced squamous cell carcinoma of the head and neck: a Radiation Therapy Oncology Group Study, *Am J Clin Oncol* 12:85, 1989.

78. Jobsis FF, Boyd JB, Barwick WJ: Metabolic consequences of ischemia and hypoxia. In Serafin D, Buncke EU, editors: *Microsurgical composite tissue transplantation,* St Louis, 1974, Mosby.

79. Johnson JL, Lane CA: Helping families respond to cancer. In Baird SB, McCorkle R, Grant M, editors: *Cancer nursing: a comprehensive textbook,* Philadelphia, 1991, Saunders.

80. Kies MS and others: Analysis of complete responders after initial treatment with chemotherapy in head and neck cancer, *Otolaryngol Head Neck Surg* 93:199, 1985.

81. Kish J and others: Clinical results in recurrent head and neck carcinoma. In Jacobs JR and others, editors: *Head and neck cancer: scientific and clinical perspectives in management and strategies for cure,* New York, 1987, Elsevier.

82. Klein S and others: Total parenteral nutrition and cancer clinical trials, *Cancer* 58:1378, 1986.

83. Komisar A: The functional result of mandibular reconstruction, *Laryngoscope* 100:364, 1990.

84. Kramer S and others: Combined radiation therapy and surgery in the management of advanced head and neck cancers: final report of Study 7303 of the Radiation Therapy Oncology Group, *Head Neck Surg* 1:19, 1987.

85. Kudsk EG, Hoffman GS: Rehabilitation of the cancer patient, *Prim Care* 14:381, 1987.

86. Lamb M: Alterations in sexuality and sexual functioning. In Baird SB, McCorkle R, Grant M, editors: *Cancer nursing: a comprehensive textbook,* Philadelphia, 1991, Saunders.

87. Leveque FG and others: A multicenter, randomized, double-blind, placebo-controlled, dose-titrated study of oral pilocarpine for treatment of radiation-induced xerostomia in head and neck cancer patient, *J Clin Oncol* 11(6):1124, 1993.

88. Levine PH and others, editors: *EBV DNA content and expression in nasopharyngeal carcinoma,* Amsterdam, 1985, Martinus Nijhoff.

89. Licciardello JT, Spitz MR, Hong WK: Multiple primary cancer of the head and neck: second cancer of the head and neck, esophagus and lung, *Int J Radiat Oncol Biol Phys* 17:467, 1989.

90. Little W, Falace DA: *Dental management of the medically compromised patient,* St Louis, 1980, Mosby.

91. Loescher LJ and others: Physiologic and psychological implications of surviving adult cancer (2 parts), *Ann Intern Med* 111:411, 1989.

92. Lukash FN, Sachs SA: Functional mandibular reconstruction: prevention of the oral invalid, *Plast Reconstr Surg* 84:227, 1989.

93. Mahon SM: Managing the psychosocial consequences of cancer recurrence: implications for nurses, *Oncol Nurs Forum* 16:39, 1989.

94. Mashberg A, Samit A: Early diagnosis of asymptomatic oral and oropharyngeal squamous cancers, *CA Cancer J Clin* 46:328, 1995.

95. McConnel FMS, Teichgraeber JF, Adler RK: A comparison of three methods of oral reconstruction, *Arch Otolaryngol Head Neck Surg* 113:496, 1987.

96. McPhetride L: Nursing history: one means to personalize care, *Am J Nurs* 68:68, 1968.

97. Medina JE, Rigual NM: Neck dissection. In Cummings CW and others, editors: *Otolaryngology–head and neck surgery,* ed 2, St Louis, 1993, Mosby.

98. Mendenhall W and others: Is elective neck treatment indicated for T2 squamous cell carcinoma of the glottic larynx? *Radiat Ther Oncol* 14:199, 1989.

99. Mendenhall W and others: The role of radiation therapy in laryngeal cancer, *CA Cancer J Clin* 40(3):150, 1990.

100. Metcalf MC, Fischman SH: Factors affecting sexuality of patients with head and neck cancer, *Oncol Nurs Forum* 12(2):21, 1985.

101. Million R, Cassisi RR, editors: *Management of head and neck cancer: a multidisciplinary approach,* Philadelphia, 1994, Lippincott.

102. Morrish RB and others: Osteonecrosis in patients irradiated for head and neck carcinoma, *Cancer* 47:1980, 1981.

103. Muldooney JB and others: Oral cavity reconstruction using the free arm radial flap, *Arch Otolaryngol Head Neck Surg* 13:1219, 1987.

104. Murphy GP, Lawrence W, Lenard RE, editors: *American Cancer Society textbook of clinical oncology,* ed 2, Atlanta, 1995, American Cancer Society.

105. Murray CG, Daly TE, Zimmerman SO: The relationship between dental disease and radiation necrosis of the mandible, *Oral Surg* 49:99, 1980.

106. Myers EN, Suen JY: *Cancer of the head and neck,* New York, 1989, Churchill Livingstone.

107. Parker RG, Enstrom JE: Second primary cancers of the head and neck following treatment of initial primary head and neck cancer, *Int J Radiat Oncol Biol Phys* 14:561, 1988.

108. Parker SL and others: Cancer statistics, 1996, *CA Cancer J Clin* 46(1):5, 1996.

109. Pennington JE: Respiratory tract infections: intrinsic risk factors, *Am J Med* 76(suppl SA):34, 1984.

110. Pomp J, Levendag PC, Putten WLJ: Reirradiation of recurrent tumors in the head and neck, *Am J Clin Oncol* 11:543, 1988.

111. Poplin E and others: Combined therapies for squamous cell carcinoma of the esophagus: a Southwest Oncology Group Study (SWOG 8037), *J Clin Oncol* 5:622, 1987.

112. Puthawala AA and others: Limited external beam and interstitial iridium-192 irradiation in the treatment of carcinoma of the base of tongue: a 10 year experience, *Int J Radiat Oncol Biol Phys* 14:839, 1988.

113. Reese JL: Head and neck cancers. In Baird SB, McCorkle R, Grant M, editors: *Cancer nursing: a comprehensive textbook,* Philadelphia, 1991, Saunders.

114. Reuther JF, Steinau H, Wagner R: Reconstruction of larger defects in the oropharynx with revascularized intestinal grafts: an experimental clinical report, *Plast Reconstr Surg* 73:345, 1984.

115. Reynolds JV and others: Arginine, protein calorie malnutrition and cancer, *J Surg Res* 45:513, 1988.

116. Rieke JW and others: Oral pilocarpine for radiation-induced xerostomia: integrated efficacy and safety results from two prospective randomized clinical trials, *Int J Radiat Oncol Biol Phys* 31(3):661, 1995.

117. Rirken M and others: Rectus abdominis free flap in head and neck reconstruction, *Arch Otolaryngol Head Neck Surg* 117:857, 1991.

118. Robson MC: The physiologic basis of reconstruction of the head and neck defect. In Jacobs JR and others, editors: *Head and neck cancer: scientific and clinical perspectives in management and strategies for cure,* New York, 1987, Elsevier.

119. Robson MC, Phillips LG: Head and neck: overview. In Moosa AR, Schimpff SC, Robson MC, editors: *Comprehensive textbook of oncology,* ed 2, Baltimore, 1991, Williams & Wilkins.

120. Rodriguez-Monge EJ, Shin DM, Lippman SM: Head and neck cancer. In Padzur R, editor: *Medical oncology: a comprehensive review,* Huntington, NY, 1995, PRR.

121. Schleper JR: Prevention, detection, and diagnosis of head and neck cancer, *Semin Oncol Nurs* 5(3):139, 1989.

122. Schuller DE and others: Analysis of disability resulting from treatment including radical neck dissection or modified neck dissection, *Head Neck Surg* 6:551, 1983.

123. Schulmeister L: Nutrition. In Otto S, editor: *Oncology nursing,* ed 2, St Louis, 1994, Mosby.

124. Schusterman MA and others: Use of the A0 plate for immediate mandibular reconstruction in cancer patients, *Plast Reconstr Surg* 88(4):588, 1991.

125. Schwartz HC: Mandibular reconstruction using Dacron-Urethane prosthesis an autogenous cancellous bone: a review of 32 cases, *Plast Reconstr Surg* 73:387, 1994.

126. Seidel HM and others: *Mosby's guide to physical examination,* ed 3, St Louis, 1995, Mosby.

127. Seligman M and others: Combined therapy for recurrent or metachronous squamous cell carcinoma of the head and neck. In Wolf T, Carey TE, editors: *Head and neck oncology research: Proceedings of the 2nd International Head and Neck Oncology Research Conference,* Arlington, Va, September 1987, Kugler.

128. Shah JP, Lydiatt W: Treatment of cancer of the head and neck, *CA Cancer J Clin* 45(6):352, 1995.

129. Shaha AR, Strong EW: Cancer of the head and neck. In Murphy GP, Lawrence W, Lenhard RE, editors: *American Cancer Society textbook of clinical oncology,* ed 2, Atlanta, 1995, American Cancer Society.

130. Shellito PC, Malt RA: Tube gastrotomy: techniques and complications, *Ann Surg* 201:180, 1985.

131. Sigler BA: Nursing care for head and neck tumor patients. In Thrawley SE, Panye WR, editors: *Comprehensive management of head and neck tumors,* Philadelphia, 1987, Saunders.

132. Sigler BA: Nursing care of the head and neck cancer patient, *Oncology* 2:49, 1988.

133. Sigler BA, Schuring LT: *Ear, nose, and throat disorders,* St Louis, 1993, Mosby.

134. Slaughter DL, Southwick HW, Smejkal W: "Field cancerization" in oral stratified squamous epithelium: clinical implications of multicentric origin, *Cancer* 6:963, 1953.

135. Smith K, Lesko IM: Psychological problems in cancer survivors, *Oncology* 2:33, 1988.

136. Sonis ST: Oral complications of cancer therapy. In DeVita VT, Hellman S, Rosenberg SA, editors: *Cancer nursing: principles and practice,* ed 2, Philadelphia, 1985, Lippincott.

137. Spitz MR: Epidemiology and risk factors for head and neck cancer, *Semin Oncol* 21(3):281, 1994.

138. Stoll BA: *Coping with cancer stress,* Dordrecht, 1986, Martinus Nijhoff.

139. Strohl RA: Radiation therapy for head and neck cancers, *Semin Oncol Nurs* 5(3):166, 1989.

140. Sweeney PJ and others: Radiation therapy in head and neck cancer: indications and limitation, *Semin Oncol* 21(3):296, 1994.

141. Szeliga D, Groenwald S, Sullivan D: Nutritional disturbances. In Groenwald S and others, editors: *Cancer nursing: principles and practice,* ed 2, Boston, 1990, Jones and Bartlett.

142. Taylor I and others: Free vascularized bone graft: plastic and reconstruction of patients with oral cancer, *Oral Surg Oral Med Pathol* 68(4):499, 1992.

143. Teichgraeber J, Bowman J, Goetert H: New test series for functional evaluation of oral cavity cancer, *Head Neck Surg* 8:819, 1985.

144. Thompson LW: Head and neck cancer: early detection, *Semin Surg Oncol* 5:168, 1989.

145. Tiwari RM: Masseter crossover flap reconstruction of oral-oropharyngeal defects. In Wolf T, Carey TE, editors: *Head and neck oncology research: Proceedings of the 2nd International Head and Neck Oncology Research Conference,* Arlington, Va, September 1987, Kugler.

146. Tiwari RM: Masseter muscle crossover flap in primary closure in oral oropharyngeal defects, *J Laryngol Otol* 101:172, 1987.

147. Tiwari RM, Snow GB: Role of myocutaneous flaps in reconstruction of the head and neck, *J Laryngol Otol* 97:441, 1983.

148. Tonenelli PM, Hume WR, Kenny EB: Chlorhexidine: a review of the literature, *J West Soc Periodont* 31:5, 1983.

149. Wallis DP: Lateral face reconstruction with the medal-based cervicopectoral flap, *Arch Otolaryngol Head Neck Surg* 114:729, 1988.

150. Wang CC, Blitzer PH, Siuit HD: Twice-day radiation therapy for cancer of the head and neck, *Cancer* 55:2100, 1985.

151. Wang CC and others: Treatment with preoperative irradiation and surgery of squamous cell carcinoma of the head and neck, *Cancer* 64:3233, 1989.

152. Weichselbaum R, Beckett MA: The maximum recovery potential of human tumor cells may predict clinical outcome in radiotherapy, *Int J Radiat Oncol Biol Phys* 13:709, 1987.

153. Weiland AJ: Vascularized bone grafts: reconstructive surgery. In Green DP, editor: *Operative hand surgery,* New York, 1988, Churchill Livingstone.

154. Wil TK, Pietrocola D, Welch HF: A new method of percutaneous endoscopic gastrotomy using anchoring devices, *Am J Surg* 153:230, 1987.

155. Wolf GT and others: Neoplasms of the head and neck: head and neck cancer. In Holland J and others: *Cancer medicine,* Philadelphia, 1993, Lea & Febiger.

156. Wong CS, Cummings BJ: The place of radiation therapy in the treatment of squamous cell carcinoma of the nasal vestibule, *Acta Oncol* 27:203, 1988.

157. Zarbo RJ, Crissman JD: The pathologist's role in diagnosis and staging of upper aerodigestive tract carcinoma. In Jacobs JR and others, editors: *Head and neck cancer: scientific perspectives in management and strategies for cure,* New York, 1987, Elsevier.

CHAPTER 12
Human Immunodeficiency Virus (HIV) and Related Cancers

CYNTHIA F. BROGDON

On June 5, 1981, the first cases of an illness later defined as *acquired immunodeficiency syndrome* (AIDS) were reported by California health care providers to the Centers for Disease Control (CDC).[5] This first cluster of five Los Angeles men presented with unusual opportunistic infections and were thought to represent a geographically localized epidemic of an unknown infectious disease. Just 4 years later, in 1985, 14,049 cases of AIDS were reported in the United States. Later that same year, the *human immunodeficiency virus* (HIV) was identified as the causative agent of AIDS; more than 7000 Americans had already died of the disease.[5]

We are now in the second decade of this epidemic, which has claimed the lives of 1.1 million people across the globe.[18] Although scientific and clinical progress has been made and new treatments and comprehensive models of care developed, HIV disease remains an incurable illness spreading rapidly throughout the United States and the world.

Nurses play a pivotal role in treatment and prevention of this disease. Patient education about risk behaviors and risk reduction techniques will help prevent new infections and will undoubtedly save countless lives. Appropriate, compassionate nursing care for those already infected may extend survival and will improve the quality of life for those afflicted with HIV disease.

HUMAN IMMUNODEFICIENCY VIRUS
EPIDEMIOLOGY

HIV infection has occurred in approximately 1.5 million Americans and progressed to AIDS in more than 500,000. This epidemic has killed 300,000 Americans, and the numbers increase daily.[4] Throughout the world, more than 12 million people are infected with HIV, and almost 2 million have progressed to an AIDS diagnosis. It is estimated that more than 1 million people have died

of AIDS worldwide. Although changes in risk behaviors have slowed the spread of HIV infection in some areas of the United States, HIV transmission has accelerated in others. More than 40,000 new infections are expected this year in the United States alone.[8] In 1991 the World Health Organization estimated 40 million infections worldwide by the year 2000. That estimate has been revised, and now many experts report that more than 110 million persons will be infected with HIV by the end of this decade.

Throughout the epidemic the numbers of those infected have steadily increased each year. Early in the U.S. epidemic, more than 80% of those infected were homosexual men. Currently, less than 50% of infections occur in this population. Those persons now at greatest risk for acquiring HIV infection in the United States include heterosexual women and their children and intravenous drug users (IDUs). Women now represent nearly 20% of new U.S. cases and IDUs almost 30%. HIV infection continues to affect racial minorities disproportionately: 38% of all U.S. HIV infections now occur in blacks and 18% in Hispanics.[4]

Worldwide, HIV continues to ravage heterosexual men, women, and their children. New infections in Asia have increased dramatically in the past 2 years, and areas of Africa have infection rates as high as 35% to 50% among the general population.

ETIOLOGY AND RISK FACTORS

Since the first description of AIDS in 1981, an extraordinary scientific adventure has ensued. In just over a decade, remarkable advancements have occurred in our understanding of the disease and its causative agent, HIV. The origin of HIV is still largely unknown, although evidence appears to support the hypothesis of an African origin. The first reports of an AIDS-like illness date back to the early 1960s in central Africa. HIV in humans probably has an animal origin, most likely nonhuman primates.

HIV is a human retrovirus and belongs to the lentivirus subfamily. Currently, five human retroviruses have been identified: human T cell lymphotrophic virus type 1 (HTLV-1), HTLV-2, HTLV-5, HIV-1, and HIV-2. HTLV-2 has not been conclusively associated with human disease. HTLV-1 and HTLV-5 have been associated with human T cell leukemia and lymphoma, conditions characterized by proliferation of CD4+ (T4) helper cells. HIV-1 and HIV-2 both cause depletion of CD4 cells, resulting in loss of cellular immunity, as characterized by AIDS. HIV-1 is the predominant cause of AIDS in the United States, accounting for more than 95% of AIDS cases. HIV-2 seems to be limited to geographic distribution and is most prevalent in West Africa.[11]

The life cycle of HIV is similar to that of the other retroviruses. Mature virions interact with specific host receptors and then use the host cell for viral replication. HIV interacts with the CD4 glycoprotein, which occurs on the membrane of specific cells, primarily the CD4+ (T4) helper lymphocytes. These specific white blood cells contain the CD4 glycoprotein on their membranes, allowing the virus to fuse. The viral core is subsequently injected into the cell cytoplasm, where the viral ribonucleic acid (RNA) genome is translated into deoxyribonucleic acid (DNA) by a retroviral enzyme called *reverse transcriptase*. Infection and subsequent viral replication eventually deplete the host's CD4 cells, resulting in a dramatic loss of the protective immune response against invading microorganisms.

The routes for transmission of HIV are well documented: (1) intimate sexual contact; (2) parenteral exposure to blood, blood-containing body fluids, and blood products; and (3) mother-to-child contact during the perinatal period. Although HIV has been identified in a variety of body fluids, those consistently shown to be infectious are blood, semen, and vaginal secretions. Transmission has also been associated with breast milk, although this appears to occur infrequently. HIV is transmitted directly from person to person by sexual contact; from direct innoculation with contaminated blood products, needles, or syringes; and from an infected mother to her newborn. HIV is not transmitted by casual contact, including sneezing, coughing, or spitting; handshakes; toilet seats, bathtubs, showers, or swimming pools; or utensils, dishes, or linens used by an infected person. HIV disease is a blood-borne, sexually transmitted disease. Although certain sexual practices may be associated with higher risks for infection than others, any practice that exposes one to infected blood, semen, or vaginal secretions carries the potential for viral transmission.

The natural history of HIV infection is associated with an unpredictable course of disease progression. Most patients undergo a prolonged period of clinically silent infection, often lasting more than 10 years.[12] Although the virus is consistently detectable throughout this time, patients typically have only subtle immunologic alterations. Once the patient becomes symptomatic, however, decreases in the number of T4 helper cells can be detected and viral replication increases.

It is postulated that several potential cofactors may be associated with HIV disease progression. These cofactors, which may be of a viral, host, or environmental nature, are thought to directly influence the replication of HIV or the severity of its pathogenic effects. Viral cofactors that may influence the progression of the disease include herpes simplex virus (HSV), cytomegalovirus (CMV), and Epstein-Barr virus (EBV). Host cofactors may include a variety of cytokines and intracellular mediators. Environmental cofactors may include repeated exposure to HIV, which may induce hyperactivation of the immune system, resulting in an expansion of the pool of HIV-replicating cells. As viral replication increases, depleting the body of T4 helper lymphocytes, the body's defense mechanisms are progressively weakened. Infections that were once disarmed by the healthy immune system are eventually able to cause serious and potentially life-threatening disease. These *opportunistic infections* (OIs) include a variety of organisms, such as viruses (HSV, EBV, CMV), protozoa (*Pneumocystis carinii, Toxoplasma*), *Mycobacterium* (*tuberculosis* and *avium [avium-intracellulare]* complex), and fungi (*Histoplasma, Cryptococcus*). In addition to the various OIs, the profound immune dysfunction also allows the development of several neoplasms, including non-Hodgkin's lymphoma, Kaposi's sarcoma, and cervical carcinomas.

PREVENTION, SCREENING, AND DETECTION

Since HIV disease is blood borne and sexually transmitted, prevention efforts must be directed toward ways to avoid exposure to contaminated blood and body fluids. With less than 3% of AIDS cases attributed to exposure to contaminated blood products, the greatest exposure risk is through sexual contact. AIDS prevention efforts must therefore focus on ways to reduce sexual transmission.

Historically, it has been difficult to talk about sexuality in the American culture. It has been a subject laden with moral judgments and an area seldom addressed in the U.S. health care system. Nurses are in an excellent position to discuss sexuality with patients. Typically, it is the nurse who has an intimate rapport with the patient, talking about sensitive subjects and related health concerns. It is usually the nurse with whom the patient feels most at ease and the nurse who is most accessible to patients. The nurse plays a major role in the education of individuals and groups in the prevention of HIV disease.

Prevention efforts must include accurate, reliable, and clear information about risk factors for HIV disease and ways to decrease these risks. Prevention education programs must include the topics of practicing safer sexual techniques and using clean drug paraphernalia, as well as public health measures such as blood product screening and perinatal counseling. Prevention efforts must focus on behaviors that put patients at risk for infection.

Safe Sex Counseling

Any exchange of blood, semen, or vaginal secretions can potentially put an individual at risk for HIV disease. Common sexual practices that are therefore risky behaviors include vaginal or anal penetration without a condom and possibly oral sexual practices. Use of barrier products such as latex condoms while engaging in these behaviors greatly reduces the likelihood of exposure to potentially infectious blood, semen, or vaginal secretions. In addition, education about condom use should include the use of prelubricated condoms. Nonoxynol 9, a frequently used spermicidal lubricant, may also have some antiviral properties. Use of condoms prelubricated with nonoxynol 9 may therefore further increase the protection afforded by condoms. Use of additional water-based lubricants should also be encouraged. Petroleum-based lubricant use should be discouraged, since these agents may cause latex breakdown. Prevention education must also include risk reduction techniques such as minimizing the number of sexual partners and engaging in a mutually monogamous sexual relationship. In addition, sexual practices that do not put the individual at risk for potentially infectious fluids should be discussed. Mutual masturbation, massage, and body rubbing are safe sexual practices with no exchange of body fluids.

Intravenous Risk Reduction

The use of contaminated needles for subcutaneous, intramuscular, or intravenous injection represents a serious risk for HIV infection. Prevention education must include ways to clean needles and other paraphernalia used to inject drugs. Educational efforts may include information about substance abuse counseling and programs, but use of a bleach solution to disinfect needles and paraphernalia must also be discussed.

Perinatal Transmission

Women who are HIV infected may pass the virus on to their newborns via three potential routes: during gestation, during delivery, and through breastfeeding. Although the exact mechanism of perinatal transmission is unknown, the current estimate of risk to the newborn from an infected mother is approximately 30% in the United States.[19] A ground-breaking study of mother-to-infant transmission was completed in 1994. This study revealed the risk of mother-to-infant transmission could be reduced by more than 67% if women were treated with AZT during the pregnancy and newborns were then treated postpartum. In this study, only 18.3% of treated mothers had infants who were HIV infected. Based on this study, the U.S. Public Health Service now recommends that HIV-positive pregnant women be advised of these results and be offered AZT.[4]

Public Health Measures

Prevention programs must also educate the public about the measures that are currently in place to screen and protect the blood supply from contamination. Currently, each unit of donated blood is tested for HIV infection and several other blood-borne infections such as hepatitis. Because HIV screening of blood products has been conducted since 1985 in the United States, only recipients of transfusions before this time are at significant risk for infection via the blood supply.

Screening

HIV antibody testing plays an essential role in prevention and treatment of this disease process. The most common form of screening for HIV disease is the use of the antibody test with the *enzyme-linked immunosorbent assay* (ELISA) technique and the *Western blot* technique. The ELISA test uses spectrophotometry to detect serum antibody reactions to specific HIV viral proteins. The ELISA is highly sensitive and specific with a sensitivity of 98.4% to 99.6%. A positive ELISA test must be confirmed by the Western blot technique.

Both the ELISA and the Western blot techniques depend on antibody formation. Approximately 90% of the population will form antibodies in response to HIV exposure within 6 weeks to 3 months after exposure. A negative antibody test may occur in the "window phase" between the dates of actual exposure leading to infection and development of detectable serum antibodies. Although approximately 90% of the population will form antibodies in response to HIV exposure within 6 weeks to 3 months after exposure, this period may be as long as 6 months.[9]

Since newborn infants maintain maternal antibodies for as long as 18 months, antibody testing is unreliable until the infant is 18 months of age. A newer test, the *polymerase chain reaction* (PCR), is now available. The PCR does not rely on antibody formation; instead, genetic subunits of the virus are identified, confirming infection. This test is relatively new and sensitivity studies are still being conducted, but it will undoubtedly prove valuable in a wide variety of patient populations such as newborns.

Maintaining patient confidentiality is essential in HIV testing. Every measure possible should be taken to ensure that privacy is guaranteed. Unauthorized disclosure, stigmatization, and discrimination against HIV-positive individuals continue to occur with unfortunate regularity.

CLINICAL FEATURES

It has been estimated that 1.5 to 2 million Americans are infected with HIV; approximately one half are unaware they carry the virus that causes AIDS. Although some (fewer than 50%) of those infected will develop a viral syndrome resembling mononucleosis or influenza within a few days or weeks of infection, most are unaware the symptoms are related to the initial infection with HIV. Acute infection is followed by a period of asymptomatic HIV infection. In these early stages of HIV disease, there are no symptoms of infection. Infected persons may remain asymptomatic for several years, with half remaining asymptomatic for 10 years or longer.[21]

As HIV depletes the body of sufficient numbers of T4 helper cells, subtle symptoms of immunodeficiency may emerge. Patients may develop persistent generalized lymphadenopathy or minor dermatologic manifestations such as seborrhea. During this time a slow, persistent destruction of the immune system occurs with a gradual decline in the number of CD4 cells.

With continued destruction of the immune system, OIs and malignancies begin to develop and cause clinical symptoms. Clinical findings that appear to predict rapid progression to end-stage HIV disease (otherwise known as AIDS) include unexplained weight loss greater than 10% of usual body weight and persistent fever, diarrhea, or night sweats of longer than a 2-week duration.

Figure 12-1 provides an explanation of the usual progression of HIV disease in the United States. Table 12-1 lists specific clinical features of various OIs.

DIAGNOSIS AND STAGING

The spectrum of HIV infection ranges from asymptomatic infection to potentially life-threatening OI. In the

Table 12-1 Opportunistic Infections (OIs)

Opportunistic infections	Clinical features
BACTERIAL INFECTIONS	
Mycobacterium avium-intracellulare	General: persistent fever, night sweats, fatigue, weight loss, abdominal pain, weakness, lymphadenopathy, hepatosplenomegaly
FUNGAL INFECTIONS	
Candidiasis	Oral: white patches on tongue or buccal mucosa
	Vaginal: vulvar pruritus, vaginal discharge
Cryptococcosis	Meningitis: headache, fever, progressive malaise, altered mental status, seizures
	Pneumonia: fever, shortness of breath, cough
Histoplasmosis	Fever, weight loss, shortness of breath, lymphadenopathy
PROTOZOAL INFECTIONS	
Cryptosporidiosis	Diarrhea, abdominal cramping, nausea, vomiting, fatigue, weight loss, dehydration
Pneumocystis carinii	Pneumonia: fever, nonproductive cough, shortness of breath, weight loss, night sweats, fatigue
Toxoplasmosis	Encephalitis: altered mental status, seizures, fever, coma
VIRAL INFECTIONS	
Cytomegalovirus	Retinitis: unilateral visual deficit or change
	Gastrointestinal: dysphagia, wasting, nausea, fever, diarrhea
Herpes simplex	Painful blisters or ulcers

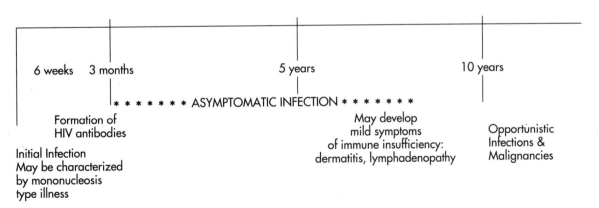

Figure 12-1   Usual progression of human immunodeficiency virus (HIV) disease in the United States.

past many clinicians used an informal staging system that put patients into one of three categories: (1) HIV positive, (2) AIDS-related complex (ARC), and (3) AIDS. In this staging system, "HIV positive" referred to patients who were completely asymptomatic but HIV positive. Those patients classified as "ARC" exhibited constitutional symptoms, including persistent generalized lymphadenopathy, persistent fevers, involuntary weight loss, and/or diarrhea. Any patient who had experienced an OI was classified as "AIDS."

Today, clinicians have become much more sophisticated about the stages of HIV disease and realize that it is a chronic, progressive illness characterized by four distinct categories. Although end-stage HIV disease is usually referred to as AIDS, most clinicians also use the staging system recommended by the CDC. The CDC Classification System for HIV Infection in Adults is currently the most widely used staging system (Table 12-2).

METASTASIS

HIV disease is a chronic, systemic infection. The infection itself primarily infects a specific group of lymphocytes (the T4 helper cells) but also has the potential for direct infection of the monocytes and macrophages and possibly muscle and nerve cells. In addition, many patients experience HIV infection directly affecting the central nervous system (CNS). As the disease progresses, almost every organ system is affected by one or more of the OIs that occur secondarily to the profound immunodeficiency that results from the original HIV infection. Most patients experience illness affecting the skin and mucous membranes, respiratory tract, gastrointestinal (GI) tract, and CNS.

TREATMENT MODALITIES
Chemotherapy

Several treatment options are now available to slow the progression of the illness, but currently no cure exists for HIV disease. However, the associated OIs that occur as a result of HIV infection can be treated and, in some patients, prevented.

In general, patients with HIV infection may remain relatively free of clinical symptoms for several years. Because of the variability of the disease progression, immune system surveillance on a regular basis is an important component of HIV treatment. It is recommended that patients with stable CD4 counts above 500 cells/mm^3 obtain a physical examination and laboratory evaluation every 3 to 6 months. Currently the CD4 count is the most important indicator in tracking progressive deterioration of immune system function in HIV-infected individuals. Studies are underway, however, to improve laboratory surveillance of the immune system with the use of PCR and branched DNA (bDNA) tests. These tests measure the viral load, and it is hoped they will provide a better analysis of a patient's clinical progression. In the meantime, however, CD4 cells are the most widely used laboratory assessment tool.

If the CD4 cell count falls below 500 cells/mm^3, initiation of antiretroviral therapy is indicated (Table 12-3). Zidovudine (Retrovir, AZT) was the first drug approved to treat HIV infection and remains the first choice of therapy for patients with fewer than 500 CD4 cells. If patients fail to tolerate zidovudine or the disease progresses despite zidovudine therapy, three other similar drugs are available: Videx (didanosine, ddI), HIVID (zalcitabine, ddC), and Stavudine (D4T). All three of these antiretrovirals belong to a class of drugs known as

Table 12-2 CDC Classification System for HIV Infections in Adults

Stage	Classification	Description
I	Acute infection	Occurs at time of initial HIV infection and may last from days to weeks; characterized by mononucleosis-like or influenza-like syndrome, with approximately 50% of patients reporting or recalling symptoms
II	Asymptomatic infection	Occurs after stage I and may last for several years
III	Persistent generalized lymphadenopathy (PGL)	Characterized by palpable lymph node enlargement of 1 cm or greater at two or more extrainguinal sites, persisting for longer than 3 months
IV	Other diseases	PGL not prerequisite
		Subgroup A: constitutional disease—fever persisting for longer than 1 month, involuntary weight loss greater than 10% of usual body weight, diarrhea persisting for longer than 1 month
		Subgroup B: neurologic disease—dementia, myelopathy, peripheral neuropathy
		Subgroup C: secondary infectious diseases—specific infectious diseases identified by CDC; typically referred to as *opportunistic infections*
		Subgroup D: secondary cancers—includes Kaposi's sarcoma, non-Hodgkin's lymphoma, primary lymphoma of brain
		Subgroup E: other conditions—includes other conditions specified by CDC (e.g., chronic lymphoid interstitial pneumonitis)

the *nucleoside analogues* and work to slow the rate of viral replication. These drugs are not cures for HIV infection.

In early 1996 a new class of antiretroviral drugs became available (Table 12-3). These new drugs, members of a class known as the *protease inhibitors,* have a different mechanism of action than the previously available *reverse transcriptase inhibitors* (AZT, ddI, ddC, D4T). The protease inhibitors include Ritonavir and Saquinavir and represent a significant breakthrough in the management of HIV disease. For the first time, patients have the option of using combination therapy with two drugs (e.g., AZT and Ritonavir), both of which have different side effects and toxicities. As in the treatment of malignancies and other infectious diseases, the most successful therapy involves the use of multiple drugs that have different mechanisms of action and different side effects.

Several other drugs are available to treat specific OIs that occur as the immune system is depleted. Various degrees of success have been achieved with these regimens in treating the OI. In some patients, prophylaxis for recurrent or even primary OIs may be effective.

Pneumocystis carinii infection is the most common OI occurring in HIV-infected patients. This protozoan is a ubiquitous organism acquired by most persons during childhood. Most often in HIV infection, *P.*

carinii causes pneumonia. Until recently, *P. carinii* pneumonia (PCP) was an almost universally life-threatening OI in patients with HIV disease. Although it remains the most common OI, occurring in as many as 85% of HIV patients, the mortality rate from PCP has been greatly reduced since the use of intravenous trimethoprim-sulfamethoxazole or pentamidine therapy. Oral trimethoprim-sulfamethoxazole has now been shown to be highly effective in preventing recurrence of PCP as well. In addition, initiation of oral PCP prophylaxis in patients known to be at high risk for PCP infection has reduced the primary occurrence rate.

Biotherapy

Anemia, leukopenia, and thrombocytopenia are part of the natural history of HIV disease. These cytopenias can result from marrow failure or cell-destructive processes. They can also be caused by drugs used to treat HIV disease and associated infections or malignancies. Several HIV drug therapies have been shown to be myelotoxic. Many drugs used to treat OIs as well as Retrovir (AZT) may have to be interrupted in certain patients secondary to myelotoxicity. Use of colony-stimulating factors (CSFs) such as granulocyte and granulocyte-monocyte CSFs (G-CSFs and GM-CSFs) has proved useful in decreasing myelotoxicity and often allows successful completion of therapy.

Erythropoietin (EPO) can be used for treatment of Retrovir-induced marrow suppression. Although this therapy has not been successful in all patients, a significant number have required fewer transfusions and have been able to continue antiviral, antiinfective, or antineoplastic therapy while receiving EPO.[14]

Future Therapies

In the early years of the AIDS epidemic, there was steadfast hope that a vaccination could be developed to stop the spread of this deadly virus. Many researchers across the United States have conducted countless trials of various vaccines, but none has yet proved to be successful. The rapid rate of mutation of HIV has made it difficult for scientists to match this with a vaccine that would stimulate appropriate antibody responses. Although vaccine research is continuing, most researchers believe that a vaccine for the general population will likely not be available before the end of the decade.[20] Vaccine research historically has focused on the prevention of infection. Much current vaccine research, however, is evaluating administration of a vaccine to patients who are already HIV infected. Through the use of an inactivated virus vaccine, researchers hope to spur the body's production of an antibody specific for fighting HIV as well as the production of CD4 cells. By stimulating the immune system's response to HIV, researchers hope that

Table 12-3 Antiretroviral Drugs for HIV Disease

Category/specific drugs	Side effects
REVERSE TRANSCRIPTASE INHIBITORS: NUCLEOSIDE ANALOGUES	
Zidovudine (azidothymidine, AZT, ZDV, Retrovir)	Bone marrow suppression, GI upset, headache, myopathy
Didanosine (dideoxyinosine, ddI, Videx)	Peripheral neuropathy, pancreatitis, diarrhea
Zalcitabine (dideoxycytidine, ddC, Hivid)	Peripheral neuropathy, pancreatitis, oral ulcers
NONNUCLEOSIDE REVERSE TRANSCRIPTASE INHIBITORS	
Nevirapine (investigational)	Rash; still investigational
Delaviridine (investigational)	Rash; still investigational
PROTEASE INHIBITORS	
Indinavir (Crixivan)	Kidney stones; side effects still being assessed secondary to rapid FDA approval
Saquinavir (Ro31)	Still being assessed secondary to rapid FDA approval
Ritonavir (ABT987)	GI upset; side effects still being assessed secondary to rapid FDA approval

GI, Gastrointestinal; *FDA,* Food and Drug Administration.

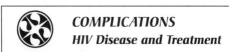

COMPLICATIONS
HIV Disease and Treatment

Disease-related complications

Profound immunosuppression
Development of various opportunistic infections/
  malignancies
Constitutional symptoms: fever, night sweats, weight loss
Persistent generalized lymphadenopathy
Financial loss, including employment, health insurance,
  housing
Societal stigmatization and discrimination

Treatment-related complications

Anemia, neutropenia, thrombocytopenia
Fatigue
Nausea, vomiting, weight loss

the vaccine might be able to halt or even reverse the spread of the virus in newly infected individuals.[7]

An increasing number of researchers now believe that *gene therapy* represents the only hope of cure for HIV disease. Gene therapy involves the insertion of a gene into a human cell. The new gene would direct the natural, antiviral human cell response. Theoretically the new gene would program the human cell to destroy HIV. Although research is now only in the early stages in this new arena, the therapy appears promising.

HIV has potential disease-related and treatment-related complications (see box above).

Prognosis

Although HIV disease appears to be a universally fatal illness, a small number of patients (less than 5%) appear to be long-term nonprogressors. These individuals are clearly infected with HIV but do not progress in the usual pattern of immunosuppression. The usual time to progression of profound immunodeficiency varies widely among patients. As more information and treatment options become available, HIV disease is likely to become a manageable, chronic illness. The nurse plays a primary role in educational efforts to prevent this disease and provide compassionate and appropriate care to those already infected.

HIV-RELATED CANCERS

The HIV epidemic has been characterized not only by the occurrence of opportunistic infections, but also by the development of specific cancers. As the patient's immune system function declines, the risk of malignancy increases. Kaposi's sarcoma and non-Hodgkin's lym-

phoma are the primary types of cancer associated with HIV infection. More recently, the occurrence of cervical and anal carcinomas has been noted in HIV-infected patients. As patients with HIV disease experience increased survival, it is anticipated that an increased frequency of HIV-related cancers will occur.[17]

KAPOSI'S SARCOMA

AIDS was first reported to the CDC in 1981 as a combined epidemic of PCP and Kaposi's sarcoma (KS). KS remains the most common neoplasm in HIV-infected patients. Although some progress has been made in understanding this malignant process, much remains to be understood.

Epidemiology

In a San Francisco cohort of gay men diagnosed with AIDS from 1981 to 1982, KS accounted for more than 75% of the AIDS-defining illnesses. By 1988, however, only 19% of patients with AIDS were diagnosed with KS as their presenting illness.[1] This curious decline in the proportion of patients having KS as their initial AIDS-defining illness is currently unexplained. Although all types of patients with AIDS have been found to have KS (heterosexual, homosexual, IDU), the incidence is greatest in homosexual HIV-positive men.

Etiology and Risk Factors

KS is a tumor of vascular origin. Although little is known of the nature of the malignant cells, KS is a multifocal neoplasm capable of arising simultaneously at multiple sites. The cause of KS in patients with HIV infection (AIDS-KS) is not yet known. It is suspected, however, that AIDS-KS may not be secondary to infection with HIV disease itself, but in fact may be another sexually transmitted infection, most likely caused by a herpes family virus.[1]

In addition to HIV disease, other immunodeficient states, such as iatrogenically induced immunosuppression, as seen in renal transplant patients, have also been the setting for KS. However, immunodeficiency may not be a prerequisite for the development of KS. The host's genetic makeup may be a factor contributing to the development of KS in AIDS patients. An increased frequency of major histocompatibility antigens DR-5 and DR-2 has been reported in some studies of HIV-associated KS. The absence of the HIV genome in the KS tumor lends further support to an indirect role for HIV in AIDS-KS.[17]

Prevention, Screening, and Detection

Since AIDS-KS is likely a result of a sexually transmitted disease, prevention must include education about risky sexual behaviors. As with prevention of HIV disease, prevention of KS must involve barrier protection such as condoms and avoidance of potentially infectious body fluids, including blood, semen, and vaginal secretions. Since HIV-infected patients are at significant risk for AIDS-KS, all HIV patients would be screened routinely for potential signs and symptoms of KS. Such screening requires visual inspection of all body surfaces, including oral mucosa. Since no laboratory test exists for KS, patients must be educated to report any suspicious lesions immediately to their health care providers.

Classification

Before the advent of the HIV epidemic, KS was seen as an indolent, cutaneous vascular tumor in elderly men, particularly of Jewish or Mediterranean descent. This classic or endemic form of KS is rarely life-threatening. AIDS-KS (also called *epidemic KS*) is usually characterized by multifocal, widespread lesions at the onset of the illness. AIDS-KS has a wide range of virulence in patients with HIV disease, ranging from limited stable involvement to fulminant disease with rapid, continuous development of new lesions. AIDS-KS is usually classified based on the site of the lesions. Nodular KS is characterized by subcutaneous nodular lesions that vary in size from several millimeters to several centimeters in diameter. Lymphadenopathic KS primarily affects the peripheral lymph nodes. Oral KS lesions can produce bleeding, tooth displacement, and pain. Visceral KS most often affects the lungs and GI tract.[6]

Clinical Features

AIDS-KS is usually characterized by multifocal, widespread lesions at the onset of illness. These lesions may involve the skin, oral mucosa, lymph nodes, or visceral organs, including the lung, liver, spleen, and GI tract. Most patients have skin lesions that appear as flat or raised plaques ranging in size from a few millimeters to several centimeters. Colors range from blue-purple to red-brown. Although lymph node involvement occurs frequently, it is often difficult to distinguish from HIV-associated lymphadenopathy. Visceral involvement may affect as many as half of reported cases.[6] GI involvement may be asymptomatic, although advanced disease may result in blood loss, diarrhea, and weight loss. Pulmonary involvement, although uncommon, may result in radiographic abnormalities and symptoms of cough, dyspnea, and fever. Although lesions from KS have been observed at autopsy in all organs, including the brain, pancreas, heart, and major vessels, these lesions remain generally asymptomatic.

Diagnosis and Staging

AIDS-KS is generally diagnosed by examining biopsies of skin or mucous membrane lesions. Although AIDS-KS has often been diagnosed without biopsy, the visual ap-

Table 12-4 Staging Classification for AIDS-KS

Stage	Definition
TUMOR (T)	
T-0	Confined to skin and/or lymph nodes
	Minimal oral KS
T-1	Tumor-associated edema or ulceration
	Extensive oral KS
	Gastrointestinal KS
	Other visceral KS
IMMUNE SYSTEM (I)	
I-0	T4 helper cells $\geq 200/mm^3$
I-1	T4 helper cells $\leq 200/mm^3$
SYSTEMIC ILLNESS (S)	
S-0	No history of opportunistic infection or thrush
	No constitutional symptoms
	Karnofsky performance score ≥ 70
S-1	History of opportunistic infection and/or thrush
	Constitutional symptoms
	Karnofsky performance < 70
	Other related HIV illness

pearance may be similar to several other dermatologic presentations, including fungal infection, lymphoma, dermatofibroma, and bacillary epithelioid angiomatosis (cat-scratch disease). AIDS-KS involving the lungs or GI tract is usually diagnosed by endoscopic examination.[15]

Several staging systems have been proposed for AIDS-KS, but none has achieved universal acceptance. The Oncology Committee of the National Institute of Allergy and Infectious Diseases (NIAID) has developed a proposal for staging criteria using a description of the tumor's extent, the status of the patient's immune system, and presence or absence of other HIV-related disease manifestations (Table 12-4).

Metastasis

Despite the overall progressive course of AIDS-KS, there may be a wide range of disease progression. A rapid course with short survival is seen in patients with opportunistic infections, systemic symptoms, and low CD4 counts. This rapid course is typically associated with aggressive, disseminated disease involving the lungs and visceral organs. In patients with no history of opportunistic infections (OIs) or systemic symptoms and in those with CD4 counts greater than 200 cells/mm³, the disease may be limited to cutaneous lesions and relatively slow progression.

Treatment Modalities

Curative therapy for AIDS-KS does not exist. AIDS-KS, however, is rarely life-threatening. Most patients with AIDS-KS ultimately die of OIs related to the profound immunodeficiency produced by HIV infection. Treatment of AIDS-KS is therefore usually instituted to relieve symptoms and to eliminate or reduce cosmetically unacceptable lesions.

In those patients who have minimal cutaneous disease, several treatment options exist. Observation alone is a possibility, since the lesions themselves are not usually painful and typically cause no morbidity or mortality. Patients, however, may choose one of the local modalities to reduce unacceptable cosmetic appearance. Local modalities include surgical excision, electrodessication, and radiation therapy.

KS is generally very responsive to *radiation therapy,* and good palliation can usually be obtained. Excellent responses can be obtained in treatment of cutaneous KS using whole-body electron beam therapy, fractionated focal x-ray therapy, or single-dose treatments. Radiation therapy is particularly useful when a prompt local response is desired. It is important to note, however, that patients with AIDS-KS seem to be unusually sensitive to radiation in specific areas, including the oral cavity, pharynx, and feet.[15]

Patients with more rapidly progressive disease may benefit from *chemotherapy.* Chemotherapy is most appropriate for patients who have relatively limited disease and for those with relatively intact immune function. Single-agent chemotherapy can produce cosmetic and symptomatic improvement with little toxicity or significant immune impairment. Overall, single-agent chemotherapy may control disease in approximately 30% of patients. Single-agent chemotherapy regimens may employ vinblastine, bleomycin, VP-16, or doxorubicin.

Combination chemotherapy has also been used successfully in the treatment of AIDS-KS. Since combination chemotherapy has not been shown to be consistently superior to single-agent chemotherapy, combination therapy is usually reserved for patients with widespread KS, which results in functional impairment secondary to edema, pain, or disfigurement. Visceral KS may also be managed with combination chemotherapy. Combination regimens may include vinblastine and vincristine; vinblastine and bleomycin; doxorubicin, bleomycin, and vinblastine; doxorubicin, bleomycin, and vincristine; or vinblastine, vincristine, and methotrexate.

Myelotoxicity and *neurotoxicity* have been the major adverse effects. However, the availability of hematopoietic growth factors (G-CSF, GM-CSF) may alleviate the myelotoxicity in a number of patients, and a survival advantage may be obtained in the future.

A number of clinical trials have confirmed the efficacy of alfa-2 recombinant interferon (IFN-2). Patients with relatively high numbers of T4 helper cells without prior OIs are more likely to respond to interferon therapy. Unfortunately, at doses required to produce responses in AIDS-KS, significant toxicities of interferon are common. Flu-like symptoms, weight loss, rash, and leuko-

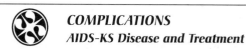

COMPLICATIONS
AIDS-KS Disease and Treatment

Potential disease-related complications

Disfigurement related to skin lesions
Airway obstruction related to pulmonary lesions
Nausea, vomiting, diarrhea related to gastrointestinal lesions

Potential treatment-related complications

Radiation
  Skin: erythema, dry/wet desquamation
  Abdomen: gastritis, nausea, vomiting
  General: fatigue
Chemotherapy
  Neutropenia
  Increased risk of opportunistic infection (OI)
  Nausea, vomiting
  Alopecia
Interferon therapy
  Flu-like syndrome
  Weight loss
  Rash
  Neutropenia and resultant increased risk of OI

penias occur in most patients. Combination therapy with IFN-2 and Retrovir may improve the chances for response to therapy, particularly in patients with CD4 cell counts greater than 200 before treatment initiation.

AIDS-KS has potential disease-related and treatment-related complications (see box above).

Prognosis

Despite significant progress in the treatment options available for patients with AIDS-KS, this unfortunately has not translated into an improvement in overall survival. Since optimal therapy of all stages is still in an early phase of development, patients are encouraged to enter into clinical trials whenever possible. Although curative therapy for AIDS-KS does not yet exist, KS is rarely life-threatening. Most patients with AIDS-KS ultimately die of OIs that develop as a result of the profound immunodeficiency that develops secondary to HIV infection.

NON-HODGKIN'S LYMPHOMA

Along with the improved survival of patients with HIV disease, new clinical complications are developing. HIV-related non-Hodgkin's lymphoma (NHL) appears to be increasing in frequency as the life span of patients with HIV disease is extended. These tumors appear most frequently at the end stages of AIDS, when the immune system is most profoundly impaired.

Epidemiology

The incidence of NHL among the population with advanced HIV infection is increasing steadily as the HIV epidemic continues. It is clear that NHL cases will continue to increase as HIV infection increases in the population and as HIV-infected individuals survive for longer periods.[10]

The epidemiology data indicate a disproportionate number of cases among HIV-infected patients, with rates nearly twice those of non-HIV-infected patients. In certain areas of the United States with high rates of HIV infection, the incidence of NHL is now five times greater than the highest pre-epidemic rate.

The median age of diagnosis in HIV-related NHL ranges from 26 to 40 years; the median age among HIV-negative patients is 56. Clearly, immunosuppression as a result of HIV infection is a risk factor in the development of NHL.

Etiology and Risk Factors

The etiology of lymphoid neoplasia in the setting of HIV infection remains unclear. Lack of similarity in the molecular characteristics of these tumors suggests that several different mechanisms may be responsible for the development of lymphoma in HIV-infected individuals. Pathogenesis of many of these lymphomas has been linked to latent infection of B lymphocytes with the *Epstein-Barr virus* (EBV). EBV does seem to be present in approximately 50% of the tumors with monoclonal origins, but not in those of polyclonal origin. In both EBV-positive and EBV-negative tumors, however, the onset of disease appears related to the degree of immunosuppression in the patient created by the original HIV infection.

Prevention, Screening, and Detection

Currently, there is no known way to prevent or screen for NHL. Clinicians should be suspicious of an NHL diagnosis in any HIV-infected patient who presents with a history of a lump or other mass. Laboratory studies are difficult to evaluate in this patient population. A complete blood count is usually normal, although anemia may be present and lymphopenia can occur in as many as 50% of patients. Erythrocyte sedimentation rate and lactic acid dehydrogenase may be elevated, although these elevations may also be attributable to HIV diseases or OI.

Classification

NHLs in HIV-infected patients are classified similarly to those occurring in noninfected patients. Rappaport introduced a classification system for the various histologic types of NHL in the late 1950s. This classification system has been formalized and is now commonly referred to as the *Working Formulation*.

In the Working Formulation classification scheme, the

HIV-associated NHLs are generally placed in the intermediate-grade and high-grade categories. Most cases of HIV-related NHL consist of high-grade NHL with B phenotype. The most represented histologies are Burkitt's lymphomas, immunoblastic lymphomas, and the otherwise nonspecified "undifferentiated" lymphomas. Diffuse large cell lymphoma, particularly of the high-grade immunoblastic type, is the most frequently diagnosed HIV-related NHL.[10]

Clinical Features

Patients presenting with HIV-associated NHL are a heterogeneous group. The most common symptom of NHL is painless lymphadenopathy that may involve the abdominal nodes. One third of patients with NHL have had preceding persistent generalized lymphadenopathy (PGL). Patients may present with systemic "B" symptoms such as fever, chills, and weight loss, although these symptoms may be difficult to differentiate from those associated with HIV infection and related OIs. Since extranodal sites such as the GI tract, bone marrow, spleen, and liver may be affected, patients may have symptoms of vague abdominal discomfort, back pain, GI complaints, or ascites.

Diagnosis and Staging

The findings of lymphadenopathy, splenomegaly, or hepatomegaly suggest lymphoma, but NHL may also present as an abdominal mass or as a discrete lesion of the lung or CNS. A complete physical examination is essential. In addition, routine tests, including a complete blood count and chemistries, should be obtained. Abnormal liver function tests may suggest involvement of the hepatic system, and liver biopsy may be indicated. Bone marrow involvement is common in HIV-associated NHL, and bone marrow aspiration and biopsy should be performed early in the diagnostic work-up. Chest x-ray evaluation may reveal mediastinal, hilar, or parenchymal involvement, and more sophisticated nuclear medicine studies such as the computed tomography (CT) scan and magnetic resonance imaging (MRI) can be used to scan the liver and spleen. The clinical value of the staging laparotomy has yet to be demonstrated, and bone marrow evaluation may provide adequate information.

Although its prognostic significance is unknown, the Ann Arbor Staging Classification is used to categorize the extent of disease, as follows:

Stage I	Involvement of a single lymph node region or of a single extralymphatic organ or site
Stage II	Involvement of two or more lymph node regions on the same side of the diaphragm
Stage III	Involvement of lymph node regions on both sides of the diaphragm
Stage IV	Disseminated involvement of one or more extralymphatic organs or tissues

Metastasis

Few patients present with stage I or II disease. In fact, most patients present with stage IV disease, which is further complicated by frequent involvement of the bone marrow and the CNS. In addition, the immunodeficiency and possible history of previous OIs may potentiate the aggressive course of the disease. Widely disseminated disease is diagnosed at the initial presentation in more than two thirds of patients. Also common to this population is the occurrence of unusual sites of lymphomatous disease, including the myocardium, adrenals, ear lobes, maxillae, gallbladder, orbit, and rectum.[6]

Treatment Modalities

Treatment of patients with HIV-related NHL is often complicated by their underlying immunodeficiency. As a group, these patients generally do not respond well to treatment. Those patients more likely to tolerate intensive therapy and to do relatively well are those without a prior history of profound immunodeficiency or OIs. Unfortunately, most patients have significant immunodeficiency at presentation. In addition, most patients have advanced stage IV disease of a high-grade type with possible involvement of the bone marrow and/or CNS. The neutropenia frequently seen in this patient population secondary to the HIV infection further complicates the use of conventional multiagent chemotherapy regimens.

Recent approaches to treatment have focused on variations in the dosing of the standard chemotherapeutic agents. Hematopoietic growth factors have also been used to alleviate the myeloid toxicity associated with chemotherapy. These trials have demonstrated that hematologic toxicity can be reduced by using reduced dosages of chemotherapy and by using myeloid growth factors with standard doses. It is still unclear, however, which of these treatment approaches will be associated with improved response and survival.[10]

In general, standard chemotherapy doses should be given to patients with CD4 counts greater than 200 cells/mm^3. Growth factor support is also recommended in this population. For patients with more compromised immune function (with CD4 cell counts less than 200), reduced-dosage chemotherapy regimens are advised because these patients are less likely to tolerate cytotoxic therapy. The most frequently used regimen is that of mBACOD, which includes methotrexate, bleomycin, doxorubicin, cyclophosphamide, vincristine, dexamethasone, and folinic acid, and CHOP, which includes cyclophosphamide, doxorubicin, vincristine, and predisone. For patients who are profoundly ill with significantly compromised immune status, the option of only palliative therapy should be considered.

Non-Hodgkin's lymphoma has potential disease-related and treatment-related complications (see box at right).

Prognosis

The prognosis for patients with HIV-associated NHL is poor. Median survival for patients with peripheral NHL treated with a variety of standard chemotherapeutic regimens ranges from 4 to 7 months in patients with less than 100 CD4 cells. For those with CNS involvement, the prognosis is even poorer, with median survival of approximately 2.5 months. Treatment for these patients, however, has a significant impact on survival, since the anticipated survival for untreated patients would be on the order of weeks.

Patients with CD4 counts greater than 100 have a median survival of 24 months. These patients are more likely to tolerate intensive therapy, since they present without prior history of OI and with higher performance status.

OTHER HIV-RELATED MALIGNANCIES

In addition to the more common HIV-related malignancies such as Kaposi's sarcoma and non-Hodgkin's lymphoma, a variety of other malignancies are also becoming evident. Unfortunately, it is becoming apparent that as patients live longer with HIV disease, more malignancies will become clinically significant.

Primary Central Nervous System Lymphoma

Primary CNS lymphoma is of B-cell origin in the majority of reported cases. It is not simply a manifestation

COMPLICATIONS
*Non-Hodgkin's Lymphoma (NHL)
Disease and Treatment*

Disease-related complications

Pain secondary to lymphadenopathy and associated dysfunction
Mental status changes secondary to central nervous system involvement
Abdominal pain secondary to hepatic, splenic, or gastrointestinal involvement
Fatigue secondary to constitutional symptoms of fever, chills, and weight loss

Treatment-related complications

Infection related to myelotoxicity of chemotherapy
Fatigue related to myelotoxicity of chemotherapy
Altered nutrition secondary to emetigenic potential of chemotherapy, mucositis, stomatitis
Pain related to mucositis associated with chemotherapy
Pain and self-care deficit secondary to peripheral neuropathy related to chemotherapy
Altered respiratory function related to chemotherapy

of systemic NHL, but instead is a discrete entity. HIV-infected individuals demonstrate an increased frequency of primary CNS lymphoma, and it is now estimated that its incidence is approaching 6% of all cases of AIDS.

It is difficult to diagnose CNS lymphoma in the setting of HIV disease because the differential diagnoses include a variety of OIs involving the CNS. Presenting signs and symptoms may include confusion, lethargy, memory loss, hemiparesis or dysphasia, seizures, or headaches.

CT brain scanning is usually nonspecific for CNS lymphoma, and lumbar puncture is rarely diagnostic. Open-brain biopsy is technically required to confirm the diagnosis. The current treatment approach includes combination radiation therapy and corticosteroids. The prognosis for these individuals remains poor, with long-term survival of only a few months.[17]

Cervical Cancer

The gynecologic problems associated with HIV infection include a variety of sexually transmitted diseases, pelvic inflammatory disease, genital ulcers, vaginal candidiasis, and cervical intraepithelial neoplasia (CIN), which can be a precursor to cervical cancer. The most common neoplasia of the cervix, squamous cell neoplasia, has been linked to early age at first sexual intercourse, multiple sexual partners, and infection with the human papillomavirus (HPV). HPV is also thought to be the causative agent for most condylomata acuminata (genital warts).

Genital warts in HIV-infected women may exist as multiple small lesions or as unusually large and profuse lesions. External warts often extend to adjacent, moist epithelium, including the vagina, cervix, urethra, and rectum. Cervical dysplasia, the premalignant changes noted on Papanicolaou (Pap) smear screening, can result from HPV infection and can progress to cervical cancer. Cervical dysplasia occurs at an unusually high rate in HIV-infected women at 5 to 10 times the expected rate. Cervical cancer caused by HPV is potentially fatal and is the most serious gynecologic disease for HIV-infected women. In addition, cervical dysplasia and cancer may be more aggressive and persistent among HIV-positive women than among uninfected women.[13]

Recently, the adequacy of the Pap smear as a screening device has been questioned. Almost 80% of HIV-infected women had normal Pap smears, but nearly half of these women were later found to have histologic evidence of CIN when they underwent colposcopy. Colposcopy evaluation should be considered for all HIV-positive women.[2]

The presence and severity of CIN correlates with both absolute number and function of CD4 cells. Women with more profound immunodeficiency are more likely to have high-grade lesions than asymptomatic HIV-positive women. Lymph node involvement is common, although greatly enlarged nodes may also result from HIV disease. Women with HIV disease also have higher recurrence and death rates with shorter intervals to recurrence.

For patients with early disease, radical hysterectomy and pelvic lymphadenectomy may be performed safely. In patients with advanced or systemic disease, chemotherapy may be used along with radiation therapy, although careful monitoring of hematologic toxicities must be performed. Drugs that are relatively sparing of the bone marrow, such as cisplatin, bleomycin, and vincristine, may be used.[19]

Anal Carcinoma

Anal carcinoma in HIV-infected men is similar to cervical carcinoma in HIV-infected women. Increasing numbers of men with concurrent HIV and HPV infection are now showing signs of intraanal cytologic abnormalities. More than 50% of patients with abnormal anal cytology have been shown to have HPV DNA on specimen. The prevalence of these abnormalities seems to increase with time in serial follow-up.[1]

Anal intraepithelial neoplasia (AIN), as with CIN, can develop into a malignant process. Among HIV-negative men, AIN is relatively uncommon. Approximately 15% of symptomatic HIV-positive men, however, have been shown to have AIN, and this number increases to about 30% over longitudinal follow-up. The risk appears to increase with advancing immunosuppression.[16] Since anal cancer may take several years to develop from AIN, it seems likely that the rate of anal cancer will continue to increase as immunosuppressed individuals live longer.

Patients with anal carcinoma have a much higher incidence of venereal warts compared with patients with carcinoma of the colon or rectum.[17] What role HIV plays in the pathogenesis of this malignancy has yet to be defined. HIV may promote the development of HPV-related malignancies or may allow a broadened expression of the latent HPV.

AIN and early stages of anal cancer usually are not associated with any symptoms. Some individuals may notice rapid growth of an external anal lesion or may develop new onset of anal pruritus or a change in bowel habits. In advanced disease, anal cancer may be associated with weight loss, pelvic pain, and even obstruction of the anal canal.

The natural history of AIN is currently under study. It is not yet known what percentage of those with AIN will go on to develop anal cancer if left untreated. It seems likely, however, that treatment of AIN will prevent the development of anal cancer. It therefore seems reasonable to perform an anal Pap test and anoscopy on any HIV-positive patient with new-onset signs or symptoms related to anal carcinoma and on those who have a history of venereal warts. Although the optimal forms of treatment have not yet been identified, fulguration or

NURSING MANAGEMENT

The nursing management of the patient with HIV disease is complex and demanding. Because the disease has such an unpredictable course, the nurse must be prepared to provide appropriate care to those with early asymptomatic disease, to those who have acute opportunistic infections (OIs), to those battling AIDS-related malignancies, and to those in the terminal stages of their illness (see box, p. 274).

NURSING DIAGNOSIS

• *Infection, risk for related to disease process, with viral destruction of T4 helper cells; neutropenia related to medication, treatment, or infection; knowledge deficit regarding infection control precautions; or impaired skin integrity*

ASSESSMENTS

Patients with HIV infection are at risk for developing infections at any stage of the disease because of a number of factors. A variety of signs and symptoms may alert the nurse to an impending or current infection: neutropenia; decreased T4 helper count; fever, chills; impaired skin integrity with or without draining wounds; shortness of breath, cough; mental status change; and nausea, vomiting, or diarrhea.

OUTCOME GOALS

• Patient will remain free of infection.
• Infections will be identified early and treatment initiated quickly.

INTERVENTIONS

• Carefully monitor vital signs and laboratory results for signs of possible infection.
• Institute a low-microbial diet for patients with an absolute neutrophil count less than 500 cells/cm^3. Patients should receive only pasteurized dairy products and no fresh fruits or vegetables.
• Perform appropriate physical assessment, including careful examination of skin integrity and respiratory and gastrointestinal status.
• Perform appropriate mental status examinations.
• Maintain asepsis when caring for patient, including appropriate handwashing and limiting infectious visitors.
• Educate patient in protective strategies, such as handwashing, diet precautions (e.g., thorough cooking of meat products), pet care precautions, and avoidance of rectal thermometers and suppositories.

NURSING DIAGNOSIS

• *Coping, ineffective individual*
Patients with HIV disease face a chronic, life-threatening illness. In addition, they face stigmatization and often overwhelming discrimination. Ineffective coping may be related to anxiety secondary to having a life-threatening illness, multiple losses secondary to the illness and resultant debilitation, changes in life-style secondary to HIV infection, or changes in self-concept.

ASSESSMENTS

Ineffective coping occurs when the individual is unable to manage stressors successfully secondary to lack of personal or external resources.[9] Ineffective coping may be evidenced by:
• Behavioral changes, including sudden mood swings, social withdrawal, anger, depression, anxiety
• Decreased self-esteem
• Inability to solve problems

OUTCOME GOALS

Patient will be able to:
• Devise new coping strategies and enhance current strategies.
• Express feelings and maintain relationships.

INTERVENTIONS

• Establish a therapeutic nursing relationship using empathy, acceptance, and support.
• Facilitate expression of patient's feelings.
• Assist patient in identification of past and current coping strategies and effective and ineffective skills.
• Identify resources available to patient, including family members, friends, clergy, and support groups.
• Utilize multidisciplinary resources, including social services, clergy, and psychiatry.

NURSING DIAGNOSIS

• *Knowledge deficit related to disease and treatment*
Patients with HIV disease often have an overwhelming amount of information to assimilate regarding their illness and treatment. Knowledge deficits may be related to disease process, various treatment modalities, infection control, or protective mechanisms.

ASSESSMENTS

Patients exhibit knowledge deficits in a variety of ways. Signs and symptoms that may alert the nurse to potential and actual deficits include new HIV diagnosis, institution of new treatment, inability to perform procedures correctly (e.g., failure to wash hands), failure to maintain infection control mechanisms (e.g., not using condoms during sexual contact), or repeated infections.

OUTCOME GOALS

Patient will be able to:
• Verbalize correct knowledge of illness and treatments.
• Practice appropriate infection control precautions for protection of self and others.

INTERVENTIONS

- Assess patient's knowledge and learning patterns.
- Provide a variety of educational resources, including videos, printed materials, and one-on-one instruction.
- Provide baseline education to patient regarding illness trajectory, infection control, protective mechanisms, laboratory evaluation, and medication administration.
- Explain all procedures and treatments to patient.
- Encourage patient and family to ask questions.

NURSING DIAGNOSIS

- *Body image disturbance related to cutaneous lesions*

ASSESSMENTS

A person's self-concept results from thoughts and feelings related to his or her identity, self-esteem, role performance, and body image.[9] Changes in physical appearance often accompany AIDS-KS and place the patient at risk for disturbance in body image and self-concept. Indications of this disturbance include social withdrawal or isolation, statements of low self-worth, and depression.

OUTCOME GOALS

Patient will be able to:
- Have an improved self-concept.
- Identify and implement strategies for coping with physical disturbance of lesions.
- Maintain social and intimate relationships.
- Verbalize statements reflecting self-worth.

INTERVENTIONS

- Establish a therapeutic nursing relationship based on acceptance and encouraging open sharing of feelings.
- Identify sources of threats to body image and self-concept.
- Educate patient in use of self-affirmation techniques.
- Facilitate incorporation of past adaptive coping behaviors.
- Involve family and significant others in support of patient.
- Utilize multidisciplinary group such as dermatology, psychology, social work, and support groups.
- Educate patient in techniques to reduce visibility of lesions.

NURSING DIAGNOSIS

- *Skin integrity, impaired*

Impairment of skin integrity may be related to KS lesions, poor nutritional status secondary to chemotherapy/radiation treatment, or radiation therapy.

ASSESSMENTS

Signs and symptoms of actual or impaired skin integrity include erythema, scaling, or broken skin resulting from:
- Draining wounds
- Radiation therapy
- Limited activity patterns

OUTCOME GOALS

- Patient will remain free of skin breakdown and associated infection.
- Breaks in skin integrity will heal.

INTERVENTIONS

- Assess skin surfaces at least every 8 hours for erythema, breakdown, excessive moisture, or other changes.
- Keep skin clean and dry; provide skin care at least every 4 hours.
- Provide appropriate beds, mattresses, or other appliances for pressure relief.
- Maintain adequate hydration and nutrition.
- Utilize multidisciplinary team, including dermatology, skin care, and speciality nurse.

NURSING DIAGNOSIS

- *Knowledge deficit related to Kaposi's sarcoma (KS) disease and treatment*

ASSESSMENTS

Signs and symptoms that may alert the nurse to potential and actual knowledge deficits include new KS diagnosis, institution of new treatment, failure to report new suspicious lesions, and altered coping skills.

OUTCOME GOALS

Patient will be able to:
- Verbalize correct knowledge of illness and treatments.
- Report suspicious lesions.
- Exhibit adequate coping skills.

INTERVENTIONS

- Assess patient knowledge and learning patterns.
- Provide a variety of educational resources, including videos, printed materials, and one-on-one instruction.
- Explain all procedures and treatments to patient.
- Encourage patient and family to ask questions.

NURSING DIAGNOSIS

- *Nutrition, altered: less than body requirements related to anorexia secondary to chemotherapy or chronic infection; nausea, vomiting, or diarrhea secondary to OI or treatment; impaired swallowing related to mucositis secondary to infection or treatment; or knowledge deficit*

Continued.

ASSESSMENTS

Patients with HIV infection in general are at risk for the development of malnutrition. The nutrition of these patients is further compromised when treatments for non-Hodgkin's lymphoma (NHL) are instituted. In addition, these treatment modalities may further compromise the immune status, resulting in GI opportunistic infections, which may further deplete the nutritional status. Signs and symptoms of altered nutritional status include weight loss; anorexia, nausea, and vomiting; dehydration; and mucositis.

OUTCOME GOAL

Patient will be able to:
• Achieve or maintain body weight.

INTERVENTIONS

• Monitor weight at least weekly with daily recording of intake and output.
• Assess for signs and symptoms of malnutrition, such as weight loss, weakness, fatigue, and decreased intake.
• Monitor laboratory data, such as serum protein, albumin, and electrolyte levels.
• Minimize anorexia, nausea, and vomiting by administering antiemetics; offering small, frequent meals at cool or room temperature; and avoiding spicy foods.
• Assist with good oral hygiene.
• Consult dietitian.
• Educate patient in nutritional needs and ways to reduce nausea, anorexia, and pain.

---

cryotherapy of anal lesions through the use of a proctoscope or sigmoidoscope seems reasonable. If the lesion has progressed to anal carcinoma, chemotherapy and possibly radiation therapy may be considered.

Other Malignancies

Although only a few cases of *malignant melanoma* have been reported in HIV-positive patients, this incidence may increase as survival is extended in this population. The incidence of malignant melanoma in renal transplant patients, a group with iatrogenic immunosuppression, is reported to be approximately four times that of the general population. Since this is probably related to immunosuppression, the same increase may occur in the HIV-infected population. The possibility of an increased incidence of *hepatocellular carcinoma* also seems likely in HIV-infected patients who are concurrently infected with chronic hepatitis B.

CONCLUSION

HIV disease has quickly become an overwhelming epidemic, claiming the lives of hundreds of thousands of people throughout the world and threatening to defeat the current health care delivery systems. It is a sexually transmitted, blood-borne viral infection that destroys the host's immune system, resulting in life-threatening opportunistic infections and a variety of malignant processes.

HIV disease is now the third leading cause of death among American women of childbearing ages and the first leading cause of death of young American men. Approximately 1.5 million people are currently infected in the United States, with a new infection occurring about every 54 seconds. It is estimated that as many as 110 million people worldwide will be infected by the end of this decade.

PATIENT TEACHING PRIORITIES
HIV and Related Cancers

Risk reduction techniques: minimize the number of sexual partners and engage in a mutually monogamous sexual relationship.

Safe sex counseling: any exchange of blood, semen, or vaginal secretions can potentially put an individual at risk for HIV disease.

Intravenous risk reduction: use of contaminated needles for any injection represents a serious risk for HIV infection.

Signs and symptoms of infectious process: these include fever, chills, shortness of breath, cough, pain, diarrhea, nausea, vomiting, skin breakdown, weight loss, and a sense of mental confusion.

Self-help care strategies: know where and when to seek medical, psychosocial, and financial assistance.

As the number of infected individuals continues to grow and as scientific advances are made with this disease, extending the life span of those infected, health care systems will be burdened even more with the ever-increasing load of patients requiring comprehensive, extended care. Caring for the patient with HIV disease is a complex issue given the life-threatening nature of the disease, the relative youth of the affected population, and the sociopolitical issues surrounding the epidemic. Nurses have played critical roles in defining the need for comprehensive, compassionate care of patients with HIV disease.

Patient teaching priorities are listed in the box above.

■ CHAPTER QUESTIONS

1. Which of the following represents a significant risk factor for transmission of HIV infection?
   a. Unprotected sexual intercourse
   b. Swimming in nonchlorinated pools
   c. Sharing drinking glasses with a person with AIDS
   d. Marijuana use
2. How long does it take after infection for an HIV test to become positive in the average adult?
   a. 24-48 hours
   b. 5-7 days
   c. 6-12 weeks
   d. 6-9 months
3. How soon does the average patient develop opportunistic infections after initial infection?
   a. 6 weeks
   b. 10 months
   c. 6 years
   d. 10 years
4. The cell most frequently infected and destroyed by HIV is:
   a. CD4 suppressor T cell
   b. CD4 helper T cell
   c. CD8 suppressor T cell
   d. CD8 helper T cell
5. The best example of combination antiretroviral therapy for HIV disease is:
   a. AZT + ddI + ddC
   b. ddC + cyclophosphamide
   c. Protease inhibitor + cyclophosphamide
   d. AZT + ddI + protease inhibitor
6. The most common AIDS-related malignancy is:
   a. Kaposi's sarcoma
   b. Non-Hodgkin's lymphoma
   c. Hodgkin's disease
   d. Cervical cancer
7. An AIDS-related malignancy characterized by multifocal, widespread lesions of the skin and oral mucosa is most likely:
   a. Kaposi's sarcoma
   b. Non-Hodgkin's lymphoma
   c. Hodgkin's disease
   d. Cervical cancer
8. AIDS-related Kaposi's sarcoma is a highly curable illness.
   a. True
   b. False
   c. True, but only in women
   d. True, but only in IDUs
9. AIDS-related non-Hodgkin's lymphoma usually:
   a. Occurs early in the HIV illness
   b. Occurs only in homosexual men
   c. Usually presents as a highly aggressive, early-stage malignancy
   d. Usually presents as a highly aggressive, late-stage malignancy
10. AIDS-related cervical cancer is most likely related to:
    a. *Toxoplasma* infection
    b. Concurrent herpes simplex infection
    c. Human papillomavirus
    d. Epstein-Barr virus

BIBLIOGRAPHY

1. Abrams DI: Acquired immunodeficiency syndrome and related malignancies: a topical overview, *Semin Oncol* 18(5):41, 1991.
2. ACOG: Human immunodeficiency virus infections, *ACOG Tech Bull* 165:1, 1992.
3. American Foundation for AIDS Research: Statistics, *AIDS Clin Care* 4(6):1, 1992.
4. Centers for Disease Control and Prevention: Zidovudine for the prevention of HIV transmission from mother to infant, *MMWR* 43(16):285, 1994.
5. Centers for Disease Control and Prevention: First 500,000 AIDS cases—United States, 1995, *MMWR* 44(46):840, 1995.
6. Errante D and others: Management of AIDS and its neoplastic complications, *Eur J Cancer* 27(3):389, 1991.
7. Food and Drug Administration: Trials sanctioned for study of potential therapeutic use of new AIDS vaccine in HIV infected individuals, Communication, March 12, 1990.
8. Friedland G: AIDS: the first decade, *AIDS Clin Care* 3(6):41, 1991.
9. Gee G: *AIDS: concepts in nursing practice,* Baltimore, 1988, Williams & Wilkins.
10. Kaplan L: HIV-associated lymphoma, *AIDS File* 6(1):6, 1992.
11. Lucey D: The first decade of human retroviruses: a nomenclature for the clinician, *Military Med* 156(10):555, 1991.
12. Lusso P, Gallo R: Pathogenesis of AIDS, *J Pharmaceut Pharmacol* 44(suppl 1):160, 1992.
13. Marte C, Allen M: HIV-related gynecologic conditions: overlooked complications, *Focus Guide AIDS Res Counsel* 7(1):1, 1991.
14. McPhedran P: Using hematopoietic hormones in HIV disease, *AIDS Clin Care* 4(6):43, 1992.
15. Northfelt D: AIDS-associated Kaposi's sarcoma, *AIDS File* 6(1):1, 1992.
16. Palefsky J: Anal cancer among HIV-positive men, *AIDS File* 6(1):9, 1992.
17. Schwartz J, Dias B, Safai B: HIV-related malignancies, *Dermatol Clin* 9(3):503, 1991.
18. Thompson D: Invincible AIDS, *Time,* Aug 3, 1992, p 30.
19. Tinkle M, Amaya M, Tamayo O: HIV disease and pregnancy, *J Obstet Gynecol Neonat Nurs* 21(2):86, 1992.
20. Torres G: Update on vaccine development, *Treatment Iss* 5(6):3, 1991.
21. Volberding P: *Management of HIV infection: treatment team workshop handbook,* New York, 1991, World Health Communications.
22. Wright M: Guide to opportunistic infections, *Project Inform Perspect* October 1991, p 11.

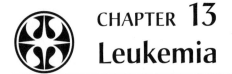

CHAPTER **13**
Leukemia

ROSANNE LUCY EBLE OSOSKI

The leukemias are a complex collection of diseases that were first described in 1845 by Virchow. He described a condition in which the relationship between red and colorless corpuscles was the reverse of normal. He coined the term *weisses blut,* or "white blood."[54]

The two major classifications of leukemia are *acute* and *chronic.* These two types of leukemia are similar in that they are the product of dysfunctional bone marrow, but they differ dramatically in disease presentation, treatment, and prognosis. Acute and chronic leukemia can be characterized by the cell line of origin: myeloid or lymphoid.

An understanding of any leukemia must begin with a knowledge of normal bone marrow function, which is described in the first section of this chapter. The chapter is then divided into three major sections: acute leukemias, chronic leukemias, and nursing management of the patient with leukemia. Hairy-cell leukemia and myelodysplastic syndromes are also discussed.

Much of the scientific knowledge of adult leukemia is derived from the studies done on pediatric leukemia. Although pediatric leukemia is referred to in this chapter, especially in the acute lymphoblastic leukemia section, the focus of this chapter is the adult patient with leukemia.

PATHOPHYSIOLOGY

Leukemia is a malignant hematologic disorder characterized by a proliferation of abnormal white blood cells (WBCs) that infiltrate the bone marrow, peripheral blood, and other organs. Leukemia may present as an acute or chronic disease process.

Elements of the blood are formed in the bone marrow, vertebrae, clavicle, scapula, sternum, ribs, skull, proximal ends of long bones, and pelvis in children. In adults, most of the blood cells are produced in the pelvis, sternum, and vertebrae. The body can be imagined to have three pools of blood cells. The first pool of cells are the *pluripotent stem cells* of the bone marrow, the most primitive form of blood cell from which all blood cells originate. The stem cell pool is responsible for the generation of new cells to meet the body's requirements throughout the person's lifetime. The pluripotent stem cell can proliferate and differentiate. The decision to proliferate or differentiate is based on the body's current needs. With every stem cell division, one daughter cell remains in the stem cell pool, so the lifetime pool of stem cells is never depleted. An injury to the stem cell pool, such as a lethal dose of radiation, prevents the production of blood cells and results in marrow aplasia. The stem cell pool cannot be assessed by a routine bone marrow examination. Studies of the stem cell population are called *colony-forming assays* and are performed by in vitro culturing. In the bone marrow, blood cells mature within a framework of supportive cells and blood vessels that supply nutrition and growth factors for proliferation and differentiation.[27] Proliferation of stem cells is mediated by specific *colony-stimulating factors* (CSFs) acting on progenitor cells to give rise to granulocytes, erythrocytes, macrophages, and megakaryocytes.[3]

The second pool of cells are *precursor cells* for red blood cells (RBCs), platelets, granulocytes, and lymphocytes. A stem cell becomes committed to a certain blood cell line when it leaves the stem cell pool. In the second pool the cells differentiate and mature. Figure 13-1 illustrates the steps of cell differentiation and maturation. The second-pool cells at the blast phase of development cannot function as mature blood cells, but they can undergo mitosis. At this stage of development the *blast cells* (the least differentiated cells without commitment as to their blood line) may be responsive to specific CSFs. As the cells divide, they differentiate, enabling them to carry out only specific functions, and they lose their proliferative response to CSFs. In the myeloid series, cells lose their proliferative ability after the myelocytic stages.

When the precursor cells of the second pool are mature, they are released into the *peripheral circulation,* the third pool. Each mature blood cell performs a specific

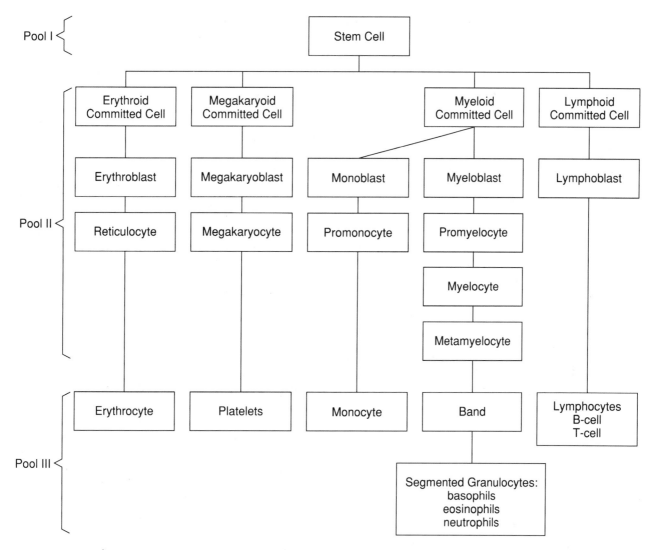

Figure 13-1 Maturation process of various blood cell lines originating from the stem cell.

function (RBCs—oxygen transport; granulocytes—phagocytosis; platelets—clotting). The mature circulating cells cannot undergo mitosis and must be replaced at the end of their life span (RBCs—120 days; granulocytes—6 to 8 hours; platelets—8 to 10 days). Mature blood cells are released from the bone marrow in response to the body's need.

In leukemia the control factors regulating the orderly differentiation and maturation of the blood cells are absent. This lack of regulatory control results in the arrest of the maturation process of a specific cell line. The involved immature cell form proliferates and accumulates in the bone marrow, resulting in crowding of the normal marrow cells. This marrow crowding impairs the production and function of normal cell lines; ultimately, the marrow is replaced by leukemic cells, which are released into the circulating blood. The leukemic cells may also invade body organs.

The specific type of leukemia depends on which stem cell line is affected (myeloid or lymphoid) and the point of maturation at which growth is arrested. Acute leukemias result from arrest of immature blood cells; chronic leukemias involve more mature blood cells. Leukemic cells actually generate more slowly than normal WBCs, but the mechanisms controlling cellular division are errant, allowing more cells to be capable of division at any point in time.

ACUTE LEUKEMIAS

Acute leukemia is a severe and aggressive disease characterized by rapid onset and a rapidly terminal course if untreated. There are two types of acute leukemia: *lymphocytic* or *lymphoblastic* (ALL) and *myelogenous* (AML).

In acute leukemia the leukemic or blast cells function abnormally and accumulate in the peripheral blood, bone marrow, reticuloendothelial system (RES), and possibly the central nervous system (CNS). The overproduction of leukemic cells in the bone marrow impairs normal hematopoiesis, resulting in anemia, granulocytopenia, and thrombocytopenia.

Acute Lymphocytic (Lymphoblastic) Leukemia

EPIDEMIOLOGY AND ETIOLOGY

The exact etiology of acute lymphocytic leukemia (ALL) is unknown. Radiation, chemicals, drugs, viruses, and genetic abnormalities have been implicated in the etiology of this disease. A causal relationship between the human T-cell leukemia virus type I (HTLV-I) and T-cell leukemias and lymphoma is suspected but not proved.[2]

An estimated 27,600 new cases of leukemia occurred in 1996, divided equally between acute and chronic leukemias. Adults are diagnosed more frequently than children (24,800 versus 2800). ALL accounts for approximately 1600 of childhood leukemias. In adults the most common are acute myelocytic (approximately 6800) and chronic lymphocytic (approximately 7200).[2] Whites are more frequently affected than blacks. Twenty percent of acute leukemias in adults is ALL.[81]

ALL has a bimodal distribution. The initial peak in children occurs at less than 5 years of age. The second peak occurs after age 60, after remaining stable from ages 20 to 60.[57]

CLINICAL FEATURES

The most common presenting complaints are a result of anemia, neutropenia, and thrombocytopenia caused by a rapidly expanding leukemic cell population. Symptoms are malaise, fatigue, bony pain, bleeding, bruising, and fever. Pain, especially in children, results from increased blasts in the bone marrow. CNS involvement is present in 10% of patients.[21,79] Most CNS manifestations involve meningeal infiltrates resulting in increased intracranial pressure and cranial nerve palsies, most frequently involving III, IV, VI, and VIII. Parenchymal involvement of the brain is rare in leukemia, as is testicular involvement at diagnosis. Enlargement of the testes may be unilateral or bilateral. Lymphadenopathy is present in almost 80% of patients. The spleen and/or liver are also involved in 70% to 75%.[21]

DIAGNOSIS

The diagnosis of acute leukemia is often indicated by the peripheral blood smear; however, a bone marrow evaluation is essential to finalize the diagnosis and provide specimens for further histochemical staining, immuno-

phenotyping, and cytogenetics. The differentiation between AML and ALL based on cell morphology is generally accurate, especially with experienced hematopathologists. However, the additional studies are still indicated on all newly diagnosed patients.

The WBC count is normal to low in most ALL patients; approximately one third have an initial leukocyte count greater than 20,000/mm³. Leukemic cells may be seen in the blood. Despite high WBC counts, absolute neutrophil counts are low.[84] Anemia is almost universal; two thirds of patients present with fewer than 50,000/ mm³ platelets.[21] The bone marrow aspirate is used to obtain the *differential* count, which quantitates the percentage of each of the hematologic components in the marrow. Lymphoblasts comprise at least 30% of the marrow cells in ALL.[85]

Smears of the bone marrow aspirate are specially stained to define the specific subtype of ALL. A portion of the bone marrow aspirate is heparinized for cytogenetic analysis. These studies may reveal certain patterns of gene translocations or rearrangements that are prognostically significant.

A core biopsy of the bone is obtained during the bone marrow procedure. This specimen is used to determine the marrow cellularity. *Cellularity* refers to the ratio of hematopoietic tissue to adipose tissue in the marrow. The amount of blood-forming, or *red,* marrow decreases with the aging process and is replaced by fat, or *yellow,* marrow. Normocellular marrow for an adult is 30% to 40% cellularity. Young adults and children have bone marrow that is much more cellular. Older adults have more fat in their marrow. These age-related changes are reflected in defining marrow cellularity: *normocellular* marrow has normal proportions of the hematopoietic cells and adipose cells; *hypocellular* marrow has a reduced number of hematopoietic cells and an increase in adipose elements; and *hypercellular* marrow has an increased number of hematopoietic cells and a decreased amount of adipose tissue.[53] A bone marrow report for a newly diagnosed ALL patient is usually hypercellular with increased lymphoblasts (e.g., cellularity = 90%; lymphoblasts = 80%).

Infiltration of the cerebrospinal fluid (CSF) by leukemic cells is seen in 5% of children and fewer than 10% of adults.[21,85] The CSF specimen is centrifuged and stained to determine the presence of leukemic cells. A low glucose level or a high protein level may indicate either leukemic infiltration or an infectious process. Platelet transfusions may be required before the procedure in thrombocytopenic patients to decrease the potential risk of bleeding. Patients with high numbers of circulating blast cells may have their CSF specimens contaminated with circulating blast cells. This may lead to an inaccurate diagnosis of CNS involvement.

Table 13-1 presents the physical findings, laboratory

Table 13-1   Physical Findings and Laboratory Results in ALL and AML Patients

	Acute lymphocytic leukemia	Acute myelogenous leukemia
PHYSICAL EXAMINATION		
Infection	Frequently present	30% have serious infections
Bleeding	Mild in 30%	30% have significant bleeding or petechiae
		75% have intracutaneous bleeding
Adenopathy	Present in 80%	Rare
Splenomegaly	Frequently present	Occurs in 25%
Gingival hypertrophy	Rare	Present with monocytic element
Neurologic findings	Headaches, visual disturbances	Rare
LABORATORY VALUES		
White blood cell count (WBC)	Normal to low	30% decreased
	10% WBC >100,000/mm^3	30% normal
	Often neutropenic	30% increased
	Most have blasts	>50,000/mm^3 in 25%
		10% have no blasts
Platelets	<50,000/mm^3 in 60%	<20,000/mm^3 common
Uric acid	Increased	Increased in 50%
Lactate dehydrogenase (LDH)	Increased	Typically increased
Bone marrow		
Cellularity	Hypercellular	Hypercellular
Blasts	30% or greater	30% or greater
Erythroid elements	Decreased	Increased
Morphology	Normal	Bizarre granulation of mature granulocytes
Cerebrospinal fluid		
Cytology: infiltration with leukemic cells at presentation	Children: 5% Adult: <10%	<5% occurrence: greater risk in M$_4$ and M$_5$, greater risk with WBC >100,000

values, bone marrow, and CSF results in ALL and AML patients.

CLASSIFICATION

Classification of leukemias at diagnosis is necessary to determine prognosis and select therapy. The *French-American-British (FAB) classification system,* developed in 1976 based on cellular morphology and histochemical staining of blast cells, is universally accepted.[26] ALLs are also subclassified according to their immunophenotypic features. Cytogenetic analysis further defines the specific clonal abnormalities found in acute leukemia. Information about the role of molecular genetic techniques and the relationship of retroviruses and oncogenes is increasing knowledge about the nature of acute leukemia.

The three FAB classes of ALL are L$_1$, L$_2$, and L$_3$.[4] The L$_1$ classification is most common in childhood leukemias (80%). Morphologically the leukemia cells are small, homogeneous, and nongranular with scanty cytoplasm. The common adult form of ALL is the L$_2$ classification.[59] Microscopically these blasts appear larger and are heterogeneous. The L$_3$ classification is very rare and resembles Burkitt's lymphoma.[60] Morphologically the

Table 13-2   Immunologic and Morphologic Classification of ALL

Immuno-phenotype	Incidence (%)		Effect on prognosis	FAB morphology
	Children	Adults		
Early pre–B cell	65-70	50-60	Favorable	L$_1$, L$_2$
Pre–B cell	15-20	15-25	Moderately favorable	L$_1$
B cell	<5	<5	Unfavorable	L$_3$
Pre–T cell	10-15	6	Unfavorable	L$_1$, L$_2$
T cell	<5	20	Favorable	L$_1$, L$_2$

L$_3$ blasts are large and homogeneous with moderately abundant cytoplasm.

Lymphoblastic leukemias originate in either B cell or T cell progenitors at various stages of differentiation and proliferation. Assessing the reactivity of leukemic cells to several monoclonal antibodies specific for different cell types establishes their expression, or *immunophenotype.* These are also called *cell surface marker studies.* Different antigens are expressed as the cell matures, which aids in identification[20] (Table 13-2).

About 75% of adult cases are of B cell lineage. Most express the *common ALL antigen,* or CALLA (CD10). They are divided into early pre–B-cell, pre–B-cell, and B-cell ALL. Approximately 25% of ALL cases are of T-cell lineage, either pre-T or T cell.[20]

PROGNOSIS

Approximately 75% of adults treated for ALL will achieve complete remission (CR), and 20% to 40% will be cured. In children, 90% will achieve CR, and 60% to 85% will be cured.[21,65]

The different response rates between adult and children are caused by differences in disease biology. Adults with ALL generally have poor prognostic indicators, and therefore their response is different from that seen in children.[20,65]

Age. Infants younger than age 1 year and children older than age 10 years have a worse prognosis than those 1 to 9 years old. Adults have a worse outcome than children, with adults older than 60 having the worst prognosis.[21]

White blood cell (WBC) count. A high initial WBC count is a poor prognostic indicator and has an adverse effect on remission duration.[45,81] A National Cancer Institute (NCI) workshop has suggested a WBC greater than 50,000/mm^3 as a poor risk for children.[21] Adults with a WBC count greater than 30,000/mm^3 have a poorer prognosis.

Time to response. Prognostic models by Hoelzer, Kantarjian, and Gaynor all list time to CR that is longer than 4 weeks as a high-risk factor.[21,59,65]

Cytogenetics. Cytogenetic characteristics are the most important prognostic factor for ALL. Abnormalities can be structural or related to the number of chromosomes. In children, *ploidy* is the most important prognostic factor; those with more than 50 chromosomes have the best prognosis.[21] In adults the *Philadelphia chromosome* (9;22) translocation is present in approximately 30% of adults and represents a poorer prognosis. Other karyotypes that signal poorer prognosis are t(8;14), t(4;11), and t(1;19).[26,81]

Gender. Males have a lower long-term survival rate in both adult and pediatric populations. Testicular relapses may account for the decreased survival of male children with ALL.[46,84]

Other risk factors. CNS leukemia is a high-risk factor, especially when associated with the L$_3$ or B cell subset.[21,85] Splenomegaly, hepatomegaly, thrombocytopenia, low lactate dehydrogenase (LDH), increased serum aspartate aminotransferase (ADH, SGOT), and weight loss have been shown to indicate a worse prognosis in single studies and require confirmation.[60,81]

Table 13-3 lists the factors affecting prognosis in ALL.

Table 13-3 Prognostic Indicators in ALL

Factor	Good	Poor
FAB	L$_1$, L$_2$	L$_3$ in adult
Cell type	T cell, CALLA positive	B cell, null cell
Age	1-9 years	>60 years
Gender	Female	Male
WBC at diagnosis	<30,000/mm^3	>30,000/mm^3
CR	<4 weeks	>4 weeks
Cytogenetics	Normal karyotype	Cytogenetic abnormalities: t(4;11), t(1;19), t(9;22)
CNS involvement	No	Yes
Immunophenotype	Early pre–B cell (usually children)	Pre–T cell Pre–B cell

FAB, French-American-British classification system; *CALLA,* common ALL antigen; *WBC,* white blood cell count; *CR,* complete remission; *CNS,* central nervous system.

TREATMENT MODALITIES

The treatment goal in ALL is to achieve a cure. Standard treatment regimens for this disease consist of two parts: induction therapy and postremission therapy. Prophylactic treatment to prevent CNS disease is incorporated into both parts of treatment.

The purpose of induction therapy is to induce a CR. A CR is documented by a bone marrow aspirate containing less than 5% lymphoblasts and the elimination of extramedullary disease. Postremission therapy is administered over 2 to 3 years after CR to eradicate completely any remaining clinically undetectable leukemia cells that may potentially cause disease relapse.

Induction Therapy

The primary chemotherapeutic agents used to induce remission are (1) vincristine, (2) a corticosteroid (usually prednisone), and (3) an anthracycline (doxorubicin, daunorubicin).[21,26,81] Remission rates range from 70% to 85%, with a low mortality rate resulting from induction. Some induction regimens use additional drugs (L-asparaginase, cyclophosphamide, methotrexate, 6-mercaptopurine, cytarabine [ARA-C]), but these do not appear to increase response rates.[20,21] An exception appears to be mature B-cell ALL, which may respond to the use of high-dose cyclophosphamide, alternating with high doses of methotrexate and ARA-C.[21,65,90]

Central Nervous System Treatment

The CNS may serve as a "sanctuary" site for leukemia cells. Leukemic involvement in the CSF at the time of diagnosis is seen in 5% of children and fewer than 10%

of adults.[21,85] However, if the CNS is not treated, as many as 50% to 75% of adults will develop CNS involvement.[21] CNS prophylaxis is a critical component of postremission therapy for leukemia-free survival. Cranial irradiation plus intrathecal chemotherapy with methotrexate or ARA-C was the standard for children with ALL. This can result in neuropsychologic deficits and endocrine dysfunction. Newer treatments include intrathecal and high-dose systemic chemotherapy with CNS penetration (e.g., high-dose methotrexate or ARA-C). The latter treatment is also used in adults.[21,26,65,90]

Patients who have CNS leukemia should be treated more aggressively. This includes intraventricular chemotherapy and cranial irradiation. An Ommaya reservoir may be inserted. The advantages of drug administration through an Ommaya include ease of access to CSF and higher and more predictable levels of the drug in ventricular CSF than when administered by lumbar puncture.[20,21]

Postremission Therapy

ALL will almost certainly recur without some form of postremission therapy. The optimal form of this therapy remains controversial, but the two most widely used types of therapy are consolidation/intensification and maintenance.

Consolidation/intensification therapy. The role of consolidation/intensification in children has improved prognosis in those with high-risk features.[90] The role in adults is less clear. One recent study has shown a response rate at 4 years of 43%.[59] The regimens may include high-dose ARA-C or methotrexate or may repeat the drugs used in induction therapy. Neither the optimal drugs nor the optimal durations of treatment are known.[20]

Maintenance therapy. An extended program of low-dose maintenance therapy using 6-mercaptopurine (6-MP) and methotrexate weekly for 2 to 3 years is effective in preventing relapse and improving survival in children.[90] Most adult maintenance therapies are based on pediatric studies, but the intensities vary. A combination of several antileukemic agents and 6-MP and methotrexate is generally used. The optimal drugs and dosage remain unknown. Newer regimens consisting of more aggressive induction and consolidation therapy for mature B-cell ALL has increased CR rates and disease-free survival rates in adults and children. This makes maintenance therapy unnecessary.[20,21,65]

Bone Marrow Transplant

The role and timing of allogeneic (marrow harvested from a histocompatible donor) bone marrow transplant (BMT) in adult ALL is controversial. It is unclear whether BMT offers an advantage for ALL patients with a favorable prognosis. ALL patients with the Philadelphia chromosome have had a 38% leukemia-free survival when they received BMT during first CR. Other high-risk ALL subgroups include t(4;11), t(1;19), high-WBC presentation, and longer than one course to achieve CR. These groups should be considered for allogeneic BMT during first CR.[20,65,81,89]

Autologous (marrow harvested from the patient) BMT or peripheral blood stem cell (PBSC) transplantation may be considered for patients too old for allogeneic BMT or without a matched donor. Results have been inferior to allogeneic BMT because of inability to effectively purge residual leukemic cells from the harvested bone marrow.[26,65,81] Clinical trials comparing allogeneic BMT (if a matched sibling is present), autologous BMT, and conventional maintenance therapy are underway that will answer crucial issues in management.[20] (See Chapter 24 for details on BMT.)

Recurrent Disease Therapy

Most ALL relapses occur within the first 2 years of remission. As many as half of relapsed patients may achieve a second remission by repeating their original induction regimen.[84] Patients who relapse after completing maintenance therapy have a better chance of attaining second remission than those patients who relapse while receiving therapy.[60]

Patients with resistant disease who fail to achieve a first remission may respond to treatment with intermediate-dose to high-dose methotrexate and leukovorin rescue or with L-asparaginase.

BMT may allow long-term survival for as many as 50% of patients after second relapse and 10% to 20% of patients after third relapse.[49] These survival rates in advanced disease may exceed those of conventional or experimental agents. In pediatric and adult patients, it is a common practice to offer allogeneic BMT for patients in second CR.

Acute Myelogenous Leukemia

EPIDEMIOLOGY AND ETIOLOGY

Specific risk factors have been identified in acute myelogenous leukemia (AML). People with certain genetic disorders, such as Down syndrome (trisomy 21), Bloom syndrome, Klinefelter's syndrome, and Fanconi's anemia, are at increased risk to develop AML.[55] Exposure to the hydrocarbon benzene also increases the risk of disease development. Benzene is an aromatic solvent and is present in unleaded gasoline, rubber cement, and cleaning solvents.[92] Leukemia has been associated with exposure to ionizing radiation from nuclear reactions and from exposure to therapeutic and occupational radiation.[55] Because some ribonucleic acid (RNA) tumor viruses (retroviruses) cause myeloid leukemias in rodents, felines, and avians, a viral etiology of AML has been suspected in humans.[43,95] Cigarette smoking may be a risk factor for acute leukemia, with rates attributed to smoking as high as 7% to 14%[8] of leukemia cases in the United States. Electromagnetic field (EMF) exposure has been implicated, but a review of all the literature to date reveals a doubtful link between EMF exposure and leukemia.[56]

Improvements in multimodality therapy over the past decade have resulted in increased survival and a potential cure for patients with a variety of cancers. Long-term survival now allows evaluation of late effects of cancer therapy. The incidence of secondary malignancies related to cytotoxic therapy and especially therapy-related acute nonlymphocytic leukemias (T-AMLs) has increased dramatically over the past decade. The median interval of occurrence of T-AML is 4 to 6 years after the original cancer treatment and is usually preceded by a preleukemic state detectable for 6 months.[25] Alkylating agents, especially prolonged use of melphalan in ovarian cancer,[31] multiple myeloma,[5] and breast cancer[86] and nitrogen mustard for Hodgkin's disease,[82] are strongly implicated. The risk of leukemia rises with increasing doses of alkylating agents so that the rise is directly related to the total dose received. Chlorambucil, busulfan, and thiotepa are also associated with an increased risk of developing a later malignancy.

The incidence of AML is 3 cases per 100,000 population, with approximately 6500 new cases each year in the United States.[2] The median age at diagnosis is about 50 years.

CLINICAL FEATURES

As with ALL, AML symptoms are related to the rapidly expanding leukemic cell population. Symptoms of anemia are also found in AML patients at presentation. In addition, a very common finding is that of recurrent infections unresponsive to standard oral antibiotics. Reports of easy bruisability, epistaxis, or gingival bleeding reflect thrombocytopenia. Unlike ALL patients, virtually all AML patients are symptomatic at presentation.

Abnormal findings on physical examination are related to leukemic infiltration of an organ, granulocytopenia, or thrombocytopenia. A thorough and systematic physical examination confirms many of the patient's complaints and is an integral part of the diagnosis. Table 13-4 lists possible physical manifestations of both ALL and AML. Gingival infiltrates and skin nodules are frequently seen in acute myelomonocytic and monocytic leukemias and may precede other manifestations by 2 to 4 weeks.

DIAGNOSIS

A diagnosis of AML is highly suspect when the examination of peripheral blood smears shows an increased number of immature blast cells associated with anemia and thrombocytopenia. The presence of Auer bodies (rods) suggests a diagnosis of AML before other diagnostic results are available. The total WBC count in AML may be normal, decreased, or increased. A small percentage of AML patients may present without peripheral blast cells. Platelet counts of less than $20,000/mm^3$ are common in AML. Abnormalities in one or more organ systems may result from leukemic cell infiltration or metabolic complications related to leukemia. Rarely a solid mass of leukemic cells will develop called a *granulocytic sarcoma*.

As with ALL, the marrow aspirate is used to obtain the differential count, and the biopsy is used to establish the percentage of cellularity. Myeloblasts comprise at least 30% of the nucleated cells in AML, and the marrow is hypercellular. A "packed" bone marrow with cellularity of 90% to 100% may be seen in AML patients.

A small sample of marrow aspirate is used for cytogenetics; the FAB stains and flow cytometry techniques are used to establish the specific subclassification.

Table 13-1 compares physical findings and laboratory results of AML patients with those of ALL patients.

CLASSIFICATION

AML is classified morphologically according to the FAB criteria by the degree of differentiation along different cell lines and the extent of cell maturation.[44] Familiarity with this system is helpful for nurses caring for AML patients because it identifies the unique features of each subtype. Table 13-5 outlines the FAB classification for AML.

PROGNOSIS

Oncology nurses should understand the factors affecting the prognosis of the patient with AML. In this disease, certain prognostic factors influence the rate of remission; other factors affect the duration of response. Patients over age 70 are less likely to survive the rigors of induction therapy, but those who do achieve remission generally survive as long as younger patients.

Age. In children, AML represents 20% of all cases of acute leukemia. Children younger than 1 year have a poor prognosis, probably related to their abnormal cytogenetics. Those ages 3 to 10 years have the best prognosis based on their favorable cytogenetics.[85] From 70% to 85% of patients achieve a CR, but more than half will relapse if treated only with chemotherapy.[90] In adults the

Table 13-4 Clinical Features in Acute Leukemias

System/region	Manifestation	Cause
Head/eyes/ears/nose/throat	Retinal capillary hemorrhage	Leukemic infiltration
	Fundic leukemic infiltration	Leukemic infiltration
	Papilledema	Leukemic infiltration
	Oropharyngeal infections	Secondary to immunocompromise
	Periodontal infections	Secondary to immunocompromise
	Gingival hypertrophy (AML)	Leukemic infiltration
	Dry mucous membranes	Overall systemic illness
	Dysphagia	Possible leukemic infiltration
	Cervical adenopathy	Leukemic infiltration
	Epistaxis	Thrombocytopenia
	Gingival bleeding	Thrombocytopenia
Cardiovascular/pulmonary	Possible tachycardia, tachypnea	Anemia or infection
	Conduction defects	Leukemic infiltration of bundle of His, valves, pericardium, or myocardium (rare)
	Murmurs	
	Pericarditis	
	Congestive heart failure	
	Abnormal lung sounds	Possible bacterial pneumonia
Abdomen	Splenomegaly (ALL)	Leukemic infiltration
	Enlarged, tender kidneys (more common in pediatric ALL)	Leukemic infiltration
	Hepatomegaly	Leukemic infiltration
	Menorrhagia	Thrombocytopenia
Genitourinary	Renal failure or anuria	Uric acid nephropathy
Rectal	Perirectal abscesses	Decreased infection-fighting capabilities
Extremities	Skin pallor	Anemia
	Ecchymosis, petechiae	Thrombocytopenia
	Leukemic skin infiltrates: small, raised, pinkish nodules	Leukemic infiltration
	Swollen joints or tenderness (most common in pediatric ALL)	Leukemic infiltration
Neurologic (CNS, central nervous system)	Headache, vomiting	Possible infiltration of CNS
	Visual disturbances	Possible CNS hemorrhage
	Cranial nerve VI, VII palsy	Infiltration of nerve sheath
Musculoskeletal	Bone or joint pain	Leukemic infiltration
	Swelling	Leukemic infiltration
	Osteolytic lesions	Leukemic infiltration

frequency of AML increases with age, with up to a tenfold increase compared with younger adults. The median age of AML patients is 60 years. In individuals older than 60 years, a combination of unfavorable cytogenetics, a higher incidence of previous myelodysplastic syndrome that has evolved into AML, and poor performance status of many elderly patients results in a poor prognosis.[19,35] Approximately 60% to 65% of adult AML patients achieve CR, with 20% maintaining a cure.[35]

White blood cell count. Of patients presenting with a WBC count greater than 100,000/mm^3, significantly more die during the first week of therapy, deaths from CNS hemorrhage are more common, overall remissions is shorter, and fewer survive, compared with those presenting with lower WBC counts.[29] Another poor prognostic factor in AML patients is prior treatment with chemotherapy or radiation therapy. This group includes patients with a treatment-related secondary leukemia and AML patients with recurring or resistant disease.

Immunophenotyping. The use of monoclonal antibodies to differentiate antigens aids in defining lineage. It is most useful in poorly differentiated AML and necessary to identify type M_0.[44]

Cytogenetics. As in ALL, the cytogenetic classification of AML is more indicative of prognosis than any other factors. As many as 60% to 90% of adults with AML have cytogenetic abnormalities. Some correspond to a specific FAB subtype: M_3 with t(15;17), M_2 with

Table 13-5   French-American-British System (FAB) Classification System of AMLs

FAB type (% of AMLs)	Bone marrow morphology	Clinical features/prognosis
M_0 (5%)	Myeloid lineage cannot be determined by conventional morphologic or cytochemical analysis; can be identified by immunophenotyping	
M_1: myeloblastic (20%)	Without maturation >90% blasts Auer bodies present	M_1 and M_2 are most common adult AML diagnoses
M_2: myeloblastic (30%)	With maturation Blasts and promyelocytes >50% of cells Auer bodies and/or granules 8;21 chromosome translocation	Most favorable prognosis High rate of cure (85%-100%) with conventional chemotherapy
M_3: promyelocytic (APL) (10%)	Most cells abnormal promyelocytes Cells filled with large granules; may be microgranular Nucleus varies in size and shape Bundles of Auer bodies 15;17 chromosome translocation	10% of adult AMLs; disseminated intravascular coagulation present in 80% of patients: May occur after treatment initiation Granules released as blasts die and initiate coagulation cascade Good duration of remission WBC usually normal to low, <3,000/mm^3
M_3: variant (M_3V)	Granules detected only on electron microscopy (microgranular variant)	
M_4: myelomonocytic (15%-20%)	Promonoblasts and monoblasts >20%, myeloblasts and promyelocytes >20% of cells	Organomegaly Lymphadenopathy Gingival hyperplasias Soft tissue infiltration CNS leukemia
M_4E (5%-10%)	Variable number of morphologically abnormal eosinophils present Inversion of chromosome 16	High rate of complete remission
M_5: monocytic *Subtype A*—poorly differentiated: all monoblasts (5%) *Subtype B*—differentiated: promonocytes predominant (5%)	Monocytic cells exceed 80% Granulocytic component rarely exceeds 10% Abnormalities with chromosome 11 Few cells may have Auer bodies	Organomegaly Lymphadenopathy Gingival hyperplasia Soft tissue infiltration CNS leukemia Short remissions
M_6: erythroleukemia (Di Guglielmo syndrome [erythroleukemia]) (<5%)	Erythropoietic component exceeds 50% of marrow cells Blasts have bizarre morphology Myeloblasts and promyelocytes >30% of erythroid cells Complex karyotypes	Occurs in <5% AMLs Prolonged prodromal period May present with rheumatic disorder; 75% have positive Coombs' test; 30% have rheumatoid factor Almost always progresses to M_1, M_2, M_4
M_7: megakaryocytic (<5%)	Reticulin and collagen fibrosis; blasts resemble immature megakaryocytes or may be quite undifferentiated Complex karyotypes	Rare variant Marrow difficult to aspirate Increased lactate dehydrogenase Intense myelofibrosis Very poor prognosis

Other poor prognostic cytogenetic abnormalities: 5q-, -F, Fq-, and +8,11q-. These patients have short durations of complete remission (median, 6 months).

t(8;21), and M_4E_0 with inv(16), which are all favorable karyotypes; and M_6 and M_7 with complex karyotypes, which are unfavorable.[21] Monosomy 5 and 7 are frequently found in T-cell AML, which carries a poor prognosis. Plans for postremission therapy rely heavily on cytogenetic analysis at diagnosis.[26]

Other risk factors. A preexisting hematologic disorder, serious infection at diagnosis, CNS leukemia, organomegaly, and lymphadenopathy are clinical features indicative of poor prognosis.[43] Laboratory findings predictive of poor response include anemia, high peripheral blast count, thrombocytopenia, elevated blood urea nitrogen (BUN) and creatinine, increased LDH, or increased fibrinogen.[43]

TREATMENT MODALITIES

The treatment goal of AML, as in ALL, is cure. Treatment is divided into two phases: induction and postremission therapy. Currently, maintenance therapy is not recommended in the treatment of AML. Postremission therapy options include the following[44]:

1. Consolidation therapy with drug regimens almost as intensive as induction therapy. Consolidation is given over a period of months after the attainment of a complete remission.
2. Intensification with a dose-intensified schedule of drugs used during induction. The most frequently used agent is high-dose ARA-C (HDAC) in combination with other antileukemic drugs.
3. Ablative therapy with allogeneic, autologous, or PBSC rescue.

A complete remission in AML is defined as less than 5% nucleated marrow blasts in a normocellular marrow. Peripheral blood counts must return to normal, and preexisting adenopathy or organomegaly must be absent.[70]

Induction Chemotherapy

Successful treatment of AML requires the control of bone marrow and systemic disease and specific treatment of CNS disease, if present. Cytarabine (ARA-C), 100 to 200 mg/m^2 continuous intravenous (IV) infusion for 7 days, plus daunorubicin, 45 to 60 mg/m^2/day IV bolus for 3 days, is the standard treatment. This 3 + 7 regimen results in CR rate of 65% to 70%. Doxorubicin has been substituted but has more severe gastrointestinal toxicities.[26]

Idarubicin has been substituted for daunorubicin, with reports of higher CR. Randomized trials have shown at least equal results with mitoxantrone and aclarubicin. Concerns have been raised that the doses of drugs were not biologically equivalent and therefore comparisons may not be accurate.[3] HDAC has been studied in various schedules, with no clear benefits over the 3 + 7 regi-

men. However, follow-up reports show a longer remission rate with HDAC.[44]

A bone marrow examination is repeated on days 10 to 14 from the first day of chemotherapy to assess for antileukemic response. A positive response is indicated by a hypocellular, aplastic marrow. Peripheral blood studies reflect marrow aplasia, with profound neutropenia and thrombocytopenia at the 14-day nadir. If the day 14 bone marrow shows persistent leukemia, a second induction is started despite severe pancytopenia. The marrow examination is repeated as the peripheral counts begin to recover. If evidence of leukemia persists 3 to 4 weeks after the start of induction and the marrow cellularity is recovered, the patient is reinduced with the same drugs and doses.

In previous studies, elderly patients were treated with reduced doses of chemotherapy. These trials showed a trend toward persistent leukemia with reduced doses. Further studies have supported the use of standard-dose chemotherapy for patients over age 60.[9]

Postremission Therapy

If further chemotherapy is not administered to the AML patient in remission, the survival time is much shorter and most patients will experience disease relapse within 6 to 8 months.[10,13] The most effective postremission therapy and the program's optimal length are not known. Studies have shown no benefit from maintenance therapy over the shorter, more intense consolidation therapies.[87,108] Other studies, however, found some benefit when comparing maintenance therapy with historical control studies.[16,30] Because this conflicting information exists, patients should enter randomized clinical trials.

Intensification with HDAC resulted in a significantly higher 4-year disease-free survival rate in patients under age 60 compared with standard doses.[77] HDAC resulted in a significantly higher response in subgroups with unfavorable cytogenetics. It also increased duration of response in both unfavorable and favorable cytogenetic groups.[3,58]

Bone Marrow Transplant

BMT may be the treatment of choice in certain AML patients in first remission. The BMT may be an autologous transplant, allogeneic transplant, or PBSC transplantation. Controversy exists whether intensification, autologous BMT, or allogeneic BMT is the treatment of choice during first remission. Patients with the favorable karyotypes inv(16), t(8;21), or t(15;17) (generally AMLM$_4$, M$_2$, and M$_3$) have long-term remission rates and should be treated with chemotherapy only. Clinical trials have compared allogeneic BMT with autologous BMT during first remission with mixed results. Purging of the marrow was used in one study but not the other.[32,103] Many centers recommend allogeneic BMT during first CR for those with unfavorable karyotypes. Patients who have human lymphocyte antigen–(HLA-)identical siblings often receive BMT during first CR, resulting in 60% leukemia-free survival versus 20% to 30% with standard chemotherapy.

Clinical trials comparing intensification, autologous BMT, and allogeneic BMT continue. The role of autologous PBSC transplantation has not been defined. Concerns include a reinfusion of a higher number of malignant cells because of the large cell dose reinfused with PBSC transplants. (See Chapter 24 for more information on transplant options in AML patients.)

Recurrent Disease Therapy

Most patients who achieve a CR later relapse with AML and die. Achieving remission after relapse is difficult, and patients with these remissions rarely survive more than a year. The likelihood of achieving a second CR depends on the length of the first CR. Those patients refractory to initial therapy or with a 6- to 12-month first remission achieve about 20% CR, compared with 60% for those with a longer first CR. For patients eligible for allogeneic transplant, this is the first choice of treatment. Those not eligible for BMT should receive investigational treatment if the first CR is less than 1 year or should repeat the original induction if longer than 1 year.[44]

Hematopoietic Growth Factors

The addition of granulocyte colony-stimulating factor (G-CSF) and granulocyte-macrophage CSF (GM-CSF) has been studied in elderly patients in four large randomized studies. Myelosuppression was decreased in all four studies, but clinical benefits such as decreased infection rates were not always seen.[3] GMCSF has been approved for use during induction and consolidation therapy in elderly patients. The growth factors are usually administered after days 10 to 14 bone marrow shows a complete clearing of leukemic cells. This avoids stimulation of leukemic cells.

Multidrug Resistance

Multidrug resistance (MDR) to chemotherapy has been attributed to the MDR1 gene and its protein product, P-glycoprotein (P-gp). P-gp functions as a pump, transporting anthracyclines, *Vinca* alkaloids, amsacrine, mitoxantrone, and etoposide in and out of malignant cells. This results in decreased chemotherapy levels in the malignant cells and affects response rate. P-gp does not affect alkylating agents or antimetabolites.[109]

A relationship between MDR1 expression and treatment outcome has been shown.[75] Patients with a high level of P-gp have a poorer prognosis. Patients may also develop increased MDR-1 expression after treatment

with chemotherapy. Many clinical trials require bone marrow aspirate specimens to determine MDR status.

Cyclosporin A (cyclosporine) has been shown to overcome MDR. List and others[75] used cyclosporine in combination with ARA-C and daunorubicin in poor-risk AML patients and reported a complete response rate of 62%. Ongoing trials with cyclosporine and cyclosporine derivatives continue.

Therapy for Acute Promyelocytic Leukemia

Acute promyelocytic leukemia (APL), or FAB type M_3, is now treated differently than the other AMLs. Its unique t(15;17) forms a PML/RAR–fusion protein that blocks differentiation of hematopoietic precursor cells.[52] All-*trans*-retinoic acid (ATRA, tretinoin), when given, promotes cell differentiation.

APL usually presents with disseminated intravascular coagulation (DIC), which exacerbates with chemotherapy and has a mortality rate from hemorrhage ranging from 8% to 47%. Conventional chemotherapy produces CR in 60% to 80% of patients, with long-term survival of 35% to 45%.[110] Induction with ATRA at 45 mg/m^2 daily is given until no more APL blasts are seen in bone marrow smears, approximately 30 to 45 days.[24] With the use of ATRA, CR rates greater than 90% and a quicker resolution of coagulopathy are seen. Induction mortality is decreased. ARA-C and daunorubicin may still be used as the primary treatment without ATRA. Once CR is achieved, consolidation is mandatory for long-term cure. Consolidations currently used include combination chemotherapy with an anthracycline and ARA-C or anthracycline alone.[24] Other studies have added ATRA as consolidation. Exposure to ATRA either as induction or after CR leads to improved 1 year disease-free survival.[104]

Complications of ATRA include retinoic acid syndrome (RAS) and hyperleukocytosis. RAS consists of fever and respiratory distress, weight gain, lower extremity edema, pleural or pericardial effusions, hypotension, and sometimes renal failure. Hyperleukocytosis can lead to pulmonary and CNS toxicity. Two different approaches are used to treat RAS. The addition of chemotherapy to patients with high WBC counts has decreased symptoms; leukapheresis may be used to control elevated counts. High-dose corticosteroids begun at the first sign of symptoms have alleviated symptoms. ATRA may be discontinued.[24]

CHRONIC LEUKEMIAS

Chronic Myelogenous Leukemia

Chronic myelogenous leukemia (CML) is a myeloproliferative disorder characterized by proliferation of the granulocyte cell series. Chronic leukemias differ from acute leukemias in that the malignant WBCs appear mature and are well differentiated. A second unique difference is the progression of CML through three stages: chronic, accelerated, and blastic transformation, or blast crisis.

EPIDEMIOLOGY AND ETIOLOGY

The incidence of CML increases with exposure to radiation but is not clearly associated with alkylating agents or hereditary factors.[51] CML occurs in less than 5% of pediatric leukemia cases. Two types of CML are seen in children. Juvenile CML occurs in children younger than 5 years and presents more like acute leukemia. It is not responsive to chemotherapy and should be treated with allogeneic BMT. If patients receive BMT, 30% to 50% become long-term disease-free survivors.[94] The adult form of CML is seen in the remainder of patients, with the same treatment options used.

The annual incidence of CML is 1 to 1.5 per 100,000 population[20]; CML is less common than chronic lymphocytic leukemia and is one-fourth as common as acute leukemia. This disease is most frequently encountered between ages 20 and 60, with the peak incidence between ages 50 and 60.[51] Males have a rate 1.7 times higher than females.[79]

Significant advances have been made in understanding the biology of CML, and therapeutic improvements have increased the length of the chronic phase.

Philadelphia Chromosome

The hallmark of CML is the presence of a Philadelphia chromosome (Ph[1]). Nowell and Hungerford[80] identified this unusually small chromosome occurring in CML patients in 1960 at the University of Pennsylvania and named the chromosome for its city of origin. Chromosome 22 is missing part of its long arm, which is translocated to the long arm of chromosome 9. A new hybrid BCR-ABL oncogene is formed. It produces abnormal RNA and results in normal hematopoietic cells changing into CML cells.[67] The presence of BCR-ABL is diagnostic and can be used to detect early relapse.

CLINICAL FEATURES AND DIAGNOSIS
Chronic Phase

The presenting symptoms of chronic phase CML are related to expansion of the granulocytic mass. Other symptoms may include fatigue, night sweats, pallor, dyspnea, anemia, anorexia, weight loss, and sternal tenderness. The most common finding at diagnosis is splenomegaly. The spleen may be only minimally enlarged or may be greatly enlarged, filling most of the abdomen.

Most patients are diagnosed during the chronic phase, which has a median duration of 3 to 5 years. The chronic phase is the initial indolent form of CML. The presenting symptoms resolve as the patient responds to therapy. Patients usually feel well and are ambulatory during this period. Presenting complaints may include symptoms related to massive splenomegaly caused by infiltration of WBCs, left upper quadrant abdominal pain, early satiety, and abdominal fullness.

A very high WBC count can cause leukostatic lesion development in the microvasculature of the lungs or CNS. Leukostasis may lead to thromboembolic episodes and pulmonary or CNS bleeding. Presentation with an excessively high WBC count is a medical emergency, and the count must be reduced rapidly with hydroxyurea and/or leukapheresis. Thrombocytosis is present in one third of patients, with platelet counts greater than 1 million/mm^3 in some patients. WBC and platelet counts may fluctuate in 30- to 60-day cycles without any therapy.[79]

Diagnosis of CML is established by hematologic evaluation. The following results of a complete blood cell count (CBC) are characteristic of CML:
- WBC count greater than 100,000/mm^3
- Mature and immature granulocytes; segmented neutrophils predominate
- Myelocytes exceeding metamyelocytes
- Increased eosinophils
- Increased basophils
- Normal or increased platelets

A bone marrow evaluation is required to assess cellularity, detect fibrosis, and obtain a specimen for cytogenetic analysis.

In addition to the presence of the Ph[1] chromosome in 95% of CML patients, the marrow is extremely hypercellular and may be devoid of fat. Myeloid elements are increased, and megakaryocytes may be excessive.[18] Cytogenetic studies to detect the Ph[1] chromosome may be performed on peripheral blood if the WBC count is sufficiently elevated.[22]

Accelerated Stage

The term *accelerated stage* is generally used to refer to patients who have been under treatment for some time and have shown a variety of signs of disease progression but who do not meet the criteria for blastic disease.[65] Progression to the accelerated phase is characteristic of 75% to 80% of patients with CML. The time of progression to the accelerated phase is variable and greatly impacts length of survival. The leukocyte doubling time (LDT) shortens to 20 days or less during this stage. The first evidence of accelerated stage may be failure to respond to drugs effective during the chronic stage. Other evidence shows peripheral blasts being 15% or more of cells, thrombocytopenia with a WBC count less than 100,000/mm^3 unrelated to therapy, and cytogenetic clonal evolution.

CLINICAL FEATURES
Comparison of Chronic Phase CML and Accelerated Phase/Blastic Transformation

Chronic phase	*Accelerated phase/blastic transformation*
Fatigue	
Pallor	Increased fatigue
Dyspnea	Increasing anemia
Anemia	Recurrence of splenomegaly
Anorexia	Thrombocytopenia
Weight loss	Fever of unknown origin
Sternal tenderness	Lymphadenopathy
Splenomegaly	Hepatomegaly
	Thrombocytosis/thrombocytopenia

Physical examination reveals increased fatigue, increasing anemia, recurrence of splenomegaly, and thrombocytopenia; occasionally, fever of unknown origin, lymphadenopathy, hepatomegaly, thrombocytosis, and basophilia are also noted. The patient may exhibit signs of hypermetabolism, including night sweats, decreased appetite, and weight loss. Periosteal infiltrates and lytic lesions may cause bony pain in addition to sternal pain.

Blood and bone marrow evaluation reveals increased promyelocytes and blasts. The onset of the accelerated phase is difficult to distinguish, and the diagnosis may be made retrospectively. The box above differentiates the clinical features in the chronic phase and the accelerated phase/blastic transformation.

Survival for patients in accelerated phase is difficult to describe because of disease heterogeneity but can be estimated at about a year.[99]

Blastic Phase

Patients with CML inevitably enter the blastic stage, an aggressive, rapidly terminal phase that is refractory to treatment. The International CML Prognosis Study Group uses any one of the following criteria to define the blastic stage[69]:
- Blasts accounting for more than 20% of cells in peripheral blood or marrow
- Blasts plus promyelocytes greater than 30% of cells in peripheral blood
- Blasts plus promyelocytes greater than 50% of cells in marrow
- Extramedullary blastic infiltrates
- Leukemic tumor masses

Two thirds of patients have cells with predominantly myeloblastic characteristics; one third exhibit lympho-

blastic features.[79] It is important to distinguish between myeloid or lymphoid transformation because patients with lymphoid disease respond better to treatment (with vincristine and prednisone) and live slightly longer. The presence of the enzyme deoxynucleotidyl transferase in blasts identifies the presence of lymphoblastic disease. The blastic stage resembles a disease similar to AML or ALL.

Median survival after blastic transformation is usually less than 6 months.[102] At least 85% of patients die during the blast phase from complications such as bleeding, infections, and cerebral or pulmonary hemorrhages.[106]

TREATMENT MODALITIES

Treatment of CML is usually initiated when the diagnosis is established. At this stage, patients under age 55 should be considered for allogeneic BMT, the only curative treatment for this disease. For those without a donor, interferon therapy should be initiated.[67] Traditional therapies include busulfan and hydroxyurea.

Chemotherapy

Until 1980, busulfan (Myleran) and hydroxyurea (Hydrea) were the most effective agents in CML therapy. The usual busulfan dose is 0.1 mg/kg/day until the WBC count decreases by 50%, and then the dose is reduced by 50%. Therapy is stopped when the count is less than 20,000/mm^3 and restarted when greater than 50,000/mm^3. Busulfan therapy is associated with lung, marrow, and heart fibrosis and can cause Addison's disease.[28]

Hydrea has a lower toxicity profile than busulfan but shorter control of WBC count and therefore needs more frequent follow-up. Starting doses of 40 mg/kg/day are adjusted based on the counts.[22] Hydrea is the drug of choice to control WBC count before BMT.

Although treatment during the chronic phase with busulfan or hydroxyurea will improve marrow cellularity and decrease splenomegaly, it does not eliminate the Philadelphia chromosome. Thus, even though the disease is controlled by these agents for an average of 3 years, all patients will progress to accelerated and blastic phases.

Intensive combination chemotherapy has been developed with the goal of reducing or eradicating the Ph[1]-positive clones to delay the onset of blast crisis and to prolong survival. Regimens appropriate for the treatment of AML have been evaluated in several small studies. The results showed conversion to a Ph[1]-negative state in as many as 25% of patients. This conversion, along with the duration of normal hematopoiesis, was transient, however, and no cures were achieved.[51]

Intensive multidrug regimens are the treatment of choice for the blastic transformation phase of CML in patients who are not BMT candidates. These regimens include ARA-C, programs with anthracyclines, amsacrine (m-AMSA, Amsidyl), 6-thioguanine (6 TG), and hydroxyurea. More recently, high doses of ARA-C (2 g/m^2) with anthracyclines and mitoxantrone have been studied. Overall response rates are low, ranging from 10% to 30%. Patients with lymphoid blast crisis, however, have a 40% to 70% response rate with ALL regimens based on vincristine and prednisone.[105]

Interferon

Interferon (IFN) has been studied in the treatment of CML since 1981. It has allowed for a complete hematologic response (CHR) in many patients and cytogenetic responses (suppression of the Ph^1-positive clone) in 10% to 15%. A randomized comparison between IFN alfa-2a (Roferon) and Hydrea showed that the overall survival of the IFN group was significantly better because of slowing of disease from chronic to accelerated or blastic phase.[62] A summary of ongoing trials shows median survival of 60 to 65 months, with 25% of patients being in durable cytogenetic remissions.[67] Current trials are studying a combination of IFN and low-dose ARA-C to improve the percentage of cytogenetic responses.[68]

The dose used in most studies is IFN 2 to 5 million IU/m^2/day. Lower doses may be needed if patients experience severe side effects. (See Chapter 23 for a complete discussion of interferon and its side effects.)

Bone Marrow Transplant

BMT after high-dose chemotherapy and radiation therapy is the only potentially curative treatment for CML.[78] Best results occur when the transplant is performed early in the chronic phase. The 5-year survival for chronic phase patients is 60%, compared with 22% in the accelerated phase and 13% in the blast phase.[107]

All patients younger than 55 years with an identical twin or with HLA-matched siblings should be considered for BMT early in the chronic phase. Many BMT centers now treat CML patients up to age 60.

Future Treatments

Combinations of chemotherapy and biologic response modifiers need be tested as the optimal treatment form for CML. Because of the limitations of allogeneic BMT in relation to patient age, donor compatibility, and graft-versus-host complications, alternative marrow ablative regimens are needed.

CML patients treated with chemotherapy have peripheral blood stem cells (PBSCs) that are predominantly Ph^1 negative. These cells have been harvested and used to autograft after high doses of chemotherapy (as in autologous BMT). Others have given IFN to achieve Ph^1-negative status, had their PBSCs harvested, and then received BMT. Further studies will validate this approach.[50]

Chronic Lymphocytic Leukemia

Chronic lymphocytic leukemia (CLL) is a malignant hematologic disorder characterized by proliferation and accumulation of relatively normal-appearing lymphocytes. The vast majority of cases (95%) are B-cell lymphoproliferative disorders with a single clone of B lymphocytes undergoing malignant transformation. The remaining 5% are T-cell lymphoproliferative disorders.[93]

EPIDEMIOLOGY AND ETIOLOGY

The development of CLL is more a result of genetic predisposition than environmental influences. A familial tendency has been suggested, as well as concordance in several identical twins, but no pattern of inheritance has been reported.[18] A strong correlation exists between CLL and autoimmune diseases such as systemic lupus erythematosus, Sjögren's syndrome, and autoimmune hemolytic anemia.

CLL is the most common leukemia in the United States, accounting for 30% or 10,000 cases of all newly diagnosed leukemias. The median age of CLL patients is 60 years.[79] The disease affects twice as many males as females.[11]

The clinical course and prognosis of B-cell CLL is variable and depends on the disease stage at diagnosis. Patients with early-stage disease may live 10 years or longer without treatment; patients with a more aggressive, advanced stage at diagnosis usually die within 2 years.[40]

CLINICAL FEATURES

CLL is discovered on routine physical examination or routine laboratory work in the 25% of patients who are asymptomatic. Because CLL is a disease of immunoglobulin-secreting cells, recurrent skin and respiratory infections may be elicited from the patient history. Nearly 50% of the bone marrow is infiltrated before peripheral blood counts are compromised. Progressive accumulation of the abnormal lymphocytes into nodal structures and the advancing marrow involvement yield symptoms of malaise, anorexia, fatigue, and lymphadenopathy in the patient with advanced disease. Gastrointestinal and genitourinary complaints are related to enlarging abdominal lymph nodes. Splenomegaly may cause abdominal discomfort or early satiety.

Physical findings may be negative or positive only for splenomegaly in the early-stage patient. Advanced patients with anemia and thrombocytopenia display the typical findings of anemia and bruising or petechiae. Lymph node enlargement may be present on examination. Hepatomegaly may be seen in addition to splenomegaly if portal obstruction is related to abdominal adenopathy.

DIAGNOSIS AND STAGING

The diagnosis of CLL is suspected in the presence of unexplained lymphocytosis on the peripheral blood examination. Monoclonal antibodies directed at specific heavy and light chains of immunoglobulins or gene rearrangement studies define the clonal nature of the disease, thus establishing the diagnosis. A bone marrow or lymph node biopsy is rarely required to establish the diagnosis but, for patients in research studies, may provide valuable information about treatment response, cytogenetics, and molecular biology.

In the diagnostic evaluation of CLL, lymphocytosis is the most consistent finding. The peripheral WBC count may exceed 50,000/mm^3, with greater than 90% mature lymphocytes.

The bone marrow is hypercellular with a diffuse infiltration of small and medium lymphocytes (more than 30% of cells) with mature morphologic features. Myeloid elements of the marrow have normal morphology and maturation.

Lymph node biopsy shows a histopathologic pattern of diffuse lymphoma with small, noncleaved lymphocytes. Immunologic studies and cytogenetics further define the disease process.

In 1975 Rai and Montserrat[91] proposed a clinical staging system based on lymphocytes, lymphadenopathy, splenomegaly, hepatomegaly, anemia, and thrombocytopenia. In 1987 it was modified to a three-stage system: low, intermediate, and high. Low risk is stage 0, intermediate is stages I and II, and high is stages III and IV, as follows:

Rai clinical staging system

Stage 0   Lymphocytosis only, in blood (>15,000/mm^3) and bone marrow (>40%). Median survival is 12+ years.

Stage I   Lymphocytosis with lymphadenopathy. Median survival is 8+ years.

Stage II   Lymphocytosis and splenomegaly with or without hepatomegaly. Median survival is 6 years.

Stage III   Lymphocytosis and anemia (hemoglobin <11 g/dl). Median survival is 1.5 years.

Stage IV   Lymphocytosis and thrombocytopenia (platelets <100,000/mm^3). Survival is 1.5 years.

Other staging systems have widespread acceptance, but the Rai system is the one used most frequently in the United States. Clinical stage at diagnosis is the most reliable predictor for response to treatment and survival.[11]

TREATMENT MODALITIES

Indications for Treatment

One of the most difficult decisions in CLL is when to initiate treatment.[40] At present, no cure exists for CLL. Treatment aims at alleviating symptoms. The absolute WBC count is not an indication for treatment. Patients with low-risk prognostic factors should not be treated. There is no survival advantage, and early treatment has had detrimental effects in some studies.

Intermediate-risk patients are treated when they show evidence of disease progression.

High-risk patients are treated with chemotherapy. Other indications for treatment include control of manifestations of progressive disease, such as fever, night sweats, weight loss, progressive anemia and thrombocytopenia, worsening lymphadenopathy, massive splenomegaly, and repeated infections.[11,34,93]

Single-Agent Chemotherapy

Chlorambucil, an alkylating agent, is the agent most frequently used in CLL patients. It is given orally in 6 mg to 14 mg doses every 2 to 4 weeks. The dose is reduced once the disease is controlled. Several months of treatment are required to obtain a complete response. Response rates range from 40% to 70%. Combinations with prednisone have revealed mixed results.[34]

Cyclophosphamide is as effective as chlorambucil, and its non-cross-resistance makes it useful in treating patients unresponsive to chlorambucil.[39]

Prednisone has been used to control leukocytosis and to treat immune-mediated hemolytic anemia and thrombocytopenia. Patients with extensive disease are often treated with steroids before initiating chemotherapy.[40]

Combination Chemotherapy

Combination chemotherapy with cyclophosphamide, vincristine, and prednisone (CVP) has been used in patients with advanced CLL.[39] The addition of doxorubicin to this regimen (CHOP) resulted in a survival advantage.[42] No survival differences were observed between patients randomized to CHOP or chlorambucil plus prednisone.[34] Currently there is little evidence of a role for maintenance chemotherapy in CLL once a response has been obtained.[39]

Nucleoside Analogues

Three nucleoside analogues that are currently undergoing trials are: fludarabine (Fludara), cladribine (2-chlorodeoxyadenosine, 2-CdA), and pentostatin (Nipent). Their major toxicity is myelosuppression; acute tumor lysis and autoimmune hemolytic anemia have also been documented.[11] Fludarabine and 2-CdA have shown complete response rates of 25% to 74% in untreated patients. Pentostatin has been less extensively studied.[93]

Fludarabine is the most studied, but its mechanism of action is unclear. It is the treatment of choice after failure with chlorambucil. In previously treated patients an overall response rate of 57% has been seen.

Splenectomy

Splenectomy has no influence on survival in CLL patients but may be indicated for autoimmune anemia or thrombocytopenia refractory to systemic therapy or for persistent symptomatic splenomegaly in a patient responding to chemotherapy.[34]

Radiation Therapy

Splenic irradiation has been used to alleviate symptoms when the surgical risk is too high. It also may be employed to palliate symptoms or relieve organ dysfunction caused by abdominal adenopathy, such as biliary tract or urinary tract obstruction.[40]

Bone Marrow Transplant

Allogenic BMT has been performed in a limited number of patients, with CRs in approximately 50%. Relapses as late as 4 years after BMT may occur.[11,93] Studies are underway to assess the effects of allologous BMT, autogeneic BMT, and PBSC therapy as curative options.

HAIRY-CELL LEUKEMIA

EPIDEMIOLOGY AND ETIOLOGY

Hairy-cell leukemia (HCL) is a rare chronic lymphoproliferative disorder of unknown etiology. There does not seem to be an association with ionizing radiation or other environmental factors. The disease is usually diagnosed in middle-aged patients and is quite rare, representing less than 2% of adult leukemias, and approximately 500 to 600 new cases in the United States yearly.[63]

CLINICAL FEATURES

Clinical manifestations of HCL are related to excessive infiltration of the bone marrow and/or spleen with "hairy cells." This results in underproduction or excessive peripheral sequestration of circulating cells, manifested as granulocytopenia, anemia, or thrombocytopenia.[7] The presenting complaints in more than half of patients are constitutional symptoms of weakness, lethargy, or fatigue. As many as one fourth of patients are diagnosed incidentally when a routine CBC reveals abnormalities. Physical findings are limited to splenomegaly, which is seen in as many as 90% of patients.[111] Patients are more susceptible to infections, usually gram-negative bacteria.[34]

DIAGNOSIS

The hallmark of HCL is the presence of the peculiar hairy cell in the blood, bone marrow, and reticuloendothelial organs. This cell is characterized morphologically by its hairlike projections. Cytochemical stains demonstrate the presence of tartrate-resistant acid phosphatase (TRAP). Patients are diagnosed based on the presence of cytopenias, hairy cells in the peripheral blood, splenomegaly, and bone marrow aspiration and biopsy. The bone marrow is frequently fibrotic and may not be aspirable.

CLASSIFICATION

Generally, no accepted staging system is useful for both prognosis and therapy. For the purpose of treatment decisions, it is best to consider this disease in two broad categories: untreated and progressive.

TREATMENT MODALITIES

HCL is a highly treatable and sometimes curable disease. Patients who are asymptomatic with acceptable blood counts can be observed until the disease progresses and requires treatment. Treatment is required when cytopenias become symptomatic, splenomegaly increases, or infectious complications exist.

The standard therapy for HCL was originally splenectomy. This procedure normalizes the peripheral blood in most patients, but virtually no change occurs in the bone marrow, and all patients have progressive disease in 12 to 18 months.[96]

Interferon-α in low, well-tolerated doses is effective in HCL.[46,72,96,98] The interferon is administered subcutaneously three times a week for 1 year and yields a 10% complete remission rate and an 80% overall response rate.[46] This treatment is not curative, however, and retreatment is necessary in most patients whose therapy is stopped.[100] Reinitiation of interferon therapy can induce second responses in at least some patients.

Deoxycoformycin (dCF), also called pentostatin, is a purine analogue first reported to have activity in HCL in 1984. This drug is given as a short infusion every other week for 3 to 6 months and produces a 57% complete response rate and an overall 83% response rate. Complete remissions are of substantial duration, and some patients appear to be cured by this agent.[14,46]

Cladribine (2-CdA), another purine analogue, has similar activity to dCF. The drug is given IV daily for 1 week and produces a total response rate of 97%, with 85% CR and 12% partial remission. Both previously treated and newly diagnosed patients have had the same results. Fever is common. Recovery of blood counts has ranged from 11 to 268 days.[84] Limited data suggest 2-CdA has greater activity than dCF, with the advantage of only one treatment. 2-CdA is emerging as the treatment of choice for HCL.[97]

MYELODYSPLASTIC SYNDROMES

EPIDEMIOLOGY AND ETIOLOGY

The myelodysplastic syndromes (MDSs) are a heterogeneous group of disorders previously referred to as "oligoblastic leukemia," "smoldering acute leukemia," or "preleukemia."[17] MDS is classified into five distinct pathologic entities: (1) refractory anemia (RA), (2) refractory anemia with ringed sideroblasts (RARS), (3) chronic myelomonocytic leukemia (CMML), (4) refractory anemia with excess blasts (RAEB), and (5) refractory anemia with excess blasts in transition (RAEB-t). These disorders vary from relatively indolent hematologic disorders to conditions indistinguishable from acute leukemia.

Myelodysplasia is a disease of elderly persons and most often affects those over age 60. The incidence may be increasing, especially secondary MDS. Males are affected more frequently than females. Although the etiology of MDS is unclear, its manifestations result from neoplastic transformation at the level of the pleuripotent stem cell.[12] Some studies have implicated exposure to benzene, radiation, chemotherapy, and alkylating agents in particular as initiating factors in the development of myelodysplasia.[74]

CLINICAL FEATURES

Patients with MDS usually have severe cytopenias or pancytopenia.[23] Infections, particularly respiratory or gram-negative septicemias, are frequently the presenting symptom. Bleeding may be present as a result of either thrombocytopenia or poorly functioning circulating platelets.[12]

DIAGNOSIS

The diagnosis of MDS is established by bone marrow aspiration and biopsy. The following blast percentages are seen: RA less than 5%; RARS less than 5%; RAEB, 5% to 20%; RAEB-t, 20% to 30%; and CMML greater than 20%, with peripheral monocytes greater than 1000/mm³. Particular morphologic changes can be seen in both the marrow and the peripheral blood. Chromosomal studies are also performed because approximately half of all MDS patients display karyotypic abnormalities.[23] The abnormalities are similar to those seen in AML karyotypes related to a poor prognosis.[32]

CLASSIFICATION

The FAB classification system developed in 1982 is used to classify the MDSs into the five groups previously listed. A 1995 MDS risk analysis workshop studied stratifying patients into high-intensity, intermediate-intensity, or low-intensity groups according to the percentage of marrow blasts, platelet count, and age. Recommendations are forthcoming.

TREATMENT MODALITIES

Because of the elderly age of MDS patients, various treatment approaches have been used, including no therapy, pyridoxine, androgens, and steroids. These options are rarely effective.[32] Patients with only RA may have an indolent disease course and can be supported by transfusion therapy for many years.

CSFs in various combinations are undergoing clinical trials. A multicenter phase III study examined different doses of GM-CSF for RA and RAEB patients. Most had an increase in neutrophil counts, but GM-CSF was discontinued because of side effects or disease progression. In 25% of patients, platelet counts decreased to less than 50% of baseline values. Therapy with GM-CSF plus low-dose ARA-C also was evaluated, with equal thirds of patients improving, remaining stable, or declining.[50] Another multicenter phase III study randomized RAEB/RAEB-t patients to observation versus long-term G-CSF therapy. Improved neutrophil counts were observed in most G-CSF patients without side effects. No difference in the incidence of or time of progression to AML was noted. The incidence of infections is being evaluated.[49]

Erythropoietin (EPO) alone has shown limited effect. However, in combination with G-CSF, 40% to 45% of patients had decreased transfusion requirements and increased hemoglobin levels. Most had neutrophil responses.[50]

Differentiating agents can transform nonfunctional immature blasts and promyeloblasts into functional mature granulocytes.[12] Various agents have been studied, including retinoic acids, low-dose cytarabine, tretinoin, interferon-α, and hexamethylmelamine bisacetamide. Thus far, none of these agents has achieved a measure of success substantial enough to consider differentiating agents to be standard therapy for MDS.

"Low-intensity" or low-risk MDS subgroups may benefit from the cytokines or differentiating agents just listed. "High-intensity" MDS subgroups may benefit from chemotherapy or BMT. Results of clinical trials will assist in determining appropriate therapies.

"High-intensity" or high-risk patients have been treated with AML-type chemotherapies, with CR rates greater than 50%. However, the CRs were not durable for most patients.[32]

Allogeneic BMT studies have shown disease-free survival rates of 41% and 55%, with a median patient age of 30 years. Again, most patients are over age 60 and will not be eligible for these therapies.[32]

Text continued on p. 307.

NURSING MANAGEMENT

The medical and nursing management of lymphocytic and nonlymphocytic leukemia patients is similar and is detailed here. Supportive care of the leukemic patient is a major contributor to increased survival and improved quality of life. The talents and resources of all members of the interdisciplinary team are required to support the patient and family through the phases of this disease process. The nurse, relying on a strong knowledge of the disease and the potential complications, uses systematic assessments to monitor physiologic homeostasis. For the person with leukemia, medical and nursing support is required in three areas: (1) to prevent or correct expected side effects of the disease and treatment, (2) to anticipate and treat unexpected or potential complications, and (3) to facilitate psychosocial adaptation of the patient and family.[64]

NURSING DIAGNOSIS

• *Knowledge deficit related to new leukemia diagnosis, disease process, treatment plan, side effects*

OUTCOME GOAL

Patient and family will be able to:
• Verbalize and demonstrate understanding of disease treatment and goals.

INTERVENTIONS

• Review disease process, treatment regimen, management and prevention of complications, and goals of treatment.
• Assess patient's preferred style of learning; identify any existing barriers to learning, including language and cultural beliefs; teach in short sessions; involve family members and significant others in teaching sessions; question patient to evaluate understanding of new information; and continue to reinforce information.
• Participate in informed consent process if patient is eligible for a clinical trial (see Chapter 25).
• Assess and discuss patient's desired level of information; explain common terminology.
• Orient patient and family to hospital unit and services (e.g., parking, accommodations, meals).
• Explain role of multidisciplinary team members and how to access their services.
• Provide information about insertion of venous access devices, and promote self-care of line after insertion.
• Provide information regarding available community resources and link where possible.
• Assist patient in developing system of treatment management through use of calendars, schedules, etc.
• In fertile patients, discuss issues of fertility (sperm banking, egg retrieval).

• Discuss issues of sexuality.
• Explain purpose of baseline testing.
• Provide a calendar of planned treatments and tests (Figure 13-2).

NURSING DIAGNOSIS

• *Anxiety related to new diagnosis, uncertain outcome of potentially fatal disease, loss of control in hospital environment, alteration in body image, alteration in interpersonal relationships.*

OUTCOME GOAL

Patient and family will be able to:
• Verbalize and/or demonstrate manageable anxiety throughout course of illness and seek out appropriate resources.

INTERVENTIONS

• Perform psychosocial assessment of patient/family; identify strengths, weaknesses, coping skills, and cultural preferences.
• Recognize increased anxiety levels that may occur while awaiting an official diagnosis, before painful or frightening procedures, before major treatments, on learning of relapse, and on anniversary dates.[71]
• Administer/offer antianxiety medications as ordered; assess effectiveness.
• Use therapeutic and healing touch.
• Use guided imagery, relaxation training, and cognitive distraction to alleviate anxiety before painful or stressful procedures.[71]
• Assist patient/family to set realistic goals concerning level of activity, work schedule, and self-care activities.[71]
• Encourage patient/family to verbalize questions, fears, and concerns.
• Involve chaplaincy services, social workers, psychologists, psychiatry, and support volunteers as needed.
• Inform patient/family of available community resources (e.g., Leukemia Society of America, American Cancer Society).

PREINDUCTION PHASE

The nurse caring for the patient with leukemia must have a thorough knowledge of the medical management of treatment-related toxicities and potential disease complications to provide effective nursing care.

The following assessments and medical interventions are performed before initiating antileukemia therapy. The nurse must incorporate the rationale for these studies into the patient teaching plan to help orient the patient and family to the plan of care.

Continued.

- Assessment of serum chemistries:
  - —Renal function: elevated creatinine may limit use of aminoglycoside antibiotics.
  - —Hepatic function: doses of anthracyclines or vincristine may require reduction for elevated liver enzymes.
  - —Electrolytes: normal electrolytes may minimize risk of certain drug side effects.
- Blood typing should be performed to ensure the availability of RBC and platelet transfusions.
- HLA typing should be performed on admission for patients who are possible bone marrow transplant (BMT) candidates.
- Baseline coagulation profile should be performed on patients with acute promyelocytic leukemia. These patients have an increased incidence of disseminated intravascular coagulation (DIC) (see Chapter 19). Patients with DIC may require heparinization or fresh-frozen plasma and platelet support before treatment initiation.
- Baseline chest x-ray film eliminates later confusion and assesses presence of possible pulmonary complications before treatment.
- Radionucleotide ventriculogram ensuring an adequate left ventricular ejection fraction before treatment requiring anthracyclines is important in patients with a questionable cardiac history or before enrollment in clinical trials.
- It is important to establish central venous access, preferably with a multiple-lumen catheter, before treatment. If patient is thrombocytopenic at diagnosis, platelet transfusion may be required before invasive procedure to reduce risk of bleeding. Catheter site must be monitored closely for postoperative bleeding.
- Decision to delay chemotherapy initiation in order to resolve an infection is determined by status of leuke-

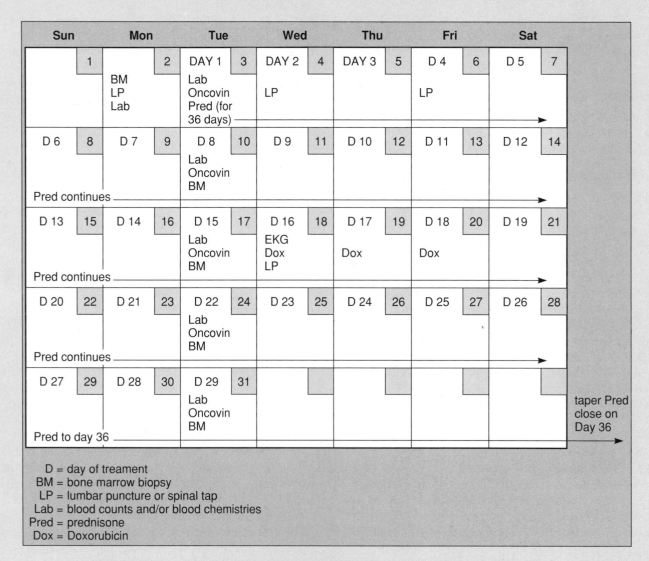

Figure 13-2   Example of patient teaching calendar outlining common induction regimen for acute lymphocytic leukemia (ALL).

mia, severity of infection, and number of circulating granulocytes.

- Acute tumor lysis syndrome occurs more often in L_2 and L_3 ALL. Patients at risk should receive high doses of allopurinol before treatment and urinary alkalinization, with sodium bicarbonate added to IV solutions.
- Although uncommon, uric acid deposits in the urinary tract may occur in patients with very high WBC counts. Again, allopurinol, 300 mg orally daily, should be instituted before starting treatment.

By monitoring the results of these studies, the nurse can assess potential patient complications. For example, an abnormal coagulation profile in a patient with acute promyelocytic (M_3) leukemia should signal the nurse to incorporate bleeding precautions and assessment for shock-like symptoms into the patient care and teaching plan.

CHEMOTHERAPY SIDE EFFECTS

Regardless of the chemotherapy regimen chosen, infection and bleeding are the most common side effects of acute leukemia therapy. Induction chemotherapy not only kills the malignant clone of leukemia cells in the marrow, but also suppresses the production of normal hematologic elements. Thus, as the platelets, WBCs, and to a lesser extent RBCs in the peripheral blood die, there are no new cells to replace them. The patient is severely immunocompromised until the normal marrow components begin to regenerate.

One of the most important considerations in the care of the leukopenic patient is the lack of the normal host responses to infection (see Chapter 30 for care of the immunosuppressed patient).

In patients who receive high-dose ARA-C (HDAC) or regimens aimed at overcoming multidrug resistance, the period of myelosuppression may last up to 3 weeks. Infection risk increases when the *absolute neutrophil count* (ANC) falls below 500 cells/mm^3 and exceeds 1 week. The ANC is calculated by multiplying the percentage of segmented and band neutrophils by the total WBCs.

Therapy with HDAC increases the risk for ocular problems and neurotoxicity. Corneal damage, burning, photophobia, decreased acuity, and conjunctivitis are reported. Corticosteroid eye drops are thought to help prevent these side effects.[109]

Increased neurotoxicity is seen in elderly patients receiving HDAC, which is not recommended in patients over age 60. Nursing interventions include a pretreatment assessment of the patient's neurologic status, gait, speech, eye movements, and ability to perform alternating movements rapidly. These assessments should be repeated daily.[109]

Asparaginase, used in ALL, often produces hypersensitivity reactions. It may occur with the first injection but generally occurs after repeated exposure. The patient must be observed for signs of an allergic reaction for 1 hour after injection. Anaphylaxis may occur, and appropriate medications should be available.

An increased temperature may be the only indication of an infectious process. Other indications may include chills, cough, burning and frequency on urination, diarrhea, or a sore that will not heal. It is important to note that corticosteroid therapy may suppress the febrile response. Also, with few WBCs, pus will not always be present in infected wounds. Astute nursing assessment is required to monitor potential sites of infection and provide appropriate interventions. The primary nurse, caring for the leukemic patient on a daily basis, is also in the best position to detect subtle changes that may be the earliest indicators of impending septic shock.

With the availability of platelet transfusion support, hemorrhage is less of a problem than in past years. Prophylactic transfusions are usually administered in asymptomatic patients when the platelet count is below 10,000 to 20,000/mm^3. Platelet counts should be checked 1 hour after transfusion to assess the increment of platelet increase. This also enables evaluation of possible alloimmunization and the need for a different platelet product. Alloimmunization occurs because the antigens on the transfused platelets react with the patient's antibodies, and the platelets are destroyed. The risk can be decreased by using platelets with few leukocytes. If a poor response still occurs, single-donor or HLA-matched platelets may be used. When patients develop fever, chills, or hives during transfusions, they may be premedicated with diphenhydramine and hydrocortisone and/or acetaminophen.

Transfusion of packed RBCs may be required to control anemia. Patients are usually transfused when their hemoglobin concentration falls below 7 to 8 g/dl because hemorrhage is more likely to occur in the severely anemic patient. Nursing assessment includes monitoring for paleness, dyspnea, dizziness, headache, and irritability. Cardiac hypoxia is indicated by tachycardia and tachypnea.

NURSING DIAGNOSIS

- *Infection, risk for, related to alteration in immune function secondary to leukemia and immunosuppressive chemotherapy*

OUTCOME GOALS

Patient will be able to:
- Demonstrate an understanding of the precautions to take to avoid infections and the signs and symptoms of possible infection.
- Seek appropriate treatment when demonstrating signs and symptoms of infection.

Continued.

INTERVENTIONS

- Teach patient/family the purpose and importance of neutropenic precautions.
- If appropriate, encourage patient to keep a chart of daily blood counts.
- Monitor temperature and vital signs every 4 hours when patient is neutropenic. Assess for changes in blood pressure, urine output, and mental status that may be early signs of septic shock.
- Have patient avoid fresh fruits and vegetables.
- Do not allow fresh flowers in patient's room.
- Avoid rectal manipulation.
- Ensure consistent handwashing by all people entering patient's room.
- Ensure consistent handwashing by patient before eating and after toileting.
- Limit number of visitors to two at a time; no visitors with colds, influenza, herpes, or recent vaccinations.
- Avoid trauma to skin and mucous membranes.
- Do not administer intramuscular or subcutaneous injections

NURSING DIAGNOSIS

- *Injury, risk for, associated with bleeding related to alteration in clotting factors, thrombocytopenia secondary to leukemia and/or treatment*

OUTCOME GOALS

Patient will be able to:
- Verbalize/demonstrate an understanding of the precautions to prevent bleeding so that risk of bleeding will be minimized.
- Seek appropriate treatment when demonstrating signs and symptoms of occult bleeding.

INTERVENTIONS

- Teach patient/family the significance of platelet function and bleeding precautions.
- Check platelet count at least every other day during immunosuppressive leukemia therapies.
- Monitor results of coagulation studies; assess for signs and symptoms of DIC.
- Assess for petechiae, bruising, epistaxis, hematuria, hematochezia, and oral, rectal, or vaginal bleeding.
- Monitor platelet transfusions.
- Apply pressure on bone marrow or venipuncture sites for 3 to 5 minutes.
- Do not administer intramuscular or subcutaneous injections.
- Avoid rectal manipulation.
- Use only electric razors.
- Do not administer aspirin-containing medications.
- Ensure safe environment: no sharp objects, bed rails up, ambulate with assistance.

- Prevent trauma to skin and mucous membranes.
- Use soft toothbrush.

NURSING DIAGNOSIS

- *Nutrition, altered: less than body requirements, related to treatment-induced nausea, vomiting, stomatitis, anorexia*

OUTCOME GOALS

Patient will be able to:
- Maintain adequate body weight and muscle mass throughout treatment.
- Verbalize/demonstrate an understanding of measures to prevent treatment-induced side effects.

INTERVENTIONS

- Monitor patient's weight.
- Refer to nutritionist if ongoing pattern of weight loss or history of eating disorder, obesity, or diabetes.
- Record intake and output every shift.
- Record calorie counts.
- Administer antiemetics for nausea, and assess effectiveness.
- Assess for diarrhea and constipation, and medicate as needed.
- Perform daily assessment of lips and oral mucosa for mucositis.
- Teach patient the purpose of oral care protocol and evaluate technique.
- Evaluate and document compliance to oral care protocol.
- Use topical analgesics in mouth and on lips if open ulcers are present.
- Encourage small, frequent meals with high-calorie, high-protein foods.
- Encourage intake of culturally preferred foods from home if unable to obtain at hospital.

DISEASE-RELATED COMPLICATIONS
Leukostasis

Patients with exceptionally high circulating blast counts are at risk to develop leukostasis. This syndrome is caused by leukemic blasts aggregating and invading capillary walls, causing rupture and bleeding. This occurs most often in the brain because of its vascularity and limited space. Intrapulmonary bleeding can also result from this "sludging syndrome." These complications are associated with significant morbidity and mortality, and this medical emergency necessitates immediate reduction of the circulating leukocytes. High doses of hydroxyurea or high-dose chemotherapy may be instituted, or leukapheresis with a filtered, continuous-flow cell separator may help reduce the cell burden. Once the danger of leukostasis is eliminated, definitive antileukemia therapy is initiated.

INTERVENTIONS

- Monitor for changes in level of consciousness; perform neurologic examinations as ordered.
- Monitor respiratory status.
- Administer high-dose chemotherapy as ordered.
- Monitor leukapheresis process.
- Monitor absolute blast counts after interventions using the following equation:

$$\text{Absolute blast count} = \frac{\text{Total WBC count} \times \text{Blasts}}{100}$$

Disseminated Intravascular Coagulation

Diffuse or disseminated intravascular coagulation (DIC) is a complex syndrome characterized by the activation of coagulation and formation of fibrin within the general circulation (see Chapter 19). Patients with acute promyelocytic leukemia (APL, FAB type M_3) are at high risk of developing DIC after the initiation of chemotherapy as the granules from the promyelocytes are released and initiate the coagulation cascade.

INTERVENTIONS

- Ensure systematic assessment for occult, overt, or sudden massive bleeding.
- Begin therapy with ATRA according to protocol for M_3 (APL).
- Initiate antileukemia therapy to correct the underlying disease pathology.
- Administer antibiotics for sepsis.
- Administer blood products (platelets, fresh-frozen plasma) as ordered.
- Apply pressure to venipuncture sites.
- Administer heparin if ordered.

Treatment for DIC must focus on eliminating the underlying cause and instituting supportive therapy with the appropriate blood products.

Typhlitis

Typhlitis, or inflammation of the cecum, is thought to be related to *Clostridia* sepsis or other bacteria, including *Pseudomonas, Escherichia coli,* or *Klebsiella*. This diagnosis should be considered in the neutropenic patient who develops severe abdominal pain. Bloody diarrhea, absence of bowel sounds, rebound tenderness, and fever may accompany the pain. An abdominal x-ray film may reveal a right lower quadrant soft tissue mass, dilated colon, or pericecal edema. The pathologic diagnosis is established by stool culture, and the identified pathogen is treated with appropriate antibiotics.

INTERVENTIONS

- Put patient on bedrest.
- Maintain intravenous fluids.
- Assess fluid and electrolyte balance.
- Ensure patient has no oral intake.
- Administer and evaluate analgesics.

Renal Failure

Renal failure in leukemia patients may result from urate nephropathy, aminoglycoside toxicity, sepsis, or leukemic infiltration of the kidneys.

INTERVENTIONS

- Hydration and urine alkalinization are used with certain regimens (e.g., high-dose methotrexate).
- Monitor BUN and creatinine values.
- Record accurate intake and output.
- Monitor vital signs and mental status.
- Assess for signs of alteration in tissue perfusion.

PATIENT AND FAMILY TEACHING

As with other types of cancer care, the teaching of leukemic patients should begin at the time of diagnosis and

---

GERIATRIC CONSIDERATIONS
Leukemia

Perform cardiovascular evaluation, including radionucleotide ventriculogram to assess left ventricular ejection fraction.

Monitor for signs and symptoms of fluid overload.

Maintain a safe environment: bed rails, call light within reach, assistance with ambulation.

Assess potential barriers to learning: decreased visual acuity, poor hearing, decreased concentration.

Assess previous bowel routines.

Assess over-the-counter drug use.

Assess visual and auditory status before treatment.

PATIENT TEACHING PRIORITIES
Leukemia

Normal hematopoiesis, purpose of red blood cells, white blood cells, and platelets

Pathophysiology of leukemia

Goals of planned treatment

Treatment schedule and method of administration

Expected side effects and related interventions

Plan for symptom management

Neutropenia and bleeding precautions

Plan for patient/family participation in treatment and shared decision making

---

Continued.

Table 13-6   Patient/Family Teaching Topics Regarding Leukemia

Topic	Pretreatment phase	Treatment phase	Outpatient/follow-up care
DISEASE DESCRIPTION	X	X	
Disease-related symptoms	X	X	
Potential disease-related complications	X	X	
TREATMENT DESCRIPTION	X	X	
Goals of treatment	X	X	
Duration of treatment	X	X	
Treatment schedule	X	X	
Chemotherapeutic agents	X	X	
TREATMENT-RELATED SIDE EFFECTS	X	X	
Immunosuppression	X	X	
Thrombocytopenia	X	X	
Nausea and vomiting	X	X	
Stomatitis	X	X	
Alopecia	X	X	
Fatigue	X	X	
Anorexia	X	X	
MULTIPLE-LUMEN TUNNELED CATHETER	X	X	
Surgical procedure	X	X	
Catheter care	X	X	
SUPPORTIVE CARE		X	
Infection precautions		X	
Bleeding precautions		X	
Red blood cell transfusions		X	
Platelet transfusions		X	
Antibiotics		X	
DISEASE-RELATED COMPLICATIONS AND TREATMENT		X	
Sepsis		X	
Disseminated intravascular coagulation		X	
Tumor lysis syndrome		X	
SELF-CARE		X	
Oral care		X	
Nutrition		X	
Care of tunneled catheter		X	
Bowel/skin care		X	
DETERMINATION OF RESPONSE		X	
Meaning of remission		X	
Continuation therapy		X	
Possible preparation for discharge		X	
PSYCHOSOCIAL ADJUSTMENT	X	X	X
Coping strategies	X	X	X
Referral to social services, psychologist/psychiatrist	X	X	X
Identification of community resources (family support groups, Leukemia Society of America, American Cancer Society)	X	X	X
Schedule for laboratory work			X
Schedule for office visits			X
Outpatient medications			X
Diet			X
Exercise			X
Return to work			X
Sexuality	X		X
Long-term side effects of treatment			X
Surveillance bone marrow biopsies			X

continue throughout the disease course. In acute leukemia, teaching is required in both the inpatient setting during the induction phase and intensive supportive care period and in the outpatient setting during continuation therapy and long-term follow-up.

A leukemia diagnosis may be a shock to patients experiencing few if any symptoms at the time of diagnosis. Some patients experiencing an acute illness or a lengthy period of medical evaluation before the discovery of the diagnosis may feel a sense of relief to know finally a definitive diagnosis. Certainly the diagnosis of any potentially fatal disease is a time of crisis for the entire family.

Table 13-6 lists teaching topics in the pretreatment period, treatment period, and follow-up period. The boxes, p. 305, list geriatric considerations and patient teaching priorities.

To provide effective care, the nurse must always be sensitive to the patient's feelings of isolation and loss of control. The patient may display the need to regain control, especially during lengthy hospitalizations. Addressing this need for control early in the hospitalization is important. Control issues can be divided into three areas as follows:

Patient controlled	No control	Nurse controlled
Antibiotic skin care regimen	Disease process	Scheduled medications
Time to bathe	Administration of blood products	Vital signs
Time for dressing change	X-ray films	Mealtimes
Oral care	Laboratory work	Weights
Dietary choices		
Analgesia		
Visiting times		

The main point to remember is that many aspects of nursing care can be flexible, and items such as when the patient will bathe can be negotiated.

Future clinical trials will continue to build on the results of current studies of MDS therapy.

CONCLUSION

Great progress has been made in the knowledge of the biologic nature and treatment of leukemia during the past decade. Advances in supportive care of the immunosuppressed patient have dramatically improved survival in leukemia patients. Much research is still required to define more effective therapies to increase disease-free survival and decrease relapse rates.

The challenges and opportunities for nurses are numerous in the field of leukemia. The acuity level of patient care for those with leukemia depends on the disease variables and practice setting. Hospital-based nurses provide care for the leukemic patient who is acutely ill. The intensity and complexity of the nursing care required for many of these patients rival those of intensive care units. Other patients with leukemia, such as those in chronic phase CML, early CLL, AML, or ALL in remission or those receiving milder continuation therapy, are seen in the clinic or outpatient setting.

Another practice setting is the BMT unit, where intensive acute care and ambulatory care are required. Historically, most leukemia patients were transferred to major metropolitan centers for treatment. In recent years, however, with improved mechanisms to transfer medical technology into the community, more patients are cared for locally.

The National Cancer Institute's Cooperative Group Outreach Program (CGOP) and, since 1983, the Community Clinical Oncology Program (CCOP) provide the opportunity to enroll leukemia patients in cooperative group clinical trials. The number of institutions performing BMT has also increased dramatically and will continue to increase over the next decades as BMT becomes a promising treatment option for many types of cancer.

The nurse in clinical practice may easily feel overwhelmed by the complexity and intensity of both learning about the disease of leukemia and providing care to the patient with leukemia. A useful strategy for learning this information and integrating it into one's nursing practice is to focus on one type of leukemia at a time. The nurse should select a patient newly diagnosed with leukemia and review the individual patient's presenting symptoms, results of the diagnostic evaluation, prognostic indicators, and treatment plan. The nurse should monitor this treatment plan, the selected drug regimen, blood counts, marrow results, and the potential side effects experienced by the patient as a result of the disease or treatment. These concepts should be incorporated into an individualized nursing plan of care. Depending on the practice setting, the nurse may want to collaborate with another inpatient or outpatient nursing colleague to follow the patient's progress. After completing this exercise a few times, the nurse will gain confidence in the knowledge of the leukemias and their treatment and thereby improve clinical practice expertise in caring for patients with leukemia.

The intensity and complexity of caring for leukemic patients are both rewarding and frustrating. Providing direct care to an acutely ill patient in a life-threatening situation fosters very close relationships with both the patient and the members of his or her support system. These relationships can be intensely rewarding. At the same time the intensity of care can lead to frustration and exhaustion when the patient does not respond to therapy or dies. Sudden and unexpected medical crisis and death do occur in this population of patients. Nurses caring for patients with leukemia must be cognizant of their own feelings and needs. The most valuable support system oncology nurses have is the support and understanding of their peers. These are the people who experience the same joys, fears, pain, and frustration of caring for the acutely ill patient. The oncology unit psychologist or psychiatrist is available not only to the patient and family, but also to the nursing staff. The most important self-care aspect of the nurse caring for the patient with leukemia is recognizing the level of investment and acknowledging the emotional peaks and valleys that accompany this investment.

■ CHAPTER QUESTIONS

1. Which of the following acute myelogenous leukemias (AMLs) is treated with all-*trans*-retinoic acid (ATRA, tretinoin)?
   a. M_1
   b. M_2
   c. M_3
   d. M_4
2. Patients with an infection may have masked symptoms because of which of the following?
   a. Antiinflammatory effect of corticosteroids
   b. Inability to produce purulent drainage
   c. Body's inability to activate the inflammatory response
   d. All the above
3. All the following tests are used to determine the classification and prognosis of acute leukemia *except:*
   a. Morphology
   b. Cytogenetics
   c. Immunophenotyping
   d. Human lymphocyte antigen (HLA) typing
4. Multidrug resistance is attributed to:
   a. Translocation of the chromosomes
   b. Changes in the cell membrane
   c. All-*trans*-retinoic acid absorption
   d. P-glycoproteins in the leukemia cell
5. Which of the following is *not* associated with chronic myleocytic leukemia (CML)?
   a. Presence of the Philadelphia chromosome
   b. Massive splenomegaly
   c. High incidence of central nervous system (CNS) involvement
   d. Only cured by bone marrow transplantation
6. Treatment in hairy-cell leukemia becomes necessary when:
   a. Bone marrow becomes fibrotic.
   b. Cytochemical staining demonstrates the presence of tartrate-resistant acid phosphatase.

   c. Cytopenia becomes symptomatic.
   d. Patient presents with splenomegaly.
7. In myelodysplastic syndrome (MDS), which of the following can transform nonfunctional immature blasts and promyeloblasts into functional mature granulocytes?
   a. Chemotherapy
   b. Differentiating agents
   c. Steroids
   d. Colony-stimulating factors
8. Which of the following life-spans is *incorrect?*
   a. Red blood cells, 120 days
   b. Granulocytes, 6 to 8 hours
   c. Platelets, 8 to 10 hours
9. All the following are true regarding acute lymphocytic leukemia (ALL) *except:*
   a. Adults are diagnosed more frequently with ALL than AML.
   b. 20% of all leukemias diagnosed are ALL.
   c. Lymphoblasts comprise greater than 30% of the bone marrow.
   d. CNS involvement occurs in less than 10% of patients.
10. Which of the following is *false* regarding bone marrow transplant (BMT)?
    a. Timing of BMT is controversial.
    b. Autologous or peripheral blood stem cell transplants may be indicated if there is no matched sibling.
    c. Patients with poor prognostic indicators at diagnosis are not good candidates for BMT when in remission.
    d. Patients with chronic myelogenous leukemia (CML) have the greatest chance of disease-free survival if receiving BMT during the chronic phase of their illness.

BIBLIOGRAPHY

1. Alkire K, Collingwood J: Physiology of blood and bone marrow, *Semin Oncol Nurs* 6:99, 1990.
2. American Cancer Society: *Cancer facts and figures—1996,* Atlanta, 1996, The Society.
3. Applebaum FR, Downing J, William C: The biology and therapy of AML. In *Hematology 1995,* American Society of Hematology.
4. Barrett AJ and others: Bone marrow transplantation for Philadelphia chromosome–positive acute lymphoblastic leukemia, *Blood* 70:3067, 1992.
5. Bergsagel DE, Bailey MB, Langley GR: The chemotherapy of plasma-cell myeloma and the incidence of acute leukemia, *N Engl J Med* 301:743, 1979.
6. Bishop JF and others: Etoposide in acute nonlymphocytic leukemia, *Blood* 75:27, 1990.
7. Bouroncle BA: Leukemic reticuloendotheliosis, *Blood* 53:412, 1979.
8. Brownson RC, Novotny TE, Perry MC: Cigarette smoking and adult leukemia: a meta-analysis, *Arch Intern Med* 153:469, 1993.
9. Buchner T: Management of acute myeloid leukemia in the elderly, *Cancer Control,* March/April 1995.
10. Buchner T and others: Intensified induction and consolidation with or without maintenance chemotherapy for AML: two multicenter studies of the German AML Cooperative Group, *J Clin Oncol* 3:1583, 1985.

11. Caguioa PB, Tansan S, McCaffrey RP: Chronic lymphocytic leukemia, *Am J Med Sci* 308:196, 1994.

12. Cain J and others: Myelodysplastic syndromes: a review for nurses, *Oncol Nurs Forum* 18(1):113, 1991.

13. Cassileth PA and others: Maintenance chemotherapy protocols remission duration in adult acute nonlymphocytic leukemia, *J Clin Oncol* 6:583, 1988.

14. Cassileth PA and others: Pentostatin induces durable remissions in HCL, *J Clin Oncol* 9:243, 1991.

15. Cassileth PA and others: Varying intensities of postremission therapy in acute myeloid leukemia, *Blood* 79:1924, 1992.

16. Champlain R and others: Postremission chemotherapy for adults with acute myelogenous leukemia: improved survival with high-dose cytarabine and daunorubicin consolidation treatment, *J Clin Oncol* 8:1199, 1990.

17. Cheson BD: The myelodysplastic syndromes: current approaches to therapy, *Ann Intern Med* 112:932, 1990.

18. Conley CL, Misiti J, Laster AJ: Genetic factors predisposing to chronic lymphocytic leukemia and to autoimmune disease, *Medicine* 5:323, 1980.

19. Conrad KJ: Cerebellar toxicities associated with cytosine arabinoside: a nursing perspective, *Oncol Nurs Forum* 3:57, 1986.

20. Copelan EA, McGuire EA: The biology and treatment of acute lymphoblastic leukemia in adults, *Blood* 85:1151, 1995.

21. Cortes JE, Kantarjian H: Acute lymphocytic leukemia. In Pazdur R, editor: *Medical oncology: a comprehensive review,* ed 2, New York, 1996, Huntington.

22. Cortes JE, Talpaz M, Kantarjian H: Chronic myelogenous leukemia. In Pazdur R, editor: *Medical oncology: a comprehensive review,* ed 2, New York, 1996, Huntington.

23. Dang CV: Myelodysplastic syndrome, *JAMA* 267(15):2077, 1992.

24. Degos L and others: All-*trans*-retinoic acid as a differentiating agent in the treatment of acute promyelocytic leukemia, *Blood* 85:2643, 1995.

25. DeGramont A and others: Preleukemic changes in cases of non-lymphocytic leukemia secondary to cytotoxic therapy: analysis of 105 cases, *Cancer* 58:630, 1986.

26. Devine SM, Larson RA: Acute leukemia in adults: recent developments in diagnosis and treatment, *CA Cancer J Clin* 44:326, 1994.

27. DiJulio J: Hematopoiesis: an overview, *Oncol Nurs Forum* 18(suppl):3, 1991.

28. Douglas IDC, Wiltshaw E: Remission induction in chronic granulocytic leukemia using intermittent high dose busulfan, *Br J Haematol* 40:59, 1978.

29. Dutcher JP, Schiffer CA, Wiernik PH: Hyperleukocytosis in adult nonlymphocytic leukemia: impact on remission rate, duration, and survival, *J Clin Oncol* 5:1364, 1987.

30. Dutcher JP and others: Intensive maintenance therapy improves survival in adult nonlymphocytic leukemia: an eight-year follow-up, *Leukemia* 2:413, 1988.

31. Einhorn N: Acute leukemia after chemotherapy (Melphalan), *Cancer* 41:444, 1978.

32. Estey EH: Treatment of acute myelogenous leukemia and myelodysplastic leukemia and myelodysplastic syndromes, *Semin Hematol* 32:132, 1995.

33. Estey EH and others: Treatment of hairy cell leukemia with 2-chlorodeoxyadenosine (2-CdA), *Blood* 79:882, 1992.

34. Fayad L, O'Brien S: Chronic lymphocytic leukemia and associated disorders. In Pazdur R, editor: *Medical oncology: a comprehensive review,* ed 2, New York, 1996, Huntington.

35. Feldman EJ: Acute meylogenous leukemia in the older patient, *Semin Oncol* 22(supp 1):21, 1995.

36. Fenaux P and others: Cytogenetics and their prognostic value in childhood and adult acute leukemia, *Hematol Oncol* 7:307, 1989.

37. Fialkow PJ and others: Evidence for a multistep pathogenesis of chronic myelogenous leukemia, *Blood* 58:158, 1981.

38. Foon FA, Todd RF: Immunologic classification of leukemia and lymphoma, *Blood* 68:1, 1986.

39. Foon KA, Gale RP: Biology of chronic lymphocytic leukemia, *Semin Hematol* 24(4):209, 1987.

40. Foon KA, Gale RP: Staging and therapy of chronic lymphocytic leukemia, *Semin Hematol* 24(4):264, 1987.

41. Fraser MC, Tucker MA: Second malignancies following cancer therapy, *Semin Oncol Nurs* 5:43, 1989.

42. French Cooperative Group on Chronic Lymphocytic Leukemia: Effectiveness of "CHOP" regimen in advanced untreated chronic lymphocytic leukemia, *Lancet* 1:1346, 1986.

43. Gale RP, Foon KA: Acute myelogenous leukemia. In Gale RP, editor: *Acute leukemia,* Boston, 1986, Blackwell.

44. Ghaddar HM, Estey EH: Acute myeloenous leukemia. In Pazdur R, editor: *Medical oncology: a comprehensive review,* ed 2, New York, 1996, Huntington.

45. Giona F and others: Adult acute lymphoblastic leukemia: description and analysis of long-term survivors, a retrospective study, *Haematologica* 74:475, 1989.

46. Golomb HM, Ellis E: Treatment options for hairy cell leukemia, *Semin Oncol* 18(suppl 7), 1991.

47. Goodman M: Managing the side effects of chemotherapy, *Semin Oncol Nurs* 5(suppl):29, 1989.

48. Green MH and others: Evidence of a treatment dose response in non-lymphocytic leukemia which occur after therapy of non-Hodgkin's lymphoma, *Cancer Res* 43:1891, 1983.

49. Greenberg P and others: Phase III randomized multicenter trial of G-CSF vs. observation for MDS, *Blood* 82(suppl 1):196a, 1993.

50. Greenberg P and others: Myelodysplastic syndromes and myeloproliferative disorders: clinical, therapeutic and molecular advances. In *Hematology 1995,* American Society of Hematology.

51. Griffin JD: Management of chronic myelogenous leukemia, *Semin Hematol* 23(suppl):20, 1986.

52. Grignani F and others: Acute promyelocytic leukemia: from genetics to treatment, *Blood* 83:10, 1994.

53. Gulati GL, Ashton JK, Hyun BH: Structure and function of the bone marrow and hematopoiesis, *Hematol Oncol Clin North Am* 2(4):495, 1988.

54. Gunz FW: Leukemia in the past. In Gunz FW, editor: *Leukemia,* Orlando, Fla, 1983, Grune & Stratton.

55. Heath CW: Epidemiology and heredity aspects of acute leukemia. In Wiernik P, editor: *Neoplastic diseases of the blood,* New York, 1985, Churchill Livingstone.

56. Heath, CW: Electromagnetic field exposure and cancer: a review of epidemiologic evidence, *CA Cancer J Clin* 46:29, 1996.

57. Hernandez JA, Land KJ, McKenna RW: Leukemias, myeloma, and other lymphoreticular neoplasms, *Cancer Suppl* 75:381, 1995.

58. Hiddeman W and others: Cytogenetic subgroups of AML and outcome from high dose versus conventional dose ARA-C as part of double induction therapy, *Blood* 86(suppl 1), abstract 1054, 1995.

59. Hoelzer DF: Therapy of the newly diagnosed adult with acute lymphoblastic leukemia, *Hematol Oncol Clin North Am* 7:139, 1993.

60. Hoezler D, Gale RP: Acute lymphoblastic leukemia in adults: recent progress, future directions, *Semin Hematol* 24(1):27, 1987.

61. Hoelzer D and others: The German Multicenter Trials for treatment of acute lymphoblastic leukemia in adults, *Leukemia* 6(suppl 2):175, 1992.

62. Italian Cooperative Study Group on Chronic Myeloid Leukemia: Interferon alpha-2a as compared with conventional chemotherapy for the treatment of chronic myeloid leukemia, *N Engl J Med* 330:820, 1994.

63. Jaiyesimi IA, Kantarjian HM, Estey EH: Advances in therapy for hairy cell leukemia, *Cancer* 72:5, 1993.

64. Johnson BL: Leukemias. In Groenwald SL, editor: *Cancer nursing: practice and principles,* Boston, 1987, Jones & Bartlett.

65. Kantarjian HM: Adult acute lymphocytic leukemia: critical review of current knowledge, *Am J Med* 97:176, 1994.

66. Kantarjian HM, Schachner J, Keating MJ: Fludarabine therapy in hairy cell leukemia, *Cancer* 67:1291, 1991.

67. Kantarjian HM and others: CML: a concise update, *Blood* 82:691 1993.

68. Kantarjian HM and others: Interferon alpha and low-dose cytosine arabinoside therapy in Philadelphia-positive CML, *Blood* 86(suppl 1), abstract 2105, 1995.

69. Karanas A, Silver RT: Characteristics of the terminal phase of chronic granulocytic leukemia, *Blood* 32:445, 1968.

70. Keating MJ, Estey E, Kantarjian H: Acute leukemia. In Devita VT Jr, Hellman S, Rosenberg SA, editors: *Cancer: principles and practice of oncology,* ed 4, Philadelphia, 1993, Lippincott.

71. Levenson JA, Lesko LM: Psychiatric aspects of adult leukemia, *Semin Oncol Nurs* 6:76, 1990.

72. Lill MC, Golde DW: Treatment of hairy cell leukemia, *Blood Rev* 4:238, 1990.

73. Linos A and others: Low-dose radiation and leukemia, *N Engl J Med* 202:1101, 1980.

74. List AF and others: The myelodysplastic syndromes: biology and implications for management, *J Clin Oncol* 8:1424, 1990.

75. List AF and others: Phase I/II trial of cyclosporin as a chemotherapy-resistance modifier in acute leukemia, *J Clin Oncol* 11:1652, 1993.

76. MacDonald JS and others: Subacute and chronic toxicities associated with nitrosurea therapy. In Prestayko AW and others, editors: *Nitrosureas: current status and new developments,* New York, 1981, Academic.

77. Mayer RJ and others: Intensive postremission chemotherapy in adults with acute myelogenous leukemia, *N Engl J Med* 331:896, 1994.

78. McGlave P and others: Therapy of chronic myelogenous leukemia with allogeneic bone marrow transplantation, *J Clin Oncol* 5:1033, 1987.

79. Mitus AJ, Rosenthal DS: The adult leukemias. In Murphy GP, Lawrence W Jr, Lenhard RE Jr, editors: *American Cancer Society textbook of clinical oncology,* ed 2, Atlanta, 1995, American Cancer Society.

80. Nowell PC, Hungerford DA: A minute chromosome in human granulocytic leukemia, *Science* 132:1497, 1960.

81. Ong ST, Larson RA: Current management of acute lymphoblastic leukemia in adults, *Oncology* 9:433, 1995.

82. Papa G and others: Acute leukemia in patients treated for Hodgkin's disease, *Br J Haematol* 309:1079, 1984.

83. Pape LH: Therapy-related acute leukemia, *Cancer Nurs* 11(5):295, 1988.

84. Piro LD, Douglas JE, Saven A: The Scripps Clinic experience with 2-chlorodeoxyadenosine in the treatment of hairy cell leukemia, *Leuk Lymphoma* 13(suppl 1):121, 1994.

85. Poplack DG and others: Leukemias and lymphomas of childhood. In Devita VT Jr, Hellman S, Rosenberg SA, editors: *Cancer principles and practice,* ed 4, Philadelphia, 1993, Lippincott.

86. Portugal MA and others: Acute leukemia as a complication of advanced breast cancer, *Cancer Treat Rep* 63:177, 1979.

87. Preisler H and others: Comparison of three remission induction regimens and two postinduction strategies for the treatment of acute nonlymphocytic leukemia: a Cancer and Leukemia Group B study, *Blood* 69:1441, 1987.

88. Preti A, Kantarjian HM: Management of adult acute lymphocyte leukemia: present issues and key challenges, *J Clin Oncol* 12:1312, 1994.

89. Preti A and others: Philadelphia-chromosome-positive adult acute lymphocytic leukemia: characteristics, treatment results and prognosis in 41 patients, *Am J Med* 97:60, 1994.

90. Pui C: Childhood leukemias, *N Engl J Med* 332:1618, 1995.

91. Rai KR, Montserrat E: Prognostic factors in chronic lymphocytic leukemia, *Semin Hematol* 24(4):252, 1987.

92. Rinsky RA and others: Benzene and leukemia, *N Engl J Med* 316:1044, 1987.

93. Rozman C, Montserrat E: Chronic lymphocytic leukemia, *N Engl J Med* 333:1052, 1995.

94. Sanders JE: Bone marrow transplantation for pediatric leukemia, *Pediatr Annu* 20:671, 1991.

95. Sandler DP and others: Cigarette smoking and risk of acute leukemia: associations with morphology and cytogenetic abnormalities in bone marrow, *J Natl Cancer Inst* 85:1994, 1993.

96. Saven A, Piro LD: Treatment of hairy cell leukemia, *Blood* 79:1111, 1992.

97. Saven A, Piro L: Newer purine analogues for the treatment of hairy cell leukemia, *N Engl J Med* 330:691, 1994.

98. Schiffer CA: Interferon studies in the treatment of patients with leukemia, *Semin Oncol* 18(suppl 7):1, 1991.

99. Silver RT: Chronic myeloid leukemia: a perspective of the clinical and biologic issues of the chronic phase, *Hematol Oncol Clin North Am* 4:319, 1990.

100. Smith JW and others: Prolonged continuous treatment of hairy cell leukemia patients with recombinant interferon-alpha 2a, *Blood* 78:1664, 1991.

101. Smith RE: Leukemia. In Thorup OA, editor: *Fundamentals of clinical hematology,* Philadelphia, 1987, Saunders.

102. Sokal JE and others: Staging and prognosis in chronic myelogenous leukemia, *Semin Hematol* 25(1):49, 1988.

103. Stuart RK: Autologous bone marrow transplantation for leukemia, *Semin Oncol* 20:40, 1993.

104. Tallman MS and others: Phase III randomized study of all-*trans* retinoic acid (ATRA) vs daunorubicin (D) and cytosine arabinoside (A) as induction therapy and ATRA vs observation vs maintenance therapy for patients with previously untreated APL, *Blood* 86(suppl 1), abstract 488, 1995.

105. Talpaz M: Clinical studies of alpha-interferons in chronic myelogenous leukemia, *Cancer Treat Rev* 15(suppl A):49, 1988.

106. Talpaz M and others: Therapy of chronic myelogenous leukemia: chemotherapy and interferons, *Semin Hematol* 25(1):62, 1988.

107. Thomas ED: Marrow transplantation for chronic myelogenous leukemia. In Gale RP, Champlin R, editors: *Bone marrow transplantation: current controversies,* San Diego, 1988, Academic.

108. Toronto Leukemia Study Group: Survival in acute myeloblastic leukemia is not prolonged by remission maintenance or early reinduction chemotherapy, *Leuk Res* 12(3):195, 1988.

109. Waldman AR: High-dose post remission therapy. In Wujcik D, editor: *Nursing care issues in adult acute leukemia,* New York, 1995, Huntington.

110. Warrell RP and others: Acute promyelocytic leukemia, *N Engl J Med* 329:177, 1993.

111. Westbrook CA, Golomb HM: Hairy cell leukemia, *Curr Concepts Oncol,* Winter 1984.

112. Winston DJ and others: Prevention and treatment of infection in leukemia patients. In Gale RP, editor: *Leukemia therapy,* Boston, 1986, Blackwell.

113. Wujcik D: Options for postremission therapy in acute leukemia, *Semin Oncol Nurs* 6:25, 1990.

CHAPTER 14
Lung Cancers

JUDITH A. SHELL
KATHLEEN R. BULSON
LINDA F. VANDERLUGT

Lung cancer is the leading cause of cancer-related deaths in men 35 years of age and older and in women 55 to 74 years of age.[92] Although lung cancer mortality continues to rise among American men, the incidence of lung cancer among males has leveled off or slightly declined for the first time.[85] Despite research and public education efforts, however, lung cancer incidence and mortality continue to rise among American women.

Most patients present with metastatic disease, which ultimately leads to death. Clinical trials using multimodality therapies or new agents are attempting to reverse this trend. In the meantime, smoking prevention remains the key to reducing lung cancer deaths and is a major focus for nursing intervention. Patients with lung cancer must learn to deal not only with the physiologic and economic effects of cancer and its treatment, but also with fears about the disease, its treatment, and dying.

EPIDEMIOLOGY

An estimated 177,000 new cases of lung cancer were reported and 158,700 deaths occurred in the United States in 1996. More men than women develop lung cancer, but the gap is narrowing. Lung cancer mortality among women has skyrocketed more than 400% during the past 30 years.[2]

In 1987 lung cancer surpassed breast cancer as the leading cause of cancer deaths in women.[77] Although not the most common cancer in either gender, lung cancer continued to be the leading cause of cancer death for both men (32%) and women (25%) in 1996.[92]

The authors would like to express their appreciation to Cindy Wadlow for her assistance with this chapter.

ETIOLOGY AND RISK FACTORS
Smoking

Death from lung cancer was relatively rare until this century. In 1912 Adler found only 374 cases of lung cancer described in world literature and questioned the value of writing about such an insignificant problem.[102] Little did he expect the abrupt increase in deaths related to lung cancer beginning around 1935 (4300 deaths) and continuing until now (158,700 deaths estimated in 1996).[2] The increased incidence in men in the 1930s and in women in the 1960s followed the pattern of increased acceptance of smoking behavior, first in men and then in women. A prospective study by Hammond[48] in 1954 first demonstrated the relationship between smoking and the risk of developing lung cancer. Observers note that lung cancer mortality rates in people who have smoked two packs per day for 10 years (20 pack-years) are 15 to 25 times higher than in nonsmokers.[88,119] It is estimated that 85% of lung cancer deaths are related to smoking.[12,77] The latency period between initiation of smoking and the development of lung cancer is about 15 to 20 years.

Air Pollution

Air pollutants have been incriminated in the etiology of lung cancer (e.g., sulfur dioxide). Nevertheless, although high rates of lung cancer occur in Los Angeles, where high levels of air pollution are a problem, no definite correlation to lung cancer incidence has been proved.[12,91]

Race and Socioeconomics

Among black males of all ages in the United States, incidence of lung cancer has decreased since 1980 and this may be associated with a corresponding drop in mortality rates.[11] Smoking prevalence among blacks is also on the decline (from 41% in the mid-1970s to 34% in the late 1980s to 26.5% in 1992).[92] Nevertheless, cancer mortality is higher among nonwhites than whites and may be related to the increased smoking and use of non-filter cigarettes by blacks.[91] Socioeconomic factors (e.g., workplace conditions, poor nutrition) might contribute to this difference, but this is only speculation. Unconfirmed studies suggest, however, that there is an increased risk of squamous cell and small cell lung cancers in men with diets low in vitamin A.[91]

Geography

Geographic clustering of lung cancer among males has been noted along the Gulf of Mexico and the southeastern Atlantic coast.[71] Whether this is related to industrial asbestos exposure from industries such as shipbuilding is not known. Mortality rates are lowest in farming areas and lower in rural versus urban counties.[113]

Industry

Industrial exposure to the following agents is believed to place persons at greater risk of lung cancer: mustard gas, radon, asbestos, radioisotopes, polycyclic aromatic hydrocarbons (present in crude petroleum, coal, tars, combustion products of most organic materials), nickel, chromium, haloethers, iron ore, inorganic arsenic, wood dust, and isopropyl oil.[12,91] Certain occupational groups at risk because of potential exposure to the above agents have been identified (see box below).

Family and Health History

The risk of lung cancer is increased in persons with a prior history of lung disease or a family history of lung cancer.[130] Recent research supports the theory that lung cancer risk is an inherited trait. A specific gene that predisposes to early-age onset of lung cancer may account for as many as 47% of cases by age 60.[108] In a recent analysis of 337 lung cancer families, a mendelian codominant inheritance that predisposed those exposed

---

OCCUPATIONAL GROUPS AT RISK FOR LUNG CANCER

Asbestos workers	Insecticide workers
Atomic energy workers	Insulation workers
Automobile maintenance	Metal material workers
Chemical workers	Nickel workers
Chloromethyl ethyl workers	Petroleum workers
	Shipyard workers
Copper smelter workers	Spray painters
Foundry workers	Steel workers
Gas workers	Uranium miners
Glass, pottery, linoleum workers	

Modified from Oleske DM: *Semin Oncol Nurs* 3:3, 1987.

---

to smoking to the development of lung cancer was the best explanation of the data.[109] If this genetic predisposition proves true, it could mean that lung cancers occur uniquely among gene carriers and would help explain why all smokers do not develop lung cancer. This would have a major impact on approaches to lung cancer prevention, screening, and early detection.

PREVENTION, SCREENING, AND DETECTION
Primary Prevention

Smoking. Of the 554,680 estimated cancer deaths in 1996, about 158,000 (29% of all cancer deaths) were caused by lung cancer. The majority (at least 85%) of lung cancer deaths are smoking related and thus preventable. As many as one third of heavy smokers (25 cigarettes/day or more) who are 35 years old will experience premature death from a smoking-related disease.[87]

Primary lung cancer prevention focuses on decreasing the number of new smokers and helping present smokers to quit. It may involve decreasing the hazards of smoking through use of low-tar and filtered cigarettes for those who continue to smoke. The risk of developing and dying from lung cancer correlates directly with the number of cigarettes smoked, and lung cancer incidence can be reduced by as much as 20% by use of low-tar and filter cigarettes, assuming no increase in number of cigarettes smoked.[91]

Studies show that the spouse of a smoker can be at increased risk of developing lung cancer, since the National Research Council reports that as many as 6000 people die annually from passive cigarette smoke.[44] Side-stream smoke contains as many, if not more, carcinogens than inhaled smoke. Many worksites where extensive smoking occurs (e.g., bars, restaurants) may also place people at risk. In a population-based case-control study of cancer risk secondary to passive smoking, the only individuals found to be at increased risk (twice the risk of an unexposed nonsmoker) were those exposed during childhood and/or adolescence to the secondary smoke of more than one smoker in the home.[60,97]

Although smokers are encouraged to stop smoking, a smoker's risk of developing lung cancer may never equal that of one who has never smoked, perhaps because of the prolonged lag time in the development of lung cancer. One study found no benefit from smoking cessation at 10 years,[90] whereas others found lung cancer risk dropping to 5.9 times by 10 years. Smokers who quit for at least 15 years may still have twice the risk of developing lung cancer as those who never smoked.[119] It may take 20 years before the risks are similar.

Smoking cessation and public education. The overall prevalence of smoking among high-school seniors has decreased from 27% when programs were instituted in the 1970s but has now leveled off at about

18% of students. By age 18, 75% of smokers have tried their first cigarette and 50% are regular smokers.[86] The trend toward recruitment of smokers in adolescence, especially among teenage girls, needs to be broken. Programs found most successful in preventing initiation of smoking among youth are school based, using peer leaders and role playing.[98] Because more than half of female smokers begin smoking before age 13, prevention efforts must be aimed at the junior-high age-group or younger.

Among adults, many avenues are available to encourage smoking cessation, but 95% of smokers who quit do not seek outside help, preferring methods that can be done on their own.[98] Nurses need to set an example in smoking cessation; their rate (23.6%) exceeds that of the general female population (21.5%).[98] Factors that distinguish those smokers who quit from those who do not include a strong motivation to quit, use of behavioral techniques, and good social support to quit. Physician advice, even if minimal, fosters quitting, particularly when the patient is experiencing increased symptoms or a new smoking-related illness, such as emphysema. (For an excellent review of smoking cessation methods, see Risser[98] and National Cancer Institute.[87])

Radon. Identification of risk groups helps to establish safety guidelines. Much media coverage has been given to the risk of lung cancer resulting from radon or asbestos exposure. Radon has been implicated as a significant cause of lung cancer.[23,126] However, even in uranium miners with high cumulative radon exposure, most lung cancers can be attributed to synergism between radon and cigarette smoking.[24,105,128] Extrapolating risks from high-level, industrial radon exposure (uranium mining) to low-level, nonindustrial exposure (home, worksite) is met with conflicting opinions. A recent review of published studies found inconsistencies in results and methodology, leaving the correlation between residential radon exposure and lung cancer weak at best.[89] There is some agreement, however, that most lung cancers attributed to indoor radon probably occur among smokers; only about 2000 of the 13,000 estimated annual lung cancer deaths attributed to nonindustrial radon exposure occur in nonsmokers.[23,64,106]

Asbestos. Before the establishment of the 1971 Occupational Safety and Health Administration (OSHA) asbestos exposure guidelines, studies done on workers in the asbestos industry (e.g., automobile maintenance, insulation, shipyard work) showed clearly that lung cancer was vastly increased if workers also smoked. Numerous studies have shown a strong synergism between smoking and asbestos exposure in the development of lung cancer.[66] Asbestos workers who did not smoke had a risk of lung cancer about five times that of nonsmokers who worked in other industries. This compared with a 10 times greater risk for smokers not working in the

asbestos industry and an 87 times greater risk for asbestos workers who were smokers. Again, extrapolating the risk from industrial to low-level asbestos exposure (school, worksite) is controversial. It appears that the risk of lung cancer related to exposure to the levels of asbestos left intact in public buildings is very small.[56] If primary prevention priorities are based on the numbers of persons expected to die of lung cancer caused by environmental exposure, efforts should focus on elimination of passive smoking, which results in about 6000 lung cancer deaths per year in Americans, rather than on reducing low-level radon, which is associated with the deaths of about 2000 nonsmokers per year, or low-level asbestos exposure, which causes far fewer deaths.[32,56]

Secondary Prevention

Secondary prevention is aimed at early diagnosis of lung cancer in populations at high risk. Populations considered at high risk generally include persons more than 45 years of age who have smoked heavily, that is, one or more packs per day. Patients who claim to be nonsmokers need to be queried as to past smoking history.

The National Cancer Institute (NCI) sponsored three large randomized, controlled trials beginning in the early 1970s to examine the benefit of radiologic examinations and sputum cytology as lung cancer screening tools in asymptomatic, high-risk individuals. None of the studies has shown a difference in the lung cancer mortality rates among screened versus control groups. It is possible that patients who undergo regular screening eventually die of their lung cancer at the same rate as others, having only been diagnosed earlier in the natural history of their disease (lead-time bias).[98] The NCI began a large-scale study in late 1992 at 15 U.S. centers and will continue over 16 years to assess the value of screening in reducing mortality in prostate, lung, and colorectal cancers.[21] There will be 37,000 men in both the screened and the control groups. It is hoped this study at last will answer the important questions about lung cancer screening. The box, p. 315, lists prevention and early detection teaching priorities.

In persons with symptoms, a history of lung disease, a family history of lung cancer, and/or a heavy smoking history, chest x-ray films and sputum cytology are the primary tools used to screen for lung cancer. Monoclonal antibodies may prove to be a valuable tool in the detection of early lung cancer by sputum cytology. Early findings showed that cells in sputum specimens that stained positive with anti–lung cancer antibodies were 91% predictive of the development of lung cancer within 2 years.[124] No useful tumor markers are currently available for screening.

Carcinoembryonic antigen (CEA), elevated in only 50% of lung cancer patients, may be useful in postop-

PATIENT TEACHING PRIORITIES
Lung Cancer: Prevention and Early Detection

1. Avoid use of tobacco.

Risks increase according to number of cigarettes/day, number of years smoking, and tar and nicotine content of cigarettes.

Passive smoking increases the risk of lung cancer in nonsmokers, especially children and adolescents.

Parental smoking habits influence children.

Pipe or cigar smoking or smokeless tobacco is not an acceptable alternative.

Smoking cessation clinics and programs and medications are available to help those who desire to quit.

Women, youth, blacks, and uneducated persons should be the focus of smoking cessation efforts.

2. Know environmental carcinogens that increase risk.

High-risk occupations have been identified that expose persons to high levels of carcinogens.

Certain toxic substances increase risk (see Oleske[91]).

The synergistic effects of environmental carcinogens (especially radon or asbestos) and cigarette smoking increase risk.

3. Personal and family history are important risk factors.

Lung cancer risk may be inherited and is greater in those with a history of lung disease.

Lung cancer is difficult to detect early, and symptoms do not appear until disease is advanced. Best advice is to *quit smoking now.*

There are currently no special tools for detecting cancer early enough to improve cure rates, even in high-risk populations.

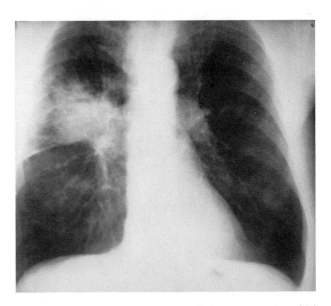

Figure 14-1 Patient with small cell lung cancer in which large tumor mass is centrally located and adjacent pleura is thickened. There is fluid in fissure and possible postobstructive signs of atelectasis. (Courtesy Dr. Norman Martin, Diagnostic Radiology, University of Kansas Medical Center.)

erative follow-up,[12] but it is not useful in lung cancer screening or for prognostic purposes.

CLASSIFICATION

The World Health Organization (WHO) has identified numerous categories of lung tumors or lesions, but the overwhelming majority (90%) consist of one of five types: (1) small cell anaplastic carcinoma, (2) squamous cell carcinoma, (3) adenocarcinoma, (4) large cell anaplastic carcinoma, and (5) mixed cell types.[50,81] The histology of a lung cancer is often suggested by the clinical signs and symptoms at presentation; adequate tissue for cytologic or pathologic examination is essential for diagnosis. This section describes some of the clinical and histologic features of the five main types of lung cancer. It is now believed that all lung cancers arise out of a common stem cell gone awry.[12]

Small Cell Lung Cancer

Small cell anaplastic carcinoma behaves biologically and clinically so differently from all other cell types that the latter are referred to as non–small cell lung cancers (NSCLCs). Although usually metastatic at the time of diagnosis (more than two thirds of the time) because of its rapid growth and aggressive nature, small cell lung cancer (SCLC) is the most sensitive of all lung cancers to chemotherapy and radiation therapy. It is thought to arise from the basal cell lining of the bronchial mucosa called a *Kulchitsky-type cell.* Because it most often arises in the central part of the chest, postobstructive pneumonia and atelectasis often occur (Figure 14-1). Frequent sites of distant metastasis are the brain, liver, and bone marrow. SCLC has sometimes been referred to as *oat cell carcinoma* because of its microscopic resemblance to oats.

Paraneoplastic syndromes in SCLC patients include Eaton-Lambert syndrome (proximal muscle weakness), syndrome of inappropriate antidiuretic hormone (SIADH, from ectopic arginine vasopressin [AVP]), and Cushing's syndrome (from ectopic adrenocorticotropic hormone [ACTH]). Although the incidence of ectopic ACTH production and Cushing's syndrome in association with SCLC may be low (4.5% in one series), its appearance has been associated with a poor response to

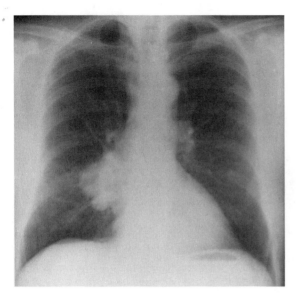

Figure 14-2 Patient with squamous cell carcinoma that developed centrally (right middle lobe) with left hilar prominence showing regional lymph node spread. (Courtesy Dr. Norman Martin, Diagnostic Radiology, University of Kansas Medical Center.)

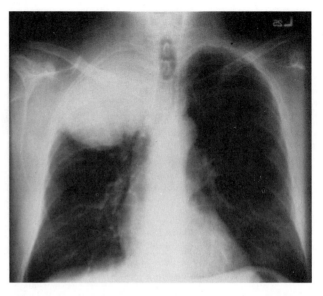

Figure 14-3 Classic Pancoast's tumor in patient with squamous cell carcinoma of lung. Large right upper apex mass with nearly complete right first rib bony destruction and right supraclavicular fullness. (Courtesy Dr. Norman Martin, Diagnostic Radiology, University of Kansas Medical Center.)

chemotherapy, a shortened survival time, and an increase in therapy-related complications.[112] Other hormones produced by SCLCs include calcitonin and gastrin-releasing peptide (GRP), or bombesin.[50,72] That SCLC cells contain neurosecretory granules and are capable of hormone production was once thought to result from neural crest embryologic origin.[50] The term *dispersed neuroendocrine cells* is now used to describe the variety of cells (carcinoid, some large cell, and small cell undifferentiated carcinomas) that share similar morphologic and immunohistochemical features and are capable of peptide hormone production.[50]

Non–Small Cell Lung Cancer

Squamous cell carcinoma may be described as well, moderately, or poorly differentiated. These cells differentiate toward stratified columnar (squamous) epithelium lining the airway and have receptors for epidermal growth factor, which stimulates the growth of epidermal tissues and is perhaps critical to malignant cell growth.[12] This carcinoma may not be visualized easily on chest x-ray films because it tends to arise in the central (medial) portion of the lung. This may delay diagnosis (Figure 14-2). Squamous cell is the most likely lung cancer to present as a *Pancoast's tumor*, which is high in the lung apex with extension to the chest wall, causing a classic shoulder pain that radiates down the ulnar nerve distribution (Figure 14-3). It is often associated with sudden onset of hypercalcemia resulting from the produc-

tion of a parathyroid hormone–like substance and is not associated with the presence of bone metastases.

Adenocarcinoma is increasing in frequency, perhaps as a result of the increasing incidence of women with lung cancer. This type is often recognized microscopically by its glandular appearance and mucin production and includes acinar, papillary, solid, and bronchioalveolar types.[50] Along with large cell carcinoma, adenocarcinoma is easily seen on chest x-ray films because it usually arises in radiographically visualized, peripheral lung tissue (Figure 14-4). Because of adenocarcinoma's highly metastatic nature, patients may present with or develop brain, liver, adrenal, or bone metastasis. Paraneoplastic syndromes frequently associated with adenocarcinomas are hypercoagulability syndromes (marantic endocarditis, disseminated intravascular coagulation [DIC], migratory thrombophlebitis) and clubbing of the fingers with hypertrophic pulmonary osteoarthropathy.[12]

Large cell anaplastic carcinoma is so named because it appears microscopically as large cells lacking any distinguishing features.[50] Clinical signs and symptoms are similar to those seen in adenocarcinoma, such as pain from pleural or chest wall invasion and lung abscesses, but this lesion is less likely to spread beyond the chest cavity.[12]

Mixed cell types are the final major lung cancer category. The theory that all lung cancers have the same stem cell origin helps explain the existence of mixed cell tumors. In a review of 100 lung cancer cases, 45%

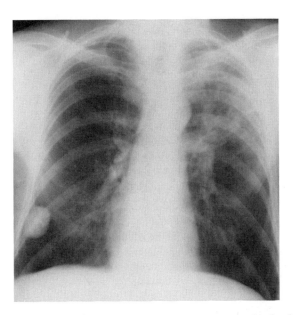

Figure 14-4 Adenocarcinomas can present as clearly defined peripheral lesions. Patient with right lower lobe lesion. (Courtesy Dr. Norman Martin, Diagnostic Radiology, University of Kansas Medical Center.)

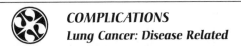

> **COMPLICATIONS**
> *Lung Cancer: Disease Related*
>
> *Direct spread or metastases*
>
> Bone marrow involvement (pancytopenia)
> Bone metastasis (pain, pathologic fractures)
> Brain metastasis
> Spinal cord compression (paralysis)
> Superior vena cava syndrome (respiratory distress)
> Pleural effusion
> Pericardial effusion (tamponade, dysrhythmias)
> Endobronchial lesion (cough, hemoptysis)
> Postobstructive atelectasis and/or pneumonia
> Liver metastasis
> Regional spread (see Clinical Features)
>
> *Indirect effects or paraneoplastic syndromes*
>
> Syndrome of inappropriate antidiuretic hormone (SIADH) (small cell) and hyponatremia
> Hypercalcemia (squamous cell)
> Cushing's syndrome and ectopic adrencorticotropic hormone (ACTH)
> Anorexia, taste changes, weight loss, cachexia
> Degenerative neuropathies
> Fever of unknown origin (multiple cultures and work-ups)
> Disseminated intravascular coagulopathies (bleeding, deep vein thromboses)
> Clubbing and hypertrophic osteoarthropathy
> Anemia
> Granulocytosis, thrombocytosis

showed two different major histologic cell types.[51] Multiple cell lines are seen in 10% to 20% of specimens.[15] In a given patient, any combination of cell types is possible within a single lesion or specimen, while the predominant cell type in different metastatic lesions may vary.[12]

BIOLOGY OF LUNG CANCER AND CLINICAL SIGNIFICANCE

Multiple genetic lesions and events may be necessary in the development of lung cancer.[109] Chromosomal mutations or deletions that appear to play a role in malignant transformation and growth involve both the activation of "up-regulating" genes (*proto-oncogenes*) and the inactivation or deletion of "down-regulating," suppressor genes (*antioncogenes*).[72] Recent research demonstrates a deletion in the 3p chromosome region of 100% of SCLCs and up to 74% of NSCLCs.[12,15] This chromosome region has become the focus of intense research to determine the exact gene and its function. Whether the deletion is the same in both SCLC and NSCLC is not known. Other chromosomal deletions common in lung cancer are in the regions of 11p, 17p (p53 gene), and the retinoblastoma (Rb) gene.[12,15] The p53 gene is frequently mutated or inactivated in all types of lung cancer.[15] Reincorporation of some of these genes in malignant cell cultures has halted cell growth,[12,15] suggesting these genes control or down-regulate cellular growth.

The box above lists the disease-related complications of lung cancer.

DIAGNOSIS

The search for a lung cancer diagnosis is undertaken only after a good preliminary evaluation, including the following:

1. History and physical examination (see box, p. 318, for clinical features common in lung cancer)
2. Chest x-ray films (anteroposterior and lateral), which may reveal peripheral lesions at least 1 cm in size, a widened mediastinum, or hilar adenopathy
3. Complete blood count (CBC) with differential and platelet count, as well as blood chemistries

Histologic diagnosis, which may be as simple as collecting early-morning sputum 3 days in a row (diagnostic 80% of the time), is most valuable in squamous cell carcinoma.[44] However, *bronchoscopy* is frequently used today because it expedites diagnosis, provides a better specimen for histologic evaluation, and aids in staging.

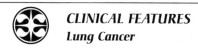

CLINICAL FEATURES
Lung Cancer

Most common symptoms at presentation

Change in cough (most have chronic smoker's cough)

Chest pain

Recurrent bronchitis or pneumonia unresponsive to
   antibiotics

Shortness of breath or wheezes

Hemoptysis

Weight loss

Fatigue

Dysphagia

Symptoms of regional tumor spread

Superior vena cava syndrome (SVCS; see Chapter 19)

Hoarseness from recurrent laryngeal nerve paralysis

Phrenic nerve paralysis with elevated hemidiaphragm and
   dyspnea

Horner's syndrome (unilateral ptosis, miosis, loss of facial
   sweat)

Pancoast's syndrome (shoulder pain radiating down arm
   along ulnar nerve distribution)

Tracheal or esophageal obstruction

Pericardial effusion and tamponade (see Chapter 19)

Pleural effusion

Hypoxia and dyspnea related to lymphangitic spread

*Evidence of metastatic disease or paraneoplastic
syndrome*

Headaches, mental status changes, or other neurologic
   findings resulting from brain metastasis or SIADH with
   hyponatremia (see Chapter 19)

Abdominal discomfort, elevated liver function tests,
   enlarged liver, and/or nausea and vomiting because of
   liver involvement

Bone pain related to bone involvement

Pancytopenia secondary to bone marrow involvement

Other paraneoplastic syndromes

Modified from Bunn PA: *Lung cancer: current understanding of
the biology, diagnosis, staging, and treatment,* monograph,
Princeton, NJ, 1992, Bristol-Myers.

Efforts to obtain adequate tissue for diagnosis become increasingly more invasive and can involve the following:

- Fiberoptic bronchoscopy with biopsy or bronchial brushings or washings for cytology (90% efficient)[12]
- Percutaneous transthoracic needle aspiration or biopsy under fluoroscopy and/or computed tomography (CT) guidance for peripheral lung lesions
- Biopsy of supraclavicular or scalene lymph nodes
- Mediastinoscopy (or mediastinotomy, if left upper chest lesions) to biopsy nodes or tissues, which aids in staging
- Biopsy of accessible metastatic sites (e.g., bone)
- Thoracentesis for cytology or pleural biopsy
- Thoracotomy as a last resort

STAGING

Obtaining a tissue diagnosis may involve use of staging procedures. The histology (SCLC versus NSCLC) will then determine how to proceed with staging. Histology and stage of disease help dictate prognosis and treatment options. When discussing treatment options with the patient, prognosis is an important consideration because risks and toxicities associated with the treatment must be balanced against potential survival benefits. Prognostic factors in lung cancer are discussed later in this chapter.

In general, a CT scan or magnetic resonance imaging (MRI) of the chest down through the adrenal glands must be done in addition to the studies just listed for either SCLC or NSCLC. Some argue that further staging in asymptomatic patients is unwarranted because it rarely reveals metastatic disease.[12,83] The incidence of "silent" metastases in asymptomatic patients who appear to be clinically stage I or II disease is low: the incidence of metastases to the brain is 2.7%; to bone, 3.4%; and to the liver, 9.3%.[83] Others note that 46% of patients with NSCLC have metastatic disease, and because of inadequate staging, as many as one fourth of patients who undergo so-called curative therapy will eventually die as a result of metastatic disease.[51] In many cases, nonresectability will still be demonstrated by the time these studies are done.[12] If NSCLC patients have evidence of bone pain, weight loss, or abnormal liver function or calcium levels, further work-up might require the following:

- Bone scan
- CT scan of the abdomen or liver
- CT or MRI study of the head
- Liver or bone marrow biopsy
- Plain films of bone

One of the greatest current controversies in the treatment of NSCLC is the resectability of stage IIIA disease (based on mediastinal lymph node involvement) with curative intent. Therefore preoperative staging of these patients has become more critical. CT scans and MRI are often inadequate in diagnosing chest wall and mediastinal involvement,[79] essential determinants of resectability and likelihood of cure. Although CT or MRI scans guide decisions regarding the necessity of invasive procedures and which procedure to perform, mediastinoscopy, mediastinotomy, and/or thoracotomy frequently are required after the scans (at least in the study setting) to document involvement histologically.[83]

If the cancer is deemed resectable, pulmonary function and blood gas studies are required to determine if the patient is able to undergo pneumonectomy or pulmonary resection.

Because two thirds of SCLC patients have metastatic disease, initial staging routinely includes the following:
- Bone scan
- CT scan of the abdomen
- Bone marrow biopsy
- CT or MRI study of the head
- With or without liver biopsy[12,22]

The American Joint Committee on Cancer's (AJCC's) tumor, node, metastasis (TNM) cancer staging system has been useful in prognosis and planning treatment for NSCLC. The TNM system classifies cancers according to the following staging designations[5] (Table 14-1):

Primary tumor (T)*

TX   Primary tumor cannot be assessed or tumor proved by the presence of malignant cells in sputum or bronchial washings but not visualized by imaging or bronchoscopy

T0   No evidence of primary tumor

Tis Carcinoma in situ

T1   Tumor 3 cm or less in greatest dimension, surrounded by lung or visceral pleura, without bronchoscopic evidence of invasion more proximal than the lobar bronchus (i.e., not in the main bronchus)

T2   Tumor with any of the following features of size or extent:
- More than 3 cm in greatest dimension
- Involvement of main bronchus 2 cm or more distal to the carina
- Invasion of the visceral pleura
- Associated with atelectasis or obstructive pneumonitis that extends to the hilar region but does not involve the entire lung

T3   Tumor of any size that directly invades any of the following: chest wall (including superior sulcus tumors), diaphragm, mediastinal pleura, parietal pericardium; or tumor in the main bronchus less than 2 cm distal to the carina; or associated atelectasis or obstructive pneumonitis of the entire lung

T4   Tumor of any size that invades any of the following: mediastinum, heart, great vessels, trachea, esophagus, vertebral body, carina; or tumor with a malignant pleural effusion

Regional lymph nodes (N)

NX   Regional lymph nodes cannot be assessed

N0   No regional lymph node metastasis

N1   Metastasis in ipsilateral peribronchial and/or ipsilateral hilar lymph node(s), including direct extension

N2   Metastasis in ipsilateral mediastinal and/or subcarinal lymph node(s)

N3   Metastasis in contralateral mediastinal, contralateral hilar, ipsilateral or contralateral scalene, or supraclavicular lymph node(s)

Distant metastasis (M)

MX   Presence of distant metastasis cannot be assessed

M0   No distant metastasis

M1   Distant metastasis

For the most part, the TNM system is not useful in SCLC. TNM takes on clinical significance only when surgery for stage I SCLC is a consideration. The Veterans Administration Lung Cancer Study Group's two-stage system is typically used for SCLC because it cor-

*Reprinted with permission from Beahrs O and others, editors: *Manual for staging of cancer,* ed 4, Philadelphia, 1992, Lippincott.

Table 14-1   Stage Grouping for Lung Cancers

Stage	Tumor	Node	Metastasis
Occult carcinoma	TX	N0	M0
0	Tis	N0	M0
I	T1	N0	M0
	T2	N0	M0
II	T1	N1	M0
	T2	N1	M0
IIIA	T1	N2	M0
	T2	N2	M0
	T3	N0, N1, N2	M0
IIIB	Any T	N3	M0
	T4	Any N	M0
IV	Any T	Any N	M1

From Beahrs OH and others, editors: *Manual for staging of cancer,* ed 4, Philadelphia, 1992, Lippincott.

relates with prognosis. Controversy exists regarding what constitutes limited versus extensive disease. A 1989 international workshop on SCLC reached the following consensus regarding staging[121]:
- *Limited*—Disease is restricted to one hemithorax with regional lymph node metastases, including hilar, ipsilateral, and contralateral mediastinal and/or supraclavicular nodes, and including ipsilateral pleural effusion regardless of cytology.
- *Extensive*—Disease is beyond the above definition and may involve metastasis to liver, bone, bone marrow, brain, adrenals, and lymph nodes.

Other authors maintain that limited disease is that which is confined to one hemithorax and can be encompassed in a single radiation port.[12] They therefore continue to assign pleural effusions to the extensive stage category because of the large volume of tissue requiring radiation to treat the pleural surface. Since pleural effusions are a poor prognostic factor, variations in staging SCLC can make comparisons of treatment response rates and survival data by stage confusing and possibly misleading.

METASTASIS

Metastasis to any site, as a consequence of lung cancer, can seriously interfere with the patient's ability to accomplish simple activities of daily living. Depending on where the metastatic lesion is located, clinical manifestations can lead to critical oncologic emergencies. Cancers of the lung find many distant sanctuaries, including bone marrow, pericardium and heart, kidney, and adrenal gland. The most common sites of metastasis of lung cancer are to the other lung and pleura, brain, bone, liver, and lymph nodes.

Because of its relevance to staging of NSCLC, only intrathoracic spread is addressed here. Other sites of metastasis are discussed later in conjunction with their treatment.

Intrathoracic Spread

As previously reviewed, various methods are employed to assess lymph node involvement. In patients with SCLC, if there is a definite diagnosis, further invasive procedures to determine lymph node involvement are usually not done. Work-up will continue to ascertain brain, bone, and liver metastasis.[25] Even in limited disease, local thoracic extension may account for chest pain, wheeze, hemoptysis, dysphagia, and hoarseness. If a pleural effusion or an abnormal lactate dehydrogenase (LDH) level is present, long-term survival is not likely.[1] The usual consensus is that a primary NSCLC tumor is incurable if nodes (high paratracheal, subcarinal, or contralateral) are replaced with tumor. When evaluating NSCLC for mediastinal involvement, some literature notes that on CT scan: (1) nodes less than 1 cm are considered normal; (2) nodes from 1 to 1.5 cm in diameter are considered suspicious; and (3) nodes greater than 1.5 cm in diameter are considered abnormal. Nodes considered normal may harbor disease, and nodes considered abnormal may just be reactive to pneumonia or other disease.[43,53]

Controversy surrounds what constitutes a "normal" node. Study results conflict on the accuracy of CT or MRI staging. Of patients with a negative CT scan, 10% to 20% will prove to have positive mediastinal lymph nodes at the time of thoracotomy, while 30% of those with enlarged nodes on CT will be negative on biopsy.[125] Mountain[83] recommends mediastinoscopy and/or mediastinotomy for patients who might otherwise be denied curative resection based on the radiologist's interpretation. Based on examination of the mediastinum by mediastinoscopy, Mountain cites the following criteria for incurable and unresectable NSCLC: (1) tumor involvement of "contralateral paratracheal lymph nodes or ipsilateral paratracheal lymph nodes in the upper half of the intrathoracic trachea"; (2) direct invasion of the trachea; and (3) evidence of gross perinodal disease.[83] If surgery is to be performed for NSCLC, Watanabe and others[127] recommend extensive nodal dissection for accurate postoperative staging. Obvious clinical contralateral lymph node involvement is associated with a much poorer 5-year survival than when only microscopic nodal involvement is discovered.[123]

TREATMENT MODALITIES
Non–Small Cell Lung Cancer

Surgery. Surgery is the treatment of choice for stages I and II NSCLC, representing 25% of all lung cancers, and the primary hope for cure.[83] Some selected stage IIIA patients may benefit from surgical resection in terms of improved survival.[44,83] Stage IIIB patients are not surgical candidates.[125] Pneumonectomy for stage II and

some stage I patients may be required unless precluded by preexisting cardiopulmonary disease. Some surgeons advocate wedge or segmental resection for small, peripheral lung lesions; others find the incidence of local recurrence too high with this limited procedure when a more aggressive approach could be curative. At the very least, lobectomy with regional lymph node dissection is most optimal for early-stage disease whenever possible.[44] Criteria for nonresectability include T4, N3, and M1 lesions (stages IIIB and IV); the presence of small cell histology; or inability of the patient to tolerate the procedure clinically.[12] A "complete" resection should mean (1) the surgeon is certain the procedure removed all known disease; (2) the proximal margins of the resected specimen are microscopically free of tumor; (3) the most distant lymph nodes within each lymphatic drainage area are microscopically free of tumor; and (4) the resected lymph node capsules are intact.[83]

Squamous cell cancer patients have the best survival rates, perhaps because of earlier diagnosis and because the disease exhibits less of a tendency to metastasize and has a slower growth rate.[44] More than 70% of patients relapse after "curative" surgery because of distant metastases rather than local lesions (less than 25%). This argues for improved methods of early detection and good systemic adjuvant therapy. Five-year survival after curative therapy is excellent for stage I patients (60% to 80%) but drops dramatically to 28% for the best stage IIIA patients.[83] Thus the potential benefit of surgery must be weighed against the risks of operative morbidity and mortality. The incidence of lung resection complications increases with age (over 70 years of age). However, age alone is not a contraindication to surgery because age may not reflect other important risk factors, such as coexisting diseases, low forced expiratory volume, weight loss, disease stage, and extent of resection.[83] Surgical resection for palliation of NSCLC metastases can help maintain a decent quality of life in patients with rapidly progressing or recurrent spinal cord compression[81] or solitary brain metastasis.[44] The box, p. 321, lists surgical treatment–related complications of lung cancer.

Laser therapy. Lung cancer patients may experience distressful symptoms or complications from endobronchial lesions, including postobstructive atelectasis and pneumonia, hemoptysis, irritating and uncontrolled cough, and hypoxemia and self-care deficit. If the endobronchial lesions involve the trachea or mainstem bronchii, laser therapy may be successfully used with palliative intent. The laser is less effective in treating obstructions of smaller airways. Treatment may be repeated and can be done entirely on an outpatient basis.[101] The procedure has been associated with a 75% success rate in advanced lung cancer. Effectiveness of the procedure is independent of other modes of therapy, patient's age, or

COMPLICATIONS
Lung Cancer: Surgical Treatment

Fever, sepsis (antibiotics, empyema, fistula formation)
Bleeding (hypotension, cardiogenic shock)
Cardiac dysrhythmias, congestive heart failure, fluid over-load
Airway obstruction, dyspnea, hypoxemia, respiratory failure
Pneumothorax
Pulmonary embolus
Pneumonia
Prolonged hospitalization, intensive care unit psychosis
Death

performance status. Patients whose airway is obstructed by an exophytic lesion of squamous cell origin may derive the greatest benefit.[100]

Radiation therapy. Optimal doses of external beam radiation for NSCLC are now believed to be about 60 Gy. Best tumor control occurs with five fractions (treatments) per week over 6 to 7 weeks without interruption (no midtherapy "rests" as in treatment known as a "split course").[10] Hyperfractionation schedules (more than one treatment per day) are currently under study, and preliminary findings suggest these achieve better responses than standard schedules.[12,51] A hyperfractionated dose-response relationship to survival appears to plateau at 69.9 Gy. Since doses in this range can be delivered by standard radiation with comparable survival, studies are now comparing hyperfractionated with standard schedules to answer the question of superior method.[10] However, tumors of greater than 6 cm are not effectively destroyed by external beam therapy, whereas tumor size less than 3 cm is associated with a favorable prognosis.[10]

Brachytherapy. Local recurrences develop in as many as 60% of patients within 15 months of standard radiation therapy to the primary chest tumor.[94] Brachytherapy, based on the known dose-response relationship to tumor control, is being used to treat these relapses. It is also indicated for the patient who cannot undergo resection because of the tumor's location, medical contraindications, or refusal of surgery. In the last two cases, patients with otherwise resectable NSCLC could be offered radiation therapy with curative intent; 5-year survival rates may be as high as 23%.[12] In some cases, brachytherapy radiation implants with iodine-125 are used to sterilize tumors 7 to 8 cm in size by delivering doses of 160 to 250 Gy to the tumor without significant damage to surrounding tissue.[51] These treatments require hospitalization while the radioactive implants are in

place. More recently, high-dose/rate (HDR) brachytherapy is used, often in combination with laser therapy, to treat recurrent and obstructing lung lesions. This technology allows for careful placement of catheters close to the tumor. Then, using computerized remote control, HDR iridium (^{192}Ir) is introduced into the catheter. Within a few minutes, while caregivers are safe from exposure, a very high dose of radiation (5 to 10 Gy/session) can be delivered to select tissue without injury to adjacent healthy tissue, which is especially critical at this anatomic site.[62] Sessions may be repeated every 1 to 2 weeks for a cumulative dose in the range of 20 to 43.6 Gy.[10,62,65] Symptoms (cough, hemoptysis, and dyspnea) can be relieved 30% to 80% of the time with minimal risk in properly selected patients.[10,62] This is experimental palliative therapy, but the role of HDR brachytherapy in primary treatment is being explored through randomized comparisons with external beam radiation therapy.[10,62]

For inoperable, locally advanced NSCLC in patients with poor prognosis, radiation alone is usually reserved for palliation of symptoms such as painful bone metastases, superior vena cava syndrome (SVCS), or those previously mentioned. Symptoms are relieved in 24% to 100% of these patients.[10,12] Some studies have shown comparable symptom relief with lower than standard radiation doses at considerably less cost and inconvenience for these terminal patients.[10]

The use of definitive radiotherapy at an unresectable early stage (stages I to IIIA) remains controversial.[58] Some recognize improved median or 5-year survival in the clinical setting.[45,58] The median survival in stage IIIA or IIIB NSCLC treated with radiation alone is less than 1 year.[47] Results of trials comparing chemotherapy plus radiation with radiation alone in unresected, locally advanced NSCLC have been contradictory. One author notes a modest survival benefit if the chemotherapy regimen is cisplatin based and no difference in survival if it is not.[12] An important Eastern Cooperative Group/Radiation Therapy Oncology Group (ECOG/RTOG) study addresses the issue of superior modality. The study randomizes patients to cisplatin-vinblastine followed by chest radiation versus standard radiation alone (60 Gy) versus hyperfractionated chest irradiation alone.[47] No randomized clinical trial has shown a survival advantage to either preoperative or postoperative radiation therapy in resected NSCLC, although it may reduce local recurrence in N1 or N2 disease.[10]

Chemotherapy. As many as 80% of all lung cancers are NSCLC; of these, 70% will present with regional or advanced disease.[92] Even in the best of cases involving surgical resection (stage I), about 20% to 40% will relapse.[12] Relapse occurs in 70% of patients with more advanced disease.[12,51] Thus the majority of lung cancer patients have frank or occult metastatic NSCLC and could benefit from effective systemic therapy. Response rates with single agents have been notoriously low (9% to 27%).[12] The most active single agents in NSCLC include mitomycin-C, vindesine, vinblastine, etoposide, ifosfamide, cisplatin, carboplatin,[12] cyclophosphamide, vincristine, doxorubicin, bleomycin, navelbine, and paclitaxel.[101] Among newer single agents showing promise are epirubicin, docetaxel, and gemsar.[46,80] Docetaxel has shown significant activity in advanced NSCLC, producing response in both untreated patients and those previously treated with a platinum-based regimen.[41] Navelbine, in controlled randomized studies, has produced an increase in survival; therefore in newly diagnosed stage IV NSCLC, this should be considered as a first-line therapy option.

Carney[16] reports on several phase II and III randomized trials of NSCLC patients and explains:

(1) With few exceptions, response rates rarely exceed 40% (usually ranging from 20% to 30%); (2) complete responses are almost never observed and, for almost all patients, chemotherapy is only palliative; (3) combinations containing cisplatin usually produce the best responses; (4) the overall impact of combination chemotherapy regimens on improved survival is modest (for all NSCLC patients, the median length of survival remains at 8 to 12 months, and the majority of patients rarely survive longer than 1 year); and (5) most combination chemotherapy regimens are associated with moderate toxicity (including alopecia and nausea and vomiting) and frequent hospital admissions for administration of chemotherapy and/or the evaluation of chemotherapy-induced side effects.

Performance status has become a major factor in deciding who should undergo chemotherapy. Patients are pathologically staged before therapy if mediastinal nodes are greater than 1 cm on CT. A Southwest Oncology Group (SWOG) study (9019), closed December 1995, will assess the role and necessity of surgery in select stage IIIA and IIIB patients when concurrent preoperative chemotherapy and radiation therapy are compared with chemotherapy and radiation alone. Outside a protocol setting, some will recommend chemotherapy to patients with NSCLC only if the patient (1) is informed of the limitations of therapy, (2) is clearly incurable by surgery or radiation, (3) has no significant symptoms that radiation could palliate, (4) has a good performance status, and (5) has measurable disease to assess any response so that treatment can be continued appropriately.[58]

In the early 1990s, Bunn[12] summarized the findings of six randomized trials comparing best supportive care with various cisplatin-based chemotherapy regimens in patients with advanced NSCLC. On the average, survival benefit in favor of the treated group was 11 weeks. This represented the first significant evidence of survival advantage with combination chemotherapy in these pa-

tients. Clearly, quality of life studies must be used to corroborate the benefit of modest 3- to 4-month gains in survival for the patient with advanced disease. An encouraging corollary to these findings is that if micrometastases respond equally well to current chemotherapy regimens, more cures may be expected in "completely resected" stages I to IIIA NSCLC, in which micrometastases are the only harbinger to failure.

Combination chemotherapy and radiation therapy. For inoperable, locally advanced NSCLC, cisplatin-based regimens in combination with radiotherapy may improve median but not long-term survival.[12,107] Postoperative cisplatin-based regimens plus radiotherapy in incompletely resected[12] or fully resected[47] stage II and IIIA patients are associated with improved median survival and a decrease in distant relapses (except for brain) but have not reduced mortality rates. Because of an apparent synergism when cisplatin is combined with radiation, studies continue to investigate this combination to achieve improved cure rates.

The best inroads seem to be occurring in the treatment of stage IIIA NSCLC with preoperative adjuvant (also known as *protoadjuvant* or *neoadjuvant*) chemotherapy with or without radiation therapy. Although results are difficult to compare because of inconsistencies in staging (lack of pretreatment pathologic staging) and absence of multiinstitutional trials, preliminary findings indicate a prolonged survival for patients receiving adjuvant therapy. Preoperative chemotherapy alone or in combination with radiotherapy is apparently rendering some patients pathologic complete remissions (CRs) at thoracotomy (9% to 11% in one series).[12,83,99] Three-year survival rates ranged from 26% to 45%. Although findings provide hope, preoperative chemotherapy in stage IIIA NSCLC is still investigational and is appropriate only in a clinical trial setting.[123] Patients should be informed of this option. If recent and upcoming trials demonstrate a survival advantage to preoperative chemotherapy and radiotherapy, those most likely to benefit are the 20% of patients having a normal CT but who are found to have positive mediastinal nodes after biopsy.

Future concerns. New, more effective chemotherapy agents and combinations are needed, especially if they are associated with a low toxicity profile. Randomized phase III trials should be carried out only in clearly defined patient groups (e.g., pathologic staging, performance status).[120]

Immunohistochemical analysis may help to identify that subgroup of NSCLCs with neuroendocrine features that may benefit from adjuvant chemotherapy. Examination of chromosomes for K-*ras* mutations may also delineate patients with adenocarcinoma of the lung who may benefit from more aggressive treatment or else should not be subjected to treatment because of the aggressive nature of their disease and guaranteed short survival. Biotherapy research is ongoing, but thus far the trial results have been disappointing.

Small Cell Lung Cancer

Surgery. In the 1960s and 1970s most surgical attempts to treat SCLC (stages I and II) met with dismal results, with less than 1% surviving at 5 years.[12] The Veterans Administration and Armed Forces Cooperative Group found an amazing 36% 5-year survival among SCLC patients who had an unknown diagnosis and a single pulmonary lesion preoperatively.[54] However, less than 5% of SCLC patients are diagnosed in the early stages of disease when it is resectable, and the chest is still the most common site of relapse.[4,12,22] Adjuvant chemotherapy after surgical resection for stage I disease results in about a 45% 5-year survival.[68]

Current recommended treatment of SCLC presenting as a single pulmonary nodule is surgery followed by adjuvant chemotherapy with or without radiation to the chest. Prophylactic cranial irradiation may be considered, but studies have not proved any survival benefit.[68] The Lung Cancer Study Group (LCSG) and ECOG recently completed a prospective randomized study to examine the benefit of surgery in patients with stages I to IIIA SCLC.[69] Patients were randomized to receive either preoperative chemotherapy plus surgery and radiotherapy or chemotherapy and radiotherapy alone. Preliminary results show no survival benefit with surgery. Unless randomized trials can demonstrate an advantage to chemotherapy plus surgery in early-stage disease, the exact role of surgery will remain unclear. However, there appears to be a small group of SCLC patients (less than 1%) with true stage I disease who may be cured by surgery with or without chemotherapy.[12,54]

Radiation therapy. In limited-disease (LD) SCLC, trials combining chest radiation and chemotherapy have now shown improved long-term survival rates (24% to 54% at 2 years; 7% to 20% at 4 years) and a decrease in local recurrences.[1,20,61,125] Concurrent radiotherapy with chemotherapy or alternating chemotherapy with radiotherapy seems to produce the best results.[1,84,125] It is too early to know whether long-term survival will translate to cures. Before etoposide-cisplatin (EP) regimens, organ toxicities from combined-modality approaches were too severe (e.g., congestive heart failure, dyspnea) and without survival benefit. Toxicities noted with EP plus radiation were myelosuppression, esophagitis, and some reports of pulmonary toxicity (possibly from the radiation port size), but none was life-threatening.[125] Use of CT guidance in radiation treatment planning, individually designed blocks, and a shrinking field help protect surrounding healthy lung, esophagus, and spinal cord tissues from unwanted radiation.

With the combined-modality approach, the most common site of failure is the chest in about 30% of LD SCLCs.[4,125] When chemotherapy is given alone in LD SCLC, however, the incidence of local chest relapse is 80%.[20] Some note that the intensity of the first chemotherapy dose may predict survival.[20] Current trials are examining the role of dose intensity and timing of modalities in preventing local recurrences and in improving long-term survival. Research in this area has increased because of the availability of hematopoietic growth factors and peripheral blood stem cell (PBSC) support.[70] In extensive SCLC, there is no advantage to combining radiation therapy with chemotherapy. The main role for radiation therapy in these patients is palliation of symptoms.[59]

The brain is a frequent site of metastasis, and the effect of most systemic chemotherapy on the central nervous system (CNS) is extremely limited. Whole-brain irradiation (WBI) is often necessary. If brain metastasis has occurred, 40 Gy is needed to prevent relapse.[125]

Unlike treatment in NSCLC, *prophylactic cranial irradiation* (PCI) has often been done to prevent CNS failure.[3] PCI can reduce the incidence of CNS relapse from 25% to 6% and has generally been reserved for patients achieving a CR to chemotherapy. PCI may be used during systemic therapy in a clinical trial involving a potential cure. However, authors are questioning the value of PCI because of the high incidence and severity of CNS toxicities.[39] Late toxicities from PCI in long-term survivors are only now being realized and may be underreported in some studies because of only incidental and retrospective reporting. Among the 7% of patients surviving beyond 5 years in one retrospective review, 22% were found to have developed probable CNS toxicity that surfaced 2 to 5 years after combination chemotherapy and radiotherapy.[1] Patients had neurologic complaints, abnormal neurologic findings, and abnormal CT scans. In some patients, progressive clinical deterioration from neurologic deficits required life-style changes or extended care.[1] Because of late toxicities, PCI is usually limited to no more than 30 Gy and is not given concurrently with chemotherapy to avoid synergistic injury to brain tissue. Many still reserve PCI until treatment of the primary tumor is completed.[27,125]

Radiation to other common sites of metastasis (e.g., liver, spine) will not prevent tumor spreading to those sites. Prompt therapy (chemotherapy or radiation) for known meningeal carcinomatosis and spinal metastases is useful and necessary, but no preventive therapy exists for these complications.

Patients with extensive disease (ED) who present with SVCS should be spared radiation because they usually will respond adequately to chemotherapy.[12,49]

Chemotherapy. Before chemotherapy, half of SCLC patients with LD died within 12 to 14 weeks, and half of those with ED died within 6 weeks without treatment.[22] Combination chemotherapy became the cornerstone of treatment in the 1980s for SCLC patients, with overall responses of up to 90% and CRs of 40% to 50%.[12,49] Long-term survival depends on achieving a CR, usually within the first months of treatment.

Since the mid-1970s, many single agents have shown response rates from 15% to 50%. These include cyclophosphamide, ifosfamide, doxorubicin, epirubicin, etoposide, teniposide, cisplatin, carboplatin, vincristine, methotrexate, and the nitrosureas.[70] Etoposide appears to produce a very dose-dependent and schedule-dependent response. There are improved response rates in SCLC when etoposide is given in multiple daily intravenous (IV) doses (for 3 to 5 days) rather than as a single bolus.[115] A study has demonstrated excellent response rates and minimal toxicities (primarily mild myelosuppression) when etoposide is given as a daily oral dose (50 mg/m^2) for 5 to 21 consecutive days every 4 weeks.[61] The optimal schedule and dose, however, have yet to be defined in SCLC. Carboplatin, with a 60% response rate in untreated patients,[59] has shown to be highly active as a single agent as well as in combination regimens. Paclitaxel, topotecan, and irinotecan (the topoisomerase I inhibitors), and the antimetabolite gemcitabine have shown some promise and warrant further studies.[13] Combination chemotherapy appears to be improving survival statistics in SCLC patients.[12]

Etoposide plus cisplatin (EP) has proved superior to cytoxan, doxorubicin (Adriamycin), and vincristine (CAV) regimens for both LD and ED in regard to responses, survival, and reduced toxicities.[12] Large cooperative group and single institution studies found improved median survival (18 to 19 months) in LD patients receiving regimens containing VP-16 plus cisplatin with or without radiation therapy to the primary tumor.[12] Current practice is to give intense chemotherapy of short duration (less than six cycles) with active agents.[13,49] Restaging should include bronchoscopy and all initial staging studies to determine response. No study has shown a survival benefit for prolonged (1 to 2 years) maintenance chemotherapy in patients achieving a CR with induction therapy. In LD patients, late-dose intensification after a CR was achieved during induction therapy proved a superior treatment to maintenance therapy. The only current maintenance studies are those evaluating the role of biologic response modifiers.

Overall, 80% to 90% of SCLCs will respond to chemotherapy.[49] Of patients who respond to chemotherapy, 50% will begin to relapse within 10 to 12 months. From 30% to 64% of SCLCs that relapse after an initial response will subsequently respond to either the same or another type (second-line) of chemotherapy.[29] About 20% to 25% of ED patients will achieve a CR with combination chemotherapy, usually without radiation therapy.[12,49] Trials using combination chemotherapy

regimens have reported survival rates of 23% at 1 year and 4% at 2 years in ED SCLC.[1] Perhaps 1% of ED patients survive beyond 5 years and may be cured, although relapse is possible beyond 5 years.[12,120] Current clinical trials using combinations of new and active agents are underway to try to improve long-term survival and reduce toxicity.[13] One SWOG study (9216) compares CODE (cisplatin, vincristine, doxorubicin, etoposide) plus thoracic radiation therapy versus alternating CAV and VP-16 in extensive-stage SCLC. Another study (LUN-11) investigates the use of paclitaxel/carboplatin with extended oral VP-16 in limited-stage or extensive-stage SCLC. Efforts to overcome drug resistance by use of alternating non-cross-resistant regimens or high-dose regimens with or without autologous bone marrow transplant in ED have not generally improved disease-free survival, although initial CRs are impressive.[13,67] Aggressive chemotherapy is currently not warranted outside a protocol setting for these SCLC patients with poor prognosis. Most patients, however, can achieve some quality time by means of standard chemotherapy regimens, with mild toxicities before eventual death as a result of their disease.

Delayed effects of treatment. Only now are there sufficient numbers of SCLC survivors to appreciate the late effects of treatment. The late toxicity of PCI with or without chemotherapy depends on total dose of radiation, port size, and concurrent therapies. Findings include cerebral atrophy, dementia, confusion, and personality changes. Efforts to decrease these effects are already in place, and research is focused on whether late toxicity from PCI is worth any survival benefit.[1,39,118]

Secondary leukemias (e.g., acute myelogenous leukemia) can occur, presumably resulting from chemotherapy.[49] This problem may be resolved by avoiding maintenance regimens and alkylating agents. Patients cured of SCLC who continue to smoke tobacco have a greater risk of developing a second primary lesion than of experiencing a relapse from SCLC.[12] These people need to be so advised and encouraged to stop smoking.

Future concerns. Controversial issues that need to be addressed focus on the best schedule and dose of etoposide and the role of radiation therapy in the long-term survival of limited disease SCLC patients. Whether chemotherapy dose intensification will lead to improved long-term survival and whether the survival benefit of PCI is worth the toxicities remain to be seen. Insights gained through genetic engineering and the discovery of genetic variations unique to SCLC (i.e., *myc*-oncogene amplification and gene deletions in chromosome 3p) may lead to improved early detection or treatment by genetic manipulation. Two trials (SWOG 8991 and an Intergroup study with ECOG) are currently being analyzed related to survival data with variant versus classic SCLC subtypes to assess the prognostic significance of these histologies. Use of granulocyte-macrophage colony-stimulating factor (GM-CSF) or granulocyte CSF (G-CSF) to prevent the frequent dose-limiting side effect of neutropenic sepsis with chemotherapy is being tested in clinical trials. Preliminary results of a SWOG study (8812) in LD SCLC suggest that patients who were randomized to the combined chemotherapy-radiotherapy plus GM-CSF group had more severe toxicity (e.g., infection, thrombocytopenia) than those who did not receive GM-CSF.

TREATMENT OF METASTASIS
Brain Metastasis

Distant metastasis rather than local chest recurrence is the most common reason for failure after curative surgery for NSCLC, and the predominant site of metastasis is the brain.[83] According to one RTOG study, 60% of all metastatic brain tumors come from lung cancers. Therefore even the most vague CNS symptoms suggest the need for follow-up with CT scan, MRI, or arteriography. Lumbar puncture (LP) should be avoided if cerebral metastasis is suspected. Wright and co-workers[129] report that 53% or more of lesions will be multifocal (Figure 14-5). Increased intracranial pressure (ICP) and cerebrospinal fluid (CSF) obstruction cause generalized symptoms such as change in level of consciousness (LOC), papillary changes and papilledema, headache and seizures, vomiting, and change in vital signs (wide pulse pressure, increased blood pressure, bradycardia, irregular pulse). Local compression or destruction of tissue from edema or encroachment of the mass can cause a multitude of problems depending on location. *Aphasia* (inability to express or understand verbal symbols), *agnosia* (inability to recognize objects), and *apraxia* (inability to execute purposeful movements) result from pressure on the right parietal lobe.[104] A tumor in the left parietal lobe can cause difficulty with the simplest of tasks, such as reading or adding up the grocery bill. Other subtle mental changes, such as recent memory loss, can occur if the limbic system is involved.

Treatment should be palliative to correct the patient's neurologic deficits, which in turn enhances quality of life.[8,18] For acute management of increased ICP, large doses of corticosteroids (Decadron or Medrol) can be administered, followed by radiation therapy to the whole brain (20 to 40 Gy).[28] Certain patients can benefit from surgical resection of solitary lesions followed by a course of radiation therapy, although some clinicians are questioning the value and necessity of radiation because of its late debilitating neurologic effects. A SWOG study (9021) is prospectively evaluating through a randomized trial the benefit of postoperative radiation in terms of

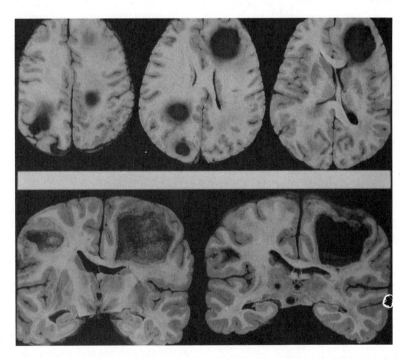

Figure 14-5 Brain metastases. *Top,* Gross specimens show metastatic deposits of an undifferentiated large cell lung carcinoma. The metastases form essentially necrotic masses with peripheral enhancement and peritumoral edema. *Bottom,* Occasionally, extensive necrosis transforms metastases into cysts lined by only a thin rim of viable tumor.

both survival and quality of life in patients with a single brain metastasis. The following factors must be considered in choosing the type of local treatment*:

- Number of lesions
- Location of lesion(s)
- Type of primary tumor (whether or not it is lung cancer)
- Patient's age and performance status
- Status of other metastatic disease and primary tumor
- Relative responsiveness to and ability to be controlled by radiotherapy
- Interval between treatment of primary tumor and development of brain metastasis

Coping with this devastating complication poses a dilemma for both patient and family. The goal of treatment is to control the neurologic deficits and promote an optimal life-style.

The following interventions may be helpful for patients with alterations in thought processes. The nurse can relate to the patient more effectively through the following measures:

- Introduce self and face patient while speaking.
- Inform patient of date, day, and time on awakening and as needed.
- Keep verbal communication simple and direct without shouting or being condescending.
- Remember that patient is thinking in slow motion.
- Speak slowly, since it takes patient a long time to process what is being said and how to respond. Use short, simple sentences.
- Present only one idea at a time.
- Ask affirmative questions rather than negative ones. "Do you want a drink?" is better than "Don't you want a drink?"
- Do not ask questions that require patient to make a choice, such as, "Do you want to stay up awhile or would you like to go back to bed?"
- Encourage the use of appropriate greetings and social exchanges.
- Do not tease or encourage patient to respond inappropriately.
- Encourage gestures and talking with hands whenever and if possible. Tell patient to describe or show you what he or she means; frequently this will enable patient to say the word itself.
- Be prepared for bizarre, inaccurate use of language and for swearing. Such responses are very common with the brain-injured patient. Accept this without amusement or anger. Help patient by providing the correct word without emotion.

*Modified from Kornblith P and others: Treatment of metastatic cancer. In DeVita VT Jr and others, editors: *Cancer: principles and practice of oncology,* Philadelphia, 1985, Lippincott.

- Decrease noise level and refrain from talking to other people over the patient.
- Keep patient's bed rails up, and avoid restraints unless necessary for patient safety.
- Supervise activities but allow as much autonomy as possible.
- Provide simple, step-by-step instructions for tasks.
- Provide positive reinforcement for accomplished tasks (e.g., bathing, self-care, eating).
- Allow patient to sleep in clothing and shoes if no injury will occur.
- Provide for rest and naps; reduce mental activity late in day.
- Check on patient at least every hour.
- Include significant other (SO) in teaching and management of patient, and refer to community resources and social services as needed.
- Encourage SO to verbalize fears and concerns, and provide support for SO.

Bone Metastasis

Characteristically, pain that becomes progressively worse over weeks or months is frequently associated with bone metastasis in the patient with lung cancer. Although this complication is rarely life-threatening, it can be disabling if pathologic fractures occur or extradural spinal disease results in spinal cord compression. Malawer and Delaney[73] report that 32.5% of all lung cancer patients will develop osseous metastasis; therefore careful evaluation with x-ray films and bone scan is required if symptoms are present. Some nonspecific chemical markers may also be used, including serum alkaline phosphatase and urine hydroxyproline secretion. When bone destruction occurs, such as from metastasis, alkaline phosphatase is elevated. As osteoblasts then remake new bone, hydroxypraline is released into the blood and in turn is secreted in the urine.

Skeletal metastasis usually occurs in the vertebra (69%), pelvis (41%), femur (25%), and skull (14%).[73] The appearance on x-ray film can vary greatly. Osteolytic lesions have ragged margins and can infiltrate an entire bone. Osteoblastic lesions are sclerotic metastatic foci characterized by increased radiographic density (Figure 14-6). Occasionally, both sclerotic and lytic patterns emerge.

Patients with widespread bony metastasis, compared with a single bony lesion, usually have decreased survival time. Management for this problem is aimed at patient comfort and prevention of additional effects such as motor paresis and sensory loss. Narcotic medications, local nonsteroidal antiinflammatory drugs (NSAIDs), and radiation therapy are frequently and successfully used to promote comfort and increase ambulation and mobility. Orthopedic management can be attempted to promote spinal stabilization and prevent cord compres-

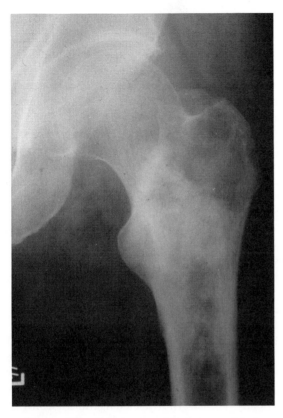

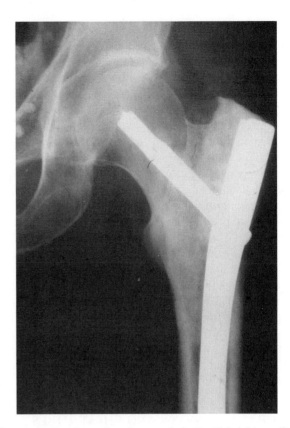

Figure 14-6 Osteoblastic metastatic lesion to hip from adenocarcinoma of lung.

Figure 14-7 Example of a prophylactic Zickel hip nailing from metastatic adenocarcinoma of lung.

sion. Prophylactic fixation of metastatic lesions in the long bones with rods (Enders) or implants (Zickel, Moore, bipolar, total hip) can prevent pathologic fractures and ensure ambulation or upper extremity control (Figures 14-6 and 14-7). Combination chemotherapy may also help alleviate or modify this painful process. Management for patients with bone metastasis, according to Carpenito's nursing diagnosis, includes surgical treatment and pain management.[17] The major problems for this patient are discomfort related to metastatic bone disease and impaired physical mobility resulting from surgical fixation to prevent or repair a pathologic fracture.

Although most lung cancer patients will not experience prolonged survival, control of painful bony metastasis remains essential.

Liver Metastasis

For the patient with lung cancer, the added diagnosis of liver metastasis is a poor prognostic sign. Current methods of treatment with systemic or intraarterial chemotherapy or radiotherapy have little to offer in terms of prolonged survival for the patient with liver metastasis from any primary tumor site.[63,96] Through improved radiologic methods, however, liver anatomy and number and location of metastasis are better appreciated by the surgeon, which leads to improved resection. Also, more refined surgical techniques have somewhat improved this patient's prognosis from a surgical standpoint.

Patients with solitary metastatic sites generally survive longer than those with widespread liver metastasis.[63] Elevated liver function tests characteristic of metastatic involvement include alkaline phosphatase, gamma-glutamyl transpeptidase (GGTP), serum aspartate aminotransferase (AST, SGOT), and lactate dehydrogenase (LDH). Hepatomegaly and liver pain denote massive end-stage liver disease.

Prophylactic treatment of liver metastasis is virtually nonexistent; palliative therapy is available through radiation or chemotherapy. Once again, in patients with lung cancer, radiation to the liver or intraarterial therapy is rarely, if ever, used. Systemic chemotherapy may be somewhat effective for a brief period of symptom control, but liver metastasis is part of the malignant process that often leads to early death.[63] If liver metastasis produces no symptoms, many clinicians believe no treatment should be initiated. Patients with painful liver involvement can usually be made comfortable with narcotics and celiac plexus blocks.

Cardiac Metastasis

Malignant involvement of the cardiac muscle produces pericardial effusion; if enough fluid accumulates in the pericardium to obstruct blood flow to the ventricle, cardiac tamponade will result.[19] The symptoms induced by pericardial effusion often mimic the cancer's overall systemic effects and include dyspnea and cyanosis, orthopnea, venous distention, leg edema, and cardiac enlargement.[93] The nurse may also observe cough, hiccups, and pain. Tamponade may develop slowly or quickly, and the severity of onset of symptoms depends on how rapidly the fluid accumulates. The nursing diagnosis would be *cardiac output, decreased.* Treatment is generally conservative and consists of pericardiocentesis, systemic chemotherapy, or intrapericardial administration of various other agents (see Chapter 19). If the patient's mean life expectancy is 9 to 13 months, active treatment should be pursued. Treatment may also be undertaken for comfort reasons. Cardiac tamponade can be treated successfully and easily with a cardiac window procedure performed using local anesthesia. This is done for palliative purposes and can improve the quality of the patient's remaining life.

PLEURAL EFFUSIONS AND CHEST TUBES

The pleural cavity consists of the space between the parietal pleura and the visceral pleura. The *parietal pleura* lines the chest, and the *visceral pleura* covers the lung. The two pleura, lubricated by a thin layer of fluid, glide over each other during inspiration and expiration. A vacuum is created by the fluid and causes the surfaces to adhere to each other. In the normal lung, no true space exists between the two pleura, and if one develops, it alters respiratory function and the lungs can no longer expand properly.[33] A pleural effusion has been created.

Lung cancer is one of the most common causes of malignant pleural effusions. About 12% of lung cancer patients have a pleural effusion that is usually tumor related.[83] Pleural fluid can accumulate as a result of obstructed lymphatic drainage and increased capillary permeability.[19] Lung expansion is impaired with poor gas exchange, and respiratory embarrassment is the outcome. Other consequences include atelectasis and recurrent infections.[74] Many months of productive life may be possible and repeated thoracentesis avoided if the effusion is properly treated.

Various methods of treatment for pleural effusion are available, including repeated thoracentesis, intrapleural instillation of chemotherapy, intracavitary radioactive colloids, and pleurectomy.[93,103] Because these patients already have a limited life expectancy, treatment should be as fast and painless as possible to control symptoms. Instillation of a sclerosing agent (antibiotic, talc, antineoplastic, radioactive) for pleural sclerosis can prevent repeated hospitalization and affords the patient good palliation.

The patient with pleural effusion who is to be sclerosed has a chest tube, and caring for patients with chest tubes in place is always cause for concern. Assessment of the tube's functioning should be done frequently and skillfully by the nurse.

When a chest tube is inserted, placement depends on whether it is to drain air only, such as pneumothorax (second or third intercostal space), or fluid, such as an effusion (fourth or sixth intercostal space). Because air rises, placement will be higher for a pneumothorax.

Once the chest tube has been inserted and sutured in place, it is connected to underwater-seal drainage (i.e., Pleur-evac; Figure 14-8). The principle is to keep the chest tube under sterile fluid (usually water) to prevent air from going back up the tube into the pleural cavity. If a pleural effusion is present, suction will remove the fluid from the pleural space. However, as the lung contracts during expiration, it is important to prevent air and the effusion fluid from returning to the chest cavity. This will not occur because the tube is sealed under water.

When a commercial drainage system such as the Pleur-evac is used, three separate chambers (formerly bottles) are usually visible. The first compartment collects the fluid from the chest, the second is the water-seal chamber, and the third is the suction control chamber. It maintains proper suction and limits the negative pressure applied to the pleura. This is usually set at 20 cm of water, negative pressure for adults.[33,34] If the flow rate is increased by turning up the suction regulator, more vigorous bubbling will occur in the suction control chamber, and air or fluid will be pulled more quickly from the chest. Because the water level is set at 20 cm H_2O, however, no increase will occur in the negative pressure applied to the pleural cavity.

A few specific factors must be assessed once the chest tube system is in place. If the patient has a pleural effusion rather than a pneumothorax, bubbling in the water-seal chamber could indicate a leak in the system. The nurse should clamp the drainage tube near the patient with a padded hemostat, and if the bubbling stops, there is probably a leak at the insertion site or inside the pleural cavity. If the bubbling does not stop when the tube is clamped, a leak is present in the system itself; the most likely place is the link between the chest tube and the drainage system. This must always be secured with adhesive tape to reduce the risk of air leakage. Great caution must be exercised when using clamps on a chest tube. If air or fluid can no longer come out of the pleural space but is still entering the space through the lung, a tension pneumothorax can ensue. This situation is serious because, with increased tension in the pleural space, the mediastinum is shifted to the opposite side and blood return to the heart is dangerously impaired. If no

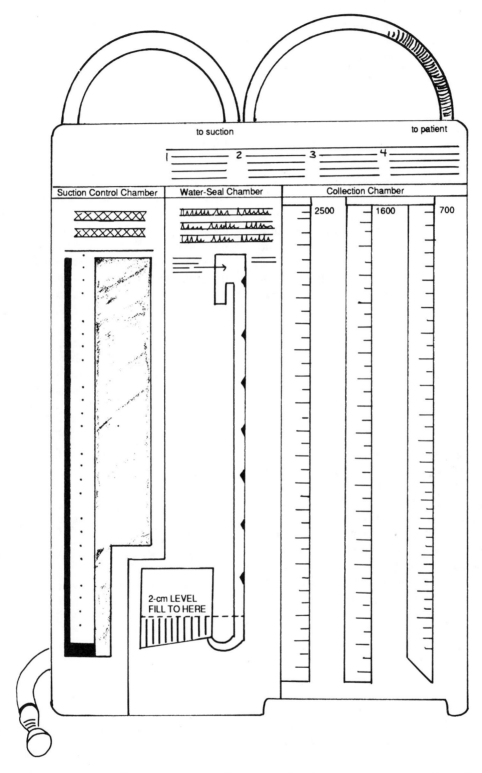

Figure 14-8   Example of Pleur-evac underwater seal drainage system. (Drawing by Julie Beets.)

blood is available for cardiac output, the blood pressure is unobtainable and the patient will be in respiratory distress.[33,34]

It is rarely necessary to clamp a chest tube. Even if the chest tube becomes disconnected from the system, it is easier to reconnect it than to clamp the tube, reconnect, and then unclamp the tube. In certain instances, the clamp may be forgotten and tension pneumothorax may result. Patients can be moved and ambulated with no problem as long as the water seal is kept intact.

Stripping and milking the chest tube can also be dangerous because suction is created, affecting the pleural space. This procedure may be done if the tube is obstructed by a blood clot or other material. Pressure as "high as 350 cm H_2O has been recorded with stripping. . . . Milking is a more gentle form of stripping; both forms use manual compression between the chest tube and drainage system."[34] To prevent obstruction, the nurse must ensure that there is good gravity drainage from the patient to the unit. Any dependent loop of tubing or tubing laid on the bed can create back pressure.

Unless fluid is within the drainage tube, raising the system above the chest causes no problem. Even if drained fluid is within the tubing, the only harm would be fluid returning to the pleural space. This may not be pleasant, but it is not an emergency. Other minor problems can develop, but usually these are not life-threatening. (For an in-depth and excellent chart on troubleshooting chest drainage problems, see Erickson.[33,34])

Because malignant pleural effusion carries a poor prognosis in lung cancer (two thirds of patients will die within 3 months), the primary management goal is to control symptoms.[93] As previously stated, an agent such as the antibiotic doxycycline can be used to sclerose the patient's lung with relatively good results. Although more expensive, some physicians prefer to use bleomycin as a sclerosing agent because little or no pain is associated with its instillation. More important than any antineoplastic activity is the sclerosis of the pleura that the agent produces to prevent fluid reaccumulation.

Sclerosing is accomplished by instilling doxycyline or talc through a thoracostomy tube. Closed-tube thoracostomy attached to water-seal drainage with gentle suction (usually 20 cm H_2O) should be in place 24 to 48 hours before pleural sclerosing to promote chest drainage. Sclerosis is usually done when the total chest tube output for 24 hours is less than 100 ml. This procedure is not nearly as painful as in the past when tetracycline was used. It has been reported that only mild chest pain was experienced when doxycycline was used as the sclerosing agent, but 4 of 18 patients needed narcotic relief; patients are usually given morphine sulfate, 5 to 10 mg IVP, 30 minutes before the procedure. Lidocaine (150 mg) can be added to the doxycycline medium, and the solution is instilled through the chest tube to sclerose the pleura. The chest tube is then clamped for 2 hours, and the patient is turned side to side, onto the stomach, and in Trendelenburg and reverse Trendelenburg positions every 15 minutes to ensure equal distribution of the doxycycline. The tube is then unclamped, left to drain for 12 to 24 hours, and removed if chest tube drainage is minimal. Sclerosing can be repeated again in 24 hours, if necessary.

ELDERLY PATIENTS WITH LUNG CANCER

The incidence and risk of developing cancer increase with age because of several related factors, including accumulation of or repeated contact with carcinogens, decreased immunologic resistance, hormonal imbalance, and age-related cell alterations that influence susceptibility to cancer.[114] Lung cancer, in particular, may be ignored because the vague symptoms can be linked with the aging process, such as fatigue, decreased appetite, nonspecific aches and pains, and even a cough.[26]

Treatment modalities associated with lung cancer can be devastating to older persons, especially if they are already debilitated. Chemotherapy not only suppresses already tired bone marrow, but also causes severe compromise to the patient's nutritional status (see box below). Many clinicians automatically reduce chemotherapy

---

IMPACT OF CANCER, CANCER TREATMENT, AND AGING ON NUTRITION

CANCER AND CANCER TREATMENT	AGING
Tumor/host competition	Impaired ability to plan/ prepare meals
Increased requirements	Psychologic/social/ sensorimotor factors
Malabsorption/obstruction	
Taste alteration (dysgeusia)	Impaired taste
	Decreased salivation
Anorexia	Slowing of digestive process
Nausea/vomiting	
Mucositis/esophagitis	Mastication difficulties
Depression/fatigue	Coexisting pathology
Early satiety	Altered hormonal secretions
Fluid and electrolyte imbalance	

INCREASED RISK OF:

Weight loss	Susceptibility to infection
Malnutrition	Depression, apathy
Cachexia	Impaired tolerance to treatment
Muscle wasting	
Impaired wound healing	Poor prognosis

From Sims S: *Nurs Times* 84:29, 1988.

doses based on a patient's age. Others examine factors such as the physiologic rather than the chronologic age and the likelihood of cure when making decisions about doses. Intensity of chemotherapy and quality of life in elderly patients have become a focus for research, particularly because of the shortened survival time associated with a lung cancer diagnosis.[95] In a retrospective review of chemotherapy for SCLC in elderly patients (age 70 or older), intensive chemotherapy (CAV regimen) was associated with more severe toxicities and deaths compared with less intensive therapy (single agent, radiation alone).[37] However, those who received more intense treatment survived about 5 months longer. The authors concluded that the small survival advantage did not justify the severe toxicities of intense chemotherapy. Johnson and others[61] cite two reports using the single agent etoposide, which was well tolerated by elderly patients. One of the trials used oral etoposide (160 mg/m^2) on days 1 to 5 every 4 weeks in previously untreated SCLC patients age 70 and older.[116] There was a 71% response rate among 35 patients, and median survival (16 months in LD and 9 months in ED) was comparable with that achieved with combination regimens. No patient required hospitalization for neutropenia and fever, and toxicities were mild. Clearly, more research is needed in defining who among elderly lung cancer patients might benefit from treatment.

Radiation therapy is notorious for causing increased fatigue, which can cause increased problems in patients who probably have other chronic diseases. One important related consequence of lung cancer in elderly persons is decreased comfort, both physical and psychologic. The attitude held by many caregivers may compromise the level of comfort afforded to elderly patients. Engelking[31] gives an example of a 70-year-old lung cancer patient and states, ". . . the caregiver who automatically anticipates reduced breathing capacity subsequent to the patient's age might underdose the patient with narcotic analgesics or hold back sleep medications because of concern about respiratory compromise." Psychosocially, these patients may want to learn how to care for themselves at home and obtain assistance with this care and may be anxious about the increased costs of treatment and decreased insurance coverage. In addition, the patient may already be caring for an ill spouse in the home.[42]

Many of these issues encompass all patients with cancer; however, the concern with patients with lung cancer is their usually limited survival time after diagnosis. For elderly patients, adjustments to change often come with greater difficulty, and the adjustment to lung cancer and its treatments must be made rapidly. Consequently, the nurse must be alerted to these particular problems so he or she can provide timely interventions for these patients' rapidly increasing nursing care needs.

REHABILITATION
Activity Maintenance

Little has been written on long-term survival of patients with lung cancer. Those who survive and complete their course of treatment may experience problems with radiation pneumonitis and pulmonary fibrosis, second malignancies, and neurologic complications (e.g., memory loss, confusion, ataxia, vision loss, dysphagia) from PCI. It is important to encourage patients and family members with supportive counseling, but the nurse must also offer some concrete suggestions for maintaining activities of daily living in the face of an altered life-style (see box below).

Pulmonary program. Patients with pulmonary fibrosis may experience exacerbation of dyspnea, which can be frightening for both the patient and the family. If this can be anticipated and measures made available to help control the physical sensations, fear and anxiety will be reduced. Family members or significant others must be aware of what to expect and what to do if breathing difficulties ensue. Most people become agitated, diaphoretic, and pale, and they gasp for breath. They may speak with short, staccato words and have a frozen appearance with large, staring eyes.[6] Patients must be educated in strategies for managing dyspnea (see box, p. 332). A grading scale for dyspnea may be helpful for

---

MODIFICATIONS OF ACTIVITIES OF DAILY LIVING FOR PATIENT/FAMILY EXPERIENCING LUNG CANCER

Do not treat patient as an invalid just because his or her activity tolerance has decreased.

Encourage the spouse/children to include patient in family decision making.

Help patient establish a new daily routine with realistic goals:
- Patient can assist with small tasks (e.g., make lunches, fold clothes, help kids with homework, pay bills if mentally alert).
- Patient should try to accomplish one major task every day, every other day, or every week.

Encourage patient to have some small activity to anticipate (e.g., visit from a friend, ride in the car, church prayer meeting, eat out at a restaurant, call a friend long distance, participate in a support group [patient can help others as well as himself or herself], enjoy nature).

If larger-scale activities are possible, encourage them but caution patient to use moderation (e.g., take a trip [there is an oncology nurse to whom patient can be referred in almost every U.S. city], participate in an activity you have always wanted to do [e.g., hot-air balloon ride], take a class).

STRATEGIES FOR MANAGING DYSPNEA

BREATHING

Teach new breathing pattern:
  Take slow, deep breaths.
  Use diaphragm.
  Exhale through pursed lips.
  Exhale longer than inhale.

POSITIONING

Have patient assume comfortable position:
  Sit on bedside, fold arms over pillow on bedside table.
  Sit on chair, feet wide apart, elbows resting on knees.
  Lean on wall, feet apart, shoulders relaxed and bent forward.
  Elevate head of bed.

EMOTIONAL SUPPORT

Do not leave patient in distress alone:
  Observe patient frequently.
  Place frequent phone call to patient on home care.
  Teach coaching and support to family or caregiver.

RELAXATION

Remember that relaxation conserves oxygen:
  Place hands on patient's shoulders and press downward.
  Dangle arms and rotate shoulders.

PLANNED ACTIVITY

Have patient conserve energy and get adequate rest:
  Assess normal life-style and activities of daily living.
  Plan chores around rest period.
  Establish support for household activities and recreation.

OXYGEN THERAPY

Provide oxygen supply and implement safety precautions.
Provide instructions regarding smoking, storage, heat, and use of equipment.

PHARMACOLOGIC AGENTS

Some agents relieve dyspnea, especially in patients who are terminally ill:
  Sedatives
  Narcotics
  Steroids
  Scopolamine

From Haylock P: *Semin Oncol Nurs* 3:293, 1987.

the patient to describe the severity of current symptoms. If instructed to grade the dyspnea on a scale from 0 to 10, with 0 being no difficulty and 10 being unable to breathe, patients can more accurately relate the problem.[40] Critical nursing assessment and identification of specific management techniques can prevent a crisis. The

patient and caregiver will feel more comfortable knowing that, although dyspnea may occur, a program is in place to manage it.

Exercise and relaxation techniques. Most patients who have been successfully treated for lung cancer or are presently undergoing treatment realize intellectually that they must begin exercising gradually, but many do not comply. Exercise is a positive reinforcer for patients in that it helps them feel good and increases their activity tolerance, but the nurse must caution the patient against too much exercise and activity too soon.

An assessment should be made of anticipated activities and activity tolerance. The patient's overall state of health will dictate level of functioning and ability to maintain an exercise program. Relaxation techniques and guided imagery also are helpful during stressful treatment regimens and the anxiety-producing posttreatment period.

Available self-help audio tapes include the following:
- *Healing Journey: The Healing Image* by Emmett Miller, MD, PO Box W, Standord, CA 94309
- *Music for Mellow Minds* by Janalea Hoffman, Mellow Minds, PO Box 6431, Shawnee Mission, KS 66206
- *Fresh Country Rain: The Essence of Relaxation* by Nature's Ensemble, Platinum Disc Corp, Canada

The effective management of short-term and long-term side effects from lung cancer treatment is essential for patient rehabilitation. The activities listed foster hope in patients with lung cancer and assure them that they are not forgotten or abandoned. However, Bernhard and Ganz[7,8] explain that although there is a high incidence of lung cancer, little is known about the various related psychosocial issues[104] (Table 14-2). Increasing the knowledge base relative to the psychosocial impact of lung cancer will assist the nurse in planning appropriate intervention programs and promoting optimal use of resources. Overcoming as many treatment barriers as possible will motivate the patient and family toward achieving increased and sustained independence.

HOME HEALTH AND HOSPICE

Most lung cancer patients will experience progressive disease with increasing symptoms and consequently increased dependency on others for self-care needs. Inherent in such a downhill trajectory is the need for frequent interventions and/or hospitalizations. In one study the most common reasons for hospital admissions of lung cancer patients were cancer therapy (primary reason), respiratory problems, gastrointestinal symptoms, pain, anemia, and thrombocytopenia.[75] At issue is how to maintain the best quality of life for these patients. Because diagnosis-related groups (DRGs) and cost containment have relegated so much care to the outpatient setting, early referral to home health is often indicated, prefer-

Table 14-2 Currently Available Data Base on Disease-Related and Treatment-Related Psychosocial Issues in Lung Cancer

Symptoms	Data availability
Psychosocial impact of surgery	Partly available
Acute side effects of chemotherapy	Well documented
Late side effects of chemotherapy	Partly available
Side effects of radiotherapy	Not available
Pain	Partly available
Dyspnea	Well documented
Cognitive changes	Well documented
Sleep disorders	Not available
Psychologic distress	Partly available
Social interaction	Partly available
Consequences for patient's next of kin	Not available
Multidisciplinary interventions in regard to:	
Anticipatory nausea and vomiting	Partly available
Learned food aversions	Partly available
Self-care of dyspnea	Not available
Pain management	Not available
Management of sleep disorders	Not available

Modified from Bernhard J, Ganz P: *Chest* 99:480, 1991.

ably to an agency that allows patients to convert to hospice care when appropriate. Early referral (within 2 months of diagnosis) of patients eligible for home health care compared with routine follow-up through a physician's office was associated with a 6-week delay in symptom distress, a longer period of independence, and a more realistic perception of declining health.[75] In addition, patients referred to specialized oncology home care rather than standard home care or routine physician's office follow-up spent fewer days hospitalized. This finding, although not statistically significant, is of economic significance and suggests that oncology specialization among registered nurses contributes to improved symptom management at home and reduction of hospitalized days.

Nurses caring for lung cancer patients in the home setting today may be involved in their actual therapy through chemotherapy administration and management of side effects. The nurse's knowledge base must include use of present technology (e.g., care of various central venous or arterial access devices, patient-controlled analgesia [PCA] pumps, epidural catheters). Nursing expertise to assist patients in understanding chronic pain management (e.g., use of scheduled versus PRN narcotics, oral dosing in preference to use of pumps when appropriate, prophylactic bowel regimens to prevent constipation) may obviate trips to the emergency room or hospitalizations. Patient and family may need assistance to understand the important role of low-dose morphine (2.5 to 5 mg every 4 hours) because it acts centrally in the brain to relieve severe dyspnea and "air hunger" associ-

ated with end-stage respiratory compromise. Compassionate nursing can assist families to know what to expect and how to deal with these events, particularly when death may be that event. Death from fatal hemoptysis, although sometimes feared, is rare; only 3.3% of patients in one large series died of exsanguination from tumor eroding through a major pulmonary vessel.[65] Historically, 60% of lung cancer patients die from tumor causing airway obstruction, postobstructive pneumonia, and sepsis.[62] Caring and knowledgeable home health and hospice nurses can do much to reduce the suffering associated with lung cancer.

PROGNOSIS
Prognostic Factors

Three factors play a major role in the prognosis of lung cancer: extent of disease, cell type, and patient's performance status. The survival rate for patients with localized disease is 37%; however, survival at 5 years is 13% for all patients regardless of stage at diagnosis.[2] This represents a slight improvement in overall survival since the early 1970s.[92] Prognosis is best for patients with well-differentiated squamous cell lung cancer, and those with SCLC have the poorest survival rate. Performance status is critical in determining the patient's treatment regimen and therefore the prognosis. Patients who are ambulatory tolerate treatment better than those who are not fully ambulatory but are out of bed 50% of the time. Prognosis continues to decline as the patient becomes more debilitated. Age, gender, weight loss, and immune status also affect the patient's response to treatment.[6] Physiologic rather than chronologic age is the important assessment factor when making treatment decisions, and age may influence treatment options and prognosis in elderly patients, as discussed earlier.

Adenocarcinoma is more predominant in female lung cancer patients, whereas squamous cell cancer is more prevalent in male patients. Overall, women with lung cancer survive longer than their male counterparts in the United States.[44] In addition to the previous prognostic factors, weight loss of greater than 10 pounds in 6 months is not a favorable sign. Patients with an intact immune system, as evidenced by a normal reaction to an immunologic challenge, will respond better.[59] Patients with SCLC have an immune deficit that may contribute to the rapid growth of this cancer.[12] Because any lung cancer patient will be exposed to multimodality treatment, it is important to be able to predict tolerance to such intense therapy.

Correlation with Histologic Cell Type and Stage

Non–small cell lung cancer. The AJCC classification system and new international staging system are used to determine the best therapy modalities for NSCLC. Successful treatment with surgery or radiation therapy is possible in most patients with stage I disease; however, only 25% to 30% of patients present with stage I or II NSCLC.[81,83] Adjuvant chemotherapy is currently being investigated for use in patients with early-stage disease.[9] For patients who present with widespread advanced disease, the administration of new combinations of chemotherapy has shown only a slight survival benefit.

Even with new treatment combinations, benefits and cure rates are modest. Five-year survival rates after resection for early-stage NSCLC are reasonably good and have continued to improve as the result of stricter patient selection and progressive nursing support.[29] These patients with later-stage disease (stage IIIa) have a better prognosis if mediastinal lymph nodes are not involved.[36]

Patients with squamous cell cancer survive longer than those with adenocarcinoma and large cell undifferentiated carcinoma. Also, patients with stage I squamous cell cancer do significantly better than those with stage II or III tumors.[81] Table 14-3 outlines the overall 5-year postoperative survival of lung cancer patients with squamous cell carcinoma and adenocarcinoma.

Depending on the TNM status and cell type of stage IIIA patients, survival ranges from 18% to 40%. The outlook for stage IIIB and IV patients remains bleak, but therapeutic strategies, including biologic response modifiers and monoclonal antibodies, are continually being pursued.[81] More successful treatments for NSCLC are being discovered, although slowly.

Small cell lung cancer. Given the great biologic and clinical difference from other lung cancer types, SCLC

is also staged differently. Patients with limited-stage disease who are treated with combination chemotherapy experience a 12- to 16-month median survival time and a 15% to 35% 2-year disease-free survival rate.[81] Recent combined radiation-chemotherapy approaches show 24% to 54% survival at 2 years in LD.[1,20,61,125] Unfortunately, patients with SCLC may still relapse 5 years after treatment.[120] Without treatment, SCLC results in death in about 3 months.[57] The best approach for long-term survival in limited-stage SCLC appears to be combination chemotherapy and radiation therapy to the chest. Researchers advocate alternating chemotherapy treatment cycles to prevent resistance to the drugs.[35] However, clinical trials have failed to demonstrate improved survival by this technique, perhaps because of the inability to define truly non-cross-resistant regimens.[49]

In stages I and II LD, patients without mediastinal node involvement who underwent surgical resection and received combination chemotherapy after surgery had a 5-year survival rate of 35%.[41] These patients represent less than 5% of SCLC patients. For patients with stage III disease, preoperative chemotherapy followed by surgery was attempted without dramatic results. Many randomized prospective studies have incorporated all the treatment modalities both alone and in combination. Although investigations continue to search for the best combination, preliminary data suggest benefit from combined therapy in limited SCLC if full doses of chemotherapy and radiation therapy are given.[1,20]

The majority of patients (70%) with SCLC have extensive disease, and the outlook for their survival is dismal. From 7% to 20% of these patients will be alive 2 years after diagnosis.[1] Radiation plays a major role in local control and in symptom management to limit or modify cranial and bone metastasis and SVCS. Many patients with extensive disease respond to therapy involving a combination of drugs and achieve notable palliation.

In a review of SWOG trials, one versus multiple metastatic sites was a predictor of survival. For patients with a single site, median survival was 12 months versus only 7 months for those with multiple metastatic sites. Other factors predictive of survival are a normal LDH and absence of a pleural effusion.[1]

Patients with extensive disease who experience a complete remission will usually survive beyond the median time frame.[22] Although initial responses can be dramatic for both limited and extensive SCLC, long-term survival is worse than that seen with NSCLC. SCLC overall survival rate at 2 years is less than 10%.[20,49] More knowledge about this disease and new agents or treatment combinations are needed to obtain better outcomes.

Table 14-3 Five-Year Postoperative Survival by TNM Groups Based on Data From Lung Cancer Study Group Trials

Classification	Percent surviving squamous cell carcinoma (*n* = 549)	Percent surviving adenocarcinoma (*n* = 572)
Stage I		
T1-N0	83	69 (*p* = 0.02)
T2-N0	64	57
Stage II		
T1-N1	75	52 (*p* = 0.04)
T2-N1	53	25 (*p* ≤ 0.01)
Stage IIIA		
T1, T2-N2	46	35
T3-N0	37	21

From Carmack Holmes E: *Staging non–small cell lung cancer,* Evansville, Ind, 1992, Bristol-Meyers Squibb.

Text continued on p. 342.

NURSING MANAGEMENT

Nursing diagnoses related to lung cancer listed below are followed by nursing interventions for various treatments and rehabilitation.

NURSING DIAGNOSES: Primary

- *Knowledge deficit related to prevention of lung cancer (see p. 315 for suggested educational guidelines)*
- *Breathing pattern, ineffective, related to loss of adequate ventilation (actual or potential)*
- *Gas exchange, impaired, related to decreased passage of gases between alveoli of lungs and vascular system (actual or potential)*
- *Knowledge deficit related to a new medical condition, new treatments, surgical procedures (preoperative and postoperative), medications*
- *Nutrition, altered: less than body requirements, related to anorexia*
- *Pain related to liver and/or bone metastasis (actual or potential)*
- *Thought processes, altered, related to brain metastasis (actual or potential)*
- *Fatigue related to treatment and treatment sequelae*

NURSING DIAGNOSIS: Secondary

- *Anxiety related to dyspnea*
- *Powerlessness related to hospitalization and feelings of lack of control*
- *Noncompliance (potential) related to negative side effects of prescribed treatments*
- *Grieving, dysfunctional, related to loss of function of body system*
- *Body image disturbance related to loss of body functions*
- *Sexual dysfunction related to change of body part, physiologic limitations*
- *Coping, ineffective individual, related to rapidly progressive disease process*
- *Coping, ineffective family: compromised, related to rapidly progressive disease process*

OUTCOME GOALS: Surgery

Patient will be able to:
- State which surgical diagnostic and operative procedures will be done (e.g., mediastinoscopy, lobectomy) and why.
- Communicate surgical discomfort and request adequate medication for relief.
- Understand the different modalities for medication administration (e.g., IV, epidural).
- Consume appropriate foods and liquids to maintain nutritional status.

- Relate importance of pulmonary hygiene and comply with necessary maintenance (cough and deep breathe [C&DB], exercise).
- Understand importance of smoking cessation before surgery and attempt to quit.
- Understand that mechanical ventilation and chest tubes may be necessary and why.
- Express concerns related to body image, life-style changes, and sexuality issues.

SURGERY

Surgical nursing care begins during the diagnostic period for those patients requiring *mediastinoscopy* (small suprasternal incision) or *mediastinotomy* (small parasternal incision that allows direct visualization of lymph nodes or through which left mediastinal lymph nodes or even a primary lung tumor may be biopsied) for tissue diagnosis and/or staging purposes. Monitoring blood pressure, pulse, and respirations and observing dressings for indication of internal or external bleeding are necessary in the immediate postoperative period. Fever can indicate mediastinitis; crepitus can indicate air leakage into subcutaneous tissues; and the development of dyspnea, cyanosis, or decreased breath sounds can be signs of pneumothorax.[71,78] Postoperative local pain requires analgesics (see box, p. 321).

In patients who undergo thoracotomy for wedge resection, lobectomy, or pneumonectomy, nursing care is more complex. Standard nursing concerns with these patients are the same as for other cancer surgeries (e.g., adequate nutritional state, coping mechanisms, risk of postoperative emboli) (see Chapter 20).

Malnutrition, hypoalbuminemia, smoking history, and chronic obstructive pulmonary disease (COPD) place lung cancer patients at higher risk of postoperative complications such as pneumonia, fistula formation, and respiratory or congestive heart failure.[76] Preoperative or postoperative total parenteral nutrition (TPN) may be necessary to improve nutritional status and promote recovery from thoracotomy. If surgery is delayed, smokers should be advised to stop smoking at least a few weeks before surgery. Although preoperative pulmonary function studies should predict patients' ability to undergo surgery, they need to know before thoracotomy that they may be placed on a ventilator and will have one or more chest tubes after the procedure.

The most common postoperative complication is *cardiac dysrhythmia*. Often asymptomatic, it is responsive to appropriate drugs.[44] The nature of drainage from chest tubes placed after partial pulmonary resection can reveal bleeding complications or development of empyema. In

Continued.

patients who become agitated, confused, and then dyspneic and hypoxic, serious alterations in ventilation and respiration are likely, and monitoring vital signs, breath sounds, and blood gases is important. Diligent aspiration of the tracheobronchial tree with frequent deep breathing and coughing can prevent mechanical obstruction and pneumonia resulting from the accumulation of secretions. However, deep suctioning that could cause trauma to the suture line must be avoided.[71]

The need for good pulmonary toilet cannot be overemphasized. Patients may experience much fear and discomfort associated with chest tubes or a ventilator, for which medication may be required. Good pain management, a major nursing concern after thoracotomy, can enhance mobility, coughing, and deep breathing. An epidural catheter to control pain may be placed during surgery; this enables the patient to recover more comfortably. Some patients may need narcotic analgesics for several months after the procedure to ease persistent pain. For prolonged postoperative pain, nerve blocks or other interventions should be considered. Depending on the amount of healthy lung tissue remaining after surgery, most patients will not experience severe respiratory compromise affecting life-style activities.[29] See the box at right for patient teaching priorities related to surgical procedures.

RADIATION THERAPY

OUTCOME GOALS

Patient will be able to:

- State which acute, site-specific side effects will occur after chest and/or brain radiation therapy (RT) (e.g., possible nausea/vomiting, radiation pneumonitis, fatigue, skin reaction, myelosuppression, difficulty swallowing, headache, hair loss) and how to treat them.
- State which long-term side effects may occur after RT (e.g., pulmonary fibrosis, sexuality concerns, radiation recall with chemotherapy, memory loss, confusion, weakness).
- Consume appropriate foods and liquids to maintain nutritional status.
- State procedure for RT treatment (e.g., simulation, blocks, treatment time).
- Communicate discomfort with swallowing and request adequate medication for relief.

Radiation to the Chest

Side effects experienced during or after radiation therapy will vary depending on (1) the organ systems or normal tissue within the radiation port (field), (2) the amount and duration of radiation, and (3) the type of concurrent or recent chemotherapy. When radiation is given to the primary tumor in the chest, portions of normal lung tissue, heart, skin, and contents of the mediastinum (major ves-

PATIENT TEACHING PRIORITIES
Surgery for Lung Cancer

Preoperative

Have patient relate knowledge of reason for surgery preoperatively.

Describe the type of procedure to be done (e.g., wedge resection, lobectomy, pneumonectomy).

Discuss need for optimal ventilation (stop smoking, cough, take deep breaths immediately after surgery).

Explain need for leg and arm exercises. Shoulder on affected side will be very sore and must be moved to prevent frozen shoulder.

Discuss different methods of pain relief (IM, IV, epidural) with patient. Encourage patient to ask for medication when needed. This promotes coughing and deep breathing.

Explain postoperative routine and that patient will most likely have a chest tube in place.

Postoperative

Reinforce need for early ambulation despite chest tube and also need to cough and deep breathe.

Reinforce all postoperative routines previously taught.

Review surgical results with patient and ensure proper follow-up.

Explore with patient the implications of altered body image:

- Changes in life-style
- Verbalization of fear of rejection and reaction of others
- Changes in relationships
- Problems with sexuality

sels, trachea, esophagus) may also receive radiation, although the dose will be much lower. By noting the tattoos or marks delineating the radiation port on the patient's chest, the nurse can make some predictions about the effects of radiation on normal tissues. Although efforts are made to block vital organs, some side effects are unavoidable. Nursing interventions focus on avoidance, relief, or management of side effects (see box, p. 337).

Skin alterations related to radiation are much less severe than in the past. Equipment has been improved so it can deliver the radiation beneath the surface of the skin and more directly to the desired depth and location. Nursing assessment of skin integrity, the patient's complaints, and knowledge of anticipated side effects form the basis of interventions. Skin damage may be only mild erythema or can progress to dry and then moist desquamation. If moist desquamation occurs, radiation treatments will likely be interrupted.[28] Therefore teaching should highlight preventive care: avoid constrictive clothing

PATIENT TEACHING PRIORITIES
Radiation Therapy for Lung Cancer

General side effects of radiation therapy

Explain measures to limit, as necessary, patient's activities during treatment to conserve energy.

Discuss measures to maintain adequate nutritional intake.

Explain measures to control radiodermatitis if necessary.

Describe rationale and measures to take following a decrease in hematopoietic function.

Discuss reasons for and measures to deal with sexuality concerns.

Site-specific side effects

Describe signs and symptoms of pneumonitis, esophagitis, and cough.

Discuss measures to maintain adequate oxygenation.

Consider forcing fluids to loosen thick secretions.

Administer antiemetics for nausea/vomiting.

Caution patient to avoid tobacco and alcohol.

Note availability of patient information booklets.

Emotional support

Educate patient/family regarding radiation therapy procedures to decrease anxiety.

Explain that side effects may last for 2 to 4 weeks after treatment completion.

Ensure understanding of anxiety or grief process because of illness and reassure patient that this is normal response.

over irradiated areas; avoid tape, perfume, deodorants, iodine, talcum, or other irritating substances on irradiated skin; wear soft cotton clothing over skin; and avoid heat, cold, or sunlight on these areas. The skin should be kept dry and open to the air when possible. For tender or dry skin, use water-based ointments (e.g., A&D Ointment, hydrous lanolin) rather than oil-based creams or ointments, which may contain heavy metals. Vigorous scrubbing or rubbing is to be avoided, but use of gentle soaps (e.g., Aveeno, Dove) is usually allowed.[110] If moist desquamation occurs, the area may be cleansed with quarter-strength hydrogen peroxide and normal saline, rinsed gently with saline, and patted dry.[28] Areas of skin breakdown should be monitored for infection. Moisture-vapor-permeable dressings (Op-site, Tegaderm) may offer protection to these areas.[111] Most patients have skin reactions by their last week of therapy. Administration of certain chemotherapeutic drugs (e.g., dactinomycin, doxorubicin) during therapy or close to the time radiation therapy starts can lead to radiation recall, and erythema or skin breakdown may occur.[28]

Sore throat resulting from esophagitis can develop by the third week of radiation therapy.[28] If the pain is severe, food and fluid intake may be decreased because of difficulty swallowing. Patients should be advised that, if this occurs, they should contact the nurse or physician. A nasogastric feeding tube or a percutaneous endoscopic gastrostomy (PEG) may be placed to assist the patient with nutrition intake. Not only can nutrition be impaired, but esophagitis may also become a source for infection. If signs of candidiasis (white, adherent plaques) are present in the oral cavity, an antifungal agent should be prescribed (Mycelex Troches, nystatin, ketoconazole). A soft, bland diet (non-citrus) and nutritional supplements (e.g., Ensure, Instant Breakfast) can be beneficial.[28,110] If weight loss resulting from esophagitis occurs, the patient should be weighed daily and evaluated for dehydration. A mixture of diphenhydramine elixir, viscous lidocaine, and Mylanta or Amphojel (depending on the consistency of the patient's stools) in a 1:1:1 ratio can be administered as a swish-and-swallow remedy when esophagitis is painful (5 ml before meals and as needed). Systemic analgesics may be required.

Nutritional status can be further compromised by *anorexia,* which occurs in most patients by the fourth week of treatment.[28] Anorexic patients should be encouraged to eat small amounts frequently. The book *Eating Hints* by the NCI may aid patients and their families in discovering types of food more tolerable to these patients. The addition of small amounts of powdered milk to appropriate foods will also increase protein intake. Good nutrition is essential to repair and heal normal tissues during radiation therapy.

Fatigue is a major problem in more than 90% of patients by the third week of treatment.[28] Patients should be so warned and guided into planning any activities with scheduled rest periods. Symptoms may persist for months after completion of radiation therapy.[28]

If more than 25% of active bone marrow is in the radiation port, *myelosuppression* may occur. Complete blood counts should be done weekly during therapy. Neutropenia and thrombocytopenia precede a drop in hemoglobin. Packed red blood cells may be transfused if the hemoglobin drops below 10 g, since effective radiation treatment depends on an adequate oxygen supply to the tumor.[110] If the white blood cell count drops below 3000/mm^3 or the platelets drop below 40,000/mm^3, radiation therapy may be temporarily discontinued.

Radiation pneumonitis occurs infrequently but is dose-limiting if it develops during radiation treatments. Since it is dose dependent, it can occur 3 to 24 weeks after therapy.[6] In acute radiation pneumonitis, a hacking cough or mild chest pain might be the first symptom. Signs and symptoms also include dyspnea and hypoxia, fever, and night sweats; evidence of interstitial or alveolar infiltrates is seen on chest x-ray films; and the sputum is negative for pathogens.[6] The severity of symptoms cor-

Continued.

relates with the dose and lung volume irradiated. In severe cases, pneumonitis may be associated with hemoptysis, fever, chills, or abscess and may even result in death.[76] Usually, doses of 45 Gy or less will not lead to severe toxicity, and pneumonitis will resolve, often within 3 to 4 weeks.[76] Patients may require temporary hospitalization for administration of oxygen, steroids, antibiotics, sedatives, and cough suppressants. Cultures are obtained to rule out infection, but antibiotics may be given empirically. Steroids are the cornerstone of therapy for radiation pneumonitis. At the start of therapy, patients should be given at least 60 mg of prednisone per day. Tapering is carried out very gradually, and the patient must be monitored for any recurrence of symptoms.

Coping strategies for *dyspnea* are often self-taught but may include position changes, moving slowly, and planning in advance for activities. If pneumonitis leads to subsequent scarring and tissue changes (pulmonary fibrosis), chest auscultation will reveal muffled and diminished vesicular sounds, rhonchi, and wheezes from airflow across narrowed airways. Late fibrotic changes resemble severe chronic obstructive pulmonary disease and can lead to anxiety and fear with dyspnea.[122]

Cardiac toxicities, although minimal today because of blocking techniques, can include pericarditis, the classic symptom for which is chest pain, or a pericardial effusion and tamponade, which involves increased central venous pressure, evidenced by jugular venous distention followed by tachycardia, dyspnea, and cough (see Chapter 19). Cardiac toxicities usually depend on delivery of at least 40 Gy to the heart.

Radiation to the Brain

Radiation to the brain can lead to hair loss, but the severity of hair loss is usually dose dependent. At doses of 15 to 30 Gy, the degree of hair loss is variable. At a dose of 50 Gy or more, permanent loss is likely.[28,55] Because PCI in SCLC is usually no more than 30 Gy, hair will begin to regrow about 3 to 4 weeks after the completion of radiation therapy. However, hair loss after PCI will be temporarily complete, including the eyebrows. (See Chapter 32 for resources and ways to deal with hair loss.)

During brain irradiation, patients receive dexamethasone to reduce the resultant edema of brain tissue. However, symptoms of neurologic impairment related to edema should be monitored and may include irritability, confusion, restlessness, headaches, memory loss, a change in personality or mental status, nausea, unequal or decreased pupil reactivity to light, elevated blood pressure, sensory or motor changes, or a drop in pulse rate. Cerebral edema can lead to obstruction of the eustachian tube with resultant local ear pain or infection.[28]

Late effects of whole-brain irradiation (WBI) in long-term survivors may be even more severe when it is given concurrently with chemotherapy. Findings reflecting neurologic injury can include memory loss, problems in judgment, parkinsonian symptoms, weakness, confusion, depression, dizziness, organic brain syndrome, abnormal gait, ataxia, intention tremors, inability to concentrate, and cerebral atrophy.[1,12] Symptoms have become so severe that one patient had to quit work and another was placed in an extended care facility.[1] Any sequelae such as these should be documented, and the physician should be notified for possible CT or MRI evaluation. Any such changes could also herald a CNS relapse. The box below lists potential radiation treatment–related complications of lung cancer.

Radiation Implant

Implants may be used to treat large and otherwise inaccessible tumor masses in the lung. Nursing care of these patients follows guidelines discussed on p. 321. For an excellent HDR brachytherapy guide regarding nursing care and patient educational material, the reader is referred to Jordan and Mantravadi.[62] Patient teaching related to radiation therapy should include the information given in the box below.

COMPLICATIONS
Radiation Treatment for Lung Cancer*

From radiation to chest

Skin erythema to wet desquamation
Esophagitis, dysphagia, strictures, weight loss
Acute pneumonitis or pulmonary fibrosis (dyspnea, hypoxemia, chronic or temporary oxygen and steroid dependency)
Pericarditis, dysrhythmias, pericardial effusion, congestive heart failure
Myelosuppression (sepsis, bleeding, fatigue)
Fatigue

From radiation to brain

Early and usually temporary effects: hair loss, skin erythema, nausea
Signs of cerebral edema that need immediate attention during radiation: irritability, confusion, restlessness, headaches, nausea, change in personality, sensory or motor changes
Late and permanent effects: memory loss, problems in judgment, parkinsonian symptoms, weakness, confusion, depression, dizziness, organic brain syndrome, abnormal gait, intention tremor, inability to concentrate, loss of self-care or work capability, cerebral atrophy

---

*Concurrent chemotherapy and radiation can augment all these effects.

Combined Radiation and Chemotherapy

Normal radiation therapy toxicities on organ systems are increased to varying degrees by concomitant or consecutive (within weeks of) administration of certain chemotherapy drugs. The severity of the toxicity depends on the drug and its dose, the radiation dose, and the timing of each in relation to the other. Damage to the target organ may be short term, permanent and life changing, or fatal. Because radiation therapy ports for lung cancer patients can involve the heart, lungs, brain, and other contents of the mediastinum, the potential severity of any synergistic drug-radiation toxicity is great. Specifically, esophagitis can lead to a stricture, CNS damage can include leukoencephalopathy or necrosis, or fatal interstitial fibrosis of large lung volumes can occur.[37] Nursing knowledge of chemotherapy agents can help predict toxicities resulting from their concomitant administration during radiation therapy. Combination chemotherapy regimens involving any of the drugs listed in the box,

---

DRUGS POTENTIATING RADIATION TOXICITY AND TARGET ORGANS

Bleomycin*: lung,* skin, mucosa
Doxorubicin*: lung,* heart,* skin, mucosa, esophagus
Etoposide (VP-16): heart
5-Fluorouracil: lung, heart, skin, mucosa
Hydroxyurea: lung, skin, mucosa, esophagus
Methotrexate*: central nervous system,* lung, skin, mucosa, bone, soft tissue
Mitomycin-C: lung, heart
Procarbazine: esophagus
Vinblastine: esophagus
Vincristine: central nervous system

Modified from McNaull F: *Semin Oncol Nurs* 3:194, 1987.
*Drugs/organ systems with potential for fatal toxicity if chemotherapy given in combination with radiation.

COMPLICATIONS
Chemotherapy for Lung Cancer

Myelosuppression (sepsis, bleeding, weakness, fatigue)
Nephrotoxicity (compromised renal function, magnesium wasting)
Hemorrhagic cystitis
Neurotoxicity
  Peripheral neuropathies (paresthesias, jaw pain, sensory loss, motor weakness, constipation or ileus, tinnitus, permanent hearing loss)
  Central nervous system toxicity (confusion, hallucinations, somnolence, coma)
Cardiac (myopathy, dysrhythmia, congestive heart failure, myocardial infarction)
Pneumonitis or pulmonary fibrosis
Nausea and vomiting (dehydration, weight loss)
Taste changes (anorexia, weight loss)
Mucositis (pain, difficulty swallowing, weight loss, diarrhea)
Anaphylaxis (death) or hypotension
Alopecia
Tissue damage and pain if vesicant extravasates
Syndrome of inappropriate secretion of antidiuretic hormone (SIADH) and hyponatremia

---

PATIENT TEACHING PRIORITIES
Chemotherapy

Chemotherapeutic agents

Review patient knowledge of chemotherapy and explain the therapeutic effects.
Provide patient/family with written information regarding all chemotherapeutic agents used.
Explain immediate and late (7 to 14 days) side effects of specific drug regimen.
Note availability of patient information booklets and community resources.

General side effects

Provide information for patient/family on self-management of stomatitis, nausea/vomiting, diarrhea and constipation, alopecia, myelosuppression, fatigue, and sexuality concerns.
Discuss which side effects must be reported to the physician/nurse immediately.

Specific side effects

Discuss specific side effects with patient/family according to prescribed drug regimen.
Explain which side effects are reversible.
Explain which medications/foods are to be avoided, if any.
Review how patient makes contact with appropriate health care team member should side effects occur that cannot be handled at home.
Review community resources available to patient.

Emotional support

Encourage patient/family to verbalize needs and questions concerning chemotherapy and its side effects.
Encourage patient to maintain activities and relationships to promote self-worth.
Encourage patient to verbalize feelings, frustrations, anger, and thoughts regarding changed life-style.
Teach patient/family problem-solving techniques.
Discuss methods of handling and addressing stress and coping with family/friends.

Continued.

upper left, p. 339, may enhance and broaden the spectrum of usual organ system toxicities.[82] Neither intrathecal therapy nor systemic chemotherapy with these agents should be given during radiation therapy to the associated target organ unless part of a specific protocol or investigational study, in which the rationale for combined radiation and chemotherapy is clearly stated and the patient understands the risks before therapy is begun.

CHEMOTHERAPY

Patients with lung cancer, especially small cell carcinoma, may receive several chemotherapy drugs having multiple potential toxicities and, in some cases, synergistic toxicities because two or more treatment modalities are being used sequentially or simultaneously (see box, lower left, p. 339).[30] These toxicities include myelosuppression, nausea and vomiting, renal damage, cardiac insult, pneumonitis/fibrosis, hemorrhagic cystitis, neurotoxicities, stomatitis, extravasation, and phlebitis.

Nursing assessment and management of these toxicities can help to greatly improve the patient's quality of life and are discussed in depth in Chapter 22. For an excellent nursing process approach to managing side effects of chemotherapy, the reader is referred to Burke and others.[14]

Tables 14-4 and 14-5 list some of the newer or investigational regimens used in small cell and non–small cell lung cancer. Some of these have been associated with significant toxicity. Tables 14-6 and 14-7 list doses and schedules of common chemotherapeutic regimens. These tables are not intended to be a comprehensive summary of all available regimens, but merely a sample of current therapies.

The box, lower right, p. 339, outlines patient teaching priorities related to chemotherapy.

OUTCOME GOALS: CHEMOTHERAPY

Patient will be able to:
- Verbalize importance of monitoring bleeding, infection, and fatigue when myelosuppressed and reporting to physician.
- Monitor intake and output.
- Monitor and report side effects (e.g., peripheral neuropathies, sensorimotor weakness, constipation, confusion, uncontrolled dry cough, mucositis).
- Understand and comply with prevention and intervention of side effects.[117]
- Communicate concerns related to body image, alopecia, and sexuality.
- Describe and use appropriate stress reduction techniques (e.g., relaxation therapy, guided imagery).

Table 14-4   New or Investigational Chemotherapy Regimens in Non–Small Cell Lung Cancer[13,21,36]

Drug regimen	Dose	Schedule
ICE		
Ifosfamide (+ Mesna)	4 g/m^2 IV day 1	Every 4 weeks
Cisplatin	250 mg/m^2 IV days 1-3	Every 4 weeks
Etoposide (VP-16)	100 mg/m^2 IV days 1-4	Every 4 weeks
or		
Ifosfamide (+ Mesna)	1500 mg/m^2 IV days 1-3	Every 4 weeks
Carboplatin	300 mg/m^2 IV day 1	Every 4 weeks
Etoposide (VP-16)	60-100 mg/m^2 IV days 1-3	Every 4 weeks
MIP		
Mitomycin-C	6 mg/m^2 IVP day 1	Every 3-4 weeks
Ifosfamide (+ Mesna)	4 gm/m^2 IV day 1	Every 3-4 weeks
Cisplatin	100 mg/m^2 IV day 2	Every 3-4 weeks
or		
Mitomycin-C	6 mg/m^2 IVP day 1	Every 4 weeks
Ifosfamide (+ Mesna)	3 g/m^2 IV day 1	Every 4 weeks
Cisplatin	50 mg/m^2 IV day 1	Every 4 weeks
TAXOL	200-250 mg/m^2 IV over 24 hours day 1	Every 3 weeks
TAXOL-CISPLATIN		
Taxol	135-170 mg/m^2 IV over 6 hours day 1 followed by	Every 3 weeks
Cisplatin	75 mg/m^2 IV day 1	Every 3 weeks

IV, Intravenous; *IVP,* IV push.

Table 14-5 New or Investigational Chemotherapy Regimens in Small Cell Lung Cancer[13,36,38,61]

Drug regimen	Dose	Schedule
CEV		
Carboplatin	300 mg/m^2 IV day 1	Every 4 weeks
Etoposide	140 mg/m^2 IV days 1-3	Every 4 weeks
Vincristine	1.4 mg/m^2 IVP days 1, 8, 15	Every 4 weeks
VIP		
Etoposide (VP-16)	75 mg/m^2 IV days 1-4	Every 3 weeks
Ifosfamide (+ Mesna)	1.2 g/m^2 IV days 1-4	Every 3 weeks
Cisplatin	20 mg/m^2 IV days 1-4	Every 3 weeks for 4 cycles
IFEX/VP-16		
Ifosfamide (+ Mesna)	5 g/m^2 IV over 24 hours day 1	Every 3 weeks
Etoposide (VP-16)	120 mg/m^2 IV days 1-2 and 240 mg/m^2 PO day 3	Every 3 weeks
ICE		
Ifosfamide (+ Mesna)	5 g/m^2 IV over 24 hours day 1	Every 4 weeks
Carboplatin	300-400 mg/m^2 IV day 1	Every 4 weeks
Etoposide	100 mg/m^2 IV days 1-3	Every 4 weeks

IV, Intravenous; *IVP*, IV push; *PO*, oral.

Table 14-6 Common Chemotherapy Regimens in Advanced Non–Small Cell Lung Cancer[12,13,36,38]

Drug regimen	Dose	Schedule
CAP		
Cyclophosphamide	500 mg/m^2 IV day 1	Every 3-4 weeks
Doxorubicin	50 mg/m^2 IV day 1	Every 3-4 weeks
Cisplatin	50 mg/m^2 IV day 1	Every 3-4 weeks
CE		
Caboplatin	100 mg/m^2 IV day 1	Every 3-4 weeks
Etoposide	3 mg/m^2 IV days 1-3	Every 3-4 weeks
	300-375 mg/m^2 IV day 1	
	100-120 mg/m^2 IV days 1-3	
BEP		
Bleomycin	25 mg/m^2 IV days 1-3	Every 4 weeks
Etoposide	100 mg/m^2 IV days 1-3	Every 4 weeks
Cisplatin	25 mg/m^2 IV days 1-3	Every 4 weeks
EP		
Etoposide (VP-16)	80-120 mg/m^2 IV days 1-3	Every 3-4 weeks
Cisplatin	80-120 mg/m^2 IV day 2	Every 3-4 weeks
MVbP		
Mitomycin-C	10 mg/m^2 IV day 1	Every 6-12 weeks
Vinblastine	6 mg/m^2 IV day 1	Every 2-3 weeks
Cisplatin	40-100 mg/m^2 IV day 1	Every 3-6 weeks
VbP		
Vinblastine	6 mg/m^2 IV days 1 and 2	Every 3 weeks
Cisplatin	120 mg/m^2 IV day 1	Every 3 weeks
VdP		
Vindesine	3 mg/m^2 IV every week for 5 weeks	Every other week
Cisplatin	120 mg/m^2 IV days 1 and 29	Every 6 weeks

IV, Intravenous.

Continued.

Table 14-7   Common Chemotherapy Regimens in Small Cell Lung Cancer[13,36,38,61]

Drug regimen	Dose	Schedule
CAV (OR CHO)		
Cyclophosphamide	750-1500 mg/m^2 IV day 1	Every 3 weeks
Doxorubicin	40-50 mg/m^2 IV day 1	Every 3 weeks
Vincristine	2 mg IV day 1	Every 3 weeks
CAE		
Cyclophosphamide	1000 mg/m^2 IV day 1	Every 3 weeks
Doxorubicin	45 mg/m^2 IV day 1	Every 3 weeks
Etoposide	50 mg/m^2 IV days 1-5	Every 3 weeks
CEV		
Cyclophosphamide	1000 mg/m^2 IV day 1	Every 3 weeks
Etoposide (VP-16)	50 mg/m^2 IV day 1	Every 3 weeks
Etoposide	100 mg/m^2 PO days 2-5	Every 3 weeks
Vincristine	2 mg IV day 1	Every 3 weeks
EVAC		
Etoposide (VP-16)	150 mg/m^2 IV days 1 and 8	Every 3-4 weeks
Vincristine	1 mg/m^2 IV days 1 and 8	Every 3-4 weeks
Doxorubicin	40 mg/m^2 IV day 1	Every 3-4 weeks
Cyclophosphamide	200 mg/m^2 PO days 3-6	Every 3-4 weeks
HANSEN'S		
Cyclophosphamide	700 mg/m^2 IV day 1	Every 4 weeks
Lomustine	70 mg/m^2 PO day 1 HS	Every 4 weeks
Vincristine	1 mg IV weekly for 4 weeks, then day 1 only	Every 4 weeks
Methotrexate	20 mg/m^2 PO days 18 and 21	Every 4 weeks
HANSEN'S VP		
Cyclophosphamide	1000 mg/m^2 IV day 1	Every 4 weeks
Lomustine	70 mg/m^2 PO day 1 HS	Every 4 weeks
Vincristine	1 mg IV weekly for 4 weeks then day 1 only	Every 4 weeks
Etoposide	70 mg/m^2 PO days 3-6	Every 4 weeks
EP		
Etoposide	80-120 mg/m^2 IV days 1-3	Every 3-4 weeks
Cisplatin	60-100 mg/m^2 IV day 1	Every 3-4 weeks

IV, Intravenous; *PO,* oral; *HS,* at bedtime.

CONCLUSION

Lung cancer remains the most common cause of cancer death for both women and men, and most patients have metastatic disease at the time of diagnosis. Their overall 5-year survival is 13%.[2] Therefore smoking prevention remains the key to reducing lung cancer disease and death. Because of the many complications, such as brain, bone, liver, and cardiac metastases and pleural effusions, nursing care can be very challenging. Compassionate and knowledgeable nursing care is of great importance to the patient with lung cancer and the family.

■ CHAPTER QUESTIONS

1. In 1996 approximately how many Americans were diagnosed with lung cancer?
   a. 300,000
   b. 177,000
   c. 158,000
   d. 125,000
2. In patients with lung cancer, which of the following prognostic factors have been found to be predictive of survival?
   a. Extent of disease
   b. Cell type
   c. Performance status
   d. All the above

3. Newer single agents showing promise in the treatment of NSCLC are:
   a. Gemsar, docetaxel
   b. Adriamycin, ifosfamide
   c. a and b
4. Eighty percent of all lung cancers are NSCLC. How many of these will present with regional or advanced disease?
   a. 35%
   b. 44%
   c. 66%
   d. 70%
5. Etoposide appears to produce a very dose-dependent and schedule-dependent response. What is the optimal schedule and dose in SCLC?
   a. Still to be defined
   b. Single bolus over 30 minutes
   c. Multiple daily IV doses for 3 to 5 days
   d. Oral dose for 5 to 21 days every 4 weeks
6. Which of the following is *not* included in the work-up for a suspected lung cancer diagnosis?
   a. History and physical examination
   b. Chest x-ray film and/or CT scan of chest
   c. Bone scan
   d. Sputum for cytology performed three times
   e. Bronchoscopy
7. What is a frequent site of metastasis in SCLC?
   a. Spleen
   b. Brain
   c. Colon
   d. Bone
8. When a patient experiences brain metastasis from lung cancer, which of the following should be considered when deciding what type of treatment the patient should receive?
   a. Number and location of lesions in the brain
   b. Patient's age and performance status
   c. Status of other metastatic disease
   d. Lesions' responsiveness to and ability to be controlled by radiation therapy
   e. All the above
   f. None of the above
9. Lung cancer is a common cause of pleural effusion. To treat effusions, a chest tube is inserted and connected to underwater-seal drainage. Which of the following is applicable to proper care of the chest tube?
   a. The nurse need not worry about leakage, and the tube may or may not be secured with adhesive tape.
   b. Clamps may be used on the tube as often as needed without fear of side effects.
   c. Unless fluid is within the tube, raising the system above the chest causes no problem.
   d. Stripping and milking the tube is a good way to unblock an obstructed tube without causing a problem of increased suction affecting the pleural space.
10. Rehabilitation is usually not associated with the lung cancer patient, but there are modifications in activities of daily living that may be helpful. The nurse can suggest that:
    a. Family members treat the patient like an invalid because recovery will be slow.
    b. The patient should be helped to establish a new daily routine with realistic goals.

    c. The patient assist with many household tasks in the morning because this is when he or she has the most energy.
    d. The patient be kept fairly well isolated and discouraged from taking trips so that he or she can conserve energy.
11. Many nursing issues arise when the lung cancer patient undergoes surgery. Which of the following is *not* one of these issues?
    a. Deep suction should be used to clear the bronchial tree of thick secretions.
    b. Preoperative or postoperative total parenteral nutrition may be needed for the high-risk, malnourished patient.
    c. The patients should be informed that he or she may return from surgery on a ventilator and with one or more chest tubes.
    d. Since cardiac dysrhythmia is one of the most common complications, the patient needs to know that he or she may receive many new medications after surgery.
12. Patients may experience several side effects from radiation treatments to the chest for lung cancer. The nurse should inform the patient about what causes these side effects and why. Which of the following should be included in the teaching?
    a. Skin reactions will be very severe and will take months to heal.
    b. A sore throat can occur because of esophagitis, and if the pain is severe, the patient may not be able to swallow food very well.
    c. Fatigue rarely occurs, and the patient is encouraged to do as much as possible each day.
    d. Radiation pneumonitis occurs frequently, and the patient may be hospitalized.

BIBLIOGRAPHY

1. Albain KS, Crowley JJ, Livingston RB: Longterm survival and toxicity in small cell lung cancer: expanded Southwest Oncology Group experience, *Chest* 99:1425, 1991.
2. American Cancer Society: *Cancer facts and figures—1996,* Atlanta, 1996, The Society.
3. Arriagada R and others: Prophylactic brain irradiation for patients with SCLC in complete remission, *J Natl Cancer Inst* 87:169, 1995.
4. Arrigado R and others: Competing events determining relapse-free survival in limited small cell lung cancer, *J Clin Oncol* 10:447, 1992.
5. Beahrs OH and others, editors: *Manual for staging of cancer,* ed 4, Philadelphia, 1992, Lippincott.
6. Belcher A: Lung cancer. In Belcher A: *Cancer nursing,* St Louis, 1992, Mosby.
7. Bernhard J, Ganz P: Psychosocial issues in lung cancer patients. Part I, *Chest* 90:216, 1991.
8. Bernhard J, Ganz P: Psychosocial issues in lung cancer patients. Part II, *Chest* 90:480, 1991.
9. Bitram J and others, editors: *Lung cancer: a comprehensive treatise,* Orlando, Fla, 1988, Grune & Stratton.
10. Bleenhen NM: The current role of radiotherapy in the treatment of non–small cell lung cancer, educational session, *Proc Am Soc Clin Oncol,* May 1992.

11. Boring CC, Squires TS, Heath CW: Cancer statistics for African Americans, *CA J Cancer Clin* 42:7, 1992.

12. Bunn PA: *Lung cancer: current understanding of the biology, diagnosis, staging, and treatment,* monograph, Princeton, NJ, 1992, Bristol-Myers.

13. Bunn P, Kelly K: New treatment agents for advanced small cell and non small cell lung cancer, *Semin Oncol* 22(3, suppl 6):53, 1995.

14. Burke MB and others: *Cancer chemotherapy: a nursing process approach,* Boston, 1991, Jones and Bartlett.

15. Carney DN: Lung cancer biology, *Eur J Cancer* 27:366, 1991.

16. Carney D: Management (chemotherapy/best supportive care) of advanced stage NSCLC, *Semin Oncol* 22(4, suppl 9):58, 1995.

17. Carpenito L: *Nursing diagnosis: application to clinical practice,* Philadelphia, 1987, Lippincott.

18. Cella D: Measuring quality of life in palliative care, *Semin Oncol* 22(2, suppl 13):73, 1995.

19. Chernecky C, Krech R: Complications of advanced disease. In Baird S, McCorkle R, Grant M, editors: *Cancer nursing: a comprehensive textbook,* Philadelphia, 1991, Saunders.

20. Chevalier TL, Arriagada R, Tubiana M: Combined chemotherapy and radiotherapy in small cell lung cancer. In Muggia FM, editor: *New drugs, concepts, and results in cancer chemotherapy,* Boston, 1992, Kluwer.

21. *Clinical Cancer Letter* 15:9, Washington, DC, 1992.

22. Comis R, Marstin G: Small cell carcinoma of the lung: an overview, *Semin Oncol Nurs* 3:174, 1987.

23. Council on Scientific Affairs: Radon in homes: Council report, *JAMA* 258:5, 1987.

24. Damber L, Larsson S: Combined effects of mining and smoking in the causation of lung carcinoma, *Acta Radiol Oncol* 21:305, 1982.

25. Delarve N, Eschapasse H: *Lung cancer: international trends in general thoracic surgery,* vol 1, Philadelphia, 1985, Saunders.

26. Dellefield M: Informational needs and approaches for early cancer detection in the elderly, *Semin Oncol Nurs* 4:156, 1988.

27. Diggs CH and others: Small cell carcinoma of the lung: treatment in the community, *Cancer* 69:2075, 1992.

28. Dow K, Hilderly L: *Nursing care in radiation oncology,* Philadelphia, 1992, Saunders.

29. Einhorn L, Loehrer P: Hoosier Oncology Group studies in extensive and recurrent small cell lung cancer, *Semin Oncol* 22(1, suppl 2):28, 1995.

30. Elpern E: Lung cancer. In Groenwald S and others, editors: *Cancer nursing: principles and practice,* ed 3, Boston, 1993, Jones and Bartlett.

31. Engelking C: Comfort issues in geriatric oncology, *Semin Oncol Nurs* 4:198, 1988.

32. Eriksen M, Lemaistre C, Newell GR: Health hazards of passive smoking, *Annu Rev Public Health* 9:47, 1988.

33. Erickson R: Mastering the in's and out's of chest drainage. Part 1, *Nursing '89* 19:36, 1989.

34. Erickson R: Mastering the in's and out's of chest drainage. Part 2, *Nursing '89* 19:46, 1989.

35. Evans W and others: Superiority of alternating non-cross-resistant chemotherapy in extensive small cell lung cancer: a multicenter, randomized clinical trial by the NCI of Canada, *Ann Intern Med* 107:451, 1987.

36. Feld R and others: Lung. In Abeloff M and others, editors: *Clinical oncology,* New York, 1995, Churchill Livingstone.

37. Findlay MP and others: Retrospective review of chemotherapy for small cell lung cancer in the elderly: does the end justify the means? *Eur J Cancer* 27:1597, 1991.

38. Fischer DS, Knobf MT, Durivage HT: *The cancer chemotherapy handbook,* ed 4, St Louis, 1993, Mosby.

39. Fleck JF and others: Is prophylactic cranial irradiation indicated in small cell lung cancer? *J Clin Oncol* 8:209, 1990.

40. Foote M and others: Dyspnea: a distressing sensation in lung cancer, *Oncol Nurs Forum* 13:25, 1986.

41. Fossella F and others: Summary of phase II data of docetaxel (taxotere), an active agent in the first and second line treatment of advanced NSCLC, *Semin Oncol* 22(2, suppl 4):22, 1995.

42. Frank-Stromborg M: Future projected trends in the care of the elderly individual with cancer, and implications for nursing, *J Oncol Nurs* 4:224, 1988.

43. Friedman P: Lung cancer: update on staging classifications, *Am J Radiol* 150:261, 1988.

44. Ginsberg R, Kris M, Armstrong J: Cancer of the lung. In De Vita VT Jr, Hellman S, Rosenberg SA, editors: *Cancer: principles and practice of oncology,* ed 4, Philadelphia, 1993, Lippincott.

45. Gradishar WJ and others: The impact on survival by adjuvant chemotherapy and radiation therapy in stage II non–small cell lung cancer, *Am J Clin Oncol* 15:405, 1992.

46. Greco F, Stronp S, Hainsworth J: Paclitaxel by 1 hour infusion in combination chemotherapy of stage III NSCLC, *Semin Oncol* 22(4, suppl 9):75, 1995.

47. Green MR: New directions in chemotherapy for NSCLC, educational session, *Proc Am Soc Clin Oncol,* May 1992.

48. Hammond E, Selikoff I, Seidman H: Asbestos exposure, cigarette smoking and death rates, *Ann NY Acad Sci* 330:473, 1979.

49. Hansen HH, Kristjansen PE: Chemotherapy of small cell lung cancer, *Eur J Cancer* 27:342, 1991.

50. Haque AK: Pathology of carcinoma of the lung: an update on current concepts, *J Thorac Imaging* 7:9, 1991.

51. Harwood K: Non–small cell lung cancer: issues in diagnosis, staging, and treatment, *Semin Oncol Nurs* 3:183, 1987.

52. Haylock P: Breathing difficulty: changes in respiratory function, *Semin Oncol Nurs* 3:293, 1987.

53. Heitzman E: The role of computed tomography in the diagnosis and management of lung cancer, *Chest* 89:237, 1986.

54. Higgins GA, Shields TW, Keehn RJ: The solitary pulmonary nodule: ten-year follow-up of Veterans Administration Armed Forces Cooperative Study, *Arch Surg* 110:570, 1975.

55. Hilderly L, Dow K: Radiation oncology. In Baird S, McCorkle R, Grant M, editors: *Cancer nursing: a comprehensive textbook,* Philadelphia, 1991, Saunders.

56. Hughes J, Weill H: Asbestos exposure—quantitative assessment of risk, *Am Rev Respir Dis* 133:5, 1986.

57. Iannuzzi M, Scoggin C: Small cell lung cancer, *Am Rev Respir Dis* 134:593, 1986.

58. Ihde DC, Minna JD: Non–small cell lung cancer. Part II. Treatment, *Curr Probl Cancer* 15:105, 1991.
59. Ihde D, Pass H, Glastein E: Small cell lung cancer. In DeVita VT Jr, Hellman S, Rosenberg SA, editors: *Cancer: principles and practice of oncology,* ed 4, Philadelphia, 1993, Lippincott.
60. Janerich DT and others: Lung cancer and exposure to tobacco smoke in the household, *N Engl J Med* 323:632, 1990.
61. Johnson DH and others: Current status of etoposide in the management of small cell lung cancer, *Cancer* 67:231, 1991.
62. Jordan LN, Mantravadi RVP: Nursing care of the patient receiving high dose rate brachytherapy, *Oncol Nurs Forum* 18:1167, 1991.
63. Kemeny N, Sugarbaker P: Treatment of metastatic cancer to liver. In DeVita VT Jr, Hellman S, Rosenberg SA, editors: *Cancer: principles and practice of oncology,* ed 4, Philadelphia, 1993, Lippincott.
64. Kerr RA: Indoor radon: the deadliest pollutant, *Science* 240:606, 1988.
65. Khanavkar B and others: Complications associated with brachytherapy alone or with laser in lung cancer, *Chest* 99:1062, 1991.
66. Kjuus H, Langard S, Skjaerven R: A case-referent study of lung cancer, occupational exposure and smoking. II. Role of asbestos exposure, *S J Work Environ Health* 12:203, 1986.
67. Klastersky J: Small cell lung cancer: can treatment results be improved further? *Semin Oncol* 22(1, suppl 2):1, 1995.
68. Kreisman H, Wolkove N, Quoix E: Small cell lung cancer presenting as a solitary pulmonary nodule, *Chest* 101:225, 1992.
69. Lad T, Thomas P, Piantadosi S: Surgical resection of small cell lung cancer: a prospective randomized evaluation, *Proc Am Soc Clin Oncol* 10:244, 1991.
70. Lima M, Khouri I, Glisson B: Small cell lung cancer. In Pazdur R, editor: *Medical oncology: a comprehensive review,* ed 2, Huntington, NY, 1995, PPR.
71. Lind J: Lung cancer. In Clark JC, McGee RF, editors: *Core curriculum for oncology nursing,* Philadelphia, 1992, Saunders.
72. Makela TP, Mattson K, Alitalo K: Tumor markers and oncogenes in lung cancer, *Eur J Cancer* 27:1323, 1991.
73. Malawer M, Delaney T: Treatment of metastatic cancer to bone. In DeVita VT Jr, Hellman S, Rosenberg SA, editors: *Cancer: principles and practice of oncology,* ed 4, Philadelphia, 1993, Lippincott.
74. Maxwell M: Malignant effusions and edemas. In Groenwald S and others, editors: *Cancer nursing: principles and practice,* ed 3, Boston, 1993, Jones and Bartlett.
75. McCorkle R and others: A randomized clinical trial of home nursing care for lung cancer patients, *Cancer* 64:1375, 1989.
76. McDonald S, Missaillidou D, Rubin P: Pulmonary complications. In Abeloff M and others, editors: *Clinical oncology,* New York, 1995, Churchill Livingstone.
77. McNaull F: Lung cancer: what are the odds? *Am J Nurs* 87:1428, 1987.
78. Miaskowski C: Knowledge deficit related to surgery. In McNally J and others, editors: *Guidelines for cancer nursing practice,* ed 2, Philadelphia, 1991, Saunders.
79. Miller JD, Gorenstein LA, Patterson GA: Staging: the key to rational management of lung cancer, *Ann Thorac Surg* 53:170, 1992.
80. Miller V and others: New chemotherapeutic agents for non–small cell lung cancer, *Chest* 107(6, suppl 1):3065, 1995.
81. Minna J and others: Cancer of the lung. In DeVita VT, Hellman S, Rosenberg SA, editors: *Cancer: principles and practice of oncology,* ed 4, Philadelphia, 1993, Lippincott.
82. Moseley J: Nursing management of toxicities associated with chemotherapy for lung cancer, *Semin Oncol Nurs* 3:202, 1987.
83. Mountain CF: Surgical treatment of lung cancer, *Crit Rev Oncol Hematol* 11:179, 1991.
84. Murray N and others: Importance of timing for thoracic radiation in the combined modality treatment of limited stage SCLC, *J Clin Oncol* 11:336, 1993.
85. National Cancer Institute: *Cancer statistics review: 1973-87,* NIH Pub No 90-2789, Bethesda, Md, 1990, US Department of Health and Human Services.
86. National Cancer Institute: *School programs to prevent smoking: the National Cancer Institute guide to strategies that succeed,* NIH Pub No 90-5000, Bethesda, Md, reprint 1994, US Department of Health and Human Services.
87. National Cancer Institute: *Self-guided strategies for smoking cessation: a program planner's guide,* NIH Pub No 91-3104, Bethesda, Md, reprint 1994, US Department of Health and Human Services.
88. National Research Council: *Environmental tobacco smoke: measuring exposures and assessing health effects,* Washington, DC, 1986, National Academy Press.
89. Neuberger JS: Residential radon exposure and lung cancer: an overview of published studies, *Cancer Detect Prev* 15:435, 1991.
90. Ockene JK and others: The relationship of smoking cessation to coronary heart disease and lung cancer in the Multiple Risk Factor Intervention Trial, *Am J Public Health* 80:954, 1990.
91. Oleske D: The epidemiology of lung cancer: an overview, *Semin Oncol Nurs* 3:165, 1987.
92. Parker SL and others: Cancer statistics, 1996, *CA J Cancer Clin* 42:19, 1996.
93. Pass H: Treatment of malignant pleural and pericardial effusions. In DeVita VT Jr, Hellman S, Rosenberg SA, editors: *Cancer: principles and practice of oncology,* ed 4, Philadelphia, 1993, Lippincott.
94. Perez CA and others: A prospective randomized study of various irradiation doses and fractionation schedules in the treatment of inoperable non–oat cell carcinoma of the lung, *Cancer* 45:2744, 1980.
95. Poplin E and others: Small cell carcinoma of the lung: influence of age on treatment outcome, *Cancer Treat Rep* 71:291, 1987.
96. Raju P and others: Treatment of liver metastasis with a combination of chemotherapy and hyperfractionated external radiation therapy, *Am J Clin Oncol* 10:41, 1987.
97. Repace JL, Lawry AH: Risk assessment, methodologies for passive smoking induced lung cancer risk, *Ann Intern Med* 10:27, 1990.

98. Risser N: The key to prevention of lung cancer: stop smoking, *Semin Oncol Nurs* 3:228, 1987.

99. Rose LJ: Neoadjuvant and adjuvant therapy of non–small cell lung cancer, *Semin Oncol* 18:536, 1991.

100. Ross DJ, Mohsenifar Z, Koerner SK: Survival characteristics after neodymium:YAG laser photoresection in advanced stage lung cancer, *Chest* 98:581, 1990.

101. Rostad M: Advances in nursing management of patients with lung cancer, *Nurs Clin North Am* 25:393, 1990.

102. Rubin SA: Lung cancer: past, present, and future, *J Thorac Imaging* 7:1, 1991.

103. Ruchdeschel J: Management of malignant pleural effusions, *Semin Oncol* 22(2 suppl 3):58, 1995.

104. Ryan L: Lung cancer: psychosocial implications, *Semin Oncol Nurs* 3:222, 1987.

105. Saccomanno G and others: Relationship of radioactive radon daughters and cigarette smoking in the genesis of lung cancer in uranium miners, *Cancer* 62:1402, 1988.

106. Samet J, Nero A: Indoor radon and lung cancer, *N Engl J Med* 320:591, 1989.

107. Scott A and others: Concurrent paclitaxel/cisplatin with thoracic radiation in patients with stage III a/b non–small cell carcinoma of the lung, *Semin Oncol* 22(4, suppl 9):34, 1995.

108. Sellers TA and others: Evidence for mendelian inheritance in the pathogenesis of lung cancer, *J Natl Cancer Inst* 82:1272, 1990.

109. Sellers TA and others: Lung cancer detection and prevention: evidence for an interaction between smoking and genetic predisposition, *Cancer Res* 52(suppl):2694s, 1992.

110. Shell J: Knowledge deficit related to radiation therapy. In McNally J and others, editors: *Guidelines for cancer nursing practice,* ed 2, Philadelphia, 1991, Saunders.

111. Shell J, Stanutz F, Grimm J: Comparison of moisture vapor permeable (MVP) dressings to conventional dressings for management of radiation skin reactions, *Oncol Nurs Forum* 13:11, 1986.

112. Shepherd FA and others: Cushing's syndrome associated with ectopic corticotropin production and small cell lung cancer, *J Clin Oncol* 10:21, 1992.

113. Silverberg B, Lubera J: Cancer statistics, *Cancer* 39:3, 1989.

114. Sims S: Cancer and aging, *Nurs Times* 84:29, 1988.

115. Slevin ML and others: A randomized trial to evaluate the effect of schedule on the activity of etoposide in small cell lung cancer, *J Clin Oncol* 7:1333, 1989.

116. Smit EF and others: A phase II study of oral etoposide in elderly patients with small cell lung cancer, *Thorax* 44:631, 1989.

117. Sommerville E: Knowledge deficit related to chemotherapy. In McNally F and others, editors: *Guidelines for cancer nursing practice,* ed 2, Philadelphia, 1991, Saunders.

118. Splinter TA: Management of non–small cell and small cell lung cancer, *Curr Opin Oncol* 3:312, 1991.

119. Sridhar KS, Raub WA: Present and past smoking history and other predisposing factors in 100 lung cancer patients, *Chest* 101:19, 1992.

120. Stahel RA: Diagnosis, staging, and prognostic factors of small cell lung cancer, *Curr Opin Oncol* 3:306, 1991.

121. Stahel RA and others: Staging and prognostic factors in small cell carcinoma of the lung: consensus report, *Lung Cancer* 5:119, 1989.

122. Strohl R: Ineffective breathing patterns. In Dow K, Hilderly L: *Nursing care in radiation oncology,* Philadelphia, 1992, Saunders.

123. Sugarbaker DJ: Non–small cell lung cancer: surgical approach to staging and therapy, educational session, *Proc Am Soc Clin Oncol,* May 1992.

124. Tockman M and others: Sensitive and specific monoclonal antibody recognition of human lung cancer antigen on preserved sputum cells: a new approach to early lung cancer detection, *J Clin Oncol* 6:1685, 1988.

125. Turrisi AT: The integration of platinum and radiotherapy in the treatment of lung cancer, *Semin Oncol* 18:81, 1991.

126. US Environmental Protection Agency: *A citizen's guide to radon: what it is and what to do about it,* OPA-86-004, Washington, DC, 1986, USDHHS Office of Air and Radiation.

127. Watanabe Y and others: Mediastinal spread of metastatic lymph nodes in bronchogenic carcinoma, *Chest* 97:1059, 1990.

128. Whittemore A, McMillan A: Lung cancer mortality among U.S. uranium miners: a reappraisal, *J Natl Cancer Inst* 71:489, 1983.

129. Wright D, Delaney T, Buckner J: Treatment of metastatic cancer to the brain. In DeVita VT Jr, Hellman S, Rosenberg SA, editors: *Cancer: principles and practice of oncology,* ed 4, Philadelphia, 1993, Lippincott.

130. Wu AH and others: Personal and family history of lung disease as risk factors for adenocarcinoma of the lung, *Cancer Res* 48:7279, 1988.

CHAPTER 15
Malignant Lymphoma

BETTY THOMAS DANIEL

Malignant lymphoma is a diverse group of neoplasms that originate in the lymphatic system. Included in this system are organs and tissues such as the thymus, lymph nodes, spleen, bone marrow, blood, and lymph. Lymph is derived from interstitial fluid and flows through lymphatic vessels so that it is eventually returned to the circulatory system by way of the thoracic duct. Along its course, lymph is filtered of particulate through lymph nodes, which are small, encapsulated organs located along the lymphatic vessels (Figure 15-1). Lymph nodes have a very specific architecture (Figure 15-2) that allows for areas of lymphocyte maturation and differentiation. Lymphocytes are the predominant cell present in lymph nodes and are the cellular element involved in malignant lymphoma.

Lymphocytes originate in the bone marrow and, through the process of maturation and differentiation, develop into several different types of mature lymphocytes (Figure 15-3). At any stage of this maturation and differentiation, the normal cell may transform into a malignant cell, giving rise to a malignancy that is specific to the stage in which the cell became transformed.

Based on the characteristics of the malignant lymphocytes, malignant lymphomas are divided into two major subgroups: Hodgkin's disease and non-Hodgkin's lymphoma. This chapter discusses the incidence, etiology, classifications, clinical manifestations, diagnosis, and treatment of Hodgkin's disease and non-Hodgkin's lymphoma and also provides guidelines for care of patients with malignant lymphoma.

HODGKIN'S DISEASE

HISTORICAL BACKGROUND

In 1832 Thomas Hodgkin described a progressively fatal disease characterized by lymphadenopathy with eventual spread to the lungs, liver, spleen, bone marrow, and other organs. Characteristic cells involved in this disease were identified microscopically by Sternberg and Reed in 1898 and 1902, respectively. The identification of these cells, now known as *Reed-Sternberg cells,* allowed for the initial classification of Hodgkin's disease. Tissues that have Reed-Sternberg cells are classified as Hodgkin's disease.

The potential curability of Hodgkin's disease was first recognized in 1939, when patients with localized tumors treated with high-dose radiation were shown to have long-term disease-free survival.[38] Because of the responsiveness of localized disease, research focused on ways to define the extent of disease before treatment. In 1969 researchers at Stanford University developed an extensive systematic way of staging and subsequently treating Hodgkin's disease based on the stage.[38] In 1970 the National Cancer Institute (NCI) reported that patients with advanced Hodgkin's disease could attain complete remission and long-term survival using a combination chemotherapy of nitrogen mustard, Oncovin (vincristine), procarbazine, and prednisone, known as MOPP.[38] These advances resulted in a standard approach to the diagnosis and treatment of Hodgkin's disease. Since the mid-1970s, development and research efforts have focused on more accurate ways of staging, initial therapies for various stages, treatment of resistance and relapsed disease, and the long-term effects of treatment regimens.

EPIDEMIOLOGY AND ETIOLOGY

Each year there are an estimated 7500 new cases of Hodgkin's disease and an estimated 1500 deaths.[33] This represents an incidence of less than 1% of all cancers. However, Hodgkin's disease is the most common cancer of young adults. Incidence peaks in the second and third decades and then gradually declines until age 45. A gradual increase in incidence is noted after age 45, with a second peak occurring in the sixth and seventh decades. Hodgkin's disease is also slightly more common in males, who may have a poorer prognosis.

The cause of Hodgkin's disease remains elusive. No strong evidence for specific etiologic factors exists.

However, clinical manifestations and epidemiologic studies have suggested a viral etiology or disturbance of the immune system. The infectious agent most frequently implicated is the *Epstein-Barr virus* (EBV).[38,43] Epidemiologic studies of clusters of Hodgkin's disease cases suggest the possibility that the disease occurs as a rare consequence of EBV infection. No conclusive evidence for a relationship between EBV and Hodgkin's disease exists.[26,32,38]

Genetic and occupational predispositions for Hodgkin's disease may also exist. Epidemiologic studies have identified an increased risk of disease among siblings of persons with Hodgkin's disease and among persons in the occupation of woodworking.[17,18] Evidence to support these ideas is inconclusive.

PREVENTION, SCREENING, AND DETECTION

Prevention of Hodgkin's disease is not applicable because there are no identified preventable risks. Early detection is important but may be hampered by the vagueness of the common symptoms. Patients should be encouraged to seek medical attention for persistent common signs and symptoms.

CLASSIFICATION

Since the identification of Reed-Sternberg cells (giant, multinucleated, transformed lymphocytes) as the diagnostic hallmark of Hodgkin's disease, histologic subtypes have been recognized. The *Rye Histopathologic Classification* identifies four subtypes of Hodgkin's disease based primarily on the microscopic features of the involved tissues. The identified characteristics help to distinguish Hodgkin's disease from other disorders. Table 15-1 lists the characteristics of the four subtypes.

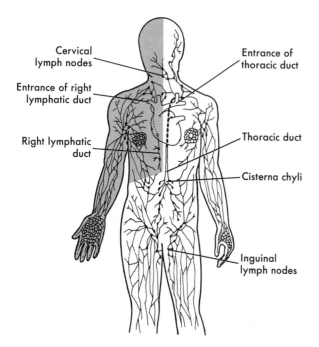

Figure 15-1 The lymphatic system. (From Beare P, Myers J: *Principles and practice of adult health nursing*, ed 2, St Louis, 1994, Mosby.)

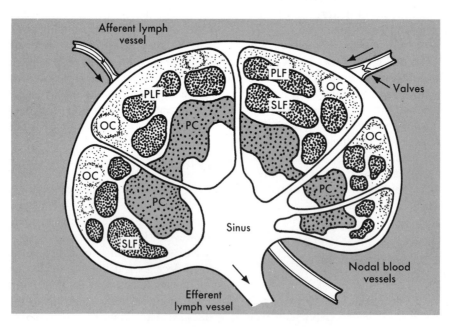

Figure 15-2 Cross-section of a lymph node. *PLF,* Primary lymphoid follicles; *SLF,* secondary lymphoid follicles; *OC,* outer cortex; *PC,* paracortical area. (From Powers LW: *Diagnostic hematology: clinical and technical principles*, St Louis, 1989, Mosby.)

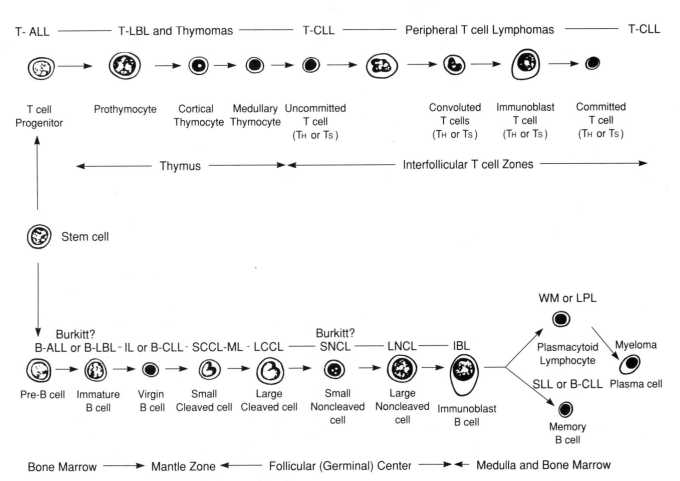

Figure 15-3 Lymphocyte differentiation. Immunologic classification of non-Hodgkin's lymphomas. This schema is based on a correlation between immunologic phenotyping and morphologic appearance of a large number of non-Hodgkin's lymphomas. *T-ALL*, T-cell acute lymphoblastic leukemia; *T-LBL*, T-cell lymphoblastic lymphoma; *T-CLL*, T-cell chronic lymphocytic leukemia; *Tн*, helper T cell; *Ts*, suppressor T cell; *B-ALL*, B-cell acute lymphoblastic leukemia; *B-LBL*, B-cell lymphoblastic lymphoma; *IL*, intermediate (mantle zone) lymphoma; *B-CLL*, B-cell chronic lymphocytic leukemia; *SCCL*, small cleaved cell (poorly differentiated lymphocytic) lymphoma; *ML*, mixed small cleaved and large cell (mixed lymphocytic-histiocytic) lymphoma; *LCCL*, large cleaved cell (histiocytic) lymphoma; *SNCL*, small noncleaved cell (undifferentiated) lymphoma, Burkitt's and non-Burkitt's subtypes; *LNCL*, large noncleaved cell (histiocytic) lymphoma; *IBL*, immunoblastic lymphoma; *WM*, Waldenström's macroglobulinemia; *LPL*, lymphoplasmacytoid lymphoma; *SSL*, small lymphocytic (well-differentiated lymphocytic) lymphoma. (Modified from Thorup O: *Fundamentals of clinical hematology,* ed 5, Philadelphia, 1987, Saunders.)

Although these subtypes predict prognosis of the natural history of the disease, they are poor predictors of prognosis when the disease is treated. Age, stage of disease, and adequacy of treatment are more important than histologic subtype in determining prognosis.

CLINICAL FEATURES

The most common signs and symptoms of Hodgkin's disease are lymphadenopathy, fever, night sweats, weight loss, pruritus, and alcohol-induced pain. Painless lymphadenopathy is evident in 70% to 90% of patients and is usually the symptom that causes patients to seek medical attention. The enlarged nodes are usually nontender, discrete, have a rubbery texture, and have been present for several weeks. Fever, night sweats, and weight loss greater than 10% of baseline weight usually signify advanced disease. Therefore noting the presence or absence of these symptoms is important. All or only one of these symptoms may occur, and their presence generally de-

Table 15-1 Rye Histopathologic Classification of Hodgkin's Disease

Type	Frequency (%)	Characteristics
Lymphocyte predominant	2-10	Predominantly found in young men Predominant cell: mature lymphocyte Reed-Sternberg cell sometimes found Localized disease in one or two nodes Most favorable prognosis
Mixed cellularity	20-40	Occurs in middle-aged to older adults More pleomorphic: plasma cells, eosinophils, neutrophils, Reed-Sternberg cells Generalized disease, including parenchymal organs Poorer prognosis; frequently with systemic signs and symptoms
Lymphocyte depleted	2-15	Predominantly affecting older adults Large numbers Reed-Sternberg cells Extensive disease Poorest prognosis
Nodular sclerosing	40-80	Often affects young women Predominantly affecting mediastinal nodes Any of the histologies, but nodes characterized by being divided into multiple nodules by bands of collagen Prognosis second to lymphocyte predominant

Data from Spivak JL, Eichner ER: *The fundamentals of clinical hematology,* ed 3, Baltimore, 1993, Johns Hopkins University Press; and Weinshel EL, Peterson BA: *CA Cancer J Clin* 43:237, 1993.

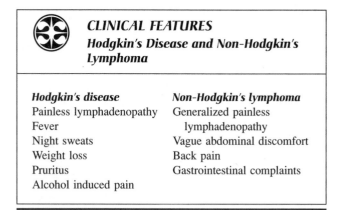

CLINICAL FEATURES
Hodgkin's Disease and Non-Hodgkin's Lymphoma

Hodgkin's disease	*Non-Hodgkin's lymphoma*
Painless lymphadenopathy	Generalized painless lymphadenopathy
Fever	
Night sweats	Vague abdominal discomfort
Weight loss	Back pain
Pruritus	Gastrointestinal complaints
Alcohol induced pain	

notes a poor prognosis. Generalized pruritus without skin lesions occurs in 10% to 15% of patients and is usually associated with mediastinal or abdominal masses. Pain in the enlarged nodes after the ingestion of alcohol occurs in about 20% of patients. Neither pruritus nor alcohol-induced pain has any pathologic or prognostic significance (see box, above right).

Less common presentations are cough, chest pain, superior vena cava syndrome (SVCS), ascites, abdominal pain or fullness, jaundice, and gastrointestinal (GI) or genitourinary (GU) problems. Almost all these signs and symptoms can be attributed to enlarged nodes or lymph tissue impinging on other structures. Respiratory symptoms or SVCS indicates intrathoracic involvement, usually mediastinal. These symptoms are more common in women because they have a higher incidence of mediastinal involvement. The abdominal-related symptoms are generally indicative of retroperitoneal node, liver, or spleen involvement.

No specific laboratory values are indicative of Hodgkin's disease. Complete blood counts (CBCs) and routine chemistry evaluations are generally within normal limits. The exceptions to this are usually seen in advanced disease. Anemia is identified in approximately 10% of patients, and increased granulocytes are noted in about 25% of patients. Decreased lymphocytes occur about 20% of the time and are a poor prognostic sign. The only laboratory study that may be a nonspecific indicator of Hodgkin's disease is the *erythrocyte sedimentation rate* (ESR). ESR is elevated in about 50% of patients with advanced disease. When a complete remission is obtained, ESR returns to normal. A subsequent rise in ESR predicts relapse 90% of the time.[38,43]

DIAGNOSIS AND STAGING

When a patient presents with clinical manifestations suggestive of Hodgkin's disease, a thorough history and physical examination must be performed. A biopsy of the enlarged node is necessary for diagnosis. However, if there is evidence of a recent infectious process, a lymph node biopsy may be delayed a short period to observe the clinical course. When feasible, the most accessible and most abnormal node should be biopsied. The entire node should be removed to ensure adequate histologic examination.

After a tissue diagnosis of Hodgkin's disease has been established, the extent of disease involvement must be determined. This process of staging is very important because it influences treatment decisions. The *Ann Arbor*

Staging Classification is used to categorize the extent of disease into four stages[10,38,43]:

Stage I Involvement of a single lymph node region or of a single extralymphatic organ or site

Stage II Involvement of two or more lymph node regions on the same side of the diaphragm

Stage III Involvement of lymph node regions on both sides of the diaphragm

Stage IV Disseminated involvement of one or more extralymphatic organs or tissues

Because Hodgkin's disease spreads in an organized, contiguous manner from one node region to another, this system of staging clearly identifies the extent of the disease. The presence or absence of fever, night sweats, or weight loss is also noted in the staging. The suffix "A" denotes the absence of these symptoms; the suffix "B" denotes the presence of these symptoms.

To stage the extent of the disease accurately, it is recommended that the following procedures be initiated as soon as possible after a definitive diagnosis of Hodgkin's disease[10,38,43]:

1. Detailed history and physical examination with emphasis on history of fever, night sweats, weight loss, and pruritus and examination of lymph node regions, liver, and spleen
2. Laboratory work-up, including CBC, differential, platelet count, ESR, liver and renal function, and cytogenetic studies
3. Radiology work-up, including a chest x-ray films; computed tomography (CT) scans or magnetic resonance imaging (MRI) of the chest, abdomen, and pelvis; and a bilateral lower extremity lymphangiogram
4. Bilateral bone marrow biopsy and aspirate
5. Skeletal survey if bone tenderness is noted on history and physical examination
6. Percutaneous liver biopsy if liver abnormalities are present on laboratory and radiology work-ups and no other abdominal disease is detected
7. Exploratory laparotomy and splenectomy if other studies do not prove abdominal disease and identification of abdominal disease will affect treatment decisions

During and after treatment, many of the same staging procedures are repeated to document response to treatment and then to document complete remission. When recurrence is suspected, the diagnostic and staging process is repeated. It is important to document disease recurrence by node biopsy and to determine the site and extent of recurrence. All these factors are as important for effective treatment of recurrence as they are for the management of new diagnoses.

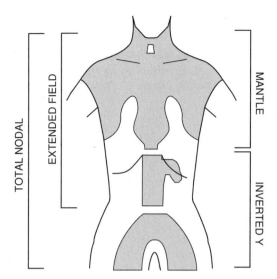

Figure 15-4 Standard radiation fields for Hodgkin's disease. *Mantle,* From mandible to diaphragm; lungs, heart, spinal cord, and humeral heads are shielded. *Inverted Y,* From diaphragm to ischial tuberosities, including the spleen if not removed; spinal cord, kidneys, bladder, rectum, and gonads are shielded. *Extended field,* Involves mantle zone and uppermost inverted Y zone; does not include the pelvic, inguinal, or femoral nodes. *Total nodal,* Mantle zone and complete inverted-Y zone.

METASTASIS

Involvement of retroperitoneal nodes, liver, spleen, and bone marrow usually occurs after Hodgkin's disease is generalized. Mesenteric lymph nodes and any organ can be involved in advanced cases.

TREATMENT MODALITIES

The appropriate use of radiotherapy and chemotherapy is required for effective treatment of Hodgkin's disease. Radiation therapy is generally given to nodal areas (Figure 15-4). A total dose of 4000 to 4400 cGy (rads) to the involved nodal areas is usually well tolerated and curative. The most common chemotherapy regimens are MOPP and ABVD (see box, p. 352). Both regimens are given in 28-day cycles for a minimum of six cycles. Chemotherapy is generally continued for two cycles after complete remission is achieved.

Initial Therapy

Because a high percentage of patients may be cured with initial therapy, it is important to select the initial therapy carefully. Proper staging, prognostic indicators, and knowledge of the toxicities of the treatment regimens are important factors considered in the selection of therapy.[6,23] Staging is the most important factor in determining if radiotherapy alone, chemotherapy alone, or

Table 15-2   Treatment for Hodgkin's Disease

Stage	Common treatment	Prognosis
IA and IIA without bulky disease	Radiation to nodal areas of known and suspected disease	70%-85% 10-year DFS*
IB and IIB without bulky disease	Radiation to nodal areas of known and suspected disease; no clear evidence that addition of chemotherapy increases DFS	40% 10-year DFS
IIA and B with bulky disease	Chemotherapy followed by radiation to bulky disease	75% 10-year DFS
IIIA and B	Optimal treatment unresolved Possibilities: Chemotherapy alone Chemotherapy with radiation to bulky disease Chemotherapy with total nodal radiation	No long-term results available
IVA and B	Chemotherapy (MOPP alternating with ABVD)	70% 8-year DFS

Data from Bonadonna G and others: *Semin Hematol* 25(suppl 2):51, 1988.
*DFS, Disease-free survival.

COMMON CHEMOTHERAPY REGIMENS FOR HODGKIN'S DISEASE

MOPP

Nitrogen mustard	6 mg/m^2 IV days 1 and 8
Oncovin (vincristine)	1.4 mg/m^2 IV days 1 and 8
Procarbazine	100 mg/m^2 PO days 1-14
Prednisone	40 mg/m^2 PO days 1-14

ABVD

Adriamycin (doxorubicin)	20 mg/m^2 IV days 1 and 15
Bleomycin	10 mg/m^2 IV days 1 and 15
Vinblastine	6 mg/m^2 IV days 1 and 15
Dacarbazine	375 mg/m^2 IV days 1 and 15

IV, Intravenous; *PO*, oral.

---

a combination of both is the treatment of choice (Table 15-2). Unfavorable prognostic factors such as number of disease sites, bulk of tumor mass, presence of "B" symptoms, age greater than 60, male gender, and lymphocyte-depleted histology also influence treatment choice. Finally, the long-term toxicities of treatment, such as secondary malignancy, sterility, cardiomyopathy, pneumonitis, and opportunistic infections, are considered when therapy is chosen.

When poor prognostic factors are present, the treatment regimen chosen is generally more aggressive. For example, a patient with stage IIA disease without a bulky mass will receive radiation alone; a patient with stage IIA disease with a bulky mass will receive a combination of radiation and chemotherapy. However, aggressive therapy must be chosen with care. The more aggressive the treatment regimen, the more severe the immediate

and long-term toxicities. Aggressive therapy may decrease the chances of retreating the patient because of toxic damage to major organs.

Recurrent Disease Therapy

After initial therapy, 20% to 50% of patients will have residual or recurrent disease. The optimal treatment regimen for these patients continues to be controversial.[40] Patients who relapse after radiation alone are generally treated with chemotherapy and, if technically feasible, with further radiation therapy. For patients relapsing after chemotherapy, several treatment approaches have been used, with varying degrees of success.[40]

When relapse occurs after chemotherapy, the length of disease-free survival is important. Patients experiencing relapse less than 12 months after initial therapy are less likely to achieve a complete remission.[40] ABVD is the most common salvage regimen used in this population. Other regimens have been developed and used, but none is any more effective than ABVD.[40] Overall, approximately 50% of patients will achieve a complete remission, and 5% to 10% will have long-term disease-free survival. Patients who experience relapse longer than 12 months after initial therapy can be retreated with the same regimen, usually MOPP. Although 70% to 80% of these patients will achieve a complete remission, only 10% to 20% will experience long-term disease-free survival.

High-dose therapy and bone marrow transplantation (BMT) is another salvage regimen that has gained increased support in the treatment of Hodgkin's disease. Autologous and peripheral blood stem cell (PBSC) transplants have shown effectiveness in patients who have failed MOPP/ABVD.[31] Patients who have received BMT in early relapse and who have not been treated with multiple chemotherapy regimens have 50% to 75% disease-

COMPLICATIONS
Hodgkin's Disease and Non-Hodgkin's Lymphoma

Disease related

Hodgkin's disease
Secondary disease development:
Childhood—osteosarcoma
Adult onset—epithelial (lung and colon)

Non-Hodgkin's lymphoma
Superior vena cava syndrome
Central nervous system involvement
Spinal cord involvement

Treatment related

Radiation therapy
Pulmonary fibrosis
Pericardial fibrosis
Hypothyroidism
Secondary malignancies
Infertility
Sterility

Chemotherapy
Myelodysplasia
Acute leukemia
Infertility
Cardiac dysfunction
Pulmonary fibrosis

free survival for 3 to 5 years.[31] (See Chapter 24 for further information.)

PROGNOSIS

Patients who achieve remission after second-line therapy have a wide range of reported long-term survival: 20% to 80%. Patients who have residual disease or who relapse after second-line therapy have diseases that are difficult to control.[23] Most oncologists do not believe these patients can be cured.

Complications from curative therapy for Hodgkin's disease can occur years after diagnosis and treatment. The major long-term complications of Hodgkin's disease and its treatment are second malignancies and gonadal dysfunction.[2] The most common second malignancies are acute nonlymphocytic leukemia, non-Hodgkin's lymphoma, osteosarcoma, and epithelial tumors. Acute nonlymphocytic leukemia is the most common second malignancy and generally occurs anytime within the first decade after treatment. The treatment regimen most often implicated as the risk factor for developing second-

ary acute nonlymphocytic leukemia is combined modality therapy.[25] The incidence of non-Hodgkin's lymphoma as a secondary malignancy is slightly less than that of acute nonlymphocytic leukemia and usually is not observed until more than 4 years after treatment.[7,24] Osteosarcoma is more common among survivors of childhood Hodgkin's disease, and the epithelial tumors (e.g., lung, colon) are more common among survivors of adult-onset Hodgkin's disease.[25] The solid tumors are generally not observed until 10 or 20 years after treatment (see box at left).

Gonadal dysfunction and sterility are common long-term effects from the treatment of Hodgkin's disease.[2] In men, chemotherapy (MOPP in particular) is the major cause of infertility. Radiation scatter from pelvic radiation can also significantly affect testicular function. Patients should be made aware of these possible effects before treatment. The testicles should be shielded during pelvic radiation.[7] Sperm banking may be offered, but many male patients with Hodgkin's disease have impaired spermatogenesis before receiving any treatment. Therefore use of sperm banking is limited.[42] In women, reproductive dysfunction after radiation or chemotherapy is usually related to primary ovarian failure. Approximately 50% of all female Hodgkin's disease patients will experience some ovarian dysfunction, and 20% to 30% will have permanent amenorrhea.[7] Women older than 25 years and those who are treated with chemotherapy and pelvic radiation have the highest incidence of ovarian failure. These possible effects should be discussed with patients, and when feasible, the ovaries should be shielded during pelvic radiation. (See Chapter 32 for further information.)

NON-HODGKIN'S LYMPHOMA

EPIDEMIOLOGY AND ETIOLOGY

As a group of neoplasms, non-Hodgkin's lymphoma (NHL) is morphologically and clinically different from Hodgkin's disease. After the Reed-Sternberg cell was identified as the characteristic cell of Hodgkin's disease, all other lymphomas were classified as non-Hodgkin's. Basically, NHL became a term to identify diseases with similarities to Hodgkin's but without the characteristic Reed-Sternberg cell.

In 1996 there were an estimated 52,700 new cases of NHL and 23,300 deaths attributed to NHL.[33] Men are at slightly higher risk than women, and whites are at higher risk than blacks. There is a preadolescent peak of incidence, then a later teenage drop-off followed by a steady increase of incidence with age.

The etiology of NHL remains unknown. However, several etiologic factors have been suggested. The most plausible one is *immune abnormality*.[38,43] The theory suggests that chronic stimulation of the immune system combined with other factors leads to the uncontrolled proliferation of the abnormal lymphocytes that occur in NHL. In support of this theory is the increased incidence of NHL that occurs with age, in patients receiving long-term immunosuppression (e.g., organ transplant recipients), and in patients with autoimmune diseases, primary immunodeficiency, or acquired immunodeficiency.[43] Patients who are human immunodeficiency virus (HIV) positive have a four times greater risk of developing NHL.[37] Viruses may also be etiologic factors by virtue of contributing to the chronic stimulation of the immune system. Two viruses linked to NHL are EBV and the human T-cell leukemia virus type I (HTLV-I). EBV is most often associated with the Burkitt's NHL; HTLV-I is implicated in the etiology of adult T-cell NHL.[13,43]

Exposure to some drugs has also been associated with an increased incidence of NHL. NHL has occurred as a secondary malignancy after chemotherapeutic treatment of acute leukemia and Hodgkin's disease.[38,43] There have also been anecdotal reports of NHL occurring secondary to treatment with diphenylhydantoin.[43]

PREVENTION, SCREENING, AND DETECTION

Prevention of NHL is not applicable because there are no identified preventable risks. Early detection is important but may be hampered by the vagueness of the common symptoms. Patients should be encouraged to seek medical attention for persistent common signs and symptoms.

CLASSIFICATION

NHL is a group of diseases with diverse histologies. Over the years, it was noted that the histology of the tumor has a significant influence on treatment and prognosis of the disease. In the late 1950s, Rappaport introduced a classification system for the various histologic types of NHL that used cell morphology, cytology, and the possible origin of the cell to categorize the diseases.[43] This system was widely accepted and used throughout the United States as a prognostic indicator.[13] As knowledge of the immune and lymphatic systems has increased over the years, the Rappaport classification has undergone alterations. These alterations were formalized into the Working Formulation.[13]

The *Working Formulation* divided the lymphomas into histologic grades based on the aggressiveness of the cell type and the observed growth pattern.[43] The histologic grades—low, intermediate, and high—generally correspond with the expected clinical course. For example, diseases with a low-grade histology are the least aggressive, and survival is measured in years. Problems developed with the Working Formulation in terms of omitted disease entities and exceptions to the prognostic categories.[13] Therefore the NCI developed a new clinical schema for NHL that closely mirrors the Working Formulation but addresses its inadequacies (see box at left). The most recent classification system is the *Revised European-American Lymphoma Classification* (REAL), proposed in 1994.[21] It attempts to overcome some of the deficiencies of earlier systems and incorporate the newer knowledge. Unfortunately, it has been met with opposition because it is not considered usable outside of major medical centers.

NATIONAL CANCER INSTITUTE CLINICAL SCHEMA FOR LYMPHOCYTIC LYMPHOMAS BASED ON NATURAL HISTORY OF UNTREATED OR PALLIATIVELY TREATED PATIENTS

INDOLENT (MEDIAN SURVIVAL MEASURED IN YEARS)

Small lymphocytic
Follicular, small cleaved cell
Follicular, mixed
Diffuse, small cleaved cells*
Diffuse, intermediately differentiated (or mantle zone)†
Cutaneous T cell†

AGGRESSIVE (MEDIAN SURVIVAL MEASURED IN MONTHS)

Follicular, large cell
Diffuse mixed
Diffuse large cell
Diffuse immunoblastic‡

HIGHLY AGGRESSIVE (MEDIAN SURVIVAL MEASURED IN WEEKS)

Diffuse small noncleaved cell (Burkitt's)
Diffuse small noncleaved cell (non-Burkitt's)
Lymphoblastic
Adult T-cell leukemia/lymphoma†

From DeVita VT Jr, Hellman S, Rosenberg SA: *Cancer: principles and practice of oncology,* ed 4, Philadelphia, 1993, Lippincott.

*Working Formulation intermediate-grade tumor with an indolent natural history.

†Omitted from Working Formulation.

‡Working Formulation high-grade tumor with an aggressive natural history.

CLINICAL FEATURES

The most common symptom of NHL unrelated to acquired immunodeficiency syndrome (AIDS) is a painless, enlarged, discrete lymph node in the neck (lymphadenopathy) similar to that of Hodgkin's disease. However, the lymphadenopathy of NHL tends to be more generalized and more frequently involves abdominal nodes and extranodal sites such as the GI tract, bone marrow, and liver. Therefore symptoms of vague abdominal discomfort, back pain, GI complaints, and ascites may be present and are usually indicative of abdominal node or GI involvement.[13,36] The "B" symptoms (fever, night sweats, and weight loss) occur 20% to 30% of the time, and although their presence signifies advanced disease, it is not as predictive of prognosis as in Hodgkin's disease (see box, p. 350).

Other possible signs and symptoms depend on the location and extent of involvement. Cough, dyspnea, and chest pain occur about 20% of the time and are indicative of lung involvement.[36] SVCS may occur, but it is rare because mediastinal involvement occurs in less than 20% of patients and is seen primarily in adult T-cell lymphoma.[13] Skin lesions that appear as isolated nodules or papules and frequently ulcerate occur in about 20% of patients and are most common in diseases of a T-cell origin, specifically cutaneous T-cell lymphoma.[13,38] Central nervous system (CNS) involvement may be primary (mass lesions) or secondary (meningeal involvement). It is most often an aggressive type of NHL and is the most common extranodal site in HIV-positive patients.[32] Manifestations of CNS involvement, such as headache, mental changes, confusion, lethargy, seizures, visual defects, cranial nerve palsies, or acute spinal cord compression, depend on the site of involvement.[13,38]

As in Hodgkin's disease, no specific laboratory studies are indicative of NHL. A CBC is normal most of the time, even if bone marrow involvement is present. Unexplained anemia may be present in about 20% of patients, and lymphopenia can occur in as many as 50%. ESR may be elevated, as occurs in Hodgkin's disease. Increased uric acid and calcium are frequent at diagnosis, and alkaline phosphatase is usually elevated when the liver is involved. When the lactate dehydrogenase (LDH) is elevated, there is generally a large tumor burden. The lymphocytes may show chromosomal abnormalities; however, the diagnostic value of such abnormalities is not known.[38]

DIAGNOSIS AND STAGING

A biopsy of an abnormal lymph node or mass is necessary to diagnose NHL. After a diagnosis of NHL, the clinical stage of the disease must be determined. Although only 15% to 20% of patients have localized disease, a staging process is necessary to identify the extent of the disease and the bulk of the tumor mass. The Ann Arbor Staging Classification is used to identify the extent of disease in NHL, although it is not as prognostically important as in Hodgkin's disease.[13]

The recommended staging procedures for NHL are as follows[10,13,38,43]:

1. Detailed history and complete physical examination with close examination of all peripheral node regions
2. Laboratory work-up, including CBC, differential, platelet count, ESR, liver function tests, renal function tests, uric acid, calcium, alkaline phosphatase, LDH, serum immunoglobulins, and serologic tests
3. Radiology work-up, including chest x-ray films and CT scan or MRI of the abdomen and pelvis if presenting signs and symptoms indicate
4. Bilateral posterior iliac crest bone marrow aspirate and biopsy
5. Diagnostic lumbar puncture, if CNS symptoms are present or if bone marrow is involved
6. Esophagogastroduodenoscopy (EGD) if GI lymphoma is suspected
7. Diagnostic thoracentesis or paracentesis if pleural or ascitic fluid is present
8. Lymphangiography, liver biopsy, and laparotomy are rarely necessary but may be done if the treatment plan would be altered by outcome

METASTASIS

The metastatic process varies with the type of lymphoma: *follicular* has bone marrow involvement and *diffuse* disseminates rapidly and involves areas such as the CNS, bone, and GI tract.

TREATMENT MODALITIES AND PROGNOSIS

The histologic type, the extent of the disease, and the patient's performance status are the most important factors in determining the treatment approach to NHL.[13,38] The histologic type as identified by the classification systems is the best indicator of the natural history of the disease. Indolent (low-grade) lymphomas have a natural history that can be measured in years, aggressive (intermediate-grade) lymphomas' natural history is measured in months, and highly aggressive (high-grade) lymphomas' natural history can be measured in weeks. Thus the treatment approach is logically dictated by the aggressiveness of the histologic type.[13]

The extent of disease is considered in conjunction with the histologic type in the determination of treatment.[5] However, histologic type is the more important factor. As mentioned, the Ann Arbor system is of limited use in staging NHL because, according to this system, most patients with NHL have widely disseminated disease at diagnosis. Although staging is considered when determining treatment, the staging for NHL needs to be modified according to histologic type to be of significant use.[13]

Performance status of the patient is important in determining treatment regimens because of the toxicities of the regimens. The patient's physical status, age, and underlying medical problems may affect the choice of therapy.[13] It is important for long-term survival that adequate treatment is given from the beginning. Therefore the extent of disease and patient's performance status need to be addressed so that treatment regimens can be modified if necessary (e.g., a patient with underlying chronic obstructive pulmonary disease should not receive regimens containing bleomycin).

The treatment of primary lymphoma in extranodal sites is the exception to determining treatment by histologic type. The GI tract and CNS are the most common extranodal sites affected by NHL. Involvement of the GI tract accounts for about 10% of all cases of NHL.[16,35] Surgery, chemotherapy, and radiation therapy may all be used to treat primary lymphoma involving the GI tract. Surgery alone is curative only in patients with truly localized disease. The addition of either radiation or chemotherapy postoperatively has improved survival.[27] However, controlled trials and longer follow-up periods are necessary.

The incidence of primary CNS lymphoma is increasing, and survival for these patients is short. Cranial radiation, usually done in conjunction with surgery, has prolonged survival but with few long-term survivors. Because of the blood-brain barrier, systemic chemotherapy is only modestly effective in these patients. Regimens providing high-dose methotrexate have shown the best results. However, these results are transient with few long-term survivors. For chemotherapy to be more effective, the drugs must be able to be delivered across the blood-brain barrier. Some current trials are investigating means of improving the drug delivery across the blood-brain barrier.[30]

Indolent Non-Hodgkin's Lymphoma

Controversy surrounds whether treatment of indolent or low-grade NHL can induce long-term disease-free survival and actually alter the disease's natural history.[13,44] Because the natural history of indolent lymphomas is such that most patients live with disease and eventually die of their disease despite treatment, the controversy is understandable. With treatment, patients will experience several episodes of remission and subsequent relapse, and the question remains whether the benefit of multiple remissions outweigh the toxicities of the treatment.

Localized (stage I or II) indolent NHL is rare and easily treated. Radiation therapy to the involved field or total nodal radiation produces 60% to 80% 5-year disease-free survival.[13] The role of chemotherapy in the treatment of localized indolent lymphoma has not been greatly explored and is therefore unclear.

Most patients with indolent NHL have disseminated (stage III or IV) disease at diagnosis. As just discussed, the optimal treatment regimen for these patients is controversial. Treatment may be deferred until symptoms become bothersome or the disease has evolved into a more aggressive type of lymphoma.[13] Patients whose histology converts to an aggressive type are then treated with curative therapy appropriate for the more aggressive histology. Patients who receive radiation tend to relapse in nonirradiated sites, and those who receive chemotherapy tend to relapse in previous disease sites. Therefore the question arises as to the efficacy of combined-modality (chemotherapy and radiation) therapy. Current clinical trials are exploring the options of deferred treatment, combination chemotherapy, and combined-modality therapy.

Aggressive Non-Hodgkin's Lymphoma

The aggressive lymphomas constitute about 60% of all NHL.[13] Thus more is known and more treatments have been tried for this group of lymphomas. In the treatment of the aggressive lymphomas, the relationship of tumor burden and bulk to prognosis is well documented. As tumor burden and bulk increase, prognosis declines. The prognostic features that signal increased tumor burden and bulk are poor performance status, more than one mass that is greater than 10 cm in diameter, presence of disease in multiple extranodal sites, presence of "B" symptoms, and elevation in LDH (greater than 500 IU/ml).[5,13] These prognostic features are important considerations in the choice of treatment regimens.

Localized disease occurs in less than 20% of aggressive lymphomas.[13] Radiation to the site of disease is the treatment of choice. However, the addition of chemotherapy to radiation regimens seems to improve results because it decreases the risk of relapse in nonirradiated sites. Little information is available on the effect of chemotherapy alone in the treatment of localized aggressive NHL.

Patients with disseminated disease and those with local disease that have one or more poor prognostic features are considered to have advanced aggressive lymphoma. Combination chemotherapy is the treatment of choice (Table 15-3). Patients with advanced aggressive lymphoma are more readily cured than those with indolent lymphomas, and more than 60% of these patients are being cured.[12] The achievement of a first complete remission is a must in achieving prolonged survival.

A variety of chemotherapy regimens have been shown to be successful in the treatment of advanced aggressive lymphomas (Table 15-3). The drawback to these regimens is the toxicity, particularly myelotoxicity, that may cause doses to be modified or courses to be delayed. When this occurs, patients are not receiving the optimal therapy and chances of achieving a complete remission

Table 15-3   Chemotherapy Regimens for Aggressive Lymphomas

ProMACE-MOPP flexitherapy	Day 1	Day 8	Day 15	Days 16-28
				No therapy
Cyclophosphamide 650 mg/m² IV	x	x		
Doxorubicin 25 mg/m² IV	x	x		
Etoposide 120 mg/m² IV	x	x		
Methotrexate 1.5 mg/m² IV			x with leucovorin rescue	
Prednisone 60 mg/m² PO	x...x			

Flexible number of cycles until complete response or decreased rate of response, then switch to:

	Day 1	Day 8	Day 14	Days 15-28
				No therapy
Nitrogen mustard 6 mg/m² IV	x	x		
Vincristine 1.4 mg/m² IV	x	x		
Procarbazine 100 mg/m² PO	x...x			
Prednisone 60 mg/m² PO	x...x			

Same number of cycles as ProMACE, then restart ProMACE.

m-BACOD	Day 1	Day 8	Day 15	Days 16-21
				No therapy
Cyclophosphamide 600 mg/m² IV	x			
Doxorubicin 45 mg/m² IV	x			
Vincristine 1 mg/m² IV	x			
Bleomycin 4 mg/m² IV	x			
Methotrexate 200 mg/m² IV		x rescue x with leucovorin rescue		
Dexamethasone 6 mg/m² PO	xxxxx			

COP-BLAM	Day 1	Day 10	Day 14	Days 15-21
				No therapy
Cyclophosphamide 400 mg/m² IV	x			
Doxorubicin 40 mg/m² IV	x			
Vincristine 1 mg/m² IV	x			
Procarbazine 100 mg/m² PO	x..............................x			
Prednisone 40 mg/m²	x..............................x			
Bleomycin 15 mg IV			x	

COP-BLAM III	Day 1	Day 2	Day 3	Day 4	Day 5
		Cycle A			
Vincristine 1 mg/m²/day IV infusion	x.......................x				
Bleomycin 7.5 mg/m² IV bolus, then 7.5 mg/m²/day IV infusion	x...x				
Cyclophosphamide 350 mg/m² IV	x				
Doxorubicin 35 mg/m² IV	x				
Prednisone 40 mg/m² PO	x	x	x	x	x
Procarbazine 100 mg/m² PO	x	x	x	x	x
		Cycle B			

As with cycle A without bleomycin and without day 2 of vincristine infusion

Week	1	3	7	10	13	16	19	22	25	28	31	34
Cycle	A	B	A	B	A	B	A	B	A	B	A	B

Continued.

Table 15-3 Chemotherapy Regimens for Aggressive Lymphomas—cont'd

CAP-BOP	Day 1	Day 7	Day 8	Day 21
Cyclophosphamide 650 mg/m^2 IV	x			
Doxorubicin 50 mg/m^2 IV	x			
Procarbazine 100 mg/m^2 PO	x...........................x			
Vincristine 1.4 mg/m^2			x	
Bleomycin 10 U/m^2 SC			x	
Prednisone 100 mg PO			x..............................x	

Cycles repeated every 3-4 weeks

ProMACE-CytaBOM	Day 1	Day 8	Day 14	Days 15-21
				No therapy
Cyclophosphamide 650 mg/m^2 IV	x			
Doxorubicin 25 mg/m^2 IV	x			
Etoposide 120 mg/m^2 IV	x			
Cytarabine 300 mg/m^2 IV		x		
Bleomycin 5 mg/m^2 IV		x		
Vincristine 1.4 mg/m^2 IV		x		
Methotrexate 120 mg/m^2 IV		x with leucovorin rescue		
Prednisone 60 mg/m^2 PO	x..x			
Co-trimoxazole 2 mg PO twice a day throughout six cycles of therapy				

MACOP-B	Week	1	2	3	4	5	6	7	8	9	10	11	12
Cyclophosphamide 350 mg/m^2 IV		x		x		x		x		x		x	
Doxorubicin 50 mg/m^2 IV		x		x		x		x		x		x	
Vincristine 1.4 mg/m^2 IV			x		x		x		x		x		x
Methotrexate 400 mg/m^2 IV*			x				x				x		
Bleomycin 10 mg/m^2 IV				x					x				x
Prednisone 75 mg/m^2 PO od		x...taper											
Co-trimoxazole 2 mg PO twice a day		x...x											

From DeVita VT Jr, Hellman S, Rosenberg SA: *Cancer: principles and practice of oncology,* ed 4, Philadelphia, 1993, Lippincott.
IV, Intravenous; *PO,* oral; *SC,* subcutaneous.
*With leucovorin rescue.

are decreased. Regimen schedules have been developed to stagger myelotoxic and nonmyelotoxic agents so that optimal doses can be given with decreased toxicity.[13]

This patient population is also at risk for CNS relapse after successful systemic therapy. The CNS is a sanctuary site for lymphomas. To minimize the risk of CNS relapse, high-dose methotrexate, which crosses the blood-brain barrier, or intrathecal chemotherapeutic agents have been added to the regimens.[13] (See box, p. 353, for complications related to NHL.)

Highly Aggressive Non-Hodgkin's Lymphoma

Highly aggressive lymphomas are almost always disseminated. Therefore staging is of questionable value. The treatment of highly aggressive lymphomas requires an intense chemotherapy regimen similar to those used to treat acute leukemia.[13] The treatment regimen should include induction, consolidation, and maintenance phases

and provide prophylactic treatment to the CNS. If complete remission is not achieved with initial therapy, the chance of any significant disease-free survival is dismal. After aggressive treatment, as many as 94% of patients with good prognostic features (LDH less than 300 IU/ml and no bone marrow involvement) can experience a 5-year relapse-free survival. More recently, clinical trials are investigating the use of BMT as a consolidation therapy for this group of patients.

Recurrent Disease Therapy

Effective treatment regimens for residual or relapsed NHL are being investigated. Patients with indolent lymphoma who relapse usually receive symptomatic treatment. Patients with relapsed intermediate-grade or high-grade lymphomas rarely achieve remission with salvage chemotherapy administered at the conventional doses. High-dose therapy followed by PBSC transfusion or BMT (autologous or allogeneic) can cure some patients.

Table 15-4 Summary of Hodgkin's Disease and Non-Hodgkin's Lymphoma (NHL)

	Hodgkin's disease	Non-Hodgkin's lymphoma
Epidemiology/etiology	Bimodal incidence pattern, predominantly males, under 40 years	Predominantly female, increased incidence in whites; median age at diagnosis, 55 years
	Higher risk associated with Epstein-Barr virus, (EBV), woodworking; familial association, linked to certain HLA antigens	Etiology unknown; association with viral infection, ionizing radiation, immunosuppression, other environmental factors
Clinical features	Cervical, supraclavicular, and mediastinal lymphadenopathy	Superficial lymphadenopathy, usually cervical and/or mediastinal involvement
	"B" symptoms in 40% of patients: fever, night sweats, weight loss	"B" symptoms less common than in Hodgkin's disease (most patients are asymptomatic)
	Occasionally pruritus and alcohol-induced pain	
Diagnosis/staging	Lymph node biopsy	Biopsy of involved lymph node
	Staging laparotomy if considering radiation therapy	Biopsy of extranodal lymph nodes if no lymphadenopathy
	Histology: Reed-Sternberg cells	National Cancer Institute (NCI) clinical schema,
	Rye Histopathologic Classification	Working Formulation for clinical use, and proposed REAL (Revised European-American Lymphoma Classification) Ann Arbor Staging System
	Ann Arbor Staging System	
Treatment*	Stages I and IIa (no mediastinal mass): radiation therapy	Low-grade lymphomas: "watch and wait" for older adults with good risks, radiation therapy for early stage, aggressive combination chemotherapy for advanced stages
	Stages I and IIA (large mediastinal mass), stages I and IIB (no mediastinal mass), and stages IIIa with upper abdominal disease: radiation therapy and ABVD or MOPP	Intermediate-grade and high-grade lymphomas: aggressive combination chemotherapy (CHOP [C, cyclophosphamide; H, doxorubicin HCl; O, Oncovin vincristine; P, prednisone] standard)
	Stages IIIA with lower abdominal disease, stage IIIB, and stage IV: MOPP/ABV, or MOPP/ABVD hybrid, and MOPP/ABV hybrid	
Salvage treatment	Failed radiation therapy: standard chemotherapy	High-dose chemotherapy with autologous or allogeneic BMT or PBSC transfusion
	Failed complete remission (CR) within months after standard chemotherapy: high-dose chemotherapy with autologous bone marrow transplant (BMT) or peripheral blood stem cell (PBSC) transfusion	Investigational combination chemotherapy
	Fail CR more than 1 year: re-treatment with same standard chemotherapy	

Data from DeVita VT Jr, Hellman S, Rosenberg SA: *Cancer: principles and practices of oncology,* ed 4, Philadelphia, 1993, Lippincott; and Handin RI, Stossel TP, Lux SE: *Blood: principles and practice of hematology,* Philadelphia, 1995, Lippincott.
*See Table 15-3 for chemotherapy regimens.

Those patients with chemotherapy-sensitive disease should be considered for BMT before being exposed to multiple chemotherapy regimens.[3,12] (See Chapter 24 for further information.)

• • •

Table 15-4 summarizes and compares Hodgkin's disease and NHL.

CONCLUSION

To provide the best patient care, nurses must be knowledgeable of the disease process and the principles of chemotherapy and radiation therapy. Nurses need to be able to provide patients and families with information regarding the disease process, treatment options, possible side effects of treatment, and consequences of treatment. This information is necessary for patients and families to make informed choices and to monitor signs and symptoms on a routine basis. Providing consistent repetition of information can help patients and families understand the abstract concepts of the disease and treatment regimen.

Psychosocial issues, such as coping, sexuality, and survivorship, also must be addressed. Malignant lymphomas, particularly Hodgkin's disease, have peak incidences in young to middle adulthood, affecting most patients at a very productive, goal-oriented time of life. Caring for lymphoma patients offers the nurse varied and exciting challenges.

Patients with malignant lymphoma can experience a broad range of physical conditions, from being mildly symptomatic to acutely ill. Patients with localized or indolent disease may be relatively asymptomatic from the disease and treatment. The majority of these patients are treated as outpatients, and the side effects from their treatments are generally not severe. Patients with extensive or aggressive disease are more often acutely ill and at risk for potentially severe side effects of therapy.

Several potential complications are specific to patients with malignant lymphoma. Nurses should monitor these so nursing care can be planned appropriately and nursing interventions can be implemented promptly. These potential complications are lymphadenopathy, myelosuppression, and central nervous system (CNS) involvement.

Lymphadenopathy is the primary symptom of malignant lymphoma. The enlarged nodes usually are nontender. However, they can cause pain or dysfunction by compressing neighboring tissues or organs. Lymphadenopathy can also cause a decrease in lymph and venous return to the heart. The flow of lymph through the affected lymph nodes is blocked because the disease process has destroyed the architecture of the nodes. Because the lymphatic system is close to the venous system, enlarged nodes may mechanically obstruct venous blood flow. The blockage of lymph and venous flow creates lymphedema in the tissues distal to the affected node region. When assessing a patient with lymphadenopathy, it is important to note the function of the surrounding tissues and organs and the presence of lymphedema. A plan must be implemented that provides for optimal mobility and drainage of the affected limb.

Myelosuppression is a common complication of cancer treatment. Patients experiencing myelosuppression are at increased risk for infection, bleeding, and anemia. As in the leukemias, myelosuppression in lymphoma can be caused by the disease as well as by the treatment regimens. This is significant in this population because patients may experience marked and prolonged myelosuppression that results in increased morbidity. Patients who have compromised bone marrow function before treatment will experience a more rapid and generally prolonged myelosuppressive period. Patients who are myelosuppressed must be monitored closely for signs and symptoms of infection, bleeding, and anemia. Thorough assessment and prompt treatment are essential to decreasing the morbidity and mortality of the myelosuppressed patient.

The degree and length of myelosuppression may also affect the treatment plan. Treatment may be delayed until bone marrow function recovers, and future chemotherapy doses may be decreased to prevent severe myelosuppression. In both instances, optimal treatment is being compromised and may affect disease response. In addition to protecting patients from infection, bleeding, and anemia, nurses must assist patients in coping with possible changes in their treatment plans.

Lymphomatous involvement of the CNS is another potential complication of malignant lymphoma. It is more common in the aggressive and highly aggressive types of non-Hodgkin's lymphoma (NHL). The involvement can occur as a space-occupying lesion in the brain or spinal cord or as an infiltration of the cerebrospinal fluid that causes irritation to the meninges. Cord compression, seizures, altered mental status, or cranial nerve palsies can occur as a result. Nurses therefore must be alert to subtle changes in patients' neurologic functioning. Nursing care must include assessment of mobility, sensory deficits or enhancements, cognitive abilities, and self-care abilities. Interventions must be appropriate to the patient's level of functioning. The ultimate goal is to assist the patient to achieve optimal functioning.

More than 50% of patients diagnosed with malignant lymphoma today will be alive in 5 years. However, complications can occur years after diagnosis and successful treatment and can have a significant impact on psychosocial functioning. Patients generally have an increased sense of vulnerability, fear of recurrence, and distress over changes in physical condition. Patients may have no apparent body changes secondary to disease and treatment but may feel less adequate, physically damaged, and less in control.

Patients and families all bring their history, experiences, and preconceived ideas into new situations. For teaching to be effective, these factors need to be identified and incorporated into the teaching plan. Because the malignant lymphomas are such a diverse group of diseases, they are often confusing. This is also a stressful time for patients and families, and it can be difficult for them to understand the abstract concepts of the disease and treatment. Consistent repetition and varying ways of providing information generally increase the ability to understand new concepts. Community resources often provide educational, emotional, or financial support and assistance. An assessment of patients' support systems, resources, and ability to communicate needs and feelings is important for nurses to be able to assist patients in maintaining or reestablishing roles and identities in school, work, and interpersonal relationships. The boxes, p. 361, list patient teaching priorities and geriatric considerations.

Examples of nursing care plans for malignant lymphoma follow.

PATIENT TEACHING PRIORITIES
Hodgkin's Disease and Non-Hodgkin's Lymphoma

Signs and symptoms of disease: fever, night sweats, weight loss, painless lymphadenopathy, generalized vague gastrointestinal discomfort, back pain

Signs and symptoms of infection: fever, chills, cough, erythema, malaise

Sexual dysfunction: infertility, sterility; discuss options for contraception and ovary and sperm banking

Discuss treatment options: chemotherapy, radiation therapy, surgery, bone marrow transplant (BMT); purpose, schedule, simulation plan for radiation therapy; monitoring weekly blood counts; chemotherapy drug side effects and schedule; BMT types (allogenic/autologus); before, during, and after transplant care components

GERIATRIC CONSIDERATIONS
Hodgkin's Disease and Non-Hodgkin's Lymphoma

Chemotherapy dose and schedule may be altered related to compromised cardiac, hepatic, renal, respiratory, and/or neuromuscular function.

Radiation therapy side effects: excessively dry skin, early skin reactions; increased fatigue; medication dose adjustment to minimize side effects; consider facilitation with transportation.

Financial considerations: fixed income—consider consultation with social services regarding housing, Meals on Wheels, medication prescriptions, and self-care needs.

NURSING DIAGNOSIS

• *Coping, ineffective individual, related to new diagnosis, potential life-style changes*

OUTCOME GOALS

Patient will be able to:

• Demonstrate evidence of adjustment to psychoemotional stressors related to new diagnosis and life-style changes

• Demonstrate positive problem-solving behaviors

INTERVENTIONS

• Assess patient's level of distress and anxiety related to:
—Uncertainty of future
—Bothersome symptoms
—Changes in self-concept
—Effect of past experiences

• Assess for signs of maladaptive or risky behaviors that interfere with responsible health practices:
—Missed appointments
—Failure to attend to symptoms
—Chronic attention to symptoms
—Loss of future orientation

• Identify patient's support system, resources, and communication patterns.

• Assess patient's problem-solving capabilities.

• Assess patient's level of knowledge regarding recurrence, development of secondary malignancy, and long-term effects of treatment.

• Listen attentively and provide support.

• Encourage verbalization of fears and concerns.

• Assist patient to recognize stressors, and assist with problem solving.

• Provide reassurance that anxiety or distress about health are common feelings among cancer survivors.

• Initiate referrals to social work, psychology, or community resources, as appropriate.

NURSING DIAGNOSIS

• *Coping, ineffective family: compromised, related to new diagnosis*

OUTCOME GOALS

Family will be able to:

• Identify stressors.

• Demonstrate effective use of coping strategies.

• Verbalize adjustments necessary in activities and roles.

INTERVENTIONS

• Assess past family relationships and coping patterns.

• Provide opportunities for expression of feelings.

• Include family/significant other in teaching sessions.

• Assist family/significant other in meeting adaptations and changes in activities and roles, as needed.

• Initiate referrals to social work, psychology, or community resources, as appropriate.

NURSING DIAGNOSIS

• *Infection, risk for, related to myelosuppression*

OUTCOME GOALS

Patient will be able to:

• Verbalize knowledge of high risk for infection.

• Demonstrate appropriate measures to minimize risk for infection.

INTERVENTIONS

• Assess for presence of risk factors:
—Bone marrow involvement
—Decreased white blood cell count

Continued.

- Assess for signs and symptoms of infection:
  —Fever
  —Cough
  —Erythema
- Institute measures to prevent exposure to potential sources of infection:
  —Meticulous handwashing
  —Meticulous hygiene
  —Avoidance of people with colds, flu
  —Good oral hygiene after meals
- Monitor laboratory values:
  —Blood counts
  —Electrolytes
  —Liver enzymes
- Minimize invasive procedures.
- Reassure patient and family that increased susceptibility to infections is temporary.

NURSING DIAGNOSIS

- *Knowledge deficit related to disease process, treatment, complications*

OUTCOME GOALS

Patient will be able to:
- State diagnosis and explain disease process.
- State rationale for treatment and identify treatment protocol.
- Identify potential treatment complications.

INTERVENTIONS

- Evaluate patient and family readiness to learn.
- Identify barriers to learning, such as language, physical deficiencies, psychologic deficiencies, and intellectual development.
- Determine patient and family level of knowledge of:
  —Function of lymph system
  —Signs and symptoms of lymphoma
  —Chemotherapy and radiation therapy
  —Side effects of treatment
  - Review information patient and family have already been given. Reinforce and clarify misconceptions.
  - Explain basic anatomy and physiology of lymphatic system and of specific body systems affected by location of disease.
  - Review and reinforce information regarding recurrence, secondary malignancy, and long-term effects of treatment.
  - Individualize information for subtype of lymphoma and extent of disease.
  - Explain symptoms of potential complications.
  - Explain radiation therapy fields and possible side effects (see Chapter 21).
  - Explain principles of chemotherapy, names of specific agents, and possible side effects (see Chapter 22).
  - Provide written materials to reinforce teaching.

- Encourage verbalization of questions, fears, and concerns.
- Listen attentively and provide support.
- Initiate referrals to other health care professionals and community resources as needed.

NURSING DIAGNOSIS

- *Mobility, impaired physical, related to CNS involvement, lymphadenopathy*

OUTCOME GOALS

Patient will be able to:
- State rationale for potential mobility problems.
- List signs and symptoms of impaired physical mobility.
- Verbalize/demonstrate measures to prevent/minimize mobility problems.

INTERVENTIONS

- Assess range of motion and strength of hands, arms, and legs.
- Assess mobility for ambulation and for self-care activities.
- Take steps to reduce environmental hazards.
- Encourage patient to perform active range of motion, perform moderate exercise, and receive adequate rest.
- Assist patient with ambulation as needed.

NURSING DIAGNOSIS

- *Self-care deficit, bathing/hygiene, dressing/grooming, feeding, related to CNS involvement, disease progression*

OUTCOME GOALS

Patient will be able to:
- Verbalize rationale for potential self-care deficit.
- Verbalize/demonstrate measures to prevent/minimize deficits.
- Perform activities of daily living within limits of functional capacity.

INTERVENTIONS

- Assess patient's abilities for:
  —Self-feeding
  —Self-bathing and self-grooming
  —Self-dressing
- Assess patient's motivation and endurance for self-care.
- Promote patient's maximum involvement in self-care activities.
- Provide assistance with self-care activities as appropriate to patient's level of functioning.

NURSING DIAGNOSIS

- *Sensory/perceptual alterations (specify) related to CNS involvement*

OUTCOME GOALS

Patient will be able to:
- Verbalize rationale for potential sensory alterations.
- Identify signs and symptoms related to sensory changes.

INTERVENTIONS

- Assess patient for level of orientation and level of activity.
- Orient patient to all three spheres as needed.
- Provide meaningful sensory input (e.g., clock, calendar, familiar objects).
- Explain all activities and request patient's perception of situation.
- If patient becomes confused, direct back to reality.

NURSING DIAGNOSIS

- *Sexuality patterns, altered, related to disease process, treatment*

OUTCOME GOALS

Patient will be able to:
- Verbalize impact of disease and treatment on sexuality.
- Maintain satisfying sexual role.

INTERVENTIONS

- Assess for physical symptoms that may affect libido:
  —Fatigue
  —Nausea and vomiting
  —Anorexia
  —Pain
- Assess for fear, anxiety, depression, and diminished self-concept.
- Promote open communication about sexual issues by bringing up the subject.
- Discuss possible effects of disease and treatment regimen on libido and sexual functioning (see Chapter 32).

NURSING DIAGNOSIS

- *Tissue perfusion, altered, related to lymphadenopathy*

OUTCOME GOALS

Patient will be able to:
- Verbalize rationale for potential lymphedema.
- State signs and symptoms of lymphedema.
- Maintain usual functional status.

INTERVENTIONS

- Assess for signs and symptoms of lymphedema:
  —Redness
  —Warmth
  —Swelling
- Assess function of surrounding tissues and organs.
- Encourage mobility of affected limb.
- Elevate affected limb.
- Assess for infection secondary to lymphedema.

■ CHAPTER QUESTIONS

1. Which is the *true* statement regarding incidence of Hodgkin's disease?
   a. Incidence peaks in the 20s and 30s.
   b. Incidence peaks in the 60s and 70s.
   c. Incidence gradually increases after age 20, then decreases after age 50.
   d. Incidence has two peaks, between ages 20 and 30 and again between ages 60 and 70.
2. According to the Rye classification system, the most common form of Hodgkin's disease is:
   a. Lymphocyte predominant
   b. Mixed cellularity
   c. Lymphocyte depleted
   d. Nodular sclerosing
3. Which of the following types of Hodgkin's disease has the best prognosis?
   a. Lymphocyte predominant
   b. Mixed cellularity
   c. Lymphocyte depleted
   d. Nodular sclerosing
4. What are "B" symptoms?
   a. Lymphadenopathy, weight loss, fever
   b. Pruritus, weight loss, fever
   c. Weight loss, fever, night sweats
   d. Lymphadenopathy, fever, night sweats
5. Which of the following is a *true* statement regarding treatment of relapsed Hodgkin's disease?
   a. Treatment of choice is radiation and combination chemotherapy with MOPP/ABVD.
   b. Treatment of choice is combination chemotherapy with MOPP/ABVD.
   c. Treatment of choice is radiation and ABMT.
   d. Treatment of choice is chemotherapy and ABMT.
6. Which is the most frequently used classification system for non-Hodgkin's lymphoma?
   a. Rappaport system
   b. NCI clinical schema
   c. Ann Arbor system
   d. Revised European-American Lymphoma system
7. The most common presenting symptom of NHL is:
   a. Mediastinal lymphadenopathy
   b. Painless, enlarged cervical lymph node
   c. Painful lymph nodes
   d. Generalized lymphadenopathy
8. Treatment plan for localized indolent NHL would include:
   a. Radiation therapy
   b. Single-agent chemotherapy

c. Combination chemotherapy

d. Radiation therapy and chemotherapy

9. Your patient was admitted last night with pain and swelling of the right leg and groin. The night nurse reports that the patient's diagnosis is lymphoblastic lymphoma. To what might you attribute the painfully swollen leg?

a. Deep vein thrombosis

b. Infection

c. Lymphedema

d. Radiation therapy

10. Your friend's mother has been diagnosed with follicular, small cleaved cell lymphoma. She is very distressed and asks if her mother will die soon. What is the prognosis for this disease?

a. Prognosis is grim; patients may live only weeks untreated.

b. Prognosis is fair; patients may live several months untreated.

c. Prognosis is fair; patients may live many months untreated.

d. Prognosis is good; patients may live years untreated.

BIBLIOGRAPHY

1. Acker B and others: Histologic conversion in the non-Hodgkin's lymphomas, *J Clin Oncol* 1:11, 1983.

2. Bakemeier RF: Recent advances in the management of Hodgkin's disease, *Curr Concepts Oncol* 3:2, 1984.

3. Bolwell BJ: Autologous bone marrow transplantation for Hodgkin's disease and non-Hodgkin's lymphoma, *Semin Oncol* 21:86, 1994.

4. Bierman P, Armitage JO: Salvage therapy for patients with relapsed or refractory aggressive non-Hodgkin's lymphoma, *Oncology* 1:11, 1987.

5. Bonadonna G, Jotti GS: Prognostic factors and response to treatment in non-Hodgkin's lymphoma (review), *Anticancer Res* 7:685, 1987.

6. Bonadonna G and others: Treatment strategies for Hodgkin's disease, *Semin Hematol* 25(suppl 2):51, 1988.

7. Bookman MA, Longo DL: Concomitant illness in patients treated for Hodgkin's disease, *Cancer Treat Rev* 13:17, 1986.

8. Canellos GP, Nadler L, Takvorian T: Autologous bone marrow transplantation in the treatment of malignant lymphomas and Hodgkin's disease, *Semin Hematol* 25(suppl 2):58, 1988.

9. Carella AM and others: High-dose chemotherapy with autologous bone marrow transplantation in 50 advanced resistant Hodgkin's disease patients: an Italian study group report, *J Clin Oncol* 6:1411, 1988.

10. Casciato DA, Lowitz BB: *Manual of bedside oncology,* Boston, 1983, Little, Brown.

11. Cohen DG: Metabolic complications of induction therapy for leukemia and lymphoma, *Cancer Nurs* 6:307, 1983.

12. Cohen SC, Krigel RL: High-dose therapy with stem cell infusion in lymphoma, *Semin Oncol* 22:218, 1995.

13. DeVita VT, Hellman S, Rosenberg SA: *Cancer: principles and practice of oncology,* ed 4, Philadelphia, 1993, Lippincott.

14. DeVita VT and others: The role of chemotherapy in diffuse aggressive lymphomas, *Semin Hematol* 25:2, 1988.

15. Eddy JL, Selgas-Cordes R, Curran M: Cutaneous T-cell lymphoma, *Am J Nurs* 84:202, 1984.

16. Gospodarowicz MK and others: Outcome analysis of localized gastrointestinal lymphoma treated with surgery and postoperative irradiation, *Int J Radiation Oncol Biol Phys* 19:1351, 1990.

17. Grufferman S and others: Hodgkin's disease in siblings, *N Engl J Med* 296:248, 1977.

18. Grufferman S, Duong T, Cole P: Brief communication: occupation and Hodgkin's disease, *J Natl Cancer Inst* 57:1193, 1976.

19. Guyton AC: *Textbook of medical physiology,* ed 7, Philadelphia, 1986, Saunders.

20. Handin RI, Lux SE, Stossel TP: *Blood: principles and practice of hematology,* Philadelphia, 1995, Lippincott.

21. Harris NL and others: A revised European-American classification of lymphoid neoplasms: a proposal from the international lymphoma study group, *Blood* 84:1361, 1994.

22. Jagannath S and others: Prognostic factors for response and survival after high-dose cyclophosphamide, carmustine, and etoposide with autologous bone marrow transplantation for relapsed Hodgkin's disease, *J Clin Oncol* 7:179, 1989.

23. Jotti GS, Bonadonna G: Prognostic factors in Hodgkin's disease: implications for modern treatment (review), *Anticancer Res* 8:749, 1988.

24. Koletsky AJ and others: Second neoplasms in patients with Hodgkin's disease following combined modality therapy—the Yale experience, *J Clin Oncol* 4:311, 1986.

25. Kushner BH, Zauber A, Tan CTC: Second malignancies after childhood Hodgkin's disease, *Cancer* 62:1364, 1988.

26. Lacher MJ: Hodgkin's disease and infectious mononucleosis: is there a causal association? *CA Cancer J Clin* 31:359, 1981.

27. Liang R and others: Chemotherapy for early-stage gastrointestinal lymphoma, *Cancer Chemother Pharmacol* 27:385, 1991.

28. List AF and others: Non-Hodgkin's lymphoma of the gastrointestinal tract: an analysis of clinical and pathologic features affecting outcome, *J Clin Oncol* 6:1125, 1988.

29. McNally JC and others, editors: *Guidelines for oncology nursing practice,* ed 2, Philadelphia, 1991, Saunders.

30. Miller TP and others: Southwest Oncology Group clinical trials for intermediate- and high-grade non-Hodgkin's lymphomas, *Semin Hematol* 25(suppl 2):17, 1988.

31. Neuwelt EA and others: Primary CNS lymphoma treated with osmotic blood-brain barrier disruption: prolonged survival and prevention of cognitive function, *J Clin Oncol* 9:1580, 1991.

32. Paffenbarger RS, Wing AL, Hyde RT: Brief communication: characteristics in youth indicative of adult-onset Hodgkin's disease, *J Natl Cancer Inst* 58:1489, 1977.

33. Parker SL and others: Cancer statistics, 1996, *CA Cancer J Clin* 46:5, 1996.

34. Rosenberg SA: Classification of lymphoid neoplasms, *Blood* 84:1359, 1994.

35. Sharma S and others: Primary gastric lymphoma: a prospective analysis of 12 cases and review of the literature, *J Surgical Oncol* 43:231, 1990.

36. Silverberg E, Boring CC, Squiries TS: Cancer statistics, 1990, *CA Cancer J Clin* 40:1, 1990.

37. Stanley H, Fluetsch-Bloom M, Bunce-Clyma M: HIV-related non-Hodgkin's lymphoma, *Oncol Nurs Forum* 18:875, 1991.

38. Thorup OA: *Fundamentals of clinical hematology,* ed 5, Philadelphia, 1987, Saunders.

39. Velasquez WS and others: Effective salvage therapy for lymphoma with cisplatin in combination with high-dose Ara-C and dexamethasone (DHAP), *Blood* 71:117, 1988.

40. Vose JM, Bierman PJ, Armitage JO: Hodgkin's disease: the role of bone marrow transplantation, *Semin Oncol* 17:749, 1990.

41. Wasserman AL and others: The psychological status of survivors of childhood/adolescent Hodgkin's disease, *Am J Dis Child* 141:626, 1987.

42. Weinshel EL, Peterson BA: Hodgkin's disease, *Ca Cancer J Clin* 43:327, 1993.

43. Williams WJ and others: *Hematology,* ed 3, New York, 1983, McGraw-Hill.

44. Young RC and others: The treatment of indolent lymphomas: watchful waiting V aggressive combined modality treatment, *Semin Hematol* 25(suppl 2):11, 1988.

CHAPTER 16

Multiple Myeloma

JANE C. CLARK

EPIDEMIOLOGY

Multiple myeloma is a rare malignancy of plasma cells that accounts for only 1% of all hematologic malignancies diagnosed in the United States. The disease accounts for an estimated 14,400 new cases and 10,400 deaths each year.[1] An increase in the incidence rate over the past decades is partially attributable to an improvement in diagnostic techniques.

Multiple myeloma is diagnosed in an equal number of men and women and occurs 14 times more frequently in blacks than whites. However, the death rates among American blacks is approximately twice that of whites. Multiple myeloma is diagnosed primarily in individuals over 40 years of age, with a peak incidence at about 70 years of age.[14]

ETIOLOGY AND RISK FACTORS

The etiology of multiple myeloma is not understood. Basic research in animal models has identified cellular factors such as chromosomal abnormalities, host-genetic factors, chronic antigenic stimulation, viruses, and growth factors as possible contributors to the development of plasma cell dyscrasias.[14] Other host factors, such as increasing age, race, and occupational exposure to petroleum products, asbestos, and radiation, may contribute to increasing risk for the disease.[3,5,11]

PREVENTION, SCREENING, AND DETECTION

No recommendations exist for the prevention or screening of asymptomatic individuals for multiple myeloma.[1,3] Detection of multiple myeloma in symptomatic individuals is based on a thorough history, physical examination, laboratory findings, and radiographic studies.

CLINICAL FEATURES

Although some individuals may be asymptomatic, most patients present to the clinician with a history of weakness, anorexia, weight loss, and fatigue. Symptoms of more advanced disease include bone pain, particularly in the back, and anemia. Depending on the sites of involvement, additional symptoms may include recurrent infection, changes in urinary patterns, and cognitive, sensory, or motor changes.[2,5,8,11] Findings on physical examination are related to the sites of involvement. Fever, redness, swelling, tenderness, and pus formation associated with bacterial infections may be present. Peripheral neuropathies may be noted. The skin may be pale, and petechiae and/or ecchymoses may be present (Figure 16-1). The boxes, p. 367, list the clinical features and disease-related and treatment-related complications of multiple myeloma.

DIAGNOSIS AND STAGING

The diagnosis of multiple myeloma is based on findings obtained from laboratory and radiographic studies. Serum and urine electrophoretic and immunologic studies reveal elevations in immunoglobulin G (IgG), IgA, and/or light-chain levels. Additional laboratory studies may demonstrate anemia, thrombocytopenia, and leukopenia in the presence of bone marrow involvement, hypercalcemia in the presence of lytic bone lesions, and proteinuria, hyperuricemia, azotemia, and elevated blood urea nitrogen (BUN), creatinine, and Bence-Jones urine protein levels with renal involvement. Radiographic studies typically include skeletal x-ray films, bone surveys, and magnetic resonance imaging (MRI) to detect the presence of osteoporosis, osteolytic lesions, or pathologic fractures.[2,3,5,11] For a diagnosis of multiple myeloma to be made, one or more of the following criteria must be met: (1) plasma cell infiltration of the bone marrow of at least 10%, (2) a monoclonal spike on serum or urine electrophoresis, (3) radiographic confirmation of osteoporosis and osteolytic lesions, and (4) soft tissue plasma cell tumors.

No universal staging system for multiple myeloma currently exists. The box, p. 368, outlines one example of a frequently used staging system based on tumor burden.

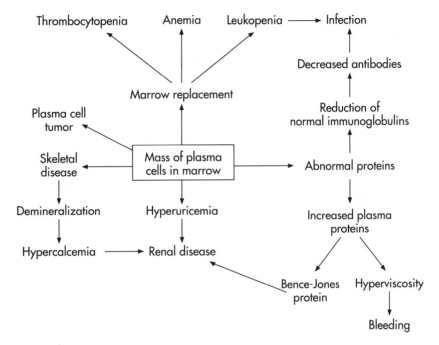

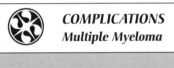

Figure 16-1   Pathogenesis of multiple myeloma. (From Megliola B: *Cancer Nurs* 3(3):221, 1980.)

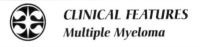

CLINICAL FEATURES
Multiple Myeloma

Anorexia, fatigue, weight loss
Back and bone pain
Recurrent infections
Changes in cognitive, sensory, and motor function and
   urinary pattern

COMPLICATIONS
Multiple Myeloma

Disease related

Thrombocytopenia
Severe anemia
Leukopenia and renal failure
Spinal cord compression
Hypercalcemia
Dehydration
Lytic bone lesions
Pathologic fractures
Repeated infections

Treatment related

Myelosuppression
Renal insufficiency
Mental status changes
Neuropathy
Cardiopulmonary toxicities

TREATMENT MODALITIES

Treatment of multiple myeloma in the early stages of the disease consists of observation if patients are asymptomatic. Patients are monitored with interval clinical examinations and laboratory and radiographic studies for signs of progressive disease such as severe anemia, thrombocytopenia and leukopenia, bone pain, osteolysis, or renal failure. Once progression of disease is documented, active treatment with antineoplastic agents or radiation therapy is initiated.

Chemotherapy

Chemotherapy usually consists of intermittent melphalan and prednisone and results in a 70% response rate.[14] Responses are generally short-term, and most patients experience progression of the disease with drug resistance. Clinicians have used combinations of prednisone,

high-dose melphalan, vincristine, carmustine (BCNU), cyclophosphamide, and doxorubicin as salvage therapy with limited success.[2,3,5,11] The use of biologic therapy with interferon-α and interleukin-2 has shown some potential when used in combination with antineoplastic agents.

MYELOMA STAGING SYSTEM

I. Multiple myeloma
  Major criteria
  A. Plasmacytoma on tissue biopsy
  B. Bone marrow plasmacytosis with > 30% plasma cells
  C. Monoclonal globulin spike on serum electrophoresis exceeding 3.5 g/dl for G peaks or 2.0 g/dl for A peaks, $\geq$ 1.0 g/24 hours of κ- or λ-light-chain excretion on urine electrophoresis in presence of amyloidosis
  Minor criteria
  1. Bone marrow plasmacytosis 10% to 30% plasma cells
  2. Monoclonal globulin spike present, but less than the level defined above
  3. Lytic bone lesions
  4. Residual normal IgM < 50 mg/dl, IgA < 100 mg/dl, or IgG < 600 mg/dl
     Diagnosis confirmed when any of following features are documented in symptomatic patients with clearly progressive disease.
     Diagnosis of myeloma requires a minimum of one major + one minor criterion or three minor criteria that must include a + b, i.e.:
     a. A + 2, A + 3, A + 4 (A + 1 not sufficient)
     b. B + 2, B + 3, B + 4
     c. C + 1, C + 3, C + 4
     d. 1 + 2 + 3, 1 + 2 + 4

II. Indolent myeloma
  Same as myeloma except:
  A. No bone lesions or only limited bone lesions ($\leq$3 lytic lesions); no compression fractures
  B. M-component levels: (1) IgG < 7 g/dl; (2) IgA < 5/dl
  C. No symptoms or associated disease features, i.e.:
    1. Performance status > 70%
    2. Hemoglobin > 10 g/dl
    3. Serum calcium normal
    4. Serum creatinine < 2.0 mg/dl
    5. No infections
III. Smoldering myeloma
  Same as indolent myeloma except:
  A. No bone lesions
  B. Bone marrow plasma cells $\geq$ 30%
IV. Monoclonal gammopathy of undetermined significance (MGUS)
  A. Monoclonal gammopathy
  B. M-component level
    1. IgG $\leq$ 3.5 g/dl
    2. IgA $\leq$ 2.0 g/dl
    3. BJ protein $\leq$ 1.0 g/24 hours
  C. Bone marrow plasma cells < 10%
  D. No bone lesions
  E. No symptoms

Modified from Salmon SE, Cassady JR: Plasma cell neoplasms. In DeVita VT Jr, Hellman S, Rosenberg SA, editors, *Cancer: principles and practice of oncology,* ed 4, Philadelphia, 1993, Lippincott.
IgA, Immunoglobulin A; *IgG,* immunoglobulin G; *IgM,* immunoglobulin M; *BJ,* Bence-Jones light chain.

Radiation Therapy

Radiation therapy may be used to treat patients with chemotherapy-resistant disease, to relieve bone pain, and to treat spinal cord compression. Although radiation therapy can greatly improve the quality of life for patients with multiple myeloma, length of survival is not enhanced.[3]

Bone Marrow Transplantation

Recently, the role of autologous bone marrow transplantation (BMT) in the treatment of patients with multiple myeloma has been explored. Success has been limited by the inability to eradicate the malignant plasma cell clone. However, researchers continue to evaluate the effectiveness of high-dose antineoplastic therapy followed by autologous BMT with marrow that has been purged with an antibody specific for plasma cells.[3] In addition, researchers are exploring the application of autologous BMT earlier in the course of the disease.[14]

The use of allogeneic BMT in the treatment of multiple myeloma has been limited by the advanced age of patients and the lack of an appropriate marrow donor. Only 5% of patients are eligible for allogeneic BMT. The mortality related to allogeneic BMT approximates 40%, with a 3-year disease-free survival of 31%.[14]

Biologic Response Modifiers

Recently, interferon-α has been used alone and in combination with conventional chemotherapy to treat patients with multiple myeloma. Response rates among patients previously untreated and among patients who were refractory to conventional therapy make interferon-α a promising second-line treatment.[14] Given the results of recent studies on the effect of interleukin-6 on disease progression, the role of biologic therapy in the treatment of patients with multiple myeloma is only beginning to be explored.[14]

PROGNOSIS

Multiple myeloma is an incurable disease.[14] The course of disease progression for patients is determined by the

NURSING MANAGEMENT

Nursing care for the patient with multiple myeloma centers on educating the patient and significant others about the disease and treatment, teaching self-care skills to minimize threats to quality of life, monitoring for signs and symptoms of complications of the disease and treatment, and coordinating implementation of an interdisciplinary plan of care that addresses complications of the disease and treatment. The teaching plan for patients with multiple myeloma and their significant others includes information about the chronic nature of the disease, rationale for observation in patients without symptoms, and health-enhancing strategies such as maintaining an adequate fluid intake of 3000 ml each day, maintaining mobility to decrease the risk of bone destruction from inactivity, and instituting safety precautions to minimize the risk of injury from thrombocytopenia, anemia, and leukopenia. Specific nursing interventions to address common nursing diagnoses among patients with multiple my

eloma are presented in other chapters in this text (see Chapters 29 and 30).

Since bony destruction is a common effect of multiple myeloma and pathologic fractures can alter the quality of life significantly, safety precautions are stressed in developing a long-term plan of care.

NURSING DIAGNOSIS

• *Injury, risk for, related to bony destruction by plasma cell tumors*

OUTCOME GOAL

Patient will be able to:
• Participate in strategies to decrease risks of pathologic fractures.

Table 16-1 Nursing Assessments for Complications of Multiple Myeloma

Complication	Nursing assessments
Renal insufficiency	Monitor BUN, creatinine, uric acid, calcium, potassium, glucose, and phosphorus levels as ordered by the physician.
	Assess for changes in the character of the urine: volume, color, and odor.
Hyperviscosity syndrome	Monitor for intermittent claudication and changes in the skin color of the extremities.
	Assess for neurologic changes, such as headache or visual disturbances.
	Monitor for changes in mental status, such as irritability, drowsiness, confusion, or coma.
	Assess for signs and symptoms of congestive heart failure.[5]
Dehydration	Monitor intake and output every 8 hours.
	Assess skin turgor each day.
	Evaluate subjective symptoms by patient, such as thirst and dry skin.

PATIENT TEACHING PRIORITIES
Multiple Myeloma

In teaching the patient with multiple myeloma, the nurse must consider critical aspects of the disease and treatment that potentially affect the quality of life for the patient. Teaching must be reinforced verbally, with written materials that are culturally sensitive, and with appropriate audiovisual resources.

Self-care activities

Create a safe environment: remove throw rugs, install safety equipment in bathrooms, keep frequently used articles within reach, and remove articles from frequently traveled paths.

Maintain range of motion, muscle strength, and endurance within limitations of bony involvement.

Monitor dietary calcium intake.

Monitor oral intake and urine output.

Symptoms to report to health care team

Signs of infection: fever, chills, pain, erythema, swelling, pus formation

Signs of dehydration: thirst, lethargy, decreased skin turgor, decreased urine output, increased urine concentration

Increased lethargy, mental confusion, apathy

Demands of treatment

Routine appointments for treatment and follow-up at regular intervals

Estimate of direct costs (e.g., drugs, supplies) and indirect costs of therapy (e.g., transportation, time away from work).

Continued.

ASSESSMENT

- Identify personal risk factors for injury: extent and sites of bony involvement, muscle strength of extremities, changes in sensation, difficulty in ambulating, type of shoes worn when ambulating, knowledge of proper body mechanics, mental status.
- Identify environmental risk factors for injury: crowded rooms, throw rugs, proximity of needed articles, or bathroom.
- Assess perceived threats to safety from patient's perspective.

INTERVENTIONS

- Consult physical therapy for instruction in proper body mechanics, transfer techniques, positioning, and use of assistive devices for development of an exercise program to maintain muscle strength and range of motion without jeopardizing risk of pathologic fractures.
- Arrange hospital room environment to decrease the risks to safety: telephone, call light, and personal articles within easy reach and clear pathway to the bathroom.
- Refer to home health agency to evaluate home environment for safety risk factors and recommended modifications before discharge.
- Encourage patient to ask for assistance from health care team or significant others, as needed, with ambulation or activities of daily living.[4,8,10]

The nurse also assumes responsibility for monitoring the patient with multiple myeloma for signs and symptoms of complications of the disease and treatment, such as hypercalcemia, pain, spinal cord compression, renal insufficiency, hyperviscosity syndrome, and dehydration. Often, early recognition and treatment of these complications will result in improvement in the patient's ability to tolerate treatment and in quality of life. Specific nursing assessments and interventions for patients at risk for or experiencing hypercalcemia, spinal cord compression, and pain are detailed in Chapters 19 and 29. Nursing assessments to monitor for renal insufficiency, dehydration, and hyperviscosity syndrome are presented in detail in this chapter (Table 16-1). Presence of any of the signs and symptoms should be reported to the physician.

The box on p. 369 and the box below list patient teaching priorities and geriatric considerations.

GERIATRIC CONSIDERATIONS
Multiple Myeloma

Peak incidence of disease: 70 years of age

Issues regarding occupation and potential for early retirement

Social and recreational activities may need adjustment to conserve energy and minimize injury risks

Potential for mental status changes

Consider environmental safety factors and abilities to meet self-care needs for hygiene, nutrition, elimination, and comfort

---

severity of organ involvement at the time of diagnosis and response to active treatment. Asymptomatic patients may live with the disease for months to years without active treatment. For symptomatic patients requiring treatment, a pattern of response has been described. During the initial 2 to 3 years of treatment, patients respond well to antineoplastic therapy. A plateau phase follows when the disease remains stable but does not respond as well as in the initial phase. During the third phase the disease becomes resistant to the antineoplastic therapy and progresses at a rapid rate.[3,5] The median survival duration ranges from 6 to 64 months.[14] A statistically significant improvement in the relative 5-year survival rate, from 12% to 28%, occurred from the 1960s to 1990s.[1]

CONCLUSION

The patient with multiple myeloma presents many challenges to the health care team during the course of the disease. Since no cure for the disease is available and its course is protracted over several years for most patients, the team's focus is to plan with the patient and significant others care that will maintain independence in activities of daily living, provide a safe living and treatment environment, and preserve an acceptable level of patient comfort. The care demands cooperation and support from significant others and members of the health care team in acute care, community, and home settings.

■ CHAPTER QUESTIONS

1. A 63-year-old male, diagnosed with multiple myeloma a year ago, reports that he has experienced increased weakness, decreased appetite, weight loss, and constipation over the past month. Which of the following laboratory tests results would be critical for the oncology nurse to evaluate?
   a. Serum potassium
   b. Serum calcium
   c. Glucose
   d. Uric acid

2. The nurse is providing discharge instructions for a patient diagnosed with multiple myeloma with extensive bony involvement. Which of the following instructions would be most important to include in the discharge teaching?
   a. Strategies for restriction of dietary calcium
   b. Techniques for monitoring urine output
   c. Safety strategies for modifying home environment
   d. Proper body mechanics for home caregiver
3. Which of the following symptoms would be most important for the patient with multiple myeloma to report immediately to a member of the health care team?
   a. Increase in the severity of pain with movement
   b. Presence of edema in the lower extremities
   c. Increase in the level of fatigue with activity
   d. Loss of sensation to pain in the lower extremities

BIBLIOGRAPHY

1. American Cancer Society: *Cancer facts and figures—1996,* Atlanta, 1996, The Society.
2. Anderson MG: The lymphomas and multiple myeloma. In Baird SB and others, editors: *A cancer source book for nurses,* ed 6, Atlanta, 1991, American Cancer Society.
3. Bubley GJ, Schnipper LE: Multiple myeloma. In Holleb AI, Fink DJ, Murphy GP, editors: *American Cancer Society textbook of clinical oncology,* Atlanta, 1991, American Cancer Society.
4. Clark JC, McGee RF, Preston R: Nursing management of responses to the cancer experience. In Clark JC, McGee RF, editors: *Core curriculum for oncology nursing,* ed 2, Philadelphia, 1992, Saunders.
5. Cook MB: Multiple myeloma. In Groenwald SL and others, editors: *Cancer nursing: principles and practice,* ed 2, Boston, 1990, Jones and Bartlett.
6. Finley JP: Nursing care of patients with metabolic and physiological oncological emergencies. In Clark JC, McGee RF, editors: *Core curriculum for oncology nursing,* ed 2, Philadelphia, 1992, Saunders.
7. Fleck A: Mobility, impaired physical, related to disease process and treatment. In McNally JC, Stair JC, Somerville ET, editors: *Guidelines for cancer nursing practice,* Orlando, Fla, 1985, Grune & Stratton.
8. Megliola B: Multiple myeloma, *Cancer Nurs* 3(3):209-218, 1980.
9. North Central New Jersey Local Chapter: Body fluid composition, alteration in hypercalcemia. In McNally JC, Stair JC, Somerville ET, editors: *Guidelines for cancer nursing practice,* Orlando, Fla, 1985, Grune & Stratton.
10. North Central New Jersey Local Chapter: Mobility, impaired physical, related to primary bone malignancy or metastatic bone disease. In McNally JC, Stair JC, Somerville ET, editors: *Guidelines for cancer nursing practice,* Orlando, Fla, 1985, Grune & Stratton.
11. Salmon SE, Cassady JR: Plasma cell neoplasms. In DeVita VT Jr, Hellman S, Rosenberg SA, editors: *Cancer: principles and practice of oncology,* ed 4, Philadelphia, 1993, Lippincott.
12. Schnipper L, Wagner H, McCaffrey R: Multiple myeloma and plasma cell dyscrasias. In Cady B, editor: *Cancer manual,* Boston, 1986, American Cancer Society.
13. Sporn J, McIntyre O: Chemotherapy of previously untreated multiple myeloma patients: an analysis of recent treatment results, *Semin Oncol* 13(3):318, 1986.
14. Varterasian M: Biologic and clinical advances in multiple myeloma. *Oncology* 9(5):417-424, 1995.
15. Willoughby S: Pain. In McNally JC, Stair JC, Somerville ET, editors: *Guidelines for cancer nursing practice,* Orlando, Fla, 1985, Grune & Stratton.

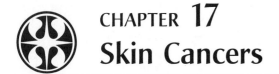

CHAPTER 17
Skin Cancers

SHIRLEY E. OTTO

Skin cancers are classified into two basic groups: non-melanoma and malignant melanoma. The two major cancers in the nonmelanoma group are basal cell and squamous cell carcinomas. Basal and squamous cell carcinomas combined account for more than one third of the 2.2 million new cases of cancer reported each year in the United States.[1,15]

Malignant melanoma is an increasingly common cutaneous malignancy. The incidence has doubled every decade since 1930. Unlike many other forms of cancer that disproportionately affect older individuals, melanoma frequently affects young people. The median age is in the early 40s. Survival of patients with malignant melanoma is directly related to early detection and prompt medical intervention.[13,15,16,26]

NONMELANOMA SKIN CANCERS
Basal Cell Carcinoma

EPIDEMIOLOGY

Basal cell carcinoma (BCC) is the most frequently occurring skin cancer and malignant tumor found in humans. This tumor most often affects whites and rarely occurs in dark-skinned persons. It is characterized by slow local growth capable of causing extensive tissue destruction. BCC is slightly more common in men than women and is usually seen in persons after age 40.[15] BCCs are becoming more common in people still in their 20s. Sun-exposed areas of the body, primarily the head and neck region, are frequent sites of BCC. Numerous types of BCC exist, including nodular, superficial, morpheaform, pigmented, and keratonic BCC syndrome. The most common form is the *nodular* type. This type of BCC frequently occurs on the face, especially the cheeks, forehead, eyelids, and nasolabial folds.[1,14,15,17]

ETIOLOGY AND RISK FACTORS

Environmental factors play an important role in the development of BCC. *Ultraviolet radiation,* primarily chronic exposure to the sun, appears to be the most important environmental risk factor.[10,12,15,24] Other environmental factors in BCC may include exposure to coal tar, pitch, creosote, and arsenic and chronic ingestion of inorganic arsenicals.[1,2] Genetic factors such as basal cell nevus syndrome, fair skin, and light-colored hair have been associated with the development of BCC. A persons' medical history is also important. An increased risk of developing BCC is present in persons who have received a deep burn or have been exposed to x-rays, especially during the first half of this century.[4,15,34]

PREVENTION, SCREENING, AND DETECTION

The primary cause of skin cancers is solar exposure. Ultraviolet (UV) radiation is divided into three different wavelengths: UVA, UVB, and UVC. *UVA waves* are longer and penetrate more deeply into the dermis than UVB waves. As a result of the deeper level of penetration, UVA radiation causes changes in blood vessels and premature aging and is linked with carcinogenesis.[15,17,26] In contrast, *UVB waves* are shorter (penetrating into the epidermis) than UVA waves. UVB radiation produces the most damage to the skin in the form of sunburns and premature aging. Exposure to UVB radiation is associated with development of malignant melanoma.[2,8,16] *UVC waves* are the shortest and rarely reach the surface of the Earth because of the blocking effect of the ozone layer and offer little threat.

Most tanning booths emit UVA radiation. Indoor tanning with UVA radiation is frequently promoted as providing protection against UVB sunburns. The deeper penetration of UVA waves into the dermis causes melanin production; however, the melanosomes are not transferred to the superficial layer of the skin, the epidermis. Persons with a UVA tan who are exposed to UVB radiation receive skin damage in the form of sunburns. The erythema associated with the sunburn is not visible because of the masking effect of the UVA suntan.[2,16,23,35] Exposure to UV radiation from tanning beds should be avoided. Up to 23% of the light from tanning devices is in the UVB range, but even with pure UVA, deoxyribonucleic acid (DNA) damage, cancer, vascular damage, and melanocyte stimulation can occur.[2]

Although it has been shown that UVB radiation is related to carcinogenesis of both melanoma and nonmelanoma skin cancer, it has not definitively been shown that stratospheric ozone depletion is translating into increasing penetrating UV radiation. The ozone depletion issue is very controversial and complex. Further studies are needed to determine the varying effects the ozone depletion has on skin cancer development and trends.[2,30]

Some experts recommend, "When you reach for the sunglasses, reach for the sunscreen."[19,27]

Protecting the cutaneous surfaces from excess solar exposure would greatly decrease the incidence of skin cancers. Solar exposure may be decreased without adversely affecting outdoor activities by employing a few simple measures. Intense sunlight should be avoided between 10 AM and 3 PM, when UV rays are the strongest. Outdoor activities, such as walking, gardening, and other hobbies, should be planned for the early morning or late afternoon to minimize exposure. Prolonged sunbathing or outdoor activities for any longer than *2½ hours per day* puts an individual at risk for skin cancer. Protective clothing, such as hats and long-sleeved shirts, helps to minimize sun exposure.

The use of sunscreens with sun protection factor (SPF) ratings of 30 or higher are preferred over those with low ratings (less than 15). Sunscreens should be applied 15 to 30 minutes before exposure and every 2 to 3 hours during exposure. Sunscreens may need to be applied more often because heat, humidity, and sweat combine to decrease the effectiveness of the sunscreens. Sunscreens should be applied liberally to sun-exposed areas of the body, especially the head and neck region, which are frequent sites of occurrence of BCC. Special attention should be paid to the nose, rim of the ears, cheeks, and forehead.[7,10,23,24,27]

CLASSIFICATION AND CLINICAL FEATURES

BCC often presents as a single, small, firm, dome-shaped, flesh-colored nodule with raised edges and pearly white borders. Telangiectatic vessels are usually prominent and easily recognizable through the thin epidermis. The center of the lesion frequently ulcerates and bleeds and may resemble a pimple that has failed to heal. Examination of all skin surfaces once a month is imperative for those persons at risk of developing new lesions or recurrences of old lesions.[34] BCC is classified according to clinical and histologic differences (see box above).

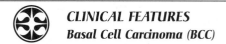

CLINICAL FEATURES
Basal Cell Carcinoma (BCC)

Nodular BCC
Bulky, nodular growth caused by lack of keratinization
Characteristics include a thinning epidermis, producing a shiny pink, translucent, pearly hue over the lesion
Early stages resemble a smooth pimple that fails to heal
As the tumor enlarges, the border edge raises and the center becomes necrotic
Lesion bleeds easily from mild injury and doubles in size every 6 to 12 months[12] at the rate of 5 mm per year[34]

Superficial BCC
Tends to develop in multiple sites, growing peripherally across the skin surface, becoming as large as 10 to 15 cm
Appears most frequently on the trunk as a well-demarcated, erythematous, scaly patch with discreet nodules[14,30]
Often confused with psoriasis[34]

Pigmented BCC
Contains melanin in the epidermis, dermis, and within the tumor itself
Often mistaken clinically as melanoma
Colors include blue, black, or brown appearance with a raised pearly border
Found in dark-complexioned persons such as Latin Americans or Japanese (not blacks)[17,30]

Morpheaform or sclerotic BCC
More aggressive lesion that appears as a flat, depressed scarlike plaque, pale yellow or white in color
Margins indistinct with nodules, ulcerations, or bleeding occurring within the plaque
Often undetected or misdiagnosed with a lower cure rate than nodular BCC[17,34]

Keratonic BCC
Appears clinically similar to nodular ulcerative form
Located in the preauricular and postauricular sulcus
Aggressive in its growth
Often recurs locally
Type most likely to metastasize[34]

DIAGNOSIS AND STAGING

Clinical diagnosis of skin cancers must be confirmed by histologic studies. A *shave biopsy* (top of lesion into depth of middermis) is performed using local anesthesia. *Punch biopsy* (sharp, small circular "punch" similar to a cookie cutter approach) is used if the tumor is suspected to be in the deeper layers of the skin. The tissue sample is examined to determine the clinical diagnosis and identifying features of the various classifications.

On determination of the clinical diagnosis, classification, and histopathologic grading, specific treatment modalities are recommended.[4,6,15,17,36]

The American Joint Committee on Cancer (AJCC) recommends the following stage grouping:

Clinical staging for nonmelanoma skin cancer (basal and squamous)*

Stage 0 (Tis-N0-M0)	Carcinoma in situ No evidence of regional lymph node or distant metastasis
Stage I (T1-N0-M0)	Primary tumor superficial and 2 cm or less at largest dimension No evidence of regional lymph node or distant metastasis
Stage II (T2-N0-M0 or T3-N0-M0)	Primary tumor greater than 2 cm but no larger than 5 cm in largest dimension, *or* primary tumor greater than 5 cm in largest dimension No evidence of regional lymph node or distant metastasis
Stage III (T4-N0-M0 or any T-N1-M0)	Primary tumor invades deep extradermal structures such as cartilage, skeletal muscle, or bone, *or* any tumor size with evidence of regional lymph node metastasis No evidence of distant metastasis
Stage IV (any T-any N-M1)	Presence of distant metastasis regardless of tumor size or nodal involvement

Clinical staging is based on the physical examination and palpation of the lesion and lymph nodes.

Pathologic staging requires resection of the entire site and confirmation of any lymph node involvement. Underlying bony structures should be imaged, especially if these lesions occur on the scalp.

Complete excision of the site and microscopic verification are necessary to determine the histologic type.

Histopathologic grading for basal and squamous cell carcinomas is similar to the grading system for other cancers. G1 signifies well-differentiated tumor cells, G2 refers to moderately well-differentiated cells, G3 signifies poorly differentiated cells, and G4 signifies undifferentiated cells. Confirmation of the extent of disease by biopsy of the suspected cutaneous or subcutaneous spread is imperative.[4,6,17,30,34]

METASTASIS

BCC metastasizes via the lymphatics or blood and is a rare occurrence. The most common predisposing factors are size of primary tumor and response to surgery and radiotherapy. Recurrence of the disease varies with the size of the tumor and length of follow-up. Recurrence rates vary; less than one-third occur in the first year; 50% occur in 2 years; almost two-thirds within the first 3 years; and 18% occur in the fifth and tenth year after treatment.[34]

*Modified from Beahrs OH, Myers MH, editors: *Manual for staging of cancer,* ed 4, Philadelphia, 1992, Lippincott.

TREATMENT MODALITIES

Treatment for both basal and squamous cell carcinomas depends on many factors: the size and location of the lesion, histologic type of cancer, extension into nearby structures, presence of metastases, previous treatment, anticipated cosmetic results, and the patient's age and condition. Multiple modalities exist for the treatment of BCC: surgery, radiation therapy, chemotherapy, and biotherapy.[4,12,32,34]

Surgery

Surgical intervention is used to treat about 90% of BCCs. The goal is the complete removal of the tumor. Most of the procedures require local anesthesia and minimal equipment and can be performed in an ambulatory setting.[4,17,30,34]

Excisional surgery. Excisional surgery is usually performed with a 4 mm margin. This is the treatment of choice in large tumors or those with poorly defined margins on cheeks, forehead, trunk, and legs. Surgical excision may also be indicated when metastasis is present.[17,34]

Cryosurgery. Cryosurgery involves tissue destruction by freezing. Liquid nitrogen is administered by a spray or the use of cryoprobes. Rapid freezing results in intracellular and extracellular ice crystallization. Cell destruction is potentiated by a rapid freeze and slow thaw cycle. This method is useful in small to large nodular and superficial BCCs but is *not* indicated for deeply invasive tumors or BCCs of the scalp. Cryosurgery is recommended for BCCs of the eyelid because the procedure preserves normal tissue and obviates the need for reconstructive surgery.[17]

Electrodesiccation and curettage. This surgical method uses heat to destroy tissue. After the tumor is marked and anesthetized, a debulking process is used to scrape away abnormal tissue within 1 to 2 mm. The base of tumor is then electrodesiccated. Curettage of the base is performed using a large and tiny curet to track any extension of the tumor. The procedure is repeated as necessary until a normal plane of tissue is reached. These interventions are useful with small (<2 cm) to medium nodular and superficial BCCs with well-defined margins. BCCs larger than 2 cm in diameter, those located in zones at high risk for recurrence, and all high-risk squamous cell carcinoma are best treated by other methods.[4,17,34]

Mohs micrographic surgery. Mohs micrographic surgery involves surgical removal of the tumor layer by layer until all margins are free of the tumor on microscopic examination. Mohs micrographic surgery permits the best histologic verification of complete removal and allows maximum conservation of tissue.[17] This is the treatment of choice for invasive squamous cell and primary basal cell carcinomas that are larger than 2 cm in diameter, have indistinct clinical margins, are located on zones of the face with a known high recurrence rate, occur in a cosmetic or functional area, such as the nose or eyelid, or are aggressive, such as morpheaform BCC.[4,17,34]

Regardless of the surgical treatment used, the cure rate for BCC after surgical intervention is nearly 95%.

Lasers. The carbon dioxide laser has advantages over conventional surgery by sealing small blood vessels and nerves. It provides a relatively bloodless surgical field and reduced postoperative pain.[17]

Radiation Therapy

Radiation therapy is a viable and effective alternative when surgical interventions are contraindicated and in elderly or debilitated persons who are unable to tolerate a surgical procedure. Tissue conservation is a benefit of radiation therapy, especially when dealing with lesions on the nose, eyelid, or lips. Cosmetic results are good with this type of treatment because surgical scars and skin grafting are eliminated. A combined approach of preoperative and postoperative radiation and surgery may be indicated for extensive tumors. Disadvantages of this treatment method are related to the administration schedule. Radiation is fractionated over multiple treatment sessions (usually 450 Gy/3 weeks in 300 cGy daily fractions) to reduce radiation-induced side effects. This schedule may pose problems for patients and their families who must travel a distance to reach the treatment center.[17,34]

Radiation therapy is not recommended for tumors located on the trunk, extremities, dorsum of the hands, or scalp; for those arising in sweat and sebaceous glands; for morpheaform basal cell and verrucous squamous cell tumors; for those larger than 8 cm; and for those located on the upper lip growing into the nostril.[17,34]

Chemotherapy and Biotherapy

Topical 5-fluorouracil (5-FU) may be used in nevoid BCC syndrome but is contraindicated in treating any of the other types of BCC. 5-FU destroys the surface tumor without affecting deeper cells, thus allowing invasion to continue at the base of the tumor.

Cisplatin, bleomycin, cyclophosphamide, 5-FU, and vinblastine have been studied; cisplatin has been the most effective and is associated with the longest remission.

The lack of an established systemic therapy for recurrent or advanced local, regional, or metastatic disease has led to the use of *biologic response modifiers* (BRMs), especially interferon-α. Systemic interferon-α has produced a 50% objective response rate in clinical testing.[4] A study of 172 patients receiving intralesional injections of interferon alfa-2b reported an 81% cure rate after a follow-up period of 1 year.[3] Other agents, specifically retinoids, have also shown some activity against BCC. Topical retinoid therapy and systemic retinoid therapy have both produced objective response rates greater than 50% in both basal and squamous cell carcinomas.[17,30,34]

PROGNOSIS

Metastatic disease is rarely seen with BCC, even though it tends to be a locally aggressive tumor. If left untreated, the tumor will locally invade vital structures such as blood vessels, lymph nodes, nerve sheaths, cartilage, bone, lungs, and the dura mater.[14,17,29,30]

BCC is highly curable with early detection and treatment. Cure rates are close to 100% in persons with lesions less than 1 cm. The overall 5-year survival rate is approximately 95% when surgical intervention or radiation therapy is used.[29]

It is imperative that patients with BCC continue defined scheduled follow-up examinations by a physician. Follow-up examinations should be performed at 6-month intervals during the first 2 years and then yearly for 5 years to detect the recurrence of previously treated or new primary BCCs while they are small enough to remove without significant cosmetic loss.[14,17,29,30,33]

Squamous Cell Carcinoma

EPIDEMIOLOGY

Squamous cell carcinoma (SCC) is less common than BCC. SCC occurs more frequently in persons with light complexions. SCC is also more common in men, and the incidence increases with advancing age. The average age of onset for SCC is approximately 60 years. Unlike BCC, this tumor frequency occurs on the hands and forearms as well as on the head and neck region,[15] especially the ears, lower lip, scalp, and upper face.[1,17,34]

ETIOLOGY AND RISK FACTORS

SCC is most often found in sun-damaged skin previously affected by actinic keratoses. All the predisposing risk factors mentioned in regard to BCC have also been associated with the development of SCC.[17,23]

PREVENTION, SCREENING, AND DETECTION

Prevention and detection methods are similar for both SCC and BCC. The avoidance of UV light and the use of sunscreens and protective clothing are important. In addition to the head and neck area, sunscreens should also be liberally applied to the hands and fore-arms.[8,10,23,24,26]

CLASSIFICATION AND CLINICAL FEATURES

SCC has a more indiscriminate method of classification. Because of the varying general characteristics and the source of tissue presentation, it is classified by presenting symptoms, tissue source, and histologic difference (see box below).

CLINICAL FEATURES
Squamous Cell Carcinoma (SCC)[17,30,34]

General characteristics

Occurs anywhere on sun-damaged skin and on mucous membrane with squamous epithelium

Appears as a round to irregular shape, with a plaquelike or nodular character covered by a warty scale, indistinct margins, and firm erythematous dome-shaped nodule with corelike center that ulcerates

Dull red in color

Grows by expansion and infiltration as well as by tracking along various tissue planes

Invades below the level of the sweat gland and has a higher degree of malignant potential

Overall invasiveness and depth of neoplasm are significant when determining risk of recurrence

Ischemic ulceration

Occurs in varicose ulcers, chronic ulcers, and poorly healed fistulas/tracks with old scars

Accompanied by increased drainage, pain, and bleeding

Bowen's disease

Associated with arsenic ingestion

Occurs on sun-exposed and non-sun-exposed areas of the skin, including mucous membrane of vulva, vagina, nose, and conjunctiva

Nodular reddish brown plaque with areas of scales and crusts

Actinic cheilitis

Rapidly growing progressive invasive lesion that occurs on the lip, often a result of smoking

Lower lip is primary site in 95% of patients

Early appearance is local thickening, progressing to a firm nodular lesion with destructive ulceration

Diagnosis is frequently missed (2 years after onset) and is usually 1 to 2 cm in diameter at initial biopsy

Reported risk of metastasis from SCC of lip has ranged from 5% to 37%

Verrucous

Well-differentiated lesion frequently seen on glans penis, vulva, scrotum, sole, back, or buttock and appears as a slowly growing, warty lesion

Surgical excision is treatment of choice

DIAGNOSIS AND STAGING

Diagnosis and staging for SCC are the same as for BCC described earlier in this chapter.[4,6,17]

METASTASIS

Overall, 2% to 3% of all patients with SCC of the skin develop metastatic disease, with death resulting in 75% of these patients. The occurrence and degree vary according to morphologic characteristics and size and depth of penetration of the tumor. Metastasis occurs late via the lymphatics (within 2 years) after the tumor has invaded the subcutaneous lymph nodes and the lymphatics of the deeper structure.[15,17,30,34]

TREATMENT MODALITIES
Surgery

SCC can be treated by procedures similar to those used with BCC. Some exceptions exist; for example, a slightly larger excisional margin should be performed surgically. In addition, it is important to examine the regional lymph nodes for the presence of tumor.

The treatment of high risk-SCC with no palpable nodes may involve local control alone, regional control with prophylactic lymph node dissection, radiation to draining nodes, or combined therapy. Metastatic SCC lymph nodes is treated surgically, with adjuvant radiation therapy given preoperatively or postoperatively.[17,30,34]

Cryotherapy

Cryotherapy for SCC is useful in selected patients. Lesions with a diameter of 0.5 to 2.0 cm and well-defined borders are amenable to this modality. This technique boasts exceptional cosmetic results and has achieved 5-year cure rates as high as 96%.[17]

Chemotherapy

Topical 5-FU is recommended for treatment of premalignant actinic keratosis. In advanced SCC, systemic retinoids have produced response rates greater than 70%.[17,30]

Radiation Therapy

Radiation therapy is used for primary SCC employing a variety of fractionation regimens, ranging from 22 Gy in a single fraction to 70 Gy in multiple fractions.[17,31]

PROGNOSIS

Of the two nonmelanoma skin cancers, metastasis is seen more often in SCC. Ordinarily, primary SCC localized to the skin has an incidence of metastasis of approximately 3%. The lesion's ability to metastasize depends on the size, degree of differentiation, and depth of invasion. SCC may metastasize to the regional lymph nodes or the lung. Primary lesions of the lip metastasize more frequently, at a rate greater than 10%.

SCC also has high cure rates (75% to 80%) when either surgery or radiation therapy is used. Because this lesion has the ability to metastasize as well as recur, it is generally considered a higher-risk skin cancer. Most of the deaths resulting from nonmelanoma forms of skin cancer can be attributed to SCC.

As in BCC, regularly scheduled follow-up is mandatory for patients with SCC. Invasive SCC can be a potentially lethal neoplasm and warrants close follow-up. The association between solar radiation and the development of SCC is firmly established, and it is important to advise patients to avoid excessive exposure to the sun and always to use a sun block with an SPF of 15 or greater. The recommended schedule is 6-month intervals during the first 2 years and then yearly for 5 years.*

MALIGNANT MELANOMA

EPIDEMIOLOGY

Melanoma, a relatively uncommon tumor, affects approximately 38,300 persons in the United States each year. The incidence of melanoma is increasing at the rate of 4% annually.[1] Estimates are that, by the year 2000, 1

*References 4, 8, 10, 17, 21, 30.

in 100 persons will develop a primary malignant melanoma during their lifetime.[15] The increase in incidence has been greater in men than women. The incidence in white males has increased 5.1% each year, 93.3% overall, while the incidence in females has increased only 3.8% per year, 67.7% overall.

Similar to the nonmelanoma skin cancers, malignant melanoma most frequently affects whites. The most common site of occurrence in dark-skinned persons are palms, soles, nailbeds, fingers, toes, and mucous membranes. Unlike basal and squamous cell carcinomas, melanoma may occur in persons in their teens and early 20s and 30s.[15] The highest incidence rates occur in persons over age 60.[36] In men the upper back and trunk are the most common sites of occurrence; the back and lower extremities are the most common sites in women (Figure 17-1).

ETIOLOGY AND RISK FACTORS

Two important environmental factors are sun exposure and geographic latitude. Intense, intermittent exposure to the sun, especially during childhood and adolescence, increases the risk for melanoma in later life.[1,2,15] A latitude gradient for melanoma also exists, with countries with areas of high solar exposure also being the areas of highest melanoma incidence. For every 1000 feet above sea level, there is a compounded 4% increase in UV radiation exposure. In short, the closer one lives to the equator, the higher the risk for developing melanoma.[5,15,16,19,36]

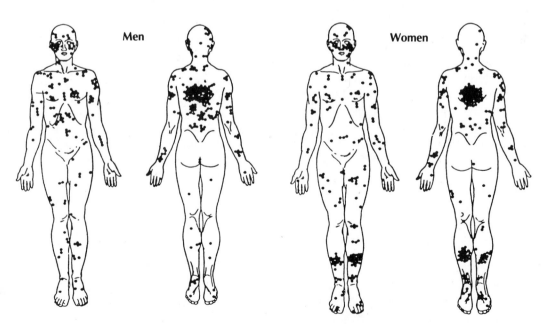

Figure 17-1 Anatomic distribution of malignant melanoma in men and women. (From Becker J, Goldberg L, Tschen JA: *Am Fam Physician* 39(5):203, 1989.)

Genetic risk factors, such as fair complexion and blond or red hair color, are similar for the development of both nonmelanoma skin cancers and malignant melanoma. A person's ability to tan seems to be a factor; persons who burn easily and are poor tanners have an increased risk.[1,2] Persons who experience intermittent heavy sun exposure are also at higher risk. In addition, a personal or family history of melanoma, dysplastic nevus syndrome, immunosuppression, or congenital nevi also increases one's risk. First-degree relatives of patients with melanoma are about two to eight times more likely than the general public to be diagnosed with melanoma.[12,13,18]

NURSING MANAGEMENT

Nursing diagnoses for basal cell carcinoma (BCC) and squamous cell carcinoma (SCC) are similar. Some variations may be necessary depending on type and location of skin cancer and method of treatment.

NURSING DIAGNOSES

- *Knowledge deficit related to prevention and early detection of skin cancer, disease process, treatment (surgery, radiation therapy, chemotherapy, biotherapy), home care management of surgical wound*
- *Skin integrity, impaired, related to skin cancer and surgical treatment*
- *Infection, risk for, related to surgical wound*
- *Mobility, impaired physical, related to surgical treatment and possible skin graft*
- *Body image disturbance related to location and surgical treatment for skin cancer*
- *Social interaction, impaired, related to location and surgical treatment of skin cancer*
- *Anxiety related to diagnosis of cancer, fear of recurrence, death, pain, disfigurement, changes in life-style*

Nursing assessment and intervention should focus on prevention, detection, and treatment methods. The nursing history should include a thorough skin assessment, which consists of information regarding patient risk factors, and a complete skin examination. Patient teaching priorities should include the prevention and detection methods discussed in this chapter (see box at right). Geriatric considerations are listed in the box, p. 379.[7,11,23,25]

Postsurgical interventions include instructing patients and families on the management of a surgical wound. Keeping the area clean and dry and observing for signs and symptoms of infection are imperative. If skin grafting is required, patients and their families should be instructed to keep the graft immobile to prevent stress on the edges of the wound. Limbs should be elevated to minimize edema. Mineral oil or lanolin may be used to remove superficial crusts, moisten the site of the skin graft, and stimulate circulation. Treatment-related complications are listed in the box, p. 379. Nursing management of complications of other treatment methods, such as radiation therapy, chemotherapy, and biotherapy, are discussed in detail in Chapters 21, 22, and 23, respectively.

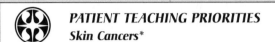

PATIENT TEACHING PRIORITIES
*Skin Cancers**

Risk factors for development of malignant melanoma

Family history of malignant melanoma
Presence of blond or red hair
Presence of marked freckling on upper back
History of three or more blistering sunburns before age 20
History of 3 or more years of an outdoor summer job as a teenager
Presence of actinic keratosis

Prevention of skin cancer measures

Avoid excessive sun exposure, particularly the hours between 10 AM and 3 PM.
Wear sunscreens and lip balm with a sun protection factor of 30 or greater.
Use available shade.
Wear protective clothing.
Refrain from using manufactured tanning devices.

Skin cancer screening and detection

Perform monthly self-examination of skin or with other person.
With good lighting, use two mirrors to visualize the abdomen, perineal area, and back.
Use blow hair dryer and mirror to visualize scalp.
Observe each body part carefully, especially hidden areas such as between toes and folds of skin.
Use of body chart facilitates documentation of changes and suspected lesions to report.
Persons with two or more family members with a history of malignant melanoma should be examined by a dermatologist every 6 months.
Recognize and report symptoms or changes in skin characteristics promptly to physician, such as:
A, Asymmetry of shape
B, Border irregularity
C, Color variegation (black, brown, white, blue, red)
D, Diameter larger than 5 mm

*References 7, 9, 10, 13, 15-19, 23, 24, 27, 33.

GERIATRIC CONSIDERATIONS
Skin Cancers*

Geriatric population has greatest incidence of precancerous and cancerous skin lesions.

Average age of onset for squamous cell, lentigo malignant melanoma, and acral lentiginous melanoma is 60 years.

Age-related sensory and muscle deficits require assistance of other person for monthly skin self-examination.

Age-related changes in skin characteristics include fair skin and easily bruised superficial tissue.

Limited access to health care system and limited health care resources may inhibit preventive health care.

Senior citizen centers should be targeted to reach those who participate in organized activities

*References 7, 11, 13, 15, 17, 26, 33.

COMPLICATIONS
Skin Cancers*

Surgery and radiation therapy

Scarring of affected tissue
Skin discoloration
Alterations in cosmetic appearance
Chronic skin ulcerations
Limited use of limb if extensive treatment

Chemotherapy and biotherapy

Nausea and vomiting
Flu-like syndrome
Myelosuppression
Paresthesia
Necrotic tissue as result of drug extravasation
Pulmonary fibrosis
Renal damage
Hot flashes
Hypersensitivity
Ototoxicity
Alopecia
Allergic reaction

General

Alteration in cosmetic appearance and body image
Loss of functional use of extremity
Scarring and skin discoloration
Metastatic disease process resulting in invasive treatment and potential ultimate death

*References 17, 19, 28, 29, 36.

The importance of early detection should be stressed with both patients and families. BCC is almost always curable. Recurrent lesions or new lesions can be successfully treated when detected early for BCC and SCC.

Patients and family members should be instructed on the procedure and the importance of periodic skin self-examination. Patients should be encouraged to keep appointments for regular follow-up examinations with their physician. Methods of prevention should also be taught, primarily the importance of avoiding intense sunlight and using protective sunscreens and clothing.*

Specific outcome goals and interventions are listed in the Nursing Management box, pp. 384-386.

*References 7, 8, 10, 16, 18, 19, 26.

PREVENTION, SCREENING, AND DETECTION

Prevention methods for nonmelanoma skin cancers and malignant melanoma are similar. The avoidance of intense sun exposure and the use of protective clothing and sunscreens are important. Children should also be protected from sunburns because an increased risk of melanoma exists in persons who have experienced traumatic sunburns as children.[2,10]

Early detection and prompt treatment are essential. Warning signs of melanoma are any unusual skin condition; scaliness, oozing, and/or bleeding of a mole or other pigmented growth; a change in color or size of a mole or any other pigmented growth or spot; a spread of the pigment beyond the normal border; a change in sensation, itchiness, tenderness, or pain; and the development of a new nodule.[13,16,36]

The early warning signs of malignant melanoma can be easily remembered by thinking of the acronym ABCD: *A*symmetry, *B*order, *C*olor, and *D*iameter. Malignant melanomas are usually asymmetric (i.e., one half of the mole does not match the other half). Early malignant melanomas tend to have irregular borders. The edges may be ragged, notched, or blurred, unlike benign lesions, which usually have regular, smooth margins. Pigmentation in malignant melanomas is not uniform. Colors may range from various hues of tan and brown to black, with red and white intermingled. Malignant melanomas are often greater than 5 mm when first identified. A sudden or continued increase in the size of a mole should be reported.[16,36]

Examination of the skin once a month by inspecting all skin surfaces for any of the above changes is imperative for those persons at risk of developing malignant melanoma (see box, p. 378). Persons previously diagnosed with malignant melanoma should also perform skin self-examination once a month because of the increased likelihood for recurrence.*

The educated patient or family member is often the first person to detect changes in skin conditions. In one study, approximately one half (53%) of 216 incident cases of melanoma in Massachusetts were self-discovered, whereas the remaining cases were detected by medical providers (26%), family members (17%), and others (3%). Compared with men, women were more likely to discover their own lesions and those of their spouses.†

CLASSIFICATION AND CLINICAL FEATURES

Malignant melanomas may arise from three types of moles, or nevi: the common acquired nevus, dysplastic nevus, or congenital melanocytic nevus. The most frequently encountered benign pigmented lesion is the *common acquired nevus* (CAN), better known as the "normal" mole. CAN are absent at birth. Nevus production begins in childhood with increased development during puberty. Production begins to taper at about 35 to 40 years of age. Most adults have about 20 to 40 nevi on their bodies. CAN are usually small (<5 mm), exhibiting uniformity in color, surface, symmetry, and regularity of borders.[5,36] The risk that any one CAN will develop into a malignant melanoma is small. See box at right for characteristics and clinical features of common benign pigmented lesions.

Dysplastic nevi (DN) are acquired pigmented lesions. These nevi are considered to be precursors of cancer as well as markers of persons at risk for development of malignant melanoma. *Dysplastic nevus syndrome* (DNS) usually manifests during young adulthood. Persons with DNS develop nevi throughout their lifetime and may have more than 100 nevi on their bodies.[5,12,13,36] Table 17-1 compares and contrasts clinical characteristics of DN with CAN. Basically, DN are larger with irregular borders and variegated colors. DN can occur anywhere on the body but are more often found on the trunk, back, breasts, buttocks, genitals, and scalp.[5,13,36]

DNS may be classified as familial or sporadic. Familial DNS is an inherited autosomal dominant trait. Persons with DN who have two or more first-degree relatives with melanoma have almost a 100% chance of developing melanoma.

Sporadic DNS is seen in persons with no family history of DN or melanoma. The risk of developing mela-

CLINICAL FEATURES
Common Benign Pigmented Lesions

Simple lentigo
Small, 1 to 5 mm, macular, pigmented lesion
Precursor to common mole
Sharply defined, round
Smooth or jagged edges that may appear on the surface of skin
More concentrated on sun-exposed areas
Junctional nevus
Small, less than 6 mm, well-circumscribed, pigmented lesion with smooth surface
Relatively uniform pigmentation that ranges from dark brown to black
Compound nevus
Well-circumscribed, less than 6 mm, raised papule
Uniform in pigmentation
Skin colored tan to various shades of brown
Solar lentigo
Small to somewhat larger macule known as a "liver spot"
Found on sun-exposed people with significant sun damage: face, chest, back, dorsa of hands
Uniform tan to brown
Seborrheic keratosis
Sharply demarcated purple that ranges in diameter
Few millimeter to several centimeter
Verrucous, round, ovid, variably raised
Surface "dull" or "warty"
Common on face, neck, trunk
Variably raised
Light brown to dark brown

noma for these persons is 5% to 26% greater than for the general population.[4,12,36]

Congenital melanocytic nevi appear as raised, dark-brown to black, oval or round macules that may contain coarse hairs. Congenital nevi are present at birth and are classified by size in diameter as small (<1.5 cm), medium (1.5 to 19.9 cm), and large (>19.9 cm). Most congenital nevi are small or medium. The risk of developing malignant melanoma from congenital nevi is controversial, with estimates as high as 22 times. Persons with congenital nevi larger than 3 to 5 cm are thought to be at even greater risk of developing malignant melanoma.[4,5,12,16,36]

Four types of malignant melanoma exist: superficial spreading, nodular, lentigo maligna, and acral lentiginous (see box, p. 381, for clinical features). *Superficial spreading malignant melanoma* is the most common form. About 70% of all cutaneous melanomas are of the superficial spreading type. Superficial spreading melanoma occurs more frequently in women than men and is usually seen in persons in the 40- to 50-year-old age-

---

*References 7, 8, 16, 18, 21, 28.
†References 18, 19, 21, 26, 32, 33.

Table 17-1 Comparison of Common Acquired Nevus (CAN) and Dysplastic Nevus (DN)

Characteristic	Common acquired nevus	Dysplastic nevus
Color	Uniformly tan or brown; one mole looks much like another	Variegated, mottled, mixture of tan, red/pink, brown, within a single nevus; nevi look very different from each other
Shape	Round; sharp, clear-cut borders between nevus and surrounding skin; may be flat or elevated	Irregular, notched border; borders may fade off into surrounding skin; always have a macular or flat component
Size	Usually <5 mm diameter (smaller than size of a pencil)	Usually >5 mm diameter
Number	Average adult has 20 to 40 scattered over body	Typically 100, although some people may have only a few nevi
Location	Usually on sun-exposed surfaces of body above waist; scalp, breast, buttocks rarely involved	Back is most common site; may occur below waist and on scalp, breast, buttocks, genitals

Modified from Lawler PE, Schreiber S: *Oncol Nurs Forum* 16(3):348, 1989.

CLINICAL FEATURES
Malignant Melanoma Pigmented Lesions[5,36]

Superficial spreading melanoma
Variegated in color with areas appearing blue, black, gray, white, or pink
Irregular pigmented plaque with areas of regression and notched borders; horizontal or radial extension
May appear scaly and crusty and itch
Increasingly more common among young adults

Nodular melanoma
Often resembles a "blood blister"
Appears as a symmetric, raised, dome-shaped lesion; vertical growth patterns
Blue-black in color
Can be amelanotic

Lentigo malignant melanoma
Appears as a large, flat, irregular lesion resembling a stain
Variegated in color, ranging from tan to black with areas of regression
Located on face and neck of elderly, severely suntanned whites

Acral lentiginous melanoma
Usually flat, irregular, with an average diameter of 3 cm
Blue or black discoloration or a tan and brown stain; occurs on palms and soles or under nailbeds

group.[5,20,36] Common sites of occurrence of this lesion are the lower extremities and back in women and the back in men.

Nodular malignant melanoma is the next most frequently occurring melanoma. This lesion occurs twice as often in men than in women and tends to affect persons in their 50s and 60s. Nodular melanoma may occur anywhere on the body; however, common sites of occurrence are the head, neck, and trunk regions.

Lentigo maligna melanoma is a rare lesion accounting for 5% to 10% of melanomas. This lesion primarily occurs after age 60. Most lesions affect the face, but they may also occur on any sun-exposed area of the body, such as lower legs and hands.[4,15,36]

Acral lentiginous melanoma is the least common, accounting for less than 10% of all melanomas. This lesion tends to occur on the palms, soles, nailbeds, fingers, toes, and mucous membranes. Acral lentiginous melanoma is the most common type of melanoma among blacks, Orientals, and Hispanics.[20,36]

DIAGNOSIS AND STAGING

When a lesion is suspected to be melanoma, a biopsy should be performed. The technique of choice is a total excisional biopsy with narrow margins. The biopsy procedure is accompanied by a thorough history and a complete physical examination. The skin should be carefully inspected and palpated for intracutaneous metastasis. Further diagnostic evaluation includes routine laboratory tests (complete blood count, lactate dehydrogenase, blood urea nitrogen, partial thromboplastin time), liver enzyme studies, urine analysis, serum creatinine, blood chemistries, and a chest x-ray film. Other essential studies (e.g., computed tomography [CT] scan or magnetic resonance imaging [MRI]) are guided by the symptomatology reported by the patient and outcome of the above tests. If lymphadenopathy is present at diagnosis and the index of metastasis is high, definitive nodal dissection may be performed without a biopsy. Radiographic studies to define the direction of the lymphatic drainage are performed before the nodal dissection.[5,19,36] Nuclear bone scans are used to evaluate recent persistent localized bone pain, with or without elevated serum alkaline phosphatase levels.

The most important prognostic factors in melanoma are depth of invasion (Clark's levels) and thickness of the tumor. Both of these factors determine the T classification and ultimately the stage grouping. If the depth of invasion (Clark's level) and the thickness of the tumor do not match, the tumor is assigned to the higher T classification (Figure 17-2).[5,25,36]

Clinical and microstaging classifications for melanoma of the skin*

Stage IA	Primary tumor invades papillary dermis
(T1-N0-M0;	Primary tumor 0.75 mm or less in thickness
Clark's level II)	No evidence of regional lymph node or distant metastasis
Stage IB	Primary tumor fills papillary dermis but does not
(T2-N0-M0;	penetrate reticular dermis
Clark's level III)	Primary tumor 0.76 to 1.5 mm thick
	No evidence of regional lymph node or distant metastasis
Stage II	Primary tumor invades reticular dermis but does
(T3-N0-M0;	not invade subcutaneous tissue
Clark's level IV)	Primary tumor 1.51 to 4.0 mm thick
	No evidence of regional lymph node or distant metastasis
Stage IIIA	Primary tumor invades reticular dermis, extending
(T4-N0-M0;	into subcutaneous tissue, and/or presence of
Clark's level V)	satellite(s) within 2 cm of primary tumor
	Primary tumor greater than 4.0 mm thick
	No evidence of regional lymph node or distant metastasis
Stage IIIB	Primary tumor invades any depth
(any T-N1 or	Evidence of regional lymph node metastasis
N2-M0)	and/or in-transit metastasis
	No evidence of distant metastasis
Stage IV	Evidence of distant metastasis regardless of tumor
(any T-any	depth or thickness or nodal metastasis
N-M1)	

*Modified from Beahrs OH, Myers MH, editors: *Manual for staging of cancer,* ed 4, Philadelphia, 1992, Lippincott.

Pathologic staging of the primary melanoma is based on a microscopic assessment of thickness and level of invasion (Clark's levels I to V). Therefore evaluation of the entire tumor is advised rather than a wedge or a punch biopsy. Regional nodes should be evaluated by a physical examination.[36]

Histopathologic grading for melanoma is identical to the grading system used for basal and squamous cell carcinoma.

METASTASIS

Malignant melanoma may spread to any organ or remote viscera. Common sites for disseminated disease are the skin (intracutaneous or subcutaneous metastasis), bone, brain, liver, and lung.[5,36]

Malignant melanomas may grow radially or vertically. All melanomas except the nodular type have an initial radial growth phase, which may last more than a decade. During this phase the melanoma cells remain confined to the epidermis. The lesion expands horizontally with only a slight increase in the tumor's depth.

The vertical phase is characterized by dermal penetration and invasion of the dermis and subcutaneous tissue by the melanoma cells. The lesion may then metastasize by way of vascular or lymphatic channels. The melanoma cells then spread rapidly to other parts of the body. Nodular malignant melanoma has no radial growth phase. These lesions are usually convex and are palpable because of the growth elevation above the level of the normal skin.[4,5,12,19,36]

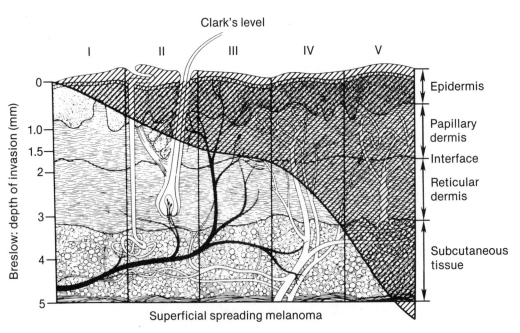

Figure 17-2   Anatomic landmarks and Clark's level of invasion. (From DiSaia PJ, Creasman WT: *Clinical gynecologic oncology,* ed 4, St Louis, 1993, Mosby.)

TREATMENT MODALITIES

Surgery

Surgical excision of the primary growth is the preferred treatment method. The shave biopsy technique should not be used. For lesions less than 1.5 mm thick, the surgeon usually makes a wide excision (approximately 2 cm), removing more normal tissue than with other skin cancer surgeries. For lesions that are greater than 1.5 mm thick, most surgeons excise margins of 5 cm including the underlying fascia.[5,36]

Elective regional node dissection (ERLAND). The rationale for performing ERLAND is based on the hypothesis that melanoma metastasizes sequentially first to the regional lymph nodes and later from the nodes to distant sites. ERLAND improves survival rates for intermediate-thickness (1.5 to 4 mm) melanomas; for melanoma 0.76 to 1.5 mm thick, there is no significant difference in survival; and ERLAND has no advantage for patients with melanoma less than 0.75 mm or more than 4.0 mm in thickness.[5,31,36]

Cutaneous melanoma spreads to four main lymph node basins: intraparotid, cervical, axillary, and ilioguinal. If metastatic disease appears first in intraparotid nodes, superficial parotidectomy in conjunction with nodal dissection is usually performed. If cervical nodes are extensively affected, a radical neck dissection is the procedure of choice. Axillary node dissection with an en bloc removal of pectoralis minor muscle is the standard procedure.[5,36]

Radiation Therapy

Melanoma has traditionally been considered relatively radioresistant. Experimental radiation therapy endeavors include radiosensitizers such as misonidazole and the use of fast neutrons. The energy released by the neutrons destroys the melanoma cells while the surrounding normal tissue are spared. Radiation therapy is useful, however, in alleviating symptoms from metastasis to the bone, brain, and other organs.[5,20,36]

Chemotherapy

Dacarbazine (DTIC) is the most extensively studied and regarded as the most effective single agent against malignant melanoma. The most common dosage schedule has been 250 mg/m^2 daily for 5 days every 4 weeks. The major side effects are severe nausea and vomiting and flu-like symptoms. Other cytotoxic agents reported to demonstrate some efficacy include carmustine (BCNU), semustine (methyl CCNU), vindesine, and cisplatin. Combination chemotherapy includes the following:
• DBPT: DTIC, BCNU, cisplatin, tamoxifen
• BELD: bleomycin, eldesin, CCNU, DTIC
• BOLD: DTIC, CCNU, bleomycin, vincristine
Responses to these regimens range from 40% to 50% with predominantly lung and or soft tissue metastasis.

Although most remissions were partial and short-lived, some have lasted several years.[5,36]

High-dose chemotherapy followed by autologous bone marrow transplant is another option for patients being explored in clinical studies. This regimen requires intensive hospitalization and is associated with significant morbidity.[5,36]

Investigational drugs such as amonafide, didemnin-B, merberone, piroxantrone, and paclitaxel (Taxol) have been developed and have shown promise in early clinical trials.[3,36]

Hyperthermic regional perfusion. Hyperthermic regional perfusion, or isolated limb perfusion, is being used for in-transit metastasis and as an adjuvant therapy. This form of therapy allows a large dose of chemotherapy to be delivered to a malignant melanoma–affected extremity with minimal systemic toxicity. The limb is usually perfused for 1 hour with a high concentration of melphalan at 39° to 41° C (102.2° to 105.8° F) with a perfusion pump and extracorporeal circulator. The hyperthermia enhances the cytotoxic effect so that the total dose of drug may be reduced. This procedure should be performed only by experts. Complications include arterial and venous thrombosis, tissue necrosis, nerve and muscle damage, and rarely, loss of the extremity.[3,36]

Biotherapy

Recombinant interferons have shown some response in selected patients with advanced disease. High-dose recombinant interleukin-2 (IL-2) has been used to treat distant metastasis with some success. This treatment is associated with a severe, toxic, vascular, hypermeability syndrome and requires intensive hospitalization. Although toxic effects of high-dose IL-2 are severe, significant response rates have been reported in many patients treated by bolus injection.

Bacille Calmette-Guérin (BCG), a form of a nonspecific immune stimulation, was one of the first agents used. It has shown tumor regression when injected intralesionally.[20,36]

Hormonal Therapy

Estrogen and progesterone receptors found on melanoma cells signify a relationship between hormones and malignant melanoma.

Hormonal therapy for malignant melanoma is under investigation. Currently, tamoxifen and diethylstilbestrol (DES) are being explored.[20,36]

PROGNOSIS

Several factors affecting prognosis are the clinical stage, location, and depth and thickness of the lesion. Currently, thickness of malignant melanoma (with local disease) is

NURSING MANAGEMENT

Nursing diagnoses, assessments, and interventions are similar for both nonmelanoma and malignant melanoma. Some variations may be necessary depending on type and location of skin cancer and method of treatment. A complete nursing history includes information regarding risk factors, previous treatment, and a thorough skin examination focusing on all moles for any suspicious changes. Nursing management of side effects of treatment methods are discussed in detail in Chapters 20 to 23. Skin grafting is common after surgical treatment of melanoma.[7,9,11]

Postsurgical interventions include instructing patients and families on the management of a surgical wound. Keeping the area clean and dry and observing for signs and symptoms of infection are imperative. If skin grafting is required, patients and their families should be instructed to keep the graft immobile to prevent stress on the edges of the wound. Limbs should be elevated to minimize edema. Mineral oil or lanolin may be used to remove superficial crusts, moisten the site of the skin graft, and stimulate circulation.

The results of treatment of both nonmelanoma and malignant melanoma may lead to rehabilitation problems. Disfigurement may occur as a result of surgical interventions. Nonmelanoma skin cancers tend to occur in sun-exposed areas of the body, especially the head and neck regions. Surgical interventions to this area of the body may affect a person's body image and self-esteem. Assisting patients to cope with alterations in body image is a prime responsibility of the nurse.[15,20,22,24]

Immobility may also occur as a result of surgical interventions. The wider margins necessary in malignant melanoma coupled with skin grafting may lead to problems of immobility. Assisting patients to maintain their level of functioning is also an important responsibility of the nurse.

Patient/family teaching for malignant melanoma is similar to the teaching for nonmelanoma skin cancers. The importance of early detection should be emphasized to both patients and family members. Patients and family members should be instructed on the importance of monthly, systematic skin self-examination. Individuals should be instructed to check the entire skin surface, paying special attention to all moles for suspicious changes. Family members can be taught to assist patients by checking the scalp and back region. Patients diagnosed with melanoma and those at risk of developing melanoma should be encouraged to keep regularly scheduled appointments with their physician.

Methods of prevention, primarily the importance of avoiding intense sunlight and the use of protective clothing and sunscreens, should also be taught. Parents should be instructed on the above-mentioned prevention measures for their children. Both patient and family members should be instructed about the ABCD rules for remembering the warning signs of melanoma.*

NURSING DIAGNOSIS

• *Knowledge deficit related to prevention and early detection of skin cancer*

OUTCOME GOALS

Patient/family will be able to:
• Define basal cell, squamous cell, and melanoma skin cancer.
• Describe risk factors: skin color, hair color, exposure to UV radiation, and chemical carcinogens.
• Recognize signs and symptoms of disease: sore that does not heal; persistent lump or swelling; bleeding from mole; freckle, birthmark, or other preexisting lesions; changes in moles or birthmarks—size, shape, outline, elevation, surface, sensation, surrounding skin changes, and color.
• State prevention measures: avoid prolonged exposure to sunlight; minimize sunburning and suntanning; and use sunscreens appropriately.

INTERVENTIONS

• Define and describe risk factors: fair complexion, sunburn easily, red or blond hair, reside in geographic region that receives high levels of UV radiation, and history of nonmelanoma/melanoma skin cancer.[23]
• Describe and discuss methods to minimize sun exposure: wear lip balm/sunscreen with SPF of 15 or higher, avoid exposure to sun between hours of 10 AM and 3 PM; wear protective clothing, maximize use of available shade, keep infants and children out of the sun, and teach and practice sun protection measures early in children's growth and developmental process.[10]
• Discuss importance of and procedure for routine skin self-examination: cover entire skin in a methodic fashion; use good lighting, mirrors, hair dryer, and another person to examine difficult-to-see areas (scalp, perineum, back); and document and report promptly any changes and or new conditions.

NURSING DIAGNOSIS

• *Knowledge deficit related to disease process*

OUTCOME GOALS

Patient/family will be able to:
• Verbalize signs and symptoms to report to physician/nurse.
• Verbalize signs and symptoms of altered skin integrity.

*References 2, 6-8, 10, 15, 18, 20, 24.

INTERVENTIONS

- Discuss clinical features related to expectations for basal cell, squamous cell, and malignant melanoma (see boxes, pp. 373, 376, and 381).[11,23,25]
- Discuss potential procedures to be used in diagnosis and treatment of the specific skin cancer.
- Discuss symptoms to report to physician regarding disease process and/or a change in recovery, such as pain, fever, redness, swelling, and drainage at the biopsy/treatment site.

NURSING DIAGNOSIS

- *Knowledge deficit related to method of treating disease (surgery, radiation therapy, chemical therapy, chemotherapy, biotherapy, isolated limb perfusion)*

OUTCOME GOALS

Patient/family will be able to:
- Verbalize selected treatment and specific side effects.
- Identify signs and symptoms to report to physician and nurse (e.g., nausea and vomiting, pain, fever, pruritus, rash, swelling, lymph node tenderness).

INTERVENTIONS

- Discuss schedule of specific therapy.
- Discuss treatment-related side effects.
- Discuss signs and symptoms related to complications from the various therapies.
- Discuss resources/alternative plans to facilitate compliance in the treatment of the disease (travel to/from physician/radiation therapy, dressings, supplies, home care assistance).
- Provide written materials explaining disease and treatment of disease.[4,11]

NURSING DIAGNOSIS

- *Knowledge deficit regarding home care management of surgical wound*

OUTCOME GOALS

Patient/family will be able to:
- Perform necessary dressing procedure.
- Demonstrate proper knowledge of medication administration.
- Identify potential complications (e.g., fever, chills, erythema, increased wound drainage).
- Demonstrates proper body mechanics for mobility purposes.

INTERVENTIONS

- Demonstrate dressing change with return demonstration of procedure.
- Have patient/family state place for purchase of supplies, resource to contact for assistance and to report symptoms, and signs and symptoms that may indicate infection.

- Ensure patient/family know procedure and can demonstrate proper body mechanics for mobility purposes, understand limitations and restrictions for elevation of extremity, and practice general hygiene.[20]

NURSING DIAGNOSIS

- *Skin integrity, impaired, related to skin cancer and surgical treatment*

OUTCOME GOALS

Patient/family will be able to:
- Verbalize/demonstrate appropriate hygiene measures.
- Maintain adequate food and fluid intake.
- Maintain normal body weight.
- Maintain normal level of activity.
- Identify protection measures to avoid sources of infection.

INTERVENTIONS

- Discuss/demonstrate hygiene (wash affected area with tepid water, pat dry); avoid pressure and irritating clothing.
- Discuss nutrition and hydration needs.
- Explain need to avoid exposure to infection.

NURSING DIAGNOSIS

- *Infection, risk for, related to skin cancer and surgical treatment*

OUTCOME GOALS

Patient remains infection free, as evidenced by:
- Temperature within normal limits
- Laboratory values within normal limits
- Absence of inflammation, tenderness, or purulent drainage
- Maintenance of skin integrity

INTERVENTIONS

- Discuss signs and symptoms of infection: pain, redness, swelling, drainage, and fever of 38° C (100.4° F); patient/family identifies when, where, and who to report information regarding infection risk.
- Provide prescribed therapies (antibiotics, analgesics, dressings).[19,20]
- Implement measures to protect skin and affected area from trauma and bleeding.

NURSING DIAGNOSIS

- *Mobility, impaired physical, related to surgical treatment and possible skin graft*

OUTCOME GOALS

Patient will be able to:
- Demonstrate measures to prevent skin breakdown.

Continued.

- Maintain optimal mobility sufficient to manage activities of daily living and independent transfers.
- Demonstrate measures to promote adequate circulation to tissues.

INTERVENTIONS

- Discuss/teach proper body mechanics when transferring to/from bed/chair/commode and when walking.
- Discuss/demonstrate restrictions and limitations for affected extremity.
- Discuss/demonstrate rationale for body position changes if immobilized in bed.
- Discuss/demonstrate body mechanics for daily hygiene, and state any restrictions on shower/tub bath.[19,20,23]

NURSING DIAGNOSIS

- *Body image disturbance related to location and surgical treatment for skin cancer*

OUTCOME GOALS

Patient/family will be able to:
- Identify/utilize appropriate community resources.
- Communicate feelings about changes in body image.
- Participate in care and ongoing decision making.

INTERVENTIONS

- Encourage patient to share feelings with physician/nurse/family regarding changes in body image.
- Arrange and/or consult with professional/lay resources (cancer survivor) if requested by patient/family.
- Provide materials and pictorial images regarding invasive procedures and reconstruction process.
- Discuss/arrange cosmetic resources to enhance positive feelings about body image changes.[20,23]

NURSING DIAGNOSIS

- *Social interaction, impaired, related to location and surgical treatment of skin cancer*

OUTCOME GOALS

Patient/family will be able to:
- Identify/utilize appropriate community resources.
- Participate in decision making.
- Verbalize/demonstrate necessary life-style adaptations.

INTERVENTIONS

- Discuss/plan selected activities patient can pursue (e.g., music, movies, reading, hobbies, crafts).
- Discuss/plan with family/significant other/home care agency resources to utilize in the community (e.g., Meals on Wheels, social contacts appropriate to age and developmental needs).
- Discuss/arrange for rehabilitation resources (e.g., physical therapy, occupational therapy).[23]

NURSING DIAGNOSIS

- *Anxiety related to diagnosis of cancer, fear of recurrence, death, pain, disfigurement, changes in life-style*

OUTCOME GOALS

Patient will be able to:
- Discuss feelings and concerns with family members/health care team.
- Identify positive coping strategies.
- Identify specific concerns related to disease and treatment.

INTERVENTIONS

- Discuss feelings and concerns related to these topics and ask what these experiences mean to patient.
- Identify patient's previous/present coping strategies when encountering difficult situations.
- Identify specific concerns and fears patient may be experiencing
- Encourage patient to share feelings with family/friends/health care team
- Demonstrate/encourage patient to use relaxation/distraction/meditation exercises to aid in other coping strategies.[23]

---

the best independent predictor of survival. The overall 5-year survival rate for melanoma is 80%. The prognosis for persons with thin lesions (less than 0.76 mm thick) is excellent, with 5-year survival of 98%. The difference in 5-year survival rates of localized (90%) versus regional disease (50%) and distant metastasis (14%) validates the importance of early diagnosis and prompt treatment to ensure high cure rates.[5,16,19,36]

CONCLUSION

More than 700,000 new cases of skin cancer occur per year, the vast majority of which are highly curable basal cell or squamous cell cancers. Malignant melanoma is the most serious skin cancer and is increasing at the rate of 4% per year. In the year 2000, malignant melanoma is expected to occur in 1 of every 100 persons.[1] Excessive exposure to the sun remains the primary risk factor for all skin cancers. Prevention, early detection, and prompt treatment are essential to effect a cure or improve survival. Nurses have a major role on the health care team in all aspects of care for the patient with skin cancer.

According to the American Cancer Society,[1] deaths related to skin cancer total 9400 each year. Of those 9400, malignant melanoma accounts for 7300, while other skin cancers account for the remaining 2000.

With continued progress and prompt surgical removal, the current death rate from malignant melanoma can be reduced to nearly zero through early detection. Clearly, if every American were completely examined yearly for malignant melanoma, death from this disease would be a rare event. However, the cost-benefit ratio of skin cancer screening and the feasibility of screening 250 million Americans for skin cancer need to be resolved.*

■ CHAPTER QUESTIONS

1. Basal cell carcinoma (BCC) types include:
   a. Nodular, superficial, pigmented, keratonic, and verrucous
   b. Morpheaform, keratonic, superficial, junctional nevi, and simple lentigo
   c. Nodular, superficial, pigmented, morpheaform, and keratonic
   d. Compound nevus, seborrheic keratosis, nodular, pigmented, and actinic chelitis
2. Ultraviolet (UV) radiation is divided into three types: UVA, UVB, and UVC. Which of the following is *true* regarding the risk of developing skin cancer from UVA, UVB, and UVC?
   a. UVA waves are shorter and do not penetrate the dermis.
   b. UVB waves are longer and penetrate into the epidermis more than UVA waves.
   c. UVC waves are the longest and cause the most severe sunburn.
   d. UVB radiation produces the most damage to skin.
3. Skin cancer prevention measures include:
   a. Avoid intense sunlight, use sunscreens with a higher than 30 SPF, wear protective attire, perform monthly skin self-examination, and know personal risk factors.
   b. Avoid intense sunlight, use sunscreens with a higher than 10 SPF, wear cool attire, perform weekly skin self-examination, and know personal risk factors.
   c. Avoid all sunlight, use sunscreens with a higher than 15 SPF, wear comfortable attire, perform weekly skin self-examination, and know personal risk factors.
   d. Avoid afternoon sunlight, use sunscreens with a higher than 30 SPF, wear comfortable attire, perform monthly skin self-examination, and know personal risk factors.
4. Squamous cell carcinoma (SCC) types include:
   a. Ischemic ulceration, Bowen's disease, actinic cheilitis, seborrheic keratosis
   b. Ischemic ulceration, Bowen's disease, actinic cheilitis, verrucous
   c. Ischemic ulceration, Bowen's disease, solar lentigo, simple lentigo
   d. Ischemic ulceration, Bowen's disease, seborrheic keratosis, nodular
5. Surgical treatment modalities for BCC and SCC include:
   a. Excisional, cryosurgery, electrodesiccation, laser, and endoscopy
   b. Excisional, cryosurgery, Mohs micrographic, photodynamic, and laser
   c. Excisional, cryosurgery, electrodesiccation, ERLAND, and laser
   d. Excisional, cryosurgery, electrodesiccation, Mohs micrographic, and laser
6. Which of the following facts are *true* for SCC metastatic disease?
   a. 6% to 10% of patients develop metastatic disease, occurrence and degree vary according to size and depth of invasion, and metastasis occurs early via the lymphatics.
   b. 2% to 8% of patients develop metastatic disease, occurrence and degree vary according to depth of invasion only, and metastasis occurs late via the lymphatics.
   c. 2% to 3% of patients develop metastatic disease, occurrence and degree vary according to size and depth of invasion, and metastasis occurs late via the lymphatics.
   d. 2% to 3% of patients develop metastatic disease, occurrence and degree vary according to size and depth of invasion, and metastasis occurs early via the lymphatics.
7. Malignant melanoma may arise from three types of moles, or nevi: common acquired nevus (CAN), dysplastic nevus (DN), or congenital melanocytic nevus. Distinguishing characteristics between CAN and DN include:
   a. Color, shape, size, number, and location
   b. Color, shape, depth, number, and location
   c. Color, shape, size, absence, and location
   d. Color, shape, depth, size, and number
8. The most important prognostic factors in melanoma include:
   a. Melanoma type, diagnostic evaluation, and treatment modality
   b. Melanoma type, size of tumor, and treatment modality
   c. Depth of invasion (Clark's level) and thickness of the tumor to determine stage grouping
   d. Depth of invasion, diagnostic evaluation, and treatment modality
9. Combination chemotherapy used in melanoma include:
   a. Doxorubicin, levamisole, cisplatin, and bleomycin
   b. Bleomycin, semustine, vincristine, and dacarbazine
   c. Bleomycin, chlorambucil, cytarabine, and vincristine
   d. Etoposide, carboplatin, thiotepa, and nitrogen mustard
10. Incidence and mortality rates for malignant melanoma in 1996 were:
    a. Incidence, 35,300; mortality, 12,300
    b. Incidence, 38,300; mortality, 12,000
    c. Incidence, 35,000; mortality, 7300
    d. Incidence, 38,300; mortality, 7300

BIBLIOGRAPHY

1. American Cancer Society: *Cancer facts and figures—1996*, Atlanta, 1996, The Society.
2. Amonette R: Tanning parlors may spread disinfomation, *Oncology News International* 4(6):16, 1995.
3. Anderson C and others: Systemic treatments for advanced cutaneous melanoma, *Oncology* 9(11):1149, 1995.

*References 10, 16, 18, 26, 28, 32, 36.

4. Arnold HL and others: Epidermal nevi, neoplasms, and cysts. In Arnold HL, Odom RB, James WD, editors: *Andrew's diseases of the skin, clinical dermatology,* ed 8, Philadelphia, 1990, Saunders.

5. Balch CM, Houghton AN, Peters LJ: Cutaneous melanoma. In DeVita VT, Hellman S, Rosenberg SA, editors: *Cancer principles and practice of oncology,* ed 4, Philadelphia, 1993, Lippincott.

6. Beahrs OH and others, editors: *Manual for staging of cancer: American Joint Committee on Cancer,* ed 4, Philadelphia, 1992, Lippincott.

7. Berwick M and others: The role of the nurse in skin cancer prevention, screening, and early detection, *Semin Oncol Nurs* 7(1):64, 1991.

8. Bolognia JL and others: Complete follow-up and evaluation of a skin cancer screening in Connecticut, *J Am Acad Dermatol* 23:1098, 1990.

9. Buller DB, Buller MK: Approach to communication preventive behaviours, *Semin Oncol Nurs* 7(1):53, 1991.

10. Buller DB, Callister MA, Reichert T: Skin cancer prevention by parents of young children: health information sources, skin cancer knowledge, and sun-protection practices, *Oncol Nurs Forum* 22(10):1559, 1995.

11. Cooley ME and others: Patient literacy and the readability of written cancer educational materials, *Oncol Nurs Forum* 22(9):1345, 1995.

12. Crijins MB and others: Dysplastic nevi occurrence in first- and second-degree relatives of patients with 'sporadic' dysplastic nevus syndrome, *Arch Dermatol* 127(9):1346, 1991.

13. Crutcher WA, Cohen PJ: Dysplastic nevi and malignant melanoma, *Am Fam Physician* 42(2):372, 1990.

14. Epstein E: Recalling basal cell carcinoma patients: a regional survey, *J Derm Surg Oncology* 20(3):180, 1994.

15. Fraser MC and others: Melanoma and nonmelanoma skin cancer: epidemiology and risk factors, *Semin Oncol Nurs* 7(1):2, 1991.

16. Friedman RJ and others: Malignant melanoma in the 1990s: the continued importance of early detection and the role of the physician examination and self-examination of the skin, *CA Cancer J Clin* 41(4):201, 1991.

17. Friedman RJ and others: Basal cell and squamous cell carcinoma of the skin. In Murphy GP, Lawrence W Jr, Lenhard RE Jr, editors: *American Cancer Society textbook of clinical oncology,* ed 2, Atlanta, 1995, American Cancer Society.

18. Geller AC and others: Practices and beliefs concerning screening family members of patients with melanoma, *J Am Acad Dermatol* 26(3):419, 1992.

19. Lawler PE: Cutaneous malignant melanoma, *Semin Oncol Nurs* 7(1):26, 1991.

20. Lawler PE, Schreiber S: Cutaneous malignant melanoma: nursing's role in prevention and early detection, *Oncol Nurs Forum* 16(3):345, 1989.

21. Limpert GH: Skin-cancer screening: a three-year experience that paid for itself, *J Fam Pract* 40(5):471, 1995.

22. Loescher LJ, Meyskens FL Jr: Chemoprevention of human skin cancers, *Semin Oncol Nurs* 7(1):45, 1991.

23. Longman A: Skin cancer. In Clark JC, McGee RF, editors: *Core curriculum for oncology nursing,* ed 2, Philadelphia, 1992, Saunders.

24. Marlenga B: The health beliefs and skin cancer prevention practices of Wisconsin dairy farmers, *Oncol Nurs Forum* 22(4):681, 1995.

25. McFadden ME: Cutaneous T-cell lymphoma, *Semin Oncol Nurs* 7(1):36, 1991.

26. Miller AB: Cancer screening. In DeVita VT, Hellman S, Rosenberg SA, editors: *Cancer principles and practice of oncology,* ed 4, Philadelphia, 1993, Lippincott.

27. Pathak MA: Broad-spectrum screens block UVA and UVB, *Oncology News International* 4(6):16, 1995.

28. Romero JB and others: Follow-up recommendations for patients with stage I malignant melanoma, *J Derm Surg Oncology* 20(3):175, 1994.

29. Rowe DE and others: Long-term recurrence rates in previously untreated (primary) basal cell carcinoma: implications for patient follow-up, *J Dermatol Surg Oncol* 15:315, 1989.

30. Safai B: Cancers of the skin. In DeVita VT, Hellman S, Rosenberg SA, editors: *Cancer principles and practice of oncology,* ed 4, Philadelphia, 1993, Lippincott.

31. Shimm DS, Wilder RB: Radiation therapy for squamous cell carcinoma, *Am J Clin Oncol* 14(5):383, 1991.

32. Sober AJ: Cutaneous melanoma: opportunity for cure, *CA Cancer J Clin* 41(4):197, 1991 (guest editorial).

33. Trizenberg DJ, Smith MA, Holmes TM: Cancer screening and detection in family practice: a MIRNET study, *J Fam Pract* 40(1):27, 1995.

34. Vargo NL: Basal and squamous cell carcinomas: an overview, *Semin Oncol Nurs* 7(1):13, 1991.

35. Volker DL: Standards of oncology practice and standards of oncology education; patient, family, and public. In Clark JC, McGee RF, editors: *Core curriculum for oncology nursing,* ed 2, Philadelphia, 1992, Saunders.

36. Urist MM, Miller DM, Maddox WA: Malignant melanoma. In Murphy GP, Lawrence W Jr., Lenhard RE Jr., editors: *American Cancer Society textbook of clinical oncology,* ed 2, Atlanta, 1995, American Cancer Society.

CHAPTER 18
Pediatric Cancers

SUSAN TOBIN RUMELHART

Over the past three decades, marked progress has been realized in the detection, prognostic staging, and treatment of childhood cancers, leading to improvements in disease-free survival. Great advances have been made with some diseases, such as leukemia and Wilms' tumor, whereas others have been more disappointing. This chapter provides a basic review of the most common childhood cancers.

LEUKEMIA

Leukemia is the most common malignancy in children younger than 15 years, representing 31.4% of all childhood cancers. The majority of leukemias in children are *lymphoblastic* (75.5%), with myeloid leukemias accounting for 15% to 40% and the largest group of these being the acute myeloid leukemias (11.4%).[85] The cause of leukemia remains unknown and is most likely a result of a combination of factors. Possible causative agents under investigation include viruses, radiation, chemical and drug exposures, chromosomal aberrations, and familial predisposition.[46]

Acute Lymphoblastic Leukemia

The incidence of acute lymphoblastic leukemia (ALL) is 40 per 1 million white children and 20 per 1 million black children in the United States annually, with 2500 cases diagnosed each year. There is a male predominance of 3 : 1 over females and a peak incidence at 4 years of age.[133] Survival has dramatically improved from 4% in the early 1960s to 78% in the early 1990s.[101]

CLASSIFICATION

Based on the French-American-British (FAB) classification system, 80% of childhood cases of ALL are L1 type, 17% L2, and 3% L3.[4] Of the immunophenotypes, 57% of childhood ALL are early pre–B cell, 25% pre–B cell, 1% transitional pre–B cell, 2% B cell, and 15% T cell.[109] (See Chapter 13 for a further discussion of the FAB subtypes and immunophenotypes.)

CLINICAL PRESENTATION

Manifestations depend on the degree to which the bone marrow has been compromised as well as the location and the extent of extramedullary infiltration. Common presenting signs and symptoms are fever, pain, bleeding, petechiae, purpura, fatigue, pallor, recurrent infection, and lymphadenopathy. These symptoms may have been present for days or weeks or, rarely, months before diagnosis. These nonspecific symptoms must be distinguished from many nonmalignant conditions and other malignant diseases that involve the bone marrow.[107]

PROGNOSIS

Multiple factors have been used to predict outcome in children with ALL and are now also used to direct treatment. Only age (younger than 1 year or older than 15 years) and hyperleukocytosis have consistently been associated with a poor outcome.[11,78,109] In general, the more mature the cell of origin, the less favorable is the prognosis, with early pre–B cell having the best prognosis and mature B cell the poorest.[20] Early pre–B-cell leukemia is more likely to have initial features predictive of a good outcome. With improvements in treatment, the prognostic distinctions among immunophenotypes decrease or disappear.[109]

The presence of the common ALL antigen (CALLA) is associated with a positive outcome, and 75% to 80% of B-cell ALL patients are CALLA positive. Hyperdiploidy is also associated with a good prognosis. Some chromosomal aberrations are associated with a poor outcome, such as Philadelphia-positive cells, t8;14, t1;19, and 14;11.[10,82,106,107]

TREATMENT MODALITIES

All protocols now include some form of four phases of therapy: induction for remission, a phase of intensification/consolidation, treatment directed toward the central nervous system (CNS), and continuation therapy.[56,109] Over the past decade the use of intensive induction therapy has greatly improved survival in children with

ALL, resulting in a remission rate of 97% to 98% in children with ALL.[109] It has been recognized that some form of intensification is necessary in the prevention of bone marrow relapse, even for those considered low risk.[10,109]

The need for CNS treatment was recognized in the 1960s. The use of radiation and intrathecal methotrexate is associated with adverse effects. It is now common practice to omit radiation for those at low risk for CNS disease but to provide CNS treatment through the use of intrathecal methotrexate or triple intrathecal therapy (cytarabine, hydrocortisone, methotrexate). Radiation is reserved for those with CNS disease or at high risk for a CNS relapse (high white blood cell count [WBC], T-cell ALL with high WBC, and Philadelphia-positive ALL).[111,121] Under investigation is the benefit for use of a second induction/intensification phase before the continuation or maintenance phase for some subgroups of patients.[111-113] The length of treatment has not been established but in general continues for 2½ to 3 years after diagnosis.[10,84]

Most relapses occur either during treatment or within 2 years after completion of therapy. Treatment of recurrent leukemia remains under investigation. Although achievement of a second remission is possible in more than 90% of patients, long-term survival remains a challenge for those patients with a bone marrow relapse. For those with an isolated CNS or testicular relapse, 50% are long-term survivors with a second course of therapy.[10,25] Many investigators now recommend the use of allogeneic bone marrow transplantation (BMT) for those that have a bone marrow relapse on or shortly after the completion of therapy.[17,107,120]

Late Effects

A major delayed effect of therapy has been the development of second malignancies. One estimate is that 2.5% of patients will develop a second cancer 15 years after diagnosis. Brain tumors were the most common second malignancy occurring in those who have received cranial radiation, followed by a second leukemia associated with the use of epipodophyllotoxins and lymphomas.[92,113] Declines in intelligence quotient (IQ) and cognitive dysfunctions, decreased reading and mathematic levels, and memory deficits have been noted. These problems are thought to be related to the use of methotrexate and radiation for CNS prophylaxis and treatment.[89,102]

Acute Myelogenous Leukemia

Acute myelogenous leukemia (AML) is less common in children then in adults, representing 15% to 25% of leukemias in children. Approximately 350 new cases are diagnosed annually in the United States.[85] AML is more common in whites and males, with a slight peak incidence in adolescence and in those younger than 4 weeks of age.[91]

ETIOLOGY

As stated earlier, the cause of leukemia in children remains unclear, but those with certain genetic disorders such as Down syndrome are at higher risk for the development of AML. A statistically significant risk was found for children who had a parent exposed to pesticides and petroleum products and those with mothers who used marijuana while pregnant.[70]

CLASSIFICATION

Several subtypes of AML become important when determining treatment and prognosis. The subtypes according to the FAB classification system are M1, myeloblastic undifferentiated; M2, myeloblastic differentiated; M3, promyelocytic; M4, myelomonocytic; M5, monoblastic; M6, erythroblastic; and M7, megakaryoblastic.[49]

CLINICAL PRESENTATION

As in ALL, the primary presenting symptoms with AML are a result of bone marrow disease: pallor, anemia, fever, infection, petechiae, and bruising or bleeding. In addition, children with AML may have symptoms of organ involvement. Splenomegaly and hepatomegaly are present in 50%, lymphadenopathy in 25%, and CNS disease in 5% to 15% of children at diagnosis.[12,83]

PROGNOSTIC FACTORS

Prognostic indicators have been extensively studied in ALL but have not been as clear-cut as in AML. Only WBC and the FAB subtype M5 have consistently been identified with a poor prognosis. Young age (younger than 2 years) has also been associated with a poor prognosis, but whether this is related to age or the most common subtypes in infants (M5, M4) is not known.[16,49,70,126]

TREATMENT MODALITIES

Induction protocols vary, but remission rates are 75% to 85%, and those who do not achieve remission die of infection, bleeding, leukostasis, or resistant disease.[12] CNS prophylaxis is often included in treatment regimens to prevent CNS relapse and consists of intrathecal cytosine arabinoside (cytarabine). Consolidation or continuation therapy is far from standardized. Some centers recommend BMT, either allogeneic or autologous, in the first remission, whereas others wait for a relapse to occur. Studies are ongoing regarding the efficacy of intensive chemotherapy versus BMT. Current long-term survival rates are 25% to 40% for all treatment regimens.[49]

Chronic Myelogenous Leukemia

Chronic myelogenous leukemia (CML) is an uncommon disease in children, representing 1% to 5% of all childhood leukemias. The two forms of CML are the *adult type,* which is usually seen in older children and adolescents but seldom seen in children younger than 6 months, and the *juvenile form,* which is almost always seen in infants younger than 24 months.[4,19] The cause of CML is unknown, as is the case with other childhood leukemias.

ADULT CML

Adult CML is usually associated with the presence of the Philadelphia chromosome, which is directly attributed to the disease process. Three phases of adult CML have been identified: chronic, accelerated, and blast. The chronic phase is an indolent phase lasting from 3 to 4 years. Most children are diagnosed in this phase either through an abnormal complete blood count (CBC) during a routine physical examination or through the development of symptoms. Common symptoms include fever, pallor, weight loss, and bone pain. Patients often have splenomegaly and/or hepatomegaly, which can be mild or severe, and an elevated WBC, eosinophilia, and basophilia.[4,40] Treatment with oral hydroxyurea or busulfan provides adequate control in the chronic phase but does not reduce the number of cells containing the Philadelphia chromosome.[63]

Eventually the chronic phase leads to the accelerated phase, with an increasing WBC and redevelopment of the presenting symptoms. Patients usually progress rapidly to the blast phase, with symptoms of bone marrow disease resembling ALL. This phase is very resistant to therapy. Multiagent regimens are used in an attempt to obtain a second chronic phase.[4,63]

JUVENILE CML

Juvenile CML is very rare and presents as well as follows a more acute course. The median survival is less then 10 months with or without treatment.[40] Presenting symptoms include bleeding, malaise, lymphadenopathy, and fever. A small number of patients have pulmonary symptoms caused by leukemic infiltrates. Abdominal distention and pain result from a rapidly enlarging spleen. Many patients have skin manifestations similar to an eczematous rash and caused by cutaneous infiltrates.[4,18,40,63]

TREATMENT MODALITIES

No real cure exists for either type of CML, and the only possible curative therapy is BMT. With the adult form the ideal time to transplant is in the chronic phase. The juvenile form is very resistive to treatment, but intensive multiagent regimens have been used to obtain short remissions, during which BMT is then employed.[4,40,63,114]

BRAIN TUMORS

Brain tumors are the most common solid tumor of childhood and are second in frequency only to leukemia. The annual incidence is 23.9 per 1 million children younger than 15 years, with 1500 to 2000 new cases diagnosed in the United States each year.[105] A peak incidence occurs from 5 to 10 years of age, with an overall equal frequency between white and black children and between males and females.[129]

CLASSIFICATION

No uniform classification system exists for brain tumors because of no uniform grading system. The histologic types differ from those in adults. The majority of tumors in children older than 1 year are infratentorial (60%), in contrast to adults, who have primarily supratentorial tumors. Supratentorial tumors predominate in those younger than 1 year and begin to increase in the adolescent years.[105]

HISTOLOGY

Approximately 50% of brain tumors in children are *astrocytomas,* with 11% high grade, 13% cerebellar astrocytomas, and 23% cerebral astrocytomas. Of the remaining tumors in children, 25% are medulloblastomas, 10% brain stem gliomas, 9% ependymomas, and 9% other subtypes.[35]

ETIOLOGY

The cause of brain tumors in children is unknown. Both hereditary and environmental factors have been implicated. Prior radiotherapy is a known cause of brain tumors.[62,128] Parental occupation in the chemical or aircraft industry have also been suspected as a risk factor.[103] Fifteen percent of those with neurofibromatosis develop brain tumors, and in patients with acquired immunodeficiency syndrome (AIDS) the Epstein-Barr virus (EBV) may initiate an aggressive form of non-Hodgkin's lymphoma of the brain.[62,128]

CLINICAL PRESENTATION

The presenting symptoms of a child with a brain tumor depend on the site and size. These signs and symptoms can range from nonspecific to characteristically localizing. The presenting symptoms are often related to increased intracranial pressure (ICP) and are often worse in the morning, improving as the child is upright with improved cephalic venous return. In one series, 86% of children with brain tumors had signs of increased ICP.[44] The child may complain of a headache, which can be diffuse, frontal, or occipital. Vomiting can be projectile or nonprojectile in nature. Lethargy, irritability, and behavior changes often occur. An increased head circumference may be noted in the infant, possibly with separation of the sutures.[2] Papilledema is often found, and the child may also experience diplopia and strabismus.[62,104,105]

Symptoms often provide clues to the tumor's location. These symptoms include ataxia, gait disturbances, seizures, focal motor or sensory abnormalities, decreased visual acuity, nystagmus, and strabismus. Growth retardation, diabetes insipidus, delayed puberty, hormonal deficits, and visual disturbances may result if the hypothalamic-pituitary axis is involved.[29,62,105,128]

DIAGNOSTIC EVALUATION

The diagnostic evaluation of a child with a suspected brain tumor begins with a thorough physical and neurologic examination. Magnetic resonance imaging (MRI) or computed tomography (CT) scan with and without contrast is the major radiologic examination. A lumbar puncture and gadolinium-enhanced MRI are necessary for detection of dissemination of tumor into the cerebrospinal fluid (CSF).

TREATMENT MODALITIES

The management of children with brain tumors involves the use of surgery, chemotherapy, and radiation. The goal of surgery is to decrease the tumor burden, thereby decreasing symptoms, and to obtain tissue for histologic evaluation. The exception is with diffuse gliomas of the brain stem, in which case MRI is usually diagnostic.[3] In general, the better the resection, the better is the prognosis.[35,36] Advances in neurosurgery have increased the cure rate, decreased perioperative complications, and decreased the postsurgical deficits. Stereotactic needle biopsies of deep-seated tumors allow diagnosis in delicate regions.[35,131]

The use of radiation has long been the major approach to management of brain tumors in children and is usually initiated as soon as the diagnosis is confirmed and the surgical would is healed. Total doses as low as 2000 to 3000 cGy or as much as 7000 cGy are given, depending on the tumor's pathology and location and the child's age. The use of hyperfractionated radiation has allowed the delivery of higher doses without increasing the adverse effects.[36,62,104,105] The use of radiation in young children often requires sedation to obtain complete im-

mobility, along with casts or molds individually designed for positioning. Radiation is not without risks, and it is now standard procedure to defer radiation by the use of postoperative chemotherapy in those younger than 2 or 3 years.[31] (See Chapter 21.)

Chemotherapy has proved to be a valuable addition to radiation and surgery in the management of brain tumors, increasing median survival. Chemotherapy protocols vary greatly in the drugs used, timing, and dose. The use of chemotherapy before radiation is becoming increasingly common as a method to evaluate tumor response separate from the response caused by the effects of radiation.[57] The use of autologous BMT or peripheral blood stem cell (PBSC) rescue is currently under investigation as a method to intensify therapy with high-grade or recurrent tumors.[35,105]

PROGNOSIS

Prognostic signs include the amount of resection, child's age, and tumor's grade.[122] Survival depends on tumor histology, amount of surgical resection, age, neurologic and physical status, and presence or absence of dissemination.[32] The 5-year survival rate for all children with brain tumors ranges from 10% to 70%.*

LATE EFFECTS

Problems with decreased cognitive function, and in some cases mental retardation, are seen after the diagnosis and successful treatment of brain tumors in children. Young age at diagnosis is an important risk factor for long-term sequelae.[88] Possibly 68% of children younger than 6 years treated for brain tumors may experience intellectual deterioration. The effects of cranial radiation have long been recognized as a risk, especially in the young child. Children with infratentorial tumors are at higher risk for long-term adverse effects than those with supratentorial tumors. Endocrine deficiencies, including growth problems and hypothyroidism, are typically seen.[34] Finally, children treated for brain tumors are at risk for the development of secondary brain neoplasms, most often from radiation.[23,41]

LYMPHOMA

Lymphomas represent the third most common cancer in children and, along with other reticuloendothelial neoplasms, 12.4% of all childhood cancers.[85] These malignancies of the lymphatic system have long been thought to have an infectious etiology. The main integrating fac-

---

*References 21, 35, 37, 96, 119, 121.

tors in these diseases include infection with EBV, genetic predisposition, and exposure to toxins.

Hodgkin's Disease

Hodgkin's disease in children is now considered similar to that in adults regarding biology, etiology, natural history, and response to treatment.[27] (See Chapter 15 for a complete discussion of Hodgkin's disease, since this section refers only to those aspects pertinent to the disease in children.)

EPIDEMIOLOGY

Hodgkin's disease accounts for 5% of all childhood cancers in the United States. The annual incidence is 7.3 per 1 million white children and 5.2 per 1 million black children in the United States.[133] It is rarely seen in those younger than 5 years, with two peaks in incidence, ages 15 to 40 years and after age 50 years. Hodgkin's disease has a higher incidence in males until the adolescent years, when a slight female predominance occurs.[26]

Of the four subtypes of Hodgkin's disease, 77% of those occurring in adolescents and 45% of those in children younger than 10 years are the nodular sclerosing subtype. The lymphocytic depletion subtype is rare under the age 10 years, but the lymphocytic predominant subtype occurs more often in this age-group than in adults. Thirty-two percent of children younger than 10 years are diagnosed with the mixed cellularity subtype.[85]

CLINICAL PRESENTATION

The diagnosis of lymphoma in a child is difficult because of the common finding of enlarged lymph nodes in children, which are most often a benign reactive process.[7] Ninety percent of children with Hodgkin's disease present with an unusual lump, which varies in size and may have been present for weeks or months.[43] Lymph nodes involved with Hodgkin's disease are usually not tender, are firm and rubbery, and are fixed or minimally movable. Location can also be a clue to malignancy in that enlarged nodes in the upper half of the neck (anterior and posterior chains or submandibular region) are often associated with upper respiratory infections in children. These nodes should be biopsied if the enlargement has not resolved within 3 to 6 weeks. The nodes of the lower cervical and supraclavicular chains are more often involved with Hodgkin's disease and should be biopsied without delay.[7] In one review, 48% of nodes biopsied from the supraclavicular and lower neck regions were involved with Hodgkin's disease.[64] From 20% to 30% of children present with the classic "B" symptoms of weight loss, fevers, and night sweats (see Chapter 15).[5,7] Almost 60% of children have mediastinal involvement.[27]

DIAGNOSTIC EVALUATION

An extensive diagnostic evaluation is necessary for staging, which plays an important role in determining treatment. (See Chapter 4 for a complete discussion of diagnostic staging evaluation, which is approached the same in children as in adults.) Alkaline phosphatase is a nonspecific indicator of disease activity but is less useful in children because of normal elevated levels from bone growth, but if elevated, a bone scan is done to detect bone disease. Serum copper levels may be elevated because of normal hormonal activity in children and is not related to the malignancy. Splenectomies are controversial in children, but it is now generally believed that they are necessary when radiation is used alone. When chemotherapy is used, however, either alone or in combination with radiation, splenectomies are not necessary and clinical staging is sufficient.[27]

TREATMENT MODALITIES

Treatment for children is similar to that for adults. Radiation doses may be reduced in young children to decrease the negative effects on bone and soft tissue growth.[42] The traditional MOPP (mechlorethamine, vincristine, procarbazine, prednisone) is used, along with other regimens that have been developed. The use of MOPP alternating with ABVD (Adriamycin [doxorubicin], bleomycin, vinblastine, dacarbazine) is under investigation.[24,71] Various chemotherapeutic regimens are being investigated for resistant or relapsed disease, including autologous BMT.

Late Effects

Hodgkin's patients are at risk for multiple complications related to chemotherapy and radiation to the chest, including cardiac, pulmonary, and gonadal dysfunctions and abnormalities in development of bone and soft tissue in the radiation field. The development of second malignancies is similar to that in other children who have received radiation and chemotherapy, especially with alkylating agents. A relationship between splenectomy and the development of leukemia has also been reported.[81]

PROGNOSIS

Young age is clearly a positive prognostic sign, as is early diagnosis. Both those younger than 10 years and those 11 to 16 years old, regardless of stage, have a projected survival of 74%, versus 34% in those age 17 years or older.[27]

Non-Hodgkin's Lymphoma

Sixty percent of all lymphomas are of the non-Hodgkin's type and represent 10% of all childhood malignancies.[85]

Non-Hodgkin's lymphoma (NHL) in children is often widespread at diagnosis.

EPIDEMIOLOGY

NHL has a peak incidence in the 7- to 11-year-old age-group, a low incidence in adolescence, and a male predominance.[45] Viruses, genetic factors, and radiation have been implicated as causative factors in several studies, along with an increased risk in those with primary immunodeficiency syndromes, immunosuppression, connective tissue diseases, and anticonvulsant therapy.[108] NHL has been increasing as a secondary malignancy after multimodal therapy.[81]

HISTOLOGY

NHL can be divided into three groups: lymphoblastic, small noncleaved cell (Burkitt's or non-Burkitt's), and large cell lymphomas. Lymphoblastic lymphomas are usually T cell in origin. Small noncleaved cell and large cell lymphomas are usually of B-cell origin. Various chromosomal abnormalities have been associated with NHL.[75]

CLINICAL PRESENTATION AND STAGING

The child with NHL often has an acute onset of symptoms and rapid progression. Lymphoblastic lymphomas typically arise in the anterior superior mediastinum, and 75% of these children have a mediastinal mass at diagnosis. They often present with symptoms of dyspnea, wheezing, or stridor. Other sites of involvement may include the skin, tonsils, lymph nodes, bone, bone marrow, CNS, and testes.[134] Eighty percent of nonlymphoblastic lymphomas originate in the abdomen, often presenting as an acute abdomen.[75]

Many different staging systems exist, and all are based on the extent of disease: localized disease, extensive thoracic or intra-abdominal disease, widespread disease without bone marrow involvement, and disease with bone marrow involvement. Controversy exists regarding whether lymphoma with bone marrow involvement is a true lymphoma or is actually a leukemia, but regardless of the classification, it is an aggressive disease requiring aggressive treatment.[75]

DIAGNOSTIC EVALUATION

The diagnostic and staging evaluation is based on tissue samples from any bulky disease, bone marrow aspirates and biopsies to evaluate bone marrow involvement, and CSF to detect CNS involvement. Appropriate radiographic studies should be done to evaluate the extent of bulky disease, and laboratory studies should include EBV titers.

TREATMENT MODALITIES AND PROGNOSIS

All children receive chemotherapy, with the exact combination and length of therapy depending on the type and extent of disease. Those with extensive disease, especially the Burkitt's and lymphoblastic types, are at high risk for tumor lysis syndrome.[6,61,75]

The overall survival rate for patients with localized disease is almost 90%, with a 60% to 70% rate for those with advanced disease.[75,108] When it occurs, relapse is usually early in treatment, although relapse toward the end or after the completion of therapy is also possible. The most common sites of relapse are the primary site, bone marrow, and CNS. Those who relapse or have resistant disease have a very poor survival rate, and autologous or allogeneic BMT is often done.[90,118]

WILMS' TUMOR (NEPHROBLASTOMA)

Wilms' tumor, an embryonal neoplasm, is the most common renal tumor of childhood and the fifth most common childhood cancer, representing 6% of all childhood cancers. It occurs in 7.5 per 1 million white children and 7.8 per 1 million black children annually under age 15 years.[67] The incidence is fairly equal between females and males, with 400 new cases diagnosed each year and a median age of 2 to 3 years.[47]

ETIOLOGY

Most cases are sporadic, but a small number are familial and are inherited in an autosomal dominant manner.[28] An association exists between Wilms' tumor and deletion or inactivation of the short arm of chromosome 11, band 13. Wilms' tumor is also associated with aniridia, Beckwith-Wiedemann syndrome, and congenital hemihypertrophy.[67]

CLINICAL PRESENTATION

Typically an otherwise healthy-appearing child has an asymptomatic abdominal mass, often noted by the parent or primary health care professional on a routine examination. Other presenting symptoms include hematuria, dysuria, hypertension, abdominal pain, fever, anemia, and malaise. Wilms' tumor is usually a nontender, firm, flank mass that is confined to one side.[48]

The lungs are the primary site of distant metastasis and recurrent disease, with 25% of patients showing metastasis at diagnosis. Other sites of metastasis include the collateral kidney, liver, bones, or brain. Lymphatic spread to regional nodes is associated with advanced disease.[48,66]

DIAGNOSTIC EVALUATION

Initially a flat plate of the abdomen will identify the primary mass, followed by an ultrasound, which can identify the site of origin. The other kidney is also examined to rule out bilateral involvement and detect extension into renal veins and the inferior vena cava. An abdominal CT scan or MRI has become the imaging modality of choice for evaluating the extent of disease before surgery. A chest CT scan and chest x-ray films are done preoperatively to detect pulmonary metastasis.[38]

A bone marrow aspirate, biopsy, and skeletal survey should be done if bone metastasis is suspected. Laboratory tests should include a serum and 24-hour urine creatinine clearance.[47] Control of hypertension is important preoperatively, and although it resolves in most children after surgery, some may require long-term antihypertensive therapy.[48] Definitive diagnosis is made at surgery, usually involving removal of the involved kidney. In bilateral disease the most involved kidney is removed and the other resected as much as possible.

STAGING AND PROGNOSIS

Wilms' tumor is generally staged according to the classification system identified by the National Wilms' Tumor Study Group (see box at right). Staging is based on surgical findings, pathology, and the presence or absence of distant metastasis. Wilms' tumor is further stratified by histologic type, designated favorable or unfavorable. Treatment and prognosis are based on stage and histologic type.

The overall cure rate for patients with Wilms' tumor, at all stages and with any histologic type, is greater then 85%. Those with favorable histology (renal embryoma without anaplasia) and without metastatic disease currently have a 90% rate of long-term survival. Those with an unfavorable histology (anaplastic, clear cell sarcoma) or those with metastatic disease have an 80% chance of long-term survival. The exception is those with rhabdoid tumors, who have a poor prognosis and a greater than 80% mortality. Twenty-five percent of those with stage IV disease and favorable histology have recurrence of their disease, and 50% of those with unfavorable histology and stage II or IV disease experience a relapse.[22]

TREATMENT MODALITIES

Through the cooperative work of the Children's Cancer Group and the Pediatric Oncology Group in the National Wilms' Study Group trials, advances have been made re-

---

STAGING OF WILMS' TUMOR

Stage I
Tumor limited to kidney and completely removed
Surface of renal capsule intact
No rupture before or during removal
No apparent residual tumor beyond margins

Stage II
Tumor extends beyond kidney but completely removed
Regional extension of tumor (i.e., penetration of renal capsule)
Vessels outside kidney infiltrated or contain tumor thrombus
Tumor may have been biopsied, or there has been spillage of tumor confined to flank
No residual tumor apparent at or beyond the margins of excision

Stage III
Residual nonhematogenous tumor confined to abdomen
Occurrence of any of the following:
Lymph nodes found to be involved in hilus, periaortic chains, or beyond
Diffuse peritoneal contamination by tumor (e.g., spillage of tumor beyond flank before or during surgery or tumor growth that has penetrated through peritoneal surface)
Implants on peritoneal surface
Tumor extends beyond surgical margins grossly or microscopically
Tumor not completely resectable because of local infiltration into vital structures

Stage IV
Hematogenous metastases (e.g., lung, liver, bone, brain)

Stage V
Bilateral renal tumors; attempt to stage both sides separately according to disease extent before biopsy

---

garding treatment intensity and duration.[22] Three trials have been completed, and a fourth is in progress. Treatment involves chemotherapy alone with or without radiation, depending on the stage and histologic type.[67,93] Recurrent disease is treated with an aggressive, multimodal approach, and many patients are cured, especially those who have an isolated pulmonary relapse.[22,50]

Late Effects

Follow-up for late effects include (1) surveillance of function of the remaining kidney, scoliosis and soft tissue growth problems related to radiation, and thyroid abnormalities after lung irradiation and (2) monitoring for second malignancies, usually in the radiation field.[48,67]

NEUROBLASTOMA

Neuroblastoma originates from neural crest tissue anywhere along the craniospinal axis and is one of the small, round, blue cell tumors of childhood. Neural crest tissue is the precursor for the adrenal medulla and sympathetic nervous system, and the tumor can present wherever nervous tissue is found. It is the most common malignant tumor in infancy and second only to brain tumors as the most frequent solid tumor in the first decade of life.[14]

EPIDEMIOLOGY

Neuroblastoma represents only 8% of all childhood malignancies but accounts for 15% of cancer deaths. The annual incidence is 9.6 per 1 million white children and 7 per 1 million black children in the United States, with 500 cases diagnosed annually.[32,85] The true incidence remains unknown because of the ability of neuroblastoma to regress spontaneously, most often in neonates and infants.[51,94] More than 50% of patients are diagnosed before 2 years of age and more than 80% before age 5 years. There is a slightly higher frequency in males.[14,74]

ETIOLOGY

The etiology of neuroblastoma remains unknown. Although most cases are probably sporadic, some evidence indicates that neuroblastoma may have an autosomal dominant pattern of inheritance. However, the risk for development of neuroblastoma in siblings or offspring is less than 6%.[65]

GENETICS

Several genetic abnormalities have been found associated with neuroblastoma and have prognostic implications. The *N-myc* oncogene is an amplified gene present in human neuroblastomas. The higher the number of *N-myc* copies present, the poorer is the prognosis.[13,115] A deletion or rearrangement on the short arm of chromosome 1 has been described, and some evidence suggests that this is associated with a very poor prognosis.[53] Deoxyribonucleic acid (DNA) content has also been analyzed, with diploid neuroblastoma carrying a poorer prognosis then aneuploid.[98,99]

CLINICAL PRESENTATION

Presenting symptoms depend on the location of the tumor and the stage of the disease. Neuroblastomas most often arise in the retroperitoneum (65%) and present as hard, nontender abdominal masses. Other common sites include the mediastinum (15%), pelvis (5%), and neck (less than 5%).[68,69] Paraspinal tumors tend to grow through the intervertebral foramina, and patients often have paralysis.[124] Those with cervical or high thoracic ganglia involvement may have Horner's syndrome. Approximately two thirds have metastasis at diagnosis, most often to the cortical bone, bone marrow, lymph nodes, liver, or subcutaneous tissue. Sphenoid bone or orbital soft tissue involvement results in the distinctive ecchymotic orbital proptosis or "raccoon eyes." Characteristic of neuroblastoma in neonates is hepatic and skin metastasis.[69]

DIAGNOSTIC EVALUATION

Serum ferritin and neuron-specific enolase are useful for prognostic purposes, with elevations indicating a poorer prognosis. More than 90% of children with neuroblastoma have elevated urine catecholamines (VMA and/or HVA).[55] The primary tumor should be evaluated with a CT scan or MRI, with MRI especially useful for intraspinal extension. Bilateral bone marrow aspirates and biopsies, a bone scan with radiographic films of abnormal sites, and a CT scan or MRI of the head and orbits, chest, abdomen, and pelvis are necessary to detect and evaluate metastatic disease.[15]

STAGING AND PROGNOSIS

Currently, four staging systems are in use, one by each of the major cooperative groups (Pediatric Oncology Group [POG], Childrens Cancer Group [CCG] and one used by St. Jude's Children's Research Hospital (SJCRH). The fourth was proposed by a group of international experts to standardize staging and direct treatment (see box, p. 397).[15]

Age and stage at diagnosis are important prognostic factors, with young age (younger than 1 year) and low stage (I, II, or IVS) associated with a favorable prognosis.[14,95] A number of biologic features of neuroblastoma are associated with a poor prognosis: amplified *N-myc* copies, chromosomal ploidy, elevated serum ferritin (greater than 150 ng/ml) and neuron-specific enolase (1000 ng/ml), and a low urine VMA/HVA ratio. Those with poorly differentiated tumors have a poor prognosis, and those with the more highly differentiated tumors have a better prognosis.[13,115]

TREATMENT MODALITIES AND SURVIVAL

Survival for patients with stage I disease is approaching 100%. For this group and others with localized disease

INTERNATIONAL NEUROBLASTOMA STAGING SYSTEM

Stage I	Localized tumor with complete gross resection, with or without microscopic disease
	Representative ipsilateral and contralateral lymph nodes microscopically negative
Stage IIA	Unilateral localized tumor with incomplete gross resection
	Representative ipsilateral and contralateral lymph nodes microscopically negative
Stage IIB	Unilateral localized tumor with or without complete gross resection
	Positive ipsilateral regional lymph nodes and enlarged contralateral lymph nodes negative microscopically
Stage III	Tumor crossing midline with or without regional lymph node involvement
	or
	Unilateral tumor with contralateral regional lymph node involvement
	or
	Midline tumor with bilateral regional lymph node involvement
Stage IV	Dissemination of tumor to distant lymph nodes, bone, bone marrow, liver, and/or other organs (except as defined for stage IVS)
Stage IVS	Localized primary tumor (as defined in stages I, IIA, and IIB), with dissemination limited to liver, skin, and/or bone marrow
	Younger than 1 year of age

(stage II), surgery may be the only treatment required. Stage IVS occurs almost exclusively in those younger than 1 year. Treatment varies: no surgery, awaiting spontaneous regression; surgery alone; and/or low-dose chemotherapy. Neuroblastoma is one of the few tumors that may demonstrate spontaneous regression. The survival rate among these treatment groups is not statistically significant and ranges from 70% to 80%. For patients with stage III disease, survival has improved dramatically to 60% to 72% with the use of intensive therapy, including radiation, surgery, and chemotherapy. The survival for stage IV patients has not improved significantly in the past 20 years and remains at 11% to 17%. New

approaches, including autologous and allogeneic BMT, are under investigation.*

RHABDOMYOSARCOMA

Rhabdomyosarcoma is the third most common extracranial solid tumor in childhood. It is the most common soft tissue sarcoma in children and accounts for 5% to 8% of all childhood malignancies.

EPIDEMIOLOGY

The annual incidence of rhabdomyosarcoma in the United States is 4.5 per 1 million white children and 1.3 per 1 million black children. Rhabdomyosarcoma occurs in two peaks: at 2 to 6 years of age and during adolescence. There is a male predominance, with a male/female ratio of 1.4:1.[79] Although most cases of rhabdomyosarcoma are sporadic, it has been associated with neurofibromatosis and with familial cancer syndromes. Rhabdomyosarcoma is included in the family cancer syndrome known as *Li-Fraumeni syndrome,* which has been associated with mutations in the p53 gene.[76] Mothers of children with rhabdomyosarcoma have an increased risk of developing breast cancer, and an increased incidence of adrenocortical cancer and brain tumors has been reported in first-degree relatives.[5,77]

HISTOLOGY

Rhabdomyosarcomas are highly malignant tumors that originate from mesenchymal cells, the precursors to striated skeletal muscle cells, and are included in the category of small, round, blue cell tumors of childhood.[86] No uniform histologic classification system exists, but efforts are underway to evaluate data from the Intergroup Rhabdomyosarcoma Studies (IRS) to establish a common histologic and clinical staging criteria for classification.[129] For the purposes of determining treatment strategies, the IRS classifies rhabdomyosarcoma as favorable histology (mixed, undifferentiated, embryonal, botryoid, other) or unfavorable histology (alveolar).[127] The box, p. 398, summarizes the clinical grouping system. Development and testing of a new, nonsurgical-based staging system are being done with IRS-IV.[77,129]

CLINICAL PRESENTATION

The most common presenting symptom is the presence of a mass, usually found by the patient or parent, but symptoms vary according to the site of origin and the presence of metastasis. The most common site of occurrence is the head and neck (38%), followed by the geni-

---

*References 14, 25, 51, 94, 116, 117.

CLINICAL GROUP STAGING SYSTEM FOR RHABDOMYOSARCOMA

Group I   Localized disease, completely resected
             A: Confined to site of origin
             B: Infiltration beyond site of origin

Group II   Total gross resection with evidence of regional spread
             A: Gross resection with microscopic disease
             B: No microscopic disease, regional disease with involved nodes
             C: Regional disease with involved nodes, gross resection with microscopic disease

Group III   A: Localized or locally extensive tumor, gross residual after biopsy only
             B: Localized or locally extensive tumor, gross residual after major resection

Group IV   Distant metastasis at diagnosis

---

tourinary tract (21%), extremity (18%), trunk (7%), and retroperitoneum (7%). Rhabdomyosarcoma most often metastasizes to the lungs, bones, bone marrow, lymph nodes, brain, spinal cord, and heart.[110,129]

DIAGNOSTIC EVALUATION

The diagnostic evaluation is also determined by the site and includes radiologic imaging of the primary tumor through both plain films and a CT scan and/or MRI. Bone scans and skeletal surveys are useful for detection of metastatic disease, followed by a CT scan or MRI of any identified areas of concern. Ultrasounds are used for tumors such as abdominal masses. A bone marrow aspirate and biopsy should be done to rule out bone marrow metastasis. A biopsy is necessary to confirm the diagnosis.

TREATMENT MODALITIES AND PROGNOSIS

Rhabdomyosarcoma is both a local and systemic disease, with most patients having metastasis at diagnosis; thus treatment must be aimed at local control and eradication of metastasis. Treatment is based on the site of origin and extent of disease but often includes surgery, chemotherapy, and radiation.[60,110]

Surgical removal of the tumor is indicated when it will

not compromise function and may reduce the amount of radiation necessary for local control. It is not indicated when there is extensive disease, since it does not improve the outcome, probably because of micrometastasis. If only partial surgical removal is possible, the initial approach should be biopsy alone.[77,110]

Various drugs have been used in the treatment of rhabdomyosarcoma in multiple combinations, with more intensive therapy and additional drugs for patients with more extensive disease or unfavorable histology. The length of treatment also depends on the extent of disease and the primary site. Radiation is used to eradicate residual cells at the primary site or to reduce bulk disease. New methods of delivery are being used, such as brachytherapy to decrease the long-term cosmetic effects of radiation, especially to the head and neck.[77,110,129]

Patients with distant metastatic disease and those with resistant or recurrent disease remain a challenge, with few significant improvements in treatment in recent years. Currently, overall survival is 60% to 70%, but of those with metastatic disease, only 20% to 25% are curable even with the most aggressive therapy. New, more intensive therapeutic regimens are being investigated, including the use of growth factors and BMT.[1,110,129]

BONE TUMORS

Malignant bone tumors represent 5% of all malignancies in children and 10% of all malignancies in adolescence.[85,122] *Osteosarcoma (osteogenic sarcoma)* is the most common bone malignancy in childhood, accounting for 60% of bone tumors. *Ewing's sarcoma* represents 30% of these tumors, and the remaining 10% are of a variety of malignancies.[9]

Osteogenic Sarcoma

Osteosarcoma occurs more frequently in males than females (1.75:1) and at a rate of 5.6 per 1 million white children under age 15 years and slightly less in black children.[8] A peak incidence occurs in the second decade of life, most often between 15 and 19 years of age.

ETIOLOGY

The etiology of osteosarcoma is unclear. A relationship appears to exist between the growth spurt of adolescence and the development of osteosarcoma. It has also been reported that those who develop osteosarcoma are taller than their peers.[39]

There is an increased risk for the development of osteosarcoma in children with the hereditary form of retinoblastoma and for those treated with radiation, especially in doses greater than 6000 cGy.[9,125] Almost all cases of osteogenic sarcoma in those over age 40 years are associated with Paget's disease, a precursor to os-teosarcoma.[30] Trauma was thought at one time to be associated with the development of osteosarcoma, but the occurrence of an injury brings the person to medical attention and the lesion is found coincidentally.

CLINICAL PRESENTATION

In order of frequency, the most common sites of occurrence are femur, tibia, humerus, fibula, scapula, ilium, radius, mandible, and clavicle.[123] Pain in the affected site is the most frequent presenting complaint. The pain can be severe, may have been present for a short time or for months, and increases with activity, often resulting in a limp. Other symptoms may include tenderness, swelling, erythema, or limited range of motion. Metastasis is present in 10% to 20% of patients at diagnosis, with 90% occurring in the lungs. Other possible sites of metastasis include bone, kidney, and brain.[72]

HISTOLOGY

Osteosarcoma is a malignant sarcoma of bone that originates from osteon. The histologic subtype is important. No uniformly accepted classification system exists, but the categories used most often are conventional (osteoblastic, chondroblastic, fibroblastic), telangiectatic, parosteal and periosteal, multifocal, and miscellaneous.[72] The conventional subtype is that seen most often in adolescents and children.

DIAGNOSTIC EVALUATION

Although a biopsy is required to confirm the diagnosis of osteosarcoma, all imaging studies should be completed before biopsy. Plain radiographic films are usually the first indication of the presence of a tumor. MRI and CT scans of the primary lesion provide information regarding extent of disease and the presence of "skip" lesions. The initial evaluation should include a bone scan to determine extent of disease and areas of metastasis. A chest x-ray film and chest CT scan are also necessary to rule out lung metastasis. These radiographic examinations are also helpful in measuring response to treatment, progression of disease, or the development of metastatic disease.

TREATMENT MODALITIES
Surgery

Treatment of osteosarcoma incorporates both surgery and chemotherapy. Advances in radiographic imaging, the use of preoperative chemotherapy to reduce the size of the primary lesion, and improvements in surgical techniques have revolutionized the treatment of osteosar-

coma. The extent of surgery depends on the location and degree of tumor involvement, with amputation no longer necessary for all patients. Limb salvage is possible only if a clear margin of 6 to 7 cm can be maintained and if the extremity will be functional postoperatively. Limb salvage procedures are not used when a pathologic fracture exists or when there is skeletal immaturity. The boxes below review common terms and techniques used in limb salvage surgery. Regardless of the procedure used, both physical rehabilitation and psychologic rehabilitation are necessary.[9]

Chemotherapy

Surgery only provides local control of the tumor. Eighty percent of those treated with surgery alone will develop

---

TERMINOLOGY FOR LIMB SALVAGE SURGERY

Allograft—graft from another individual (usually a cadaver)
Autograft—graft taken from patient
Vascularized graft—graft implanted with vessels supplying it intact
Arthroplasty—surgical formation or reformation of a joint
Arthrodesis—surgical fusion of a joint
Endoprosthesis—artificial replacement of a joint or bone by a metallic implant

Modified from Hockenberry MJ, Lane B: *Cancer Nurs* 11:2, 1988.

LIMB SALVAGE TECHNIQUES

Distal femur
  Autologous arthrodesis (with tibia or femur intermedullary rod graft)
  Segmental prosthesis to restore skeletal continuity
  Prosthetic knee replacement for lesions involving diaphysis
  Tibial rotation plasty
Proximal femur
  Endoprosthesis—long-stem Moore prosthesis with acrylic cement
  Total joint prosthesis—hip replacement or arthroplasty
Proximal tibia
  Resection arthrodesis
Proximal humerus
  Tikhoff-Linberg procedure
  Total shoulder replacement
  Endoprosthesis
  Proximal humerus allograft

Modified from Hockenberry MJ, Lane B: *Cancer Nurs* 11:2, 1988.

and die of metastatic disease.[8,72] Prior clinical trials have documented the efficacy of a variety of drugs in various combinations.[123] With the use of adjuvant chemotherapy and the improvement in surgical technique, survival rates are now 65%.[73] Intraarterial infusions directly to the tumors, thus avoiding systemic effects of the drugs, is now possible.[122]

Preoperative chemotherapy provides not only reduction in tumor size before resection, but also evaluation of tumor response, allowing for changes in therapy if efficacy is unsatisfactory. Osteosarcoma is highly radioresistant, and radiotherapy is reserved primarily for reduction before surgery or for palliation for those with unresponsive disease.

Late Effects

In addition to long-term follow-up to detect adverse effects resulting from chemotherapy, osteogenic sarcoma patients need ongoing evaluation regarding limb or prosthesis function. In general, osteosarcoma patients have less risk of second malignancies than those with other childhood tumors.[52,80]

PROGNOSIS

Tumors localized to the axial skeleton (e.g., trunk, pelvis) and the presence of symptoms for more then 6 months are considered poor prognostic signs.[122] In general, the more distal the lesion, the better is the prognosis, which corresponds to the likelihood of complete surgical resection. The most important prognostic factor is the extent of disease at diagnosis, and metastasis is a poor sign. Other relevant factors include age (younger than 10 years, worse; older than 20 years, better), tumor size (less than 15 cm, negative factor), gender (female more favorable), elevated alkaline phosphatase and lactate dehydrogenase (LDH) levels (both poor prognostic signs), and histology, with telangiectatic associated with the poorest outcome.[72]

Ewing's Sarcoma

Ewing's sarcoma is second only to osteosarcoma as the most common malignant bone tumor in children and adolescence, representing 1% of all childhood cancers. The differential diagnosis includes all the common solid tumors of childhood when they present in their primitive or undifferentiated form. These small, round, blue cell tumors of childhood include small cell osteosarcomas, rhabdomyosarcomas, neuroblastomas, lymphomas, and primitive neuroectodermal tumors. The extraosseous origin of some Ewing's sarcoma is consistent with current evidence that suggests the cell of origin of most tumors is neural and not mesenchymal as previously believed.[59]

EPIDEMIOLOGY

Ewing's sarcoma occurs in 2 or 3 per 1 million white children, with a low incidence in black children.[58] There is a slight male predominance, with females having a slightly better prognosis. Sixty-five percent of patients are diagnosed in the second decade of life, and the disease is rarely seen before age 5 years or after age 30.[87] As in osteosarcoma, there is a sightly increased incidence in taller adolescents, with the typical patient 15 years old, tall, white, and male.

CLINICAL PRESENTATION

The most common symptom is pain with or without swelling at the primary site. Two thirds of patients have a palpable mass, and one fifth have fever and leukocytosis, leading to a misdiagnosis of osteomyelitis.[130] Presenting symptoms are also related to site of occurrence. The duration of symptoms can be days, months, or even years as in those with pelvic tumors. Systemic symptoms of weight loss, fatigue, and fever are present in only one third of patients and are most often associated with metastatic disease.[87] The most common sites of occurrence are the pelvis, tibia, fibula, and femur, but Ewing's can occur in any bone.

DIAGNOSTIC EVALUATION

The most important step in the diagnosis of Ewing's sarcoma is the biopsy, securing adequate tissue for evaluation. The diagnostic work-up includes plain films of the primary lesion, and MRI or CT scan of the primary tumor site allows for detection of extent of soft tissue involvement. A chest x-ray film and CT scan are necessary to rule out metastatic lesions. To detect distant metastasis, a bone scan is usually included in the initial work-up. Bilateral bone marrow aspirate is used to detect bone marrow involvement.

STAGING AND PROGNOSIS

No widely accepted staging system exists for Ewing's sarcoma. The tumors are often characterized by site of presentation, size, and the presence or absence of metastasis. Twenty-five percent of patients have metastasis at diagnosis, most often to the lung, bone, and bone marrow.

The most important prognostic indicator is extent of disease and metastasis. Large tumor size and volume are also associated with a poor prognosis.[59,97] Most primary lesions in unfavorable sites tend to be large. An elevated LDH level is a poor sign and correlates to the extent of disease. Tumors of the proximal extremities, pelvis, and axial skeleton carry the poorest prognosis.[54] Histologic response to therapy is also a prognostic indicator, with less than 10% viable tumor at the time of surgery a positive sign.[97]

NURSING MANAGEMENT

NURSING DIAGNOSES

- *Coping, ineffective individual, related to situational crisis, ineffective coping methods, inadequate support systems*
- *Anxiety related to unmet informational needs about health condition and treatment*
- *Self-esteem disturbance related to life-threatening, acute or chronic illness*

OUTCOME GOALS

The patient/family will be able to:
- Ask for assistance.
- Participate in decision making with regard to health care, activities of daily living, and family interaction.
- Identify, cultivate, and utilize available resources.
- Openly communicate feelings related to disease, treatment, and prognosis.
- Identify alternative resources when present coping strategies do not provide support.

INTERVENTIONS

- Recognize individual needs and developmental level of child:
  —Infant: dependent on parents' presence and support
  —Toddler: separation from parent is major issue; fear of bodily injury and pain; loss of control related to loss of routine, physical restriction, and dependency; benefits from play therapy
  —Preschooler: parents' presence of primary importance; fear of mutilation related to surgery or injections; hospital viewed as punishment or rejection, treatment as punishment or hostile; benefits from play therapy
  —School-age child: concerned with lack of body control and mastery; anxiety handled through knowledge
  —Adolescent: focus on peers and separation from them/family; hospital/treatment a threat to independence; anxiety handled through knowledge and participating in decision making
- Determine patient/family learning needs and knowledge levels pertaining to specific disease process, treatment modalities, and diagnostic testing.
- Assess patient's/family's views and beliefs about cancer.
- Observe patient's/family's coping mechanisms.
- Assess cultural background and belief systems.
- Assess readiness of patient/family to learn.
- Determine what patient/family believe is important to know.
- Provide and discuss information related to specific type of cancer, diagnostic testing, and treatment.
- Teach about emotional reactions to cancer and possible developmental regression.
- Initiate referrals to other health team members: child life therapy, physical therapy, dietitian, and social services.
- Promote normalcy through attending in-hospital classroom, maintaining schoolwork, and providing opportunities for play and recreation.
- Foster maintenance of peer relationships and reentry into the community through school reentry intervention and continued contact while hospitalized or at home.

The box below lists patient teaching priorities for the pediatric patient with cancer and the family.

 PATIENT TEACHING PRIORITIES
Pediatric Cancers

Assess patient/family learning needs for:
  Specific disease process (e.g., leukemia, lymphoma, Wilms' tumor, osteosarcoma)
  Specific diagnostic testing (e.g., arteriography, bone marrow biopsy, MRI)
  Specific treatment modalities (e.g., chemotherapy, radiation therapy, surgery)
Assess and monitor developmental and psychosocial responses to cancer.
Initiate referrals to multidisciplinary health care team: physical therapist, dietitian, social services, occupational therapist, rehabilitation services, and school system.

TREATMENT MODALITIES

Marked progress has occurred in the treatment of Ewing's sarcoma since the late 1960s, resulting in a 2-year disease-free survival rate of 70% for those with localized tumors.[97] Ewing's sarcoma has been described as a systemic disease that initially presents as a local problem, making it necessary to employ not only local control with radiation and surgery, but also systemic treatment with chemotherapy. Large doses of radiation are necessary, with 5000 to 6000 rads to the whole bone and a 1000 rad boost to the primary lesion, which can be associated with functional impairment of the extremity. Portal radiation is being investigated to spare limb function further. Surgery is usually done if the bone is resectable and expendable or for children in whom radiation will cause unacceptable morbidity.[58]

The Intergroup Ewing's Sarcoma Study (IESS) protocols have documented the efficacy of a variety of drugs in varying combinations and doses.[59,97] Chemotherapy often is given, followed by radiation and resection of the primary lesion, and then further chemotherapy. For those with localized disease treated in this way, the 2-year survival rate is 60% to 70%.

Historically the survival for those considered high risk has been 20%. Under examination is a more intensive therapy employing autologous BMT in the treatment regimen, with a projected disease-free survival at 2 years of 80%.[97] Those with metastasis and recurrence still have a bleak prognosis, and late relapse continues to be a problem.

Long-term surveillance includes issues similar to those associated with osteogenic sarcoma. In addition, radiation-induced malignancies constitute a risk, especially for those who have received multiagent therapy.[58]

CONCLUSION

Nurses play a major role in caring for the child with cancer. Multimodality diagnostics and therapies may be used, which creates a strong need for teaching. Many of these patients are treated in multiple settings, so it is imperative that ongoing communication exits between all the health care staff in these various settings. Great strides have been made in the past decade with imaging techniques, laboratory studies, combination chemotherapy, radiation therapy, and new surgical interventions. Significant advances have been made with some diseases, such as leukemia and Wilms' tumor, whereas others have been more disappointing. Continued research and commitment to providing conscientious care for the child with cancer and the family are essential to their quality of life.

■ CHAPTER QUESTIONS

1. The most common cancer in children is:
   a. Lymphoma
   b. Leukemia
   c. Brain tumors
   d. Bone tumors
   e. None of the above
2. All children with acute lymphoblastic leukemia (ALL) receive cranial radiation.
   a. True
   b. False
3. Which of the following are included in the family cancer syndrome associated with mutations in the p53 gene?
   a. Osteosarcoma
   b. Brain tumors
   c. Rhabdomyosarcoma
   d. Burkitt's lymphoma
   e. None of the above

4. The most common solid tumor in children is:
   a. Bone tumors
   b. Neuroblastoma
   c. Wilms' tumor
   d. Brain tumors
5. Ewing's sarcoma or osteogenic sarcoma results from trauma or injury to a bone.
   a. True
   b. False
6. All the following are classified as small, round, blue cell tumors of childhood *except*:
   a. Neuroblastoma
   b. Rhabdomyosarcoma
   c. Ewing's sarcoma
   d. Wilms' tumor
   e. All the above
7. Late effects of radiation include:
   a. Second malignancy
   b. Soft tissue and growth problems
   c. Learning problems
   d. Thyroid abnormalities
   e. All the above
8. CNS prophylaxis is necessary for all but which of the following diseases?
   a. Lymphoma
   b. ALL
   c. AML
   d. None of the above
9. All enlarged lymph nodes in children should be biopsied.
   a. True
   b. False
10. Which of the following typically presents with a mediastinal mass?
    a. ALL
    b. AML
    c. Lymphoblastic lymphoma
    d. None of the above

BIBLIOGRAPHY

1. Adamson PC and others: The child with recurrent solid tumors, *Pediatr Clin North Am* 38:489, 1991.
2. Albright AL: Pediatric brain tumors, *CA Cancer J Clin* 43:272, 1993.
3. Albright AL and others: Magnetic resonance scans should replace biopsies for the diagnosis of diffuse brain stem gliomas: a report from the Children's Cancer Group, *Neurosurgery* 33:1026, 1993.
4. Altman AJ: Chronic leukemias of childhood. In Pizzo PA, Poplack DG, editors: *Principles and practice of pediatric oncology,* ed 2, Philadelphia, 1993, Lippincott.
5. Altman AJ, Schwartz AD: *Malignant diseases of infancy, childhood and adolescence,* ed 2, Philadelphia, 1983, Saunders.
6. Anderson JR and others: Childhood non-Hodgkin's lymphoma: results of a randomized therapeutic trial comparing a four drug regimen (COMP) with a ten drug regimen, *N Engl J Med* 308:559, 1983.
7. Bestak, M: Hodgkin disease, *Pediatr Rev* 16:456, 1995.

8. Betcher D: New trends in osteogenic sarcoma, *J Pediatr Oncol Nurs* 8:70, 1991.

9. Betcher D: Bone tumors. In Foley GV, Fochtman D, Mooney KH, editors: *Nursing care of the child with cancer,* ed 2, Philadelphia, 1993, Saunders.

10. Bleyer WA: Acute lymphoblastic leukemia in children, *Cancer* 65:689, 1990.

11. Bleyer WA and others: The staging of childhood acute lymphoblastic leukemia: strategies of the Children's Cancer Study Group and a three-dimensional technic of multivariate analysis, *Med Pediatr Oncol* 14:271, 1986.

12. Boulad F, Kernan N: Treatment of childhood acute nonlymphoblastic leukemia: a review, *Cancer Invest* 11:534, 1993.

13. Bourhis J and others: *N-myc* genomic content and DNA ploidy in stage IVS neuroblastoma, *J Clin Oncol* 9:1371, 1991.

14. Brodeur GM, Castleberry RP: Neuroblastoma. In Pizzo PA, Poplack DG, editors: *Principles and practice of pediatric oncology,* ed 2, Philadelphia, 1993, Lippincott.

15. Brodeur GM and others: Revisions of the international criteria for neuroblastoma diagnosis, staging, and response to treatment, *J Clin Oncol* 11:1466, 1993.

16. Brunin NJ, Puim CH: Differing complications of hyperleucocytosis in children with acute lymphoblastic or acute nonlymphoblastic leukemias, *J Clin Oncol* 3:1590, 1985.

17. Butturini A and others: Which treatment for childhood acute lymphoblastic leukemia in second remission? *Lancet* 1:429, 1987.

18. Castro-Malaspina H and others: Subacute and chronic myelomonocytic leukemia in children (juvenile CML), *Cancer* 54:675, 1984.

19. Clark RH and others: Congenital juvenile chronic myelogenous leukemia: case report and review, *Pediatrics* 73:324, 1984.

20. Cohen DG: Acute lymphocytic leukemia. In Foley GV, Fochtman D, Mooney KH, editors: *Nursing care of the child with cancer,* ed 2, Philadelphia, 1993, Saunders.

21. Cohen ME and others: Prognostic factors in brain stem gliomas, *Neurology* 36:602, 1986.

22. D'Angio and others: Treatment of Wilms' tumor, *Cancer* 64:349, 1989.

23. Danoff BF and others: Assessment of long-term effects of primary brain tumors in children, *Cancer* 49:1580, 1982.

24. DeVita VT, Hubbard SM: Hodgkin's disease, *N Engl J Med* 328:560, 1993.

25. Dini G and others: Myeloablative therapy and unpurged autologous bone marrow transplantation for poor-prognosis neuroblastoma: report of 34 cases, *J Clin Oncol* 9:962, 1991.

26. Donaldson SS, Link MP: Combined modality treatment with low-dose radiation and MOPP chemotherapy for children with Hodgkin's disease, *J Clin Oncol* 5:742, 1987.

27. Donaldson SS, Link MP: Hodgkin's disease: treatment of the young child, *Pediatr Clin North Am* 38:457, 1991.

28. Drigan R, Adrokites AL: Wilms' tumor. In Foley GV, Fochtman D, Mooney KH, editors: *Nursing care of the child with cancer,* ed 2, Philadelphia, 1993, Saunders.

29. Duffner PK and others: Referral patterns of childhood brain tumors in the state of Connecticut, *Cancer* 50:1636, 1982.

30. Enneking WE, Conrad EU: Common bone tumors, *Clin Symp* 41:2, 1989.

31. Epstein F: A staging system for brain stem gliomas, *Cancer* 56:1804, 1985.

32. Evans AE: Natural history of neuroblastoma. In Evans AE, editor: *Advances in neuroblastoma research,* New York, 1980, Raven.

33. Evans AE and others: The treatment of medulloblastoma: results of a prospective randomized trial of radiation therapy with and without CCNU, vincristine, and prednisone, *J Neurosurg* 72(4):572, 1990.

34. Finlay JL, Goins SC: Brain tumors in children. III. Advances in chemotherapy, *Am J Pediatr Hematol Oncol* 9:264, 1987.

35. Finlay JL and others: Progress in the management of childhood brain tumors, *Hematol Oncol Clin North Am* 1:753, 1987.

36. Finlay JL and others: Brain tumors in children. II. Advances in neurosurgery and radiation oncology, *Am J Pediatr Hematol Oncol* 9:256, 1987.

37. Finlay JL and others: High-dose multiagent chemotherapy followed by bone marrow "rescue" for malignant astrocytomas of childhood and adolescence, *J Neurooncol* 9:239, 1990.

38. Fletcher BD, Platt CB: Evaluation of the child with a suspected malignant solid tumor, *Pediatr Clin North Am* 38:226, 1991.

39. Fraumei JF Jr: Stature and malignant tumors of bone in childhood and adolescence, *Cancer* 20:967, 1967.

40. Freedman MH and others: Juvenile chronic myelogenous leukemia, *Am J Pediatr Hematol Oncol* 10:261, 1988.

41. Friedman HS and others: Medulloblastoma: tumor biological and clinical perspectives, *J Neurooncol* 11:1, 1991.

42. Gehan EA and others: The international group Hodgkin's disease in children: a study of stages I and II, *Cancer* 65:1429, 1990.

43. Gilchrist GS, Evans RG: Contemporary issues in pediatric Hodgkin's disease, *Pediatr Clin North Am* 32:721, 1985.

44. Gjerris F: Clinical aspects and long-term prognosis of intracranial tumors in infancy and childhood, *Dev Med Child Neurol* 18:145, 1976.

45. Graham M: Non-Hodgkin's lymphomas, *Pediatr Ann* 17:192, 1988.

46. Greaves M: A natural history for pediatric acute leukemia, *J Am Soc Hematol* 82:1043, 1993.

47. Green DM and others: Wilms' tumor. In Pizzo PA, Poplack DG, editors: *Principles and practice of pediatric oncology,* ed 2, Philadelphia, 1993, Lippincott.

48. Green DM and others: Wilms' tumor, *CA Cancer J Clin* 46:46, 1996.

49. Greier HE, Weinstein HJ: Acute myelogenous leukemia. In Pizzo PA, Poplack DG, editors: *Principles and practice of pediatric oncology,* ed 2, Philadelphia, 1993, Lippincott.

50. Grundy P and others: Prognostic factors for children with recurrent Wilms' tumor: results from the second and third national Wilms' tumor study, *J Clin Oncol* 7:638, 1989.

51. Haas D and others: Complete pathologic maturation and regression of stage IVS neuroblastoma without treatment, *Cancer* 62:818, 1988.

52. Hawkins MN: Longterm survival and cure after childhood cancer, *Arch Dis Child* 64:798, 1989.

53. Hayashi Y and others: Similar chromosomal patterns and lack of *N-myc* gene amplification in localized and IV-S stage neuroblastomas in infants, *Med Pediatr Oncol* 17:111, 1989.

54. Hayes FA and others: Therapy for localized Ewing's sarcoma of bone, *J Clin Oncol* 7:208, 1989.

55. Helson L: Neuroblastomas: detection and diagnosis, *Oncol Rounds* 4:10, 1987.

56. Hockenberry MJ and others: Childhood cancers: incidence, etiology, diagnosis, and treatment, *Pediatr Nurs* 16:239, 1990.

57. Horowitz ME and others: Brain tumors in the very young child, *Cancer* 61:428, 1988.

58. Horowitz ME and others: Ewing's sarcoma, *Pediatr Clin North Am* 38:365, 1991.

59. Horowitz ME and others: Ewing's sarcoma family of tumors: Ewing's sarcoma of bone and soft tissue and the peripheral primitive neuroectodermal tumors. In Pizzo PA, Poplack DG, editors: *Principles and practice of pediatric oncology*, ed 2, Philadelphia, 1993, Lippincott.

60. Houghton PJ and others: Rhabdomyosarcoma: from the laboratory to the clinic, *Pediatr Clin North Am* 38:349, 1991.

61. Jenkins RDT and others: The treatment of localized non-Hodgkin's lymphoma in children: a report from the Children's Cancer Study Group, *J Clin Oncol* 2:443, 1984.

62. Kadota RP and others: Brain tumors in children, *J Pediatr* 114:511, 1989.

63. Kantarjian HM and others: Treatment of advanced stages of Philadelphia chromosome-positive chronic myelogenous leukemia with interferon-α and low-dose cytarabine, *J Clin Oncol* 10:772, 1992.

64. Knight PJ and others: When is lymph node biopsy indicated in children with enlarged peripheral nodes? *Pediatrics* 69:772, 1982.

65. Knudson AG, Strong LC: Mutation and cancer: neuroblastoma and pheochromocytoma, *Am J Hum Genet* 24:514, 1972.

66. Kobrinsky NL and others: Wilms' tumor, *Pediatr Ann* 17:241, 1988.

67. Kobrinsky NL and others: Wilms' tumor, *Hematol Oncol Annu* 1:174, 1993.

68. Kushner BH, Cheung NV: Neuroblastoma, *Pediatr Ann* 17:269, 1988.

69. Kushner BH, Cheung NV: Neuroblastoma: an overview, *Hematol Oncol Ann* 1:189, 1993.

70. Lamkin BC and others: Biologic characteristics and treatment of acute nonlymphocytic leukemia in children, *Pediatr Clin North Am* 35:743, 1988.

71. Leventhal BG: Management of stage I-II Hodgkin's disease in children, *J Clin Oncol* 8:1123, 1990.

72. Link E, Eilber F: Osteosarcoma. In Pizzo PA, Poplack DG, editors: *Principles and practice of pediatric oncology*, ed 2, Philadelphia, 1993, Lippincott.

73. Link MP and others: The effect of adjuvant chemotherapy on relapse-free survival in patients with osteosarcoma of the extremity, *N Engl J Med* 314:1600, 1986.

74. Lopez-Ibor B, Schwartz AD: Neuroblastoma, *Pediatr Clin North Am* 32:755, 1985.

75. Magrath IT: Malignant non-Hodgkin's lymphoma in children. In Pizzo PA, Poplack DG, editors: *Principles and practice of pediatric oncology*, ed 2, Philadelphia, 1993, Lippincott.

76. Malkin D and others: Germ line p53 mutations in a familial syndrome of breast cancer, sarcomas, and other neoplasms, *Science* 250:1233, 1990.

77. Malogolowkin MH, Ortega JA: Rhabdomyosarcoma of childhood, *Pediatr Ann* 17:251, 1988.

78. Mastrangelo R and others: Report and recommendations of the Rome workshop concerning poor prognosis acute lymphoblastic leukemia in children: biologic bases for staging, stratification, and treatment, *Med Pediatr Oncol* 14:190, 1986.

79. Maurer HM and others: The Intergroup Rhabdomyosarcoma Study: a preliminary report, *Cancer* 40:2015, 1977.

80. Meadows AT and others: Second malignant neoplasms in children: an update from the Late Effects Study Group, *J Clin Oncol* 3:532, 1985.

81. Meadows AT and others: Second malignant neoplasms following childhood Hodgkin's disease: treatment and splenectomy as risk factors, *Med Pediatr Oncol* 17:477, 1989.

82. Meyers P: Malignant bone tumors in children: Ewing's sarcoma, *Hematol Oncol Clin North Am* 1:667, 1987.

83. Miller DR and others: Central nervous system involvement at presentation in acute granulocytic leukemia, *Am J Med* 68:691, 1980.

84. Miller DR and others: Three versus five years of maintenance therapy are equivalent in childhood acute lymphoblastic leukemia: a report from the Children's Cancer Study Group, *J Clin Oncol* 7:316, 1989.

85. Miller RW and others: Childhood cancer, *Cancer* 75:396, 1995.

86. Miser JS, Pizzo PA: Soft tissue sarcomas in childhood, *Pediatr Clin North Am* 32:779, 1985.

87. Miser JS and others: Ewing's sarcoma and nonrhabdomyosarcoma soft tissue sarcomas of childhood. In Pizzo PA, Poplack DG, editors: *Principles and practice of pediatric oncology*, Philadelphia, 1989, Lippincott.

88. Mulhern RK and others: Neuropsychological sequelae of childhood brain tumors: a review, *J Clin Child Psychol* 12:66, 1982.

89. Mulhern RK and others: A prospective comparison of neuropsychologic performance of children surviving leukemia who received 18-Gy, 24-Gy, or no cranial irradiation, *J Clin Oncol* 9:1348, 1991.

90. Nachman J: Therapy for childhood non-Hodgkin's lymphoma non-lymphoma-blastic type, *Am J Pediatr Hematol Oncol* 12:359, 1990.

91. Neglia JP, Robinson LL: Epidemiology of the childhood acute leukemias, *Pediatr Clin North Am* 35:675, 1988.

92. Neglia JP and others: Second neoplasms after acute lymphoblastic leukemia in childhood, *N Engl J Med* 325:1330, 1991.

93. Nesbit ME: Advances and management of solid tumors in children, *Cancer* 65:699, 1990.

94. Nickerson HJ and others: Comparison of Stage IV and IV-S neuroblastoma in the first year of life, *Med Pediatr Oncol* 13:261, 1985.

95. Nitschke R and others: Localized neuroblastoma treated by surgery: a Pediatric Oncology Group Study, *J Clin Oncol* 6:1271, 1988.

96. North CA and others: Low-grade cerebral astrocytomas: survival and quality of life after radiation therapy, *Cancer* 66:6, 1990.

97. O'Connor ME, Pritchard DJ: Ewing's sarcoma: prognostic factors, disease control, and the reemerging role of surgical treatment, *Clin Orthop* 262:78, 1991.

98. Oppedal BR and others: Prognostic factors in neuroblastoma: clinical, histopathologic and immunohistochemical features and DNA ploidy in relation to prognosis, *Cancer* 62:772, 1988.

99. Oppedal BR and others: *N-myc* amplification in neuroblastoma: histopathological, DNA ploidy, and clinical variables, *J Clin Pathol* 49:1148, 1989.

100. Packer RJ and others: Hyperfractionated radiation therapy (72cGy) for children with brain stem gliomas: a Children's Cancer Group Phase I/II trial, *Cancer* 72:1414, 1993.

101. Parker SL and others: Cancer statistics, 1996, *CA Cancer J Clin* 65:5, 1996.

102. Peckham VA and others: Educational late effects in long-term survivors of childhood acute lymphocytic leukemia, *Pediatrics* 81(1):127, 1988.

103. Peters JM and others: Brain tumors in children and occupational exposure of parents, *Science* 213:235, 1981.

104. Petriccione MM: Central nervous system tumors. In Foley GV, Fochtman D, Mooney KH, editors: *Nursing care of the child with cancer,* ed 2, Philadelphia, 1993, Saunders.

105. Pollack IF: Brain tumors in children, *N Engl J Med* 331:1500, 1994.

106. Poplack DG: Acute lymphoblastic leukemia. In Pizzo PA, Poplack DG, editors: *Principles and practice of pediatric oncology,* ed 2, Philadelphia, 1993, Lippincott.

107. Poplack DG, Reaman G: Acute lymphoblastic leukemia in childhood, *Pediatr Clin North Am* 35:903, 1988.

108. Poplack DG and others: Leukemia and lymphoma in childhood. In DeVita VT Jr, Hellman S, Rosenberg SA, editors: *Principles and practices of oncology,* ed 3, Philadelphia, 1989, Lippincott.

109. Pui CH, Crist WM: Biology and treatment of acute lymphoblastic leukemia, *J Pediatr* 124:491, 1994.

110. Raney RB and others: Rhabdomyosarcomas and the undifferentiated sarcomas. In Pizzo PA, Poplack DG, editors: *Principles and practice of pediatric oncology,* ed 2, Philadelphia, 1993, Lippincott.

111. Reiter A and others: Favorable outcome of B-cell acute lymphoblastic leukemia in childhood: a report of three consecutive studies of the BFM group, *Blood* 80:2471, 1992.

112. Reiter A and others: Chemotherapy in 998 unselected childhood acute lymphoblastic leukemia patients: results and conclusion of the multicenter trial ALL-BFM 86, *Blood* 84:3122, 1994.

113. Rivera GK and others: Treatment of acute lymphoblastic leukemia, *N Engl J Med* 329:1289, 1993.

114. Sanders JE and others: Allogenic marrow transplantation for children with juvenile chronic myelogenous leukemia, *Blood* 71:1144, 1988.

115. Seeger RC and others: Association of multiple copies of the *N-myc* oncogene with rapid progression of neuroblastomas, *N Engl J Med* 313:1111, 1985.

116. Seeger RC and others: Intensive chemoradiotherapy and autologous bone marrow transplantation for poor prognosis neuroblastoma, *Adv Neuroblastoma Res* 3:527, 1991.

117. Shuster JJ and others: The prognostic significance of autologous bone marrow transplant in advanced neuroblastoma, *J Clin Oncol* 9:1045, 1991.

118. Smith S and others: Non-Hodgkin's lymphoma in children, *Semin Oncol* 17:113, 1990.

119. Sposto R and others: The effectiveness of chemotherapy for treatment of high grade astrocytoma in children: result of a randomized trial: a report from the Children's Cancer Study Group, *J Neurooncol* 7:165, 1989.

120. Streinherz PG: Radiotherapy vs. intrathecal chemotherapy for CNS prophylaxis in childhood ALL, *Oncology* 3:47, 1989.

121. Sutton LN and others: Prognostic factors in childhood ependymomas, *Pediatr Neurosurg* 16:57, 1991.

122. Tebbi CK: Osteosarcoma in childhood and adolescence, *Hematol Oncol Annu* 1:203, 1993.

123. Tebbi CK, Gaeta J: Osteosarcoma, *Pediatr Ann* 17:285, 1988.

124. Traggis DG and others: Prognosis for children with neuroblastoma presenting with paralysis, *J Pediatr Surg* 12:419, 1977.

125. Tucker MA and others: Bone sarcomas linked to radiotherapy and chemotherapy in children, *N Engl J Med* 317:588, 1987.

126. Van Wering ER, Kamps WA: Acute leukemia in infants: a unique pattern in acute nonlymphocytic leukemia, *Am J Pediatr Hematol Oncol* 8:220, 1986.

127. Van Wezel-Bolen G: Rhabdomyosarcoma. In Foley GV, Fochtman D, Mooney KH, editors: *Nursing care of the child with cancer,* ed 2, Philadelphia, 1993, Saunders.

128. Walker RW, Allen JC: Pediatric brain tumors, *Pediatr Ann* 12:383, 1983.

129. Wexler LH, Helman LJ: Pediatric soft tissue sarcomas, *CA Cancer J Clin* 44:211, 1994.

130. Wilkens RM and others: Ewing's sarcoma of bone, *Cancer* 58:2551, 1986.

131. Yasargi NG and others: Surgical approaches to "inaccessible" brain tumors, *Clin Neurosurg* 34:42, 1986.

132. Young JL, Miller RW: Incidence of malignant tumors in the U.S. children, *J Pediatr* 86:254, 1975.

133. Young JL Jr and others: Cancer incidence, survival and mortality for children younger than age 15 years, *Cancer* 58:598, 1986.

134. Ziegler JL: Burkitt's lymphomas, *CA Cancer J Clin* 32:144, 1982.

CHAPTER 19
Oncologic Complications

SANDRA LEE SCHAFER

Cancer involves a multiplicity of tissues in a wide range of locations with metabolic diversities and various metastatic potentials that can result in a variety of oncologic complications.[12] The complex nature of the disease, together with patients with cancer living longer because of improvements in the diagnosis and treatment of cancer and its sequelae, results in an increase in the frequency of cancer-related complications. This trend will probably continue, since cancer is the second leading cause of death in the United States. Most patients with cancer die of metastatic disease and related complications of the disease, which can occur at any time during the course of the disease. Therefore prevention, early recognition, adequate decision making, and prompt treatment of oncologic complications are of paramount importance when delivering care to patients with cancer.

Once the oncologic complication is analyzed, the decision whether to treat or not and to what degree to treat can be made. Treatment may be aggressive when potential exists for a cure or prolonged survival. On the other hand, in advanced disease the treatment may be given to palliate symptoms and restore functional status. Finally, withholding treatment and providing supportive care may be the most appropriate decision in the presence of disseminated metastatic disease.[14,57,102] Quality of life should always be the driving force in any decision regarding care of the patient with cancer. The overall goal is to prevent, reverse, or minimize life-threatening oncologic complications through prophylactic measures, early detection, and effective management.

Management of an oncologic complication depends on many important factors related to the patient and the underlying disease (see box, p. 407). These factors must be given thorough consideration before the initiation of treatment.

Decisions regarding who, how, when, and where to treat the patients with oncologic complications have become more difficult in light of the many changes in health care delivery systems. Patients are more acutely ill and have shorter hospitalization periods. There are fewer inpatient beds for medical/surgical and critical care patients. According to Shoemaker,[141] "As our resources and knowledge have increased, so have indications." Utilization of critical care interventions for patients with cancer has increased for a variety of reasons: new hopes for cure or long-term remission, increased ability to treat certain complications, and consumer demands. The newer therapies are more aggressive and cause increased organ toxicity, prolonged aplasia, and various complications that may be life-threatening. Depending on the type and status of the underlying primary malignancy, the complications may occur at diagnosis, during treatment, and with progressive disease. A team approach is necessary to avoid bias of independent thinking. A framework for decision making should be developed and used within the organization. This should be supported by a multidisciplinary ethics committee. The goal is the provision of accurate information and appropriate options to patients and families.[141]

Nursing care of the patient with a potential for or an oncologic complication or with a complication is multifaceted and challenging regardless of the clinical setting. The patient status may be anywhere along a continuum, from being at high risk for the development of a problem through manifestations of it in various degrees (mild, moderate, severe). Striking similarities exist among these patients despite the extreme individual differences.

These common nursing care themes are not addressed in this chapter. Instead, the focus is on selected nursing diagnoses related to specific problems. However, it is important to review these similarities for purposes of comprehensive care planning. Common nursing diagnoses for patients with oncologic complications include the following:
- Pain
- Nutrition, altered: less than body requirements
- Anxiety
- Knowledge deficit
- Coping, ineffective individual
- Coping, ineffective family: compromised

MANAGEMENT FACTORS IN THE EVALUATION AND TREATMENT OF AN ONCOLOGIC EMERGENCY

SYMPTOMS AND SIGNS

1. Are the symptoms and signs caused by the tumor or by complications of treatment?
2. How quickly are the symptoms of the oncologic emergency progressing?

NATURAL HISTORY OF THE PRIMARY TUMOR

1. Is there a previous diagnosis of malignancy?
2. What is the disease-free interval between the diagnosis of the primary tumor and the onset of the emergency?
3. Has the emergency developed in the setting of terminal disease?

EFFICACY OF AVAILABLE TREATMENT

1. No prior therapy versus extensive pretreatment
2. Should treatment be directed at the underlying malignancy and/or the urgent complication?
3. Will the patient's general medical condition influence the ability to administer effective treatment?

TREATMENT AND GOALS

1. Potential for cure
2. Is prompt palliation required to prevent further debilitation?
3. What is the risk versus benefit ratio of treatment?
4. Should treatment be withheld if the patient is terminal with minimal chance of response to available antitumor therapies?

From Glover D, Glick JH: Oncologic emergencies. In Holleb AI, Fink DJ, Murphy GP, editors: *American Cancer Society textbook of clinical oncology,* Atlanta, 1991, American Cancer Society.

These diagnoses, along with those listed for specific problems, assist in the nursing management of these patients (see Chapters 28, 29, and 31). Assessment is essential because a change in the patient's condition may be subtle or dramatic. Two key concepts when caring for people with cancer are (1) the identification of patients at risk for developing an oncologic complication and (2) the involvement of the family and significant other(s). The patient and family require considerable education and support. Time limits are the greatest enemy, creating great anxiety. Explanations of tests and procedures and the rationale for changes in patient care or setting must be kept simple. Treatment options and goals of therapy must be explained and discussed. This is especially important when the realistic outcome is palliation. Anticipatory guidance and discharge planning may be necessary because some therapies may last several weeks or longer.

DISSEMINATED INTRAVASCULAR COAGULATION

DEFINITION

Disseminated intravascular coagulation (DIC) is considered to be a bleeding disorder. In the past it was referred to as a "consumptive coagulopathy." Bleeding disorders are classified as congenital or acquired. DIC is one of the acquired disorders. It is not a disease entity but rather an event that can accompany various disease processes. DIC is an alteration in the blood-clotting mechanism, with abnormal acceleration of the *coagulation cascade* (activates the vasomotor reactions and inhibits fibrinolysis), resulting in thrombosis, and hemorrhage may occur consecutively and/or simultaneously.[60,127,157]

ETIOLOGY AND RISK FACTORS

DIC is not a primary independent disorder. An underlying pathology, benign or malignant, is responsible for DIC. The pathology creates the triggering mechanism or initiating event necessary for the activation of thrombin, which is responsible for the cascade of blood clot formation and clot dissolution, thus producing DIC.* A variety of pathologies involve a triggering event, which can cause either endothelial tissue injury or blood vessel injury.

- Endothelial injuries include the following[71]:

Shock or trauma—head injury, burns

Infections—aspergillosis, gram-positive sepsis or gram-negative sepsis

Obstetric complications—abruptio placentae, amniotic fluid embolism

Malignancies—acute promyelocytic myelogenous leukemia (APML), acute myelogenous leukemia (AML), mucin-producing gastrointestinal (GI) adenocarcinomas, cancers of the lung, colon, breast, and prostate

- Blood vessel injuries include the following:

Infectious vasculitis—Rocky Mountain spotted fever, certain viral infections, severe glomerulonephritis

Vascular disorders—aortic aneurysm, giant hemangioma, angiography

Intravascular hemolysis—hemolytic transfusion reaction, multiple whole-blood transfusions, massive trauma, extracorporeal circulation devices (e.g., cardiopulmonary bypass machine, aortic balloon pump), heatstroke, peritoneovenous shunting

Miscellaneous—pancreatitis, liver disease (e.g., obstructive jaundice, acute hepatic failure), snakebite

In patients with cancer the incidence of DIC is less than 10% to 15%. It is usually related to the disease process or the treatment of the cancer and often occurs concomitantly with sepsis.[40,46,107]

---

*References 3, 40, 102, 103, 127, 133.

Patients with leukemia often have some of the characteristics of DIC without having the complete DIC syndrome. Occurrence of DIC in patients with leukemia is 1% to 2%. Approximately 85% of the patients with APML will develop DIC.[13,29] The blast cells in APML are hypergranular and release a procoagulant substance similar to factor III. This release may occur at any time, such as at diagnosis or after chemotherapy.[34]

PATHOPHYSIOLOGY

Body hemostasis depends on an intricate balance between blood clot formation and blood clot dissolution. The fibrin blood clot is the end product of the blood-clotting mechanism.[40,46,107] Normally this mechanism is initiated when tissues sustain an injury. Disruption of the vascular endothelium exposes collagen fibers to blood. Smooth muscle spasm then occurs, releasing serotonin. Vasoconstriction follows, which slows the flow of blood and causes circulating platelets to change shape and adhere to the rough surface of injured vessels within 1 to 2 seconds.[33,70] More platelets aggregate and form a loose plug at the site of injury, creating a seal on the vessel wall to control bleeding. The injured vascular tissue also releases a phospholipid called *thromboplastin,* which initiates the clotting reaction.[1,3,33,70]

The fibrin blood clot is formed through a series of sequential reactions that are protein activated (Figure 19-1). This protein activation occurs through two different cascades of reactions known as the intrinsic and extrinsic pathways, which operate jointly to form the blood clot. The *intrinsic pathway* is activated by injury to the blood vessel wall. The *extrinsic pathway* is activated after tissue injury. Central to each pathway is the conversion of prothrombin to thrombin through a series of reactions involving various blood factors (phospholipids, proteins, calcium). The thrombin then acts as a catalyst to convert fibrinogen (monomer) to fibrin (polymer).[33,70] The fibrin polymers form a mesh of fibrin strands, which trap platelets, red blood cells (RBCs), and leukocytes, making an occlusive clot.

The series of reactions that forms the clot is balanced by a series of reactions that limits the size of the clot and later dissolves it. Therefore clot dissolution occurs in conjunction with clot formation. When the clot is no longer needed, it is converted from a polymer back to a monomer by *fibrinolysin (plasmin).* Fibrinolysin is formed in the presence of thrombin during coagulation when preactivators come in contact with a tissue enzyme known as *kinase.*[33,70] Fibrinogen and fibrin are broken down by fibrinolysis, resulting in *fibrin degradation products* (FDPs) or *fibrin split products* (FSPs). As these fragments circulate, they interfere with the formation of fibrin and coat the platelets, thus decreasing their adhesive ability. The result is anticoagulation along with the process of fibrinolysis; the body forms *antithrombins,* natural anticoagulants that also interfere with thrombin (clotting) activity. Hemostasis is therefore balanced between fibrin clot formation *(coagulation)* and clot dissolution by fibrinolysis *(anticoagulation).*[80,161]

DIC is a disruption of body hemostasis. One of the triggering mechanisms from the underlying pathology initiates the process (Figure 19-2), which results in the formation of thrombin and fibrinolysin (plasmin).

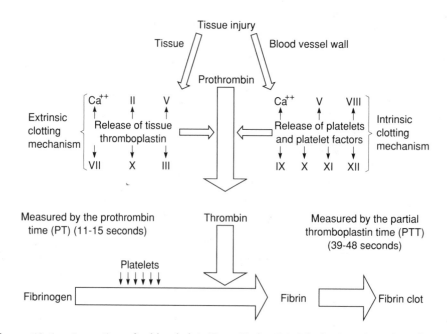

Figure 19-1 Formation of a blood clot. (From Yasko JM, Schafer SL: Disseminated intravascular coagulation. In Yasko JM, editor: *Guidelines for cancer care: symptom management,* Reston, Va, 1983, Reston.)

Thrombin acts to convert fibrinogen to fibrin to form clots. At the same time, fibrinolysin degrades some of the fibrin into a soluble monomer form; this initiates clot dissolution. The remaining portion of fibrin is an insoluble polymer, which continues to form clots. These clots may be deposited in the extremities or in organs such as the lungs, kidneys, and brain. Capillary clots slow the blood flow, resulting in tissue ischemia, hypoxia, and necrosis.[33,70] The clots also trap circulating platelets in the microvasculature, which results in the thrombocytopenia. As the fibrinolysin continues to degrade fibrin, the byproducts FDPs are produced. These FDPs disrupt the conversion of fibrin to a polymer; coat platelets, decreasing their adherence; and degrade factors V, VIII, and X, which leads to capillary hemorrhage.[1,40,46,70,127]

If the underlying pathology with its triggering mechanism is not treated or otherwise eliminated, it will promote further coagulopathy. The term *consumptive coagulopathy* has been used to describe this increased use (consumption) of platelets and clotting factors, leading to a continuation of thrombocytopenia and a further decrease of clotting factors and resulting in bleeding. Thus the abnormal activation of thrombin in DIC results in a cyclic paradox of thrombosis or hemorrhage or both (Figure 19-2).

CLINICAL FEATURES

The onset of DIC may be acute, chronic, or somewhere between acute and chronic. The clinical manifestations and laboratory findings depend on the triggering event and the body tissues involved. The presenting signs and symptoms result from disseminated clotting and bleeding, which may be overt or occult. Bleeding usually predominates.[33,70]

Signs of bleeding are multiple and may be seen from any body orifice. Bleeding may range from oozing to frank bleeding or hemorrhage. Patients may have overt oozing from venipuncture sites, mucous membranes, needle puncture sites, or incisions. Petechiae, ecchymoses, purpura, or hematomas may be evident. Profound menstrual or GI bleeding may occur, as well as epistaxis or hemoptysis.

Less dramatic but equally critical is the possibility of occult internal or intracerebral bleeding. Abdominal distention, blood in stools, blood in urine or skin, and scleral changes may be observed. Other signs of occult bleeding may be mental status changes, orthopnea, and tachycardia. Clotting resulting from fibrin deposits in the microcirculation will impede blood flow and can cause severe tissue ischemia and lead to tissue necrosis. Multiple system changes may be observed. Observation of the skin may show acrocyanosis, also known as *Raynaud's sign* (generalized sweating with symmetric mottling of the nose, fingers, toes, and genitalia), and other ischemic changes, which can lead to superficial gangrene. Pulmonary signs, such as severe, sudden dyspnea at rest with tachypnea and progressive rales and rhonchi, are similar to those observed with adult respiratory distress syndrome (ARDS).[1] The GI tract may have an ischemic insult appearing as an ulceration, and tubular necrosis of

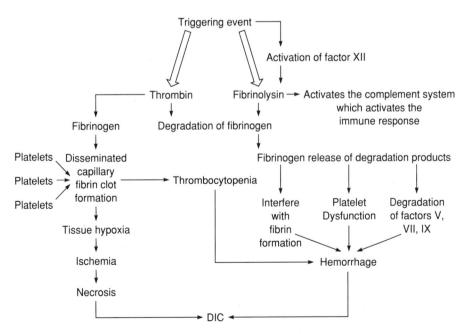

Figure 19-2 Pathophysiology of disseminated intravascular coagulation *(DIC)*. (From Yasko JM, Schafer SL: Disseminated intravascular coagulation. In Yasko JM, editor: *Guidelines for cancer care: symptom management*, Reston, Va, 1983, Reston.)

the kidney may lead to renal failure. If microcoagulation occurs in the brain, multifocal cerebrovascular accidents (CVAs, strokes), mental change, delirium, and coma may result.[5] The associated symptoms of bleeding or clotting will vary depending on the system sustaining the ischemic insult or bleeding. Complaints include malaise, weakness, air hunger, altered sensorium, visual changes, and headaches. The presence and magnitude of these disturbances depend on the extent of the clotting and bleeding.

A major concern for a person experiencing DIC is the possibility of a life-threatening syndrome known as *multiple organ dysfunction syndrome* (MODS).[17] This is a phenomenon described as a progressive, sequential deterioration of two or more organ systems occurring over a brief time. Tissue injury or illness produces intravascular inflammation. This triggers a nonspecific systemic response mediated by a number of cellular, humoral, and biochemical reactions. This response is usually seen in conjunction with a septic focus that is considered essential for the occurrence of MODS.[17,102,103]

DIAGNOSIS

Laboratory findings substantiate a diagnosis of DIC (Table 19-1). No single blood test can confirm or exclude a diagnosis of DIC; instead, a classic triad of screening tests is used, which includes platelet count, prothrombin time (PT), and fibrinogen level. The abnormal results of these tests reflect the consumption of clotting factors and the occurrence of fibrinolysis, resulting in the production of FDPs or FSPs that further interfere with clotting, as follows[1,33,46,126]:

- Platelet count is decreased. This indicates *thrombocytopenia,* which is the cardinal laboratory finding. More than 90% of patients with DIC have abnormal platelet count and PT.[1] In about 50% of these patients, the platelet count is less than 50,000/mm^3 (normal: 150,000 to 400,000/mm^3).

- PT is prolonged (normal: 10 to 13 seconds). This evaluates the extrinsic coagulation system, reflecting decreased levels of clotting factors II, V, and X and of fibrinogen.
- Fibrinogen level is decreased (normal: 200 to 400 mg/dl). This results from the consumption of fibrinogen by thrombin-induced clotting and excessive fibrinolysis.[58] Fibrinogen levels less than 150 mg/dl are found in 70% of patients with DIC.[143]

Other laboratory indicators for DIC include the following:

- Partial thromboplastin time (PTT) is prolonged (normal: 39 to 48 seconds). This evaluates the intrinsic coagulation system. However, during DIC, PTT is less sensitive than PT.
- Thrombin time (TT) is usually prolonged, indicating depression of clotting factors (normal: 10 to 13 seconds).
- FDPs or FSPs are increased (normal: less than 10). A D-dimer test is a recent semiquantitative analysis for FDPs. Although this study has extreme sensitivity, it is not exclusive for DIC.
- Factor assays, especially V and VIII, are decreased.
- Protamine sulphate precipitation test (thrombin activation test) is strongly positive (normal: negative).
- Antithrombin III levels are decreased (normal: 89% to 120%).

Laboratory tests for DIC can be complicated by underlying conditions. Patients with liver disease have abnormal clotting studies and often thrombocytopenia. Laboratory findings in these patients show prolonged PT and decreased fibrinogen levels. Fibrinogen levels, usually elevated in the presence of sepsis, pregnancy, or malignancy, may fall within the normal range if DIC is present concurrently. Finally, multiple transfusions may cause alteration in the levels of clotting factors or platelets.

Table 19-1 Disseminated Intravascular Coagulation (DIC) Laboratory Profile

Diagnostic test	Normal value	Expected value in DIC
Prothrombin time (PT)	10-13 seconds	Prolonged
Partial thromboplastin time (PTT)	39-48 seconds	Usually prolonged
Thrombin time (TT)	10-13 seconds	Usually prolonged
Fibrinogen level	200-400 mg/dl	Decreased
Platelet level	150,000-400,000/mm^3	Decreased
Factor assay (II, V, VII, VIII, IX, X, XI, XII)		Decreased levels of factors VI, VIII, and IX
Fibrinogen/fibrin degradation products	<10	Increased
Protamine sulfate test (soluble fibrin monomer)	Negative	Strongly positive
Antithrombin III levels (AT-III) (used to monitor response to therapy)	89%-120%	Decreased

From Yasko JM, Schafer SL: Disseminated intravascular coagulation. In Yasko JM, editor: *Guidelines for cancer care: symptom management,* Reston, Va, 1983, Reston.

TREATMENT MODALITIES

No specific medical treatment exists for DIC. Instead, the goal of therapy is to eliminate or alter the triggering event. Common examples are the treatment of sepsis with antibiotics and treatment of cancer with surgery, chemotherapy, and radiation therapy. If the DIC is chronic, only supportive measures may be necessary until the DIC is resolved. Depending on the progression of the DIC and the success of treating the triggering event and the predominant signs and symptoms, therapy is directed at stopping the intravascular clotting process and controlling the bleeding. When bleeding is severe, blood component therapy is necessary to achieve hemostasis. It is used to correct the clotting deficiencies caused by the consumption of blood components during the DIC process. Common blood products used in treating DIC are as follows:

- Platelets contain platelet factor III, which strengthens the endothelium, prevents petechial hemorrhage, facilitates the conversion of prothrombin to thrombin, and functions as a mechanical plug by adhering to the vessel wall.[127] The amount and frequency of platelet replacement depend on the patient's platelet count and physical condition. Spontaneous hemorrhage is of concern especially when the platelet count falls below 20,000/mm^3. Usually, 8 to 10 U is given once or twice a day. One unit of infused platelets should increase the platelet count by 5000 to 8000/mm^3.
- Fresh frozen plasma (FFP) is used for volume expansion. It contains clotting factors V, VIII, XIII, and antithrombin III. Usually, 2 to 4 U of FFP is given once or twice a day. Each unit of infused FFP raises each clotting factor by 5%.
- Packed red blood cells (PRBCs) are used to increase RBCs and clotting factors. PRBCs are used instead of whole blood to reduce the development of antibodies and fluid overload. Usually, 2 U is given when the hematocrit drops below 28%. Each unit of PRBCs should raise the hemoglobin count by 1.
- Cryoprecipitate contains fibrinogen (approximately 200 mg/U) and factor VIII.[135] It is used for patients with severe hypofibrinogenemia. Usually, 2 U of cryoprecipitate is given every 6 hours when the fibrinogen level is below 50 mg/dl. A total of 10 U of cryoprecipitate are administered. Each unit of cryoprecipitate increases the level of fibrinogen and factor VIII by 2%.

Heparin therapy, which inhibits thrombin formation, has met with controversy for the treatment of DIC. Research is lacking to support its utilization or withholding.[143] The anticoagulation effects of heparin result from its prevention of the platelet aggregation that initiates the intrinsic pathway of the coagulation cascade.[133] Heparin interferes with thrombin and stops the conversion of fibrinogen to fibrin, which prevents clot formation. It does not lyse those clots that are already formed; that requires thrombin to activate fibrinogen.

Usual doses of heparin are 2500 to 5000 U subcutaneously (SC) every 8 to 12 hours, 50 U/kg of body weight by intravenous (IV) bolus every 4 to 6 hours, or 100 to 200 U/kg every 24 hours by IV infusion. Effective heparin therapy produces cessation of clot formation, a rise in platelet count and fibrinogen levels, and a decrease in the level of FSPs. PTT is monitored to assess the patient's response to heparin. A therapeutic level is reached when the patient's PTT is 1.5 to 2 times the normal level.

Failure to respond to heparin therapy has been attributed to a depletion of antithrombin III (AT-III). AT-III is a blood component factor that inhibits the competitive action of thrombin during heparin therapy.[133] Therefore, in patients with low AT-III levels and no response to heparin therapy, AT-III is administered along with heparin. The usual dose is 1500 to 1725 U in 50 ml of distilled water infused over 10 hours concurrently with 500 to 1500 U of IV heparin/hour. This form of therapy is still considered experimental.[161]

Finally, in addition to the control of clotting, medical attention is given to the control of bleeding. Usually, heparin therapy produces anticoagulation and at the same time controls fibrinolysis. In 5% of patients, however, fibrinolysis continues and uncontrolled bleeding results.[133] In these patients, antifibrinolytic therapy may be administered, using a drug called ε-*aminocaproic acid* (EACA). EACA interferes with the intrinsic fibrinolytic process, which can lead to further clot formation. Therefore EACA is used only when heparin is effectively controlling intravascular clotting. The usual dose is 5 to 10 g given by IV slow bolus followed by 2 to 4 g every 1 to 2 hours for 24 hours or until bleeding stops. Patients receiving EACA must be closely monitored for hypotension, hypokalemia, cardiac dysrhythmias, and increased intravascular coagulation.[40] This drug is rarely used and is considered controversial.

PROGNOSIS

The prognosis of the patient with DIC depends on the underlying cause, the degree of disruption of the coagulation system, and the effects of bleeding and clotting.[1] Most patients with cancer who develop DIC experience hemorrhage. A smaller number demonstrate thromboembolism. The estimated mortality rate for DIC is 54% to 68%. Mortality from DIC has decreased in the past decade. This is attributed to new antileukemia agents, combinations of anticancer therapies, and advances in blood component therapies.[68,84] Increasing age, severity of laboratory abnormalities, and number of clinical manifestations increase the mortality from DIC.[31,70,86,133] In the DIC patient a minor injury can have a fatal consequence.

See pp. 412-413 for nursing management of DIC.

NURSING MANAGEMENT

The nursing management of patients with disseminated intravascular coagulation (DIC), as in the condition itself, is extremely complex. Depending on the onset and severity of DIC, the nurse's role may vary from watchful waiting to intensive participation in treatment.[74,78,143] Nursing care focuses on minimizing the multitude of potentially life-threatening problems associated with DIC. Therefore care must be directed toward astute and ongoing assessment to detect bleeding (overt or occult) or thrombosis, provision of care for bleeding and thrombosis, prevention of further complications, and support of other needs.

NURSING DIAGNOSIS

• *Injury (bleeding, thrombosis), risk for, related to fibrous clot formation in the microcirculation, clotting factor consumption and decreased platelets, fibrinolysis or clot dissolution*

OUTCOME GOAL

Patient will be able to:
• Exhibit resolution of signs and symptoms of DIC, as evidenced by cessation of bleeding, return of hematologic values to normal range, return of coagulation and fibrinogen levels to normal, and absence of cyanosis to extremities.

INTERVENTIONS: *Observation for Signs of Bleeding and Thrombosis*

• Assess organ systems for evidence of bleeding and thrombosis:
  —Integumentary: observe skin for evidence of bleeding (petechiae, ecchymosis, purpura, pallor, frank blood, oozing). Closely examine the mouth, including the mucous membranes of the palate and gums; sclera; nose; ears; urethra; vagina; and rectum. Check all venipuncture and puncture sites and wound sites.
  —Pulmonary: auscultate lungs for crackles, wheezes, and stridor. Observe for dyspnea, tachypnea, cyanosis, hemoptysis, and chest pain.
  —Cardiovascular: monitor for tachycardia, hypotension, and changes in peripheral pulses. Assess for palpitations and angina.
  —Renal: measure intake and output. Observe for peripheral edema and oliguria.
  —Gastrointestinal: palpate abdomen for pain. Measure abdominal girth daily.
  —Neurologic: observe for irritability or changes in mental status. Assess frequently for headache, blurred vision, and vertigo.
• Monitor vital signs (temperature, pulse, blood pressure, respirations) every 4 hours.
• Test all excreta (urine, stool, sputum, vomitus) for blood.
• Assess for fatigue, lethargy, muscle weakness, and pain.
• Monitor laboratory values closely for abnormalities indicative of bleeding or infection, including complete blood count (CBC), platelet count, prothrombin time (PT), and fibrinogen level.

INTERVENTIONS: *Measures to Prevent Further Tissue Trauma*

• Prevent further bleeding.
• Prevent skin breakdown.
• Institute safety measures:
  —Keep bed rails up at night.
  —Pad bed rails and any sharp objects.
  —Instruct patient to ambulate with assistance.
• Perform activities that decrease risk of bleeding:
  —Provide adequate hydration and soft diet.
  —Avoid administration of aspirin or products that contain aspirin.
  —Discourage activities that increase intracranial pressure (ICP) or intraabdominal pressure (Valsalva's maneuver).
  —Administer stool softeners as ordered.
• Prevent further clotting:
  —Provide adequate hydration.
  —Avoid constrictive clothing and devices.
  —Use prescribed elastic support hose.
  —Discourage dangling of legs, sitting for long periods, and crossing legs.
  —Elevate legs at intermittent intervals to prevent venous stasis when sitting or lying.
  —Perform range-of-motion (ROM) exercises for legs.
  —Encourage deep breathing and coughing.
  —Administer heparin therapy as ordered using an infusion-controlling device.

NURSING DIAGNOSIS

• *Skin integrity, impaired*

OUTCOME GOALS

Patient/family/caregiver will be able to:
• Describe measures to prevent further trauma to damaged skin.
• State signs and symptoms that must be reported to health care team.
• Ensure patient's skin heals without development of infection.
• Perform necessary treatments and procedures to promote skin integrity.

INTERVENTIONS

- Observe skin and mucous membranes for changes in integrity, color, and moisture.
- Provide meticulous skin care and lubrication.
- Maintain skin and mucosal integrity:
  - —Limit venipunctures, and when necessary, use small-gauge needles.
  - —Avoid subcutaneous (SC) and intramuscular (IM) injections.
  - —Apply pressure to puncture sites for 5 minutes.
  - —Administer medications orally (PO) or intravenously (IV).
  - —Avoid rectal manipulation (rectal suppositories, thermometers, digital examinations).
  - —Use electric razors instead of straight-edged razors.
  - —Avoid indwelling catheters, and when necessary, keep them well lubricated and without tension.
  - —Avoid vaginal manipulation (tampons, douches).
  - —Use paper tape instead of adhesive tape and remove gently.
  - —Use Montgomery straps on wound dressings.
  - —Suction with care.
- Perform frequent gentle oral hygiene:
  - —Use soft-bristled toothbrush or sponge toothettes.
  - —Avoid mouthwashes with high alcohol content.
  - —Lubricate mucous membranes and lips.

NURSING DIAGNOSES

- *Fluid volume deficit related to bleeding*
- *Fluid volume deficit, risk for, related to bleeding*

OUTCOME GOAL

- Patient's fluid balance will be restored, as evidenced by blood pressure and pulse within patient's normal range, lungs clear to auscultation, absence of neck vein distention, absence of edema, normal sodium and serum osmolarity, and urine output within patient's normal range.

INTERVENTIONS

- Observe for signs of active bleeding, hypocalcemia, and hypoxia (decreased blood pressure, tachypnea, tachycardia, restlessness, irritability, confusion, dizziness, decreased urine output).
- Measure intake and output.
- Administer fluids, blood, and blood products as ordered.

NURSING DIAGNOSIS

- *Tissue perfusion, altered, related to bleeding, thrombosis*

OUTCOME GOAL

Patient will be able to:
- Maintain adequate perfusion through critical period, as evidenced by absent or diminished bleeding, adequate urine output, maintenance of circulation, and adequate respiratory function.

INTERVENTIONS

- Assess organ systems for malfunctions resulting from ischemia.
- Monitor laboratory values closely.
- Measure intake and output.
- Provide oxygen therapy as prescribed.
- Administer vasoactive drugs as ordered.
- Administer pain medications as ordered.

The management of a patient with DIC is complex and difficult. The experience is often terrifying for the patient and family and frustrating for the nurse. The patient's condition can change rapidly. Everyone must be alert to and prepared for all possible sequelae of DIC.

HYPERCALCEMIA

DEFINITION

A metabolic condition referred to as hypercalcemia occurs when the serum calcium level rises above the normal level of 9 to 11 mg/dl. Hypercalcemia is a frequent complication of certain types of malignancies and metastatic disease. It is a potentially life-threatening problem because the onset is variable and often goes unnoticed until the problem becomes severe. With prompt recognition and adequate treatment, this condition can be reversed.

ETIOLOGY AND RISK FACTORS

A variety of conditions can cause hypercalcemia. The common malignancies associated with this condition include cancers of the breast and kidneys, squamous cell cancers of the lung, head, neck, or esophagus; lymphoma, leukemia; and multiple myeloma. Patients with metastatic cancers being treated with estrogens or antiestrogens may experience progression of hypercalcemia, possibly from hormonal stimulation of the tumor.[5,41] Bony metastasis from any malignant primary tumor may also be a causative condition. Nonmalignant conditions that can induce or worsen hypercalcemia include primary hyperparathyroidism, thyrotoxicosis, prolonged immobilization, vitamin A and D intoxication, renal failure, and diuretic therapy with thiazide preparations.[41,144] Dehydration, volume depletion, and hypoalbuminemia may contribute to or aggravate hypercalcemia.[144]

Hypercalcemia is considered the most frequent complication in oncology, occurring in 10% to 20% of patients with cancer.* Solid tumors, lung cancer, and breast cancer account for 80% of malignancy-related hypercalcemia. The remaining 20% include causes from multiple myeloma, leukemia, and lymphoma.[34,78,144]

PATHOPHYSIOLOGY

Calcium is an essential inorganic element in the body. Most of it (99%) is found in skeletal tissue, providing strength and durability. The remaining 1% is in the serum. One half of the serum calcium (0.5%) is ionized and one half (0.5%) is bound to circulating albumin. Laboratory reports reflect the total serum calcium level, which includes both the ionized portion and the protein-bound portion.[5] Under normal conditions the ionized calcium is in equilibrium with the protein-bound calcium. Changes in serum albumin level directly affect serum calcium levels.

Serum calcium levels in the presence of hypoalbuminemia may not be representative of the true value for ionized calcium. Reduction of serum albumin, which is often seen in very ill patients or elderly patients, may result in a greater proportion of ionized calcium because of the unavailability of albumin for binding. Therefore the severity of hypercalcemia in a patient with hypoalbuminemia may be underestimated.[5,26,160] The box at right provides a formula to correct for decreased serum albumin. The ionized portion of calcium is capable of physiologic function. Calcium is responsible for bone and tooth formation, normal clotting mechanism, and cellular permeability. Calcium ion concentration regulates the contractility of the cardiac, smooth, and skeletal muscles and the excitability of nerve tissue.[74,78]

Normal serum calcium levels are maintained in a state of equilibrium through a dynamic relationship among all three forms of calcium (stored, ionized, albumin bound), with a constant shifting from one form to another. Homeostasis is maintained through several body processes: GI calcium absorption, renal calcium reabsorption, and a balance of bone resorption (absorption or removal) of calcium and deposition of calcium through new bone formation.[56,57] Metabolism of calcium is controlled by a negative feedback mechanism between calcium ion concentration and three hormones: parathyroid hormone (PTH, parathormone), activated vitamin D, and calcitonin.[15,53,82]

---

*References 15, 74, 78, 97, 112, 122.

CALCULATION OF ESTIMATED IONIZED SERUM CALCIUM

Formulas to correct for changes in serum albumin concentrations (allow 0.8 mg/dl for each g/dl change in serum albumin):

1. Corrected serum calcium = Measured total serum calcium value (mg/dl) + [4.0 − Serum albumin value (g/dl)] × 0.8
2. Corrected serum calcium = Measured total serum calcium value (mg/dl) − Serum albumin value (g/dl) + 4.0

A decrease in serum calcium stimulates an increase in PTH secretion (Figure 19-3). PTH enhances calcium absorption from the GI tract and renal tubular reabsorption of calcium with increased excretion of phosphorus. Calcium ions and phosphorus ions have a directly inverse relationship: when the amount of one is increased, the amount of the other is decreased. PTH also promotes osteoclastic activity. *Osteoclasts* are multinucleated bone cells, which function to remove damaged bone tissue. This results in the destruction of bones, releasing calcium into the bloodstream.[56,57]

Vitamin D is activated by PTH and increases calcium absorption from the GI mucosa. Calcitonin is released by the thyroid gland in response to an increased serum calcium level and inhibits bone resorption of calcium. The effect of calcitonin is short lived. In general, hypercalcemia is the result of increased bone resorption of calcium, which exceeds renal ability to excrete the calcium overload. Hypercalcemia resulting from malignancies occurs through several different mechanisms, depending on the location and action of the cancer cells, as follows[62,63,78]:

- Direct bony destruction by tumor cells, which causes osteoclastic activity, resulting in the release of calcium from the bone into the serum
- Prolonged immobilization, which increases osteoclastic activity
- Ectopic PTH production by tumor cells, which enhances calcium resorption; secretion continues despite an elevated serum calcium level
- Metabolic substances produced by the tumor, such as osteoclastic activating factor (OAF), prostaglandin, or prostaglandin-like substances, all of which enhance osteoclastic activity[23,45]

Other contributing conditions include the following:
- Dehydration or volume depletion or both
- Hypervitaminosis of A and D (excessive use of vitamin A and D supplements)
- Excessive use of calcium supplements

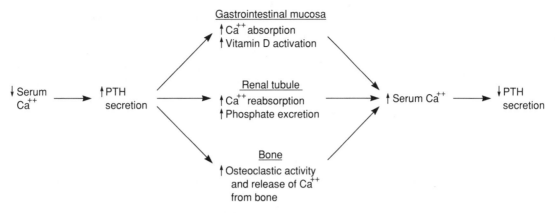

Figure 19-3   Effects of parathyroid hormone *(PTH)* on serum calcium levels.

Table 19-2   Degrees of Hypercalcemia: Signs and Symptoms*

Body system affected	Mild (<12 mg/dl)	Moderate (12-15 mg/dl)	Severe (>15 mg/dl)
Gastrointestinal	Anorexia, nausea, vomiting, vague abdominal pain	Constipation, increased abdominal pain, abdominal distention	Atonic ileus, obstipation
Neurologic	Restlessness, difficulty in concentrating, depression, apathy, lethargy, clouding of consciousness	Confusion, psychoses, somnolence	Coma, death
Muscular	Easily fatigued, muscle weakness (generalized or involving shoulders and hips), hyporeflexia	Increased muscular weakness, bone pain	Profound muscular weakness, ataxia, pathologic fractures
Renal	Nocturia, polyuria, polydipsia	Renal tubular acidosis, renal calculi	Oliguric renal failure, renal insufficiency, azotemia
Cardiovascular	Hypertension (may or may not be present)	Cardiac dysrhythmias, electrocardiographic (ECG) abnormalities (shortening of QT interval on ECG, coving of ST-T wave, widening of T wave)	Cardiac arrest, death

From Poe CM, Radford AI: *Oncol Nurs Forum* 12(6):29, 1985.
*Signs and symptoms regardless of serum calcium levels may vary from person to person.

• Hyperparathyroidism
• Prolonged use of thiazide diuretics

Historically, malignancy-related hypercalcemia has been closely associated with tumor invasion into the bone by direct tumor extension or metastasis. This skeletal process, *local osteolytic hypercalcemia* (LOH), is no longer considered the most common mechanism of hypercalcemia. Approximately 80% of hypercalcemic malignancies are caused by a humoral response: the tumor production of PTH-related peptide (PTHrP).[80] The humoral agents have a normal physiologic function in the body but can be induced by and released from malignant cells.[24,43]

CLINICAL FEATURES

Hypercalcemia disrupts normal cellular functions and adversely affects various organs. Clinical manifestations vary tremendously, depending on the level of serum calcium, the rate of onset, the underlying cause, and the patient's general condition. Patients may be asymptomatic or mildly symptomatic or may have severe problems (Table 19-2). Onset may be insidious or acute. Diagnosis is often difficult because of multisystem involvement making it resemble other disorders.[78,102,103] The box, p. 416, lists clinical features of hypercalcemia.

Signs and symptoms are directly related to cellular activity of the involved body system (Table 19-2). Normal cell membranes are lined with calcium ions, which control the permeability of the cell. This gating mechanism allows sodium ions to enter the cell and depolarization to occur. Increased calcium ions decrease cellular permeability and subsequently alter cellular function. This decreases neuron permeability, resulting in a depressive effect on the central nervous system (CNS) and peripheral nervous system (PNS).[160]

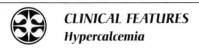

CLINICAL FEATURES
Hypercalcemia

Clinical signs
Lethargy
Change in mental status (restlessness, confusion, stupor, coma)
Vomiting
Dysrhythmias
Polyuria
Electrocardiographic changes
Renal calculi
Renal failure
Symptoms
Anxiety
Fatigue and weakness
Anorexia
Nausea
Polydipsia
Constipation

Symptoms may include restlessness, agitation, lethargy, and confusion and may lead to coma. Skeletal muscles become hypotonic with decreased or absent deep tendon reflexes, ataxia, and fatigue. The smooth muscle action of the GI system slows, leading to decreased motility, anorexia, nausea, vomiting, constipation, possible abdominal distention, and later, ileus. Impaired cardiac muscle conduction and contractility can result in dysrhythmias or even cardiac arrest.

Compensatory renal mechanisms increase urinary calcium reabsorption, leading to an inability to concentrate urine. This causes a syndrome similar to nephrogenic diabetes insipidus and manifested by polyuria and polydipsia. The polyuria and hypercalciuria result in dehydration and a decrease in glomerular filtration rate (GFR). Dehydration from this event or from nausea and vomiting produces a further decline in the GFR of the kidney. The lowered GFR in turn increases reabsorption of sodium in the proximal tubules in an attempt to retain water. Since sodium and calcium work closely, calcium is also reabsorbed. This can further potentiate the hypercalcemia. Elevation of serum calcium levels produces a supersaturation of calcium and then precipitation. Precipitation in the kidneys can lead to calcium renal stones and possible renal failure, as evidenced by an elevated blood urea nitrogen (BUN) and creatinine.

The clinical syndrome of hypercalcemia is complex because of the extreme variability in its manifestation of signs and symptoms. In addition, the symptomatology

does not always correlate with serum calcium levels. These must be closely correlated with an in-depth history, physical examination, and laboratory profile. Diagnosis can be confusing, but because of its frequency in patients with cancer, hypercalcemia of malignancy should be one of the first differential diagnoses in patients who develop a change in mental status.[70,82,112]

DIAGNOSIS

The diagnostic work-up for hypercalcemia begins with laboratory determination of the serum calcium level. Normal values are 9 to 11 mg/dl. The procedure for obtaining a serum calcium level should include the following measures[16,22]:
• Two determinations to ensure accuracy
• A fasting specimen to avoid postprandial changes
• Removal of tourniquet before 2 minutes because of a possible 10% elevation in level thought to be caused by oxidation of fluid from increased venous pressure

Urinary calcium should be measured. Hypercalciuria may be detected before an elevation in serum calcium.[5] Other serum laboratory testing should include phosphorus, alkaline phosphatase, BUN, creatinine, electrolytes, and PTH. Patients with no bony involvement (e.g., squamous cell cancer of the head and neck) and whose tumor is producing PTH-like substances may have a normal serum phosphorus level. Hypercalcemia resulting from direct bony involvement (e.g., breast cancer, myeloma, renal cell carcinoma) often results in increased serum phosphorus levels. Furthermore, within this subset of patients, only those with breast cancer and bone metastasis usually have an elevated alkaline phosphatase. Serum albumin should be tested, since patients may be more hypercalcemic than serum levels indicate as a result of hypoalbuminemia, as discussed earlier.[78,82]

Radiographic examinations can be helpful in differential diagnosis. A chest x-ray film may suggest tumor, sarcoidosis, or bony changes associated with hyperparathyroidism.[126] Plain x-ray film or a radioisotope bone scan may demonstrate bone metastases or multiple myeloma. Electrocardiograms (ECGs) may show tachycardia, increased PR segment, shortened QT interval, and widening of the T wave. However, these changes may be subtle and difficult to detect.[82]

TREATMENT MODALITIES

Decisions concerning whether and how to treat hypercalcemia caused by malignancy depend on the clinical situation.[78,82] The degree of serum calcium elevation, the symptomatology, the patient's condition, and the ability to treat the underlying disease are determining factors in the decision-making process. Untreated cancer-induced hypercalcemia is usually progressive, and death is usually inevitable. Death from hypercalcemia may be a reasonable way to die for the patient with advanced cancer, since most people become comatose and do not experience pain.[114] However, death may not be rapid, and unpleasant symptoms (anorexia, nausea, vomiting, sedation, confusion) may occur. Patients with advanced disease must be evaluated carefully. Although the only effective long-term treatment for hypercalcemia is antineoplastic therapy directed at the underlying malignancy, very potent, well-tolerated therapies now exist to readily correct hypercalcemia.[82] The choice of treatment for the patient whose cancer cannot be eradicated is therefore a difficult one. If quality of life will not be improved, the decision may be to provide no treatment. When a decision is made to treat the hypercalcemia, the medical treatment is based on two principles: reduction of bone resorption of calcium and promotion of urinary excretion of calcium.

Successful treatment of the underlying malignancy is the preferred modality and is often likely to accomplish these principles.

Hydration

Adequate hydration is usually the primary treatment for hypercalcemia. Increased fluids by mouth and intravenously rehydrate the patient and dilute the urine, which prevents supersaturation with calcium ions.[82] Large volumes of isotonic saline (Table 19-3) restore plasma volume and promote urinary calcium excretion through sodium diuresis. Calcium loss follows sodium loss. Fluid volume in the range of about 5 to 8 L/day is common for the first 24 hours, followed by 3 L/day thereafter. Infusions of large volumes of fluids may necessitate central venous pressure monitoring to avoid fluid overload. Accurate recordings of intake, output, and weight and laboratory studies should be done to prevent hyponatremia, hypomagnesemia, and hypokalemia.[78,82]

Mobilization

Immobilization should be avoided because it will increase resorption of calcium from the bones. Activity should be appropriate for the patient's physical condition. Weight bearing through standing and ambulation produces physical stress at the ends of long bones, resulting in osteoblastic activity. Osteoblasts synthesize the collagen and glycoproteins to form a matrix and develop into osteocytes, which are mature bone cells.[21] Muscle activity produces acid end products needed to assist in the production of acid urine. Physical therapy may be helpful to establish a program of active exercises with resistance. A pain management program may be necessary to support activities.[21,131]

Dialysis

Patients who are in renal failure secondary to hypercalcemia but who have a relatively good prognosis with their malignancy could benefit from renal dialysis. Saline diuresis is precluded in these patients so that dialysis will remove both excess calcium and phosphate. Serum phosphate levels should be measured and phosphates replaced as necessary.[40,53,82]

Dietary Manipulation

Little attention is given to dietary restriction of calcium, since the increase in calcium is caused by resorption from the bones rather than GI absorption of calcium.[40] However, excessive volumes of milk and dairy products should be discouraged. Furthermore, a diet low in calcium may also lack phosphate, which would promote an increase in serum calcium.[122]

Pharmacologic Therapy

The first pharmacologic consideration in the treatment of increased serum calcium is the discontinuation of any medications known to precipitate hypercalcemia, such as estrogens, antiestrogens, thiazide diuretics, high doses of vitamin A and D, and calcium supplements.

The second measure involving medications is the administration of chemotherapy to treat patients with underlying hematologic malignancies such as multiple myeloma or lymphoma. In patients with breast cancer, chemotherapy or hormonal therapy may produce a remission. However, the initial use of hormonal therapy, especially tamoxifen (Nolvadex), may worsen the hypercalcemia. Some patients receiving hormonal therapy for breast cancer metastatic to the bone may experience episodes of increased serum calcium. This is often referred to as a "flare," which is indicative of tumor response to the hormone. These patients need to be monitored closely. Diuretics have been given in addition to saline infusions to increase calcium excretion. Furosemide (Lasix) and ethacrynic acid (Edecrin) are frequently used, since their mechanism of action on the kidney decreases reabsorption of calcium and sodium.[78,82,122] During diuresis, serum levels of potassium and magnesium should be monitored closely and cardiac medication given cautiously.

The use of *oral phosphates* (Table 19-3) is somewhat limited. It has been shown that patients with renal failure or patients with serum phosphorus levels greater than 3.8 mg/L will not benefit from the use of phosphates.[112] However, patients with low serum phosphorus levels may benefit from oral phosphorus administered in doses of 0.5 g four times a day. The mechanism of action, although uncertain, appears to be the reduction of bone resorption of calcium and impairment of the absorption of calcium from the intestine. Diarrhea, which can result at

Table 19-3 Therapy for Hypercalcemia of Malignancy

Therapy	Dosage	Comments
Saline; add loop diuretics such as furosemide	5-8 L IV during the first 24 hours, then 3 L/day of normal saline; diuretic dose 20 mg every 4-6 hours; calciuretic dose 80-100 mg every 1-2 hours	Restores plasma volume, increases glomerular filtration rate, promotes renal calcium excretion; loop diuretics block calcium reabsorption in loop of Henle; especially important when hypercalcemia is severe and patient is dehydrated; should not be used as sole therapy
Pamidronate disodium (Aredia)	60-90 mg IV infusion over 4 or 24 hours for 1 day	Interferes with osteoclast activity by absorbing to calcium crystals in bone, blocking dissolution of calcium; this inhibits bone resorption; safe in patients with renal failure
Gallium nitrate (Gallium)	200 mg/m²/day IV 24-hour infusion for 4-5 days	Inhibits bone resorption without compromising bone strength; nephrotoxicity is a potential toxicity; discontinue this drug if serum creatinine exceeds 2.5 mg/dl
Etidronate (Didronel, Didronel IV)	7.5 mg/kg/day IV infusion over 2 hours for 4-5 days, then 10 mg/kg/day PO for up to 3 months	Inhibits bone resorption; limits calcium absorption from gut; promotes soft tissue and skeletal calcification; returns serum calcium level to normal within 3 to 5 days; contraindicated in patients with renal failure; given with saline hydration
Calcitonin (salmon)* (Calcimar, Miacalcin) plus a glucocorticoid	Calcitonin—salmon, 200 MRC U every 12 hours SC; hydrocortisone, 100 mg IV every 6 hours	Impairs bone resorption and increases renal calcium excretion; especially effective in patients with hematologic malignancies; safe in patients with renal or cardiac failure
Plicamycin (Mithracin)	15-25 μg/kg/day by slow IV infusion over 4 hours for 1 day	Inhibits bone resorption by direct injury to osteoclasts; calcium-lowering effects not seen for 24-48 hours; potentially dangerous in patients with renal or hepatic failure
Phosphate	Up to 0.5 g PO 4 times daily	Reciprocal relationship between calcium and phosphorus; useful when hypercalcemia is associated with low serum phosphorus level; diarrhea may be a problem; contraindicated in patients with renal failure or serum phosphorus levels >3.8 mg/dl; often used as maintenance therapy

Modified from Mundy G: *Hosp Ther,* February 1988, p 52; and Zimberg M, Mahon S: *Qualify Life Nurs Challenge* 1(1):3, 1992.
IV, Intravenously; *PO*, orally; *SC*, subcutaneous; *MRC U*, Medical Research Council units.
*Calcitonin (human) (Cibacalcin) has not yet been approved for use in hypercalcemia but is expected to be as effective as calcitonin (salmon) for this condition.

these high oral doses, may hamper the use of oral phosphorus. Large IV doses may cause precipitation of calcium in the heart, lung, or soft tissues, which can lead to renal failure; therefore they are rarely indicated.

Glucocorticoids have been used to treat hypercalcemia associated with breast cancer, myeloma, and lymphoma. Prednisone, 40 to 60 mg/day, has been given.

Steroids may have some direct effect on the tumor itself, but the exact mechanism is unknown. Increasing the dose of the steroids does not increase their effectiveness.[57,78] The effect of steroids may be delayed by a week, and chronic use enhances immunosuppression, which can result in osteolytic activity. Steroids are not recommended for long-term maintenance in view of the possible toxicities associated with chronic administration.[5]

Nonsteroidal antiinflammatory drugs (NSAIDs) such as indomethacin (Indocin) or aspirin appear to inhibit prostaglandin synthesis and thus mediate bone resorption. Although their role in treating hypercalcemia may be minor, they may be of value in patients with refractory hypercalcemia who are unable to tolerate other agents or if NSAIDs are part of a regimen for cancer pain control. The usual dose of indomethacin is 75 to 100 mg/day in divided doses. Gastric upset is a frequent side effect of this drug.[5]

Prostaglandin synthesis inhibitors such as indomethacin and aspirin have rarely been effective in lowering the serum calcium. However, they are sometimes useful for patients who cannot tolerate any other agent and when nonsteroidal drugs are part of a palliative pain management team.[78]

Recently, *cisplatin,* a widely used antineoplastic agent with broad spectrum of antitumor activity, has demonstrated efficacy in reducing serum calcium levels. The calcium-lowering effect was delayed (10 days) and prolonged (mean duration: 38 days) and independent of antitumor activity because the decrease in calcium levels occurred in patients who experienced no tumor regression. The toxicities (GI, renal, neurologic) associated with cisplatin may limit its consideration for antihypercalcemic therapy.[5]

Currently, five parenteral medications with similar mechanisms of action are used to treat hypercalcemia (Table 19-3). Each drug impairs bone resorption and increases renal calcium excretion. *Calcitonin (salmon)* (Calcimar) appears to have a transient effect in lowering serum calcium.[57,78,82] A usual dose is 200 MRC U given intramuscularly (IM) or subcutaneously (SC) every 12 hours. One benefit of this drug is its safety in patients with renal failure. The addition of a glucocorticoid to calcitonin has prolonged its effect in lowering serum calcium. The current recommendation is hydrocortisone sodium succinate, 100 mg IV every 6 hours. The combination of calcitonin and a glucocorticoid has been especially efficacious in patients with hematologic malignancies.[82,112]

Plicamycin (Mithramycin) has calcium-lowering effects that may not appear for 24 to 48 hours.[13,82,112] The usual dosage is a slow infusion of 15 to 25 μg/kg/day. Disadvantages of plicamycin are venous irritation, myelosuppressive effects, liver toxicity, and potential danger in patients with renal failure.

Etidronate (Didronel) has shown efficacy in more than 80% of patients with cancer-induced hypercalcemia. Lowered serum calcium is seen in 3 to 5 days after a regimen of 7.5 mg/kg/day IV for 4 to 5 days. The daily dose of etidronate is diluted in 250 ml of normal saline and administered over at least 2 hours. Intravenous administration can be followed with oral doses of 10 mg/kg/day for 7 to 10 days, which may be continued for up to 3 months. However, the oral efficacy of this agent is still under study. Etidronate is contraindicated in patients with a serum creatinine level greater than 5 or those with renal failure.[13,15,112] Hyperphosphatemia may result from etidronate therapy.[5]

Gallium nitrate (Gallium) is an antineoplastic agent noted to have hypocalcemic effects by directly inhibiting bone resorption without causing toxicity to bone cells. It is administered over 24 hours daily for 5 days at a dose of 100 to 200 mg/m^2 mixed in 1 L of 0.9% normal saline or 5% dextrose in water. Adequate hydration must be maintained throughout the treatment period. Nephrotoxicity is the major side effect of gallium nitrate. The requirement of continuous infusion potentially limits its usefulness, especially in the outpatient setting.[5]

Pamidronate (Aredia) is a highly effective second-generation bisphosphonate derivative. Dosage is not based on body surface area, but rather on the severity of the hypercalcemia. The recommended dosage of pamidronate in moderate hypercalcemia (corrected serum calcium 12 to 13.5 mg/dl) is 60 to 90 mg given as a single IV infusion over 24 hours. For patients with severe hypercalcemia (corrected serum calcium greater than 13.5 mg/dl), 90 mg should be given as the initial treatment. The drug is usually mixed in 0.45% or 0.9% normal saline or 5% dextrose in water. One liter is infused over 24 hours or 250 ml is infused over 4 hours. The 90 mg dose has normalized serum calcium in 95% of the patients.[80] The single parenteral therapy can be repeated weekly. Fever is a common side effect, occurring in 17% of patients, and is successfully treated with prophylactic acetaminophen.[98] Adequate hydration is necessary during treatment. Hypocalcemia and hypophosphatemia have occurred after therapy. However, nephrotoxicity does not appear to be a problem. Current studies of multiple low doses (15 mg/day) and single doses (5 to 90 mg) have shown significant activity and the possibility of a dose-response relationship. Oral preparations of pamidronate, etidronate, and clondronate are currently being evaluated.[80]

The use of pamidronate in a group of patients with advanced multiple myeloma resulted in significantly fewer skeletal-related events per year. These events were defined as pathologic fractures, spinal cord compression, radiation therapy, and surgery to the bone. Furthermore, treatment with pamidronate in these patients decreased the occurrence of new pathologic fractures, prevented early hypercalcemia, alleviated bone pain, and improved quality of life. No healing of bone lesions was observed, but bone mineral density was not measured. Finally, a small subset of patients showed a significant trend toward increased survival.[13,15,100]

The choice of therapy for hypercalcemia depends on how fast a response is desired, the functional status of the renal system and other major organ systems, potential for side effects, ease of administration, and cost of therapy.[15,78,82] Response to treatment, a decrease in serum calcium, is usually seen within 24 hours, peaking at 48 hours.[82] Consideration must also be given to long-term therapy, since it is easier to lower the serum calcium level than to keep it low.

PROGNOSIS

Cancer-induced hypercalcemia is a common complication of certain cancers and has the potential to be life-threatening. Clinical manifestations and onset vary greatly, but the course is usually progressive and can worsen quickly. Hypercalcemia is reversible in 80% of episodes if it is recognized and prompt aggressive therapy initiated. It has been shown that the more severe the hypercalcemia, the poorer the prognosis, and vice versa.[24] Without prompt treatment, it is associated with a 50% mortality rate.[21,40,97] After the diagnosis of hypercalcemia, median survival is 3 months. No treatment of hypercalcemia alone has been demonstrated to improve the increased mortality rate associated with this complication.[82]

Nursing management of the patient with hypercalcemia is outlined on pp. 421-422.

MALIGNANT PLEURAL EFFUSION

DEFINITION

Pleural effusion, the abnormal accumulation of fluid in the pleural cavity, is a common complication of malignancy. Effusions in any body cavity are a potential problem with cancer, and the pleural space is the most frequent site, followed by the pericardial and the peritoneal spaces. Abnormal fluid accumulation results when the balance between secretion and reabsorption is altered. Malignant pleural effusion is debilitating and life-threatening because the increased pleural fluid affects respiratory function by restricting lung expansion, decreasing lung volume, and altering gas exchange.[110,135,146]

ETIOLOGY AND RISK FACTORS

Abnormal fluid accumulation in the pleural space may be the result of a benign or neoplastic process. Benign causes of pleural effusion include congestive heart failure (CHF), pericarditis, respiratory infections (pneumonia, tuberculosis), superior vena cava syndrome (SVCS), mediastinal irradiation, ascites, hypoalbuminemia, and nephrosis. Patients with cancer often develop pleural effusions in the course of their disease, especially if their disease involves primary or secondary intrathoracic malignancies. This may be the first sign of their cancer, a complication of existing disease, or a late manifestation in metastatic disease, or it may be related to a nonmalignant process.[58] Regardless of etiology, malignant pleural effusion causes alterations in ventilation and perfusion, hypoxia, pain, and hemorrhage and may lead to atelectasis, infection, and death.[142]

The reported incidence of malignant pleural effusion varies greatly, from 25% to 53%. The true incidence remains unknown, since there has been no recent report on the incidence in the general hospital population.[116,134]

At least one third to one half of all pleural effusions are thought to be caused by cancer.[111,142] Exudative pleural effusion in patients over age 60 years is caused by malignancy.[138] Malignant pleural effusion is the result of metastatic disease of the pleura or mediastinal lymph nodes. Approximately one half of patients with lung cancer or breast cancer will develop pleural effusions at some point during the course of their disease. In the early 1980s, breast cancer was the leading malignancy associated with pleural effusion, but more recent studies report that lung cancer is the most common primary site to develop pulmonary metastases.[66,116] This probably reflects the increased incidence and death rate from lung cancer in this decade. The anatomic proximity and frequent invasion of the pulmonary vasculature with the embolization of the visceral pleural space from the lung cancer make it the most common cause of metastatic pleural malignancy.[142] Lung cancer is followed by breast cancer, lymphomas and leukemias, gastric cancer, and ovarian cancer as causes of pleural effusions. Together, these account for 80% of malignant pleural effusions.[138,142] Less frequent causes include malignant mesothelioma (primary pleural tumor), genitourinary cancers, and sarcomas. Interestingly, many malignant pleural effusions are caused by pulmonary adenocarcinomas of unknown primary origin.[110] In essence, all types of cancer have the potential to cause malignant pleural effusion.

PATHOPHYSIOLOGY

The pleura is a thin serosal membrane that envelops the lungs and lines the interior of the thoracic cavity (Figure 19-4). There are two portions of the pleura, a visceral surface and a parietal surface lined by two thin layers of mesothelial cells. The *visceral pleura* adheres to the lung, encases each lobe, and extends within the interlobar fissures. Capillaries of the visceral pleura originate from the bronchial circulation. Lymphatic channels are present and coincide with the capillary bed. No nerve endings for pain are present. The *parietal pleura* lines the mediastinum, diaphragm, and chest wall. Capillaries of the parietal pleura are supplied by the intercostal arteries. Nerve endings for pain are present and, when stimulated,

NURSING MANAGEMENT

Nursing care of the patient with hypercalcemia is directed at early detection and support through treatment. A thorough nursing assessment should include a history of the patient's cancer and cancer treatment and a review of all medications. Drugs that may cause or potentiate hypercalcemia, such as lithium carbonate, thiazide diuretics, vitamins A and D, and large doses of calcium supplements, should be reported and discontinued. Drugs whose action may be altered by high serum calcium, such as digitalis and some antihypertensive agents, should also be noted. Physical examination results should be correlated with potential symptomatology of hypercalcemia.[42,74,97,100,122] This is often difficult because of the varying possibilities and degrees of clinical manifestations. However, the initial assessment will dictate the intensity of nursing care.

NURSING DIAGNOSES

• *Fluid volume deficit related to effects of the disease (impending renal failure with increased polyuria; fluid loss related to nausea and vomiting), effects of treatment (increased urine output secondary to diuretic therapy; fluid loss related to diarrhea)*
• *Fluid volume excess related to effects of treatment (hydration)*

OUTCOME GOALS

Patient/family/caregiver will be able to:
• Demonstrate knowledge related to hypercalcemia.
• Identify signs and symptoms.
• Identify factors that influence serum calcium levels.
• Identify potential complications.
• Achieve serum calcium level within normal limits.
• Achieve fluid balance, as evidenced by adequate hydration and elimination status, diminished or absent nausea and vomiting, and vital signs and body weight within patient's normal range.

INTERVENTIONS

• Assess for signs and symptoms of alterations in fluid volume:
  —Excess: rales, shortness of breath, neck vein distention, weight gain, edema of sacrum and lower extremities
  —Deficit: dry mucous membranes, poor skin turgor, weight loss, rapid thready pulse, orthostatic hypotension, restlessness
• Auscultate lungs for breath sounds every 4 hours.
• Monitor intake and output closely:
  —Encourage oral fluids.
  —Maintain IV fluids per physician orders (usually 6 to 8 L/day of saline).

  —Monitor IV infusions carefully using flow regulator.
  —Accurately measure urine output (maintain output at least at 50 ml/hour).
• Obtain daily weight.
• Monitor laboratory values (serum BUN, creatinine, sodium, potassium).
• Administer diuretics as ordered. Thiazide diuretics are contraindicated because they inhibit urinary excretion of calcium and therefore may potentiate hypercalcemia.
• Obtain urine pH. An acidic urine should be maintained to prevent calcium precipitation, which can lead to renal calculi.

NURSING DIAGNOSES

• *Mobility, impaired physical, related to bone breakdown secondary to metastasis*
• *Injury, risk for, related to bone destruction*
• *Trauma, risk for, related to bone destruction*

OUTCOME GOALS

Patient will be able to:
• Maintain activity and mobility appropriate to physical status.
Patient/family/caregiver will be able to:
• Identify/demonstrate measures to manage alteration in mobility.
• Demonstrate proper positioning and transfer techniques.
• Perform necessary treatments and procedures.
• Maintain good skin integrity and optimal level of physical activity.
• Identify signs and symptoms to report to health care team.

INTERVENTIONS

• Assess patient for presence of spinal cord compression (signs and symptoms: pain, sensory loss or paresthesia, motor weakness or dysfunction, changes in patterns of elimination).
• Establish activity and exercise regimen according to patient's physical ability and physician orders:
  —Change patient's position every 2 hours.
  —Stand patient at bedside for short periods (several minutes) at least 4 to 6 times a day.
  —Use isometric exercises each hour while awake.
  —Institute passive ROM exercises if patient is on bedrest.
• Provide a footboard for bedridden patients, and use a tilt table several times a day.
• Check for evidence of venous thrombosis in lower extremities caused by immobilization (redness, swelling, warmth, positive Homans' sign, pain, dorsiflexion).

Continued.

- Monitor skin integrity and provide skin care.
- Promote and assist with regulation of elimination.
- Provide pain control as needed.
- Consult with physical therapy and occupational therapy for evaluation and assistance.
- Discuss and teach the use of assistive and supportive devices as needed.
- Use safety precautions:
  —Move patients with care (use lift sheets and support joints).
  —Assist patient with transfer and ambulation as needed.
  —Place all articles within patient's reach.
  —Pad bed rails.
  —Modify bed surface with approved pressure-reducing mattress.
  —Use bed rails at night.
  —Closely monitor restless, anxious, or confused patients.
  —Employ restraints as necessary.

NURSING DIAGNOSIS

- *Thought processes, altered, related to hypercalcemia*

OUTCOME GOALS

Patient will be able to:
- Remain orientated to person, place, and time.
- Maintain mental and psychologic function at optimal level.

INTERVENTIONS

- Assess level of consciousness and check for changes in mentation and behavior.
- Closely observe for restlessness or anxiety.
- Orient patient frequently to time and place.
- Allow time for verbalization of feelings regarding condition.
- Teach patient and family about changes caused by hypercalcemia, potential for its recurrence, and appropriate measures to be taken.

NURSING DIAGNOSIS

- *Cardiac output, decreased, related to changes in serum calcium and electrolytes*

OUTCOME GOAL

Patient will be able to:
- Maintain adequate fluid volume, as evidenced by serum electrolytes and serum calcium within patient's normal limits, vital signs and body weight within patient's normal limits, and return of cardiac function to patient's optimal level.

INTERVENTIONS

- Assess for changes in cardiac function:
  —Monitor for presence of dysrhythmias, bradycardia, and tachycardia.
  —Observe ECG for shortened QT intervals or prolonged PR intervals.
  —Take pulse and blood pressure every 4 hours.
- Monitor serum calcium and electrolytes.
- Administer oral potassium as ordered (hypokalemia frequently occurs in the presence of hypercalcemia).
- Monitor effects of digitalis and digoxin, if given to patient, since hypercalcemia potentiates their action. The dose is usually reduced in the presence of hypercalcemia.

NURSING DIAGNOSIS

- *Diarrhea related to treatment for hypercalcemia*

OUTCOME GOAL

Patient will be able to:
- Demonstrate regular and normal pattern of elimination, as evidenced by stools of normal frequency and consistency, normal bowel sounds, absence or minimal abdominal pain and cramping, and absence or minimal skin breakdown.

INTERVENTIONS

- Monitor status of bowel elimination daily (color, texture, frequency of stools).
- Assess the abdomen daily:
  —Observe for distention.
  —Auscultate for the presence of bowel sounds.
  —Palpate to determine any painful areas.
- Provide perianal hygiene and skin care, and use anesthesia and lubricants as ordered.
- Monitor perianal skin integrity.
- Avoid administration of antidiarrheal agents, since calcium is excreted via stool.
- Provide explanation of diarrhea to patient and family.

Hypercalcemia is one of the most common oncologic problems seen in patients with cancer. Therefore nurses practicing in all areas of cancer care should be educated regarding this problem. Nursing assessment of patients with cancer, especially those cancers typically associated with hypercalcemia (breast, lung, head and neck, lymphoma, myeloma, bony metastases), should focus on the potential manifestations of this problem.

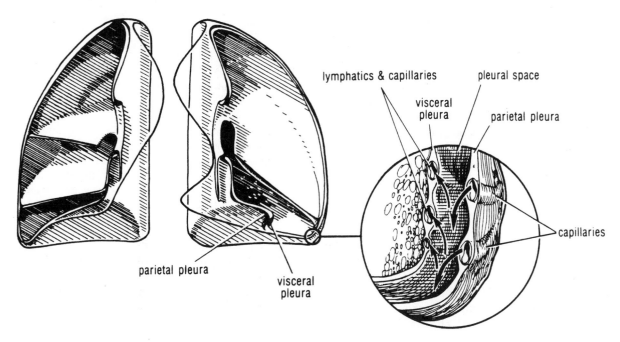

Figure 19-4 Right and left pleural membranes. Inset shows fluid movement from parietal pleura across pleural space to visceral pleura. (From Miller SE, Campbell DB: Pleural effusions in malignant disease. In Polomano RC, Miller SE, editors: *Understanding and managing oncologic emergencies,* monograph, Columbus, Ohio, 1987, Adria Laboratories.)

produce referred pain to the adjacent chest wall, shoulder, or abdomen.[58] The right and left pleura have no communication.[58,98]

A potential space exists between the two layers of pleural membrane, referred to as the *pleural space* or *pleural cavity.* Within the pleural space is a small amount of relatively protein-free transudative fluid produced by the mesothelial cells of the pleura, which flow across, from one pleura to the other, lubricating, moistening, and cushioning the pleural surfaces during respiration and providing lung movement without friction. Normally, 5 to 10 ml of fluid is present in the pleural space. Fluid is continuously produced and shunted to the pleural space from the systemic capillaries of the parietal pleura. Approximately 80% to 90% of the fluid is then reabsorbed by the pulmonary capillaries of the visceral pleura. The remaining 10% to 20% of the pleural fluid, which contains large molecular substances, proteins, and erythrocytes, is reabsorbed through the lymphatic channels of the visceral pleura.[128,138,142]

Equilibrium of pleural fluid movement is regulated by five dynamic forces (Figure 19-4): capillary permeability, hydrostatic pressure (capillary and interstitial), colloidal osmotic pressure (plasma protein and interstitial protein), negative intrapleural pressure, and lymphatic drainage. The *Starling hypothesis* of fluid movement from intravascular to extravascular space also applies to

formation and removal of pleural fluid.[66,111,116,138] The lymphatic channels regulate fluid and protein reabsorption. It is estimated that 5 to 10 L of fluid passes through the pleural space in 24 hours, but only 5 to 10 ml remains in the space at any given time.[58,66] Abnormal fluid accumulation occurs when the regulating forces are disrupted, causing excessive fluid production or decreased fluid reabsorption. Cancer will disrupt one or more of the five processes that are relative to the dynamics of fluid exchange in the pleural space, causing excess fluid accumulation. Malignant pleural effusions will result by several different mechanisms: pleural implants, tumor cell suspensions, lymphatic metastasis with blockage, venous obstruction, necrotic malignant cell shedding, and obstruction with tear of the thoracic duct.[58,116] Malignant tumors may produce *pleural implants,* which are tumor cells found in either the parietal or the visceral pleura. These implants are caused by seeding of the primary tumor by direct extension or by metastasis via the pulmonary artery. This is a common finding with lung cancer and mesothelioma.[58] The presence of implants causes irritation and an inflammation that makes the capillaries more permeable to fluid and protein and leads to increased fluid in the pleural space.

Malignant cells shed from the pleura and may grow freely in the pleural space, forming *tumor cell suspensions.* These collections of malignant cells are similar to pleural implants in origin and nature of growth. The difference between a tumor cell suspension and an implant is the greater number of cells found on cytologic examination. A tumor cell suspension may have cell counts higher than 4000 cells/ml, which is more than an implant. Ovarian cancer and lung cancer are often associated with tumor cell suspension.[58,128]

Lymphatic blockage or venous obstruction interferes with drainage of fluid and large molecules from the pleural space, resulting in an overaccumulation of fluid. Lymphatic blockage is seen with lymphoma and metastasis from breast or lung cancer. Disruption of the capillary endothelium changes hydrostatic pressure gradients and allows fluid and protein to leak into the pleural space.

Necrotic malignant cells may shed into the pleural space, which raises its colloid osmotic pressure, thus reducing absorption of fluid by the visceral pleural capillaries. This occurs often in patients with lung or breast cancer. Obstruction and tearing of the thoracic duct may produce a true chylous pleural effusion, as seen with lymphoma.[116]

Finally, other pathologies may contribute to the development of malignant pleural effusion. These include SVCS, postobstructive pneumonitis, pericardial effusion, bronchial obstruction with atelectasis, hypoalbuminemia, and CHF. Any condition in which fluid formation in the pleural space exceeds fluid removal will lead to fluid accumulation. The space between the two pleural surfaces will then expand to accommodate the fluid (pleural effusion). Expansion of the pleural space leads to compression or collapse of the lung with decreased lung volume.

CLINICAL FEATURES

Alterations in pulmonary function by a pleural effusion produce clinical signs and symptoms related to impairment of lung expansion and hypoxia. The onset of a malignant pleural effusion may be slow or rapid. Insidiously developing effusions can produce a moderate to large amount of fluid overaccumulation before diagnosis. Thus 25% of patients may be asymptomatic on presentation.[58,111,135]

Physical examination will disclose abnormal findings if more than 300 ml of fluid has accumulated in the pleural space.[58,159] Pleural effusion frequently causes atelectasis, which predisposes the patient to respiratory infection with signs such as fever, chills, and night sweats.

Symptoms expressed by a patient with malignant pleural effusion are related to alterations in pulmonary function, which result from impairment from the effusion, and baseline respiratory status. *Dyspnea* is the most common reported symptom and is caused by alveolar collapse in the affected lung.[142] In addition, decreased chest wall compliance, contralateral mediastinal shift, and loss of ipsilateral lung volume occur. This increases the dys-

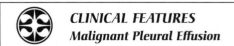

CLINICAL FEATURES
Malignant Pleural Effusion

Clinical signs
Labored breathing
Tachypnea
Restricted chest wall expansion
Decreased tactile fremitus on palpation
Dullness or flatness to percussion on affected side
Decreased diaphragmatic excursion with percussion
Diminished or absent breath sounds over affected area during auscultation
Pleuritic rub over affected area during auscultation
Egophony (change in transmitted sound) with auscultation just above level of effusion: the letter "e" spoken by the patient becomes higher pitched and sounds like an "a"[147]
If the effusion is large, additional signs could include:
  Bulging of intercostal spaces on affected side
  Splinting of chest on affected side
  Cyanosis
  Chest tenderness
  Shift in point of maximum intensity (PMI) to the left if effusion is on the right
  Tracheal deviation to unaffected side[135]

Symptoms
Dyspnea on exertion or at rest
Dry, nonproductive cough
Shortness of breath
Chest pain, often described as a "heaviness" or dull and aching rather than pleuritic[135]
Desire to lie on the affected side[135]
Malaise
Weight loss
Anxiety, fear of suffocation

pnea with any physical exertion. The degree of symptomatology depends on the rapidity of fluid accumulation rather than the amount of fluid present.[142] The box above lists clinical features of malignant pleural effusion.[47,53]

Physical findings of a pleural effusion are often not enough to make a differential diagnosis from a pleural or pulmonary mass or to determine a malignant versus benign underlying process. Further work-up is necessary to confirm a diagnosis of pleural effusion.[159]

DIAGNOSIS

Pleural effusion is usually detected by chest x-ray films. The lateral and decubitus views are most helpful and reveal as little as 100 ml of pleural fluid. Accumulation must be about 300 ml to be seen in the upright anteroposterior position on chest x-ray film, where they appear as opacity in the lower lung field or hemithorax on the affected side.[48,110] Additional radiographic studies could include an ultrasound of the chest or a computed tomography (CT) scan of the thorax. These two tests, as well as serial chest x-ray films, are especially helpful in identifying a site for thoracentesis and demonstrating the mobility of fluid and absence of loculation that indicate the fluid is separated into cavities by adhesions.[48] Confirmation of a pleural effusion in a patient with cancer does not necessarily indicate a malignant process. Aspiration and cytologic examination of the pleural fluid are required to identify the nature of the effusion. The mechanism of fluid accumulation should be ascertained, since it will guide treatment decisions.

Thoracentesis is a procedure in which a needle is introduced into the pleural space and fluid is aspirated. This procedure is indicated for diagnostic and therapeutic reasons. It is performed at the bedside. The patient is placed in the upright position with neck and dorsal spine flexed and arms extended and raised, usually over a bedside table. In this position, fluid will shift down into the dependent portion of the pleural space and the intercostal spaces will widen. A needle puncture is made, under local anesthesia, through the second intercostal space below the scapula on the affected side. The needle is directed inferiorly to avoid the neurovascular bundles located beneath and along the lower borders of the ribs.[110] Fluid is removed by a syringe or vacuum drainage collection, depending on the amount present. A minimum of 25 to 50 ml of fluid is needed for laboratory examination, but usually more than 250 ml is sent for analysis. Several puncture sites may be necessary if the fluid is loculated.[20,48,58,66]

Initially, large volumes of fluid can be removed rapidly. However, this should not exceed 1500 ml because it could result in hypotension, circulatory collapse, or pulmonary edema. The effusion should never be tapped dry. Leaving a small amount of fluid facilitates the placement of a chest tube.[48] At an initial thoracentesis and when malignancy is suspected, 500 to 1000 ml of the fluid is usually aspirated. This amount will remove mesothelial cells, which may interfere with a definitive cytologic evaluation. The removal of amounts more than 1000 ml will encourage new fluid formation containing freshly shed malignant cells.[137] Although thoracentesis is a relatively safe procedure, other potential complications include pneumothorax, if the lung is lacerated; hemorrhage, if a blood vessel is lacerated; vasovagal symptoms; and infection.[110] To rule out complications, a chest x-ray film is done after the thoracentesis. Thoracentesis alone will not prevent fluid reaccumulation. Recurrence of pleural effusion is seen within a few days in as many as 87% of patients.[110] Repeated therapeutic thoracenteses for symptom relief may be warranted, but they

are expensive and painful. In addition, they place the patient at risk for electrolyte imbalance, hypoproteinemia, pneumothorax, fluid loculation, and infection and may damage underlying lung parenchyma.[47,128,159]

Pleural fluid analysis helps establish the underlying mechanism of fluid accumulation. Normal pleural fluid is straw colored. Fluid from an effusion is either a transudate or an exudate. A *transudate fluid* is a clear fluid usually attributed to an increased leakage of water. It is found in diseases characterized by sodium and water imbalances, such as CHF, cirrhosis, nephrotic syndrome, peritoneal dialysis hypoalbuminemia, and constrictive pericarditis.[138] Although most diseases associated with transudate fluid are benign, 10% to 20% are malignant. An *exudate fluid* usually occurs with an excessive accumulation of protein in the pleural space. This is typically seen when the pleural surface is irritated or seeded with tumor. Although an exudate fluid does not specify neoplastic involvement in the pleural space, the most common cause is a malignancy. Other causes of an exudative effusion are tuberculosis, pneumonia, systemic lupus erythematosus (SLE), pancreatitis, chylothorax, sarcoidosis, Meig's syndrome, prior radiation therapy, and mesothelioma. Most malignant effusions are exudative. The color of the pleural fluid can further define the type of exudate, as follows[58,116,138]:

- Purulent fluid—emphysema or infection (tuberculosis or pneumonia)
- Chylous fluid (milky)—blockage of the thoracic duct with involvement of the mesenteric or retroperitoneal lymph nodes (lymphoma or benign disease process)
- Bloody fluid (more than 100,000 erythrocytes/mm^3)—usually indicates malignancy. A pleural fluid hematocrit higher than 50% than that of the blood characterizes hemothorax.

Malignant pleural effusions are always classified as an exudate. They usually have a bloody color and also must meet one of the following conditions: lactate dehydrogenase (LDH) level greater than 200 U, ratio of pleural fluid LDH level to serum LDH level greater than 0.6, or ratio of pleural fluid protein to serum protein greater than 0.5.[128]

Other less sensitive markers in the fluid that indicate a malignant effusion include the following:
White blood cell count (WBC) greater than 1000/mm^3
RBC count greater than 100,000/mm^3
Low pH
Low glucose
High specific gravity
High amylase
Carcinoembryonic antigen (CEA) level greater than 12 ng/ml[128]

Approximately one third of malignant pleural effusions have a pleural fluid pH of less than 7.3. If there is also a low glucose level, less than 60 mg/dl; low oxygen tension; and a high LDH concentration, the prognosis is poorer. These types of effusions are associated with large tumor burdens and fibrosis of the pleural space. The effusion tends to be chronic and may have been present for months. These patients with a low-pH malignant effusion respond poorly to pleurodesis, and survival is only 2½ months.[138]

Cytologic examination, which determines cell count and cell composition of fluid, is considered the most specific test for malignancy. Malignant cells tend to exfoliate more readily than normal cells. Approximately 60% to 80% of pleural specimens have been positive for malignant cells. A negative cytology does not exclude malignancy as the cause of the effusion. Repeated negative cytology is more common with lymphoma and warrants a pleural biopsy. In general, however, the patient with a malignant effusion will have other convincing evidence of cancer. Therefore a pleural biopsy may not be required.[48,110,111]

In situations with a false-negative finding, however, other procedures can be done to make a differential diagnosis if necessary and if the patient can tolerate the work-up. Testing would include bronchoscopy, mediastinoscopy, thoracoscopy, transcutaneous needle biopsy, open-lung biopsy, or thoracotomy. Future techniques that may prove to be beneficial in identifying malignant cells are those involving monoclonal antibodies and various types of chromosomal analysis.[14]

TREATMENT MODALITIES

Once a diagnosis of malignant pleural effusion has been confirmed and the cause established, therapy is determined by the underlying cancer (Figure 19-5). The goal of treatment is related to the patient's overall medical condition, the degree of respiratory impairment and underlying pulmonary status, the extent and nature of the malignancy, the cause of the pleural effusion, prior or concurrent tumor therapy, and the patient's life expectancy.[125] Treatment may be focused on systemic therapy, local therapy, a combination of both systemic and local, or no therapy.

Systemic Therapy: Chemotherapy

If the underlying cancer is treatable, therapy is directed at the primary malignancy and not the effusion. After diagnostic thoracentesis and lung reexpansion, systemic chemotherapy is initiated to prevent fluid reaccumulation. If the patient has a new diagnosis of lung cancer, a pleural effusion does not rule out surgery unless the cytology is positive. In that instance the tumor would be inoperable, and therapy would be determined by the responsiveness of the tumor. Treatment options (Figure 19-5) could be chest tube drainage with or without scle-

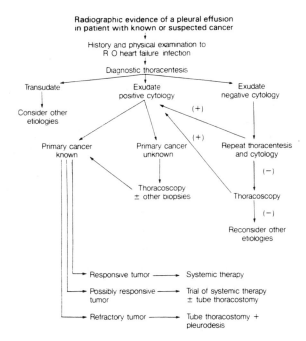

Figure 19-5 Clinical algorithm for prompt diagnosis and management of malignant pleural effusions. *RO,* Rule out; +, positive; −, negative. (From Ruckdeschel JC: *Semin Oncol* 15[suppl 3]:27, 1988.)

rosis, local radiation therapy, systemic chemotherapy, or any combination of these.[110]

Local Therapy: Radiation Therapy

Local radiation therapy may be used to treat malignant pleural effusions when the cause is a lymphoma. It may also be indicated in certain types of lung cancer. Radiation therapy in these two diseases may be the primary treatment or may be combined with other types of treatment, such as chest tube drainage, pleurodesis, or systemic chemotherapy.

Chest tube drainage is considered a more appropriate means of controlling pleural effusion than repeated thoracenteses, which can lead to complications. A thoracostomy tube inserted into the pleural space will not prevent fluid recurrence but will facilitate drainage and then pleural sclerosing. The procedure can be performed at the patient's bedside. The patient should be premedicated with a systemic analgesic such as meperidine or morphine sulfate.

With the patient under local anesthesia the chest tube is inserted through the fifth intercostal space on the anterior or lateral chest wall. These sites are usually chosen for patient comfort when lying and to prevent occlusion or kinking of the tube. After insertion the tube is connected to a water-seal drainage system under suction. This restores negative pressure in the pleural space, removes the fluid, and allows the lung to reexpand.[110] A chest x-ray film is done immediately after insertion of the chest tube to confirm its placement and to rule out a pneumothorax. Drainage usually requires 2 to 3 days, and subsequent chest films will be done, usually daily, to monitor fluid level and status of the lungs. Patients often complain of a cough as the lung reexpands.

Chest tube insertion may cause complications similar to those from thoracentesis, including pneumothorax, hemorrhage, infection, and damage to the lung parenchyma. An additional problem may be subcutaneous emphysema, or air under the subcutaneous tissues, although this is unusual unless the lung was injured.[110] Fluid or air may leak around the insertion site, which would require future stitching at the insertion site and/or a more occlusive petroleum-based gauze dressing. Malfunctions of the drainage system are possible, so frequent monitoring of the drainage system for patency is required.

Pleurodesis (Chemical Sclerosing)

Needle thoracentesis and chest tube drainage can successfully remove fluid from the pleural cavity. However, neither procedure can consistently prevent recurrence of fluid accumulation. Therefore chest tube drainage is usually followed by pleurodesis (Figure 19-5), which is the chemical sclerosing of the two pleural membranes. The goal is to obliterate the pleural space by instilling an irritating chemical into the space, causing the formation of adhesions that prevent fluid accumulation around the lung. These chemical agents damage the alveolar membrane and permeability, allowing clotting proteins such as fibrinogen to leak into the pleural space. Fibrinogen converts to fibrin, which accumulates and forms a lattice. Fibroblasts deposit collagen on the lattice and create the pleural adhesions.[50] Pleurodesis can be done at the bedside after the effusion has been drained by the chest tube, producing less than 100 ml of fluid in 24 hours. Drainage of the effusion is confirmed by a chest x-ray film showing lung reexpansion. If larger quantities of fluid continue to drain, pleurodesis may be less effective and may require a repeat procedure.

Pleurodesis is initiated by selecting the sclerosing agent. Many different agents have been used, including talcum powder, an antimalarial agent called quinacrine, radioisotopes of gold or phosphorus, antineoplastic agents, and antibiotics. The antineoplastic agents were employed with the hope that there would be a cytotoxic effect, as well as sclerosing effect. Findings show that the effectiveness of neoplastic agents when used as sclerosants depends on the ability to cause irritation and not on their antineoplastic activity. Thiotepa, 5-fluorouracil (5-FU), nitrogen mustard, doxorubicin (Adriamycin), and bleomycin were researched with varying results.[39,118,138] Continued research with bleomycin or talc as a sclerosant have shown it to be as effective as or su-

perior to tetracycline for pleurodesis. Many studies have demonstrated an overall response rate of 50% to 90%. The major disadvantage is the high cost. Problems of systemic absorption, bone marrow suppression, and other toxicities have limited the use of most of these agents.[49,111,134,138] Tetracycline had been the most frequently used sclerosing agent to date, with 80% being its highest reported response rate.[138] However, injectable tetracycline was discontinued by its manufacturer, and as a result, alternative efficacious and safe sclerosing agents are now being tested.[49] Minocycline and doxycycline may be alternatives to tetracycline because there are analogues putting them in the same drug class; they all have a similar pH in solution, are readily available, do not cause bone marrow suppression, and are inexpensive. However, doxycycline requires multiple instillations, and bleomycin may be cost prohibitive. Ongoing research and new drug development are needed.[49,111,134,138]

Because the sclerosing agents work by irritation of the pleura, patient preparation for pleurodesis may involve sedation with an IV sedative (e.g., diazepam) or narcotic analgesic (e.g., meperidine, morphine sulfate). Even with intrapleural lidocaine, the pain may be quite severe. Therefore bleomycin, which is much less painful and better tolerated, has gained popularity as a sclerosant. Doses vary from 60 U in 100 ml of 5% dextrose in water to 120 or 150 U in 100 ml normal saline.[135]

Most recently, sterile talc has been used for the sclerosing process because of the less desirable outcomes with other agents. The significant problem with talc is the sterilization process. Once sterilized, the talc is administered in one of two methods; a sterile mixture is sprayed into the pleural cavity via thoracoscopy or chest tube and/or with sterile 0.9% sodium chloride via a chest tube. Success rates with talc as a sclerosing agent have been reported as high as 90% to 100%, defined as no return of fluid after 30 and 90 days on a chest x-ray film. Sclerosol is a new agent used in clinical trials and is currently approved by the Food and Drug Administration (FDA).[47,138] The chest tube is unclamped by the physician, who then slowly injects the prepared sclerosing mixture into the pleural cavity. The chest tube is clamped, and the patient is asked or helped to turn from side to side to allow contact between the sclerosing agent and the entire surface of the pleura. Repositioning is continued every 15 to 30 minutes for 2 to 6 hours. The chest tube is then opened to drainage and the amount of drainage monitored. The chest tube remains in place for approximately 24 hours. The drainage of pleural fluid usually decreases over a few days, and when the amount is less than 50 ml in an 8-hour period, the chest tube is removed.[110] Expansion of the lung permits contact between the irritated vesical and parietal pleural surfaces. The inflammatory response of these membranes predicts total pleurodesis. A chest x-ray film is repeated to evaluate the success of the pleurodesis and to rule out a pneumothorax after chest tube removal.[47,138]

Surgery

Pleurectomy (mechanical pleurodesis). Surgical intervention for the management of pleural effusion is usually reserved for those situations when other treatment options fail to resolve the accumulation of fluid in the pleural cavity (Figure 19-5) and the patient has a life expectancy that makes the procedure worth the time and energy expenditure. Pleurectomy is the surgical removal of the parietal pleura with concomitant abrasion of the visceral pleura. Thus it is referred to as a mechanical pleurodesis.[110] The goal of either type of pleurodesis is the same: obliteration of the pleural space. Both require adequate lung expansion to meet the chest wall. Therefore drainage of the pleural space by a chest tube is done preoperatively.

Removal of the parietal pleura involves the same considerations as for any other thoracotomy procedure. It is done in the operating room with the patient under general anesthesia. A thoracotomy incision is established, and the parietal pleura is separated and removed from the chest wall. The visceral pleura, on the lung, is then swabbed with dry gauze, which causes granulation and the formation of adhesions. Chest tubes are inserted and kept in place initially during the postoperative period to allow effective sclerosing. In certain cases of chylous effusions caused by neoplastic obstruction of the mediastinal lymphatics, the surgical procedure may include ligation of the thoracic duct at the level of the diaphragm.[110]

Pleurectomy has produced excellent results; however, it has been accompanied by a morbidity rate of 20% or more and a 10% mortality rate.[58] Complications include air leaks, bleeding, and infection (pneumonia, empyema). Surgical removal of the pleura is a radical procedure usually reserved for patients in good physical condition and with a good life expectancy.

Pleuroperitoneal shunts. Another surgical treatment is available for intractable effusions when chemical pleurodesis is not feasible or has failed or when pleurectomy is not a viable option. The procedure involves the shunting of fluid from the pleural cavity into the abdominal cavity (Figure 19-6). With the patient under local anesthesia in the operating room, a commercially available device with one-way valve tubing is placed subcutaneously on the lateral chest wall. One end is inserted into the pleural cavity and the other into the abdominal cavity.

Early shunting devices were manually operated and required manual activation of the pump approximately 50 times a day.[66] More recent devices are heparinized systems that drain spontaneously by positive pressure in the pleural cavity created by the effusion. This can be supplemented manually by applying pressure on the subcutaneous device (Figure 19-6). Patients are often taught to activate the device themselves.[110] Success of the device depends on the amount and rate of fluid accumulation and proper pump function.

Long-term thoracotomy access and drainage. A final alternative for the control of pleural effusion is long-term thoracotomy access and drainage. This approach is used for palliation. Patient selection is based on patient performance status and degree of disability, general health condition with attention to past and present pulmonary status, extent of underlying malignancy, and estimated life expectancy.[64,125] Eligible patients include those with debilitating symptoms who have been unsuccessfully treated for pleural effusion by thoracentesis, chest tube drainage, pleurodesis, radiation therapy, or chemotherapy and those patients who are not candidates for surgery.

Access to the pleural cavity is accomplished by either a long-term access device, such as an implantable subcutaneous port, or by a chest tube. The subcutaneous port, with attached catheter or drainage tube, is placed into the pleural cavity by surgical implantation. The port

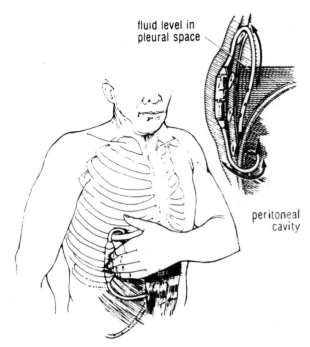

fluid level in pleural space

peritoneal cavity

Figure 19-6 Pleuroperitoneal shunt procedure. Inset shows position of device on rib cage. Arrows indicate direction of flow. (From Miller SE, Campbell DB: Pleural effusions in malignant disease. In Polomano RC, Miller SE, editors: *Understanding and managing oncologic emergencies,* monograph, Columbus, Ohio, 1987, Adria Laboratories.)

is accessed through the usual subcutaneous method and fluid withdrawn intermittently. This can be done as often as deemed necessary but usually is done twice a week. Complications include infection, bleeding, occlusion, and device malfunctions.[66,111,116]

Continuous long-term drainage can be accomplished by using either a standard chest tube or a small-bore catheter such as a Foley catheter placed into the pleural space. The smaller catheters are less traumatic to insert, may be sewn in place onto the skin, and will not cause splinting of the ribs, which is sometimes a complication with larger tubes. The principles and procedures of long-term drainage represent modifications of those for the standard short-term chest tube drainage system.[66] The two necessary components of a long-term drainage system include the drainage tube and the collection equipment. Options are available, and choices depend on the patient's status. The following comparisons may help the decision process:

Standard chest tube	Small-bore catheter
Drainage tube	
Large, allows view of fluid	Small, may or may not give view of fluid
Rigid, uncomfortable	Flexible, more comfortable
Anchored by sutures only	Inflatable bulb available in addition to sutures
Collection equipment	
Drainage under water seal	Drainage without water seal (continuous urinary drainage bag or system may be used)
Large and cumbersome	Smaller and easier to handle
Expensive	Less expensive
May or may not be portable	Usually portable
Noisy, requires suction	Quiet, drains by gravity

A one-way valve (Heimlich valve) may or may not be used between the drainage tube and collection equipment. It is usually indicated when there is a risk of pneumothorax, since it allows the drainage of fluid and escape of air from the thorax but prevents their return. An advantage of the one-way valve is that the collection equipment can be kept at any level below or above the chest without adverse effects. However, if the one-way valve is not used, all collection equipment must be at or below the chest tube insertion site for adequate drainage and to prevent complications.[66,146]

Long-term thoracotomy access drainage provides an important alternative method for managing intractable pleural effusions. It can reduce cost by decreasing the number of procedures and hospitalizations. Many patients can be managed at home using this method. This long-term treatment can provide comfort through relief of respiratory distress and control of associated symptoms. Most important, it can improve quality of life, the primary goal of any treatment.

PROGNOSIS

Patients with pleural effusion have a variable prognosis depending on the extent of the effusion and the success of treatment for the underlying disease. Malignant pleural effusion is usually an indication of advanced disease. Survival rates vary from 3 months to 4 years, with the longest survival in patients with lymphoma.[66,146] Results from several studies indicate that mean survival from time of diagnosis of the effusion is about 6 months for lung cancer and 1 year for breast cancer.[66] Treatment efforts must be aimed at the underlying disease; however, they are always accompanied by measures to improve the patient's quality of life. With improving technology, earlier diagnosis and better interventions may increase survival rates.

Nursing management of the patient with malignant pleural effusion is outlined on pp. 430-431.

NEOPLASTIC CARDIAC TAMPONADE

DEFINITION

Neoplastic cardiac tamponade is the compression of the cardiac muscle by pathologic fluid accumulation under pressure within the pericardial sac. Fluid accumulates because the pericardium is constricted by a tumor or by the presence of postirradiation pericarditis.[159] Compression of the myocardium interferes with dilation of the heart chambers, which prevents adequate cardiac filling during diastole. This in turn reduces blood flow to the ventricles and reduces stroke volume, which results in decreased cardiac output. Other pressures are then affected, including an elevated central venous pressure (CVP) and a lowered left atrial pressure (Figure 19-7). Two compensatory mechanisms initiated by adrenergic stimulation attempt to counteract these pressures to increase cardiac output and maintain peripheral perfusion.[83] An increase in heart rate (tachycardia) helps maintain cardiac output at low stroke volumes and increases systolic emptying. Peripheral vasoconstriction maintains arterial pressure and venous return.[139] If cardiac output is not increased by compensatory mechanisms, this can cause circulatory collapse, which is fatal if untreated.[8,57,85,139]

ETIOLOGY AND RISK FACTORS

A variety of nonmalignant or malignant conditions may be responsible for the development of cardiac tamponade. Nonmalignant causes include the following[40,85,110]:
- Cardiovascular causes: heart surgery, chest trauma, aneurysm, rupture of the great vessel, cardiac procedures (angiography, insertion or removal of pacer wires), insertion of central venous catheter

NURSING MANAGEMENT

Nursing care of a patient with pleural effusion depends on the extent of the effusion, the underlying disease, and the patient's overall condition. The problem is serious, and nursing care will be diverse, as with other oncologic complications. However, pleural effusions usually have a more gradual and detectable onset. This fact, coupled with a high recurrence rate, places great emphasis on the nurse's assessment skills. Objective and subjective data must be collected systematically.[47,66,75,111,116]

NURSING DIAGNOSES

- *Breathing pattern, ineffective, related to limited lung expansion secondary to pleural effusion*
- *Gas exchange, impaired, related to ineffective breathing patterns and pleural effusion*

OUTCOME GOALS

Patient will be able to:
- Exhibit improved respiratory status, as evidenced by reduction in abnormal breath sounds, laboratory values and respiratory function tests approaching normal limits, ability to participate in self-care activities, and maintenance of normal respiratory rate and function.
- Identify/demonstrate emergency measures for acute respiratory distress.
- Maintain/return to activity tolerance levels.

INTERVENTIONS

- Determine current respiratory status:
  —Observe for signs and symptoms of respiratory difficulty (dyspnea, shortness of breath, tachypnea, increased sputum production, change in color of sputum, hemoptysis, persistent cough, decreased activity tolerance, headache, chest, arm, or shoulder pain).
  —Assess lungs. Observe ventilatory movements (rate, depth), patency of the airway, use of accessory muscles, clubbing of fingernails, and discoloration of nailbeds or mucous membranes.
  —Palpate chest for fremitus, crepitance, deviation of trachea, or nonsymmetric chest expansion. Percuss chest for density or consolidation and displacement of organs. Auscultate chest for breath sounds.
  —Monitor laboratory and other respiratory function tests: complete blood count (CBC), electrolytes, arterial blood gases (ABGs), chest x-ray film, pulmonary function studies, and scans.
- Assist with breathing and pulmonary toilet:
  —Positioning for comfort and enhanced chest expansion
  —Deep breathing and coughing every 2 hours
  —Pursed-lip breathing
  —Postural drainage
  —Mouth care frequently
  —Suctioning if necessary
- Provide oxygen therapy as indicated.
- Consult with physician regarding need for more aggressive pulmonary toilet measures (incentive spirometry, ultrasonic nebulizer, chest physical therapy).
- Administer respiratory medications as ordered.
- Provide mechanical ventilation if necessary.
- Teach measures to maintain optimal respiratory abilities:
  —Use of oxygen therapy
  —Pursed-lip breathing
  —Breathing exercises
  —Scheduled rest periods
  —Humidification
  —Adequate hydration and nutrition
  —Use of incentive spirometry and/or inhalers
  —Smoking cessation if indicated
  —Measures to decrease anxiety and stress (environmental manipulation, relaxation techniques, antianxiety medications)
- Make referrals to other health care professionals in the hospital and community as needed.
- Monitor chest tube drainage if indicated, as outlined in hospital procedure.
- Assist with pleurodesis if ordered, as outlined in hospital procedure.

NURSING DIAGNOSIS

- *Tissue perfusion, altered, related to impaired gas exchange from pleural effusion*

OUTCOME GOALS

Patient will be able to:
- Maintain adequate pulmonary function, as evidenced by vital signs and activity tolerance within patient's normal limits.
- Identify strategies for optimal pulmonary health.
- Develop plan for behavioral and life-style changes.

INTERVENTIONS

- Assess organ systems for malfunction related to ischemia.
- Evaluate skin color of extremities.
- Note any change in mental status.
- Monitor laboratory values closely.
- Measure intake and output.
- Provide oxygen therapy as prescribed.
- Administer vasoactive drugs as ordered.

If the treatment used is surgery, the usual postoperative nursing care is implemented. The goal is to prevent or minimize complications. Patient assessment, pain management, oral hygiene, skin care, nutrition, and passive/active exercising are important aspects of surgical nursing care planning. When the patient is undergoing chemotherapy or radiation therapy, the nurse manages any side effects that may occur, such as fatigue, skin changes, alopecia, nausea, vomiting, diarrhea, and bone marrow suppression.

Discharge planning for patients treated for pleural effusion depends on their status after treatment. Some patients may be discharged symptom free and need only follow-up care to monitor for recurrence. Some patients may need support at home for intermittent or continuous pleural drainage. Other patients may require a hospice or extended care facility to continue management of the pleural effusion. The nurse is responsible for the transition from the hospital setting (see Chapter 27).

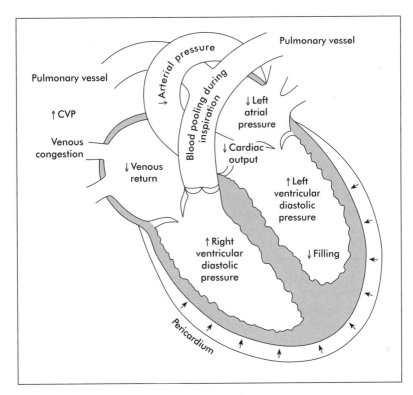

Figure 19-7   Cardiovascular effects of increased intrapleural pressure. Intraventricular diastolic pressure rises as a result of higher intrapericardial pressure. This prevents adequate filling of the ventricle, causing venous congestion, decreased cardiac output, lowered left atrial pressure, and elevated central venous pressure *(CVP)*. ↑, Increased; ↓, decreased. (From Dietz KA, Flaherty AM: Oncologic emergencies. In Groenwald SL, others, editors: *Cancer nursing: principles and practice*, ed 2, Boston, 1990, Jones and Bartlett.)

- Infectious pericarditis; bacterial, fungal, viral, or tubercular infections
- Connective tissue disorders: SLE, scleroderma, rheumatoid disease
- Myxedema
- Uremia
- Pharmacologic therapy: anthracyclines (doxorubicin, daunomycin), anticoagulants (heparin, sodium warfarin), hydralazine (Apresoline), procainamide (Procan SR, Pronestyl)

Malignant causes include the following[110,159]:

- Neoplastic pericarditis with effusion: primary tumors of the pericardium (mesotheliomas, sarcomas), metastatic tumors of the pericardium (lung cancer, breast tumors, leukemias, lymphomas, melanomas, sarcomas)
- Neoplastic constrictive pericarditis (metastatic tumor infiltration)
- Radiation pericarditis (exposure of the heart to 400 Gy or more)

Pericardial effusion with tamponade is a life-threatening problem whether the cause is malignant or nonmalignant. Open-heart surgery is the leading cause of cardiac tamponade, which occurs postoperatively in approximately 3% to 8% of patients.[8,74] Malignant pericardial tamponade occurs in approximately 10% to 20% of patients with a neoplasm that involves the heart. The high estimates of this complication are based on compilations of autopsy data regarding cardiac (including pericardial) metastasis, which range from 0.1% to 21%.[74,83] The majority of these patients are asymptomatic, with only 20% to 30% showing clinical evidence of cardiac disease before death.[74]

Most cases of neoplastic cardiac tamponade represent metastatic invasion of the pericardium. Pericardial metastasis is unusual without documentation of other metastases. Only rarely is the cause primary disease of the myocardium (mesothelioma, angiosarcoma, fibrosarcoma, malignant teratoma).[75] Any cancer has the potential for metastatic spread to the pericardium via direct tumor extension, lymphatic invasion, or hematogenous dissemination. Patients with pericardial effusions are at risk for tamponade. Pericardial effusions caused by metastatic disease are present in 5% to 50% of patients with cancer. However, cancers at greatest risk for the development of neoplastic cardiac tamponade include breast cancer, lung cancer, lymphoma, and leukemia, which account for 80% of this complication. Other malignant causes are melanoma, GI cancers, and oronasopharyngeal carcinoma. Approximately 5% of patients who re-

ceive radiation therapy to the mediastinum (400 Gy or more) develop acute pericarditis with or without pericardial effusion during treatment or chronic constrictive pericarditis up to 20 years after treatment. More than 90% of the cases occur in the first year after radiation treatment.[74,75,83,116,118]

PATHOPHYSIOLOGY

The heart and a portion of the great vessels are encased in a thin, tough, double-layered fibrous sac called the *pericardium,* which contains little elastic tissue. The inner layer, or sheath, is known as the *visceral pericardium.* It is a delicate serous membrane that lines the interior of the fibrous sac and is continuous with the surface of the heart.[57] The outer layer of the pericardium is called the *parietal pericardium.* This sheath is fibrous and provides strength and protection. The left sternal portion is in direct contact with the chest wall. Between the two layers of the pericardium is a cavity that contains 10 to 20 ml of a clear serous lubricating fluid, originating from the lymphatic channels surrounding the heart, and serves to cushion the myocardium.

The pathophysiology of pericardial tamponade is a progressive accumulation of fluid in the pericardial sac

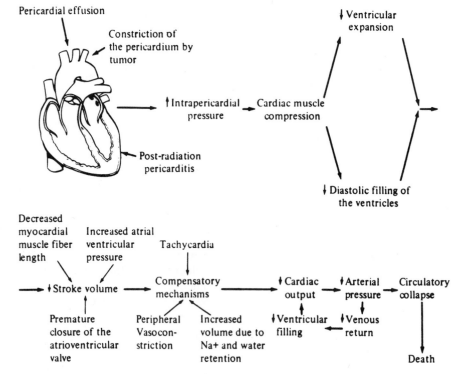

Figure 19-8 Development of neoplastic pericardial tamponade. (From Yasko JM, Schafer SL: Neoplastic pericardial tamponade. In Yasko JM, editor: *Guidelines for cancer care: symptom management,* Reston, Va, 1983, Reston.)

(Figure 19-8), which leads to compression of the heart, hampering dilation of its chambers and thus limiting diastolic atrial filling: intrapericardial pressure rises, and bilateral ventricular stroke volume decreases. Initially the sac will stretch to accommodate increases in fluid, and compensatory mechanisms—an increased heart rate (tachycardia) and increased peripheral vascular tone (peripheral vasoconstriction)—maintain adequate cardiac output. However, as these temporary adaptive responses begin to fail, a vicious cycle of increased fluid with decreased atrial pressure, decreased cardiac output, and decreased venous return will progress to circulatory collapse and, if untreated, to shock, cardiac arrest, and death.

The severity of cardiac tamponade depends on the amount of fluid in the pericardium, the rate of accumulation, and the degree of pericardial and organic compromise. Usually there will be no change in cardiac activity with the addition of 50 ml or less of fluid in the pericardial space. Gradual fluid accumulation permits the pericardium to stretch and accommodate. As much as 2 L or more can accumulate without producing signs of cardiac compromise.[57,58,75,93,110] However, 100 to 200 ml of fluid may cause severe cardiac impairment if the accumulation occurs rapidly.[75] Whether gradual or acute, the fluid accumulation that leads to cardiac tamponade in the presence of malignant disease is the result of one of the following mechanisms:

- Direct tumor (primary or metastatic) extension and blockage of the lymphatic drainage
- Malignant lymphatic engorgement and impairment of drainage
- Tumor (primary or metastatic) implantation in or around the pericardium with inflammation and fluid production
- Radiation-induced pericarditis of the pericardium with fluid accumulation

Retrograde lymphatic dissemination is thought to be the main pathway of pericardial metastasis, creating fluid seepage through the visceral pericardium and into the pericardial space.[93] Neoplastic cardiac tamponade related to malignant pericardial effusion, whether resulting from a constricting tumor, lymphatic dissemination, or postirradiation pericarditis, is a medical emergency and must be recognized and treated promptly.

CLINICAL FEATURES

Patients with neoplastic cardiac tamponade manifest a wide variety of clinical signs and symptoms, directly related to the degree of fluid accumulation (amount and rapidity of onset) and subsequent disruption of normal hemodynamics (see box at right). Figure 19-8 outlines the related stages of a progressive pericardial effusion.

Identification of neoplastic cardiac tamponade de-

pends greatly on a clinical diagnosis based on a detailed history and thorough physical examination. The presence or absence of any of the signs and symptoms depends on the stage of cardiac tamponade. A current or past history of cancer and cancer treatments should be noted. Occasionally, neoplastic cardiac tamponade is the first sign of a malignancy. Beck's triad has been considered a hallmark of cardiac tamponade. These three signs include an elevated CVP, distant heart sound, and arterial hypotension. However, these signs may not be found in all patients, and their appearance usually marks an advanced stage of tamponade. Therefore Beck's triad is not a sufficient clinical indicator of cardiac tamponade.[8,9,85]

DIAGNOSIS

A differential diagnosis of neoplastic cardiac tamponade is often difficult; in a patient with cancer it becomes even more complex. With no known history of cancer, other

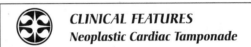
CLINICAL FEATURES
Neoplastic Cardiac Tamponade

Clinical signs
Tachycardia
Low systolic blood pressure
Tachypnea with normal breath sounds
Vasoconstriction
Thready, diminished pulse pressure or pulsus paradoxus
Increased central venous pressure (CVP)
Arterial hypotension
Cardiomegaly
Precordial dullness to percussion
Distant weak heart sounds
Pericardial friction rub
Engorged neck veins
Ascites
Hepatomegaly
Hepatojugular reflux
Peripheral edema
Cool, clammy extremities or peripheral cyanosis
Oliguria secondary to decreased renal perfusion
Apprehension, anxiety
Clouded sensorium or impaired consciousness
Symptoms
Dyspnea or shortness of breath
Retrosternal chest pain
Diaphoresis
Anxiety
Cough
Hoarseness, hiccups
Nausea, vomiting
Abdominal pain

possible diagnoses must be ruled out, such as right ventricular heart failure, hydropericardium, rapid blood volume expansion, CHF, and pulmonary edema.[9,58]

Patients with cancer present a challenge for differential diagnosis because of the different malignant and nonmalignant pathophysiologic processes that can cause pericarditis and result in cardiac tamponade.[8,9,110] Patients who have received radiation therapy to the mediastinal area may develop cardiac tamponade secondary to pericardial constriction. This process is more difficult to diagnose than malignant tumor invasion and requires a different treatment. Cardiac function may also be affected without fluid accumulation by cancer-related or treatment-related processes, such as radiation fibrosis, heart muscle metastasis, coronary artery occlusion, or drug-induced CHF.[8,9,85]

Two clinical findings that are classic features of cardiac tamponade are pulsus paradoxus and hepatojugular reflux. Testing for these two manifestations can be performed at the bedside. *Pulsus paradoxus* (Figure 19-9) is an abnormal finding of a weaker pulse during inspiration, resulting from a greater than normal (10 mm Hg) decrease in systolic blood pressure during the inspiratory phase of normal respiration. Cardiac tamponade constricts the myocardium, and during inspiration the diaphragm exerts additional pressure on the pericardial sac. The left ventricle receives less blood, and stroke volume is decreased, which is seen as a decrease in systolic blood pressure during inspiration. The arterial pulse may also be absent during inspiration.[57,75,93,110,140]

Pulsus paradoxus can be determined in one of two ways (Figure 19-9). Patients with an indwelling arterial catheter can have their blood pressure monitored during inspiration. Patients without invasive equipment can have their blood pressure evaluated by routine sphygmomanometry. A blood pressure cuff is placed around the arm and inflated to greater than 20 mm Hg above systolic pressure. The cuff is deflated slowly until the first systolic sound (Korotkoff sound) is auscultated, and the reading is noted. This occurs during expiration, and the sounds disappear during inspiration. The cuff is further deflated until sounds can be heard throughout the respiratory cycle (expiration and inspiration). This reading is also noted. The difference in mm Hg between the two readings is the value of the paradox. If the difference is more than 10 mm Hg between the two readings, pulsus paradoxus is present.[58,75,93,140]

Inaccurate results may occur when assessing for pulsus paradoxus. Mechanical ventilation can artificially mimic paradoxic pulse.[58] If hypotension is present, pulsus paradoxus may not be found by auscultation. In this situation the inspiratory decline in blood pressure can be noted by close examination of the carotid or femoral pulse. Pulsus paradoxus may disappear during extreme tamponade, when the systolic pressure may decrease below 50 mm Hg. Finally, other conditions may be manifested with pulsus paradoxus. These include obesity, severe obstructive respiratory disease, acute cor pulmonale, right ventricular infarction, and hypovolemic shock.[45,48,58,93]

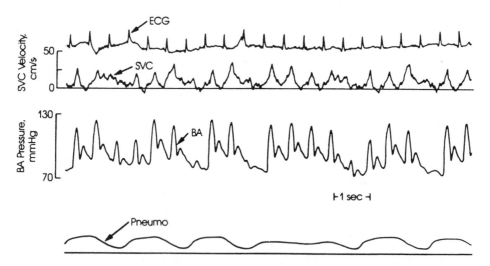

Figure 19-9 Simultaneous recording of electrocardiogram *(ECG),* blood flow velocity in the superior vena cava *(SVC),* brachial arterial *(BA)* pressure, and the pneumogram *(Pneumo)* in a patient with cardiac compression and paradoxic pulse (pulsus paradoxus). A downward deflection of the pneumogram denotes inspiration, when SVC blood velocity rises and arterial pressure falls (paradoxic pulse). Arterial pressure is maintained during prolonged expiratory pause. (From Braunwald E: Pericardial disease. In Braunwald E and others, editors: *Harrison's principles of internal medicine,* ed 11, New York, 1987, McGraw-Hill.)

Hepatojugular reflex is an elevation in jugular venous pressure by 1 cm or more. Testing for this abnormal condition is accomplished by placing the patient in the supine position with the head of the bed elevated to a level where jugular venous pulsations are visible. Pressure is then exerted continuously over the right upper quadrant of the abdomen for 30 to 60 seconds, and jugular pressure is observed. An increase in the pressure represents a positive reflex arising from venous congestion associated with a prolonged elevation of the CVP.[58,93,140]

Tests ordered by the physician will include a chest x-ray film, ECG, and an echocardiogram. A routine chest x-ray film is not a specific diagnostic tool, since it cannot differentiate among possible causes of an enlarged heart shadow. Fluid accumulation of 100 ml will not change the cardiac silhouette on a film, but this amount of fluid can produce tamponade if onset is rapid. More than 250 ml of fluid within the pericardial sac will enlarge the cardiac silhouette. A "water bottle heart" is seen on the x-ray film as a result of the disappearance of the normal contours between the great vessels and the cardiac chambers.[48,93,110] More than half the patients with cardiac tamponade have cardiac enlargement, mediastinal widening, or hilar adenopathy.[85] Lung fields on chest x-ray films are usually normal because pulmonary bed capacity has not been impaired.

The electrocardiogram provides a limited amount of useful information. Elevated ST segments, nonspecific T wave changes, decreased QRS voltage, and sinus tachycardia may be seen.[85,93,110] *Electrical alternans,* which is the alternation of amplitude and direction of the P wave and QRS complexes on every other beat, is the most specific although infrequent abnormality in patients with neoplastic cardiac tamponade. This heart block, appearing at every other beat, is thought to result from variations in cardiac position at the time of electrical depolarization. In rare cases, atrial fibrillation has been present.*

Echocardiography, both M mode (motion mode) and two dimensional, is the most specific and sensitive technique for establishing the presence of pericardial effusion. This noninvasive, reliable test should always be done when cardiac tamponade is suspected. The presence, location, and approximate quantity of fluid can be determined by the cardiac ultrasound. Normal findings on the echocardiogram show the posterior left ventricular wall in contact with the posterior pericardium and pleura and the anterior right ventricular wall in close approximation to the chest wall.[8,18] In tamponade, echo-free spaces that separate the moving walls from the immobile pericardium indicate the presence of fluid.[48,140] The spaces appear first posteriorly and then anteriorly. The absence of pericardial fluid usually rules out cardiac

tamponade. Although an echocardiogram cannot determine the cause of the pericardial fluid, it is extremely helpful in the evaluation of an effusion, as well as in site selection for pericardiocentesis.[85]

The echocardiogram is especially useful for differential diagnosis if cor pulmonale is a possibility, since it can mimic cardiac tamponade. Cor pulmonale can present with a huge globular heart, hypertension, decreased pulse pressure, and pronounced pulse paradoxus.[74]

Recent advances in echocardiography have added new dimensions to diagnostic testing, including transesophageal echo (TEE), stress echo, and intraarterial echo. TEE has been used in critically ill patients as a diagnostic tool in hypotensive crisis. Pericardial tamponade has been correctly diagnosed in these patients. The esophagus is the closest structure to the heart. Positioning the TEE scope with its transducer in that location permits high-resolution images of the cardiac structure. The TEE scope is a modification of the endoscope, and its tip can be moved antegrade, retrograde, and laterally to obtain tomographic views of cardiac structures using a biplane or omniplane transducer. This procedure can be done at the bedside, in the operating room, or as an outpatient procedure.[74,85,134]

Other testing that may be performed during a diagnostic work-up for neoplastic cardiac tamponade includes cardiac catheterization, various types of scanning, and laboratory blood work. Catheterization of the heart can confirm a diagnosis of tamponade and determine the size and exact location of the pericardial fluid. In the presence of tamponade, intracardiac pressure is increased, and diastolic pressures are abnormal but almost equal in all chambers of the heart (10 to 25 mm Hg), as measured during catheterization.

Recent improvements in technology have assisted in the diagnosis of cardiac tamponade. CT and magnetic resonance imaging (MRI) have been useful in the assessment of a thickened pericardium and the diagnosis of constrictive pericarditis with effusion versus radiation fibrosis. The CT scan of the chest is the most sensitive test to visualize cardiac metastasis.[139] These specific differential diagnoses are crucial because treatment differs in each situation.

Laboratory blood tests ordered during the diagnostic work-up for neoplastic cardiac tamponade may include hematocrit, potassium (K^+), calcium (Ca^{++}), and arterial blood gases (ABGs). These tests are not conclusive for cardiac tamponade, but they can support a differential diagnosis. Pericardial fluid sent for cytologic examination has been diagnostic in about 80% of patients, but there is a significant percentage of false-negative reports. Certain malignancies (e.g., lymphoma, leukemia) make cytologic diagnosis more difficult. Pericardial biopsy has a 55% diagnostic yield.[139,140]

---

*References 9, 48, 75, 85, 93, 140.

Testing for neoplastic cardiac tamponade varies greatly in scope and depth, as determined by the patient's clinical appearance, including tolerance for various procedures. Time is of the essence. Clinically evident neoplastic effusions are usually large enough to be evaluated by echocardiography.[74,85,139,140]

TREATMENT MODALITIES

Neoplastic cardiac tamponade is a life-threatening situation that requires immediate medical intervention as soon as the diagnosis is confirmed. The immediate goal of treatment is the removal of pericardial fluid to relieve impending circulatory collapse. After symptomatic relief of tamponade, the longer-range goal is management of the underlying disease.

Pharmacologic Therapy

Mild neoplastic cardiac tamponade may be treated with drug therapy using corticosteroids and diuretics. Supportive measures during cardiac tamponade are aimed at maintaining blood pressure and cardiac functioning.[75] Common prescriptions include prednisone (40 to 60 mg/day) with furosemide (Lasix) (40 mg/day) or Aldactazide (spironolactone and hydrochlorothiazide, 25 to 200 mg/day). Radiation pericarditis is often effectively treated with high-dose steroids or NSAIDs. However, when these drugs are discontinued, the pericarditis often recurs.[118,159] If an effusion recurs or tamponade becomes acute, more aggressive treatment is indicated.[48,140] Infusions of blood products and IV fluids will expand volume and increase ventricular filling pressures. Vasoactive drugs (e.g., nitroprusside, isoproterenol, dopamine) may be useful.[85] Isoproterenol can increase heart rate and contractility, and low-dose dopamine may improve contractility. However, α-adrenergic medications will likely increase afterload and adversely affect cardiac output. The use of diuretics at this point will decrease volume and further impair ventricular filling.[75]

Pericardiocentesis

Pericardiocentesis, which is a percutaneous needle pericardiotomy with aspiration, is done for both therapeutic and diagnostic reasons. Indications for this approach include a slow leak, diagnostic confirmation, rapid relief of acute tamponade, or symptomatic relief when deterioration of the patient's condition is evidenced by cyanosis, dyspnea, changes in mental status, or shock.[74,85,139] Another indicator for an aggressive approach to relieve tamponade is the "rule of 20," or a decrease in pulse pressure of more than 20 mm Hg, pulsus paradoxus greater than 20 mm Hg, and CVP greater than 20 cm H_2O before pericardiocentesis.

When aspiration is delayed, treatment may be initiated along with pharmacologic measures to improve hemo-dynamic status. Temporary interventions include the administration of volume expanders such as plasma blood or other colloid solutions that help to increase ventricular filling pressure. Vasoactive drugs (e.g., isoproterenol, epinephrine, dopamine) are used to improve cardiac contractility and filling. Oxygen therapy may also be given. These combined measures are often continued during the pericardiocentesis.

The technique most often used for pericardiocentesis is the introduction of a large-bore needle into the pericardial space through a small stab incision by a subxiphoid approach. The needle is angled toward the left shoulder.[139] The safety of this procedure depends on attention to the underlying disease and the amount and exact location of the fluid present. An echocardiogram done before pericardiocentesis can be of great assistance in site selection. There is less risk with larger volumes of fluid accumulation because of the increased distance between the pericardium and the surface of the heart. To reduce the risks associated with pericardiocentesis, the procedure is performed with continuous monitoring of CVP and ECG using the V lead directly attached to the metal hub, or shaft, of the needle.[74,85,139]

Possible complications of pericardiocentesis include puncture of the right atrium or ventricle, laceration of the coronary artery, accidental introduction of air into the chambers of the heart, dysrhythmias, vasovagal reaction with bradycardia, and infection. Although the subxiphoid approach avoids the pleural space, pneumothorax or other injury to the lungs can occur.[48,140] Throughout the procedure, equipment must be available for emergency surgery and cardiopulmonary resuscitation.

Successful penetration of the pericardial sac during pericardiocentesis is often confirmed by a palpable "pop."[74,85,139] This is accompanied by an increase in the QRS-complex voltage on the ECG, resulting when the pericardium is touched. If there is an acute elevation of the ST and PR segments, premature atrial contractions (PACs), or premature ventricular contractions (PVCs), there has been contact between the needle and the myocardium, and the needle should be withdrawn.[58] After confirmation of needle location, fluid is aspirated slowly over 10 to 30 minutes. Although there is dramatic improvement in the patient with the removal of 25 to 50 ml of fluid, as much of the fluid as possible should be removed.[9,85]

Fluid return from the pericardium is normally clear and straw colored. In the presence of a malignancy, it is often bloody. This fluid should be immediately tested for hematocrit and fibrinogen to distinguish between a bloody effusion and penetration of the heart. Bloody effusions have lower levels of hematocrit and fibrinogen than circulating blood.[74,85,139]

Malignant effusions are usually serosanguineous; however, clear fluid does not rule out a neoplastic disease. Fluid studies include specific gravity, protein, cell count, stains, cultures, and cytologic analysis. Cytologic examination of pericardial fluid is essential to assist with diagnosis. With metastatic cancer the cytologic identification is 80% to 90% accurate, with essentially no false-positive results. The results with lymphomas, sarcomas, and primary mesotheliomas of the pericardium are much less sensitive. Although a positive cytology may define the histopathology of the neoplastic disease, it may not identify the primary site.[140]

Pericardiocentesis is usually effective in relieving signs and symptoms of neoplastic cardiac tamponade, but fluid generally reaccumulates in 24 to 48 hours. In some instances the elevated venous pressure associated with cardiac tamponade may remain despite pericardiocentesis. This situation may result from SVCS, CHF, or effusive-constrictive pericardial disease caused by radiation therapy (400 Gy or more), tuberculosis, or extensive malignancy. This condition can be confirmed by measuring simultaneous pressures in the pericardial sac and the right atrium.[110,140] Therefore further local or systemic therapy is required after any pericardiocentesis. The choice of treatment depends on the etiology and extent of the underlying disease and the patient's overall condition.

Multiple taps and placement of an indwelling catheter have been helpful in controlling fluid accumulation; however, these measures are temporary. Long-term catheter placement is contraindicated because of the high risk of infection. A short-term indwelling pericardial catheter with multiple holes for drainage can be easily inserted with an introducer over a flexible guide wire. Once it is in place, a stopcock is placed at the distal end of the catheter. The catheter is drained each shift and may be irrigated daily with a small volume (5 to 10 ml) of saline or heparinized saline (100 U/ml). Irrigation may be useful if the tamponade is caused by a coagulopathy. In the presence of neoplastic fluid it is probably not necessary, since fibrinogen levels of the fluid are low.

Surgery

Surgical procedures can provide prolonged palliation of recurrent neoplastic cardiac tamponade. The type and extent of the surgery depends on the amount and cytology of the pericardial fluid and the patient's overall condition. A pericardial "window" *(partial pericardiectomy)* is created by means of a small, left anterior thoracotomy. Through this subxiphoid approach, a piece of the pericardium measuring several square centimeters is removed. The open window permits drainage of the pericardial fluid into the pleural space.[110,140]

A more extensive surgical procedure is a *total pericardiectomy* (Figure 19-10), in which most of the visceral pericardium is removed. A median sternotomy is performed, which provides excellent exposure and visu-

alization of the pericardium. The pathology can be observed and biopsied. Large rectangular pieces of the pericardium are removed from both the left and right sides. The phrenic nerves define the boundaries of the procedure and remain intact. For several days a chest tube is left in each side to assist with drainage.[85,140]

Total pericardiectomy is the treatment of choice for patients with radiation-induced effusive-constrictive pericardial disease, or fibrosis, and also for those with pericardial mesothelioma. It is usually contraindicated in patients with extensive metastatic disease.[140]

These surgical procedures are usually effective in controlling pericardial effusions by allowing the pericardial fluid to drain into the pleural cavity, which provides greater surface area for reabsorption. Pericardial effusions and tamponade rarely recur after these surgical procedures. However, in some instances the windows have closed. Several potential complications are associated with these procedures, including the usual risks associated with general anesthesia and the possibility of dysrhythmias, bleeding, infection, and hemothorax. Pulmonary edema can occur with postoperative diuresis in patients who were heavily hydrated before surgery.[140]

Radiation Therapy

Radiation therapy may be the treatment of choice for neoplastic cardiac tamponade of gradual onset caused by a radiosensitive tumor of the lung or breast or a hematopoietic malignancy. Generally, external beam radiation therapy (200 to 400 Gy) is delivered to a port that includes the heart and pericardial structures and the lower mediastinum. Careful assessment of any previous radiation therapy is important to establish tissue tolerance. Cardiac tolerance is 350 to 400 Gy, beyond which a complication of pericarditis may develop.[109] External beam radiotherapy is most often employed, but internal radiation therapy has been done using radioactive phosphorus, yttrium, or gold instilled into the pericardial space.[159]

Chemotherapy

The use of local or systemic chemicals to treat neoplastic cardiac tamponade has had varying degrees of success. Local treatment with chemotherapy involves the instillation of antineoplastic agents or sclerosing substances into the pericardial space through an indwelling pericardial catheter after drainage. Chemotherapeutic agents used include bleomycin, nitrogen mustard, 5-FU, methotrexate, and thiotepa. Tetracycline and quinacrine have also been instilled for their sclerosing properties. All these substances cause local inflammation and then fibrosis, which prevents collapse of the pericardial sac.[110,140,159] Lidocaine is usually instilled into the pericardial cavity before sclerosis for pain control.

The sclerosing technique most frequently used in-

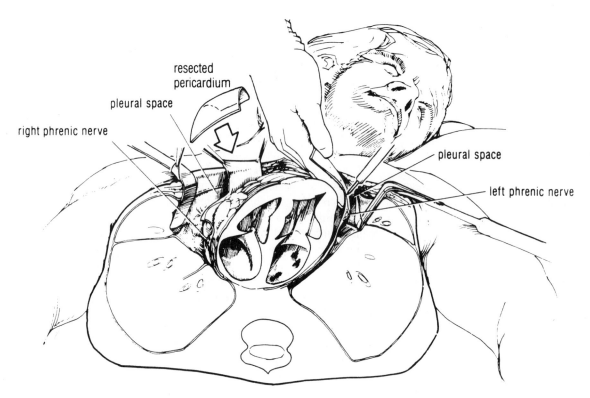

resected
pericardium

pleural space

right phrenic nerve

pleural space

left phrenic nerve

Figure 19-10   Pericardiectomy through a median sternotomy approach. (From Miller SE, Campbell DB: Malignant pericardial effusions. In Polomano RC, Miller SE, editors: *Understanding and managing oncologic emergencies,* Monograph, Columbus, Ohio, 1987, Adria Laboratories.)

volved the instillation of tetracycline (500 to 1000 mg) through the indwelling catheter. This is followed by a flush of normal saline. The procedure is repeated every 2 to 3 days. Sclerosis is considered successful when there is no drainage for a 24-hour period. Response to tetracycline sclerosing has not proved to be as effective as obliterative treatment for pleural effusions.[140,159]

Currently, injectable tetracycline has been discontinued by its manufacturer. Other sclerosing agents, such as bleomycin, minocycline, and doxycycline, have been used to treat malignant pleural effusion. However, few studies have been published regarding pericardial effusions. Recent reports have shown effective pericardial sclerosing with one instillation of bleomycin (30 to 60 mg) through a pericardial catheter 24 hours after the fluid has been evacuated. The tube is then clamped for 10 minutes and then withdrawn. No major side effects were noted except transient temperature elevation. Severe fibrosis of the pericardial sac was not reported or found at autopsy.[49,57,134]

Systemic chemotherapy may be given to responsive tumors such as lymphoma, breast cancer, or small (oat) cell carcinoma of the lung. This may be the initial treatment of a pericardial effusion when it is slow and the patient is asymptomatic. However, in acute neoplastic cardiac tamponade, systemic chemotherapy is done when the patient is clinically stable after pericardiocentesis.

PROGNOSIS

Survival of the patient with neoplastic cardiac tamponade depends on the cause of the primary malignancy, the stage of cancer at the time of intervention, tumor responsiveness to radiation therapy or chemotherapy, hemodynamic significance of the tamponade, effectiveness of therapy, and general medical condition of the patient. Response rate with local therapies is 50%, with duration of remission approximately 4 to 6 months.[110,139] Average survival, regardless of neoplastic cause, is reported at 16 months. Patients with breast cancer or Hodgkin's disease may survive for more than 2 years.[139] Even without tamponade, most patients with neoplastic-related pleural effusions do not live beyond 12 to 18 months.[72] Patients with effusions and tamponade related to radiation therapy may survive longer than any others. Although the overall prognosis of the patient may be poor, the spectacular response that is usually seen with the removal of pericardial fluid warrants aggressive action.

Nursing management of the patient with neoplastic cardiac tamponade is outlined on pp. 439-440.

NURSING MANAGEMENT

Nursing interventions for the patient with neoplastic cardiac tamponade are multifaceted and highly variable, depending on the acuteness of the patient's condition. Onset of tamponade may be impending and insidious or rapid and life-threatening. Knowledge of the patient's current and past history, coupled with astute physical assessment skills, is necessary.

Patients may be in a routine hospital unit or in the critical care area. Close monitoring of vital signs is of paramount importance. Nursing care is directed at maintaining optimal cardiopulmonary function and preventing circulatory collapse through immediate identifications and treatment of neoplastic cardiac tamponade.*

NURSING DIAGNOSES

- *Cardiac output, decreased, related to diastolic filling of the ventricles from compression of the heart*
- *Tissue perfusion, altered, related to decreased cardiac output*

OUTCOME GOAL

Patient will be able to:
- Maintain optimal cardiac output, as evidenced by relief of chest pain, vital signs within patient's normal limits, cardiac rhythm without dysrhythmias, central venous pressure (CVP) and pulmonary capillary wedge pressure (PCWP) within patient's normal limits, adequate intake and output, and laboratory values and diagnostic tests approaching normal levels.

INTERVENTIONS

- Assess hemodynamic and cardiovascular status:
  —Monitor blood pressure, pulse, CVP, and cardiac output.
  —Observe cardiac rhythm continuously (note abnormalities associated with cardiac tamponade: ST segment elevation, T-wave inversion, and electrical alterations).
  —Monitor heart sounds.
  —Assess extremities for color, temperature, and pulses.
- Assess respiratory status:
  —Observe breathing patterns (note abnormalities associated with cardiac tamponade: pulsus paradoxus, respiratory alkalosis, Kussmaul's sign, and hypoxemia).
  —Auscultate lungs for breath sounds.
- Observe skin temperature, color, and turgor.
- Monitor intake and output.
- Assess gastrointestinal status:
  —Measure abdominal girth and note any ascites.
  —Determine positive hepatojugular reflux.

---

*References 71, 79, 89, 108, 110, 140, 145, 146, 150.

- Assess neurologic status:
  —Determine orientation to person and place.
  —Assess responses to verbal and tactile stimuli.
  —Report any changes in level of consciousness.
- Monitor laboratory values and test results:
  —Electrolytes, with attention to Ca^{++} and K^+ because of the risk of cardiac dysrhythmias
  —ECG for changes
  —Echocardiogram
  —Chest x-ray film
- Reposition patient to enhance circulation. This must be done slowly to allow compensation for decreased cardiac output.
- Perform measures to reduce the workload of the heart:
  —Assist with all activities.
  —Schedule rest periods.
  —Use comfort measures (analgesics, repositioning, relaxation techniques, antianxiety medications).
- Administer vasoactive drugs as ordered.
- Be prepared for cardiac arrest and emergency resuscitation.

NURSING DIAGNOSIS

- *Gas exchange, impaired, related to decreased circulation and pulmonary congestion*

OUTCOME GOAL

Patient will be able to
- Achieve/Maintain adequate pulmonary function, as evidenced by vital signs within patient's normal limits, breath sounds and respiratory stable/improved, and activity tolerance within patient's normal limits.

INTERVENTIONS

- Monitor respiratory status:
  —Observe for signs and symptoms of respiratory difficulty (dyspnea, tachypnea, Kussmaul's sign, shortness of breath, air hunger).
  —Auscultate chest for breath sounds.
  —Monitor laboratory values (arterial blood gases, electrolytes, chest x-ray film).
- Assist with breathing and pulmonary toilet:
  —Position for comfort and enhanced chest expansion
  —Deep breathing and coughing every 2 hours
  —Frequent mouth care
  —Suctioning if needed
- Administer oxygen therapy and mechanical ventilation as prescribed.

NURSING DIAGNOSES

- *Injury, risk for, related to invasive procedures/surgery*
- *Trauma, risk for, related to invasive procedures/surgery*

Continued.

OUTCOME GOAL

Patient will be able to:
• Experience minimal side effects related to invasive procedure, as evidenced by adequate skin integrity, absence of or minimal bleeding, adequate respiratory function, and absence of infection.

INTERVENTIONS

• Assess patient for complications: bleeding, infection, atelectasis, pneumothorax, and pleural effusion.
• Check vital signs every 15 minutes for the first hour after procedure/surgery and continue frequently as indicated.
• Monitor respiratory status closely:
—Observe respirations for rate, rhythm, and depth.
—Note any difficulties.
—Auscultate chest for breath sounds and expansion.
• Observe monitoring equipment frequently for changes.
• Assess all catheters for patency and drainage, and observe site for signs of infection.
• Assess patient with care but encourage as much independence as possible.

SEPTIC SHOCK

DEFINITION

Shock comprises a group of diverse life-threatening syndromes that result from different pathophysiologic circumstances: decreased cardiac function, hemorrhage, trauma, antigen/antibody reaction, and sepsis. There are three major classifications of shock: hypovolemic, cardiogenic, and distributive or vasogenic. *Hypovolemic shock* is a result of decreased intravascular volume. *Cardiogenic shock* results from the heart's impaired ability to pump blood adequately. *Distributive shock* or *vasogenic shock* is the result of an abnormality in the vascular system. Included under distributive shock is neurogenic, anaphylactic, and septic shock.[129] The progression of septic shock produces a severe maldistribution of blood flow in the microcirculation. This leads to inadequate tissue perfusion, cellular ischemia, cellular hypoxia, and organ or system failure.[119,129] If not immediately treated and reversed, shock will result in death.[10,129,151]

Sepsis and its sequelae are a complex compilation of related pathophysiologic processes. In an attempt to elucidate information, concepts, and issues, a consensus conference was held in 1992 to formulate and publish a new set of definitions. The two groups involved were the American College of Chest Physicians and the Society of Critical Care Medicine. These combined efforts will provide education and structure for infection and sepsis management.[30,76]

Septic shock is a shock syndrome in response to sepsis. *Septicemia* is usually the result of a gram-negative bacterial infection or toxins produced by the bacteria. It is accompanied by a disseminated inflammatory response unrelated to the causative organism. Infection and sepsis are common causes of morbidity and the leading causes of death in patients with cancer. Approximately 30% to 90% of deaths in America's intensive care units are related to infection and sepsis.[17,64,76]

ETIOLOGY AND RISK FACTORS

Septic shock as a consequence of gram-negative bacteremia has been documented extensively in the literature.[10,64,76] The incidence of gram-negative sepsis in the United States is estimated at 300,000 to 800,000 cases per year, with a 75% mortality rate. When gram-negative sepsis progresses to septic shock, mortality increases to 85% to 90%.[30] Various microorganisms are responsible for the invasion of the bloodstream leading to sepsis and septic shock. The most predominant pathogens in patients with cancer are three gram-negative bacilli: *Escherichia coli, Klebsiella pneumoniae,* and *Pseudomonas aeruginosa.* Other bacteria (*Staphylococcus aureus, S. epidermidis*), viruses, fungi, protozoa, and rickettsiae are all potential pathogens for septicemia.[64,105] Mortality from septic shock has been estimated at 25% to 60% of reported cases of septicemia.[64] Among patients with cancer, the rate is 30% to 80%.[10,64,151] Infectious processes are the cause of death in at least 50% of patients with solid tumors.[151] In patients with uncontrolled leukemia and lymphoma who develop septic shock, death almost always follows 80% of the time.[105]

Patients with cancer are at increased risk of developing infection and subsequent septicemia because of the profound suppression of their normal body defense mechanisms. This suppression is caused by both host-related and treatment-related factors.[10,27,76] A decrease in host resistance permits tissue invasion by endogenous or exogenous flora.[4,27] Gram-negative bacteria, which are the most common infective microorganisms, are normally found in the mouth and GI tract, vagina, and feces and on the skin.[14]

Patterns of bacterial infections have changed over the years because of improved antibiotic therapy. β-Lactamase-resistant penicillins provided highly effective therapy against *S. aureus,* a gram-positive organism most frequently identified in immunocompromised patients in the 1950s and 1960s. Today the use of empiric combination antibiotic therapy, including third-generation cephalosporins, has greatly reduced the number of gram-negative infections. A recent resurgence of gram-positive infections is thought to be related to a prevalence of methicillin-resistant strains of *Staphylococcus.*

A particular infectious life-threatening condition seen in patients with cancer is *neutropenic enterocolitis,* also called *typhilitis,* an inflammation of the small intestine or colon. The exact pathologic etiology is unclear. However, it is proposed to be initiated by direct cytotoxic damage from chemotherapy, radiation therapy, or neoplastic infiltration. Disruption of mucosal integrity, alteration of normal gut flora, and lack of neutrophil response lead to invasion of the GI tract by bacteria, viruses, and fungi. The implicated organisms include gram-negative bacilli such as *Klebsiella, Pseudomonas, Escherichia coli, Candida,* and *Clostridium septicum.* Although *C. septicum* is not a flora, which is normally found in the gut, it may appear after the use of multiple antibiotics, which alter the normal gut flora. Neutropenic enterocolitis can lead to septic shock. Mortality rates have been estimated to be greater than 50%.[147]

The factors that predispose a patient with cancer to infection and sepsis can be categorized according to the precipitating event, site of infection, and pathogen (Table 19-4; see box, p. 443).[62,64,76] Each of the events that may initiate an infection leading to septic shock is a consequence of the underlying cancer and/or its treatment. All four treatment modalities (surgery, radiation therapy, chemotherapy, biotherapy) can result in profound suppression of host defense mechanisms. Monitoring the patient for effects of tumor growth and side effects of therapy is crucial to preventing septic shock.

PATHOPHYSIOLOGY

Septic shock is a complex interaction of hemodynamic, humoral, cellular, and metabolic abnormalities.[10,22,23] This is a result of the effects of the proliferation of gram-negative bacteria and/or the release of endotoxins by those bacteria (Figure 19-11). *Endotoxin* is a component of the cellular wall of gram-negative bacteria and, when released, activates the coagulation complement and kinin systems.[10,64] This toxin-induced reaction activates the humoral cellular and immunologic defense mechanisms, leading to a generalized inflammatory response.[22,23,64] Evidence of this response is the production of various chemical mediators, such as prostaglandins, endorphins, and kinins, which modulate the variety of multisystem alterations seen in septic shock.[64,105]

Current research has been better able to delineate several of the endogenously produced biochemical mediators and their associated mechanism of action that results in the deleterious effects of sepsis. *Tumor necrosis factor* (TNF) appears to be one of the more important mediators. Other newly discovered endogenous mediators include the cytokines Interleukin-1 (IL-1), IL-2, IL-3,

IL-4, IL-6, and IL-8 and *macrophage-derived procoagulant and inflammatory cytokine* (MPIC). Most of these mediators have a useful function in homeostasis. Investigators are just beginning to understand the reason for their adverse effect in sepsis and septic shock.[17] The pathophysiology of septic shock (Figure 19-12) are summarized next.[10,22,23,64,105]

Hemodynamic Instability

Abnormal coagulation occurs through a variety of processes initiated by the gram-negative bacteria. It damages the endothelial lining of the capillaries, which is the site of thrombus formation. The bacteria attach to the erythrocytes (RBCs), producing an antigen-antibody reaction. Hemolysis results, and microhemorrhagic lesions appear in major organs. Clotting factor XII (Hageman factor) is activated by the bacteria. This initiates the clotting mechanisms, causing the formation of microthrombi and, at the same time, fibrinolysis for clot dissolution. The result is consumption of clotting factors (consumptive coagulopathy) and platelets (thrombocytopenia). The final outcome of all of these processes is *disseminated intravascular coagulation* (DIC)—simultaneous hemorrhage and thrombosis.[105]

Cardiovascular alteration is present during shock in two different patterns. Initially, cardiac output is higher than normal but still inadequate to supply the peripheral blood vessels because of massive vasodilation. Later, cardiac output is low, accompanied by severe vasoconstriction.[64]

Humoral and Cellular Alterations

The microcirculation is grossly altered through a variety of mechanisms attributed to the production of several vasoactive mediators: bradykinin, histamine, and serotonin (see Figure 19-11). The bacterial endotoxin is responsible for the activation of factor XII, which in turn initiates the release of bradykinin, a potent vasodilator. The complement system is also activated by the endotoxin, which causes the release of histamine and serotonin. These substances produce vasodilation or vasoconstriction depending on the status of the circulation.[17,21-23]

Changes in the microcirculation occur as the arterioles dilate and the venules constrict, resulting in increased vascular permeability. In response to this, the internal cellular sodium-potassium pump is hampered, and water accumulates in the cells, causing them to swell. Secretion of antidiuretic hormone (ADH) and aldosterone increases sodium and water retention. Capillary pressure increases, and plasma oncotic pressure changes and allows intravascular fluid to leak to the extravascular space. This fluid shift into the interstitial spaces occurs throughout the body. Insufficient blood perfusion to peripheral tissues results from the impaired microcirculation. This leads to cellular hypoxia and death. The lungs

Table 19–4 Factors Predisposing Cancer Patients to Infection

Precipitating event	Common site of infection	Common organism
Local effects of tumor growth or treatment		
Skin or mucous membrane breakdown	Cancer or treatment of skin, head and neck, gastrointestinal tract, female genital tract	Locally colonizing organisms
Obstruction of natural passages (obstructive phenomenon)	Solid tumors or treatment of cancer (especially pulmonary, biliary, and urinary tracts)	Locally colonizing organisms
Alterations in microbial flora	All cancer sites or treatment of cancer (especially pulmonary, gastrointestinal)	Locally colonizing organisms
Stasis of blood and body fluids secondary to obstruction or inactivity	All cancer sites or treatment of cancer	Locally colonizing organisms
Central nervous system dysfunction (brain tumors, spinal cord tumors, metabolic abnormalities)	Pulmonary (aspiration pneumonia) Urinary tract	Locally colonizing organisms
Hyposplenism secondary to neoplastic infiltration or splenectomy	Disseminated	Bacteria: *Streptococcus pneumoniae, Neisseria meningitidis, Escherichia coli, Haemophilus influenzae, Clostridium difficile, Staphylococcus* species
Granulocytopenia (neutropenia) prevalent with acute leukemia	Skin lesions, thrombophlebitis, pulmonary (pneumonia), sinuses, pharynx, esophagus, colon, perianal	Gram-negative bacilli: *E. coli, Pseudomonas aeruginosa, Klebsiella pneumoniae, Staphylococcus aureus* Yeasts: *Candida* Filamentous fungi: *Aspergillus* species, agents of mycomycosis
Cellular immune dysfunction (T-cell immune alteration) prevalent with lymphoma	Disseminated	Bacteria: *Listeria monocytogenes, Salmonella* species, *Mycobacterium* species, *Nocardia asteroides, Legionella* Fungi: *Cryptococcus neoformans, Histoplasma capsulatum, Coccidioides immitis* Viruses: *Varicella zoster,* cytomegalovirus, herpes simplex Protozoa: *Pneumocystis carinii, Toxoplasma gondii, Cryptosporidium* Helminths: *Strongyloides stercoralis*
Humoral immune dysfunction (B-cell immune alteration) prevalent with multiple myeloma	Disseminated	*S. pneumoniae, H. influenzae*
Iatrogenic factors (invasive procedures, devices, equipment) Diagnostic procedures (barium enema, endoscopies), urinary catheterization Genitourinary tract manipulations Bone marrow aspirations Biopsies Placement of shunts, stents, and tubes Venipuncture Long-term venous access devices Respiratory assist devices	Skin Mucous membranes	*Staphylococcus epidermidis* Locally colonizing organisms
Nosocomial sources		
Air	Pulmonary	*Aspergillus* species
Surface contact	Skin and mucous membranes	*S. aureus*
Food (fresh fruits and vegetables)		Bacteria, fungi
Water (humidifiers, respiratory devices, flowers, water pitchers, faucet aerators, skin drains, shower heads, ice machines)	Disseminated	*P. aeruginosa, Serratia marcescens*
Medical personnel (illness, organism transmission or cross-contamination, poor handwashing)	Various	Locally colonizing organisms
Extended prophylactic use of broad-spectrum antibiotic therapy (superinfection secondary to overgrowth of resistant strains)	Disseminated	Bacteria

FACTORS PREDISPOSING TO INFECTION IN PATIENTS WITH CANCER

GRANULOCYTOPENIA (E.G., ACUTE LEUKEMIA)
Sites of infection

Pneumonia
Perianal lesions
Pharyngitis
Skin lesions
Esophagitis

Most common pathogens

Gram-negative bacilli
  Escherichia coli
  Pseudomonas aeruginosa
  Klebsiella pneumoniae
  Staphylococcus aureus
Yeasts
  Candida
Filamentous fungi
  Aspergillus species
  Agents of mucormycosis

CELLULAR IMMUNE DYSFUNCTION (E.G., LYMPHOMA)
Common organisms

Bacteria
  Listeria monocytogenes
  Salmonella species
  Mycobacterium sp
  Nocardia asteroides
  Legionella
Fungi
  Cryptococcus neoformans
  Histoplasma capsulatum
  Coccidioides immitis
Viruses
  Varicella zoster
  Cytomegalovirus
  Herpes simplex
Protozoa
  Pneumocystis carinii
  Toxoplasma gondii
  Cryptosporidium
Helminths
  Strongyloides stercoralis

HUMORAL IMMUNE DYSFUNCTION (E.G., MULTIPLE MYELOMA)
Common organisms

Streptococcus pneumoniae
Haemophilus influenzae

OBSTRUCTIVE PHENOMENA (E.G., SOLID TUMORS)
Common sites

Respiratory tract
Biliary tract
Urinary tract

Common organisms

Locally colonizing

CENTRAL NERVOUS SYSTEM DYSFUNCTION (E.G., BRAIN TUMORS)
Common sites

Pneumonitis
Urinary tract infection

Common organisms

Locally colonizing

IATROGENIC PROCEDURES

Disruption or bypassing of anatomic barriers
Indwelling venous or arterial catheters
  Bacteremia
Indwelling urinary catheters
  Urinary tract infection
Respiratory assist devices
  Pneumonia
  Immunosuppression
  Chemotherapy, surgery, radiation

ALTERATIONS IN MICROBIAL FLORA

Underlying illness
Stasis
Antibiotics

ACQUISITION OF POTENTIAL PATHOGENS

Air
  Aspergillus species
Water
  P. aeruginosa
  Serratia marcescens
Contact
  S. aureus

From Joshi J: *Mediguide Infect Dis* 9(2):2, 1989.

are a target organ for dysfunction because of the fluid shifts and cellular hypoxia. Marked changes occur in lung compliance and gas exchange. Consequently, patients in septic shock may develop pulmonary edema and adult respiratory distress syndrome (ARDS).

Metabolic Dysfunction

A variety of metabolic alterations take place during septic shock (Figure 19-12). There is a mobilization of energy stores, producing a conversion of carbohydrate (glucose), fat, and protein to energy. Gluconeogenesis (en-

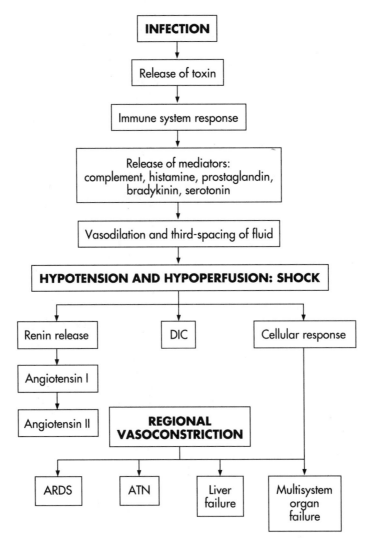

Figure 19-11   Pathophysiology of septic shock. (From McMorrow ME, Cooney-Daniello M: *RN* 54[10]:32, 1991. [Published in *RN*; copyright (c) 1991, *Medical Economics,* Montvale, NJ].)

dogenous production of glucose) occurs, but there is a progressive inability to utilize the energy stores. Protein catabolism leads to a negative nitrogen balance. Tissues are unable to receive oxygen or nutrients because of impaired blood flow. There is a shift from oxidative metabolism to anaerobic metabolism. Lactic acid accumulates in the blood and leads to metabolic acidosis. To compensate, hyperventilation occurs, leading to respiratory alkalosis. The depletion of cellular energy and inhibition of protein synthesis lead to cellular death and major organ failure.[17,21-23]

Septic shock results from a maldistribution of blood flow. Microcirculatory alterations are caused by endotoxin produced by the invading pathogen, which is usually gram-negative bacteria. As shock progresses, there is inadequate tissue perfusion of somatic cells of major systems or organs. System malfunction can result in DIC,

ARDS, and acute tubular necrosis (ATN). When capillary occlusion occurs for longer than 2 hours, the cells in that area do not receive adequate nutrition or oxygen, and cellular death results.[119] Cellular death causes organ failure and is ultimately fatal.

The process of septic shock is complex and its progress can be rapid (Figure 19-12). The progression of shock depends on several factors, including the following[51,119]:

- The patient's physical condition before the onset of the incident
- Duration of the shock state
- Effectiveness of treatment
- Correction of reversible causes (infection and sepsis)

Although sepsis is a triggering process that can lead to shock, attention should be given to several other treatable causes of shock: hemorrhage, trauma, or a reduc-

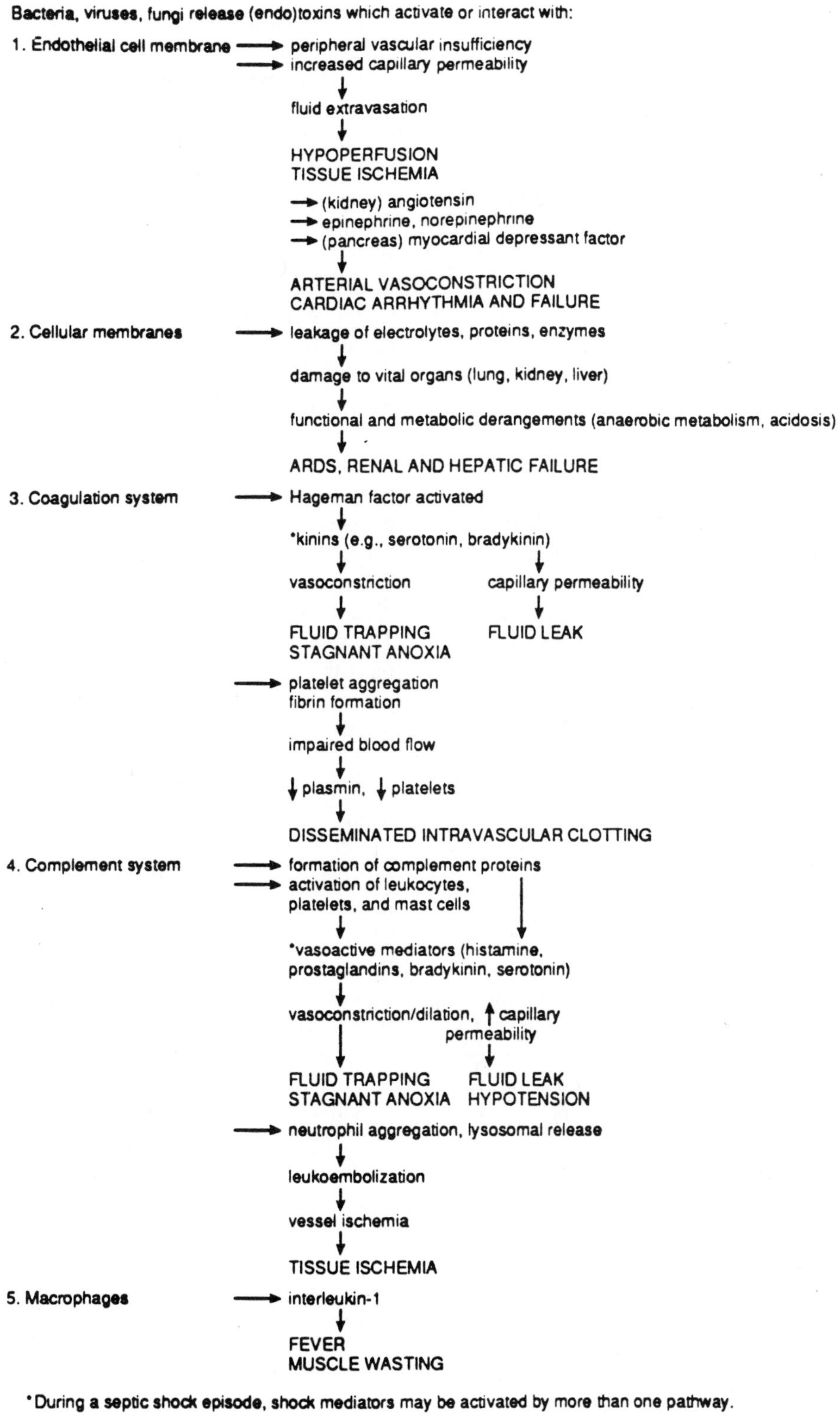

Bacteria, viruses, fungi release (endo)toxins which activate or interact with:

1. Endothelial cell membrane ⟶ peripheral vascular insufficiency
⟶ increased capillary permeability
↓
fluid extravasation
↓
HYPOPERFUSION
TISSUE ISCHEMIA

⟶ (kidney) angiotensin
⟶ epinephrine, norepinephrine
⟶ (pancreas) myocardial depressant factor
↓
ARTERIAL VASOCONSTRICTION
CARDIAC ARRHYTHMIA AND FAILURE

2. Cellular membranes ⟶ leakage of electrolytes, proteins, enzymes
↓
damage to vital organs (lung, kidney, liver)
↓
functional and metabolic derangements (anaerobic metabolism, acidosis)
↓
ARDS, RENAL AND HEPATIC FAILURE

3. Coagulation system ⟶ Hageman factor activated
↓
*kinins (e.g., serotonin, bradykinin)
↓   ↓
vasoconstriction   capillary permeability
↓   ↓
FLUID TRAPPING   FLUID LEAK
STAGNANT ANOXIA

⟶ platelet aggregation
fibrin formation
↓
impaired blood flow
↓
↓ plasmin, ↓ platelets
↓
DISSEMINATED INTRAVASCULAR CLOTTING

4. Complement system ⟶ formation of complement proteins
⟶ activation of leukocytes,
platelets, and mast cells
↓
*vasoactive mediators (histamine,
prostaglandins, bradykinin, serotonin)
↓
vasoconstriction/dilation, ↑ capillary
permeability
↓   ↓
FLUID TRAPPING   FLUID LEAK
STAGNANT ANOXIA   HYPOTENSION

⟶ neutrophil aggregation, lysosomal release
↓
leukoembolization
↓
vessel ischemia
↓
TISSUE ISCHEMIA

5. Macrophages ⟶ interleukin-1
↓
FEVER
MUSCLE WASTING

*During a septic shock episode, shock mediators may be activated by more than one pathway.

Figure 19-12 Pathophysiology of septic shock. (From Harnett S: *Cancer Nurs* 12[4]:191, 1989.)

tion in cardiac function. Consideration should also be given to other situations that are frequently overlooked as possible causes of shock, including the following[99,119]:

- Inadequate infusion of fluids
- Inadequate ventilation
- Unrecognized pneumothorax
- Pulmonary emboli
- Previous prolonged treatment with antihypertensive drugs
- Cardiac tamponade
- Acid-base abnormalities
- Adrenal insufficiency
- Hypothermia

CLINICAL FEATURES

The signs and symptoms of septic shock vary with the stage of shock manifested by the patient. Some patients progress from early to late shock; others appear in late shock initially.[1,2,40] Complications and major organ failure may be prevented if shock is detected early and treated immediately.

There are several ways to classify the stages of shock. A three-stage classification is particularly useful.[17] The box, p. 447, lists the clinical findings associated with each stage. Once a patient has entered stage three shock, he or she will not respond to treatment. Multiple organ failure occurs, leading to death.

DIAGNOSIS

The diagnosis of septic shock depends critically on astute observations of the patient. Sepsis may or may not have been confirmed. An initial finding could be a subtle patient complaint of "just not feeling right." Physical assessment of all systems is crucial and should be correlated with a brief recent history highlighting any changes and noting any possible sources of infection. Continuous assessment and monitoring of the patient is essential. This includes taking vital signs, observing tissue perfusion, watching for signs of bleeding, checking mental status, and assessing heart, lung, and kidney function.[21,64,136]

Initial testing includes a chest x-ray film, 12-lead ECG, and blood work (CBC, chemistry panel). Other laboratory tests should include coagulation studies, cardiac and liver enzymes, urinalysis, ABGs, and various culture and sensitivity testing (e.g., blood, urine, sputum, wound).

Blood samples should be drawn *before* the initiation of antibiotic therapy. Usually, three samples are ordered to be drawn at 15-minute intervals from two different sites. Multiple interval sampling is based on the theory that bacteria are released into the bloodstream in bursts,

and this method increases the chances that bacteria will appear in the sampled blood specimen. Dual-site sampling decreases the possibility of a contaminated venipuncture procedure.[136]

The following findings could assist in the diagnosis of sepsis:
Chest x-ray film—pulmonary infiltrates
ECG—dysrhythmias
Urine—glycosuria, elevated specific gravity, increased urinary sodium
WBC count—low (leukopenia)
Platelet count—low (thrombocytopenia)
Coagulation profile—fibrinogen levels decreased, FDPs elevated, PT and partial PT prolonged
Serum glucose—elevated
Serum lactate—elevated

Careful evaluation of the febrile patient is important. *Fever* is classically the telltale sign of infection. Contrary to popular myth, fever is present in immunocompromised and neutropenic patients, including those with cancer. Elevated temperature is produced in the body by the monocytes, not the neutrophils. Some monocytes migrate into body tissue, where they become macrophages. The monocyte secretes an endogenous pyrogen that affects the thalamus, which houses the body's temperature control, resulting in a rise in temperature[62,136] (see Chapter 30).

Infections are especially difficult to evaluate in the presence of neutropenia. When organisms have been isolated from these patients, 80% are from their own body flora.[139] Patients with neutropenia and an infection or sepsis have fever, but they may not have other signs of inflammation, such as ulceration, fissure, and exudate. These signs are greatly diminished, since there are little to no granulocytes (WBCs) to produce the inflammatory process. Erythema and pain will be present if the infection is localized. However, fever is the most important clinical sign of infection in a patient with neutropenia.[62,139]

Febrile episodes in the patient with granulocytopenia or neutropenia are indicative of infection 60% to 80% of the time.[62,74,76] In patients with cancer whose granulocyte counts are normal, fever usually results from causes other than infection. These include tumor-associated fever (hepatoma, renal cell carcinoma, childhood sarcoma), chemotherapeutic agents (bleomycin, cytosine arabinoside [cytarabine, ARA-C], high-dose methotrexate), blood product transfusions, radiation therapy, and TNF.[74]

TREATMENT MODALITIES

The identified stage of septic shock will dictate the necessary medical interventions. Prompt medical treatment is essential to prevent progression of shock syndrome to

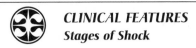

CLINICAL FEATURES
Stages of Shock

Stage one: hyperdynamic stage (early shock, warm shock)
Decreased tissue perfusion: 10% reduction in blood volume
Usually lasts less than 24 hours
Feelings of anxiety, apprehension, nervousness
Complaints of nausea
Altered mental status, restlessness, irritability, disorientation, inappropriate euphoria
Temperature normal, below normal, or above normal
Skin warm and flushed because of arteriole dilation
Peripheral cyanosis
Tachycardia and bounding peripheral pulses
Normal or slightly elevated blood pressure with a widening pulse pressure
Tachypnea, hyperventilation
Rales and decreased breath sounds
Respiratory alkalosis: decreased oxygen pressure
Renal output normal or elevated (polyuria)
Blood urea nitrogen and creatinine may be slowly increasing
Hyperglycemia
Urine may test positive for sugar (glycosuria)
Urine specific gravity normal
No signs of bleeding
Coagulation profile normal
Stage two: normodynamic stage (intermediate shock, cool shock)
Decreased tissue perfusion: 15% to 20% reduction in blood volume
Usually lasts a few hours
Complains of thirst
Altered mental status: lethargy, confusion
Skin pale, cool, and clammy because of peripheral vasoconstriction and diversion of blood to vital organs
Peripheral edema possible because of increased secretion of antidiuretic hormone and aldosterone leading to sodium and water
    retention
Temperature normal or subnormal
Tachycardia continues
Blood pressure decreases with a narrow pulse pressure because of decrease in cardiac output
Respirations slow and shallow
Respiratory acidosis
Renal output decreased (oliguria)
Urine specific gravity elevated
Abdominal distention because of air swallowing and decreased peristalsis
Hemorrhagic lesions may be apparent
Stage three: hypodynamic stage (late shock, refractory shock, irreversible shock, cold shock, "classic" shock)
Decreased cardiac output, decrease in blood volume
Altered mental status, stupor, coma
Skin cold, possible cyanosis of digits and mottling
Temperature subnormal
Tachycardia
Weak or absent pulses because of decreased myocardial contractility: "pump failure"
Hypotension
Respiratory depression
Pulmonary edema, or "shock lung," because of decreased oxygen pressure and decreased pulmonary microcirculatory adult
    respiratory distress syndrome
Metabolic acidosis because of anaerobic metabolism and increased levels of lactic acid
Hypoglycemia
No renal output (anuria)
Renal failure: acute tubular necrosis
Hemorrhagic lesions

the irreversible stage and subsequent death. Most patients in septic shock are transferred to the intensive care unit (ICU) for close observation and invasive hemodynamic monitoring. Recognition of the signs and symptoms of shock and the determination of sepsis are the first medical interventions.

The underlying infection, if determined, should be treated. Initial antibiotic therapy is tailored to the specific organisms identified in the culture and sensitivity reports. Various procedures, including surgery, may also be indicated to treat the infection. Antibiotic therapy should be initiated within 1 hour of the appearance of the signs and symptoms of shock.[64,74] Broad-spectrum antibiotics (cephalosporins, gentamicin, aminoglycosides) are the drugs of choice until the specific pathogens responsible can be identified, which usually takes at least 24 hours.

Regardless of the infection site, antimicrobial therapy should be initiated at the earliest possible time. Generally, two broad-spectrum antibiotics are the initial treatment because (1) the causative microorganisms are often unidentified at the start of therapy; (2) the patient may harbor more than one organism; and (3) a synergistic effect often occurs between the antimicrobials agents.[17,72] Two-drug therapy may not always be warranted, such as if the patient has not been recently hospitalized and nosocomial infections are not an issue. Then a single extended-spectrum penicillin or a first- or second-generation cephalosporin may effectively control the infection.[72] The current recommended drug combination is an aminoglycoside and either an antipseudomonal penicillin or a third-generation cephlasporin. Antipseudomonal penicillins are effective against most bacteria, but some may not cover the penicillin-producing or methicillin-resistant staphylococci. Also, the higher the generation of cephalosporin, the less effective is the drug against gram-positive organisms.[17,74]

Additional blood work is ordered depending on the stage of shock. The first stage of shock would indicate testing for elevated catecholamine and cortisol levels. Later stages would indicate screening for the coagulopathies related to DIC.

Restoration of hemodynamic status is a major challenge in the treatment of septic shock.[4,10] Blood volume replacement is achieved through the use of IV fluids and plasma expanders. Blood transfusions may be warranted. Blood pressure and cardiac output are restored with the administration of vasoactive drugs and inotropic agents. The progress of therapy is determined by clinical aspects of the patient's status through intensive observation and monitoring.

The provision of optimal oxygenation often requires respiratory assistance.[64] Oxygen and respiratory therapy may be ordered. Mechanical ventilation may be necessary. These measures manage the metabolic acidosis seen in septic shock. The blood gas level of pH should be 7.35 to 7.45, and the oxygen partial pressure (Po_2) should be kept at 80 to 100 mm Hg.

Fluid and electrolyte balance must be maintained and any metabolic abnormalities corrected. Urine output should be at least 50 ml/hour. Serum chemistry levels are done at least daily to evaluate renal function. Aminoglycoside antibiotics and various chemotherapeutic agents can compromise renal function, warranting a potential change in therapy.[4,27]

Aggressive nutritional support is necessary for the patient with metabolic abnormalities and helps prevent tissue breakdown.[22,23] Recent studies have demonstrated close association between TNF and cachexia.[81] Close attention must be paid to the monitoring and administration of glucose because glucose uptake may be impaired. The body's compensatory mechanisms hamper glucose uptake as a result of insulin inhibition by the hormones responding to the stress response.[136] Protein and nutrient supplements are needed to meet the high energy demands of septic shock and to promote the healing process.

Steroid therapy is often administered to the patient in septic shock. The doses are extremely high, and it is important to observe the patient closely for potential side effects, especially GI bleeding and mental changes. The steroids are given to decrease the inflammatory response, neutralize the endotoxin, protect the cell membrane and structure from the endotoxin, increase cardiac contractility, and enhance cellular glucose metabolism.[21,22]

The administration of hematopoietic growth factors, which mediate the production, maturation, regulation, and activation of various blood cells (granulocytes, monocytes, macrophages, lymphocytes, erythrocytes, platelets), may help to prevent septicemia. These growth factors are commonly referred to as colony-stimulating factors (CSFs) because they stimulate the growth of colonies of maturing blood cells from these hematopoietic precursors. Classified as cytokines, the CSFs are a group of naturally occurring glycoproteins. Each CSF affects a major cell lineage and has been given the following respective name:

- Granulocyte-macrophage colony-stimulating factor (GM-CSF)
- Granulocyte colony-stimulating factor (G-CSF)
- Macrophage colony-stimulating factor (M-CSF)
- Pleuripoietin interleukin-3 (IL-3) or multicolony-stimulating factor (multi-CSF)
- Erythrocyte colony stimulating factor (erythropoietin)

The exact mechanism of action of the CSFs is unknown. However, the effects of one factor appear to cross over on the others. The growth factors hold a promising future in the treatment of immunosuppression, anemia, and thrombocytopenia that result from disease states (neoplasia, myelodysplasia, congenital neutropenia, acquired immunodeficiency syndrome [AIDS]) and treatment-induced states (high-dose chemotherapy and radiation therapy). Improving bone marrow recovery may decrease infection-related morbidity and mortality. Dosage, route, and schedule for the administration of the CSFs are being investigated (see Chapter 23).[25,37,81]

The use of investigational agents such as naloxone (an opiate antagonist), human antiserum, and endotoxin has been reported.[62] However, results are preliminary. More research is needed on these agents and on the role of shock mediators such as prostaglandins, complement, and TNF.[64]

Experimental nonantibiotic therapies are being investigated as possible adjunctive treatment for septic shock, including the following[21-23,30,92]:
- Opioid antagonists
- NSAIDs
- Prostaglandin E_1
- Pentoxifylline
- Leukotriene inhibitors
- Protease inhibitors
- Phosphodiesterase inhibitors
- IL-1 receptor antagonist
- Surfactant replacement antagonists
- Antioxidants
- Antibodies to endotoxins
- Platelet activating factor (PAF)
- Monoclonal antiendotoxins
- Monoclonal antibodies to TNF

The mainstay of treatment for septic shock is antibiotic therapy. Additional treatment for septic shock has been summarized by the acronym VIP: *V,* ventilate (provide oxygen); *I,* infuse (administer solutions to maintain an adequate blood pressure); and *P,* perfuse (administer vasopressor therapy to improve cardiac output).[108] In the late stages of shock, additional management measures are aimed at the treatment of DIC, ARDS, and ATN.

PROGNOSIS

Mortality from septic shock is as high as 75% despite advanced technology and new treatment modalities.[10,27,51] Survival depends on preventing or reversing the process of shock and on the status of the underlying disease (nonfatal, ultimately fatal, rapidly fatal). Remarkably, 60% of all patients survive warm shock, and 40% survive cool or cold shock.[64] Prompt recognition and treatment of septic shock can mean the difference between life and death.

Nursing management of the patient in septic shock is outlined on pp. 450-452.

SPINAL CORD COMPRESSION

DEFINITION

A neoplasm in the epidural space can encroach on the spinal cord or cauda equina and result in spinal cord compression (SCC). SCC is a medical emergency requiring early detection and prompt treatment. Although it is rarely fatal, it can result in permanent neurologic deficits or other complications that increase mortality.[114,120]

ETIOLOGY AND RISK FACTORS

A malignant tumor compressing the spinal cord can be a primary or secondary etiology. *Primary* spinal cord tumors arise from the parenchyma of the spinal cord or from tissues that constitute or are contained within the surrounding spinal canal (e.g., bone, meninges, nerves, fat, blood vessels). This group makes up 34% of all spinal growths and *only 3% of SCC. Secondary* spinal cord tumors account for 66% of spinal tumors and arise from metastatic deposits from other body sites.[7,113,120] The common mechanisms by which neoplasms impinge on the spinal cord are metastatic, extramedullary, and osteogenic. Although collapsed vertebrae can cause spinal cord compression, the most frequent process to occur is metastasis to the bone resulting in bone erosion, which allows tumor growth to compress directly the spinal cord or the spinal roots. Metastatic hematopoietic mechanisms account for a much smaller portion of SCC.[7,20]

Bone metastases in patients with cancer are extremely common, second only to pulmonary metastases in frequency of occurrence. The overall incidence of bony metastases is approximately 85%.[25] Cancers of the lung, breast, and prostate account for most skeletal involvement. Following closely are renal carcinoma, lymphoma, and myeloma.

Although lymphoma has a high incidence of SCC, it has declined over the past decade because of the use of aggressive radiation therapy early in the treatment of lymphoma. Lymphomas compress the cord by direct extension through the intervertebral foramina, which is the target area for radiotherapy.[40]

Metastatic bony lesions most frequently involve the thoracic and lumbar spine. The location of epidural metastasis and cord compression is related to the origin of the primary cancer and influenced by vascular supply and venous drainage.[38,40] The ribs, sternum, humerus, femur, and skull are also common areas of disease spread.[6] It has been noted that in 35% of all patients with SCC, this complication was the first evidence of cancer.[7]

The frequency of SCC in patients with systemic cancer is approximately 5% to 10%.[7] This figure may be rising because of the prolongation of life and the increased incidence of the cancers responsible for its occurrence.

Primary small cell lung cancer is the most common cause of SCC in men; in women it is breast cancer. Therefore those at risk for SCC are those with a known bone metastasis or with a cancer that has a greater potential for skeletal involvement (lung, breast, prostate,

NURSING MANAGEMENT

The nursing care of a patient with sepsis varies with the identified stage of septic shock. Infection and sepsis have a high correlation with neutropenia.[4,27,64] Patients at highest risk are those whose neutrophil count is less than $100/mm^3$ for more than 3 weeks.[4,64] Therefore the first nursing goal in the management of septic shock is prevention of infection. The following general measures outline the nursing care for the patient with neutropenia. Complete reverse isolation, although it reduces exogenous colonization, is no longer recommended for patients with neutropenia, since endogenous flora are the major source of infection. Thus current practice is to use protective isolation.

NURSING DIAGNOSIS*

- *Infection (sepsis), risk for, related to neutropenia*

OUTCOME GOALS

Patient will be able to:
- Remain infection free, as evidenced by temperature within normal limits, laboratory values within normal limits, and absence of inflammation.
- Demonstrate knowledge related to prevention of infection.
- Identify/demonstrate adequate nutrition and fluid intake.
- Identify/demonstrate appropriate hygenic measures.
- Alter environmental risk factors.
- Verbalize signs and symptoms to report to health care team.

INTERVENTIONS

- Observe for signs and symptoms of infection:
  —Monitor vital signs at least every shift. An elevated temperature and changes in blood pressure, pulse, and respiration may be the only sign of an impending infection, since neutropenic patients have a diminished inflammatory response.[4,27]
  —Observe for other general signs and symptoms of infection/sepsis: nausea, abdominal discomfort, changes in renal status, irritability, and changes in mental status.
  —Assess blood counts daily or every other day to determine the onset of infection, recovery of the bone marrow, status of renal function, and possible need to change antibiotic regimen. This should include complete blood count (CBC) with differential, platelet count, and chemistry panel.[4,27]

- Prevent cross-contamination:
  —Place patient in a disinfected private room.
  —Provide care first to patients with neutropenia before caring for other patients.
  —Do not care for both patients with neutropenia and patients with infection.
  —Wash hands consistently and thoroughly after each patient contact.
- Prevent disease transmission:
  —Educate patient, staff, and visitors on all aspects of infection prophylaxis.
  —Screen personnel and visitors. Patient should not be exposed to anyone with an infection, recent vaccination, or recent exposure to a communicable disease (e.g., bacterial infections, herpes, colds, influenza, chickenpox, measles).[4,27]
  —Limit the number of visitors.
- Eliminate possible sources of infection.
  —Provide a neutropenic diet (microbiotic diet) that eliminates unpared fresh fruits and raw vegetables. All food items should be cooked.
  —Avoid the placement of fresh fruits, flowers, or plants in patient's room.
  —Change water to prevent stagnation (e.g., denture cups, water pitchers, humidifiers, respiratory equipment, irrigation containers).
- Maintain integrity of the skin and mucous membranes:
  —Inspect patient's body daily with attention to the mouth, all orifices, all skin folds, and any site of an IV catheter insertion, a tube insertion, or a wound. Change dressings at least every other day using occlusive materials.
  —Instruct patient and provide assistance in meticulous skin and mouth care. Provide lubrications to prevent dryness and cracking. Female patients should also keep the vaginal area clean and lubricated.
  —Prevent trauma to the skin and mucous membranes by avoiding intramuscular or subcutaneous injections whenever possible; rectal manipulations, as with enemas, suppositories, or thermometers; urinary catheterization; and douching and using tampons with the female patient. If urinary catheterization is necessary, maintain a closed sterile drainage system.
  —Avoid rectal trauma by preventing constipation with dietary measures or stool softeners.
- Assess respiratory status:
  —Auscultate lungs at least every shift.
  —Encourage mobility and frequent deep breathing and coughing.
- Provide nutritional support:
  —Assess patient's food preferences.

---

*References 21, 22, 51, 72, 129, 132.

—Administer nutrition (oral, tube feeding, or parenteral) to meet increased nutrition demands.

—Encourage and provide high-calorie, high-protein food items.

—Obtain dietitian consultation.

—Measure weight every day.

—Monitor laboratory values to assess for protein wasting, with particular attention to serum albumin level. Encourage fluid intake up to 3000 ml/day.

—Ensure patient conserves energy.

NURSING DIAGNOSES

• *Tissue perfusion, altered, related to response to release of endotoxins*
• *Cardiac output, decreased, related to decreased cardiac function*

OUTCOME GOALS

Patient will be able to:
• Maintain adequate tissue perfusion, as evidenced by vital signs within patient's normal limits, laboratory values and diagnostic tests approaching normal levels, and respiratory function within patient's normal limits.
• Maintain optimal cardiac output, as evidenced by relief of chest pain, vital signs within patient's normal limits, cardiac rhythm without dysrhythmias, central venous pressure (CVP) and pulmonary capillary wedge pressure (PCWP) within patient's normal limits, and adequate intake and output.

INTERVENTIONS

• Monitor vital signs (temperature, pulse, blood pressure, respirations) every 4 hours.
• If hypotension is present, place patient flat in bed or in Trendelenburg position.
• Assess skin color, temperature, and moisture every 4 hours.
• Assess organ systems for malfunctions from ischemia.
• Monitor ECG for evidence of dysrhythmias.
• Monitor laboratory values closely.
• Obtain specimens for cultures and sensitivities as ordered:
  —Blood samples are usually taken two times, 4 hours apart.
  —Check urine, stool, throat, and sputum or any draining wound, intravenous catheter, or tube insertion site.
• Administer antibiotics as ordered. Observe patient closely for possible toxicities; nephrotoxicity and neurotoxicities are prevalent with the use of aminoglycosides (e.g., tobramycin, gentamicin).
• Provide oxygen therapy as prescribed.
• Administer vasopressive drugs as ordered.

• Administer pain medication as ordered
• Control fever:
  —Administer antipyretic medications such as acetaminophen.
  —Lower room temperature.
  —Use sponge bath with tepid water.
  —Use hypothermia blanket.
• Monitor laboratory values with attention to K^+, blood urea nitrogen, and creatinine.

NURSING DIAGNOSES

• *Breathing pattern, ineffective, related to pulmonary edema and metabolic acidosis*
• *Gas exchange, impaired, related to circulatory collapse and pulmonary edema*

OUTCOME GOALS

Patient will be able to:
• Maintain effective breathing pattern, as evidenced by chest clear to auscultation, laboratory values approaching patient's normal limits, respirations regular and nonlabored, and reduced signs and symptoms of respiratory impairment.

Patient/family/caregiver will be able to:
• Demonstrate measures to manage impaired ventilation.
• Perform necessary treatments and procedures.
• Demonstrate proper knowledge and administration of medication and oxygen.
• Identify/demonstrate emergency treatments for management of acute respiratory distress.
• Maintain vital signs within patient's normal limits.

INTERVENTIONS

• Observe ventilatory function for difficulties: shallow respirations, tachypnea, dyspnea, frothy secretions, and jugular vein distention.
• Auscultate lungs for evidence of impairment: rales, chronic and diminished breath sounds.
• Monitor intake and output.
• Measure CVP.
• Obtain or assist with measurement of arterial blood gases (ABGs).
• Adjust position accordingly:
  —High Fowler's position enhances lung expansion.
  —Turn patient every 1 to 2 hours to mobilize secretions and prevent atelectasis, but keep most congested lung up to prevent further ventilation/perfusion problems.
• Administer humidified oxygen therapy by mask if ordered.
• Administer diuretics and decrease fluid intake as ordered.
• Suction nasopharynx and lungs as ordered.

Continued.

NURSING DIAGNOSIS

• *Fluid volume deficit related to capillary dilation or leakage leading to third spacing of fluid*

OUTCOME GOAL

Patient will be able to:

• Maintain adequate fluid volume, as evidenced by laboratory values within normal limits; skin turgor, mucous membranes, and tongue hydration normal; daily intake and output balanced and adequate; absence of thirst or dry mouth; and vital signs within patient's normal limits.

INTERVENTIONS

• Monitor intake and output every 30 to 60 minutes.
• Measure urine specific gravity.
• Insert indwelling urinary catheter as ordered.
• Measure CVP.
• Monitor blood pressure every 30 to 60 minutes.
• Administer crystalloids, colloids, and blood products as ordered to maintain circulating fluid volume.

The nursing management of a patient with septic shock is extremely complex and challenging. It requires astute assessment and often quick decision making. Since septicemia is the triggering event, infection prophylaxis is crucial.

---

kidney, lymphoma, myeloma). However, SCC can occur at any time, even during active treatment for cancer.

PATHOPHYSIOLOGY

The adult human vertebral column, or backbone, is a versatile arrangement of 26 separate bony segments joined in series and supported by ligaments. The 26 vertebrae include 7 cervical, 12 thoracic, 5 lumbar, 1 sacral, and 1 coccyx. The vertebrae support the body by strength and rigidity while also providing flexibility and mobility. In addition, the column surrounds and protects the spinal cord, which is enlarged in the cervical and lumbar areas. The cord itself is covered by three protective meninges, or membranes.

These *meninges* originate as coverings for the brain and extend downward over the spinal cord. The outermost membrane is the *dura mater* (hard mother), which is made up of dense fibrous connective tissue. The space between the walls of the vertebral column and the outer surface of the dura mater is referred to as the *epidural, or extradural, space.* Within that space can be found blood vessels and connective and adipose tissue. No lymph nodes are located within this space.[132] The *subdural space* follows next, between the inner surface of the dura mater and the underlying arachnoid membrane. Below the arachnoid membrane is the *subarachnoid space.* It lies between the arachnoid membrane and the innermost membrane, the *pia mater* ("gentle mother"), which is closely attached to the spinal cord. The subarachnoid space contains liquid referred to as spinal fluid. However, it is more accurately called *cerebrospinal fluid* (CSF), since the subarachnoid space begins in the brain and follows down the cord. Prevertebral lymph nodes are also located in this space.[40,61]

Bone metastasis involves the vertebral column and invades the epidural space (Figure 19-13). It is estimated that 95% of SCCs result from tumor in the epidural space or outside the spinal cord.[25,40,61] The destruction taking place in the bone is one of two types: osteolytic or osteoblastic. The more common *osteolytic lesions* cause bone destruction as tumor cells stimulate bone reabsorption by the osteoclasts (cells developing bone that absorb bony tissue). Stimulation of the osteoblasts (cells that develop into bone or secrete substances producing bony tissue) by the tumor cells causes formation of new bone, resulting in the less common *osteoblastic lesions.* Both processes are problematic. They can be differentiated by radiographic studies.[6]

The epidural space is invaded by tumor by one of three mechanisms[40,57,61,153]:

1. Direct extension of the tumor into the space after bony erosion of the vertebral body. Carcinoma of the lung, breast, and prostate are mostly responsible for this mechanism, and it occurs with the greatest frequency.
2. Lymph node growth through the foramina into the epidural space by adjacent prevertebral lymph nodes. Lymphomas usually grow in this manner.
3. Hematogenous spread by means of an embolic process through the paravertebral and extradural venous plexus. Intramedullary metastases are one such process resulting from vascular dissemination, but they are rare, with an occurrence of 1% to 3%.[139]

Neurologic deficits result from these three mechanisms of metastases by three different processes:

1. Direct compression of the spinal cord or cauda equina by the tumor itself.
2. Interruption of the vascular supply to neural structure by the tumor.
3. Compression caused by vertebral collapse resulting from a pathologic fracture or dislocation. The bone may extrude onto the cord and produce pressure that compresses the nerve roots.

The severity of the compression can increase in the presence of edema from obstruction of the venous plexus, which supplies the spinal cord.

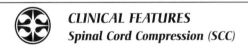

Fasciculus gracilis

NORMAL **ABNORMAL**

Tumor

Fasciculus
cuneatus

Lateral
corticospinal
tract

Tumor

Lateral
spinothalamic
tract

Anterior
spinothalamic tract

Tumor

Figure 19-13 View of spinal cord at thoracic level with effects of epidural tumor shown in several locations. (From Nissenblatt M: *Am Fam Physician* 20[2], 1979.)

CLINICAL FEATURES

The clinical presentation of SCC is similar in all patients, regardless of the origin of the tumor. Symptomatology is directly related to the location of the compression. The distribution of spinal metastases with SCC correlates with the number of vertebrae and size of the epidural space in each segment, with 10% in the cervical area, 70% in the thoracic, and 20% in the lumbosacral.[38,70,154]

The cardinal signs and associated symptoms of SCC are well documented and usually follow an established pattern of appearance, which includes pain, motor weakness, sensory loss, and finally autonomic dysfunction (see box at right).

Back pain is the presenting complaint in 97% of patients.* It is related to SCC and may occur weeks or months before the compression takes place. It is either localized or radicular. Localized pain is classically the initial symptom and results from stretching of the periosteum of the afflicted bone or from vertebral collapse. Pain that is radicular in nature is caused by nerve root

*References 38, 40, 44, 61, 73, 77, 139.

> ### CLINICAL FEATURES
> ### *Spinal Cord Compression (SCC)*
>
> ***Clinical signs***
> Muscle weakness (unsteadiness, footdrop, paralysis)
> Sensory impairment (paralysis, loss of bowel and bladder control, paraplegia)
> ***Symptoms***
> Pain
> Tingling and/or numbness in extremities
> Diminished pain and temperature sensation
> Sexual dysfunction

compression from a pathologic fracture and compression of the vertebrae (Figure 19-13). The distribution of radicular pain depends on the level of spinal involvement. It may move along the dermatomal distribution and is aggravated by movement such as coughing, sneezing, straining as with Valsalva's maneuver, or straight leg raising. Thoracic radicular pain, which is most common, radiates in a band around the chest or abdomen.[3,75]

The pain associated with SCC is usually intense, persistent, and progressive, although thoracic compression is often felt as a constriction.[3,73,77] Any pain of SCC may be accompanied by vertebral tenderness on percussion at or near the level of compression. It is often unilateral when the compression is in the cervical or lumbosacral area and usually bilateral in the thoracic region. The pain is usually worse at night because the spine lengthens when recumbent. A key to early detection is a detailed assessment for any changes in pain. Patients may have been suffering with pain from bony metastasis for a time. With the onset of SCC, the pain often changes its location and intensity.

Although weakness is rarely a presenting complaint, 75% to 86% of patients have subtle evidence of motor defect on initial clinical examination.[7] Initially, motor symptoms are asymptomatic. Compression in the cervical spine causes impairment of the arm, then the ipsilateral and contralateral legs, and finally the opposite arm. If the compression is thoracic, one leg is weak and stiff before the opposite leg.[74,139] The development of pain is followed by motor weakness. The time frame is variable, from hours to days, weeks, or months.[6,57,77,154] Common patient complaints include stiffness and heaviness of the affected extremity. It may manifest itself as an unsteady gait or ataxia with a favoring or dragging of the affected extremity or extremities.

Sensory loss usually follows motor weakness but precedes actual motor loss. These sensory losses progress in the same pattern as motor symptoms.[139] Symptoms of sensory loss include numbness, tingling, paresthesia, and feelings of coldness in the affected area. Loss of sensation to light touch first, then loss of pain, followed by loss of thermal sensation, occur in 80% of patients.[41] Concurrent loss of proprioception, deep pressure, vibratory sense, and position sense indicates a severe compression. After the release of SCC, neurologic functions return in the reverse order of how the dysfunctions appeared.[139] If the motor weakness and sensory loss progress rapidly to motor loss, the prognosis is poor.

Autonomic dysfunction appears if the compression progresses. Urinary disturbances include hesitancy and retention, followed by overflow and incontinence. Early changes may be as subtle as an increased postvoiding residual volume.[77] Lack of urge to defecate and inability to bear down are initial bowel disturbances, which may lead to constipation, obstipation, and finally incontinence. Loss of sphincter control is a later sign and is associated with a poorer prognosis. Sexual dysfunction may be manifested as impotence.[139,154]

DIAGNOSIS

When SCC is suspected in any patient, a diagnosis should be confirmed immediately because of the potential for rapid progression and possible permanent neurologic dysfunction. Figure 19-14 provides an algorithm for evaluating possible epidural metastasis.[55,61] A good history and physical examination should be accompanied by thorough neurologic testing. Physical findings include

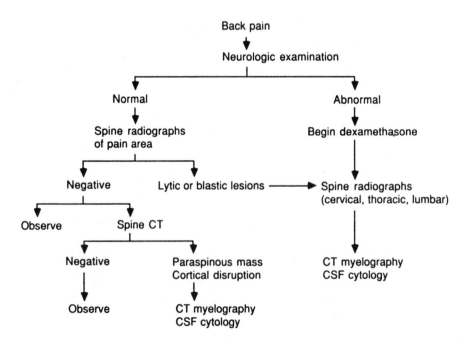

Figure 19-14 Algorithm of epidural spinal cord compression. (From Gilbert MR: Epidural spinal cord compression and carcinomectous meningitis. In Johnson RT, editor: *Current therapy in neurologic disease,* ed 3, St Louis, 1990, Mosby.)

percussion tenderness at the level of compression. If radicular pain is present, it will increase with spinal movement on straight leg raises. Motor and sensory involvement is manifested by hyperactive reflexes, positive Babinski signs, variable spastic weakness, and bilateral sensory loss below the level of the compression. Absence of sweating below the level of involvement may be noted.[139] Bowel and bladder dysfunction may also be detected. Corresponding subjective data should be elicited because differences could be significant.

Testing for a patient with suspected SCC begins with plain x-ray films and a radioisotope bone scan. Both are positive in 85% of patients with SCC.[57,139] X-ray findings reveal osteolytic lesions with loss of a pedicle, vertebral body destruction, or collapse of vertebral body. Intervertebral disks are not affected by neoplastic disease because they have an insufficient blood supply.[7] A problem with plain x-ray films is that if the tumor grows paraspinally, with invasion of the epidural space through the foramina, the bone film may be normal. This is common with lung tumors and lymphoma. Another concern is that a tumor can be present for 6 months without x-ray changes. A bone scan is often more sensitive and may be positive 6 months before plain films.[77] Osteoblastic lesions show new bone formation that may extend into the epidural space.[6,154]

A lumbar puncture (LP) may be performed; however, examination of the CSF may be helpful but is not diagnostic. CSF protein elevations greater than 100 mg/ml have been noted in most patients with SCC. Glucose is normal, cell count is unremarkable, and cytology is usually negative.[125] Progression of symptomatology has been reported after LP and may interfere with the performance of myelography.[139]

CT may identify early destructive lesions not seen on plain films, differentiate tumor from osteoporosis, and define paraspinal tumors that may extend epidurally.[77,154]

Myelography is often considered the most definitive diagnostic procedure for SCC. In 85% of patients the blockage revealed on myelography corresponds to the site of known vertebral involvement by physical examination or x-ray findings.[55,57,67] The flow of the contrast material injected at the lumbar region will be partially or completely obstructed at the level of compression. If a complete blockage is demonstrated, additional contrast material will be injected into the cisterna magna to locate the upper margin of the obstruction.[57,139] Accurate visualization of the location, extent of compression, and upper and lower borders of a block are crucial for planning treatment by either decompressive laminectomy or radiation therapy. The usual contrast material used for these myelograms is Pantopaque (iophendylate) because of its ability to be left in the subarachnoid space for repeat fluoroscopy to evaluate response to therapy or re-

currence at another site. A CSF sample can be obtained during the procedure. New imaging technology such as MRI is gaining increasing use for the evaluation of neurologic problems. Today, MRI is chosen over CT scan as a diagnostic procedure for spinal diseases.[25,38,57,61] The definitive role for MRI in SCC has been established with further clinical studies comparing MRI with myelography in terms of sensitivity, specificity, and accuracy. Current practice uses them in a complementary manner. The major benefits of MRI are as follows*:

- It is sensitive to neurologic tissue.
- It is noninvasive.
- It is helpful in patients with severe contrast allergies.
- It images the entire spine, providing various views.
- It is helpful in patients with brain metastasis.
- It may show multiple epidural deposits of tumor that may not be obvious on initial myelogram.
- It avoids the risk of neurologic deterioration after LP, which occurs in as many as 14% of patients with complete block.[38]

New open MRI machines have provided an option for people with claustrophobia and those who are too large to fit into a closed machine.

The disadvantages of MRI are as follows:

- The need for the patient to lie still in one position, which may be difficult for someone with central back pain.
- Claustrophobia has been a common problem.

TREATMENT MODALITIES

The choice of treatment for patients with SCC depends on the primary tumor, the rapidity of onset of the compression, and the level, severity, and duration of the blockage. The two most frequent treatment modalities for SCC are surgery and radiation therapy. The goal of therapy is symptom relief from metastatic disease and improvement of quality of life.

Patients are initially treated nonsurgically, except in the following three situations that would warrant a decompressive laminectomy[77,125,158]:

1. Prior maximum-tolerance radiation at the site of compression precludes further irradiation.
2. The cause for SCC is questionable, or there is no known primary malignancy.
3. Neurologic deterioration occurs during radiation therapy. In most other situations, radiation therapy is the initial treatment.

Laminectomy with decompression of the spinal cord and nerve roots will relieve compression and improve symptoms, but it rarely achieves complete removal of the tumor. Surgery affords diagnostic and therapeutic benefits. It may provide a diagnosis for a patient with no

---

*References 25, 38, 53, 57, 61, 139.

known history of cancer. As a treatment modality it allows tumor debulking, decompression of the spinal cord, and possibly bone grafting at the location of erosion.[41,44] In select patients, surgery may be done to remove a tumor or bone from the area of compression, followed by stabilization with hardware and methyl methacrylate placed into the space. However, the surgical technique is difficult and poses a potential risk of major complications.[25,38,44] Technical difficulties can arise because the surgical approach may be posterior and most tumors present in the vertebral body and invade the epidural space anteriorly. Therefore, in addition to incomplete tumor removal, the removal of the posterior elements of the vertebrae can produce an unstable spine, necessitating postoperative therapy and back braces.[6,44]

After surgery, radiation therapy is administered to treat the remaining tumor. Portal size depends on residual tumor and extends one to two vertebrae above and below the level of involvement to ensure an adequate dosage and field. Irradiation may be initiated a few days after surgery and continues for 2 weeks, with total dose approximately 2700 to 3000 cGy.[55,77] Caution should be used during and after radiation therapy, since normal osteocytes will be destroyed along with tumor cells. This disrupts the balance of osteoblastic (formation) and osteoclastic (absorption) processes. Wound separation may occur, and delay in healing is possible. Therefore complete normal bone repair is rare, and support to the spine may be necessary until radiation therapy is completed.[6,44]

Radiation therapy alone as primary treatment for SCC has been gaining increased attention. Studies comparing surgery with radiation therapy to radiation therapy alone have shown them to have equal efficacy.[6] However, response may depend on the radiosensitivity of the tumor.[77] When radiation therapy is the treatment choice, it should begin immediately after definitive diagnosis. The total dose given is 2700 to 4000 cGy over a 2- to 4-week period; margins are generous (two spinal segments above and below the lesion).[40,77] Neurologic examinations should be done frequently to assess patient response.

The use of steroids in the management of SCC is advocated to decrease edema, relieve symptoms, and control pain. Pain relief in most patients will occur within a few hours.[25,68,77] However, the presence of edema related to compression is not well substantiated. Most evidence is clinical at diagnosis of SCC or during administration of radiation therapy. Current recommendations vary among clinicians. The drug most frequently ordered is Decadron (dexamethasone), and but the dosage is either high (100 mg by IV push, initial dose) with tapering or low conventional (16 to 24 mg/day) with tapering.[68,77]

Chemotherapy has a role as adjuvant therapy in the treatment of SCC. In most instances, alkylating agents alone or combined with radiation therapy are used to treat SCC resulting from lymphoma.[40,57] Chemotherapy may be given concomitantly or after radiation therapy as systemic treatment for the primary underlying malignancy. Small cell lung cancer and breast cancer are very responsive to chemotherapy.

PROGNOSIS

Response to therapy for SCC depends on the severity and rapidity of onset of symptoms more than on their duration. Patients with intramedullary metastasis usually have a rapid progression of dysfunction and therefore a poorer prognosis.[20] Surgical intervention results in 5% mortality.[33] The amount of functional recovery after radiation therapy is often predictable when one half of the total dose is delivered.[6] Overall the best prognostic predictor is the patient's functional status before treatment.[120,139] If patients are ambulatory at the initiation of therapy, 80% will retain the ability to walk after treatment, whereas only 30% to 40% of patients with pretreatment motor dysfunction are ambulatory after treatment.[40,132] If the underlying malignancy is lymphoma, chances for continued ambulation are 80%, compared with 60% in patients with carcinomas, since these patients often experience late SCC.[120] Patients who are paraplegic before therapy have a 5% to 7% chance to become ambulatory.[120] This statistical picture of response emphasizes the crucial role of early detection of SCC.[139]

Nursing management of the patient with SCC is outlined on pp. 457-459.

SUPERIOR VENA CAVA SYNDROME

DEFINITION

The superior vena cava is a major venous vessel that returns blood to the right atrium of the heart from the head, upper thorax, and upper extremities. Obstruction of the venous flow through this vessel results in impaired venous drainage, with engorgement of the vessels from the head and upper body torso. As the venous pressure rises in the superior vena cava, blood is shunted to collateral venous pathways to facilitate return to the right atrium. The result is a characteristic constellation of physical findings known as superior vena cava syndrome (SVCS).[40,42]

ETIOLOGY AND RISK FACTORS

The causes ascribed to SVCS have changed over the years as information has increased regarding the cancer process. SVCS was first described by William Hunter in 1757 in a patient with a syphilitic aneurysm.[42] Over the

NURSING MANAGEMENT

Spinal cord compression (SCC) is a true oncologic emergency requiring immediate attention. The primary aspect of nursing care is early detection, since response to therapy is directly related to the patient's functional status at diagnosis. An in-depth history and data collection are essential in those patients who are at risk for SCC. Nursing assessment should focus on pain, motor and sensory status, and bowel and bladder functions. The nursing care of these patients is extremely variable, depending on the presence and severity of the compression and the medical treatment. Very subtle changes in patient status are significant and should be reported.[6,25,67,108]

NURSING DIAGNOSIS

• *Mobility, impaired physical, related to spinal cord compression*

OUTCOME GOALS

Patient will be able to:
• Demonstrate measures to maintain optimal mobility and prevent complications.
• Identify factors that influence maintenance or disruption in mobility.
• Perform necessary treatments and procedures.
• Demonstrate necessary life-style changes.
• Demonstrate safety measures.
• Achieve/maintain optimal mobility consistent with disease process.

INTERVENTIONS

• Assess patient's level of function/mobility:
  —Check for the presence of sensory loss and paresthesia by noting sensation and deep tendon reflexes in extremities.
  —Monitor serum calcium level for potential increase from immobility.
  —Determine motor weakness and dysfunction by checking gait, range of motion (ROM), and coordination.
  —Determine bowel, bladder, and sexual function.
• Check for evidence of venous thrombosis from immobilization:
  —Determine the presence of redness, swelling, warmth, positive Homans' sign (pain on dorsiflexion), and venous streaking and erythema.
  —Use antiembolic stockings as ordered.
  —Measure calves each day and note any edema.
• Implement pain management program as indicated.
• Establish activity regimen according to patient's physical status and physician order:
  —Institute passive ROM exercises as ordered.
  —Assist patients with transfer and ambulation as needed.

—Provide back brace for patients with unstable spines as ordered.
  —Move bedridden patients with extreme care and maintain proper body alignment. Use lift sheets and assistive devices (e.g., trapeze, Hoyer lift). Support joints. Turn patient by log-rolling method.
• Obtain consultations with physical and occupational therapy for evaluation and assistance.
• Implement safety measures as appropriate:
  —Place all articles within patient's reach.
  —Keep bed rails up and pad them if necessary.
  —Assist patient with all movements or encourage use of assistive devices.
• Encourage and assist patient to perform self-care when possible.
• Discuss and teach the use of assistive and supportive devices.
• Arrange consultation or referral to rehabilitative services as needed.

NURSING DIAGNOSIS

• *Breathing pattern, ineffective, related to the level of compression and/or immobility*

OUTCOME GOAL

Patient will be able to:
• Demonstrate absence of complications of impaired mobility, as evidenced by respiratory status and vital signs within normal limits and skin integrity intact.

INTERVENTIONS

• Assess respiratory status:
  —Observe breathing for distress (respiratory rate, rhythm, amplitude).
  —Auscultate lungs for breath sounds every shift.
  —Obtain arterial blood gases (ABGs) as ordered.
• Encourage and assist patient with pulmonary hygiene every 2 hours:
  —Reposition every 2 hours.
  —Facilitate deep breathing and coughing.
• Consult with physician regarding need for more aggressive pulmonary measures (incentive spirometry, ultrasonic nebulizer, chest physical therapy).
• Provide mechanical respiratory support, if necessary.

NURSING DIAGNOSIS

• *Skin integrity, impaired, risk for, related to immobility*

OUTCOME GOALS

Patient will be able to:
• Maintain good skin integrity and optimal level of physical activity.

Continued.

- Identify/demonstrate measures to promote skin integrity.
- Verbalize/demonstrate appropriate hygiene measures.
- Identify signs and symptoms to report to the health care team.
- Verbalize/demonstrate adequate nutritional and fluid intake.
- Verbalize/demonstrate position change and transfer techniques.

INTERVENTIONS

- Assess skin integrity, with special attention to areas over bony prominences; note any redness, discoloration, swelling, or breakdown.
- Culture any suspicious drainage.
- Institute skin care protocol specific to assessment.
- Modify bed surface with approved pressure-reducing mattress.
- Change patient's position every 2 hours and massage pressure areas.

NURSING DIAGNOSIS

- *Constipation related to decreased activity or immobility*

OUTCOME GOALS

Patient will be able to:
- Demonstrate measures to promote adequate bowel elimination.
- Verbalize/demonstrate adequate nutritional and fluid intake.
- Use prophylactic stool softeners as indicated.
- Follow schedule for defecation.
- Demonstrate knowledge of bowel training program techniques.
- Show absence of fecal impaction.

INTERVENTIONS

- Obtain history of bowel elimination, including laxative use and other aids for elimination.
- Assess abdomen each day (observe for distention, auscultate for bowel sounds, perform rectal examination for impaction).
- Monitor bowel movements (frequency, amount, odor, consistency).
- Encourage fluids as appropriate.
- Increase bulk and fiber in diet as indicated.
- Administer stool softeners, laxatives, bulk products, and lubricants as ordered.
- Initiate bowel training program as necessary, and encourage compliance.

NURSING DIAGNOSIS

- *Urinary elimination, altered, related to neurogenic bladder, loss of voluntary control of micturition*

OUTCOME GOALS

Patient will be able to:
- Maintain adequate urinary control and elimination.
- Express desire to void.
- Follow pattern of fluid intake and voiding.
- Void before activities that are prolonged.
- Check bladder for overdistention when appropriate.
- Use appropriate measures to initiate voiding when necessary.
- Maintain socially acceptable bladder-emptying program.
- Verbalize signs and symptoms of bladder distention.
- Identify signs and symptoms to report to the health care team.

INTERVENTIONS

- Obtain history of bladder elimination patterns.
- Assess abdomen (observe for distention, percuss area above symphysis pubis).
- Monitor urine output (frequency, amount, odor, color).
- Check for residual after each voiding as ordered.
- Monitor laboratory values (urinalysis, serum blood urea nitrogen, creatinine).
- Assess for signs and symptoms of a urinary tract infection (elevated temperature, changes in odor or color of urine, frequency and dysuria, complaints of burning and/or urgency).
- Culture urine as ordered.
- Observe for presence of hyperreflexia (reaction that occurs with blocks at the sixth thoracic vertebra or above in which there is increased production of norepinephrine in an attempt to cause evacuation of the bowel or bladder). Signs and symptoms include increased blood pressure, pounding headache, vasodilation, flushing, increased temperature, profuse sweating, chest pain, bradycardia, nausea.[25,54]
- Obtain order for indwelling urinary catheter if repeated catheterization is necessary to relieve distention or continued urinary residual.
- Initiate bladder training program as necessary and encourage compliance.

NURSING DIAGNOSIS

- *Sexual dysfunction related to disease process and treatment*

OUTCOME GOALS

Patient will be able to:
- Demonstrate knowledge related to alteration in sexuality.
- Identify alterations in sexual function.
- Identify factors that influence sexual identity.
- Identify/demonstrate behaviors and measures to promote acceptance of self as sexual being.

INTERVENTIONS

- Examine own attitudes, knowledge, and skills in the area of sexuality, sexual function, and sexual counseling.
- Provide a therapeutic environment that demonstrates acceptance of sexual behavior and allows patient to feel comfortable to discuss sexual concerns.
- Elicit a sexual history as appropriate.
- Be respectful of social, cultural, and religious factors that may influence patient's perceptions of sexuality, sexual function, and sexual identity, and assure confidentiality.
- Use the Plissit model to develop relevant nursing interventions.[54] Use levels with which you feel comfortable:
  —*P*, Permission: convey permission to have (or not have) sexual thoughts, concerns, feelings (assure patient that concerns regarding sexual function after cancer diagnosis are legitimate).
  —*LI*, Limited information: provide limited information relative to patient's problem while acknowledging that other individuals experience similar concerns (e.g., many individuals have concerns about type of birth control recommended while receiving chemotherapy).
  —*SS*, Specific suggestions: offer specific suggestions relevant to patient's problems (e.g., use of pillows and coital positions that minimize or allay threat of pathologic fractures).
  —*IT*, Intensive therapy: refer to appropriate resource for longer-term therapy or rehabilitation (e.g., sex therapist for continued erectile dysfunction, surgeon for reconstructive surgery).
- Discuss the potential impact of disease and treatment on sexuality and sexual function.
- Identify available resources, and make referrals as appropriate.

NURSING DIAGNOSES

- *Body image disturbance related to physical dysfunction, disease process, immobility*
- *Role performance, altered, related to physical dysfunction, disease, mobility*

OUTCOME GOALS

Patient will be able to:
- Demonstrate successful positive coping and adaptation.
- Recognize when current coping mechanisms are not working.
- Ask for assistance.
- Initiate and perform self-care tasks.
- Identify, cultivate, and use available resources.

INTERVENTIONS

- Assess patient's past and present coping abilities through interview, observation of physical and verbal participation in self-care, and discussion.
- Promote and observe interaction with family, friends, and staff.
- Encourage verbalization of feelings and concerns.
- Assist and support the establishment of goals and adaptive coping mechanisms.
- Make referrals as appropriate for counseling and rehabilitative services.

Nursing care of a patient with SCC is complex and challenging, reflecting the extreme variability among patients. Situations exist along a continuum from early detection and alarm through emergency and rehabilitation. The role of the nurse in coordinating care is crucial.

---

years, benign conditions such as aortic aneurysms, thyroid goiter, tuberculous mediastinitis, and infectious diseases were most frequently considered to be the cause of SVCS. Today, only 3% of the cases of SVCS have a benign cause; cancer is responsible for more than 97% of all cases. Any tumor, primary or metastatic, can block the blood flow of the superior vena cava. Three fourths of all malignant cases of SVCS are caused by bronchogenic cancer, particularly small cell carcinoma of the lung. Lymphomas account for approximately 15% to 20% of SVCS cases.[57,142,156] This includes both Hodgkin's disease and non-Hodgkin's lymphoma. Most frequent in the latter group is diffuse histiocytic lymphoma. Other malignancies associated with SVCS have been Kaposi's sarcoma, adenocarcinoma of the breast, thymoma, and primary or metastatic seminoma and other germ cell tumors.[142] SVCS may be present in patients with no known diagnosis of cancer.[55,118,156]

Innovations in therapeutic interventions for cancer have added two new causes. Venous thrombosis related to indwelling central venous catheters has been observed in patients with SVCS. Several authorities ascribe this to be the most common nonmalignant cause of SVC obstruction.[40,57,142] Radiation-induced fibrosis can result in the narrowing of the superior vena cava and produce the same clinical picture. SVCS occurs in approximately 3% to 4% of patients with cancer.[53,139] Most patients with SVCS are in the fourth to seventh decades of life. The ratio of men to women is approximately 3:1.[117] However, as lung cancer incidence and death rates change, especially among women, so will the incidence and age and gender distribution of SVCS.

PATHOPHYSIOLOGY

The superior vena cava is a thin-walled, low-pressure vessel about 7 cm in length (Figure 19-15). It extends from the junction of the right and left innominate veins to the right atrium. Location in the thorax is to the right of the arteries of the trachea and right mainstem bronchus and posterior to the sternum. The thorax is a rigid anatomic compartment with little ability for expansion. In its space within the thorax/mediastinum, the superior vena cava is extremely vulnerable to displacement and compression because it has a thin wall, low venous pressure, and is surrounded by the rigid structures of the sternum, trachea, vertebrae, lymph nodes, aorta, pulmonary artery, and right bronchus.[73] Therefore obstruction of the superior vena cava can be a consequence of three physiologic events.[43,73,80,108]

1. External compression by an extrinsic mass, solid tumor, or enlarged lymph node
2. Intravascular obstruction by tumor or thrombosis
3. Intraluminal reaction to tumor invasion or inflammation

Impedance of venous flow through the superior vena cava and subsequent development of SVCS depends on several factors: the degree and location of the blockage, growth rate of the tumor, patency of the azygos vein, and proliferation of collateral circulation. The azygos vein (Figure 19-15) plays a pivotal role in the flow of blood through the superior vena cava, entering it just above the pericardial reflection and making it a major tributary. There are three places where the superior vena cava may be obstructed relative to the azygos vein.[156]

1. Above the azygos vein, allowing patency of the proximal vena cava. In this situation, venous return from the upper body continues through the subclavian vein to the azygos, on to the proximal vena cava, and finally into the right atrium. Obstruction above the azygos vein is the least serious.
2. Proximal to the entrance of the azygos vein. Venous return is accomplished through blood shunting to the inferior vena cava by way of the azygos vein.[142]
3. At the junction of the azygos vein with the superior vena cava. All blood flow through the superior vena cava is blocked. This necessitates rerouting of the blood flow to the inferior vena cava by way of the azygos vein. Blockage at the junction of the azygos vein is the most complex.

Impairment of the venous circulation through the superior vena cava reduces blood flow to the right atrium, which results in venous hypertension with venous stasis and a decrease in cardiac output. If untreated, the progression is from vascular congestion to thrombosis, cerebral edema, pulmonary complications, and death.

CLINICAL FEATURES

The clinical picture seen in SVCS is directly related to obstruction of venous drainage in the upper body (Figure 19-15). Onset is usually insidious, but when fully developed, it requires immediate attention. The onset and severity of signs and symptoms vary directly with the underlying disease and related pathophysiology. Compression of intrathoracic structures, vascular congestion,

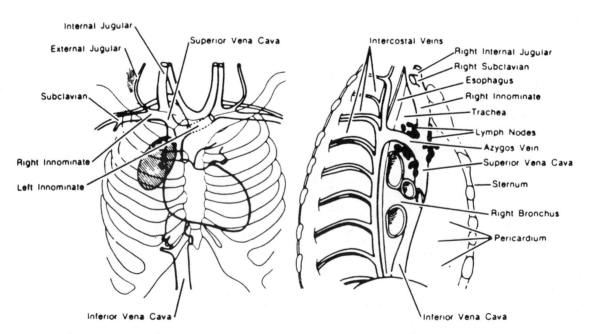

Figure 19-15 Schematic representation of the thorax, frontal and lateral views. Shaded areas indicate typical site of obstruction. (From Lockich J, Goodman R: *JAMA* 231[1]:58, 1975.)

and venous hypertension present distinguishing clinical features. The presentation may be unilateral or bilateral. Since pressures in the head are higher in the supine than in the standing position, a person with early SVCS may initially have signs and symptoms only in the morning. Symptomatology may also vary greatly depending on the underlying pathophysiology. Early detection of SVCS hinges on a careful in-depth history and physical assessment. The box below lists clinical features of SVCS.[6,139,142]

Progression of symptoms may lead to severe respiratory obstruction, paralyzed vocal cord, cyanosis of the upper torso, "wet brain syndrome" (manifested by drowsiness, stupor, unconsciousness, and seizures), and possible coma.[142]

DIAGNOSIS

The diagnostic evaluation of a patient with SVCS depends greatly on the patient's physical condition. If SVCS onset is insidious, the diagnostic work-up can proceed slowly, and treatment will not be initiated until a diagnosis is confirmed. If the onset is rapid and symptoms are acute, however, a definitive diagnosis may be deferred and treatment (usually radiation therapy) is begun immediately, especially with a known diagnosis of cancer. SVCS may be considered one of the rare occasions when treatment can be started even before a tissue diagnosis is confirmed. In this life-threatening situation, chest radiography, the results of which rarely appear normal, and clinical presentation are considered diagnostic. A tissue biopsy to determine a primary lesion and further work-up for metastases can proceed during the course of treatment.

Chest films are abnormal in 80% of patients with SVCS.[125,156] In 50% of patients, findings are a lung or mediastinal mass, most frequently on the right side because the superior vena cava enters from the right. Also, 25% of patients may have mediastinal widening and pleural effusion.[74] CT scan and MRI may further define the lesion and its location. Important information obtained by radiographic findings includes more detailed information about the SVC and its tributaries as well as the source, size, and exact location of the mass in relation to the azygos vein.[43] This information also provides anatomic detail necessary to establish the portals for radiation therapy.[6,43,139,142]

Further diagnostic procedures must be evaluated for their risk versus benefit to the patient. Biopsy of palpable superficial lymph nodes, sputum for cytology, and bone marrow biopsy are associated with low risk and may provide information about the primary tumor. Invasive procedures such as bronchoscopy, mediastinoscopy, thoracoscopy, thoracotomy, or supraclavicular lymph node biopsy may be necessary but are associated with signifi-cant morbidity and the risk of fatal thrombosis or bleeding as a result of increased venous pressure. On the other hand, immediate radiation therapy may impede later tissue biopsy because of radiation-induced tissue changes.[43,139,142]

Bronchoscopy has established a diagnosis in approximately 70% of patients.[142] Percutaneous needle biopsy, mediastinoscopy, and thoracotomy are associated with increased risk of bleeding and, if necessary, should be deferred until venous pressure is reduced. Superior venacavography is infrequently done. However, it can be most helpful in determining location and degree of obstruction, measuring venous pressure through the catheter, distinguishing between vascular and nonvascular lesions, evaluating collateral circulation, and assessing operability.[148] To establish the extent of obstruction and determine the hemodynamics of the vessel, venacavography has also been used in early diagnosis when SVCS is only suspected. Recently, CT-guided fine-needle biopsies have yielded diagnostic specimens from the lung mass with few complications.[6,43,139,142]

TREATMENT MODALITIES

Four therapeutic modalities should be considered in the treatment of SVCS: radiation therapy, chemotherapy, sur-

---

 CLINICAL FEATURES
Superior Vena Cava Syndrome (SVCS)

Clinical signs
Edema of the face, neck, upper thorax, breasts, and upper extremities
Periorbital edema and/or edema of the conjunctivae, with or without protrusion of the eye
Horner's syndrome (sinking of eye with ptosis of eyelid)
Plethora of the face
Increased pressure of the jugular veins
Dilation and prominence of collateral vessels in upper thorax and neck
Telangiectasia (capillary dilation)
Compensatory tachycardia
Symptoms
Respiratory compromise (dyspnea, shortness of breath, tachypnea, cough, orthopnea)
Feeling of facial fullness
Headache
Visual disturbances
Dizziness
Hoarseness
Chest pain
Stokes' sign (tightness of shirt collar)
Swelling of fingers (difficulty removing rings)

gery, and pharmacologic therapy. The goals are relief of symptoms and reduction of the obstructing lesion. Cure may be the goal when the primary diagnosis is small cell lung cancer, non-Hodgkin's lymphoma, or a germ cell tumor, which account for nearly half the malignant causes of SVCS.[156]

The choice of treatment depends on the rate of onset, the causative process (benign or malignant), and the type of mass (intraluminal or extraluminal).

Radiation Therapy

Radiation therapy has been the treatment of choice for SVCS because of its local therapeutic response and minimal toxicities. Treatment is begun immediately in acute and life-threatening situations. The total dose, dose fractionation, and size and type of field depend on tumor histology, patient condition, radiologic response, and symptom relief. Delivery of radiation begins initially with high-dose fractionation at 3 to 4 Gy/day for the first 3 days, followed by a reduction of the daily dose to 1.5 to 2 Gy/day, for a total dose of 500 to 600 Gy in 5 to 7 weeks.[40,42,43,118] The higher initial doses are favored because of an apparently more rapid tumor response. Patients with lymphoma require a lower total dose of 300 to 400 Gy, unless bulky masses are present, which may necessitate a total dose of 500 Gy.*

Tumor reduction usually occurs with radiation therapy, especially in patients with lymphoma and small (oat) cell lung cancer. Less tumor response is seen in patients with non–small cell lung cancer (epidermoid, adenocarcinoma, large cell). Subjective improvement has been noted in 3 to 4 days in 75% of patients, regardless of tumor histology. Within 7 days, 91% obtain relief.[43] Objective response, with decrease in facial swelling and plethora, reduction of venous engorgement, and shrinkage of tumor mass, is evident in 7 to 14 days.[43,117]

Chemotherapy

The use of chemotherapy to treat SVCS has come to the forefront of the treatment regimen. It is an effective primary treatment when the cause of SVCS is small cell lung cancer lymphoma or a germ cell tumor.[158] Chemotherapy may be used alone if the mediastinal area has received a maximum of radiation or when reduction of tumor mass will provide a smaller radiation treatment field.

The choice of chemotherapeutic agents is based on the malignant cause of SVCS. After the selection of agents, consideration must be given to IV administration. Edema and dilation of the veins in the upper extremities lead to impaired circulation. Limited venous access, poor drug distribution, and increased risk of venous irritation and

extravasation of medications may contraindicate use of the upper extremities for therapy. In some situations the lower extremities may be used to administer chemotherapy by a central IV catheter placed in the femoral vein; however, this practice is highly controversial.

Surgery

Specific surgical approaches to SVCS include superior vena cava bypass or stent placement. These approaches are used very judicially because postoperative morbidity is high. Bypass surgery is indicated when the tumor could be completely removed if the superior vena cava were excised with it; when venous return is inadequate despite collateral circulation; and when the obstruction results from venous thrombosis, fibrosis, or a benign cause. This operative procedure is delicate and precise and depends on the same factors as in arterial grafts. The graft may be constructed using a synthetic Dacron prothesis or the patient's own saphenous vein. The graft creates a new vessel, which rechannels blood flow around the obstruction. One end of the graft is sutured to the right atrium, and the other is sutured to either the internal jugular or innominate vein.[11,156]

Patency of the bypass graft depends on the size of the anastomotic site, internal venous pressure, and blood flow. External rigidity of the graft is helpful to prevent collapse but is not required. Postoperatively, patients usually receive anticoagulation therapy and aspirin for an indefinite period to assist with graft patency.[2,43,139,142] When patency is maintained for several weeks, it increases the likelihood of long-term function. Reports demonstrate patency beyond a year.

The placement of a wire stent offers an alternative for the palliation of symptoms in patients with SVCS. Use of a stent may be indicated when other treatments for SVCS are unusable or ineffective. The most common situation is recurrence of SVCS after maximum-tolerance radiation. The stainless steel stent was designed by Gianturco and is usually referred to as the *Gianturco expandable wire stent* (GEWS).[142]

The stent is placed using a small balloon catheter inserted percutaneously with fluoroscopy with the patient under local anesthesia. The catheter is introduced into the vessel with the stent in a compressed form. When the stent is released, it expands and dilates the narrowed venous lumen. If the expansion is insufficient, the balloon is used to enlarge the stent to the desired diameter. A period of about 4 weeks is necessary for the stent to become incorporated into the endothelium of the venous wall.[139,142] The stent may remain patent for long periods because of its relatively low thrombogenicity.

One study has indicated some prognostic factors for longer-term palliation using the stent. It was found that patients with postirradiation fibrosis or slowly progres-

---

*References 40, 42, 43, 57, 118, 156.

sive pressure from a recurrent extrinsic tumor had longer relief of symptoms than patients whose symptoms resulted from direct tumor invasion.[142] The use of GEWS looks promising, but further clinical studies using the stent are necessary to define its role in the treatment of SVCS.[142]

Pharmacologic Therapy

Thrombus formation in patients with SVCS has gained increasing attention over the years. Autopsy reports have demonstrated thrombosis of the superior vena cava in patients who died during treatment of SVCS.

The increased use of indwelling central venous catheters has contributed to a rise in the incidence of SVCS.[40,57,142] Whatever the cause, irritation and inflammation of the superior vena cava related to an intraluminal or extraluminal lesion produce platelet aggregation, leading to clot formation. Fibrinolytic therapy with streptokinase or urokinase has been used to treat intraluminal thrombosis.*

Recent research has demonstrated that fibrinolytic therapy is most likely to succeed in patients with SVCS caused by a central venous catheter if urokinase is used and if therapy is initiated within 5 days of the onset of symptoms.[59]

Anticoagulation therapy is indicated for SVCS because of venous stasis. It may be used alone to resolve thrombus obstruction secondary to a central venous catheter or following initial fibrinolytic therapy. It is also used as a maintenance treatment to reduce the extent of the thrombus and prevent its progression. Removal of the central venous catheter should also be followed by anticoagulation to avoid embolization.[57,142]

During the administration of radiation therapy or chemotherapy, anticoagulants may be given concomitantly as a preventive treatment. Other medical interventions may be instituted as adjunctive therapy for SVCS. Diuretics may be given to reduce edema of the head and neck, which could improve cerebration and breathing. Caution should be used when giving diuretics because venous return to the heart is low and hypovolemia resulting from diuresis may induce shock. Steroids may be administered during active treatment to reduce inflammation related to the obstruction, to radiation, or to chemotherapy and resulting tumor necrosis.[153] Oxygen therapy may be necessary for the management of respiratory complications.

PROGNOSIS

Patients usually respond to treatment for SVCS, showing regression of the tumor.

*References 14, 59, 80, 142, 156.

The prognosis of patients with SVCS strongly correlates with the prognosis of the underlying disease.[142] Some patients have not responded to treatment. This has been attributed to poor general condition, presence of thrombosis in the superior vena cava, and metastatic disease.[142] Overall, patient survival is not good, since most patients are diagnosed in an advanced stage and die from metastatic disease. Recurrence is not a problem in general, but this is probably because of the relatively short survival time after initial diagnosis.

The best responses are seen in patients with lymphoma and small cell lung cancer. Other types of lung cancer have fewer long-term responses. Only 20% to 25% of all patients survive for 12 months after therapy, probably because of the nature of the underlying malignancies. Of patients with lymphoma, 45% have survived to 30 months, compared with 10% of patients with lung cancers.[74,117,118,142]

Although a diagnosis of SVCS may not offer long-term survival, with prompt diagnosis and treatment, it can be managed and therefore improves the patient's quality of life.

Nursing management of the patient with SVCS is outlined on pp. 464-465.

SYNDROME OF INAPPROPRIATE ANTIDIURETIC HORMONE SECRETION

DEFINITION

The syndrome of inappropriate antidiuretic hormone secretion (SIADH) is a disorder of water balance. Antidiuretic hormone (ADH), also called arginine vasopressin, regulates the body's water balance. SIADH is characterized by elevated serum blood levels of ADH, excessive water retention, and hyponatremia.[91,101,123,144]

ETIOLOGY AND RISK FACTORS

SIADH develops in 1% to 2% of patients with cancer.[53,57,142,144,160] Approximately two thirds of patients with documented SIADH have a neoplasm. The most common malignant disease associated with this syndrome is lung cancer, and 87% of these cases are small (oat) cell carcinoma. In fact, 50% of patients with small cell lung cancer have impaired water excretion.* As many as to 10% of these patients develop clinically evident SIADH.[50] SIADH may be the presenting symptom in patients with small cell lung cancer.[53] Other cancers associated with SIADH include cancer of the duodenum, pancreas, and bladder; acute myelogenous leukemia; lymphoma; thymoma; mesothe-

*References 35, 40, 57, 101, 108, 123, 125.

NURSING MANAGEMENT

The nursing care of patients with superior vena cava syndrome (SVCS) begins with astute assessment skills. Identification should be made of those patients considered to be at risk, followed by close observation and baseline data collection. Documentation of vital signs, mental status, appearance, and level of activity are essential to facilitate detection of changes. Subtle changes in subjective complaints or objective parameters should be reported to the physician. Once a diagnosis of SVCS has been established, the role of the nurse continues to be important.[28,70,79,89,108]

NURSING DIAGNOSIS

• *Breathing pattern, ineffective, related to venous congestion in the upper torso*

OUTCOME GOALS

Patient will be able to:
• Demonstrate knowledge related to ineffective breathing.
• Identify signs and symptoms of altered respiratory status.
• Identify factors that influence respiratory function.
• Exhibit effective breathing pattern, as evidenced by chest clear by auscultaion, respirations regular and non-labored, laboratory values and diagnostic tests approaching normal levels, and vital signs within patient's normal limits.

INTERVENTIONS

• Determine current respiratory status:
  —Observe for signs and symptoms of respiratory distress (dyspnea, shortness of breath, tachypnea, air hunger, stridor, orthopnea).
  —Assess lungs. Observe ventilatory movements (rate and depth), patency of airway, use of accessory muscles, clubbing of fingernails, and discoloration of nail bed or mucous membranes.
  —Palpate chest for fremitus, crepitance, deviation of the trachea, or nonsymmetric chest expansion.
  —Percuss chest for density/consolidation and displacement of organs.
  —Auscultate chest for breath sounds.
  —Monitor laboratory and other respiratory function tests, CBC, electrolytes, ABGs, chest x-ray films, and scans.
• Assist with breathing and pulmonary toilet:
  —Positioning for comfort and enhanced chest expansion
  —Deep breathing and coughing every 2 hours
  —Pursed-lip breathing

  —Frequent mouth care
  —Suctioning if necessary
• Provide oxygen and mechanical ventilation as indicated.
• Administer respiratory medications and steroids as prescribed.

NURSING DIAGNOSES

• *Cardiac output, decreased, related to decreased venous return related to vena cava obstruction*
• *Gas exchange, impaired, related to venous congestion caused by vena cava obstruction*

OUTCOME GOALS

Patient will be able to:
• Maintain optimal cardiac output, as evidenced by relief of chest pain, vital signs within patient's normal limits, cardiac rhythm without dysrhythmias, and adequate intake and output.
• Maintain adequate pulmonary function, as evidenced by laboratory values and diagnostic tests approaching patient's normal values and activity tolerance within patient's normal limits.
• Develop plan for behavioral and life-style changes.

INTERVENTIONS

• Assess patient for changes in cardiac function:
  —Check blood pressure and pulse every 2 to 4 hours as indicated.
  —Observe patient for signs of impedance of venous blood flow from the upper torso (plethora of the face; thoracic and neck vein distention; facial, trunk, and arm edema, especially in the morning; dyspnea, tachypnea, cough; cyanosis; mental status changes).
  —Monitor laboratory values (CBC, ABGs, chest x-ray films, ECG, scans).
• Provide oxygen therapy as ordered.
• Position patient for comfort and enhancement of venous drainage from upper torso:
  —Elevate and support upper extremities, especially if edematous.
  —Avoid constrictive clothing.
  —Maintain a cool room temperature.
  —Avoid closed-in areas if possible.
• Prevent activities that increase intrathoracic or intracerebral pressure (Valsalva's maneuver, vomiting, bending over, stooping).
• Assist patient with physical activities as needed.
• Provide measures to decrease anxiety:
  —Relaxation techniques
  —Antianxiety medications

NURSING DIAGNOSES

- *Cerebral tissue perfusion, altered, related to upper torso venous stasis and decreased cardiac output*
- *Thought processes, altered, related to decreased cerebral tissue perfusion and impaired gas exchange*

OUTCOME GOAL

Patient will be able to:

- Maintain adequate cardiac function, as evidenced by regular pulse, regular and nonlabored respirations, laboratory values within patient's normal limits, chest x-ray film showing no mediastinal mass, and ABGs within patient's normal limits.

INTERVENTIONS

- Assess organ systems for malfunction related to ischemia.
- Note any changes in mental status.
- Monitor laboratory values closely.
- Administer vasoactive drugs as ordered.
- Provide oxygen as prescribed.
- Institute safety measures as indicated.

NURSING DIAGNOSIS

- *Skin integrity, impaired, risk for, in the chest/thorax area related to the effects of SVCS, radiation therapy*

OUTCOME GOAL

Patient will be able to:

- Demonstrate strategies to promote optimal skin integrity.

INTERVENTIONS

- Explain effects of SVCS and radiation on skin and prepare patient for temporary changes (edema, discoloration, pruritus).
- Outline proper skin hygiene:
  —Use mild soap and tepid water and pat dry.
  —Avoid use of lotions, creams, ointments, powders, and perfumes on skin in the treatment field.
- Wear loose cotton clothing on the chest.
- Protect chest from direct sunlight.
- Avoid application of heat to the area being treated.
- Report any discomfort to physician and nurse.

NURSING DIAGNOSIS

- *Swallowing, impaired, related to inflammation of the esophagus caused by vena cava obstruction, effects of radiation therapy*

OUTCOME GOALS

Patient will be able to:

- Identify signs and symptoms of difficulty swallowing and reports these to the health care team.
- Identify measures to improve swallowing ability.
- Exhibit stable nutritional status.

INTERVENTIONS

- Assess patient's ability to swallow liquids and solids.
- Observe closely for aspiration.
- Provide analgesics as indicated.
- Change diet to avoid irritating foods (spicy or coarse).
- Avoid alcohol and tobacco use.
- Provide frequent mouth care.
- Alter medication schedule and form or rate (decrease pill size, liquids, etc.) as needed.
- Provide adequate hydration and nutrition.

As the acute phase of SVCS passes, the patient will be ready to become more involved in self-care, and anticipatory guidance can be given to facilitate continued therapy and detection of any changes in the patient's condition.

lioma; and carcinoid tumors. Several chemotherapeutic agents—cisplatin, cyclophosphamide, vinblastine, and vincristine—have demonstrated the inappropriate release of ADH.[40,53,123,142,144]

The incidence of SIADH is rising because of the increased incidence of small cell lung cancer and other cancers associated with the ectopic production of ADH.[40]

Nonmalignant conditions that can account for SIADH are CNS disorders, pulmonary infections, asthma, the use of positive-pressure respirators, the administration of certain medications, hypoadrenocorticism, lupus erythematosus, and acute intermittent porphyria.[101]

PATHOPHYSIOLOGY

All body fluids are solutions containing various concentrations of solute (salt) and solvent (fluid or water). The concentration of salt in body fluid creates an osmotic pressure. Measurement of osmotic pressure is referred to as *osmolality* or *osmolarity*. It is expressed in osmols (Osm) or milliosmols (mOsm) per kilogram of either water (osmolality) or solution (osmolarity). In a steady state, normal osmolality is maintained at a constant level of 280 to 300 mOsm/kg of body weight.[156] The osmolarity and volume of the extracellular fluid and the urine are maintained by a balance of fluid intake and urinary excretion.

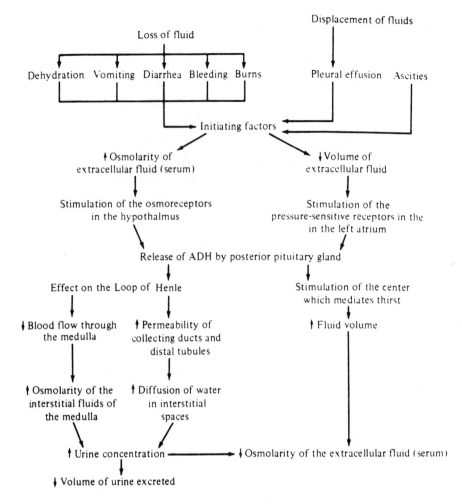

Figure 19-16   Feedback mechanism regulating the release of antidiuretic hormone *(ADH)*. (From Yasko JM: Syndrome of inappropriate antidiuretic hormone secretion. In Yasko JM, editor: *Guidelines for cancer care: symptom management,* Reston, Va, 1983, Reston.)

Fluid intake is maintained by the thirst mechanism located in the hypothalamus (Figure 19-16). Lack of water increases the osmolality of the extracellular fluid, which activates the sensation of thirst. Fluid intake is then increased to restore the fluid balance. If excess fluid is ingested, it is excreted to maintain the balance.[101]

The second portion of the osmolarity-regulating system is urinary excretion. The amount of urine excreted by the kidneys depends on how much fluid is reabsorbed and circulated throughout the body.[88,123] This regulation of fluid intake and output through the kidneys is controlled by the presence of ADH in the kidneys.

ADH is produced by the hypothalamus and transported to the posterior pituitary, where it is stored. Changes in ADH production and secretion (increase or decrease) are controlled by receptors in the kidneys, heart, and brain in response to extracellular or intravascular volume[57,88,123] (Figure 19-16). ADH secretion is extremely sensitive and responds to a 1% to 2% change in osmolality.

When plasma osmolarity is increased or plasma volume is decreased, ADH is secreted from the pituitary gland. Once in the kidneys, ADH increases the permeability of the distal tubule and the collection duct, which allows more water reabsorption. This enhanced amount of water enters the vascular system, diluting solutes, lowering plasma osmolarity, and resulting in concentrated urine excretion. Decreased plasma or blood volume also stimulates ADH secretion. A moderate increase in ADH occurs with a 10% blood loss, and a 25% blood loss can produce 20 to 50 times the normal rate of ADH secretion.[88] This response maintains arterial blood pressure.

If plasma osmolarity is decreased, as in the presence of excessive water intake, ADH secretion is halted. This decreases the permeability to water of the renal distal tubule and the collecting duct, allowing more water to be excreted as dilute urine. An increase in plasma or blood volume also stops the release of ADH. Drinking alcohol also inhibits ADH secretion. In summary, the thirst mechanism and the ADH feedback mechanisms (Figure 19-16) regulate body fluids and maintain a constant osmolality.[101,123]

A variety of conditions can disrupt the body fluid–regulating system and cause SIADH. The following three pathophysiologic mechanisms are responsible for SIADH:

- Inappropriate secretion of ADH from the supraoptic-hypophyseal system. This mechanism results from CNS disorders such as head trauma, CVA (stroke), meningitis, brain abscess, CNS hemorrhage, CNS tumors (both primary and metastatic), encephalitis, and Guillain-Barré syndrome. Postoperative patients; patients in shock; patients experiencing status asthmaticus, pain, or high stress levels; and patients on positive-pressure breathing may also experience SIADH through this mechanism. These conditions increase intrathoracic pressure and/or decrease venous return to the heart. Cardiac output decreases, leading to decreased plasma volume, stimulating ADH secretion.[101]
- ADH or an ADH-like substance is secreted by cells outside the supraoptic-hypophyseal system, referred to as *ectopic secretion*. Infections within the pulmonary system such as those caused by bacteria or viruses may release ADH by this mechanism. This may also be one process leading to SIADH seen in patients with a malignancy.
- The action of ADH on the renal distal tubules is enhanced. Various drugs can stimulate or potentiate the release of ADH. These include narcotics such as morphine, nicotine, tranquilizers, barbiturates, general anesthetics, potassium supplements, thiazide diuretics, hypoglycemic agents such as chlorpropamide (Diabinese), clofibrate (Atromid-S), acetaminophen (paracetamol, Tylenol), isoproterenol, and four antineoplastic agents: cisplatin (Platinol), cyclophosphamide (Cytoxan), vinblastine (Velban), and vincristine (Oncovin).[101,123]

Patients with cancer may have SIADH resulting from any one of these three mechanisms. Intrathoracic or mediastinal tumors can increase intrathoracic pressure, resulting in a decreased venous return and decreased cardiac output, which stimulates the release of ADH. Patients with small (oat) cell lung cancer (50%), pancreatic cancer, lymphomas, and thymomas have demonstrated synthesis and secretion of ADH or an ADH-like substance from the neoplastic tissue.[101,144] Patients receiving chemotherapy that includes cisplatin, cyclophosphamide, vinblastine, or vincristine (Oncovin) have the potential to develop SIADH.

SIADH is associated with water excess and results from the ectopic production of ADH. ADH increases the permeability of the kidney to water, promoting water reabsorption and decreasing urine output. This may be associated with hyponatremia. Hyponatremia may be caused by excessive loss of sodium or excessive gain of water. It is always a result of a relatively greater water concentration than sodium concentration.[40]

However, hyponatremia is not solely diagnostic of SIADH. Some other disorders may also stimulate SIADH. In hypothyroidism and hypoadrenocorticism, the hormone deficiency is responsible, but the exact mechanism is unknown. Finally, SIADH can also be seen with hyponatremia secondary to sodium depletion (renal disease, vomiting, diarrhea, diabetic acidosis) hypokalemia, glucocorticoid deficiency, third spacing, and dilutional hyponatremia related to CHF, renal failure, or ascites related to liver disease.[40,53,57,91,123]

Two other particular situations will elicit hyponatremia. First, hyponatremia also occurs when nonsodium solutes accumulate in the extracellular space because they do not freely diffuse across cell membranes. This causes an osmotic gradient that allows water to move from the intracellular to the extracellular space. Two conditions can produce this phenomena. Hyperglycemia is the most common cause of this disorder. The calculated and measured plasma osmolality will be the same, which is elevated because of hyperglycemia. IV mannitol therapy also demonstrates an elevated plasma osmolality, but the calculated level is lower than the measured value. In either situation, these are *not* true hypoosmolar states.

Second, *psuedohyponatremia* may occur, also called *factitious hyponatremia*. These terms describe a low serum sodium concentration secondary to volume-displacing effects that can occur with hyperproteinemia and hyperlipidemia. Large macromolecules (proteins, lipids) are present and fictitiously lower plasma sodium levels, as measured in the clinical laboratory. However, measured plasma osmolality is normal.[101]

These interesting situations must be evaluated in the presence of hyponatremia. Diagnostic work-up for any patient with hyponatremia requires determination of the existence of a hypoosmolar state.

CLINICAL FEATURES

The clinical syndrome resulting from inappropriate secretion of ADH has the following features[40,53,123,144]:

- Hyponatremia (serum sodium less than normal level of 135 to 147 mEq/L)
- Decreased osmolality of serum and extracellular fluid (less than normal level of 280 to 300 mOsm/kg)
- Excessive water retention (water intoxication)
- Urine osmolarity greater than appropriate for plasma osmolarity, producing less than maximally dilute urine (abnormally high urine specific gravity)
- Continued urinary excretion of sodium (sodium in

urine greater than 20 mEq/L) (washing of sodium in urine)
- Absence of fluid volume depletion (normal skin turgor and blood pressure)
- Suppression of plasma renin
- Normal renal, adrenal, and thyroid function
- BUN possibly low because of volume expansion

Hypouricemia and hypophosphatemia may be present because of decreased proximal tubular reabsorption.[53] The symptomatology experienced by the patient with SIADH depends on the degree of duration of water retention and hyponatremia. Excessive water retention continues despite a decrease in the osmolality of serum and extracellular fluid. Urine is concentrated, the extracellular fluid expands, and this results in hyponatremia. Patients complain of thirst, anorexia, nausea, and vomiting. Weight gain, lethargy, and muscle weakness occur. Irritability, personality changes, and mental confusion may occur and lead to seizures and coma.*

DIAGNOSIS

A differential diagnosis of SIADH is sometimes difficult because any one of the clinical features may be absent. Therefore the presence of all the features is not required for diagnosis. To support a clinical diagnosis of SIADH, a water-loading test may be performed safely if the serum sodium is greater than 125 mEq/L and if the patient is asymptomatic.[101] Patient preparation for the test requires nothing by mouth and no nicotine for 12 hours. Serum osmolality levels and serum, BUN, creatinine, Na^+, K^+, and Cl^- levels are obtained. The patient also is weighed.

The water-loading test is performed in the following manner[101]:
- Instruct the patient to remain recumbent during the duration of the test, which is 5 to 6 hours.
- Administer 300 ml of water 1 hour before test begins to replace insensible fluid losses during the period of nothing by mouth.
- Administer water (20 ml/kg) within 30 minutes.
- Collect urine hourly for 5 hours.
- Monitor patient for nausea, abdominal pain, feeling of fullness, desire to defecate, fatigue, shortness of breath, and chest pain.
- Calculate urine volume, osmolality, and specific gravity as follows:

	Normal results	Results seen with SIADH
Urine volume	80% excreted	Less than 40% excreted
Urine osmolality	100 to 1000 mOsm/kg	Less than 100 mOsm/kg
Specific gravity	1.015 to 1.025	Less than 1.003

Serum and urine levels of ADH, which would be elevated in the presence of SIADH, can also be measured.

*References 40, 53, 57, 101, 123, 125.

TREATMENT MODALITIES

The primary treatment of choice for SIADH is to treat or eliminate the underlying cause. Other medical orders include the following:
- Discontinue any medications that might cause SIADH.
- Restrict fluids to 500 to 1000 ml/24 hours depending on the severity until the plasma osmolality increases. This may take 4 to 10 days. The slowest response is seen in patients with ADH-secreting tumors.[101]
- Administer pharmacologic agents that interfere with the action of ADH on the renal tubules and induce polyuria, such as lithium carbonate (300 mg/day) or demeclocycline, a tetracycline derivative (600 mg to 1200 mg/day) (greater renal toxicity is seen with 1200 mg/day).[144] The total drug dose is divided and given two or three times a day. Doses should be reduced in patients with hepatic or renal dysfunction.
- If symptoms of water intoxication are severe, administer hypertonic (5% NaCl, 3% if hypercalcemic) solution with or without furosemide (Lasix) via volumetric pump.

Currently, no drugs are available that directly suppress the synthesis or release of ADH from malignant tissue, but effective tumor treatment and the use of lithium carbonate or demeclocycline have produced a resolution of the syndrome. Lithium carbonate disrupts the action of ADH on the kidneys, resulting in polyuria. Demeclocycline interferes with the action of ADH, producing an isotonic or hypotonic urine and an increase in serum sodium.[40,53]

Serum sodium levels should be monitored very closely during treatment for SIADH. Correction of the serum sodium should be limited to a rate of rise of 0.5 to 1 mEq/L/hour, not to exceed 130 meQ/L in the first 24 hours to minimize the risk of brain damage, including central pontine myelinolysis leading to long-lasting neurologic damage.[40,53,57]

PROGNOSIS

SIADH can be successfully treated, as evidenced by a return to normal levels of serum and extracellular osmolality, serum sodium and urine osmolality, and specific gravity. The rapidity and duration of response depend greatly on the underlying cause.

SIADH usually resolves with tumor regression, but it can persist despite control of the tumor. It may recur, suggesting tumor progression, but recurrence is sometimes seen with stable disease during the maintenance phase of therapy. Neurologic impairment from water intoxication is usually reversible and does not require long-term rehabilitation.[40]

If the underlying cause is not eliminated, the SIADH may be a chronic problem and require ongoing intermittent management.[40,57]

Nursing management of the patient with SIADH is outlined on p. 469.

NURSING MANAGEMENT

The primary nursing intervention for a patient diagnosed with the syndrome of inappropriate secretion of antidiuretic hormone (SIADH) is patient education and emotional support to facilitate patient compliance.[51,53,84,108,124]

NURSING DIAGNOSES

• *Fluid volume excess related to fluid retention (from SIADH), possible hyponatremia*
• *Fluid volume deficit related to fluid restriction as treatment for SIADH*

OUTCOME GOAL

Patient will be able to:
• Demonstrate resolution of SIADH, as evidenced by decreased or absent signs of SIADH, serum sodium range within normal limits, serum and urine osmolality within normal limits, normal urine output of at least 1500 ml/24 hours, and normal body weight for patient.

INTERVENTIONS

• Assess for signs or symptoms of alteration in fluid volume:
  —Excess: rales, shortness of breath, neck vein distention, weight gain, edema of sacrum and/or lower extremities
  —Deficit: dry mucous membranes, poor skin turgor, weight loss, rapid thready pulse, orthostatic hypotension, restlessness
• Auscultate lungs for breath sounds every 4 hours.
• Monitor cardiac function and tissue perfusion.
• Monitor intake and output closely:
  —Restrict fluids as ordered (500 to 700 ml/24 hours).
  —Allocate fluids per shift as per discussion with patient.
  —Give pills and medications with meals to allow flexibility with fluid rations.
  —Monitor IV infusions carefully using a flow regulator.
  —Accurately measure urine output. Intake and output should be almost equal until serum sodium is within normal limits.
• Obtain a daily weight.
• Monitor laboratory values (serum electrolytes, BUN, creatinine, calcium, magnesium) with special attention to the following:
  —Serum plasma osmolality: as SIADH progresses, plasma osmolality decreases, which causes the brain to swell and level of consciousness (LOC) to decrease. Therefore serum osmolality can predict LOC.
  —Serum sodium: hypernatremia may result from overcorrection of low serum levels. Accompanying signs and symptoms of hypernatremia include thirst, dry mucous membranes, irritability, lethargy, and seizures.

• Obtain urine osmolality and specific gravity.
• Monitor skin integrity and provide skin care.

NURSING DIAGNOSIS

• *Oral mucous membrane, altered, related to fluid restriction*

OUTCOME GOAL

Patient will be able to:
• Exhibit oral cavity, gums, and lips free of irritation, as evidenced by pink, moist mucosa and tongue; moist, soft lips with undisrupted integrity; pink, firm gingiva; watery saliva; and maintenance of adequate oral intake.

INTERVENTIONS

• Thoroughly assess the oral cavity daily.
• Provide oral care every 2 to 4 hours as needed:
  —Use mouthwashes with little to no alcohol.
  —Discourage smoking and drinking alcohol.
  —Avoid spicy and mechanically harsh foods.
  —Use mouth moisturizers and artificial saliva as needed.

NURSING DIAGNOSIS

• *Thought processes, altered, related to low serum sodium level*

OUTCOME GOALS

Patient will be able to:
• Remain oriented to person, time, and place.
• Demonstrate safety-related behaviors.

INTERVENTIONS

• Assess neurologic status:
  —Determine LOC, noting any changes in sensorium.
  —Check muscles and tendon reflexes for twitching.
  —Monitor for seizure activity if serum sodium level less than 120 mEq/L.
• Initiate safety precautions:
  —Monitor patient activities.
  —Assist patient with transfer and ambulation.
  —Use bed rails at night.
• Increase safety measures if change in LOC or serum sodium level less than 120 mEq/L:
  —Orient frequently to time and place.
  —Pad bed rails.
  —Use restraints as necessary.
  —Implement seizure precautions (e.g., padded tongue blade and airway at bedside, no oral thermometers).

Many patients with extreme hyponatremia cannot recollect much of their experience during the SIADH event. This points out the need to provide measures to ensure safety and to reduce anxiety.

CONCLUSION

Successful management of patients with oncologic complications requires expertise from all members of the health care team. It requires in-depth knowledge in oncology but also in many related areas, such as immunology, pharmacology, cardiopulmonary care, and critical care. The nurse is in a pivotal role as coordinator of the care and as patient advocate to help the patient and family deal with the impact of the illness on their lives.

■ CHAPTER QUESTIONS

1. Etiology and risk factors for disseminated intravascular coagulation (DIC) include:
   a. Shock, infection, nausea and vomiting, diarrhea
   b. Shock, infection, acute leukemia, diarrhea
   c. Shock, infection, acute leukemia, intravascular hemolysis
   d. Shock, infection, skin cancer, intravascular hemolysis
2. Components of the DIC laboratory test profile include:
   a. Complete blood count (CBC), serum aspartate aminotransferase (AST, SGOT), prothrombin times (PTs), fibrinogen levels
   b. PTs, fibrinogen levels, platelet levels, protamine sulfate
   c. PTs, fibrinogen levels, CBC, type and cross-match
   d. PTs, fibrinogen levels, platelet levels, HLA antigens
3. Clinical features for hypercalcemia include:
   a. Polyuria, polydipsia, diarrhea, lethargy
   b. Anuria, change in mental status, constipation, anorexia
   c. Polydipsia, constipation, change in mental status, increased appetite
   d. Polyuria, polydipsia, change in mental status, absent deep tendon reflex
4. Treatment modalities for hypercalcemia include:
   a. Hydration, dialysis, pharmacologic therapy, mobilization
   b. Hydration, dialysis, pharmacologic therapy, bedrest
   c. Hydration, pharmacologic therapy, radiation therapy, mobilization
   d. Hydration, dialysis, pharmacologic therapy, biotherapy
5. Malignant pleural effusion is life-threatening because the:
   a. Decreased pleural fluid affects respiratory function.
   b. Increased pleural fluid affects respiratory function.
   c. Increased pericardial fluid affects respiratory function.
   d. Decreased pericardial fluid affects respiratory function.
6. The lymphatic channels regulate fluid and protein reabsorption. Normally how much fluid passes through the pleural space in 24 hours? How much fluid remains in the pleural space at any given time?
   a. 1 to 5 L; 10 to 20 ml
   b. 3 to 10 L; 10 to 20 ml
   c. 10 to 20 L; 5 to 10 ml
   d. 5 to 10 L; 5 to 10 ml
7. Two clinical findings that are classic features of cardiac tamponade are:
   a. Pulsus paradoxus, bradycardia
   b. Hepatojugular reflux, elevated systolic blood pressure
   c. Pulsus paradoxus, hepatojugular reflux
   d. Hepatojugular reflux, vasodilation

8. Septic shock may be classified by hyperdynamic stage (early), normodynamic stage (intermediate), and hypodynamic stage (late). Usual progression of the clinical features for these stages are:
   a. Tachycardia, decreased respirations, hypotension, anuria
   b. Tachycardia, increased respirations, decreased urine output, altered mental status
   c. Tachycardia, respirations slow and shallow, hypertension, altered mental status
   d. Tachycardia, respirations slow and shallow, hypertension, renal failure
9. In which area of the spinal column are the majority of spinal metastases that cause spinal cord compression (SCC)?
   a. Cervical
   b. Thoracic
   c. Lumbosacral
10. Symptomatology is directly related to the location of the SCC. What is the *most* common presenting symptom of SCC?
    a. Pain
    b. Motor weakness
    c. Sensory loss
    d. Sexual dysfunction
11. What is the first therapeutic measure after a confirmed diagnosis of superior vena cava syndrome (SVCS)?
    a. Biotherapy
    b. Chemotherapy
    c. Radiation therapy
    d. Surgery
12. Syndrome of inappropriate antidiuretic hormone secretion (SIADH) is *most* common in which type of cancer?
    a. Breast
    b. Colorectal
    c. Multiple myeloma
    d. Small cell lung cancer

BIBLIOGRAPHY

1. Abraham J, Polomano R: Disseminated intravascular coagulation. In Polomano RC, Miller SE, editors: *Understanding and managing oncologic emergencies,* monograph, Columbus, Ohio, 1987, Adria Laboratories.
2. Anderson RP, Li W: Segmental replacement of superior vena cava with spiral vein graft, *Ann Thorac Surg* 36(1):85, 1983.
3. Bailes BK: Disseminated intravascular coagulation: principles, treatment, nursing management, *AORN J* 55(2):517, 1992.
4. Baird S, editor: Prevention and management of neutropenia in the cancer patient, *Oncol Nurs Forum Suppl* 17(1):3, 1990.
5. Bajorunas DR, editor: Advances in the hypercalcemia of malignancy, *Semin Oncol* 17(suppl 5):1, 1990.
6. Baldwin PD: Epidural spinal cord compression secondary to metastatic disease: a review of the literature, *Cancer Nurs* 6(6):441, 1983.
7. Barbiere CC: Are you listening? Cardiac tamponade: diagnosis and emergency intervention, *Crit Care Nurse* 10(4):7, 1990.
8. Barbiere CC: Cardiac tamponade: diagnosis and emergency intervention, *Crit Care Nurse* 10(4):20, 1990.

9. Barry S: Septic shock: special needs of patients with cancer, *Oncol Nurs Forum* 16(1):31, 1989.
10. Bass J and others: Superior vena cava syndrome: report of a new operative technique, *J Natl Med Assoc* 72(11):1105, 1980.
11. Beattie S, Meinhardt SL: Transesophageal echocardiography: advanced technology for the cardiac patient, *Crit Care Nurse* 12(8):42, 1992.
12. Berger NA: Introduction: an overview of oncologic emergencies, *Semin Oncol* 16(6):461, 1989.
13. Bick R: Disseminated intravascular coagulation and related syndromes: etiology, pathophysiology, diagnosis and management, *Am J Hematol* 5(3):265, 1978.
14. Bockheim CM: What is the role of etidronate in the treatment of hypercalcemia? *Highlights Antineoplast Drugs* 7(3):59, 1989.
15. Boh D, VanSon A: The water load test, *Am J Nurs* 82(1):112, 1982.
16. Bradof J, Sands MJ, Lakin PC: Symptomatic venous thrombosis of the upper extremity complicating permanent transvenous pacing: reversal with streptokinase infusion, *Am Heart J* 104(5):1112, 1982.
17. Brandt B: A nursing protocol for the client with neutropenia, *Oncol Nurs Forum* 11(2):24, 1984.
18. Braunwald E: Pericardial disease. In Braunwald E and others, editors: *Harrison's principles of internal medicine,* ed 11, New York, 1991, McGraw-Hill.
19. Briening EP: Septic shock: tough cases that teach the most, *RN* 51(9):36, 1988.
20. Britton D, Yasko JM: Hypercalcemia. In Yasko JM, editor: *Guidelines for cancer care: symptom management,* Reston, Va, 1983, Reston.
21. Bruckman JE, Bloomer WD: Management of spinal cord compression, *Semin Oncol* 5(2):135, 1978.
22. Buchsel PC: Managing infections in the neutropenic oncology patient. In *Challenges in treatment and management,* Proceedings of the Sixth National Conference on Cancer Nursing, Atlanta, 1992, American Cancer Society.
23. Byrne TN: Spinal cord compression from epidural metastases, *N Engl J Med* 327:614, 1992.
24. Calafato A, Jessys AL: Body fluid composition, alteration in: hypercalcemia. In McNally JC and others, editors: *Guidelines for oncology nursing practice,* ed 2, Philadelphia, 1991, Saunders.
25. Carlson A: Infection prophylaxis in the patient with cancer, *Oncol Nurs Forum* 12(3):56, 1985.
26. Cawley M: Alteration in cardiac output, decreased: related to superior vena cava syndrome. In McNally JC and others, editors: *Guidelines for oncology nursing practice,* ed 2, Philadelphia, 1991, Saunders.
27. Ciszewski M: Spinal cord compression. In Brown MH and others, editors: *Standards of oncology nursing practice,* New York, 1986, Wiley & Sons.
28. Clark JC, McGee RF, Preston R: Nursing management of responses to the cancer experience. In Clark JC, McGee RF, editors: *Core curriculum for oncology nursing,* ed 2, Philadelphia, 1992, Saunders.
29. Colman RW, Rubin RN: Disseminated intravascular coagulation due to malignancy, *Semin Oncol* 17(2):172, 1990.
30. Concilus EM, Bohachick PA: Cancer: pericardial effusion and tamponade, *Cancer Nurs* 7(5):391, 1984.
31. Coward D: Cancer-induced hypercalcemia, *Cancer Nurs* 9(3):125, 1986.
32. Cowcher K, Hanks GW: Long-term management of respiratory symptoms in advanced cancer, *J Pain Symptom Manage* 5(5):320, 1990.
33. Culpepper RN, Porter GA, Roddam RF: Why is the serum sodium low? *Patient Care* 20(7):94, 1986.
34. Dangel RN: Injury, potential for, related to disseminated intravascular coagulation (DIC). In McNally JC and others, editors: *Guidelines for oncology nursing practice,* ed 2, Philadelphia, 1991, Saunders.
35. Deisseroth A, Wallenstein R: Use of hematopoietic growth factors. In DeVita VT Jr, Hellman S, Rosenberg AS, editors: *Cancer: principles and practice of oncology,* ed 4, Philadelphia, 1993, Lippincott.
36. Delaney TF, Oldfield EH: Spinal cord compression. In DeVita VT Jr, Hellman S, Rosenberg SA, editors: *Cancer: principles and practice of oncology,* ed 4, Philadelphia, 1993, Lippincott.
37. Desser RK, Brown CM, Bitran JD: *The management of malignant pleural effusions,* monograph, Evansville, Ind, 1984, Bristol-Myers.
38. Dietz K, Flaherty AM: Oncologic emergencies. In Groenwald SL and others, editors: *Cancer nursing: principles and practice,* ed 2, Boston, 1990, Jones and Bartlett.
39. Donoghue M: Spinal cord compression. In Yasko JM, editor: *Guidelines for cancer care: symptom management,* Reston, Va, 1983, Reston.
40. Donoghue M: Superior vena cava syndrome. In Yasko JM, editor: *Guidelines for cancer care: symptom management,* Reston, Va, 1983, Reston.
41. Dutcher JP: Bleeding and coagulopathy. In Dutcher JP, Wiernik PH, editors: *Handbook of hematologic and oncologic emergencies,* New York, 1987, Plenum.
42. Dyck S: Surgical instrumentation as a palliative treatment for spinal cord compression, *Oncol Nurs Forum* 18(3):515, 1991.
43. Einzig AI: Hypercalcemia in malignancy. In Dutcher JP, Wiernik PH, editors: *Handbook of hematologic and oncologic emergencies,* New York, 1987, Plenum.
44. Ellerhorst-Ryan JM: Septic shock: understanding and managing a crisis. In *Challenges in treatment and management,* Proceedings of the Sixth National Conference on Cancer Nursing, Atlanta, 1992, American Cancer Society.
45. Epstein C, Bakanauskas A: Clinical management of DIC: early nursing interventions, *Crit Care Nurs* 11(10):42, 1991.
46. Estes ME: Management of the cardiac tamponade patient: a nursing framework, *Crit Care Nurse* 5(5):17, 1985.
47. Fingar BL: Sclerosing agents used to control malignant pleural effusions, *Hosp Pharm* 27:622, July 1992.
48. Finley JP: Nursing care of patients with metabolic and physiological oncological emergencies. In Clark JC, McGee RF, editors: *Core curriculum for oncology nursing,* ed 2, Philadelphia, 1991, Saunders.
49. Frommel L, Mesa D, Outlaw E: Septic shock. In Brown MH and others, editors: *Standards of oncology nursing practice,* New York, 1986, Wiley & Sons.
50. Fuen LG, Thurer R: *Tube drainage and intrapleural therapy for malignant pleural effusions: a portfolio of case reports,* monograph, Evansville, Ind, 1990, Bristol-Myers.

51. Gentzch P: Mobility, impaired physical, related to spinal cord compression. In McNally JC and others, editors: *Guidelines for oncology nursing practice,* ed 2, Philadelphia, 1991, Saunders.

52. Gilbert MR, Grossman SA: Incidence and nature of neurologic problems in patients with solid tumors, *Am J Med* 81:951, 1986.

53. Gilbert RW, Kim J, Posner JB: Epidural spinal cord compression from metastatic tumor: diagnosis and treatment, *Ann Neurol* 3(1):40, 1978.

54. Glover DJ, Glick JH: Managing oncologic emergencies involving structural dysfunction, *CA Cancer J Clin* 35(4):238, 1985.

55. Glover DJ, Glick JH: Oncologic emergencies. In Holleb AI, Fink DJ, Murphy GP, editors: *American Cancer Society textbook of clinical oncology,* Atlanta, 1991, American Cancer Society.

56. Gobel BH, Lawler PE: Malignant pleural effusions, *Oncol Nurs Forum* 12(4):49, 1985.

57. Gray BH and others: Safety and efficacy of thrombolytic therapy for superior vena cava syndrome, *Chest* 99:54, 1991.

58. Griffin J: Be prepared for the bleeding patient, *Nursing '86* 16(6):34, 1986.

59. Grossman SA, Lossignol D: Diagnosis and treatment of epidural metastases, *Oncology* 4(4):47, 1990.

60. Gulcap R, Dutcher JP: Fever and infection. In Dutcher JP, Wiernik PH, editors: *Handbook of hematologic and oncologic emergencies,* New York, 1987, Plenum.

61. Gulcap R and others: Comparative study of pamidronate disodium and etidronate disodium in the treatment of cancer-related hypercalcemia, *J Clin Oncol* 10(1):134, 1992.

62. Harnett S: Septic shock in the oncology patient, *Cancer Nurs* 12(4):191, 1989.

63. Henry P, Seery R, Outlaw EM: Hypercalcemia. In Brown MH and others, editors: *Standards of oncology nursing practice,* New York, 1986, Wiley & Sons.

64. Hewitt JB, Janssen WR: A management strategy for malignancy-induced pleural effusion: long-term thoracostomy drainage, *Oncol Nurs Forum* 14(5):17, 1987.

65. Hilderley LJ: Spinal cord compression: the nurse's role in early detection and rehabilitation. In *Challenges in treatment and management,* Proceedings of the Sixth National Conference on Cancer Nursing, Atlanta, 1992, American Cancer Society.

66. Hilton G, Frei J: High-dose methylprednisolone in the treatment of spinal cord injuries, *Heart Lung* 20(6):675, 1991.

67. Hogan CM: Sexual dysfunction related to disease process and treatment. In McNally JC and others, editors: *Guidelines for oncology nursing practice,* ed 2, Philadelphia, 1991, Saunders.

68. Hunter JC: Nursing care of patients with structural oncological emergencies. In Clark JC, McGee RF, editors: *Core curriculum for oncology nursing,* ed 2, Philadelphia, 1992, Saunders.

69. Hydzik CA: Alteration in cardiac output, decreased: related to cardiac tamponade. In McNally JC and others, editors: *Guidelines for oncology nursing practice,* ed 2, Philadelphia, 1991, Saunders.

70. Jenkins J: Pleural effusion. In Baird SB, editor: *Decision making in oncology nursing,* Philadelphia, 1988, Decker.

71. Jennings BM: Improving your management of DIC, *Nursing '79* 9(5):60, 1979.

72. Johndrow PD, Thornton S: Syndrome of inappropriate antidiuretic hormone: a growing concern, *Focus Crit Care* 12(5):29, 1985.

73. Joiner GA, Kolodychuk GR: Neoplastic cardiac tamponade, *Crit Care Nurse* 11(2):50, 1991.

74. Joshi J: Epidemiology of infections in cancer patients, *Mediguide Infect Dis* 9(2):1, 1989.

75. Kanner R: Epidural spinal cord compression. In Dutcher JP, Wiernik PH, editors: *Handbook of hematologic and oncologic emergencies,* New York, 1987, Plenum.

76. Kern L, Omery A: Decreased cardiac output in the critical care setting, *Nurs Diagn* 3(3):94, 1992.

77. Khandheria BK, Oh J: Transesophageal echocardiography: state-of-the-art and future directions, *Am J Cardiol* 69:61H, June 1992.

78. Klein DM, Witek-Janusek L: Advances in immunotherapy of sepsis, *Dimens Crit Care Nurs* 11(2):75, 1992.

79. Kliger A, Lovett D: Electrolyte abnormalities in cancer patients. In Yarbro J, Bornstein R, editors: *Oncologic emergencies,* New York, 1981, Grune & Stratton.

80. Kraemer K: Superior vena cava syndrome. In Johnson BL, Gross J, editors: *Handbook of oncology nursing,* New York, 1985, Wiley & Sons.

81. Kralstein J, Frishman W: Malignant pericardial disease: diagnosis and treatment. In Dutcher JP, Wiernik PH, editors: *Handbook of hematologic and oncologic emergencies,* New York, 1987, Plenum.

82. Kratcha-Sveningson L: Body fluid composition, alteration in: syndrome of inappropriate antidiuretic hormone (SIADH). In McNally JC and others, editors: *Guidelines for oncology nursing practice,* ed 2, Philadelphia, 1991, Saunders.

83. Lane G, Peirce AG: When persistence pays off, *Nursing '82* 12(1):44, 1982.

84. Larkin M, Benson LM: Ineffective airway clearance. In Clark JC, McGee RF, editors: *Core curriculum for oncology nursing,* ed 2, Philadelphia, 1992, Saunders.

85. Lazarus HM, Creger RJ, Gerson SL: Infectious emergencies in oncology patients, *Semin Oncol* 16(6):543, 1989.

86. Lind JM: Ectopic hormonal production: nursing implications, *Semin Oncol Nurs* 1(4):251, 1985.

87. Lindaman C: SIADH: is your patient at risk? *Nursing '92* 22(6):60, 1992.

88. Littleton M: Pathophysiology and assessment of sepsis and septic shock, *Crit Care Nurs Q* 11(1):30, 1988.

89. Lokich J, Goodman R: Superior vena cava syndrome, *JAMA* 321(1):58, 1975.

90. Mahon SM: Signs and symptoms associated with malignancy-induced hypercalcemia, *Cancer Nurs* 12(3):153, 1989.

91. Mangan CM: Malignant pericardial effusions: pathophysiology and clinical correlates, *Oncol Nurs Forum* 19(8):215, 1991.

92. Marcus SL, Fuks JZ: Syndrome of inappropriate antidiuretic hormone secretion and hyponatremia. In Dutcher JP, Wirnik PH, editors: *Handbook of hematologic and oncologic emergencies,* New York, 1987, Plenum.

93. Mayer DK: Cardiac tamponade. In Baird SB, editor: *Decision making in oncology nursing,* Philadelphia, 1988, Decker.

94. Mayer DK: Spinal cord compression. In Baird SB, editor: *Decision making in oncology nursing,* Philadelphia, 1988, Decker.

95. Mayer DK: Superior vena cava syndrome. In Baird SB, editor: *Decision making in oncology nursing,* Philadelphia, 1988, Decker.

96. Mayer DK: Disseminated intravascular coagulation. In Baird SB, editor: *Decision making in oncology nursing,* Philadelphia, 1988, Decker.

97. Mayer DK: Hypercalcemia. In Baird SB, editor: *Decision making in oncology nursing,* Philadelphia, 1988, Decker.

98. Mayer DK: Inappropriate antidiuretic hormone syndrome. In Baird SB, editor: *Decision making in oncology nursing,* Philadelphia, 1988, Decker.

99. Mayer DK: Septic shock. In Baird SB, editor: *Decision making in oncology nursing,* Philadelphia, 1988, Decker.

100. McFadden ME, Sartorius SE: Multiple system organ failure in the patient with cancer. Part I. Pathophysiologic perspectives, *Oncol Nurs Forum* 19(5):719, 1992.

101. McFadden ME, Sartorius SE: Multiple system organ failure in the patient with cancer. Part II. Nursing implications, *Oncol Nurs Forum* 19(5):727, 1992.

102. McGillick K: DIC: the deadly paradox, *RN* 45:41, 1982.

103. McMorrow ME, Cooney-Daniello M: When to suspect septic shock, *RN* 54(10):32, 1991.

104. Meriney DK: Application of Orem's conceptual framework to patients with hypercalcemia related to breast cancer, *Cancer Nurs* 13(5):316, 1990.

105. Meriney DK: Diagnosis and management of acute promyelocytic leukemia with disseminated intravascular coagulopathy: a case study, *Oncol Nurs Forum* 17(3):379, 1990.

106. Mersky C: DIC: identification and management, *Hosp Pract* 17:83, 1982.

107. Miaskowski C: Oncologic emergencies. In Baird SB, McCorkle R, Grant M, editors: *Cancer nursing: a comprehensive textbook,* Philadelphia, 1991, Saunders.

108. Miller SE: Superior vena cava syndrome. In Polomano RN, Miller SE, editors: *Understanding and managing oncologic emergencies,* monograph, Columbus, Ohio, 1987, Adria Laboratories.

109. Miller SE, Campbell DB: Malignant pericardial effusions. In Polomano RC, Miller SE, editors: *Understanding and managing oncologic emergencies,* monograph, Columbus, Ohio, 1987, Adria Laboratories.

110. Miller SE, Campbell DB: Pleural effusions in malignant disease. In Polomano RC, Miller SE, editors: *Understanding and managing oncologic emergencies,* monograph, Columbus, Ohio, 1987, Adria Laboratories.

111. Mizock B: Septic shock—a metabolic perspective, *Arch Intern Med* 144(3):579, 1984.

112. Moores DWO: Malignant pleural effusion, *Semin Oncol* 18(suppl 2):59, 1991.

113. Morse LK, Heery ML, Flynn KT: Early detection to avert the crisis of superior vena cava syndrome, *Cancer Nurs* 8(4):228, 1985.

114. Mundy G: Options for correcting hypercalcemia of malignancy, *Hosp Ther,* February 1988, p 52.

115. Nissenblatt M: Oncologic emergencies, *Am Fam Physician* 20(2):104, 1979.

116. Olopade OI, Ultmann JE: Malignant effusions, *CA Cancer J Clin* 41(3):167, 1991.

117. Parish J and others: Etiologic considerations in superior vena cava syndrome, *Mayo Clin Proc* 56(7):407, 1981.

118. Perez CA, Presant CA, VanAmburg AL: Management of superior vena cava syndrome, *Semin Oncol* 5(2):123, 1978.

119. Perry A: Shock complications: recognition and management, *Crit Care Nurs Q* 11(1):1, 1988.

120. Pilapil F: Disseminated intravascular coagulation (DIC). In Brown MH and others, editors: *Standards of oncology nursing practice,* New York, 1986, Wiley & Sons.

121. Pizzo PA, Myers J: Infections in the cancer patient. In DeVita VT Jr, Hellman S, Rosenberg SA, editors: *Cancer: principles and practice of oncology,* ed 4, Philadelphia, 1993, Lippincott.

122. Poe CM, Radford AI: The challenge of hypercalcemia in cancer, *Oncol Nurs Forum* 12(6):29, 1985.

123. Poe CM, Taylor LM: Syndrome of inappropriate antidiuretic hormone: assessment and nursing implications, *Oncol Nurs Forum* 16(3):373, 1989.

124. Portlock C, Goffinet D: *Manual of clinical problems in oncology,* ed 2, Boston, 1986, Little, Brown.

125. Rahko PS, Shaver JA: Superior vena cava syndrome, *Hosp Med* 21(7):83, 1985.

126. Ratnoff OD: Hemostatic emergencies in malignancy, *Semin Oncol* 16(6):561, 1989.

127. Reichel J, Menon L: Pulmonary emergencies in oncology. In Dutcher JP, Wiernik PH, editors: *Handbook of hematologic and oncologic emergencies,* New York, 1987, Plenum.

128. Rice V: Shock, a clinical syndrome: an update. Part 1. An overview of shock, *Crit Care Nurse* 11(4):20, 1991.

129. Rice V: Shock, a clinical syndrome: an update. Part 2. The stages of shock, *Crit Care Nurse* 11(4):74, 1991.

130. Rice V: Shock, a clinical syndrome: an update. Part 3. Therapeutic management, *Crit Care Nurse* 11(4):34, 1991.

131. Rice V: Shock, a clinical syndrome: an update. Part 4. Nursing care of the shock patient, *Crit Care Nurse* 11(7):28, 1991.

132. Rodriquez M, Dinapoli RP: Spinal cord compression, *Mayo Clin Proc* 55(7):442, 1980.

133. Rooney A, Haviley C: Nursing management of disseminated intravascular coagulation, *Oncol Nurs Forum* 12(1):15, 1985.

134. Rosch J and others: Gianturco expandable wire stents in the treatment of superior vena cava syndrome recurring after maximum tolerance radiation, *Cancer* 60(6):1243, 1987.

135. Rosetti A: Nursing care of patients treated with intrapleural tetracycline for control of malignant pleural effusion, *Cancer Nurs* 8(2):103, 1985.

136. Ruckdeschel JC: Management of malignant pleural effusion: an overview, *Semin Oncol* 15(suppl 3):24, 1988.

137. Ruckdeschel JC and others: Intrapleural therapy for malignant pleural effusions: a randomized comparison of bleomycin and tetracycline, *Chest* 10(6):1528, 1991.

138. Sahn SA: Diagnosis pleural effusion, *Hosp Med* 28(9):66, 1992.

139. Schruber JA: Impaired gas exchange. In Clark JC, McGee RF, editors: *Core curriculum for oncology nursing,* ed 2, Philadelphia, 1992, Saunders.

140. Sculier JP and others: Superior vena cava obstruction syndrome in small cell lung cancer, *Cancer* 57(4):847, 1986.

141. Shoemaker WC: Early diagnosis and management of pericardial tamponade, *Hosp Med* 14(11):7, 1978.

142. Siegrist C, Jones J: Disseminated intravascular coagulopathy and nursing implications, *Semin Oncol Nurs* 1(4):237, 1985.

143. Silverman P, Distelhorst CW: Metabolic emergencies in clinical oncology, *Semin Oncol* 16(6):504, 1989.

144. Siskind MM: A standard of care for the nursing diagnosis of ineffective airway clearance, *Heart Lung* 18(5):477, 1989.

145. Smith EL: Dyspnea and quality of life, *Quality Life Nurs Challenge* 1(1):31, 1992.

146. Smith LH, Van Gulick AJ: Management of neutropenic enterocolitis in the patient with cancer, *Oncol Nurs Forum* 19(9):1337, 1992.

147. Spain RC, Wittlesey D: Respiratory emergencies in patients with cancer, *Semin Oncol* 16(6):471, 1989.

148. Spross J, Stern R: Nursing management of oncology patients with a superior vena cava obstruction syndrome, *Oncol Nurs Forum* 6(3):3, 1979.

149. Theologides A: Neoplastic cardiac tamponade, *Semin Oncol* 5(2):181, 1978.

150. Tripp A: Hyper and hypocalcemia, *Am J Nurs* 769(7):1143, 1976.

151. Trounson LW: Nursing diagnosis and the syndrome of inappropriate antidiuretic hormone, *J Postanesth Nurs* 1(4):244, 1986.

152. Truett L: The septic syndrome, *Cancer Nurs* 14(4):175, 1991.

153. Utley JR: Relief of superior vena cava syndrome with spiral vein bypass grafting, *J SC Med Assoc* 81:489, 1985.

154. Varricchio CG, Jassak PF: Acute pulmonary disorders associated with cancer, *Semin Oncol Nurs* 1(4):269, 1985.

155. Warrell RP, Bockman RS: Metabolic emergencies. In DeVita VT Jr, Hellman S, Rosenberg SA, editors: *Cancer: principles and practice of oncology,* ed 4, Philadelphia, 1993, Lippincott.

156. Wilson JK, Masaryk TJ: Neurologic emergencies in cancer patients, *Semin Oncol* 16(6):490, 1989.

157. Wood HA, Ellerhorst-Ryan JM: Ineffective breathing pattern. In McNally JC and others, editors: *Guidelines for oncology nursing practice,* ed 2, Philadelphia, 1991, Saunders.

158. Yahalom J: Superior vena cava syndrome. In DeVita VT Jr, Hellman S, Rosenberg SA, editors: *Cancer: principles and practice of oncology,* ed 4, Philadelphia, 1993, Lippincott.

159. Yasko JM: Septic shock. In Yasko JM, editor: *Guidelines for cancer care: symptom management,* Reston, Va, 1983, Reston.

160. Yasko JM: Syndrome of inappropriate antidiuretic hormone secretion. In Yasko JM, editor: *Guidelines for cancer care: symptom management,* Reston, Va, 1983, Reston.

161. Yasko JM, Schafer SL: Disseminated intravascular coagulation. In Yasko JM, editor: *Guidelines for cancer care: symptom management,* Reston, Va, 1983, Reston.

162. Yasko JM, Schafer SL: Neoplastic pericardial tamponade. In Yasko JM, editor: *Guidelines for cancer care: symptom management,* Reston, Va, 1983, Reston.

163. Zehner LC, Hoogstraten B: Malignant effusions and their management, *Semin Oncol Nurs* 1(4):259, 1985.

164. Zimberg M, Mahon SM: Understanding delirium: an impediment of quality of life, *Quality Life Nurs Challenge* 1(1):3, 1992.

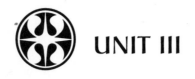

UNIT III

CANCER TREATMENT MODALITIES

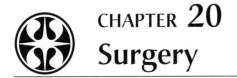

CHAPTER 20
Surgery

KAREN A. PFEIFER

The four primary modalities for the treatment of cancer are surgery, chemotherapy, radiation therapy, and biotherapy. Surgery can be the initial and preferred treatment of choice for many cancers. As a result of advances in surgical techniques, a better understanding of the metastatic patterns of individual tumors, and intensive postoperative care, tumors now can be removed from almost any part of the body.[14,23,24]

If cancer is diagnosed early enough and remains localized, surgery can effect a cure. Of the 40% of cancer patients treated by surgery alone, one third are cured. However, the key is finding the cancer while it is still localized. Surgical treatment failures are caused primarily by the presence of metastasis at the time of initial diagnosis. Metastasis has occurred in 50% of cancer patients by the time their tumor is of sufficient size to be clinically detected.[12,15,24,46,53]

Approximately 90% of cancer patients undergo some type of surgical intervention for diagnosis, initial treatment, or management of complications.[12] The nurse may encounter the cancer patient anywhere along this continuum. It is imperative that the nurse have a strong fundamental knowledge of surgical oncology upon which comprehensive plans of care can be designed and evaluated.

HISTORICAL PERSPECTIVE

Surgery is the oldest recorded form of curative treatment for cancer. At one time, surgery was the only effective method of diagnosing and treating cancer. The first recorded surgical excision of a tumor is found in the Edwin Smith Papyrus, which dates from Egypt's Middle Kingdom (approximately 160 B.C.). However, Ephraim MacDowell is credited with describing modern surgical approaches to cancer in the United States. In 1809 he excised a 22-pound ovarian tumor from Mrs. Jane Todd Crawford, who survived and lived 30 more years. This was the first of 13 ovarian resections performed by MacDowell, and it served as a great stimulus to the advancement of elective surgery. Another important individual in the evolution of surgical oncology was Albert Theodore Billroth; between 1860 and 1890, he performed the first laryngectomy, gastrectomy, and esophagectomy. In the 1890s William Stewart Halsted clarified the principles of en bloc tumor resection by his development of the radical mastectomy.[14,23,27,28,30]

However, in the early days of cancer surgery, surgical conditions were not optimal and the operative procedures often resulted in severe postoperative disfigurement, rapid local recurrence of the cancer, or death. These outcomes were largely the result of undeveloped surgical techniques and intraoperative and postoperative problems (e.g., excessive blood loss, difficult anesthesia). Modern advances such as asepsis, improved anesthesia techniques, blood transfusions, use of antibiotics, tracheostomy to alleviate airway obstruction, and nasogastric decompression of the stomach have much improved the safety of surgical oncology.[14,27]

For many years the preferred treatment was to remove the cancer and as much of the surrounding tissue as possible; therefore most surgical procedures were radical in nature. In the mid-1950s it was noted that despite the technical sophistication of these radical procedures, the mortality rates associated with certain cancer sites (e.g., breast cancer) were not improving. Many cancers thought to be local processes were discovered to be systemic diseases with metastatic lesions. It became evident that surgery alone, regardless of the magnitude of the procedure, was not effective for all cancers.[36]

APPLICATIONS FOR SURGICAL ONCOLOGY

Surgery has several applications in oncology, and these are described on p. 478 (Figure 20-1).

Diagnosis of Disease

A histologic diagnosis is critical to planning treatment, because it is the only definitive diagnostic method and different types of cancer respond differently to treatment.

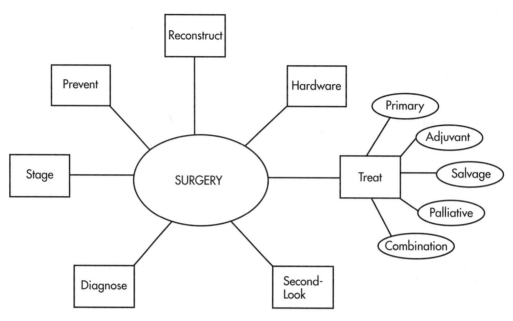

Figure 20-1   Applications for surgical oncology.

The surgeon must obtain a tissue sample for histologic study when appropriate. Surgical techniques used to obtain tissue samples for examination include incisional biopsy (a wedge of tissue is taken from tumors larger than 3 cm in diameter), excisional biopsy (the entire tumor mass, usually less than 2 to 3 cm in diameter, and a margin of surrounding normal tissue are removed), needle biopsy (core tissue samples are aspirated through a needle), or endoscopy (small portions of the tumor are removed with forceps after visual examination). The technique used depends on the tumor's location, size, and growth characteristics (Table 20-1).[24,27,30,55]

The biopsy site should be in an area that will be removed at the time of surgery, or the biopsy should contain the total tumor. Incision lines should be made in cosmetically acceptable areas or skin folds, if possible. The specimen obtained for examination must contain both normal tissue and tumor tissue for comparison by the pathologist. It must be intact and must not be crushed or contaminated. Only positive findings are definitive.[14,24,27]

The current trend is a two-step process. The biopsy is done first, followed by a period of time (usually about 2 weeks), before the surgical procedure is performed. This accomplishes two things: (1) it allows the patient and/or significant others to begin adjusting to the diagnosis, and (2) it allows the patient and/or significant others additional time to make decisions about treatment options.[24]

Staging of Disease

Diagnosis includes determining the type and extent of cancer at one point in time, a process known as staging the disease. The tumor's stage provides information re-

lating to the extent and location of disease and the prognosis.

Surgical staging is reserved for tumors that are inaccessible, difficult to evaluate, or incorrectly staged by any other means. A staging laparotomy (or diagnostic laparotomy) may be performed before radical surgery so that hidden intraperitoneal, lumboaortic, or liver metastasis can be ruled out. A staging laparotomy also can be done to obtain tissue samples and determine disease sites. In lymphoma, a staging laparotomy involves an exploratory laparotomy with splenectomy and biopsy of the liver and retroperitoneal lymph nodes. Metal clips sometimes are placed on organs to define the tumor and mark specific areas for future radiation therapy.[24,29]

Treatment of Disease

Surgical treatment of the cancer process focuses on five principal areas: primary treatment, adjuvant treatment, salvage treatment, palliative treatment, and combination treatment.

Primary treatment. Primary treatment involves removal of a malignant tumor and a margin of adjacent normal tissue. The goal is to achieve a cure by reducing the patient's total body tumor burden. Cure can be accomplished through several types of intervention. Local excision, for example, is the simple excision of a tumor and a small margin of normal tissue. This technique is often used to treat skin cancer. Wide excision or en bloc dissection involves removal of the primary tumor, regional lymph nodes, intervening lymphatic channels, and involved neighboring structures. Examples include radical mastectomy, radical neck dissection, and abdominal-perineal resection. Extended wide excision,

Table 20-1 Biopsy Techniques*

Type	Purpose	Technique	Advantages	Disadvantages
Incisional biopsy	Histologic study	Removal of a portion of tumor Secures a wedge of tumor tissue Usually performed at the tumor margin Done on tumors larger than 3 cm in diameter	Usually requires only local anesthesia Simple method of obtaining diagnosis	Negative report does not eliminate possibility of cancer Specimen may not be large enough Tumor margins may not be defined Additional surgery is required to remove tumor
Excisional biopsy	Histologic study Cure/control	Removal of entire tumor mass with a margin of surrounding normal tissue Most common type of biopsy Performed on small (2 to 3 cm), accessible tumors	Usually requires only local anesthesia Can be definitive therapy (tumors of the lip, nose, ear, and breast) Quick, simple removal of tumor at time of biopsy Decreased costs	Cells may be implanted in tissue and incision, causing local recurrence
Needle biopsy	Histologic study	Aspiration of core tissue samples through special needle inserted into tumor Either tissue or fluid samples can be obtained Performed during surgery or via percutaneous route	Simple to perform Reliable Inexpensive Causes little disturbance of surrounding tissue Done using local anesthesia Does not require hospitalization	Specimen may not be large enough Needle may miss tumor Improper handling may distort cells Technique poses risk of injury to adjacent structures; perforation and hemorrhage are additional risks
Endoscopy (bite biopsy)	Histologic study	Removal of small portions of tumor with forceps after visual examination Often used to diagnose tumors of the gastrointestinal, genitourinary, and pulmonary tracts	Allows access to tumors that might not otherwise be accessible except by laparotomy or thoracotomy Causes little disturbance of surrounding tissue Flexible instruments have made endoscopy more tolerable for patient and easier for surgeon	Tumor cells may be seeded along needle tract

*References 14, 24, 27, 30, 48, 55.

another form of wide excision, involves removal of wide tumor infiltration in a particular region. Cancer in situ is treated surgically by means of several special techniques, which result in little or no mutilation.[23,30,53,55]

Adjuvant treatment. Adjuvant treatment involves removal of tissues to reduce the risk of incidence, progression, or recurrence of cancer. Adjuvant treatment includes cytoreductive therapy, also known as debulking, which is surgery to remove a large tumor burden. If the quantity of cancer cells can be reduced to a very small number by surgical intervention, any remaining cancer cells are more likely to be destroyed by other systemic treatment. Cytoreductive therapy is commonly used in the treatment of ovarian cancer and for neuroblastomas and other childhood tumors. Adjuvant therapy also includes prophylactic surgery, or surgery performed on organs with underlying conditions marked by a high incidence of subsequent cancer. For example, ulcerative colitis carries with it a high incidence of cancer of the colon. Approximately 40% of patients with total involvement of the colon will ultimately die with colon cancer. A colectomy may very well be warranted. The decision to perform surgery is based on (1) the statistical risk of cancer based on the medical and family history, (2) the presence or absence of symptoms, (3) the degree of difficulty in diagnosing a cancer early should it develop, and (4) the patient's probable postoperative appearance and functioning.*

Salvage treatment. Salvage treatment involves use of an extensive surgical approach to treat local recurrence after a less extensive primary approach has been implemented (e.g., mastectomy after lumpectomy and radiation therapy).[55]

Palliative treatment. Surgical cures are not always possible. Nevertheless, advances in technology and research have lengthened survival for many cancer patients. However, prolonged survival brings with it the complications of disease or treatment. In these cases surgery is then redirected from cure to palliation. Palliative surgery is used to ameliorate disease- or treatment-related symptoms without trying to cure the cancer surgically. It is performed to prolong the patient's life and to ensure a better, more comfortable quality of life for the patient and significant others. The benefit of palliative treatment depends on the biologic pace of the cancer, the patient's projected life expectancy, and expected treatment outcomes. Examples of palliative procedures include:

- Bone stabilization
- Relief of life-threatening obstruction or bleeding
- Removal of solitary metastasis (e.g., cerebral, hepatic)
- Treatment of oncologic emergencies (e.g., perforation, abscess, spinal cord compression, hypersplenism)
- Treatment of complications from chemotherapy and radiation therapy (e.g., skin breakdown, fistulas, perforation, radiation proctitis)
- Ablative surgery (removal of a hormone source) to alter the hormonal environment that encourages development and growth of a tumor (e.g., oophorectomy, orchiectomy, adrenalectomy)
- Management of cancer pain (e.g., nerve blocks, cordotomy, neurectomy, rhizotomy, sympathectomy, lobotomy, thalamotomy, tractotomy)

The goals of palliative surgery are to cure or relieve distressing symptoms, to make the patient more comfortable, and to prevent symptoms that will occur if the patient goes untreated.†

Combination treatment. Combination treatment involves using surgery with other treatment modalities with the goals of improving tumor resectability, reducing the extent of tumor removed, limiting the change in the patient's physical appearance and functional ability, and improving treatment outcomes. Examples include preoperative chemotherapy, radiation therapy, or biotherapy; intraoperative chemotherapy or radiation therapy; and postoperative chemotherapy, radiation therapy, or biotherapy. Current research in this area is focused on the timing and sequencing of combination therapies and on identifying the combination therapies that are most effective in controlling cancer while producing minimal effects.[5,55]

Insertion and Monitoring of Therapeutic/Supportive Hardware

Therapeutic/supportive hardware can be surgically implanted to improve the patient's comfort and/or to ease delivery of treatment[55] (see Table 20-2 for additional information on this hardware).

Second-Look Procedures

Second-look procedures involve follow-up surgery within a predetermined time frame after the original surgery and/or adjuvant treatment to check for the presence or absence of disease. Sites and volume of residual tumor are identified and resected when possible. Second-look procedures usually are done for cancers that tend to recur locally (e.g., ovarian cancer). They also may be done to assess the response to other treatment modalities or to evaluate residual disease after other treatment modalities. Second-look procedures are used less often than in the past because other laboratory tests, diagnostic procedures, and tumor markers are available to assess the response to treatment.[55]

Reconstruction

The need to remove a sufficient margin of normal tissue around a tumor's border sometimes involves extensive surgical resection, bringing with it disfigurement and considerable impairment of function. Reconstructive surgery involves reconstruction of anatomic defects caused by cancer surgery; its purpose is to improve function or cosmetic appearance, or both.[24,29,55]

Reconstructive surgery may be immediate and permanent or immediate and temporary, or it may be postponed for safety reasons or until suitable graft tissue can be prepared and transferred. The cancer surgeries requiring the largest number of subsequent reconstructive surgeries are surgery of the head and neck (facial reconstruction), breasts (breast reconstruction after mastectomy), and superficial tissues of all sites (skin graft after resection for melanoma). The choice of method depends on several factors: the site and extent of the tumor or tumors, the loss of substance, the chance of permanent cure, the patient's age and psychologic and general condition, the availability of free skin grafts, and suitable internal prostheses.[29]

Patient teaching about options for reconstruction and counseling usually is begun before primary surgical

---

*References 12, 14, 23, 27, 29, 30, 53, 55, 60.
†References 2, 12, 21, 23, 27, 29, 30, 53, 55.

Table 20-2 Therapeutic Hardware[33,55,56]

Type	Advantages	Disadvantages
Ventricular reservoir	Increases patient's comfort and reduces anxiety because of easy access Convenient to use in the home Improves medication tolerance Often lengthens duration of remission	Infection Catheter occlusion Catheter displacement
Central venous catheter Short-term use	Multiple-lumen catheters permit simultaneous delivery of potentially incompatible medications and fluids Provides easy access to vascular system for delivery of intravenous fluids, medications, parenteral hyperalimentation, and blood/blood products, and for obtaining blood samples Increases patient's comfort by reducing number of venipunctures required	Infection, especially with devices lacking a cuff and with subcutaneous tunnel Catheter displacement Severed catheter Possible restriction of patient's activity Possible body image disturbance Requires sterile dressing changes, which often prevents patient from learning to care for catheter at home Requires frequent maintenance
Long-term use	Multiple-lumen catheters permit simultaneous delivery of potentially incompatible medications and fluids Provides easy access to vascular system for delivery of chemotherapy, intravenous fluids, other medications, parenteral hyperalimentation, and blood/blood products, and for obtaining blood samples Increases patient's comfort by reducing number of venipunctures required Can be connected to internal or external pumps for continuous drug delivery With proper instruction can be cared for by patient and/or significant other, permitting in-home use	Infection Catheter occlusion Catheter displacement Severed catheter Possible restriction of patient's activity Possible body image disturbance Requires frequent maintenance
Implantable vascular access device	Has no external component, which means less disturbance in body image, less chance for infection, and greater comfort Provides easy access to vascular system for delivery of chemotherapy, intravenous fluids, other medications, parenteral hyperalimentation, and blood/blood products, and for obtaining blood samples Creates less interference with clothing Places fewer restrictions on activities Requires minimal care (infrequent need for irrigation) Has no dressings, caps, or clamps Can be connected to external pumps for continuous drug delivery	Catheter occlusion Catheter displacement Port/catheter disconnection Can access system only through skin; needle stick is still required Improper surgical placement of port (too deep or angled) can make access difficult Rotation of port

Modified from Szopa TJ: Surgery. In Clark JC, McGee RF, editors: *Core curriculum for oncology nursing,* ed 2, Philadelphia, 1992, Saunders.

therapy is initiated. Patients often fear that family, friends, and health care personnel will interpret their desire for reconstructive surgery as vanity. They must be helped to see that reconstruction is desirable, positive, and sometimes necessary for achieving an optimal level of functioning.[24]

Prevention of Disease

Cancer prevention can entail preventive surgery. Surgery is the preferred treatment for precancerous and in situ lesions of all epithelial surfaces (e.g., skin, oral cavity, cervix). Benign polyps of the cervix, bladder, colon, and stomach often are removed surgically to reduce the risk of future cancer. Although rare, a second mastectomy sometimes is performed on women with a high potential for developing a second breast cancer.[23]

PRINCIPLES OF SURGICAL ONCOLOGY

When considering surgery for a patient with cancer, the surgeon critically evaluates three main elements: tumor factors, tumor cell kinetics, and patient variables.

Tumor Factors

Anatomic location. The tumor's location can prevent or impede access for removal. The surgeon must decide whether the area of tumor can be encompassed by regional excision. Some tumors cannot be surgically treated because an adequate margin of normal tissue cannot be removed. Tumors that involve or are attached to vital structures usually do not benefit from surgical resection; superficial, well-encapsulated tumors are the type most easily removed by surgery.[23,24,27]

Histologic type. Certain histologic types of cancer are not treated by surgery because they are disseminated at the outset of diagnosis. Examples of these are lymphomas, leukemias, and small cell cancer of the lung.[27]

Tumor size. Smaller tumors are less likely to have spread, and the patient is more likely to be cured by surgery. However, patients with larger tumors respond more favorably to surgery than to other treatment modalities. Whereas chemotherapy and radiation therapy require an excellent blood and oxygen supply to cause cell destruction, surgery does not. Therefore surgical removal of large, localized tumors that have a necrotic center and a poor blood supply also is an effective treatment procedure.[23,27]

Tumor Cell Kinetics

Growth rate or biologic aggressiveness. Well-differentiated, slow-growing tumors consisting of cells with long cell cycles lend themselves best to surgical resection. These tumors are more likely to be confined locally and to have a smaller chance for invasion and dissemination. Poorly differentiated, rapid-growing tumors are less amenable to surgery.[23,24]

Invasion. Any cell that remains after cancer therapy carries with it the potential for recurrence if that cell can reproduce. Therefore any surgery intended to be curative must include resection of normal tissue around the tumor to ensure removal of all cancer cells. Some cancers (e.g., melanomas) invade tissues deeply, thereby either requiring radical surgery or eliminating surgery as a treatment option.[23]

The first operation performed for removal of a cancer has a better chance for success than subsequent operations after recurrence. Therefore the surgeon's knowledge of invasive tumor patterns is critical for planning the most effective treatment.[23]

Metastatic potential or pattern and extent of metastatic spread. Some tumors metastasize late or not at all. Even when advanced, these tumors may be cured by aggressive surgery. Other tumors are known to metastasize to certain regional lymph nodes, and cure may be achieved by removing the tumor-bearing organ and its nearby lymph nodes. Other tumors predictably metastasize early. Surgery may not be warranted for these tumor types, or, alternatively, it may be done to remove all visible tumor before the patient begins adjuvant treatment or to resect remaining diseased tissue after several courses of chemotherapy.[24,50]

Evidence of spread into the blood or lymph vessels indicates a poorer prognosis, and less favorable results are achieved with surgery. If a patient has widespread metastatic disease, surgical resection alone usually results in a 50% or greater probability of local recurrence. Such a patient may require more treatment than simple surgical resection of a tumor.[23,27]

Patient Variables

General health. The patient's general health state plays a major role in determining the efficacy of surgery. As with any treatment, the surgical risk must be compared with the probability of long-term recovery. Cancer patients clearly are at greater risk of developing complications postoperatively and/or of succumbing to clinical problems.[23]

Host resistance or immune competence. The patient's ability to initiate an immunologic response to the cancer cells that remain after surgery is critical. A person with cancer is less likely to be able to mount an effective immune response. However, the ability to resist infection has been shown to be closely related to the total body tumor burden. Surgery can reduce the patient's tumor burden, thus improving the immune status.[23,24]

Desire for treatment. The surgeon must carefully assess the patient's desire for treatment. Even though surgery may be the most effective measure for tumor control, it is not appropriate for a patient who does not want an operation.[27,39]

Quality of life. Research has shown that some radical surgeries are not justified. Either they do not improve the end result, or they interfere with the patient's welfare. Selecting surgery as a treatment choice must include consideration of the quality of the patient's life when treatment is complete.[24]

Evaluation of tumor factors, tumor cell kinetics, and patient variables permits establishment of the following fundamental principles to guide the surgical oncologist[24,27,30,53,55]:

- Wide surgical incisions are usually made. Surgical excision of a tumor includes removal of the tumor and a wide margin of normal tissue surrounding it. The surgeon's goal is to ensure a tumor-free border.
- Removal of the tumor-bearing organ and adjacent

lymph nodes is preferable if serious morbidity or disfigurement can be avoided. Surgery is done in a manner that will produce satisfactory appearance and function.

- The surgeon will do as much surgery as necessary to eliminate the tumor and as little surgery as possible to accomplish that purpose.
- Careful surgical techniques are used to prevent the escape of tumor cells into the general circulation (seeding). These techniques include glove and instrument changes when a second area of the body requires surgery, early ligation of blood vessels and lymphatics that supply the tumor, and wound irrigation with tumoricidal solutions (0.5% formaldehyde or sterile water). Such measures reduce the risk of recurrence.
- Human tissue is friable, especially if the area has been irradiated previously. Minimal palpation and manipulation of the tumor (no-touch technique) minimize damage to tissue and seeding and local recurrence.
- The best chance for a surgical cure is at the time of the first surgical intervention.
- Slow-growing, localized tumors are more amenable to surgical intervention than are rapidly-growing ones that have metastasized early.
- A bloodless surgical field is important for gross observation of the tumor at all times.
- Surgical removal of a primary tumor can change the growth patterns of metastatic lesions, probably by changing residual tumor cell kinetics.
- Reconstruction and rehabilitation are essential components of comprehensive cancer therapy.
- Surgery is being used more frequently in conjunction with other treatment modalities (combination treatment).

SPECIAL SURGICAL TECHNIQUES

Several special surgical techniques are used in the treatment of cancer. These include electrosurgery, cryosurgery, chemosurgery, lasers, video-assisted thoracoscopy, intraoperative radiation therapy, and photodynamic therapy.

Electrosurgery

Electrosurgery eliminates cancer cells by using the cutting and coagulating effects of a high-frequency electrical current applied by needles, blades, or electrodes. This technique may be an alternative treatment for certain cancers of the skin, oral cavity, and rectum.[23,53]

Cryosurgery

Cryosurgery involves application of liquid nitrogen probes to selectively destroy tumor tissue; it therefore is the therapeutic, in situ destruction of tumor using subzero temperatures. Cryosurgery is believed to cause cell death by dehydration. The cryosurgical system produces

temperatures below $-166.2°$ F $(-200°$ C), which are immediately lethal to some cells in the target area. Freezing the cells produces hypovolemia and a subsequent toxic level of electrolytes in the affected cells. As the freezing continues, cell membranes rupture. Indirect destruction of the microcirculation from the freezing of small blood vessels in the target area further contributes to hypoxic celluar death. The treated site then thaws naturally and becomes gelatinous, healing spontaneously. Most healing is complete within 6 to 8 weeks. Cells that are not frozen internally at the time of treatment become necrotic and subsequently die during the thawing process. Carbon dioxide, Freon, and nitrous oxide are the three common gaseous freezing agents used. Whereas original cryoprobes limited cryosurgery to the treatment of surface lesions (skin cancer and precancerous and cancerous gynecologic lesions), newer cryoprobe systems and innovative intraoperative radiology and ultrasound techniques allow detection and treatment of lesions deep within the body, most notably metastatic liver cancer and prostate cancer. Most patients require only one treatment; however, cryosurgery permits retreatment of recurrent lesions.*

Chemosurgery

Chemosurgery, the combined use of layer-by-layer surgical resection of tissue and topical application of chemotherapeutic agents, was first described by Dr. Frederic Mohs in 1941. It is performed today in only a few centers in the United States. Chemosurgery (also known as Mohs' technique), involves mapping excised tissue in location to the wound; this allows the surgeon to remove mostly malignant tissue and little or no normal tissue, minimizing disfigurement.[30,55]

Lasers

The term "laser" is derived from a description of the process that creates laser light (*light amplification by stimulated emission of radiation*). In this process, photons are emitted and amplified by atoms and molecules. Safe, efficient use of lasers in surgical oncology requires an understanding of the various laser-tissue interactions. Incident laser radiation can be absorbed at the tissue surface, or light energy can be absorbed throughout the bulk of the tissue, with distribution dependent on the degree of tissue transparency. When transmitted into deeper layers, the laser radiation is redirected by reflection and scattering. Specific categories of laser-tissue interaction include photocoagulation, vaporization, photochemical ablation, and photochemical interactions. In photocoagulation, proteins, enzymes, and other biologic molecules in tissue are heated to temperatures well above $932°$ F $(500°$ C). The immediate result is denaturation of the treated

---

*References 7, 8, 23, 30, 53, 55.

tissues. Photocoagulation is used to prevent blood loss when heavily vascularized tissue is surgically incised.

Vaporization, or photothermal ablation, occurs at temperatures above 1832° F (1000° C), when the tissue water boils. The production and emission of steam result in removal of tissue in the form of microscopic particles. Vaporization is used for incision and removal of diseased tissue.

The term "photochemical ablation" was coined to specifically describe the unusually clean-cut incisions possible with short-wavelength, ultraviolet, pulsed excimer lasers. Short-wavelength photons have sufficient energy to break molecular bonds and have proved very useful when extremely thin layers must be removed, as in skin cancer. The explosive force by which molecules are thrown off the surface results from a combination of photochemical breakdown and high surface temperatures. Photochemistry occurs when visible or ultraviolet radiation interacts with molecules. However, in most instances of laser use, the photochemical effects are dwarfed by temperature increases sufficient to cause thermal denaturation of tissue. With low dose rates, photochemistry may be the dominant mechanism, as occurs in photodynamic therapy (discussed later in this section). Coagulation and tissue ablation are two features of the laser, which make it attractive to surgical oncologists.

Lasers have demonstrated their worth in removing tumors in difficult-to-access areas and those in vascularized tissues by minimizing blood loss during surgical procedures. The ability of the carbon dioxide (CO_2), Nd:YAG, frequency-doubled Nd:YAG (KTP), argon, and dye lasers to cut tissue and coagulate during incision as a means to reduce blood loss have increased their popularity, especially in the treatment of head and neck cancer. The highly vascular nature of tissues in the head and neck has favored the use of lasers because of their hemostatic properties. The laser's advantages are heightened because the restricted area within the nasal and oral cavities has required that many procedures be performed via rigid and flexible endoscopes or with the operating microscope. Both techniques lend themselves well to laser surgery.

Established uses include local excision of head and neck cancer with the CO_2, argon, and KTP lasers. Nd:YAG has been used to debulk nasopharyngeal carcinomas. CO_2, argon, and Nd:YAG lasers also have been used in microsurgery with ultrasound to ablate or remove tumor tissue that is extremely close to critical neural tissue that must not be disturbed. Removal of tumors of the bladder, urethra, and external genitalia, as well as prostatic ablation, are current clinical applications of laser use by urologists. Argon, CO_2, Nd:YAG, and KTP lasers have been used in urologic cancer surgery with both fiberoptic and cystoscopic delivery systems. It is important to remember the potential for transmural damage to the small bowel when using a laser on the bladder wall, particularly when the Nd:YAG laser is used because of the deep penetration of its wavelength.*

Video-Assisted Thoracoscopy

Video-assisted thoracoscopy is fast revolutionizing a field once associated with long incisions and longer, painful recoveries. Endoscopes permit smaller incisions, sparing many patients the trauma of extensive surgery. Thoracoscopy is not an entirely new technique. First introduced in 1910 by Hans Christian Jacobaeus, a Swedish physician, it was popular in the treatment of tuberculosis (TB). However, the treatment was largely abandoned after the advent of successful chemotherapy for TB in the 1950s. Until recently, thoracoscopy consisted of inserting a small, lighted tube into the chest cavity, where, under direct vision, the surgeon performed pleural biopsies. However, the tube was inflexible and therefore limited in its surgical applications. Today, thoracoscopy is a different story. A multichip minicamera, accompanied by intense lighting, magnifies the image and transmits it to a video monitor (Figure 20-2). Video-assisted thoracoscopy can replace approximately 70% of the thoracic procedures that previously required a standard thoracotomy; these include pulmonary wedge excisions, diagnosis and treatment of pleural effusions and pleural masses, biopsy or resection of mediastinal

---

*References 3, 4, 16, 30, 35, 51, 54, 55.

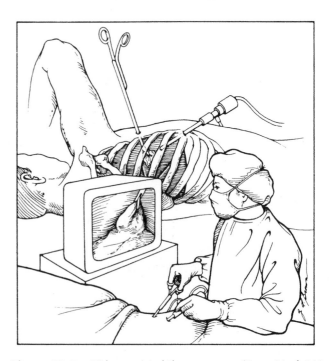

Figure 20-2 Video-assisted thoracoscopy. (From Mack MJ and others: *Ann Thorac Surg* 54(3):403, 1992.)

tumors, and, occasionally, sympathectomies, vagotomies, and thymectomies.

Video-assisted thoracoscopy is performed using general anesthesia with single-lung ventilation. Instead of the standard 20 cm thoracotomy incision, the surgeon makes three 1 cm incisions. A rigid telescope and camera are introduced through the first incision, and the endoscopic surgical instruments are introduced into the remaining incisions. Operating time can range from 15 to 20 minutes to 2 to 3 hours, depending on the complexity of the surgery. Video-assisted thoracoscopy has opened the doors of treatment to patients previously unable to withstand a standard thoracotomy because of severe emphysema or a generally debilitated state. Contraindications include extensive pleural adhesions and bleeding disorders (which obstruct the camera lens) and recent myocardial infarction. Chest wall resections and tumors larger than 3 cm in diameter still require thoracotomy. Complications with video-assisted thoracoscopy are uncommon but include atelectasis, pneumonia, and postoperative air leaks that usually resolve within the first 24 postoperative hours. Other reports have mentioned trocar injuries to the lung and other thoracic viscera, which usually are discovered and corrected during surgery.[1,32,40,45]

Intraoperative Radiation Therapy

External-beam radiation therapy has been extensively investigated for patients with unresectable, locally advanced cancer and for patients with early stage cancer who, for medical reasons, cannot undergo surgery. Generally, the radiation field includes the primary tumor and the lymph nodes that drain the area. However, the proximity of tumors to radiosensitive organs (lung, spinal cord, and heart) often limits the dose of radiation to suboptimal levels. Previous studies have suggested that local control of cancer with radiation therapy is dose related; therefore techniques that allow intensification of the radiation dose to the tumor without exceeding the tolerance of radiosensitive organs are needed.

One such technique is intraoperative electron-beam radiation therapy (IOEBRT). Using IOEBRT, tumoricidal doses of radiation can be delivered to tumors at the time of surgery while the dose to adjacent normal tissues is minimized. Dose-limiting normal tissues are protected by surgically placed lead shields or by physical displacement from the treatment field.

The first reports on IOEBRT, published in 1977, described the cases of five lung cancer patients. Three patients were alive 1 year after treatment and had no evidence of disease. No details were given about the tissues in the intraoperative radiation therapy field, nor was the toxicity of the treatment stated. To date, IOEBRT, alone or in combination with preoperative or postoperative external-beam irradiation or neoadjuvant chemo-

therapy, has been used to treat various sites, including the stomach, bile duct, pancreas, retroperitoneum, and rectum. IOEBRT of the thorax is limited to a small number of clinical trials and several studies done on large animals. For unresectable tumors inaccessible to the treatment cone of IOEBRT, intraoperative high-dose-rate brachytherapy (IOHDR) offers an alternative approach. IOEBRT is preferred for accessible tumors because the treatment and setup times are shorter and it is more convenient for treating larger tumor beds (up to 12 cm); however, it is unsuitable for treating sites deep in the inferior pelvis, subpubic locations, some lateral pelvic side walls, anterior abdominal walls, the anterior chest wall, and narrow cavities. For IOHDR, treatment time depends on the total area to be treated and the activity of the source because a single source is used to treat the tumor. Because of the complex presentations of patients who are candidates for IOHDR and the fact that most patients have received intensive multimodal therapy, it is difficult to differentiate surgical from radiation toxicities.

Lastly, stereotactic radiosurgery is worthy of mention. "Stereotaxy" refers to surgical techniques that rely on specialized instrumentation, including stereotactic frames, to perform procedures at precise intracranial locations. Typically, a coordinate system associated with a stereotactic frame attached to a patient's skull is used to reference the location of specific intracranial structures with radiologic studies and to direct intervention, such as biopsy, craniotomy, or brachytherapy. With stereotactic radiosurgery, convention is replaced by multiple narrow radiation beams that are directed toward a common point to produce highly localized radiobiologic effects, such as blood vessel thrombosis.[10,25,26,34,43]

Photodynamic Therapy

Photodynamic therapy involves intravenous injection of a photosensitizing drug with uptake by cancer cells, followed by exposure to a laser light within 24 to 48 hours of injection. This results in fluorescence of cancer cells and cell death. Most clinical experience with photodynamic therapy comes from using the porphyrin variants, HPD (hematoporphyrin derivative) and DHE (dihematoporphyrin ethers and esters). It is important to note that, although photodynamic therapy involves use of a laser, the laser's mechanism of action does not involve cutting, cauterizing, or vaporizing (the more common uses associated with lasers). Photodynamic therapy has been used with varying success to treat basal and squamous cell cancers, malignant melanoma, Kaposi's sarcoma, recurrent breast cancer, head and neck cancer, bladder cancer, and endobronchial cancer. Clearly, some cancers are more suitable than others with regard to whether complete eradication is possible. Bulky lesions and tumors that are inaccessible to light irradiation cannot be treated by photodynamic therapy. However, the development of resistance to this therapy has not been noted in any patient tumors, and long-term morbidity does not restrict the number of repeat treatments.[20,55,58]

EQUIPMENT USED IN SURGICAL ONCOLOGY

Several types of equipment and hardware are used in surgical oncology.

Ventricular Reservoir (Ommaya Reservoir)

A ventricular reservoir consists of a mushroom-shaped silicone dome that provides direct access to ventricular cerebrospinal fluid. The dome, which is approximately 3.4 cm in diameter, is attached to a silicone catheter. Ventricular reservoirs have three primary uses: (1) to more predictably and consistently deliver medication (e.g., chemotherapy drugs, pain medication) directly into the subarachnoid space and cerebrospinal fluid (intrathecal administration); (2) to permit cerebrospinal fluid to be sampled for pathologic examination; and (3) to permit measurement of cerebrospinal fluid pressure (Figure 20-3; also see Table 20-2).[33]

Central Venous Catheters

Central venous catheters are available for short- and long-term use. In short-term use, central venous catheters are used for brief intermittent or continuous administra-tion of intravenous fluids, medications, parenteral hyperalimentation, or blood/blood products. They also may be used for obtaining blood samples. Most short-term central catheters are inserted via the subclavian or jugular vein and terminate in the superior vena cava near the right atrium. Most catheters have no cuff and do not pass through a subcutaneous tunnel (see Table 20-2).[33,56]

Long-term central venous catheters are used when a prolonged course of parenteral therapy is expected. The silicone catheter is surgically placed percutaneously or by venous cutdown. The catheter is implanted via the subclavian or jugular vein, with the tip terminating in the superior vena cava near the right atrium. The catheter is then threaded subcutaneously to an exit site in the chest, usually to the right or left of midline. The procedure usually is done using local anesthesia. A Dacron cuff forms a seal around the catheter; this cuff also stabilizes the catheter and reduces infection by preventing retrograde migration of organisms. The catheter may also be sutured in place to secure its placement. Central venous pressure can be measured by connecting the catheter's lumen to a manometer. Examples of this type of catheter are the Hickman, Broviac, and Groshong catheters[33,56] (Figure 20-4; also see Table 20-2.)

Implantable Vascular Access Device (IVAD)

The IVAD system consists of a self-sealing silicone rubber septum enclosed in a metal or plastic port that is attached to a silicone catheter (Figure 20-5). The port is surgically implanted beneath the skin, generally in the chest region. The catheter is then threaded subcutaneously and terminates in a body cavity, organ, epidural space, or blood vessel (e.g., peritoneal cavity, heart, hepatic artery) (Figure 20-6). The procedure may be done on an inpatient or outpatient basis. Chemotherapy, intravenous fluids, pain medications and other drugs, and

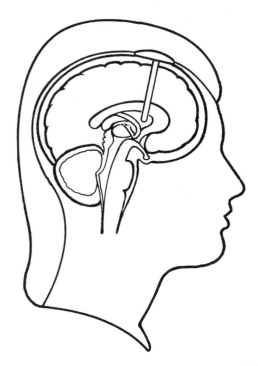

Figure 20-3   The Ommaya reservoir. (From Brager B, Yasko J: *Care of the client receiving chemotherapy*, Reston, Va, 1984, Reston.)

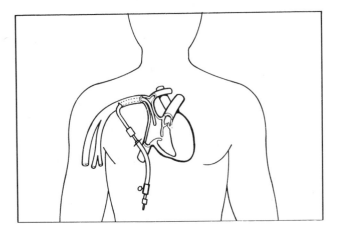

Figure 20-4   Anatomic location of long-term central venous catheter. (From LaRocca JC, Otto SE: *Pocket guide to intravenous therapy*, ed 3, St Louis, 1997, Mosby.)

blood/blood products can be given intermittently or continuously via the port. The system is accessed by a needle puncture through the skin into the port's septum. Noncoring needles must be used when accessing the port to prevent damage to the silicone septum (Figure 20-7). Intravenous fluids are administered only through a venous port. Several commercially made ports are available in single or double lumens and lower profile ports for the smaller patient. Examples are the Infuse-A-Port, Port-A-Cath, and LifePort.[33,56] This technology also extends to the peripheral vasculature, with a peripheral access port available for patients whose disease prevents the use of a traditional central venous access device (see Table 20-2).

Arterial Catheter

An arterial catheter can be surgically placed for the purpose of delivering higher concentrations of chemotherapy to a localized region (regional chemotherapy). This alleviates some of chemotherapy's systemic side effects.

Regional chemotherapy can be divided into two types. With the first type, a catheter is inserted percutaneously into the arterial system to perfuse an entire region, usually a limb. The vessel is isolated from the general circulation by a pump oxygenator that provides extracorporeal circulation. Ten times the amount of chemotherapy that can be given systemically is infused into the region. The drug is cleared from the isolated circulation by infusing dextran, followed by whole blood. An example of this use is regional intraarterial limb perfusion for melanoma or soft tissue sarcoma.

In the second type of regional chemotherapy, a catheter (e.g., an IVAD) is inserted into the tributary artery of the region where the tumor is located. An example of this use is intraarterial infusion of the liver by intrahepatic placement of a catheter using an ambulatory infusion pump for continuous infusion chemotherapy.[6,29,30]

Tenckhoff Catheter

The Tenckhoff catheter may be surgically placed for the treatment of malignant ascites, as often occurs with lymphomas and cancers of the ovary, colon, or stomach. In such cases the Tenckhoff catheter is used for administration of intraperitoneal chemotherapy. The catheter is inserted into the peritoneal cavity, using local anesthesia, and has an internal Dacron cuff (Figure 20-8).[6]

Implanted Infusion Pumps

Implanted infusion pumps are used for continuous regional infusion of chemotherapy or of pain medications

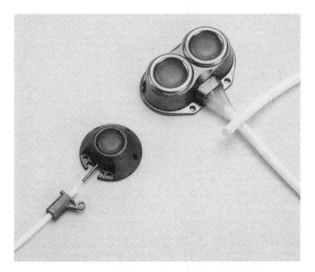

Figure 20-5 LifePort II dual-lumen and Lo-Profile ports. (Courtesy Strato Medical Corp., Beverly, Mass.)

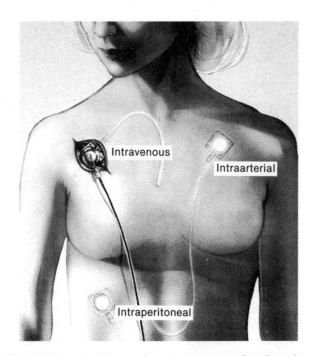

Intravenous

Intraarterial

Intraperitoneal

Figure 20-6 Location and termination sites of implanted infusion ports. (Courtesy Pharmacia Deltec, Inc., St. Paul, Minn.)

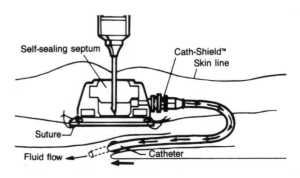

Self-sealing septum

Cath-Shield™ Skin line

Suture

Fluid flow

Catheter

Figure 20-7 Cross-section of implantable port with needle. (Courtesy Pharmacia Deltec, Inc., St. Paul, Minn.)

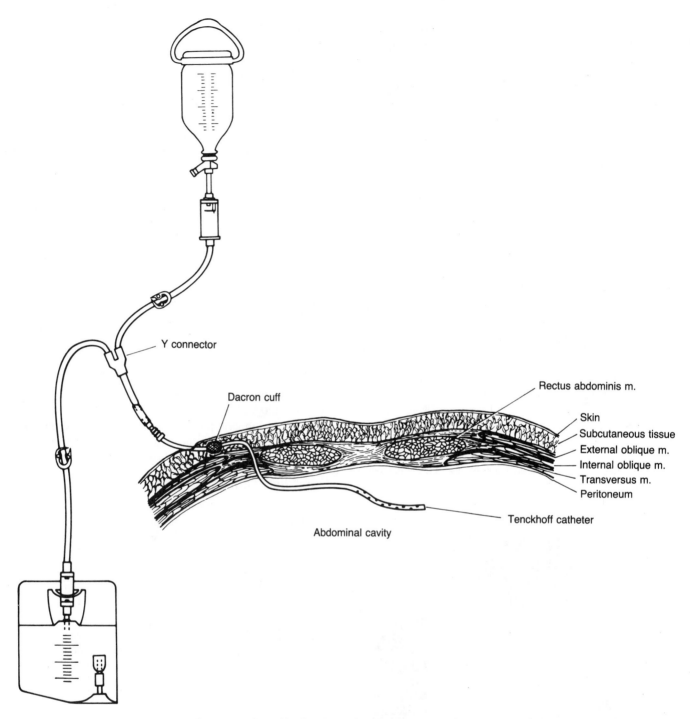

Figure 20-8 Placement of Tenckhoff catheter for administration of intraperitoneal chemotherapy. (From DeVita VT Jr, Hellman S, Rosenberg SA, editors: *Cancer: principle and practice of oncology*, ed 3, Philadelphia, 1989, Lippincott.)

or other drugs to specific body sites by way of an artery or vein or the spinal fluid. Bolus injections also may be given by the pump's side port. Examples of these ports are the Infusaid Model 400, SynchroMed Infusion Pump, and Therex 3000 (Figure 20-9).

These pumps have no external components and are accessed percutaneously. The pump is placed in a subcutaneous pocket of tissue, usually in the left lower quadrant of the abdomen. The pump may also be placed in a pocket of tissue in the right or left subclavian fossa. The

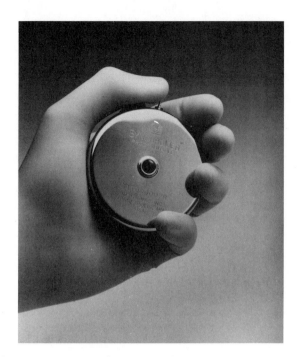

Figure 20-9 SynchroMed Infusion Pump. (Courtesy Medtronic, Inc., Minneapolis, Minn.)

silicone catheter (outlet catheter) most commonly terminates in the hepatic artery for treatment of liver cancer or liver metastasis; in the superior vena cava for systemic infusion of chemotherapy; or in the spinal fluid for pain management.[56]

SPECIAL CONSIDERATIONS IN SURGICAL ONCOLOGY
Nutrition

Protein-calorie malnutrition is a common problem in hospitalized cancer patients. Approximately 30% to 50% of hospitalized cancer patients show moderate to severe degrees of malnutrition resulting from the primary tumor and/or from the diagnostic or treatment regimens used in the management of their disease. Protein-calorie malnutrition generally results from (1) a decrease in oral intake, (2) an increase in enteral losses as a result of malabsorption or development of intestinal fistulas, and/or (3) an increase in nutritional requirements caused by hypermetabolism or the presence of a tumor.[11,12,37,59]

A nutritionally compromised cancer patient is a poor surgical risk. When subjected to the stress of surgery, the patient is unable to preserve lean body mass, and negative nitrogen balance ensues. The results are (1) poor wound healing, (2) anemia, (3) infection, (4) sepsis, (5) pneumonia, (6) further malnutrition, and (7) increased morbidity. Nutritional management is aimed first at reversing protein-calorie malnutrition and preventing weight loss. Once this has been accomplished, the nutrition plan can be as aggressive as the cancer treatment plan. The optimal duration of nutrition support varies with each cancer patient.[12,24,38,49]

Blood Disorders

Preoperative nursing management of the cancer patient must include an accurate assessment of hemodynamic parameters and an understanding of abnormal clotting factors.[24]

Anemia is common among cancer patients and should be corrected preoperatively with packed red cell transfusions to a hematocrit of 35% or above. In addition, some conditions (e.g., liver failure, uremia, leukemia) are associated with platelet dysfunction. It is generally accepted that 50,000 functionally active platelets per cubic millimeter are sufficient for surgery. An insufficient preoperative platelet count can result in postoperative bleeding and fatal hemorrhage, especially if the patient receives large volumes of blood products.[5]

The cancer patient is highly susceptible to changes in the hemostatic system, particularly hypercoagulability and thrombosis. Shortened partial thromboplastin and prothrombin times and elevated clotting factors have been observed. Postoperative deep vein thrombosis is more likely to develop in cancer patients than in other surgery patients; therefore early postoperative ambulation is critical. Cancers commonly associated with recurring deep vein thrombosis are cancers of the brain, pancreas, stomach, and lung.[24,31]

Complications of Multimodal Therapy

Radiation can cause fibrosis and obliteration of lymphatic and vascular channels, resulting in long-term damage to underlying tissues. Postoperative wound healing thus is affected in a patient who was irradiated previously in the same area. Tissue that has been irradiated is not biologically normal, and once surgery disrupts tissue integrity, infection, wound dehiscence, and necrosis can occur.[24,47,61]

Certain chemotherapy drugs (methotrexate, cyclophosphamide, 5-fluorouracil, and doxorubicin) change the histology of healing surgical incisions and reduce the tensile strength of wounds at specific times during the postoperative period. Wound strength is significantly impaired when chemotherapy is administered within the first 4 days of surgery. This highlights the need for nonabsorbable sutures and for delaying chemotherapy when extensive surgical resection is required.[19,24,47,52]

Chemotherapy drugs often reduce the cancer patient's red blood cell, white blood cell, and platelet counts. The nadir may not occur for 10 to 14 days after initial administration of the drug. Monitoring the patient's blood counts and a knowledge of the drug's schedule and effects can alert the nurse to potential complications of wound infection and bleeding.[24]

Some chemotherapy drugs are toxic to specific organ systems, producing long-term side effects that can increase the cancer patient's risk of surgical complications. For example, preoperative administration of bleomycin can predispose the patient to postoperative acute adult respiratory distress syndrome. Interstitial fibrosis can occur with bleomycin and can increase surgical pulmonary complications. Diuretics, aggressive pulmonary hygiene, and fluid restriction can prevent interstitial pulmonary edema associated with preoperative bleomycin therapy. Preoperative administration of adriamycin or daunomycin (cumulative dose of 500 mg/m^2 or higher) increases the risk of intraoperative and postoperative congestive heart failure and pulmonary edema. The patient's fluid balance must be carefully monitored and controlled during surgery. Digitalis may be given preoperatively to increase ventricular contractility. A Swan-Ganz catheter may be inserted to monitor physiologic parameters in the intraoperative and postoperative phases.[24]

Surgical Risks in Older Patients

All surgical procedures must be considered high risk for the older cancer patient. Careful preoperative assessment of physiologic parameters and correction of nutritional deficits and fluid and electrolyte imbalances should begin as early as possible. If a careful baseline assessment is completed preoperatively and if the older patient is thoroughly instructed about postoperative management, many complications can be avoided. Hypoxemia is the most common anesthesia-related problem in the older cancer patient. Age, obesity, and preexisting pulmonary disease all predispose the patient to hypoxemia, with the

Table 20-3 Physiologic Changes Related to the Aging Process

Physiologic changes	Effects	Potential postoperative complications
CARDIOVASCULAR SYSTEM		
Decreased elasticity of blood vessels	Decreased circulation to vital organs	Shock (hypotension), thrombosis with
Decreased cardiac output	Slower blood flow	pulmonary emboli, delayed wound
Decreased peripheral circulation		healing, postoperative confusion,
		hypervolemia, decreased response to
		stress
RESPIRATORY SYSTEM		
Decreased elasticity of lungs and chest wall	Decreased vital capacity	Atelectasis, pneumonia, postoperative
Increased residual lung volume	Decreased alveolar volume	confusion
Decreased forced expiratory volume	Decreased gas exchange	
Decreased ciliary action	Decreased cough reflex	
Fewer alveolar capillaries		
URINARY SYSTEM		
Decreased glomerular filtration rate	Decreased kidney function	Prolonged response to anesthesia and
Decreased bladder muscle tone	Stasis of urine in bladder	drugs, overhydration with intravenous
Weakened perineal muscles	Loss of urinary control	fluids, hyperkalemia, urinary tract
		infection, urinary incontinence
MUSCULOSKELETAL SYSTEM		
Decreased muscle strength	Decreased activity	Atelectasis, pneumonia, thrombophlebitis,
Limitation of motion		constipation or fecal impaction
GASTROINTESTINAL SYSTEM		
Decreased intestinal motility	Retention of feces	Constipation or fecal impaction
METABOLIC SYSTEM		
Decreased gamma globulin level	Decreased inflammatory response	Delayed wound healing, wound dehiscence,
		or evisceration
IMMUNE SYSTEM		
Fewer killer T cells	Decreased ability to protect against	Wound infection, wound dehiscence,
Decreased response to foreign antigens	invasion by pathogenic microorganisms	pneumonia, urinary tract infection

Modified from Phipps WJ and others, editors: *Medical-surgical nursing: concepts and clinical practice,* ed 4, St Louis, 1991, Mosby.

potential postoperative outcomes of pulmonary edema, myocardial infarction, decreased cardiac output, pulmonary thromboembolism, and aspiration pneumonia.[13]

Emergency surgery for cancer in the older patient carries greater risk than elective surgery. The older patient is at risk during emergency surgery because of declines in organ function and an increase in accompanying disease (e.g., cardiovascular disease). In addition, the increased morbidity after emergency surgery is associated with a decline in immune system competency in the older patient.[13,30]

One of the major problems facing the oncology nurse is early detection of postoperative problems that arise in the older patient because of lack of recognition that the patient's condition has changed. Continuity of nursing care and thorough assessment from the preoperative phase to the postoperative phase prevent such problems.[44]

Table 20-3 presents additional information on the physiologic changes related to the aging process that can affect the surgical outcome.

Text continued on p. 500.

NURSING MANAGEMENT

Nursing care of the surgical cancer patient is very similar to the nursing care required for any surgery patient. However, the nurse must be aware of the problems that are unique to the cancer disease process. Unlike with other surgery patients, the cancer patient's comprehensive plan of care must include nursing management of the psychosocial and existential aspects of and complications specific to the cancer.[24]

PREOPERATIVE CARE

Preoperative nursing care of the cancer patient focuses on assessment and intervention. To accomplish these tasks effectively, the nurse must know the answers to the following questions[30]:

- What is the purpose of the surgery? Is it diagnosis, staging, cure, or palliation? Each purpose has a different meaning for the patient. By knowing the purpose of surgery, the nurse can better comprehend the patient's behavior. A patient who recently has been diagnosed as having cancer will exhibit different behaviors than will the patient with metastatic disease who undergoes palliative surgery for relief of intractable pain.
- What kind of surgery will be performed? The nurse must know what preoperative preparation or care is required (e.g., bowel preparation, nutritional supplementation); where incisions will be made and how long they will be; and what devices will be attached to the patient (e.g., catheters, drains, chest tubes).
- What has the patient and/or family been told about the surgery, diagnosis, and possibilities for future treatment? Patients often hear only the words "cancer" and "surgery"; everything else is a blur. Therefore information needs to be repeated frequently.

Once answers to these questions have been obtained, preoperative nursing care of the cancer patient can focus on reducing anxiety, enhancing physical well-being, and teaching.[53]

Reducing Anxiety

Cancer has a profound psychologic impact on patients and their significant others. Complex emotional responses are evoked, often resulting in hopelessness, powerlessness, and severe depression. Patients often react to the idea of surgery with apprehension and may be resentful, angry, anxious, and even panicky about the impending operation. The basis for these powerful reactions lies in the patient's fear of death from surgery or anesthesia and the fear of pain and mutilation.[23,41]

Misconceptions and fears about surgery may be influenced by others close to the patient. Patients often expect outcomes similar to those of friends and relatives, especially if the outcome of their surgery was negative. The patient's prior experience with surgery also affects the preoperative outlook and recovery; if previous operations were difficult, problems often are encountered in subsequent ones.[41]

Tumors that are visibly evident to the patient and, more important, to others, have a greater effect on the patient's psychologic response to cancer. Cancer patients often believe that tumors located away from vital organs are less serious than those in vital structures. Tumors that involve the sex organs cause patients to question their sexuality and their ability to function sexually and reproduce.[30]

Some preoperative fear is normal, even positive, because it encourages the patient to take the surgery seriously and to make realistic plans for coping with it. For some, the question, "How do you think this surgery will change your life?" encourages the patient to explore fears, talk about related anxieties, and begin planning for change. This type of communication forms the basis for a supportive, trusting, and therapeutic relationship that will endure throughout subsequent readmissions to the hospital.[23,41,53]

Continued.

Enhancing Physical Well-Being

The cancer patient may be debilitated as a result of advanced disease or because of the type of symptoms and/or length of time symptoms have been present. Enhancement of the patient's physical well-being in the preoperative period includes alleviating physical symptoms such as pain, diarrhea, nausea and vomiting, fatigue, bowel obstruction, and malnutrition. Stress-related symptoms, such as insomnia and headaches, also can be minimized. Side effects of preoperative chemotherapy or radiation therapy increase the patient's chances of developing postoperative physical or emotional problems, or both. Proper preoperative treatment and management of these side effects will directly affect the patient's response postoperatively.[53] See Table 20-4 for information specific to preoperative assessment of physiologic parameters in the surgical oncology patient.

Teaching

Anxiety appears to be more severe in patients who do not have accurate information about their impending sur-gery. During the preoperative period, concern about the disease or diagnosis often is replaced by concern about the impending surgery. Nurses are in a primary position to correct misconceptions and fill in the gaps about surgical procedures. Honestly and clearly answering questions about the site, type, and extent of surgery, as well as probable pain, discomfort, or any body changes, often reduces rather than increases the patient's level of anxiety. Information should be provided and repeated as needed.[53]

Preoperative patient teaching will be most successful if the nurse develops an individually tailored teaching plan based on a thorough assessment of knowledge deficits. These deficits must be handled as with any other nursing diagnosis, and the nursing process must serve as the basis for developing the teaching plan. Learning needs and goals or outcomes must be mutually identified and agreed on by the patient and/or family and the nurse. See the box, p. 494, for preoperative teaching priorities and desired outcomes.[9,53]

Table 20-4 Preoperative Assessment of Physiologic Parameters[6,57]

Physiologic parameters	Factors that increase surgical risk	Assessment factors	Laboratory tests/others
Nutritional status	Debilitation and malnourishment as a result of disease and/or previous therapy	Anorexia Eating habits Special diets Food restrictions Food preferences Availability of food Supplementation Nausea Vomiting Stomatitis Smell or taste changes Recent weight loss	Decreased serum albumin
Cardiovascular system	Congestive heart failure as a result of previous and prolonged chemotherapy	Dyspnea Fatigue Anorexia Nausea Vomiting Abdominal distention Right upper quadrant pain Tachycardia Weak, thready pulse Hypotension Rapid, labored respiration Frothy, blood-tinged sputum Moist rales Displaced apical pulse Weight gain Peripheral edema Dilation of peripheral veins	Increased pulmonary capillary pressure Decreased cardiac output Increased right atrial pressure

Table 20-4   Preoperative Assessment of Physiologic Parameters[6,57]—cont'd

Physiologic parameters	Factors that increase surgical risk	Assessment factors	Laboratory tests/others
Pulmonary system	Pulmonary edema and/or fibrosis as a result of previous and prolonged chemotherapy	Nasal flaring Retractions Tachypnea Labored, noisy breathing Diaphoresis Rales Wheezing Persistent cough Frothy, blood-tinged sputum Restlessness Confusion Hypotension Tachycardia Lethargy Intake and output Sudden weight gain Swollen feet or ankles Chest pain	Decreased vital capacity Decreased minute volume Decreased cardiac output $Paco_2$ Pao_2 pH K^+ Na^+ Pulmonary capillary wedge pressure Pulmonary artery pressure Sputum specimens for culture and sensitivity Serial chest x-ray film reports
Genitourinary system	Renal insufficiency as a result of previous and prolonged chemotherapy	Frequency of voiding Dysuria Anuria Infection Urine (color, clarity)	Decreased creatinine clearance Increased blood urea nitrogen (BUN) Increased uric acid levels Increased serum creatinine levels
Fluid and electrolyte status	Dehydration and electrolyte imbalance as a result of disease and/or previous therapy Hypovolemia as a result of disease	Intake and output Vomiting Diarrhea Bleeding	K^+ Mg^{++} Ca^{++} H^+
Liver function status	Metastatic liver disease	Jaundice Ascites Vague upper abdominal pain Anorexia Weight loss Splenomegaly Esophageal varices Fever of unknown origin Dependent edema	Total bilirubin
Hematologic factors	Platelet dysfunction as a result of disease and/or previous therapy Hypercoagulability as a result of disease Anemia as a result of disease	Easy bruising Excessive bleeding Dyspnea Fatigue Previous thrombophlebitis	Prothrombin time Partial thromboplastin Platelet count Red blood cell (RBC) count White blood cell (WBC) count Hemoglobin Hematocrit
Potential for postoperative complications	Preoperative infection as a result of immunocompetence and/or previous therapy Previous radiation therapy	Sneezing Cough Sore throat Fever Skin lesions Rashes Radiation skin damage in relation to anticipated surgical incision	WBC count Throat culture Sputum culture

Continued.

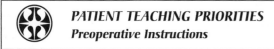

PATIENT TEACHING PRIORITIES
Preoperative Instructions

Include information about:

Surgery to be performed

General preoperative activities and the reasons for them

General postoperative behaviors expected of the patient and the reasons for them

Techniques such as turning, coughing, and deep breathing (TCDB), incisional splinting, range-of-motion (ROM) exercises, and incentive spirometry

Types of equipment to be used before and after surgery

Plan of care and rationales for procedures

Anticipated care settings, and equipment and experiences related to surgery

Self-care strategies to prevent and minimize complications of surgery

Outcomes of preoperative teaching:

Patient and/or significant other is able to:

State that anxiety about surgery has lessened

Demonstrate an understanding of preoperative procedures and routines through return demonstration, verbal feedback, and other means

Demonstrate an understanding of postoperative procedures and routines by return demonstration, verbal feedback, and other means

Participate in postoperative procedures and care

POSTOPERATIVE CARE

Postoperative nursing care of cancer patients depends on the type of cancer, the type of surgery performed, previous treatment, and preexisting physiologic deficits. Like preoperative care, postoperative care focuses on the patient's physical and psychologic needs.[30]

Physical Needs

All surgery patients' immediate postoperative needs are primarily physical. From the moment the patient arrives in the recovery room or special care unit, certain definitive goals act as guides throughout the remaining postoperative course: to prevent postoperative complications and to promote cardiovascular function, tissue perfusion, respiratory function, nutrition and elimination, fluid and electrolyte balance, renal function, rest and comfort, wound healing, and early movement and ambulation.[6,30] The reader is referred to any general surgical nursing text for a thorough discussion of these common postoperative goals.

Psychologic Needs

As patients are roused from anesthesia, their first questions are often ones such as, "Do I have cancer? Did the

doctor get all of it? Did the cancer spread? Did the doctor remove my (e.g., colon, leg, breast)?" The patient's questions should not be answered until recovery from the effects of anesthesia is complete and the surgeon or referring physician has had time to see the patient and offer an adequate explanation. However, the nurse must ensure that a supportive environment is provided when test results are shared with the patient and family.[30]

All cancer patients must make psychologic changes. For some patients, the diagnosis of cancer may mean changes in life-style, occupation, or school or job attendance and performance. The threat of change can be so great that, occasionally, the cancer patient may become psychologically immobilized. If necessary psychologic changes are not incorporated, the cancer patient is at risk of not complying with the demands of therapy. The new sick role may also be incompatible with the patient's self-concept, making it difficult for the patient to temporarily rely on others for needed care.[30,53]

After surgery, patients slowly come to the realization that they have cancer. This may initiate feelings of helplessness, depression, and grief. Patients often grieve over real or imagined changes in body image and self-worth. Changes in body image may be difficult for the cancer patient to positively incorporate. When the patient is unable to fully accept the physical changes after surgery, conflict occurs between the way the body actually looks and the way the patient mentally pictures the body. This form of denial usually is followed by recognition of reality, grief, and depression. Patients who attach great psychologic significance to the lost body part may believe that the surgery has compromised the body's internal structure and complain of frailty. These patients frequently restrict their physical and sexual activities unnecessarily, feeling their bodies are vulnerable. Appropriate nursing measures help the patient adapt to changes in body image. The nurse can assist patients by acknowledging the painfulness of the loss and by ensuring that they grieve in a safe, nonjudgmental environment.[30,41,53]

For most patients, the words "cancer" and "death" are synonymous and all cancers are considered one disease. This attitude reflects a lack of knowledge about different types of cancer. The diagnosis initially can isolate such patients from others. The patient's ability to make decisions may be affected by this same lack of knowledge. After the diagnosis is confirmed, most patients strive to regain their decision-making power. One way of doing this is by learning about the diagnosis, therapy, and hospital routines.[30]

It is important that the nurse assess the type and degree of support that significant others provide the patient. The patient's postoperative anxiety level often declines when the nurse encourages family support and availability. However, the nurse must remember that cancer and surgery are crisis situations for the entire family. Initially the family may be emotionally and psychologically immobilized by the diagnosis, and family members may neglect themselves or may not know where to turn for services. The nurse can share information on motel accommodations and restaurants and make other referrals as necessary. Sometimes, even simple decision making is overwhelming for the family in crisis. Often family members want to support the patient but do not know what to say or do. The nurse can guide them by aiding them in identifying what they can do to help.[30,41]

Nurses must be aware of the psychologic issues affecting cancer surgery patients in order to provide the most appropriate care and to encourage their patients to adapt positively to the demands of the disease and of therapy. (Also see Chapters 27, 31, and 32.)

NURSING DIAGNOSIS

• *Body image disturbance related to surgical removal of body part and to diagnosis of cancer*

OUTCOME GOAL

Patient will be able to:
• Verbalize impact of surgery and diagnosis on self-image.

INTERVENTIONS

• Encourage patient to discuss feelings and concerns with health care providers and significant others.
• Help patient identify, label, and express feelings about significance of lost body part, treatment modalities, and anticipated progress.
• Promote acceptance of a positive/realistic body image.

NURSING DIAGNOSIS

• *Coping, ineffective family: compromised related to diagnosis of cancer*

OUTCOME GOAL

Family will be able to:
• Demonstrate effective coping strategies for living with cancer.

INTERVENTIONS

• Provide opportunities for expression of feelings.
• Provide information to assist patients and their families in working through emotional reactions to the diagnosis, treatment, and prognosis.

NURSING DIAGNOSIS

• *Coping, ineffective individual, related to diagnosis of cancer and to potential life-style changes*

OUTCOME GOAL

Patient will be able to:
• Demonstrate effective coping strategies for living with cancer.

INTERVENTIONS

• Provide opportunities for patient to express feelings about diagnosis and prognosis.
• Assist patient in meeting adaptations or changes in activities and relationships.

NURSING DIAGNOSIS

• *Fluid volume deficit: risk for, related to surgical procedure, to excessive fluid loss from abnormal routes (indwelling tubes) and postoperative nausea/vomiting, and to inability to receive or absorb fluids*

OUTCOME GOAL

Patient will be able to:
• Demonstrate no evidence of fluid volume deficit.

INTERVENTIONS

• Monitor vital signs.
• Assess capillary refill time.
• Measure intake and output.
• Monitor electrolyte values.
• Measure urine specific gravity.
• Monitor hemoglobin and hematocrit.
• Assess oral mucous membranes.
• Assess skin turgor.
• Administer intravenous or oral fluids as ordered by physician.
• Administer antiemetics as ordered by physician.

NURSING DIAGNOSIS

• *Fluid volume deficit related to surgical procedure (loss of 15% to 20% of total blood volume during surgery)*

OUTCOME GOAL

Patient will be able to:
• Demonstrate adequate fluid volume within 72 hours of surgery.

INTERVENTIONS*

• Maintain strict bed rest, with patient supine and head of bed elevated slightly.
• Limit all activities.
• Monitor vital signs every 5 to 15 minutes.
• Administer drugs as ordered to maintain blood pressure (BP) and increase cardiac output.
• Maintain patent intravenous line for administration of drugs.
• Administer fluids and volume expanders as ordered.
• Monitor urine output.
• Assess skin for color, temperature, and elasticity.

---

*Modified from Friel M: Concepts related to the nursing care of surgical oncology patients. In Vredevoe D, Derdiarian A, Sarna L, editors: *Concepts of oncology nursing,* Englewood Cliffs, NJ, 1981, Prentice Hall; and Thompson JM et al: *Mosby's clinical nursing,* ed 3, St Louis, 1993, Mosby.

Continued.

- Maintain accurate input and output records.
- Monitor arterial blood gases.
- Administer oxygen as ordered.
- Monitor respiratory rate and pattern.
- Monitor hemodynamic parameters as ordered.

NURSING DIAGNOSIS

- *Gas exchange, impaired, related to embolization of thrombus*

OUTCOME GOAL

Patient will be able to:
- Demonstrate no evidence of pulmonary embolus.

INTERVENTION

- Observe for signs/symptoms of pulmonary embolus:
  —Chest pain
  —Dyspnea
  —Tachypnea

NURSING DIAGNOSIS

- *Infection: risk for, related to preoperative immunocompromised status stemming from disease and/or previous therapy*

OUTCOME GOAL

Patient will be able to:
- Demonstrate no evidence of infection.

INTERVENTIONS*

- Assess for risk factors.
- Obtain cultures as ordered and report results.
- Monitor vital signs; check for increased pulse rate and signs of low-grade, intermittent fever.
- Inspect body secretions, excretions, and exudates for signs of infection; report abnormalities.
- Monitor hydration and electrolyte balance.
- Monitor changes in white blood cell (WBC) count.
- Wash hands before and after contact with patient.
- Make sure patient is not exposed to infected visitors or staff.
- Turn patient frequently; instruct in deep breathing.

NURSING DIAGNOSIS

- *Infection: risk for, related to break in skin's integrity (surgical incision)*

OUTCOME GOAL

Patient will be able to:
- Demonstrate no evidence of wound infection.

INTERVENTION

- Monitor wound site for edema, redness, and undue pain.

NURSING DIAGNOSIS

- *Infection: risk for, related to urinary retention as a result of surgical procedure*

OUTCOME GOAL

Patient will be able to:
- Demonstrate no evidence of urinary tract infection.

INTERVENTIONS

- Check urine output for amount, color, specific gravity, and odor.
- Administer antibiotics as ordered.
- Assess for abdominal pain.
- Force fluids.

NURSING DIAGNOSIS

- *Injury: risk for, related to peritonitis secondary to breakdown of anastomosis, which occurs because of diminished tissue healing as a result of chemotherapy, radiation therapy, poor nutritional status, and/or tumor*

OUTCOME GOAL

Patient will be able to:
- Demonstrate no evidence of peritonitis.

INTERVENTIONS*

- Assess for signs/symptoms of peritonitis:
  —Moderate to severe abdominal pain
  —Burning ache aggravated by any motion, even respiration
  —Anorexia
  —Nausea
  —Vomiting
  —Fever within 48 hours after surgery
  —Chills, thirst, scant urine output
  —Inability to pass feces or flatus
  —Abdominal distention
  —Tachycardia with weak, thready pulses
  —Rapid, shallow respirations
  —Tachypnea

NURSING DIAGNOSIS

- *Injury: risk for, related to postoperative intestinal obstruction secondary to adhesions from radiation therapy*

OUTCOME GOAL

Patient will be able to:
- Demonstrate no evidence of intestinal obstruction.

INTERVENTION

- Assess for signs/symptoms of intestinal obstruction:
  —Vomiting

---

*Modified from Friel M: Concepts related to the nursing care of surgical oncology patients. In Vredevoe D, Derdiarian A, Sarna L, editors: *Concepts of oncology nursing,* Englewood Cliffs, NJ, 1981, Prentice Hall; and Thompson JM et al: *Mosby's clinical nursing,* ed 3, St Louis, 1993, Mosby.

—Abdominal cramping
—Constipation

NURSING DIAGNOSIS

• *Injury: risk for, related to hypercoagulability and post-operative inactivity*

OUTCOME GOAL

Patient will be able to:
• Demonstrate no evidence of thrombophlebitis.

INTERVENTIONS

• Assess calves daily.
• Observe for signs/symptoms of thrombophlebitis:
—Calf pain
—Calf tenderness
—Homans' sign
—Dilated superficial veins
—Edema of involved extremity
• Encourage early ambulation.

NURSING DIAGNOSIS

• *Knowledge deficit related to such areas as self-care, activities related to health care regimen, and decision making about health*

OUTCOME GOAL

Patient will be able to:
• Express an understanding of and demonstrate important self-care and daily activities resulting from diagnosis and surgical procedure.

INTERVENTIONS*

• At every interaction, assess for knowledge deficits.
• Use patient's theories about illness as a starting point for teaching, and continually elicits patient's perception.
• During interactions, assess frequently to see if patient understands and accepts diagnosis.
• Simplify information to conform to patient's terms, thought patterns, and daily routines.
• Give explicit directions.
• Be available to patient for questions.
• Demonstrate to patient and family how to use information.
• Reinforce correct use of information.
• Teach patient how to mentally rehearse a necessary health action.
• Make sure patient is actively involved in decisions about care.
• Offer access to a peer support network and opportuni-

ties for patient to watch other successfully mastering similar health care problems.
• Provide instruction in several forms (visual, written, discussion), so that patient will remember it in various ways.
• Provide materials for patient to take home for review and to use what was learned. (See box below.)

NURSING DIAGNOSIS

• *Mobility, impaired physical, related to surgical removal of limb*

OUTCOME GOAL

Patient will be able to:
• Demonstrate activities that encourage adaptation to changes in physical mobility resulting from surgical procedure.

INTERVENTIONS*

• Help patient with ambulation; control distance.
• Have patient use walker, cane, or wheelchair as needed as assistive devices.

 PATIENT TEACHING PRIORITIES
Postoperative Instructions

Include information about:

Changes in self-care and other activities as a result of surgery
Progressive return to maximum activity level
Anticipated discharge medications
Wound management
Proper use of assistive or prosthetic devices
Symptoms to watch for: fever, pain, vomiting, diarrhea, bleeding, malnutrition
When and whom to call if problems arise
Where to get additional information about cancer or its treatment
How to contact support groups (e.g., Reach to Recovery, Make Today Count)
Resources or agencies that might be helpful to patient: physical therapy, occupational therapy, speech therapy, ostomy outpatient clinics, sources of prosthetic fitting devices, home care agencies
Sources of medical supplies
Possible follow-up care
Return to work
Any necessary job retraining
Resumption of driving
Resumption of sexual activity

---

*Modified from Friel M: Concepts related to the nursing care of surgical oncology patients. In Vredevoe D, Derdiarian A, Sarna L, editors: *Concepts of oncology nursing,* Englewood Cliffs, NJ, 1981, Prentice Hall; and Thompson JM et al: *Mosby's clinical nursing,* ed 3, St Louis, 1993, Mosby.

Continued.

- Minimize environmental barriers.
- Encourage use of involved limb.
- Change patient's position slowly.
- Encourage moderate physical exercise, adequate rest, and ROM exercises.
- Balance nutritional intake; supplement protein.
- Discuss "phantom" pain with patient and family.

NURSING DIAGNOSIS

- *Nutrition, altered: less than body requirements related to surgical procedure for cancer that interferes with mechanical process of eating and with absorption of essential salts and nutrients*

OUTCOME GOAL

Patient will be able to:
- Demonstrate no evidence of protein-calorie malnutrition.

INTERVENTIONS*

- Assess for signs/symptoms of protein-calorie malnutrition:
  —Edema
  —Hair dyspigmentation
  —Easily pluckable hair
  —Muscle wasting
  —Dermatosis
- Review results of anthropometric test, dietary analysis, and clinical examination.
- Perform nutrition assessment:
  —Assess problem area, food preferences, patterns and behaviors related to food intake, intake and output, and calorie count.
- Encourage good mouth care.
- Provide relaxed, pain-free environment.
- Observe presentation of food.
- Encourage family to bring in favorite foods when allowed.
- Confer with dietitian about diet and supplements that meet patient's needs.
- Provide proper care for and monitor intravenous total parenteral nutrition.
- Provide proper care for feeding tubes.
- Before discharge, provide nutrition teaching for patient and family.

NURSING DIAGNOSIS

- *Pain related to surgical procedure and to complications at insertion sites of therapeutic hardware*

OUTCOME GOAL

Patient will be able to:

- Express and demonstrate successful control of pain related to diagnosis and surgical procedure.

INTERVENTIONS*

- Incorporate the following when assessing patient's level of pain:
  —Location and characteristics
  —Onset
  —Frequency
  —Intensity (scale of 0 to 5)
  —Quality
  —Effective pain control measures
  —Ineffective pain control measure
  —Pain expression style
  —Movement
  —Muscle tone
  —Emotional distress
  —Effect of pain on postoperative activities
  —Effect on sleep/wake pattern
- Identify strategies that eliminate or control pain.
- Explore strategies that have been successful in the past.
- Identify strategies that patient considers essential for reducing pain.
- Administer medication per physician's orders and protocols using appropriate delivery system:
  —Monitor effect frequently.
  —Graph pain assessment data.
  —Provide physician with evidence of need to change medication.
- Intervene at onset of pain.
- Position for comfort.
- Provide distraction.
- Instruct patient in relaxation techniques; for acute pain, use short, simple techniques with nurse directing.
- Pace activities, and plan activities ahead of time.
- Provide supportive environment.
- Use several pain reduction strategies.

NURSING DIAGNOSIS

- *Skin integrity, impaired, risk for, related to tissue damage and/or poor tissue healing resulting from chemotherapy, radiation therapy, and/or poor nutritional status*

OUTCOME GOAL

Patient will be able to:
- Demonstrate no evidence of tissue damage or poor tissue healing.

INTERVENTIONS*

- Inspect incision site for hematomas (swelling, discoloration).

---

*Modified from Friel M: Concepts related to the nursing care of surgical oncology patients. In Vredevoe D, Derdiarian A, Sarna L, editors: *Concepts of oncology nursing,* Englewood Cliffs, NJ, 1981, Prentice Hall; and Thompson JM et al: *Mosby's clinical nursing,* ed 3, St Louis, 1993, Mosby.

- Assess patency of drains.
- Assess for signs/symptoms of dehiscence:
  —Rapid onset of serosanguineous drainage
  —Popping sensation
- Assess for signs of impending evisceration.
  —Separation of incision
  —Protrusion of abdominal contents
- Check use of abdominal binders for obese patients.

NURSING DIAGNOSIS

- *Skin integrity, impaired, related to tissue damage and/or poor tissue healing resulting from chemotherapy, radiation therapy, and/or poor nutritional status*

OUTCOME GOAL

Patient will be able to:
- Show adequate healing of affected tissues after appropriate medical and nursing intervention.

INTERVENTIONS*

- Assess for signs/symptoms of dehiscence:
  —Monitor amount and color of drainage.
- If dehiscence occurs:
  —Call physician immediately.
  —Obtain vital signs.
  —Prepare patient for surgery.
- Assess for signs of evisceration.
  —Separation of incision
  —Protrusion of abdominal contents
- If evisceration occurs:
  —Apply sterile, moist towels over extruded intestine or omentum.
  —Prepare patient for surgery.

NURSING DIAGNOSIS

- *Tissue perfusion, altered (peripheral), related to lymphedema secondary to dissection of lymph nodes*

OUTCOME GOAL

Patient will be able to:
- Demonstrate no evidence of lymphedema.

INTERVENTIONS

- Do not use affected limb to check BP, perform venipunctures, withdraw blood, or inject medications.
- Assess affected limb for signs/symptoms of lymphedema:
  —Redness
  —Warmth
  —Unusual hardness
  —Swelling

- Use pillows to elevate affected limb above level of the heart.
- Observe for infection occurring secondary to lymphedema.
- Teach importance of good hygiene.
- Encourage progressive exercise of affected limb.

NURSING DIAGNOSIS

- *Tissue perfusion, altered (peripheral), related to hypercoagulability and postoperative inactivity*

OUTCOME GOAL

Patient will be able to:
- Demonstrate no evidence of peripheral edema.

INTERVENTIONS*

- Keep patient on bed rest.
- Limit self-care activities.
- Raise affected limb above level of right atrium.
- Do not use knee gatch.
- If patient complains of pain, assess its quality and location.
- Administer analgesics as ordered.
- Measure calf or thigh (or both) daily and record findings.
- Assess circulation of affected extremity, and check pulses in all extremities. Use Doppler sensor if pulses seem to be absent.
- Use elastic stockings as ordered.
- Check vital signs every 4 to 8 hours.
- Administer anticoagulant therapy as ordered.
- Monitor results of prothrombin time (PT) and partial thromboplastin time (PTT) studies.
- Initiate a progressive exercise program.
- Instruct patient to put on support stockings before ambulating and to avoid standing for long periods.

DISCHARGE PLANNING

The goal for the cancer patient is to develop or regain independence. This can be achieved by encouraging patients to participate in activities of daily living and to learn new self-care measures early in their hospitalization in preparation for discharge. However, in their eagerness to help patients, family members often try to do everything for them. This response serves only to foster dependence in patients and contributes to their feelings of helplessness. The nurse must guide the patient and family in understanding the significance of the patient's early steps toward independence.[30]

Nurses sometimes mistakenly assume that, once the patient is discharged from the hospital, the patient will receive the care, attention, and support needed at home.

---

*Modified from Friel M: Concepts related to the nursing care of surgical oncology patients. In Vredevoe D, Derdiarian A, Sarna L, editors: *Concepts of oncology nursing,* Englewood Cliffs, NJ, 1981, Prentice Hall; and Thompson JM et al: *Mosby's clinical nursing,* ed 3, St Louis, 1993, Mosby.

Continued.

However, some patients dread discharge from the hospital almost as much as admission to it. Some patients become very dependent on the hospital and their new sick role, particularly if their home life is unstable. A supportive home environment probably will remain so after the patient's discharge from the hospital. However, an unstable home environment (e.g., marked by poor communication, strained relationships) is likely to worsen after surgery. Whether the patient is able to adjust to changes in physical appearance or function is largely determined by the family's reaction to these same issues. If the patient feels rejected at home, the patient may fear rejection from society at large.[41]

Discharge planning therefore must begin when a patient is admitted to the hospital and continue throughout the hospital stay. The nurse's assessment must include information about the family and family situation; the patient's knowledge about the disease, its treatment, and available resources; the social setting; school and/or work; and diet. The health care team then can begin to make appropriate plans to ease the transition from hospital to home. Many times, preparing the home to receive the patient takes longer than the hospitalization. Members of the health care team must be consulted for their evaluations of the family's ability to care for the patient. Evaluation may reveal that home care by private or visiting nurses or admission to an extended care facility may be needed when the patient leaves the hospital. If the family is experiencing communication problems and emotional difficulties, the health care team might consider referral to family therapy or a family support group.[30,41]

Most cancer patients have not completely recovered from their surgery at the time of discharge from the hos-

GERIATRIC CONSIDERATIONS

Include information about:

Physiologic changes: the cardiovascular, respiratory, renal, GI, immune, metabolic, and musculoskeletal systems may be compromised (see Table 20-3)

Anesthesia risk for hypoxemia

Postoperative risk for pulmonary edema, myocardial infarction, diminished cardiac output, pulmonary thromboembolism, and aspiration pneumonia

Discharge plan requires assessment of patient's need of additional resources (e.g., home care agency, American Cancer Society, social services)

pital. Therefore the information identified in the box on p. 497 and the box above should be given to the patient in writing before discharge.

An astute nurse institutes and documents discharge planning based on a thorough admission assessment and history and makes every attempt to involve family members early in the process. If needed, referrals are made to appropriate members of the health care team so that all possible issues are addressed well before the patient's discharge from the hospital.

Discharge planning allows patients and their families to prepare for living with cancer outside the hospital. The nurse anticipates postoperative needs and concerns early, allowing the cancer patient and family to face the challenges that lie ahead.[30]

FUTURE DIRECTIONS AND ADVANCES IN SURGICAL ONCOLOGY

State-of-the-art surgical approaches of the future will reflect movement away from today's invasive procedures. By the twenty-first century, the long incisions and visceral manipulation once considered necessary for adequate visualization, comprehensive resection, and anastomosis will be uncommon. Cancer surgery of the future will combine refined endoscopic equipment, videography, lasers, microscopes, and three-dimensional imaging devices, allowing surgeons to localize tumor tissue for ablation by microendoscopic resection or targeted intraluminal radiation. Current research with radiotagged antibodies, it is hoped, will lead to earlier detection of tumors, which will facilitate surgical cures for certain cancers. This process, combining biologic, radiologic, and surgical interventions, involves preoperative injec-

tion of monoclonal antibodies for intraoperative detection and tagging of tumor sites with handheld gamma probes; this localizes the tumor and spares noncancerous tissue. In the future, molecular surgery, the use of gene therapy for preoperative tumor debulking, may be used to treat localized head and neck cancer and ovarian cancer. The day may even come when organs damaged by chemotherapy or radiation, such as the heart, liver, and lungs, may be replaced in patients who demonstrate no evidence of disease after a period of time.[18,24]

CONCLUSION

Current trends in tumor biology and interdisciplinary cancer management have changed our previous reliance on surgery as the only curative form of cancer therapy and precipitated changes in the extensiveness of surgical resections. By combining surgery, radiation therapy, chemotherapy, and biotherapy, disease-free intervals have been significantly expanded.[24]

In spite of known limitations, surgery continues to be an important treatment modality for cancer. The nurse may encounter the cancer surgery patient at the time of initial diagnosis or when the patient returns for reconstructive surgery after several years of disease-free existence. This demands flexibility on the part of the nurse and a strong understanding of the foundations and principles of surgical oncology nursing.

■ CHAPTER QUESTIONS

1. Mastectomy for local recurrence after a previous lumpectomy and radiation therapy would be classified as:
   a. Palliative therapy
   b. Primary therapy
   c. Salvage therapy
   d. Combination therapy
2. Wide excision or en bloc dissection involves:
   a. Removal of a tumor, regional lymph nodes, and lymphatic channels, and any involved neighboring structures
   b. Removal of a large tumor burden
   c. Excision of a tumor and a small margin of normal tissue
   d. Removal of a wedge of tumor tissue from a large tumor
3. Photodynamic therapy:
   a. Destroys precancerous or cancer cells by deep-freezing them
   b. Combines surgical resection of tissue with topical application of chemotherapy
   c. Destroys cancer cells by intensive thermal energy
   d. Involves intravenous injection of a light-sensitizing agent, followed by exposure to a laser, a process that kills the cancer cells
4. Surgical techniques that prevent tumor cells from escaping into the general circulation include all of the following *except:*
   a. Early ligation of blood vessels and lymphatics
   b. Irrigation of wounds with tumoricidal solutions
   c. Frequent glove and instrument changes
   d. Frequent handling and manipulation of the tumor
5. Cytoreductive (debulking) surgery is considered what type of treatment?
   a. Salvage
   b. Adjuvant
   c. Palliative
   d. Primary
6. Protein-calorie malnutrition in a preoperative cancer patient generally results from all of the following *except:*
   a. A decrease in oral intake
   b. An increase in enteral losses as a result of malabsorption
   c. An increase in nutritional requirements as a result of hypermetabolism
   d. A decrease in nutritional requirements as a result of tumor activity
7. Surgical removal of benign polyps from the colon is considered:
   a. Preventive
   b. Definitive
   c. Reconstructive
   d. Palliative
8. The advantages of an implantable vascular access device (IVAD) include all the following *except:*
   a. Need for frequent irrigation
   b. Less disturbance in body image
   c. Fewer restrictions on activities
   d. Less interference with clothing

BIBLIOGRAPHY

1. Allen MS: Video-assisted thoracoscopy. In Morris PJ, Malt RA, editors: *Oxford textbook of surgery,* vol 2, New York, 1994, Oxford Medical Publications.
2. Anseline PF and others: Radiation injury of the rectum, *Ann Surg* 194:716, 1981.
3. Arbour R: Laser and ultrasound technology in aggressive management of central nervous system tumors, *J Neurosci Nurs* 26(1):30, 1994.
4. Aronoff BL: Lasers in surgical oncology. I, *Semin Surg Oncol* 11(4):281, 1995.
5. Baird RM, Rebbeck PA: Impact of preoperative chemotherapy for the surgeon, *Recent Results Cancer Res* 103:79, 1986.
6. Black JM, Matassarin-Jacobs E, editors: *Luckmann and Sorensen's medical-surgical nursing: a psychophysiologic approach,* ed 4, Philadelphia, 1993, Saunders.
7. Brandt BT and others: Hepatic cryosurgery for metastatic colorectal carcinoma, *Oncol Nurs Forum* 23(1):29, 1996.
8. Brenner ZR, Krenzer ME: Update on cryosurgical ablation for prostate cancer, *AJN* 95(4):44, 1995.
9. Brown MH and others: *Standards of oncology nursing practice,* New York, 1986, Wiley & Sons.
10. Bucholtz JD: Implications of radiation therapy for nursing. In Clark JC, McGee RF, editors: *Core curriculum for oncology nursing,* ed 2, Philadelphia, 1992, Saunders.
11. Butler J: Nutrition and cancer: a review of the literature, *Cancer Nurs* 3:131, 1980.
12. Calabresi P, Schein PS, Rosenberg SA, editors: *Medical oncology: basic principles and clinical management of cancer,* ed 2, New York, 1993, McGraw-Hill.
13. Derby SA: Cancer in the older patient. In Ashwander P and others, editors: *Oncology nursing: advances, treatments and trends into the 21st century,* Rockville, Md, 1990, Aspen.
14. DeVita VT Jr, Hellman S, Rosenberg SA, editors: *Cancer: principles and practice of oncology,* ed 4, Philadelphia, 1993, Lippincott.
15. DeVita VT Jr, Hellman S, Rosenberg SA, editors: *Important advances in oncology,* ed 11, Philadelphia, 1995, Lippincott.
16. Dixon J: Current laser applications in general surgery, *Ann Surg* 207(4):355, 1988.
17. Duke JH, Miller TA: Salt and water: fluid and electrolyte problems. In Condon R, DeCosse J, editors: *Surgical care,* Philadelphia, 1980, Lea & Febiger.

18. Engelking C: New approaches: innovations in cancer prevention, diagnosis, treatment, and support, *Oncol Nurs Forum* 21(1):62, 1994.

19. Falcone RE, Nappi JF: Chemotherapy and wound healing, *Surg Clin North Am* 64:779, 1984.

20. Fisher AMR, Murphree AL, Gomer CJ: Clinical and preclinical photodynamic therapy, *Lasers Surg Med* 17:2, 1995.

21. Forbes J: Principles and potential of palliative surgery in patients with advanced cancer, *Recent Results Cancer Res* 108:134, 1988.

22. Friel M: Concepts related to the nursing care of surgical oncology patients. In Vredevoe D, Derdiarian A, Sarna L, editors: *Concepts of oncology nursing,* Englewood Cliffs, NJ, 1981, Prentice Hall.

23. Griffiths MJ, Murray KH, Russo PC: *Oncology nursing: pathophysiology, assessment, and intervention,* New York, 1984, Macmillan.

24. Groenwald SL and others, editors: *Cancer nursing: principles and practice,* ed 3, Boston, 1993, Jones & Bartlett.

25. Haibeck S: Intraoperative radiation therapy, *Oncol Nurs Forum* 15(2):143, 1988.

26. Harrison LB, Enker WE, Anderson LL: High-dose-rate intraoperative radiation therapy for colorectal cancer, *Oncology* 9(8):737, 1995.

27. Haskel CM, editor: *Cancer treatment,* ed 4, Philadelphia, 1993, Saunders.

28. Hill G: Historic milestones in cancer surgery, *Semin Oncol* 6(4):409, 1979.

29. Holland JF, Frei E III, editors: *Cancer medicine,* ed 3, Philadelphia, 1993, Lea & Febiger.

30. Howland WS: Preoperative evaluation of the cancer patient for emergency surgery. In Turnbull AD, editor: *Surgical emergencies in the cancer patient,* Chicago, 1987, Mosby.

31. Howland WS, Groeger JS, editors: *Critical care of the cancer patient,* ed 2, St Louis, 1991, Mosby.

32. Landreneau RJ and others: The potential role of video-assisted thoracic surgery in the patient with lung cancer. In Pass HI and others, editors: *Lung cancer: principles and practice,* Philadelphia, 1996, Lippincott-Raven.

33. LaRocca JC, Otto SE: *Pocket guide to intravenous therapy,* ed 3, St Louis, 1997, Mosby.

34. Larson DA, Flickinger JC, Loeffler JS: Stereotactic radiosurgery: techniques and results, *PPO Updates* 7(4):1, 1993.

35. Lehr P: Surgical lasers: how they work, current applications, *AORN J* 50(5):972, 1989.

36. Lewis SM, Collier IC, Heitkemper MM, editors: *Medical-surgical nursing: assessment and management of clinical problems,* ed 4, St Louis, 1996, Mosby.

37. Lindsey A, Piper B, Stotts N: The phenomenon of cancer cachexia: a review, *Oncol Nurs Forum* 9(2):38, 1982.

38. Mullen J: Consequences of malnutrition in the surgical patient, *Surg Clin North Am* 61(3):465, 1981.

39. Murphy GP, Lenhard RE, Lawrence W Jr, editors: *American Cancer Society textbook of clinical oncology,* ed 2, Atlanta, 1995, American Cancer Society.

40. Nicholson C and others: Are you ready for video thoracoscopy? *AJN* 93(3):54, 1993.

41. Office of Cancer Communications: *Coping with cancer: a resource for the health professional,* Bethesda, Md, 1982, US Department of Health and Human Services.

42. Pack R, Lynds BG: Surgical intervention. In McIntire SN, Cioppa AL, editors: *Cancer nursing: a developmental approach,* New York, 1984, Wiley & Sons.

43. Pass HI and others, editors: *Lung cancer: principles and practice,* Philadelphia, 1996, Lippincott-Raven.

44. Patterson WB: Surgical issues in geriatric oncology, *Semin Oncol* 16:57, 1989.

45. Polomano R and others: Surgical critical care for cancer patients, *Semin Oncol Nurs* 10(3):165, 1994.

46. Schwartz SI and others, editors: *Principles of surgery,* ed 6, New York, 1994, McGraw-Hill.

47. Shamberger R: Effect of chemotherapy and radiotherapy on wound healing: experimental studies, *Recent Results Cancer Res* 98:17, 1985.

48. Sherman CD: Principles of surgical oncology. In Kahn SB and others, editors: *Concepts in cancer medicine,* New York, 1983, Grune & Stratton.

49. Shiplacoff TA: Concepts in surgical oncology. In Vredevoe D, Derdiarian A, Sarna L, editors: *Concepts of oncology nursing,* Englewood Cliffs, NJ, 1981, Prentice Hall.

50. Silberman AW: Surgical debulking of tumors, *Surg Gynecol Obstet* 155(3):577, 1982.

51. Sliney DH, Trokel SL: Medical lasers and their safe use, New York, 1993, Springer-Verlag.

52. Smith RW, Sampson MK, Lucas CE: Effects of vinblastine, etoposide, cisplatin and bleomycin in rodent wound healing, *Surg Gynecol Obstet* 161(4):323, 1985.

53. Snyder CC: *Oncology nursing,* Boston, 1986, Little, Brown.

54. Summers JL, Bollard GA: Visual laser-assisted prostatectomy, *J Urol Nurs* 13(4):861, 1994.

55. Szopa TJ: Implications of surgical treatment for nursing. In Clark JC, McGee RF, editors: *Core curriculum for oncology nursing,* ed 2, Philadelphia, 1992, Saunders.

56. Tenenbaum L, editor: *Cancer chemotherapy and biotherapy: a reference guide,* ed 2, Philadelphia, 1994, Saunders.

57. Thompson JM and others: *Mosby's clinical nursing,* ed 3, St Louis, 1993, Mosby.

58. Tootla J, Easterling A: PDT: destroying malignant cells with laser beams—photodynamic therapy, *Nurs* 19(11):48, 1989.

59. Willard MP, Gilsdorf RB, Price RA: Protein-calorie malnutrition in a community hospital, *JAMA* 243:1720, 1980.

60. Wong RJ, DeCosse JJ: Cytoreductive surgery, *Surg Gynecol Obstet* 170(3):276, 1990.

61. Yasko J: *Care of the client receiving external radiation,* Reston, Va, 1982, Reston.

CHAPTER 21
Radiation Therapy

RYAN IWAMOTO

Radiation therapy is a localized treatment that is used alone or in conjunction with other treatments such as surgery or chemotherapy, or both. In certain situations, combining radiation therapy with other therapies maximizes cure rates because of the effect of the other therapies on radioresistant cells.[45] Radiation therapy may be administered before surgery to treat undisturbed tissues and to reduce the tumor's size to make resection feasible. Radiation therapy may also be delivered after surgery to treat cancer cells that may have been disseminated beyond the surgical margins or that may have remained in the tumor bed. In other instances, radiation is used before and after surgical resection. Chemotherapy may be combined with radiation therapy to control subclinical disease and enhance the local effect of radiation.

Radiation therapy is used for several purposes[11]: to cure by eradicating disease, allowing the person to live a normal life span; to control the growth and spread of the disease, allowing the person to live for a time without symptoms; to prevent microscopic disease, as with cranial irradiation for certain types of lung cancers; and to improve a person's quality of life by relieving or diminishing symptoms associated with advanced cancer. These symptoms include pain from bone metastasis; uncontrolled bleeding from the tumor; tumor obstruction around major blood vessels, gastrointestinal tract, kidneys, ureters, and trachea; spinal cord compression; and symptoms related to brain metastasis.[11] The box, p. 504, summarizes the uses of radiation therapy.

DEFINITION

Radiation therapy is the use of high-energy ionizing rays or particles to treat cancer. Approximately 60% of all persons with cancer will be treated with radiation therapy at some point during their illness.

HISTORICAL PERSPECTIVE

Since the late nineteenth century when radium, radioactivity, and x-rays were discovered, radiation has been used to treat cancer. Radiation was one of the earliest ways cancer was treated. The first successful radiation treatment for cancer was reported in 1898. At that time, large doses were delivered in a single treatment, which resulted in many complications. Between 1920 and 1940, studies were conducted to evaluate the effects of radiation on tissues, and fractionation of the dose (dividing the total dose into several small increments) was started.

With the invention of the vacuum tube, treatment with higher energies to deeper tissues was possible. In 1952 the first patient was treated with cobalt. Linear accelerators were developed in the mid-1950s and provided treatment rays with deeper penetration and less scatter to normal tissues. Over the past 100 years, the specialty of radiation oncology has advanced with the use of computer technology, the refinement of treatment machines, and advancements in radiobiologic science.

PRINCIPLES OF RADIATION THERAPY

High-energy ionizing radiation destroys the cancer cell's ability to grow and multiply. Some cells are directly damaged by the ionizing rays or particles. However, more cells are indirectly affected when the ionizing rays or particles penetrate the cell's nucleus and interact with the water content of the nucleus to form oxygen radicals. These unstable radicals then cause damage to the cell's deoxyribonucleic acid (DNA), with breakage of one or both chromosomal strands. Immediate cell death may occur if the chromosomal damage is irreparable. Some cells survive in spite of the chromosomal damage. However, these cells are unable to divide and die at the time of mitosis. As a result of radiation, some cells become giant cells, which continue to function but are unable to divide. These cells gradually degenerate and die.

The radiosensitivity of cancer cells depends on several factors:
- Type of cell (see Table 21-1)
- Phase of cell life—cells in the resting stage are less sensitive to radiation than those in active cellular division

USES OF RADIATION THERAPY

RADIOCURABLE CANCERS

Skin

Hodgkin's disease—early stages

Breast—early stage after lumpectomy

Seminoma

Uterine cervix—stage II

Larynx—disease confined to vocal cords; with or without surgery

Prostate

Bladder

Anal canal

ADJUVENT THERAPY

Bladder—preoperative radiation therapy

Breast—later stages; chest wall recurrence

Head and neck

Brain

Lung

Esophagus

Rectum

Soft tissue sarcoma

PROPHYLACTIC THERAPY

Whole brain for lung cancer

PALLIATIVE THERAPY

Pain from bone metastasis

Bleeding—uncontrolled from tumor

Pressure—superior vena cava syndrome, spinal cord compression, brain metastasis

Table 21-1 Radiosensitivity of Various Tumors and Tissues

Tumors	Relative radiosensitivity
Lymphoma, leukemia, seminoma, dysgerminoma	High
Squamous cell cancer of the oropharyngeal, glottis, bladder, skin, and cervical epithelia; adenocarcinomas of the alimentary tract	Fairly high
Vascular and connective tissue elements of all tumors, secondary neurovascularization, and astrocytomas	Medium
Salivary gland tumors, hepatomas, renal cancer, pancreatic cancer, chondrosarcoma, and osteogenic sarcoma	Fairly low
Rhabdomyosarcoma, leiomyosarcoma, and ganglioneurofibrosarcoma	Low

From Rubin P: Principles of radiation oncology and cancer radiotherapy. In Rubin P, editor: *Clinical oncology for medical students and physicians,* New York, 1983, American Cancer Society.

- Division rate of the cell—rapidly dividing cells are more sensitive to radiation than slowly dividing cells because more cells will be in the active cellular division stage
- Degree of differentiation—poorly differentiated cells are more sensitive to radiation therapy than well-differentiated cells
- Oxygenation—well-oxygenated tissues are more sensitive to radiation therapy because oxygen is needed to form the chemically active substances

Normal cells are also affected by the ionizing radiation. The sum total of the effects on each cell in the tissue accounts for the side effects of radiation therapy. However, normal cells are generally better able to repair the chromosomal damage done by the radiation. The treatments are delivered to kill as many cancer cells as possible while minimizing the damage to normal cells. Body tissues have limits to the amount of radiation that can be tolerated. Exceeding those limits can result in serious complications[5] (Table 21-2).

Radiation dose is recorded as the absorbed energy per unit mass.[45] The Systeme Internationale Unit for radiation dosage, the Gray, has replaced the rad (radiation absorbed dose). One Gray (Gy) equals 100 rad; 1 cGy equals 1 rad.

ADMINISTRATION OF RADIATION THERAPY

Radiation therapy can be delivered in many ways. External-beam radiation (teletherapy) uses a treatment machine placed at some distance from the body. Radiation can also be delivered by implanting a sealed radioactive source in or near the cancerous area to provide a localized treatment; this is called *brachytherapy*. The radioactive source may be placed in the body temporarily or permanently, depending on the situation. For brachytherapy patients receiving a temporary implant, isolation in a hospital room may be required while the implant is in place.

In other circumstances radioactive materials are injected intravenously or taken orally for a systemic effect (nonsealed sources). The radioactive substance travels to areas of the body requiring treatment. Thyroid cancer is frequently treated with radioactive iodine in this manner.

Coupling tumor-specific antibodies with radioactive isotopes combines the science of immunology with radiation therapy to maximize tumor treatment while minimizing normal tissue toxicity.[13,93] These antibodies are designed to be attracted to specific antigens on certain tumor cells while sparing normal tissues. They are pro-

Table 21-2 Minimal and Maximal Tolerance Dose of Various Organs

Organ	Injury	Minimal tolerance dose TD$_{5/5}$* (cGy)	Maximal tolerance dose TD$_{50/5}$† (cGy)	Whole or partial organ (field size or length)
Bone marrow	Aplasia, pancytopenia	250	450	Whole
		3000	4000	Segmental
Liver	Acute and chronic hepatitis	2500	4000	Whole
		1500	2000	Whole (strip)
Stomach	Perforation, ulcer, hemorrhage	4500	5500	100 cm
Intestine	Ulcer, perforation, hemorrhage	4500	5500	400 cm
		5000	6500	100 cm
Brain	Infarction, necrosis	5000	6000	Whole
Spinal cord	Infarction, necrosis	4500	5500	10 cm
Heart	Pericarditis, pancarditis	4500	5500	60%
		7000	8000	25%
Lung	Acute and chronic pneumonitis	3000	3500	100 cm
		1500	2500	Whole
Kidney	Acute and chronic nephrosclerosis	1500	2000	Whole (strip)
		2000	2500	Whole
Fetus	Death	200	400	Whole

From Rubin P, Cooper R, Phillips TL, editors: Radiation biology and radiation pathology syllabus. I. Radiation oncology, Chicago, 1975, American College of Radiology.

*TD$_{5/5}$, minimal tolerance dose; the dose that, when given to a population of patients under a standard set of treatment conditions, results in a 5% rate of severe complications within 5 years of treatment.

†TD$_{50/5}$, maximal tolerance dose; the dose that, when given to a population of patients under a standard set of treatment conditions, results in a 50% rate of severe complications within 5 years of treatment.

duced in animals and injected intravenously into the patient. When the radiolabeled antibodies are administered in the bloodstream, they seek out the tumor and the radioactivity attached to the antibody directly treats the cancer cells. Few acute side effects are associated with antibody administration. Allergic reactions may be noted during or soon after injection of the antibodies. Bone marrow suppression, particularly thrombocytopenia, may be noted 4 to 6 weeks after antibody administration.[13]

EXTERNAL RADIATION THERAPY
Treatment Planning

Before radiation treatments can begin, a plan is developed to determine the best way to deliver the treatments. A major part of the planning process is the localization procedure, which uses a simulator (Figure 21-1). A *simulator* is a machine that simulates the treatment machine in its movement and positioning. Depending on the area being treated, a variety of radiographic studies, such as computed tomography (CT) scans, magnetic resonance imaging (MRI) studies, barium enemas, and intravenous pyelograms help define the exact area within the body that needs treatment (Figure 21-2). Marks or small tattoos placed on the body are used to position the patient for treatment. These marks ensure that treatment delivery will be consistent. Special plastic or plaster forms or molds may be constructed to help support and assist the patient to maintain a precise position during each treat-

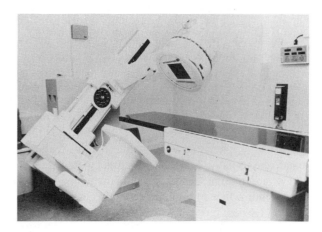

Figure 21-1 The simulator, which simulates the movement and positioning of the treatment machine, is used during the localization procedure. (Courtesy Virginia Mason Medical Center, Seattle, Wash.)

ment (Figure 21-3). The area of treatment is shaped with special shielding devices called blocks. These blocks, which are made of lead or high-density alloys, help minimize radiation exposure to normal tissues near the treatment area. A compensating filter may be used to differentially absorb the radiation beam to provide a uniform dose to the treatment volume. The treatment planning session usually lasts 1 to 2 hours.

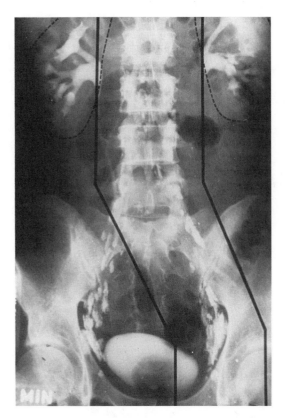

Figure 21-2   Simulation film. The radiation oncologist determines the treatment area using radiographic studies. The treatment area for this patient is the paraaortic and left inguinal lymph nodes. (Courtesy Virginia Mason Medical Center, Seattle, Wash.)

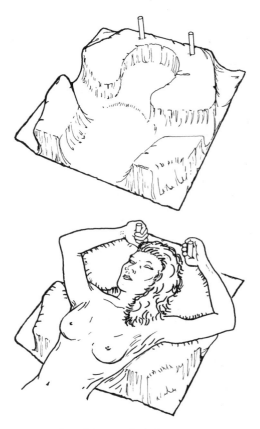

Figure 21-3   The Alpha-cradle helps a woman maintain the correct position for radiation therapy to the breast. Because the cradle is individually sized, the woman is able to conform to the exact position necessary for treatment.

Advances in the planning of radiation therapy include the use of CT scans and MRI studies to three-dimensionally recreate the treatment volume. With these specialized scans, the dose to the tumor volume can be more accurately calculated so as to maximize the dose to the tumor while minimizing the dose to normal surrounding tissues.[89]

Treatment Delivery

External radiation treatments are administered daily, Monday through Friday, for 2 to 8 weeks. Palliative treatments, such as for pain from bone metastasis, may be delivered at higher daily doses for fewer numbers of treatment. The actual treatment takes 2 to 5 minutes. More time is spent carefully positioning the patient on the treatment table.

A variety of machines are used in radiation therapy, depending on the type and extent of the tumor. These machines vary according to the energy produced and the ionizing particles delivered (Table 21-3). Linear accelerators are commonly used in cancer therapy (Figure 21-4). The higher the energy produced by the machine, the greater the depth of penetration of the radiation beam.

With higher energies, the maximum effect of the radiation occurs below the skin's surface and the dose to the skin is minimized; thus the term "skin-sparing effect." There is also less radiation scatter with higher energies (Figure 21-5).

The number of treatments delivered during a course of radiation therapy depends on the type and extent of cancer, the area treated, and the dose. Because a single large dose of radiation is too toxic for normal tissues, the total radiation dose is divided into small daily doses or fractions to be given over time. This process is called *fractionation*. The dose is usually the same each day. With fractionation of the total dose, more radiation can be delivered to the tumor while damage to normal tissues is minimized, because fractionation allows normal cells to repair the sublethal damage after each treatment.[45] Fractionation also increases damage to the tumor because of reassortment of cells into radiosensitive phases of the cell cycle and an increased oxygenation in the tumor.[38] Large tumors usually contain cells that are far from a capillary network and as a result are hypoxic. As the tumor shrinks over time, oxygenation increases within the tumor as more cells have access to the capil-

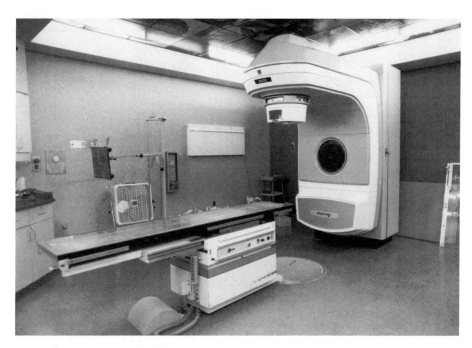

Figure 21-4 The linear accelerator delivers supervoltage treatment. (From Belcher AE: *Cancer nursing,* St Louis, 1992, Mosby.)

Table 21-3 Treatment Machines

Machine	Treatment beam	
KILOVOLTAGE		
Mechanical	X-rays	Low-level energy; superficial treatment; scatter of radiation beam; intracavitary therapy
MEGAVOLTAGE		
Cobalt 60 radioactive source is in head of machine; replaced every 5 to 10 years because of decay of the isotope	γ-rays (1-4 MeV)	Deeper penetration than kilovoltage; below skin level; less scatter
SUPERVOLTAGE		
Linear accelerators	X-rays and electrons (4-35 MeV)	Less scatter; deep tumors
Betatron	Electrons	More DNA double-strand injury; less oxygen
Cyclotron	Protons, neutrons, or electrons	dependent; less cell cycle specific

MeV, million electron volts; the energy of an electron accelerated across 1 million volts.

lary blood flow. As a result, the radiation's effectiveness is improved.

Some treatment schemes deliver treatments two to three times a day with at least 5 to 6 hours between each fraction. This is called *hyperfractionation.* Hyperfractionation may improve the treatment of large tumors, tumors with excessive bleeding, and brain tumors.[93] The increased fractionation theoretically affects more mitotically active cells each day.

The administration of radiation therapy depends on the reproducibility of the treatment setup. For most adults, teenagers and older children, this is easily accomplished. However, when working with young children and infants, special techniques are used to stabilize and sedate the patient to allow successful delivery of radiation therapy. "Body casts" can be created to immobilize the body or body part. However, these devices can cause even greater anxiety in a young child. Table 21-4 lists the medications commonly used for sedating young children for radiation therapy.[12,68] Chapter 18 further discusses issues in pediatric oncology nursing.

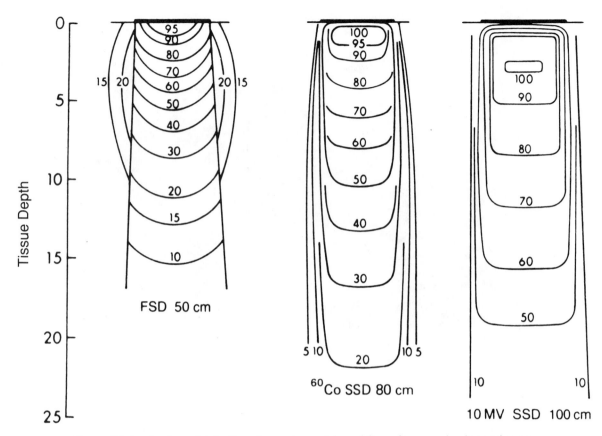

Figure 21-5   Isodose distributions (percentage of dose delivered) comparing increasing energies: kilovoltage (250 kVp), megavoltage (cobalt), and supervoltage (10 mV). *FSD* is the focal skin distance, or the distance from the focal spot in the x-ray tube to the patient's skin. *SSD* is the source-surface distance, or the distance from the front surface of the radiation source to the surface of the patient. As energy increases, the superficial tissues are spared, with the maximal radiation dose being delivered below the skin's surface; this results in fewer skin reactions and less side scatter. (From Keller BE, Rubin P: Basic concepts of radiation physics. In Rubin P, editor: *Clinical oncology for medical students and physicians,* New York, 1983, American Cancer Society.)

INNOVATIONS IN RADIATION THERAPY
Total Body Irradiation

Leukemic cells are radiosensitive. In conjunction with bone marrow transplantation, supralethal radiation in the form of total body irradiation and chemotherapy are administered to reduce the tumor volume and provide immunosuppression to prevent the rejection of the marrow graft.[32] A variety of techniques provide a homogeneous dose of radiation to the entire body (Figure 21-6). Doses range from 8 to 14 Gy, depending on fractionation. Acute side effects include nausea and vomiting, parotitis, anorexia, diarrhea, and fatigue.[29] Effects such as stomatitis, pancytopenia, and interstitial pneumonitis occur during the weeks following total body irradiation. Delayed effects of total body irradiation include gonadal insufficiency and cataracts.[4]

Half-Body Irradiation

When patients have numerous painful areas from bone metastasis located in the upper or lower half of the body, half-body irradiation may be used to provide expedient pain relief. This procedure delivers a single treatment to the upper or lower half of the body and frequently results in dramatic pain relief.[93] When the upper body is treated, premedication with antiemetics is necessary. Hypotension, fever, and chills can occur and may require brief hospitalization after the treatment. With midbody irradiation, bone marrow depression and diarrhea as well as nausea and vomiting can occur. Lower body irradiation can result in bone marrow depression and diarrhea.

Hyperthermia

The use of heat, or *hyperthermia,* with radiation therapy has shown some promise in the treatment of locally ad-

Table 21-4 Medications Commonly Used for Sedation during Radiation Therapy

Drug	Action	Dose range	Route	Comments
Chloral hydrate	Sedative	50-100 mg/kg	Oral, rectal	Contraindicated with marked liver or kidney impairment May cause gastric irritation Bitter taste with oral preparation Minimal effect upon respiration No amnesic effect Maximum 2 g Especially useful with small infants Inexpensive
Pentobarbital	Sedative, hypnotic	2-6 mg/kg	Oral, rectal, IV	May cause cardiovascular depression and hypotension IM route not used because of local irritation IV administered as slow drip Not recommended for small infants
Fentanyl	Analgesic, amnesic	0.5 μg/kg every 2-3 minutes Max: 2 μg/kg	IM, IV	Rapid onset of action Short acting Administered as slow IV push May cause respiratory depression
Fentanyl	Analgesic, amnesic	1-2 μg/kg	IM, IV	Administered in combination with other drugs Respiratory effects may outlast amnesia
Midazolam	Sedative, tranquilizer	0.01 mg/kg every 3-5 minutes Max: 0.1 mg/kg	IM, IV	Severe, life-threatening cardiorespiratory effects can occur Partially reversible with naloxone
Meperidine	Analgesic	2 mg/kg	IM, oral, rectal	Hypotension, respiratory depression and excessive sedation can occur
Promethazine	Sedative	1 mg/kg	IM	No amnesic effect Administered as deep IM injection in single syringe
Chlorpromazine	Sedative	1 mg/kg	IM	May titrate doses maintaining 2:1:1 ratio Maximum doses: meperidine, 50 mg; promethazine, 25 mg; chlorpromazine, 25 mg
Droperidol	Tranquilizer, sedative	0.12 mg/kg	IM, IV	Hypotension, orthostatic hypotension Fluids and measures to manage hypotension should be readily available Safe use in children under 2 years of age not established

From Bucholtz JD: *Oncol Nurs Forum* 19:649, 1992.
IM, Intramuscular; *IV,* intravenous.

vanced solid tumors.[27,70,71,84] Heat is cytotoxic by affecting the cell membranes and causing damage of lysosomal vesicles within the cell, which in turn release digestive enzymes that cause cell death. Hyperthermia enhances the effects of radiation therapy on certain radioresistant and hypoxic tumor cells, because heat affects more S-phase (synthesis) cells and poorly vascularized tumors are less able to dissipate the heat. The heat may also help to make permanent the radiation-induced chromosomal damage within the tumor cells, rendering them unable to repair the damage.

Hyperthermia is usually applied immediately after a radiation treatment. The number of treatments depends on the tumor site and its extent. Approximately 72 hours between treatments provide maximum benefits from hyperthermia.[70]

Hyperthermia is applied locally or regionally. Local hyperthermia may be accomplished with microwaves, ultrasound, deep heating with electromagnetic wave applicators, and interstitial hyperthermia with probes implanted in or near the tumor. Regional hyperthermia involves perfusing heated solutions through a part of the

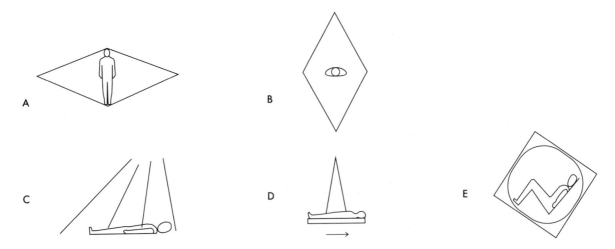

Figure 21-6   Methods of delivering total body irradiation. **A**, Lateral opposed beams. **B**, Floor and ceiling parallel opposed beams. **C**, Supine and prone technique using three matching fields. **D**, Supine and prone technique: patient moves horizontally through treatment beam field. **E**, Horizontal shrinking field technique: patient is in sitting position. (From Quast U: *Radiother Oncol* 9:95, 1987; and Novack DH, Kiley JP: *Front Radiat Ther Oncol* 21:69, 1987.)

body. The optimal therapeutic temperature is 105° to 113° F (41° to 45°C) for approximately 45 minutes.[70] Interstitial temperature probes are usually inserted within the body part as well as placed superficially to monitor the heat. Close monitoring of the heat is required to obtain optimal heating with minimal discomfort and side effects. Side effects associated with hyperthermia include local discomfort and skin reactions ranging from transient erythema to edema and blisters. Hyperthermia enhances the skin reactions associated with radiation therapy.[93] Careful assessments for signs of infections are necessary. Hyperthermia with ultrasound has occasionally been associated with substantial pain, requiring the procedure to be stopped.[90]

Hyperthermia is also being used with interstitial brachytherapy to treat tumors of the head and neck, breast, prostate, and rectum.[8] After catheters are placed within the tissues, hyperthermia is applied for approximately 1 hour. The catheters are then immediately loaded with the radioactive sources for a prescribed length of time. A second 1-hour treatment with hyperthermia is administered after the radioactive sources have been removed.

The use of hyperthermia can compound the patient's anxiety about radiation therapy. The fears of "being heated" and "being burned" are frightening perceptions that nurses can help patients confront and understand.

Intraoperative Radiation Therapy

Intraoperative radiation therapy (IORT) provides direct visualization and treatment of tumors to control local recurrence of cancer.[2,34] After surgical exposure, a targeting cone is placed directly on the tumor site. This cone

helps to displace normal tissues and thus minimize toxicities.[14] The treatment machine is carefully aligned with the cone. All persons leave the treatment room for the 15 to 25 minutes it takes to deliver the fairly large dose of electron irradiation (approximately 2000 cGy). Anesthesia personnel monitor the patient through a closed-circuit television.

Newer techniques using high-dose-rate (HDR) remote afterloading equipment to deliver intraoperative radiation are being explored.[39,40] A dedicated and shielded surgical suite with HDR remote afterloading equipment is used to perform the surgery and to deliver the HDR brachytherapy. This setup improves the convenience of providing IORT by avoiding the need to transport the patient from the surgical suite to the radiation therapy department, thus saving time, energy, and expense.

Intraoperative radiation is used to treat locally advanced abdominal cancers such as gastric, pancreatic, colorectal, bladder, cervical, and retroperitoneal sarcomas. Complications and side effects, no greater than with radiation therapy or surgery, may include nausea, vomiting, and anorexia.[34,37] No increased risk for poor wound healing or postoperative infection has been reported, and severe complications, such as neuropathy, have been few.[17] Coordination between departments and disciplines is required to provide this complex therapy.[2,3,14,37]

Radiosensitizers

Chemical radiosensitizing compounds are used to increase the lethal effects of radiation therapy in the treatment of gastrointestinal and bladder cancers.[23,38,75] Nonhypoxic sensitizers such as iododeoxyuridine (IUdR) incorporate into the DNA and increase the susceptibility of the cell to radiation damage. Hypoxic cell sensitizers (e.g., metronidazole, misonidazole, SR2508, Ro-03-8799) increase oxygen to hypoxic cells and promote damage of the DNA, preventing cell repair. Depending on the agent, side effects include peripheral neuropathy, nausea and vomiting, and skin rashes. Certain chemotherapeutic agents, such as cyclophosphamide or cisplatin, are also being used as radiosensitizers and are given in conjunction with radiation therapy.

Stereotactic External-Beam Irradiation

Stereotactic external-beam irradiation involves high-dose treatment of relatively small intracranial volumes with a three-dimensional distribution of the treatment beam.[60] This technique minimizes the radiation dose to normal tissues. Benign conditions, such as arteriovenous malformations, and malignancies, such as astrocytomas and brain metastases, are treated with stereotactic external-beam irradiation. Various machines are used, such as gamma units using cobalt ("gamma knife") and modified cobalt or linear accelerator units. To perform this treatment, a stereotactic frame is fixed to the patient's skull and used to target the treatment beam. The treatment dose may be fractionated or given in a single fraction. Steroid medications are used to minimize cerebral edema.

Strontium 89

Strontium 89, a radiopharmaceutical, has proved effective in treating pain from multiple osteoblastic bony metastases from prostate or breast cancer.[77] Pain relief from strontium 89 may be noted within 1 to 2 weeks, or this relief may be delayed for up to 5 weeks. The pain relief may last for several months. Repeated doses of strontium 89 may be given at the physician's discretion approximately every 3 months. However, toxicities increase. Strontium 89 may be used in conjunction with external-beam radiation therapy.[73]

Four millicuries of Strontium 89 are delivered intravenously to the patient in the outpatient setting. The strontium seeks out areas of bone metastases and provides radiation to the bony metastatic site. After administration of strontium 89, assessment of pain and the use of analgesics is important. Consistently using a pain analog scale (e.g., asking the patient to rate the level of pain from 1 to 10) and reviewing the record of pharmacologic and nonpharmacologic methods of pain relief, the nurse monitors the efficacy of strontium 89 and teaches the patient and family ways to improve pain control.

Side effects of strontium 89 include a temporary "flare" reaction of pain, which occurs approximately 3 to 5 days after administration of the radionuclide and lasts approximately 5 days, and mild myelosuppression. Because strontium 89 is a beta-particle emitter and very

---

STRONTIUM 89: PATIENT AND FAMILY PRECAUTIONS

1. Flush toilet twice after use.
2. Wipe up spilled urine with a paper tissue and discard in the toilet before flushing.
3. Wash hands after using the toilet.
4. Immediately wash linen and clothes that become soiled with urine or blood. Wash these items separately from other laundry.
5. If an injury occurs and blood is spilled, wash away any spilled blood with water and a paper tissue and flush the paper tissue in the toilet.

---

little radiation is distributed outside of bone, the patient does not pose a risk of radiation exposure to others and contact with others is not limited. However, because strontium 89 is administered systemically, radioactive precautions for body fluids are necessary for approximately 7 days after administration. Patients and families must be taught these precautions (see box above).

Patients should be advised that a flare reaction of pain may occur. They are instructed to continue taking prescribed analgesics and even increase the dose of medications as necessary during the time of the flare reaction. After administration of strontium 89, complete blood counts are monitored every 2 to 3 weeks for approximately 8 to 12 weeks.

PHOTODYNAMIC THERAPY

Photodynamic therapy (PDT) involves the use of light-sensitive molecules, or photosensitizers, which are activated by light to form oxygen radicals, which in turn affect cell membranes, the cytoplasm, and the DNA, resulting in cell damage and death.[62] Porfimer sodium is the most studied photosensitizer. Patients are hospitalized and given porfimer sodium. Approximately 48 hours after administration of the photosensitizer, light treatment with the appropriate wavelength is given. It takes approximately 48 hours for the tumor to reach the optimal concentration of porfimer sodium. Cutaneous photosensitivity can occur and can last for 6 weeks. Photodynamic therapy is used in clinical trials; in the treatment of superficial bladder, skin, lung, and esophageal cancers; and for bone marrow purging for the treatment of leukemias and lymphomas.

INTERNAL RADIATION THERAPY
Brachytherapy

Radioactive implants deliver relatively large amounts of radiation to a specific site over a short time.[41] Tumors

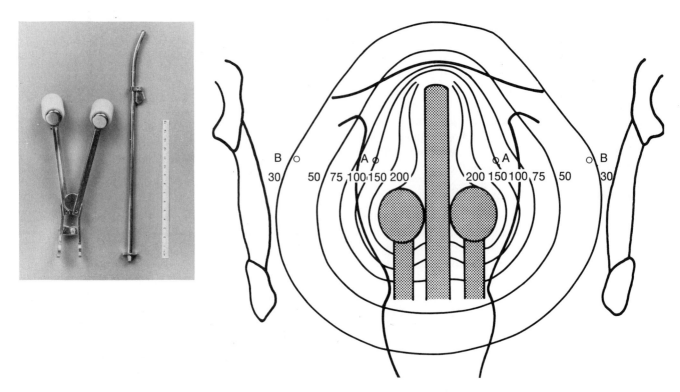

Figure 21-7   The Fletcher-Suit applicator is one of many kinds of applicators used to deliver intracavitary irradiation for carcinomas of the cervix and endometrium. The long central tandem is placed in the uterine cavity. (To the right is a section of tubing used to hold the radioactive sources and place them in the hollow tandem.) The movable sleeve on the tandem marks the cervical os, permitting localization of the os on x-ray film as a reference point for computerized dosimetry. The colpostats are placed in the lateral fornices. The entire apparatus is held in place with vaginal packing. After the applicator is in place, x-ray films are taken to confirm the accuracy of placement. Computerized dosimetry is then done to determine the best loading pattern and the time required for treatment. Finally, the radium or cesium sources are put into place. (Photograph courtesy Virginia Mason Medical Center, Seattle, Wash.; drawing from DiSaia P, Creasman W: *Clinical gynecological oncology*, ed 4, St Louis, 1993, Mosby.)

may be treated with an implant alone, but more commonly, an implant is done after a course of radiation therapy to provide a boost of radiation to the tumor.[93] Cancers of the brain, tongue, lips, esophagus, lung, breast, vagina, cervix, endometrium, rectum, prostate, and bladder may be treated with brachytherapy. Implants are usually placed temporarily within the body cavity or structure with specifically designed applicators (Figure 21-7). Because the radioactive material, ribbons, wires, seeds, capsules, needles, or tubes are encapsulated (sealed), body fluids are not contaminated. The radioactive isotopes are usually placed in the body with an afterloading technique of placing the applicators (needles, plastic or metal tubes) in the body in the operating room or under fluoroscopy. The applicators are sutured in or near the tumor. After the patient returns to the hospital room, the radioactive isotopes are placed within the applicators. With this procedure, exposure of staff members to radiation is minimized. The implant remains in the body for the prescribed length of time.

Intracavitary placement of implants within the vagina or uterus is performed using general or spinal anesthesia.[41] The vagina is packed with gauze to stabilize the applicator and separate the bladder and rectum from the radioactive source. Patients usually have a bowel cleansing before the applicator placement and are placed on a low-residue diet and diphenoxylate atropine to prevent a bowel movement while the implant is in place. Postoperative pain is managed with oral or parenteral medications.

With cervical and vaginal implants, the patient may experience fatigue and dysuria after implantation. Women may resume sexual intercourse within 2 to 3 weeks after implantation.[41] Since a decrease in normal vaginal secretions may occur, use of a water-based lubricant is recommended. Vaginal stenosis can also oc-

Text continued on p. 521.

NURSING MANAGEMENT

Understanding the principles of radiobiology is the key to understanding symptom management. The side effects associated with radiation therapy are localized and depend on the area treated, volume of tissue irradiated, fractionation, total dose, type of radiation, and individual differences. Variations of side effects will be observed among people receiving similar courses of treatment. A delay between the time of radiation exposure and the time the effects are seen can vary from days to weeks to months, depending on the cell's metabolic activity. Early reactions occur during or within weeks after treatment. Some symptoms do not subside until 2 or more weeks after treatment has ended. Delayed reactions occur months to years after therapy. Because radiation therapy has its greatest effect on rapidly dividing cells, the epithelial tissues, such as mucous membranes and the skin, are most susceptible to its effects. Selected nursing diagnoses related to radiation therapy include:

NURSING DIAGNOSES

- *Skin integrity, impaired, related to radiation therapy*
- *Infection, risk for, related to skin breakdown*
- *Activity intolerance related to radiation therapy*
- *Nutrition, altered: less than body requirements, related to anorexia*
- *Oral mucous membrane, altered, related to head and neck irradiation*
- *Sensory/perceptual alterations: gustatory, related to head and neck irradiation*
- *Swallowing, impaired, related to esophagitis*
- *Pain related to cough*
- *Nutrition, altered: less than body requirements, related to nausea and vomiting*
- *Diarrhea related to pelvic irradiation*
- *Urinary elimination, altered, related to pelvic irradiation*
- *Coping, ineffective individual, related to alopecia*
- *Self-esteem disturbance related to alopecia*
- *Anxiety about radiation therapy*
- *Knowledge deficit about radiation therapy and self-care measures*

OUTCOME GOALS

Patient and/or significant other will be able to:
- Maintain or restore skin integrity.
- Prevent skin breakdown and infection.
- Minimize fatigue and maintain activities of daily living.
- Maintain nutritional status and weight.
- Maintain integrity of oral mucous membranes.
- Control pain from pharyngitis/esophagitis and maintain nutritional intake.
- Minimize cough.
- Prevent or control nausea and vomiting and maintain nutritional status.
- Prevent or control diarrhea.
- Minimize cystitis.
- Successfully cope with alopecia.
- Control or minimize anxiety.
- Understand the use of radiation therapy for cancer and the self-care behaviors used to manage side effects of radiation therapy.

GENERAL SIDE EFFECTS
Skin

Certain skin reactions are normal and expected with radiation therapy.[43] The skin overlying the areas being treated may develop a reaction as soon as 2 weeks into the course of treatment.[22,47,48,86,92] Skin erythema may range from mild, light pink to deep and dusky.[47] Increased skin sensitivity and slight edema may also appear. As treatment continues, the skin reaction can progress, with the skin becoming slightly to moderately dry, itchy, and flaky (dry desquamation). In some cases the skin develops mild to severe moist desquamation, in which the epidermal layers of the skin slough, leaving a raw, painful area that may drain serous exudate.[22,43] Areas of moist desquamation generally heal within several weeks.[86]

Skin reactions vary but tend to be greater in those receiving large doses of radiation.[92] Also, treatments with electron beams usually produce more intense skin reactions because of the superficial concentration of the radiation dose. Some treatments involve the use of a bolus material placed on the skin to increase the skin dose. In addition, certain treatments are given from a tangential angle as opposed to perpendicular to the treatment site.[47,67,86] Certain areas of the skin, such as areas covering bony prominences or surgical wounds, tend to be more sensitive to the effects of radiation than others.[42] Areas having skin folds (e.g., the axillae, under the breasts, perineum, groin, gluteal folds) are also at increased risk for developing a skin reaction because of increased warmth and moisture and lack of aeration.[47,86] The skin on the face is particularly sensitive to the effects of radiation. Skin reactions may also occur where the radiations exit; that is, on the opposite side of the body from where the treatment is delivered. Evaluating the angle of the treatment beam will help determine where these reactions may occur. When chemotherapy is used in conjunction with radiation therapy, the patient is at higher risk of developing a skin reaction.[69]

Special consideration needs to be given to patients re-

Continued.

ceiving pelvic irradiation after low anterior or anterior-posterior resection for rectal cancer. The surgical wound site is at increased risk for skin breakdown because the perineum is generally within the treatment field. The radiation oncologist may have the buttocks taped apart during the actual radiation treatment to minimize the skin reaction.[42] If a stoma (e.g., colostomy, ileostomy) is included in the treatment field, the stoma appliance and skin barrier can act as a bolus material and enhance the skin reaction. Daily assessments of the skin are necessary, and removal of the skin barrier and appliance may be required during the actual treatment to minimize peristomal skin breakdown.[42]

Before beginning radiation therapy, instruct the patient to protect the skin and minimize sources of irritation and trauma. Nursing diagnoses related to skin care include *actual or risk for impaired skin integrity* and *risk for infection related to skin breakdown.* Assess the patient's usual skin care. Unintentional enhancement of skin reactions may occur if patients use products contraindicated during radiation therapy. These include compresses, ointments, and other remedies prescribed before diagnosis and treatment.[47] Plan to educate the patient and family about skin care during radiation therapy. Cleanse the skin with lukewarm water as needed, and pat rather than rub the skin with a towel to dry. Avoid using soaps. When soap is necessary, use only nondeodorant, unperfumed soaps. Powders, perfumes, and deodorants should not be applied to the irradiated skin, as they can dry and irritate the skin. Avoid the use of cornstarch in the axilla, groin, and gluteal folds.[48,87] Shaving with a razor blade within treatment areas should be avoided. An electric razor may be used if there is no skin irritation. Protect the treated skin from cold, heat, and sun. Only loose-fitting, cotton clothing should be worn close to the skin.[22,48] Tight, restrictive clothing, such as bras and belts, over the treated area may chafe the skin and should not be worn.[43] In addition, avoid placing adhesive tape over the irradiated skin, because this will further irritate the skin.

If the skin becomes dry, the patient may complain of tenderness and pruritus. A nonperfumed hydrophilic moisturizing lotion that contains no heavy metal ions may be applied to the skin on the recommendation of the radiation oncologist or radiation oncology nurse. Avoid having lotion on the skin during treatment, because the lotion may increase the skin reaction. Remove excess lotion with a soft washcloth before treatment. Although topical steroids can help reduce pruritus and tenderness because of vasoconstriction, they must be used with extreme caution. Steroid creams and ointments can cause thinning of the skin and delay skin healing.[42] Fluorinated preparations are not recommended because they cause more vasoconstriction and thinning of the skin.[42,47] Steroid preparations should not be used for moist skin reactions.[87]

For moist desquamation, normal saline irrigations or cool compresses may be applied to the affected area three to four times a day to soothe the skin. Cleansing with half-strength to third-strength hydrogen peroxide and saline followed by a rinse with saline may be used also.[11,43,92,100] Caution with use of ointments and salves is important to avoid increasing the skin reaction. A thin layer of A&D ointment, lanolin, or Aquaphor may be applied to the moist desquamation.[38,47,48] In some instances, treatment is stopped and zinc oxide or silver sulfadiazine cream is applied directly on the skin or onto a nonadherent dressing (Telfa pad or combine dressings), which is then applied to the moist reaction.[47] Hydrocolloid dressings have been found effective to heal dermatitis and moist desquamation.[64,78] These dressings may be left on the skin reaction for up to 5 days to provide comfort. No increase in infection rates has been reported. Assess for signs of infection, and culture suspicious lesions and drainage.[97] With painful skin reactions, systemic analgesics are sometimes necessary, especially at bedtime, to allow the patient to rest.

If moist desquamation occurs in the perineum, sitz baths, perineal compresses, and protective emollients may all be used.[42] A hand-held blow dryer may be used on the cool setting to dry the perineum. These reactions are painful, and treatment is frequently stopped for a time to allow the tissues to heal.

Once radiation therapy is completed, the skin usually heals within a few weeks. Although the acute tenderness and erythema diminish within 2 weeks, the patient may be left with a tanned skin within the treatment field, which will usually subside.[22] The irradiated skin may also remain more sensitive to heat or cold and develop a sunburn more readily than untreated parts of the body.[43,49,87] The patient should continue to protect the irradiated skin by avoiding direct sun exposure by using clothing such as scarves and hats. A sunblock with a high sun protection factor (SPF) should be used when sun exposure is unavoidable. Delayed effects to the skin from radiation include fibrosis and atrophy of the skin, telangiectasia, and lymphedema as a result of fibrosis of the lymph glands.[97] These delayed effects occur because of changes in the vascular component of the skin, which lead to tissue damage.[86] Recall phenomenon occurs months to years after a course of radiation therapy. In this phenomenon, skin, mucous membrane, or pulmonary reactions occur within the treated area when certain chemotherapeutic agents, such as dactinomycin and doxorubicin, are given systemically. These reactions, which may be more severe than the skin reactions seen during radiation therapy, subside within 2 weeks.[43] Evaluate the patient's and family's understanding of potential and actual skin reactions and appropriate care and protection of the skin. Table 21-5 summarizes guidelines for skin care.

Table 21-5 Nursing Care of Irradiated Skin

When treatment begins:	Assess skin integrity.
	Instruct patient to minimize trauma and protect skin within treatment field:
	Cleanse skin with lukewarm water as needed.
	Avoid use of soaps, powders, perfumes, and deodorants.
	Avoid shaving.
	Protect skin from cold, heat, and sun.
	Wear loose-fitting clothing over treatment site.
	Avoid adhesive tape on irradiated skin.
If dry desquamation occurs:	Use a hydrophilic moisturizing lotion two to three times a day (e.g., Aquaphor).
	Remove excess lotion from skin before daily treatment.
If moist desquamation occurs:	Saline irrigations or cool compresses may be used three to four times a day.
	Apply hydrocolloid dressing for comfort (e.g., DuoDerm).
	If treatment is withheld, zinc oxide or silver sulfadiazine may be applied to skin reaction and covered with a nonadherent dressing.
	Culture suspicious lesions and drainage.
	Use analgesics as necessary.
When treatment is completed and skin is healed:	Instruct patient to protect irradiated skin by avoiding exposure to sun, heat, or cold.
	Advise patient to use sunblock when sun exposure is unavoidable.

Fatigue

Fatigue, the subjective feeling of tiredness, is experienced by many people receiving radiation therapy.[44,56,72] The etiology of fatigue is not well understood.[100] Fatigue may result from tumor breakdown, which releases byproducts into the bloodstream. Another theory suggests an increased basal metabolic rate, which quickly uses the body's energy stores. Fatigue may occur after treatment each day and become chronic as treatment continues.[44,56,92] Variations, including less fatigue on Sundays because there is no treatment over the weekend, have been reported.[44] Fatigue is compounded by pain, depression, anorexia, infection, anemia, and dyspnea.[1] Although the level of fatigue varies among individuals, most people are able to continue their work and usual activities. Fatigue may persist weeks to months after completion of radiation therapy and disappear gradually.[56]

Nursing diagnoses of *actual or risk for activity intolerance* can be made for the person receiving radiation therapy. Assess for the presence and pattern of fatigue. Evaluate factors that increase or decrease fatigue. Monitor blood counts for anemia, which can compound fatigue.

Assist patients and families to understand that fatigue can occur with radiation therapy. Help patients evaluate their activities so they can pace themselves throughout the day and plan for rest periods or naps as needed. Determining the times of the day when extra energy is needed can help a person plan rest periods through the day and evening. Taking a nap immediately after returning home from treatment helps some have energy for the rest of the day.[48,49,100] Plan for assistance with transportation, purchase and preparation of food, child care, and other activities of daily living. Evaluate the need for assistive devices, such as a cane or walker. These measures can help minimize exertion with certain activities and reduce fatigue.[1,48,100] If the patient is experiencing pain, ensure adequate pain management with pharmacologic and nonpharmacologic measures. In addition, make sure the person is maintaining an adequate nutritional intake.[100] People with recent weight loss who are undergoing therapy will need additional nutritional supplementation. This supplementation will help the patient maintain or improve nutritional status and minimize fatigue. A dietitian is an excellent resource to help plan the patient's nutritional program. Evaluate the patient's and family's understanding of the causes of fatigue and their ability to modify activities to maintain or improve function. (See Chapter 26.)

Anorexia

Loss of appetite, or anorexia, sometimes is a result of cancer itself but also may be caused by cancer therapy. As with fatigue, the mechanisms that cause anorexia are unclear. Contributing factors include inactivity, medications, and inability to ingest and digest foods.[49] The patient has a loss of appetite, which can result in weight loss and progressive fatigue.

Assess the loss of appetite in patients receiving radiation therapy. The nursing diagnosis *altered nutrition: less than body requirements* is made for the person with anorexia. Discuss with the patient and family the fact that anorexia sometimes occurs in people undergoing radiation therapy, and suggest ways to overcome this problem. Assist the patient and family to plan ways to im-

Continued.

prove appetite to help the patient eat adequately and maintain body weight.

Frequent small meals rather than three large ones can help make eating less overwhelming and allow more food to be consumed throughout the day. Instruct the patient and family to have high-calorie, high-protein foods readily available at all times. Specially prepared nutritional supplements and carefully selected convenience foods can provide additional calories and protein. Because radiation treatments are given daily and considerable time is spent commuting to and from treatments, suggest that the patient carry snacks to consume during the commute. Some patients have found that having a meal at a restaurant each day is a special treat to look forward to. Consult a dietitian to determine the nutritional needs of the patient, and plan additional ways to meet those needs. Help the patient and family understand the importance of nutrition during therapy. Evaluate their ability to utilize suggestions to enhance appetite and maintain optimal nutrition (see Chapter 28).

Bone Marrow Suppression

When large volumes of active bone marrow are treated with radiation, a decrease in bone marrow function occurs.[100] These treatment areas include the pelvis, spine, sternum, ribs, metaphyses of long bones, and skull.[49] Blood counts must be monitored routinely. The fall in blood counts usually develops slowly. However, if chemotherapy is combined with radiation therapy, the blood counts can fall precipitously and must be closely followed. Table 21-6 presents guidelines for frequency of blood counts. Factors affecting the frequency of obtaining blood counts include the treatment site, use of other myelosuppressive therapies, the stage of disease, and the patient's age.

Assess for infections, bleeding, and fatigue. Plan and implement education for the patient and family about precautions for neutropenia, thrombocytopenia, and anemia.[21] Transfusions of blood products are sometimes used, and in some cases radiation therapy is withheld for a while to allow the blood counts to recover. Evaluate the patient's and family's understanding and use of self-care measures and precautions for bone marrow suppression (see Chapter 30).

SITE-SPECIFIC SIDE EFFECTS
Head and Neck

Radiation therapy is given to the head and neck regions for cancers of the mouth, tongue, and larynx. Some problems that develop are stomatitis, xerostomia, dental caries, taste changes, osteoradionecrosis, and hypopituitarism.[99]

Stomatitis

Stomatitis, or irritation of the mucosa in the mouth and oropharynx, can occur as the radiation affects the rapidly dividing cells of the oral mucosa. The patient may first note a tenderness in the mouth. This tenderness may be accompanied by mild to moderate erythema and edema of the mucosa. A whitish pseudomembrane may form on the surface of the mucosa; this membrane should be left undisturbed. Eventually this membrane pulls away from the underlying tissue, leaving a painful and friable ulcer.[6] Bleeding often results when stomatitis is severe. Superimposed bacterial, fungal, and/or viral infections can also occur. The mucosal reaction may be enhanced by metallic tooth restorations in adjacent areas, which cause electron back scatter of radiation. During treatments, a material with a low atomic number, such as a piece of gauze or an oral stent made of dental acrylic, sometimes is placed between the tooth and mucosa to minimize this reaction.[53,57]

Table 21-6   Guidelines for Frequency of Blood Counts—Joint Center for Radiation Therapy

Site	No prior chemotherapy	Previous chemotherapy <1 year	Previous chemotherapy >1 year	Concomitant chemotherapy
Breast	Baseline, 3 weeks later if taking tamoxifen	Weekly—every other week	Every 3 weeks	Biweekly—weekly
Head/neck	Every 3 weeks	Every other week	Every 3 weeks	Biweekly—weekly
Whole brain	Baseline only	Weekly	Every 3 weeks	Weekly
Hodgkin's	Weekly	Weekly	Weekly	Biweekly
Lung/esophagus*	Weekly—every other week	Weekly—every other week	Weekly	Biweekly—weekly
Spine†	Weekly—every other week	Weekly	Weekly	Biweekly—weekly
Pelvis* Prostate	Every other week	Every other week	Weekly—every other week	Weekly
Colon	Every other week	Weekly	Weekly	Biweekly—weekly
GYN	Every other week	Weekly	Weekly	Biweekly—weekly

From Hirshfield-Bartek J et al: *Oncol Nurs Forum* 15:547, 1988.
*Depends on field size, history of previous irradiation.
†Depends on the presence and extent of metastatic disease.

Mouth care is crucial for the person receiving radiation therapy for head and neck cancer. Tooth brushing and flossing, if tolerated, after meals and at bedtime will help remove debris from the teeth and gingiva. If tooth brushing becomes too painful, warm saline rinses and gentle swabbing with moistened gauze or a tooth sponge may be better tolerated. Instruct the patient and family in mouth care, including inspecting the oral cavity each day. Poorly fitting dental prostheses should not be worn until evaluated by a dentist; nor should the prosthesis be used when the mouth and gingiva become painful, because the prosthesis can cause more irritation and lead to mucosal breakdown. Oral pain is controlled with topical anesthetics or systemic analgesics. Viscous lidocaine, dyclonine hydrochloride, diphenhydramine, and Mylanta provide topical pain relief. Nonsteroidal antiinflammatory agents provide topical pain relief as well as antiinflammatory action.[82]

Instruct the patient to eat a soft, bland diet to make chewing and swallowing easier, allowing the patient to maintain nutritional intake. Topical thrombin can be applied to control minor areas of bleeding in the mouth and topical or systemic antibiotics are used to control oral infections.[74]

Xerostomia

Xerostomia, or dryness of the mouth, may occur 1 to 2 weeks into therapy. When the treatment field includes the salivary glands, the saliva changes from a thin fluid to a thick, sticky, acidic one that is unable to cleanse the mouth. As a result, debris adheres more readily to the teeth. The patient may note difficulty speaking, problems with retention of dentures, and difficulty eating certain foods such as crackers, breads, and peanut butter. With higher doses of radiation, xerostomia may remain a chronic problem.[25] Older patients are at higher risk for xerostomia because of normally decreased levels of oral secretions.

Instruct the patient to perform mouth care before meals to help relieve xerostomia. Assist the patient and family to assess food choices and preparation to appropriately modify the patient's diet. Sauces, gravies, and other liquids taken with meals can moisten dry and thick foods. Frequent sips of fluids and atomizer mists are helpful. Sucking on sugarless sour candies can help stimulate salivation. Commercially available saliva substitutes such as Moi-Stir, Oralbalance, and Mouth Kote provide temporary relief of xerostomia. Two to three milliliters of solution are placed in the mouth and swished to coat the mucosal surfaces. Products containing lemon or glycerin should be avoided, as these may cause further irritation and drying of the mucosa.[95,98] Lemon juice also decalcifies teeth.[98] Commercial mouthwashes should be avoided because many contain alcohol and/or flavoring agents that further irritate the mucosa. Patients may find a room humidifier used at bedtime helps decrease mucosal dryness and minimize the frequency with which they awaken to drink fluids.[58]

Tooth decay and caries

Tooth decay and caries become rampant as a result of xerostomia.[25] Cariogenic bacteria adhere to the teeth and flourish in the acidic environment. Before treatment, a dentist evaluates the patient and provides prophylaxis, including extraction of teeth with extensive decay. A daily program of fluoride application on debris-free teeth is important to prevent caries.[25,49,100] The fluoride is applied once or twice a day using specially constructed trays. These trays are filled with fluoride gel and placed over the teeth for approximately 5 to 10 minutes. The patient may expectorate the excess gel but should not rinse the mouth or drink fluids for at least 30 minutes. Because xerostomia often becomes a chronic problem, the use of fluoride must be continued even after radiation therapy is completed to prevent tooth decay.

NURSING DIAGNOSES: *Head and Neck Irradiation (Floor of Mouth): Pretreatment Phase*

- *Anxiety related to radiation therapy*
- *Knowledge deficit related to radiation therapy and self-care measures*

INTERVENTIONS: *Pretreatment Phase*

- Allow verbalization of fears, concerns, and questions.
- Provide education:
  —Use of radiation therapy for cancer of the floor of the mouth.
  —Potential side effects (stomatitis, taste changes, xerostomia, fatigue, and skin changes) and appropriate self-care measures.
- Consult dentist for evaluation and fluoride prophylaxis.
- Inspect mouth.

NURSING DIAGNOSES: *Treatment Phase*

- *Oral mucous membrane, altered, related to head and neck irradiation*
- *Sensory/perceptual alterations (gustatory) related to head and neck irradiation*
- *Skin integrity, impaired*
- *Activity intolerance*

INTERVENTIONS: *Treatment Phase*

- Inspect mouth daily: assess for stomatitis and infections.
- Review mouth care:
  —Brush and floss teeth if tolerated.
  —As stomatitis progresses, use moistened gauze instead of toothbrushing and flossing to clean teeth.
  —Rinse with normal saline at least four times a day.
- Provide soft, bland diet.

Continued.

- Maintain hydration.
- Use saliva substitute and moisten foods when xerostomia occurs.
- Offer topical anesthetics or analgesic medications before meals to relieve oral pain.
- Monitor weight.
- Instruct patient to perform mouth care before and after meals.
- Experiment with different foods and tastes, such as cold cooked chicken.
- Review skin care measures:
  —Protect skin.
  —Avoid using soap on the skin within treatment fields.
  —Avoid constricting clothing or jewelry around the neck.
  —Avoid shaving.
  —Use moisturizing lotion if dryness occurs.
- If moist desquamation occurs:
  —Burow's compresses four times a day.
  —Hydrocolloid dressings applied to desquamated areas.
- Evaluate activities.
- Plan rest periods during the day.
- Assist in using community resources:
  —Transportation to and from treatment center.
  —Food purchasing and preparation.

NURSING DIAGNOSIS: *Posttreatment Phase*

- Oral mucous membrane, altered, related to head and neck irradiation

INTERVENTIONS: *Posttreatment Phase*

- Assess oral status (xerostomia, taste changes); inspect mouth.
- Review importance of oral hygiene and frequent visits to dentist.
- To prevent osteoradionecrosis, continue prophylactic fluoride treatments.
- Review importance of minimizing alcohol and tobacco intake to reduce risk of oral complications.

Taste change

Taste changes occur as the taste buds are affected by the radiation.[20] Occasionally patients report a bad or peculiar taste in the mouth. For instance, certain red meats may taste rancid or coffee may taste extremely bitter. In other cases there is a decrease in some or all taste sensations.[16] This can be very frustrating for patients who already have a loss of appetite and are trying to increase their nutritional intake. Although some recovery of taste may occur, alterations can persist 7 years or longer.[66] Therefore follow-up assessments of taste changes and their influence on nutrition should be ongoing.[91]

Mouth care should be performed before and after each meal. Experimenting with different foods and using ad-

ditional seasonings, if tolerated, can help make food more palatable.[30] If red meats are a problem, use other sources of protein such as fish and poultry. Marinating meats in wine or sweet and sour sauce before and during cooking can mask unpleasant tastes. Serving foods cold or at room temperature also blunts peculiar tastes.

Osteoradionecrosis

Osteoradionecrosis, a late and chronic effect of radiation therapy, usually occurs in the mandible. Trauma to the bone such as tooth decay and infections heals poorly because of compromised bone structure and can lead to necrosis of the bone. Patients who continue to use tobacco and/or drink alcohol are at a greater risk for developing this serious complication.[25] Another risk factor is poorly fitting dentures, which abrade the mucosa. The mucosal breakdown can eventually reach the mandible. Treatment of osteoradionecrosis may include antibiotic therapy, surgical removal of the necrotic bone, and hyperbaric oxygen therapy to promote healing of the bone.[3,4,18,65,97]

Nursing care includes teaching and reinforcing the need to maintain good oral hygiene with frequent visits to the dentist for evaluation. Minimizing mouth irritants such as tobacco and alcohol and evaluating the fit and comfort of dentures will help decrease risk factors associated with osteoradionecrosis.

The nursing diagnoses *altered oral mucous membrane related to head and neck irradiation* and *sensory-perceptual alterations: gustatory, related to head and neck irradiation* are used when patients have alterations in the oral cavity as a result of radiation therapy. Assess mouth care practices and inspect the oral cavity for mouth changes. Evaluate the patient's ability to perform appropriate mouth care, minimize irritation, and prevent infections. (See Chapter 11.)

Hypopituitarism

The symptoms of hypopituitarism are associated with decreased secretions of cortisol, thyroxine, and sex hormones [83] (see Table 21-7). The symptoms may develop slowly within the first year after radiation therapy or up to 24 years after treatment. During times of stress, such as surgery or acute illness, the consequences of hypoadrenalism can be life threatening.[83] Adrenal insufficiency is treated with adrenocortical replacement, and sex hormone deficits are replaced with appropriate hormone therapy.

Chest

Radiation therapy is given to the chest for lung cancer; lymphoma; cancers involving the mediastinum, including the esophagus; and breast cancer. Common side effects of radiation therapy to the chest are esophagitis and cough. Late effects include pneumonitis and, in rare cases, lung fibrosis. With current tissue-sparing tech-

Table 21-7 Signs and Symptoms of Hypopituitarism

Pituitary deficiency	Target organ deficiency	Signs and symptoms
ACTH	Cortisol	Fatigue, weakness, weight loss, anorexia, nausea, postural dizziness, muscle weakness, hypoglycemia
TSH	Thyroxine	Dry skin and hair, fatigue, edema, pallor, cold intolerance, hoarseness, weight gain, delayed deep tendon reflexes, alopecia, lethargy, mental and physical slowness, constipation
LH, FSH	Estrogen	Amenorrhea, decrease in sexual libido
	Testosterone	Decrease in sexual libido
GH		Short stature in children Asymptomatic in adults
PRL		Failure of lactation

From Schultz PN: *Oncol Nurs Forum* 16:823, 1989.

niques for treating breast cancer, the dose to the lung and esophagus is minimized and these patients have few if any of the just-mentioned effects.

Esophagitis

Esophagitis occurs if part of the esophagus is within the treatment field. Approximately 2 to 3 weeks from the start of therapy, the patient may note difficulty or pain with swallowing and may complain of a "lump in the throat." Esophagitis can become so severe that radiation treatments must be withheld for a short time. The nursing diagnosis of *impaired swallowing related to esophagitis* is made when the patient experiences esophagitis. Assist the patient and family to plan a soft, bland, or liquid diet that provides a high-calorie, high-protein intake. Use of anesthetic and coating mouth rinses before meals can reduce the discomfort associated with eating and allow the patient to continue with therapy. Hilderley[46] described the beneficial use of a mouthwash containing viscous lidocaine, diphenhydramine elixir, and Mylanta taken 15 minutes before meals to relieve esophagitis. Other oral liquid pain medications may be used to numb the throat and relieve dysphagia.[26] Occasionally, systemic analgesics taken half an hour to an hour before meals are needed to obtain an acceptable level of pain relief. Evaluate the patient's and family's understanding and use of measures to relieve esophagitis and maintain an optimal nutritional intake.

Cough

A cough may develop or increase if lung tissue is within the treatment field, as with treatment for lung cancer. Initially the cough may be productive as trapped material is released by the previously blocked alveoli.[92] However, as treatment continues, the mucosa dries out and the cough becomes nonproductive. Assess the character, intensity, and frequency of cough, and monitor changes in lung sounds. The nursing diagnosis *pain related to cough* is made if the patient develops a cough. Assist the patient to plan measures to relieve the cough. Make sure the patient has an adequate fluid intake. Humidification of the air and avoiding irritants such as smoke can reduce the cough. Use of cough preparations that contain codeine may be indicated for severe, dry, hacking coughing that results in fatigue or disrupts sleep. Monitor for signs and symptoms of respiratory infection, and instruct the patient to avoid sources of infection. Evaluate the patient's use of measures to minimize cough and risk of respiratory infections.

Radiation pneumonitis

Radiation pneumonitis can occur approximately 1 to 3 months after radiation therapy to the lung.[49,92] At first there may be an unproductive cough that eventually becomes productive. The symptoms include fever and dyspnea. The effect is similar to the adult respiratory distress syndrome (ARDS). Radiation pneumonitis is treated with steroids, bed rest, and antibiotics for any superimposed infections.[92,100]

Radiation fibrosis

Radiation fibrosis may occur 6 to 12 months after treatment is completed. This consequence of radiation therapy is a restrictive disease of the lung. Lung fibrosis is seen primarily within the treated area of the lung and usually develops in areas of previous pneumonitis.[71] The primary symptom is shortness of breath. Treatment of radiation-induced lung fibrosis is limited to symptomatic control of dyspnea and supportive care.

ABDOMEN

Gastritis may occur if part of the stomach is within the treatment field. A soft, bland diet is tolerated best. Antacids may be used if needed.

Altered nutrition: less than body requirements, related to nausea and vomiting is a likely nursing diagnosis if a large part of the abdomen, including the stomach, paraaortic area, and/or small bowel is within the treatment field. Nausea and vomiting usually occur within the first 6 hours after treatments and may last for 3 to 6 hours.[100] In rare instances nausea may persist for longer periods. Assess patients for occurrence and pattern of nausea and vomiting. Prophylactic use of antiemetics before treatment each day and as needed after treatment can

Continued.

minimize and relieve nausea and vomiting from radiation therapy. For severe nausea and vomiting, around-the-clock antiemetics are recommended.

Relaxation techniques and distraction such as listening to soothing music and engaging in an enjoyable activity can help control nausea.[11] Using relaxation techniques before and after treatments helps minimize the anxiety that can exacerbate nausea.[100] Plan dietary modifications to minimize nausea and vomiting. A diet that is low in fat, low in sugar, and easily digested is best tolerated. Soups, broths, and other fluids should be consumed to maintain fluid intake and prevent dehydration (see Chapter 28). Evaluate the patient's and family's understanding of the potential and actual causes of nausea and vomiting. Also evaluate their ability to use appropriate measures to reduce or relieve nausea and vomiting and maintain the patient's nutritional status.

Pelvis

Diarrhea and cystitis commonly occur when the pelvis is being treated for gynecologic cancer, prostate cancer, testicular cancer, rectal cancer, or lymphomas. Diagnoses include *diarrhea related to pelvic irradiation* and *altered patterns of urinary elimination related to pelvic irradiation.*

Diarrhea

Diarrhea occurs as the bowel lining atrophies and resorption of fluids from the colon is decreased.[100] Malabsorption of bile salt may also cause diarrhea.[67] Diarrhea can occur 2 to 3 weeks into treatment and may last throughout the course of therapy. Some patients produce an increased number of stools; others produce loose, watery stools with cramping.[49] In certain instances treatment may be interrupted to allow the bowel to recover. Occasionally chronic enteritis develops.

Assess the patient's usual bowel pattern. If diarrhea occurs, help the patient and family plan measures to minimize diarrhea. Instruct the patient and family in the use of a low-residue diet. Reducing the amount of fat in the diet can also be helpful because fats are difficult to digest. If milk products are not tolerated, they should be avoided. If the diarrhea persists while the patient is on a low-residue diet, antidiarrheal medication such as diphenoxylate atropine or loperamide HCl may be indicated. If diarrhea tends to occur after meals as a result of the gastrocolic reflex, the antidiarrheal medication should be taken before meals. Tenesmus of the anal sphincter is controlled with antispasmodic and anticholinergic medications.[49] Evaluate the patient's and family's understanding and use of measures to minimize diarrhea and tenesmus in order to maintain the patient's usual pattern of elimination.

Cystitis

Cystitis occurs if the bladder is within the treatment field. Symptoms include dysuria, small bladder capacity, urinary frequency and urgency, nocturia, and urinary hesitancy. In rare cases bleeding occurs. Hyperbaric oxygen therapy has shown therapeutic benefits in treating chronic radiation-induced cystitis that is refractory to conventional therapy.[81,96] Hyperbaric oxygen therapy increases tissue oxygenation and promotes vascularization and formation of granulation tissue. Patients sit in a hyperbaric oxygen chamber and receive 100% oxygen for approximately 2 hours. One or two treatments a day are delivered for a total of as many as 60 treatments during the hyperbaric therapy treatment schedule.

Assess and monitor symptoms of cystitis, including signs of hematuria. Instruct the patient to maintain an adequate fluid intake.[49] As symptoms occur, bladder infections must be ruled out or treated. Obtain urine specimens for analysis and culture. Bladder analgesics such as phenazopyridine can relieve cystitis. Antispasmodic medications can provide some relief from bladder spasms. Evaluate the patient's understanding of the causes of cystitis and ways to relieve symptoms.

Erectile dysfunction

Erectile dysfunction after pelvic radiation may occur in men as a result of fibrosis of the pelvic vasculature and damage of pelvic nerves. A decline in the ability to attain and maintain an erection occurs gradually and may be permanent. Allow the patient and his partner to discuss concerns and feelings regarding changes in sexual functioning and body image. Consultation with a urologist may include a discussion of pharmacologic interventions and prostheses that may be used.

Vaginal stenosis

When the vaginal vault is included in the treatment field, vaginal stenosis may develop and cause dyspareunia and difficulties with pelvic examinations. Vaginal stenosis can be minimized or prevented by use of a vaginal dilator. With the patient lying supine with knees bent, the well-lubricated dilator is inserted into the vagina, withdrawn, and reinserted for 5 to 10 minutes.[41] Vaginal dilation needs to be performed three times a week for at least 1 year.

Ovarian failure

Ovarian failure occurs with small amounts of radiation and produces symptoms associated with menopause; hot flashes, amenorrhea, decreased libido, and osteoporosis.[28,100] Older women are at a higher risk of ovarian failure than younger women. Replacement hormonal therapy with midcyclic estrogens and progesterone reverses the clinical effects of early menopause. In certain circumstances the ovaries can be shielded from radiation.[100] In one technique, oophoropexy, the ovaries are surgically placed outside the treatment field.

Testicles

The testicles are usually shielded from radiation. However, if exposure is needed or unavoidable, spermatogenesis will stop and usually results in permanent sterility.

Sexuality

Issues related to sexuality need to be explored with sensitivity. As physical changes occur, the patient and his or her partner need to explore ways to satisfyingly express their sexuality and feelings (see Chapter 32).

Brain

Cerebral edema

When the brain is treated for a primary brain tumor or brain metastasis, assessment for symptoms of cerebral edema is crucial. Cerebral edema occurs as tissues around the tumor become inflamed. These symptoms include headaches, nausea, vomiting, seizures, vision changes, motor function disabilities, slurred speech, and changes in mental status. Steroids are usually indicated during the course of treatment to minimize cerebral edema. If symptoms occur or increase, an evaluation is needed and may indicate a need to adjust the steroid dosage. Steroids may be needed on a continuing basis to control edema. Plan to ensure the patient's safety in the home and work place as well as during transportation to and from the treatment center. Evaluate the patient's and family's understanding of the cause of cerebral edema and the signs and symptoms they should monitor and report.

Alopecia

Alopecia, which occurs within the treatment area, depends on the dose and extent of radiation to the scalp.

The hair loss may be regional or patchy, depending on the treatment technique. Alopecia starts when the dose to the scalp reaches 2500 to 3000 cGy, and the hair gradually thins over 2 to 3 weeks.[49] With large doses of radiation (>4000 cGy), as in the treatment for primary brain tumors, the hair loss is permanent.[100] With small doses such as those given for palliative purposes, alopecia is more variable. Hair loss may occur directly opposite the treatment site, where the x-rays exit. Regrowth of hair may start 2 to 3 months after completion of therapy.[67,86]

Hair texture and color

Changes in hair texture and color may also occur. The scalp may develop pruritus and become very dry or peel. The scalp needs protection along guidelines for skin care outlined earlier in this chapter. Gentle brushing and combing of hair is recommended. Permanent waves and hair coloring are contraindicated because they can irritate the scalp.[49] Using a scarf, turban, hat, or cap to protect the scalp from the wind, cold, and sun is advisable. A wig may be worn. Make sure the wig lining is comfortable and does not further irritate the scalp. A mild shampoo may be used, but excessive shampooing should be avoided. The potential or actual loss of hair can be traumatic for the patient. Nursing diagnoses are *ineffective individual coping related to alopecia* and *self-esteem disturbance related to alopecia*. Help the patient cope with the psychologic effects by recognizing the importance of alopecia, approaching the patient with gentleness, honesty and caring, and allowing verbalization of fears, grief, and anger. Prepare the patient and family in advance for alopecia. Assess its significance. Provide information on what can be done to cover and care for the scalp. These activities communicate understanding of the loss and offer support to the patient as she or he adapts to the change in body image.[100]

cur. Routine vaginal dilation is recommended to maintain the integrity of the vaginal walls.

Interstitial radioactive implants with needles, wires, seeds, or catheters are placed directly into the tissues. These implants may be temporary or permanent. Head and neck cancers are commonly treated with temporary interstitial implants. Goals of nursing care include minimizing airway obstruction and instructing the patient to perform oral care with saline irrigations every 3 to 4 hours. Nasogastric tube feedings are used to provide a high-protein, high-calorie liquid diet. Since talking is difficult and should be avoided, the patient communicates with a writing pad or specially created flash cards. With

head and neck implants, the patient is permitted to get out of bed but must remain in the hospital room. Elevating the head of bed to 30 to 45 degrees will help minimize tissue swelling and aspiration of oral secretions.

Temporary interstitial implants of the breast are performed approximately 2 weeks after a course of external-beam radiation therapy to provide more radiation to the site of tumor excision. Catheters are placed using general anesthesia, and radioactive sources are placed within the catheters once the woman returns to her hospital room.

Interstitial brain implants for recurrent brain tumors allow treatment of a highly localized area within the brain.

Catheters are placed using a stereotactic frame with CT guidance.[59]

In some instances permanent low-level radioactive implants may be placed percutaneously or intraoperatively in or near tumor masses. Because the level of radioactivity is low, radiation precautions are usually not required. Permanent interstitial implants with radioactive iodine seeds are placed intraoperatively or with transrectal ultrasound guidance within the prostate gland to treat prostate cancer.[35] The radioactive source has a short half-life, and the patient's body tissues effectively shield any radiation. Patients are instructed to filter urine for radioactive seeds that may pass through the urine, to use condoms when having sexual intercourse, and to avoid close contact with pregnant women and children while the radioactive source decays.

Radioactive isotopes that deliver a high dose rate of radition to a limited volume of tissue allow site-specific treatments over a shorter period. Treatments can be delivered within a few hours and can be done in the outpatient setting. Use of a remote afterloading brachytherapy device reduces staff exposure to the high-dose isotopes used during therapy.[55] If the patient requires direct care, the sources can be momentarily removed through the applicators by remote control before nurses enter the room.

Educating patients about the implant, the process, its effects, and how to manage those effects is crucial. Brandt[7] studied the informational needs of 22 patients receiving brachytherapy and found that most patients desired the maximum information about their illness. Symptom management, activity restrictions while the implant is in place, the causes of their current symptoms, and how the implant could affect those symptoms were subjects that the patients identified as important to know

before implantation. After implantation, the patients identified information about when to call the doctor, the potential side effects of treatment, and how to manage those side effects as most important.

Nonsealed Radioactive Therapy

When radioactive isotopes are injected intravenously or taken orally (nonsealed sources), the patient and the body secretions may be radioactive and nursing care must follow specific radiation safety precautions.[33] Depending on the isotope used, the patient usually must be isolated because of radioactivity for approximately 3 to 4 days. The amount of radioactivity emitted is carefully monitored during the patient's hospitalization. Table 21-8 describes the different radioactive isotopes used in cancer therapy.

MINIMIZING THE NURSE'S EXPOSURE TO RADIATION

Nurses play a major role in dispelling the patient's and family's fears and misconceptions about radiation therapy. When working with patients with internal radiation therapy, nurses need to be aware of their own concerns so that care can be provided thoroughly and effectively while minimizing radiation exposure.[85] Nursing inservices about radiobiology and radiation safety principles, combined with discussions and practice laboratories, can help clarify how nurses can protect themselves and still provide comprehensive nursing care. Fear is highly contagious, and nurses need to develop awareness of their behavior and its impact on patients. National and state regulations keep individual exposure below levels that produce somatic or genetic damage.[33,85]

When the nurse works with patients with a radioac-

Table 21-8   Radioactive Isotope Chart

Isotope	Emission	Half-life*	Source	Use	Administration
^{131}I (iodine)	Gamma rays†	8.05 days	Unsealed	Thyroid cancer	Oral, intravenous
^{32}P (phosphorus)	Beta particles‡	14.3 days	Unsealed	Malignant pleural or peritoneal effusion	Intrapleural; intraperitoneal in colloid form
^{192}Ir (iridium)	Beta particles Gamma rays	74.4 days	Sealed	Cancers of head and neck, breast, bronchus, brain; sarcomas	Interstitial and intracavitary
^{125}I (iodine)	Gamma rays	60.2 days	Sealed	Cancers of prostate, bladder, brain, bronchus	Interstitial
^{137}Cs (cesium)	Beta particles Gamma rays	30.0 years	Sealed	Gynecologic cancers	Intracavitary in an applicator
^{226}Ra (radium)	Beta particles Gamma rays	1602 years	Sealed	Head and neck cancer	Intracavitary and interstitial

Modified from Gillick M: *Cancer Nurs* 2(4):314, 1979.

*Time required for isotope to lose 50% of its radioactivity.

†Gamma rays: highly ionizing electromagnetic radiation emitted from radioactive isotopes; patient's body does not effectively shield gamma rays.

‡Beta particles: ionizing particles with moderate penetrating ability; the patient's body effectively shields the radiation when the isotope is injected.

tive implant or systemic radiation, he or she should anticipate the patient's needs and use the principles of time, distance, and shielding to minimize radiation exposure.[33,41]

- Time
  - —Minimize time spent in close proximity to the patient. Radiation exposure is directly related to the time spent within a specific distance of the source of radioactivity.
  - —Use time efficiently by organizing patient care activities and assembling necessary supplies before entering the patient's room. Before leaving the patient's room, place personal items within reach of the patient to avoid needing to reenter the room. Direct care is usually limited to one-half hour per person per shift. Encourage the patient to perform self-care activities.
- Distance
  - —Maximize the distance from the radioactive material. The amount of radiation decreases according to the inverse square law (see box at right). Visit frequently with the patient at the door to the patient's room.
- Shielding
  - —When appropriate, use shielding to decrease exposure to radiation. With radium or cesium implants, a 1-inch thick lead shield is positioned next to the bed

---

INVERSE SQUARE LAW

Radioactive
Source

Meters	0	1	2	3	4	5	6	7	8
Exposure rate		$\frac{1}{1}$	$\frac{1}{4}$		$\frac{1}{16}$				$\frac{1}{64}$

If the exposure at 1 m from the radioactive source is *x*, the exposure at 2 m is one fourth of *x*, and at 4 m, one sixteenth.

According to the inverse square law, exposure decreases as the distance from the radioactive source increases.

$$\text{Exposure rate} = \frac{1}{(\text{distance})^2}$$

---

to attenuate the radiation. Most nursing care is provided from behind the shields. The lead aprons used in diagnostic radiology are not sufficiently thick to stop gamma rays and therefore are not recommended.[49]

Table 21-9 presents some general guidelines for working with patients receiving internal radiation therapy.

Table 21-9 Guidelines for Internal Radiation Therapy

	Sealed sources	Unsealed sources
Preparation of the patient	Instruct patient and family on procedure and visitation restrictions. Isolation is a temporary requirement and the nursing staff is available for all needs, but, by necessity, the nurse will work quickly and remain in the room for essential activities only. Preoperatively, patients may require bowel cleansing or placement of a Foley catheter, as with cervical/vaginal implants.	
Room assignment	Private room usually required.	Private room only.
Restrictions on staff and visitors	No one under 18 years of age and no one who is or may be pregnant. Time spent close to the patient must be limited as much as possible. Visits with the patient from the doorway are usually permitted for longer periods.	
Shielding	Stay behind lead shields. Lead aprons are not effective.	Lead aprons are not effective.
Level of patient's activity	Patient remains in room. Depending on location of implant, the patient's activities may be limited to bed rest. In some instances raising the head of the bed may also be limited.	Patient remains in room. Bathroom privileges if tolerated. Patient should care for self.
	Diversional activities such as watching television or reading a book are recommended.	
Body fluid precautions	Body fluids and materials are not radioactive. No special precautions are necessary for handling these materials.	Secretions from the patient may be radioactive: • Wear gloves when handling equipment or objects that may have come in contact with body fluids or materials (e.g., urinals, bedpans, and emesis basins).

Continued.

Table 21-9 Guidelines for Internal Radiation Therapy—cont'd

	Sealed sources	Unsealed sources
		• Wash gloves before removing and place in designated waste container.
		• Wash hands thoroughly with soap and water after removing gloves.
		• Disposable shoe covers may be put on before entering the patient's room and removed before exiting. Shoe covers should be used if patient is incontinent.
		• Disposable items such as eating utensils, cups, and plates should be used.
		• Nondisposable items such as equipment and linens should not be removed from the patient's room until checked for radioactivity. Soiled items should be placed in a plastic bag, sealed, and left in the patient's room until checked for radioactivity.
		• Stool, urine, and emesis are usually discarded in the toilet in the patient's room. Instruct the patient to flush the toilet two or three times after each use.
		• Vomiting, stool or urinary incontinence, and excessive sweating may produce radioactive contamination of the room and linen. Use gloves to dispose of the material in the toilet, if appropriate, or in plastic bags, which are left in the patient's room for monitoring.
		• If skin becomes contaminated, wash affected area immediately with soap and water.
		• If clothing becomes contaminated, have level of radioactivity evaluated before leaving the immediate area.
		• Take special room preparation and additional precautions according to specific institution's policies.
Special precautions	• Check linens, clothing, and bedpans for signs of dislodged implant. If implant is dislodged, do not touch it; notify the physician immediately. If forceps are available, the radioactive source may be picked up with the forceps and placed in an available container, such as an emesis basin. The container should be placed in a corner of the room distant from the door. Immediately notify the physician. • Dressings and packings should not be changed unless ordered by the physician.	
Discharge of patient from the hospital	The patient is no longer radioactive once the implant has been removed and placed in a lead-lined container.	The patient is discharged when total body retention of the radioactive isotope is at a safe level. After the patient is discharged, the patient's room and all items in it are surveyed for any residual radioactivity.

HELPING PATIENTS AND FAMILIES COPE WITH RADIATION THERAPY

Radiation therapy can sound frightening, and many patients approach it with apprehension. The nurse is in a vital position to help the patient and family cope with this treatment and its sequelae.[50] Since most patients receive radiation therapy as an outpatient, self-care is supported by nurses through assessment, symptom management, and education.[94,99] Education can increase the patient's treatment-related knowledge while decreasing anxiety and general emotional distress during treatment.[76] The nursing diagnoses *anxiety related to radiation therapy* and *knowledge deficit related to radiation therapy and self-care measures* may be used. Support and counsel the patient who may need help to sort through his or her feelings about radiation therapy. Specifically assess the patient's expectations and concerns about therapy.

Patients are very interested in learning about their disease and treatment and ways to minimize symptoms and care for themselves.[61] Dodd[24] studied the self-care behaviors of patients receiving radiation therapy and found that patients identified themselves and physicians as the most frequent source of information about self-care behaviors.

Patient education is challenging because of limited time to provide the education and because of patient and family variables such as anxiety, symptom distress, and lack of resources.[19] Identifying the major teaching needs and tailoring the education for the patients so that it is provided over a period of time helps make the information less overwhelming. A weekly patient newsletter is one way that information can be given to patients and families throughout treatment.[36,88]

Concrete, objective information describing the common physical sensations experienced, the environmental surroundings, and information about timing of events helps to decrease the amount of disruption to the patient's usual activities during and after radiation therapy.[52] Educate the patient and family about the therapy and its side effects: what occurs, when it may occur, how long it lasts, and what they can do to manage the problem. Describe to the patient what he or she may experience.[92]

- The patient may be in the treatment room for about 20 minutes, but the actual treatment lasts only 2 to 5 minutes.
- The patient must lie on a hard table.
- The patient must remain alone in the room for the actual treatment.
- The patient may hear a buzzing, clicking, or whirring sound from the treatment machine.

PATIENT TEACHING PRIORITIES
External-Beam Radiation Therapy

Instruct patient and family about:
  Use of radiation therapy to treat cancer.
  Events that occur before, during, and after a course of radiation therapy: consultation, simulation, daily treatment, routine evaluations during course of therapy, and follow-up.
Time factors: length of simulation, length of daily treatment, length of course of radiation therapy.
Environmental information: description of surroundings, treatment room, and machine.
Effects and side effects of radiation therapy (general and site specific):
  That radiation therapy is a localized treatment and expected side effects are general as well as site specific.
  What happens, why it occurs.
  When these effects are experienced.
  How long these effects last and when they resolve.
  That patient is *not* radioactive; there is no need to isolate the patient from family and friends.
Measures that patients and families can use to minimize or prevent side effects:
  General effects: skin care, nutrition, energy conservation.
  Site-specific effects.
Delayed effects to monitor: skin care, fatigue, site-specific effects.
Follow-up care: routine follow-up with health care providers and adherence to recommendations for healthy living.

- The machine may rotate around the patient, depending on how the treatment is delivered.
- The treatment itself is painless.

Many myths, fears, and anxieties surround radiation therapy. Many patients have heard from others about someone else's experience with radiation—the burns, disfigurement, and pain. Explain to the patient and family that not all treatments cause the same problems and that as technology advances, some side effects have become less common and less severe.

The treatment machines are large and can be intimidating as they hover closely over the patient. Some patients fear being crushed by the machine or parts of it. For some patients, being alone in the treatment room during the treatment reinforces the loneliness of having cancer.

A common misconception about external radiation therapy is the fear of radioactivity. Many people mistak-

Continued.

PATIENT TEACHING PRIORITIES
Internal Radiation Therapy–Sealed and Nonsealed Sources

Instruct the patient and family about:

Use of internal radiation therapy to treat cancer.

Patient preparation before therapy.

Procedures involved in the therapy.

Visitation restrictions: no one under 18 years of age, no one who is or may be pregnant.

Isolation requirements: temporary isolation, patient remains in room, nursing care for essential activities only, time spent in close proximity will be limited. If the patient with nonsealed radioactive source has bathroom privileges, the patient is instructed to flush the toilet two or three times after each use.

Patient activity may be restricted, depending on the procedure; diversional activities such as watching television or reading a book are recommended.

Discharge from the hospital: monitor for delayed effects such as fatigue; pelvic implants: diarrhea, urinary symptoms such as bladder infections, women are instructed to perform vaginal dilation three times a week for up to 1 year after implantation.

GERIATRIC CONSIDERATIONS

Compromised body systems in the elderly place them at risk for developing side effects sooner and with greater severity:

Skin: monitor for excessive dryness and early skin reactions.

Energy stores may be depleted and increase fatigue.

Medications prescribed for symptom management may need dosage adjustments to minimize adverse reactions.

Head and neck irradiation: normally decreased oral secretions predispose the elderly for oral complications.

Check the fit and comfort of oral prostheses.

Taste acuity may be altered before start of irradiation.

Sexuality: assess changes experienced. Provide education about the effects of radiation therapy. Because of the importance of preventing vaginal stenosis so that vaginal intercourse and pelvic examinations are feasible, instruct women who have received radiation therapy involving the vaginal vault to perform vaginal dilation three times a week for up to 1 year. Radiation therapy further decreases vaginal secretions. Women are instructed to use water-based lubricants for comfort. Some men experience erectile dysfunction with aging as a result of vascular changes. Pelvic irradiation may further damage the pelvic vasculature and cause nerve damage. Provide counseling or referral to specialist.

Social concerns:

Radiation therapy is usually delivered Monday through Friday for up to 7 weeks. The elderly may need to rely on public transportation or family and friends for daily transportation. In many situations, the patient is caring for a spouse or child and being away from home is difficult without a caretaker. Many elderly are on fixed incomes, and the added expense of therapy, transportation, out-of-town housing, and additional medications needed during therapy is a hardship.

enly believe that the patient is radioactive. Reassure the patient and family that with external radiation, the patient is *not* radioactive. There is no residue of radiation on the patient, and therefore the patient should not be isolated from family or friends.

Community resources are available and can be gathered to assist the patient and family. These resources include a variety of services through the American Cancer Society, visiting nurses, home parenteral nutritional services, Meals on Wheels, accommodations for out-of-town patients, and transportation assistance for daily treatment.

Patient-teaching priorities for external and internal beam radiation therapy are given in the box, p. 525, and the box above. Geriatric considerations are shown in the box at right.

CONCLUSION

Nurses have always been involved in the development of radiation oncology as a specialty, whether being at the bedside of the patient receiving radiation therapy, delivering the treatment, or helping to calm a confused or frightened patient on the treatment table. The fears and concerns of patients have changed very little, and the impact of the diagnosis of cancer remains profound.

In a collaborative role with the radiation oncology team, the nurse provides continuity and quality patient care.[9,10] The nurse is in a prime position to assess, plan for, and evaluate interventions to prevent, minimize, or relieve side effects associated with radiation therapy.[9,10] In working with nurses in the hospital, home care and ambulatory settings, and with patients and families, the nurse helps to improve the patient's quality of life throughout treatment and rehabilitation.

■ CHAPTER QUESTIONS

1. Radiation therapy is used to treat cancer by:
   a. Increasing the temperature of the cell's cytoplasm
   b. Damaging the cell's DNA
   c. Altering the cell's membrane permeability
   d. Forming cellular abnormalities
2. Patient education for a 70-year-old man about to start radiation therapy for prostate cancer should include information about:
   a. Diarrhea
   b. Headaches
   c. Nausea and vomiting
   d. Taste changes
3. When strontium 89 is used for palliation of bone metastases, which of the following should be monitored?
   a. Bone scans
   b. Blood chemistries
   c. Complete blood counts
   d. Chest x-ray films
4. Which of the following lists the most to least radiosensitive tumors?
   a. Lymphoma, astrocytoma, salivary gland tumor
   b. Laryngeal cancer, leukemia, leiomyosarcoma
   c. Pancreatic cancer, seminoma, bladder cancer
   d. Osteogenic sarcoma, prostate cancer, stomach cancer
5. With unsealed sources of radiation, patient care involves:
   a. Using a lead apron with all patient contact
   b. Daily bed baths to promote excretion of radioactive isotopes
   c. Removing radioactive sources from the patient before discharge
   d. Observing radiation precautions with the patient's secretions
6. In radiation oncology, fractionation refers to:
   a. Dividing the daily dose into smaller fractions
   b. Dividing the total dose into smaller doses
   c. Administering one fraction per day
   d. Administering one dose per day
7. Compared with the reactions that occur when lower energies are used to treat an internal organ, the skin reactions seen with higher energies are:
   a. More frequent
   b. Less frequent
   c. No different
   d. Variable
8. Hypoxic tumors are:
   a. Well encapsulated
   b. More vascularized
   c. Less radiosensitive
   d. More radiosensitive
9. At the start of therapy, skin care includes using:
   a. Warm, moist compresses
   b. Zinc oxide
   c. Warm water to cleanse the skin
   d. Oil-based lubricants
10. Which of the following should not be used on irradiated skin?
    a. Fluorinated steroid creams
    b. Nonfluorinated steroid creams
    c. Aloe-based creams
    d. Hydrocolloid creams
11. Bone marrow suppression:
    a. Usually occurs with irradiation
    b. Rarely occurs with irradiation
    c. Depends on nutritional status
    d. Depends on the treatment field
12. Mouth care for a person receiving radiation therapy for head and neck cancer includes:
    a. Lemon-glycerin swabs
    b. Saliva substitutes
    c. Commercial antibacterial mouthwashes
    d. Breath freshener sprays

BIBLIOGRAPHY

1. Aistars J: Fatigue in the cancer patient: a conceptual approach to a clinical problem, *Oncol Nurs Forum* 14:25, 1987.
2. Bane C, Rich TA: Intraoperative radiation therapy, *AORN J* 37(5):835, 1983.
3. Bane CL, Shurkus LM: Caring for intraoperative radiation patients, *AORN J* 37(5):840, 1983.
4. Barrett A, Nicholls J, Gibson B: Late effects of total body irradiation, *Radiother Oncol* 9:1131, 1987.
5. Bentel GC, Nelson CE, Noell KT: Elements of clinical radiation oncology. In Bentel GC, Nelson CE, Noell KT, editors: *Treatment planning and dose calculation in radiation oncology,* ed 4, New York, 1989, Pergamon.
6. Beumer J, Curtis T, Harrison RE: Radiation therapy to the oral cavity: sequelae and management. I, *Head Neck Surg* 1:301, 1979.
7. Brandt B: Informational needs and selected variables in patients receiving brachytherapy, *Oncol Nurs Forum* 18:1221, 1991.
8. Brandt BB, Harney J: An overview of interstitial brachytherapy and hyperthermia, *Oncol Nurs Forum* 16:833, 1989.
9. Bruner DW: Report on the radiation oncology nursing subcommittee of the American College of Radiology task force on standards development, *Oncology* 4:80, 1990.
10. Bruner DW and others, editors: *Manual for radiation oncology nursing practice and education,* Pittsburgh, 1992, Oncology Nursing Society.
11. Bucholtz J: Radiation therapy. In Ziegfeld CR, editor: *Core curriculum for oncology nursing,* ed 2, Philadelphia, 1992, Saunders.
12. Bucholtz JD: Issues concerning the sedation of children for radiation therapy, *Oncol Nurs Forum* 19:649, 1992.
13. Bucholtz JD: Radiolabeled antibody therapy, *Semin Oncol Nurs* 3:67, 1987.
14. Campbell C, Iwamoto R: Intraoperative radiation therapy, *Todays OR Nurse* 14:1, 1992.
15. Campbell-Forsyth L: Patients' perceived knowledge and learning needs concerning radiation therapy, *Cancer Nurs* 13:81, 1990.
16. Conger A: Loss and recovery of taste acuity in patients irradiated to the oral cavity, *Radiat Res* 53:338, 1973.
17. Cromack DT and others: Are complications in intraoperative radiation therapy more frequent than in conventional treatment? *Arch Surg* 124:229, 1989.

18. Davis JC and others: Hyperbaric oxygen, *Arch Otolaryngol* 105:58, 1979.
19. DeMuth JS: Patient teaching in the ambulatory setting, *Nurs Clin North Am* 24:645, 1989.
20. DeWys W, Walters K: Abnormalities of taste sensation in cancer patients, *Cancer* 36:1888, 1975.
21. Dietz KA: Radiation therapy: external radiation, *Cancer Nurs* 2(2):129, 1979.
22. Dietz KA: Radiation therapy: external radiation, *Cancer Nurs* 2(3):233, 1979.
23. Dische S: Chemical sensitizers for hypoxic cells: a decade of experience in clinical radiotherapy, *Radiother Oncol* 3:97, 1985.
24. Dodd MJ: Patterns of self care in cancer patients receiving radiation therapy, *Oncol Nurs Forum* 11:23, 1984.
25. Dreizen S and others: Prevention of xerostomia-related dental caries in irradiated cancer patients, *J Dent Res* 56:99, 1977.
26. Dunne CF: Oral analgesics to relieve radiation-induced esophagitis, *Oncol Nurs Forum* 18:785, 1991.
27. Emami B, Perez CA: Combination of surgery, irradiation, and hyperthermia in treatment of recurrences of malignant tumors, *Int J Radiat Oncol Biol Phys* 13:611, 1987.
28. Feldman JE: Ovarian failure and cancer treatment: incidence and interventions for the premenopausal woman, *Oncol Nurs Forum* 16:651, 1989.
29. Ford R, Ballard B: Acute complications after bone marrow transplantation, *Semin Oncol Nurs* 4:15, 1988.
30. Gallucci BB, Iwamoto RR: Taste alterations in patients with cancer: nursing care of the cancer patient with nutritional problems, Report of the Ross Oncology Nursing Roundtable 40, 1981.
31. Gillick K: Radiation therapy: internal radiation, *Cancer Nurs* 2:314, 1979.
32. Glasgow G: Total body irradiation for bone marrow transplantation. In Withers HR, Peters LJ, editors: *Innovations in radiation oncology,* New York, 1988, Springer-Verlag.
33. Godwin CL, Bucholtz JD, Wall SC: Hidden hazards on the job. III, Radiation, *Nursing Life* Nov/Dec:43, 1985.
34. Goldson AL: Past, present and prospects of intraoperative radiotherapy, *Semin Oncol* 8:59, 1981.
35. Greenburg S and others: Interstitially implanted I-125 for prostate cancer using transrectal ultrasound, *Oncol Nurs Forum* 17:849, 1990.
36. Hagopian GA: The effects of a weekly radiation therapy newsletter on patients, *Oncol Nurs Forum* 18:1199, 1991.
37. Haibeck SV: Intraoperative radiation therapy, *Oncol Nurs Forum* 15:143, 1988.
38. Hall EJ: *Radiobiology for the radiologist,* ed 3, Philadelphia, 1988, Lippincott.
39. Harrison LB, Enker WE, Anderson LL: High-dose-rate intraoperative radiation therapy for colorectal cancer: part I, *Oncology* 9:679, 1995.
40. Harrison LB, Enker WE, Anderson LL: High-dose-rate intraoperative radiation therapy for colorectal cancer: part II, *Oncology* 9:679, 1995.
41. Hassey K: Demystifying care of patients with radioactive implants, *Am J Nurs* 85:788, 1985.
42. Hassey KM: Skin care for patients receiving radiation therapy for rectal cancer, *J Enterostom Ther* 14:197, 1987.
43. Hassey KM, Rose CM: Altered skin integrity in patients receiving radiation therapy, *Oncol Nurs Forum* 9:44, 1982.
44. Haylock PJ, Hart LK: Fatigue in patients receiving localized radiation, *Cancer Nurs* 2:461, 1979.
45. Hendrickson FR, Withers HR: *Principles of radiation oncology.* In Holleb AI, Fink DJ, Murphy GP, editors: *American Cancer Society textbook of clinical oncology,* Atlanta, 1991, American Cancer Society.
46. Hilderley L: Relieving radiation esophagitis, *Oncol Nurs Forum* 13:71, 1986.
47. Hilderley L: Skin care in radiation therapy: a review of the literature, *Oncol Nurs Forum* 10:51, 1983.
48. Hilderley LJ, Hassey KM, Dudjak LA: Nursing management of the patient receiving radiation therapy, Pub No 3480.04-PE, Atlanta, 1988, American Cancer Society.
49. Hilderley LJ: Radiotherapy. In Groenwald SL, editor: *Cancer nursing principles and practice,* ed 2, Boston, 1990, Jones & Bartlett.
50. Hilderley LJ: The role of the nurse in radiation oncology, *Semin Oncol* 7:39, 1980.
51. Hirshfield-Bartek J and others: Monitoring the myelosuppressive effects of radiation therapy, *Oncol Nurs Forum* 15:547, 1988.
52. Johnson JE and others: Reducing the negative impact of radiation therapy on functional status, *Cancer* 61:46, 1988.
53. Jones D, Hafermann MD: A radiolucent bite-block apparatus, *Int J Radiat Oncol Biol Phys* 13:129, 1986.
54. Jordan LN, Buck SS: A teaching booklet for patients receiving high dose rate brachytherapy, *Oncol Nurs Forum* 18:1235, 1991.
55. Jordan LN, Mantravadi RVP: Nursing care of the patient receiving high dose rate brachytherapy, *Oncol Nurs Forum* 18:1167, 1991.
56. King KB and others: Patients' descriptions of the experience of receiving radiation therapy, *Oncol Nurs Forum* 12(4):55, 1985.
57. Klevenhagen SC, Lambert GD, Arbabi A: Backscattering in electron beam therapy for energies between 3 and 35 MeV, *Phys Med Biol* 27:363, 1982.
58. Ladd L: The dry mouth dilemma, *Oncol Nurs Forum* 18:785, 1991.
59. Lamb S, Gutin PH: Interstitial radiation for treatment of primary brain tumors using the Brown-Roberts-Wells stereotaxic system, *J Neurosurg Nurs* 17:22, 1985.
60. Larson DA and others: Stereotactic external-beam irradiation. In Perez CA, Brady LW, editors: *Principles and practice of radiation oncology,* ed 2, Philadelphia, 1992, Lippincott.
61. Lauer P, Murphy SP, Powers MJ: Learning needs of cancer patients: a comparison of nurse and patient perceptions, *Nurs Res* 31:11, 1982.
62. Levy JG: Photosensitizers in photodynamic therapy, *Semin Oncol* 21:4, 1994.
63. Mansfield MJ and others: Hyperbaric oxygen as an adjunct in the treatment of osteoradionecrosis of the mandible, *J Oral Surg* 39:585, 1981.
64. Margolin SG and others: Management of radiation-induced moist skin desquamation using hydrocolloid dressing, *Cancer Nurs* 13:71, 1990.

65. Marx RE: A new concept in the treatment of osteoradione-crosis, *J Oral Maxillofac Surg* 41:351, 1983.
66. Mossman K, Shatzman A, Chencharick J: Long term effects of radiotherapy on taste and salivary function in man, *Int J Radiat Oncol Biol Phys* 8:991, 1982.
67. Mulkerin LE: *Practical points in radiation oncology,* Garden City, NY, 1979, Medical Examination Publishing.
68. Oski FA and others: *Principles and practice of pediatrics.* Philadelphia, 1990, Lippincott.
69. O'Rourke ME: Enhanced cutaneous effects in combined modality therapy, *Oncol Nurs Forum* 14:31, 1987.
70. Overgaard J: The current and potential role of hyperthermia in radiotherapy, *Int J Radiat Oncol Biol Phys* 16:535, 1989.
71. Perez CA and others: Hyperthermia. In Perez CA, Brady LW, editors: *Principles and practice of radiation oncology,* ed 2, Philadelphia, 1992, Lippincott.
72. Piper BF, Lindsey AM, Dodd MJ: Fatigue mechanisms in cancer patients: developing nursing theory, *Oncol Nurs Forum* 14:17, 1987.
73. Porter AT and others: Results of a randomized, phase III trial to evaluate the efficacy of strontium 89 adjuvant to local field external beam irradiation in the management of endocrine resistant metastatic prostate cancer, *Int J Radiat Oncol Biol Phys* 25:805, 1993.
74. Preston FA: Management of oral bleeding caused by thrombocytopenia, *Oncol Nurs Forum* 10:59, 1983.
75. Pu AT, Robertson JM, Lawrence TS: Current status of radiation sensitization by fluoropyrimidines, *Oncology* 9:707, 1995.
76. Rainey L: Effects of preparatory patient education for radiation oncology patients, *Cancer* 56:1056, 1985.
77. Robinson RG and others: Strontium 89 therapy for the palliation of pain due to osseous metastases, *JAMA* 274:420, 1995.
78. Roof LM: The use of Vigilon primary wound dressing in the treatment of radiation dermatitis, *Oncol Nurs Forum* 18:133, 1991.
79. Rubin P: Principles of radiation oncology and cancer radiotherapy. In Rubin P, editor: *Clinical oncology for medical students and physicians,* New York, 1983, American Cancer Society.
80. Rubin P, Cooper R, Phillips T, editors: *Radiation biology and radiation pathology syllabus. I, Radiation oncology,* Chicago, 1975, American College of Radiology.
81. Schoenrock GJ, Ciani P: Treatment of radiation cystitis with hyperbaric oxygen, *Urology* 27:271, 1986.
82. Schubert MM, Newton RE: The use of benzydamine HCl for the management of cancer therapy–induced mucositis: preliminary report of a multicentre study, *Int J Tissue React* 9(2):99, 1987.
83. Schultz PN: Hypopituitarism in patients with a history of irradiation to the head and neck area: diagnoses and implications for nursing, *Oncol Nurs Forum* 16:823, 1989.
84. Scott R and others: Hyperthermia in combination with definitive radiation therapy: results of a phase I/II RTOG study, *Int J Radiat Oncol Biol Phys* 15:711, 1988.
85. Sedhom LN, Yanni MIY: Radiation therapy and nurses' fears of radiation exposure, *Cancer Nurs* 8:129, 1985.
86. Sitton E: Early and late radiation-induced skin alterations. I, Mechanisms of skin changes, *Oncol Nurs Forum* 19:801, 1992.
87. Sitton E: Early and late radiation-induced skin alterations. II, Nursing care of irradiated skin, *Oncol Nurs Forum* 19:907, 1992.
88. Sporkin E: A newsletter for radiation therapy patients, *Oncol Nurs Forum* 14(suppl):149, 1987 (abstract).
89. Stephenson JA, Wiley AL: Current techniques in three-dimensional CT simulation and radiation treatment planning, *Oncology* 9:1225, 1995.
90. Storm FK, Morton DL, Bull JMC: Hyperthermia, Pub No 3364-PE, Atlanta, 1984, American Cancer Society.
91. Strohl R: Taste sensations after radiation therapy, *Oncol Nurs Forum* 10:80, 1983.
92. Strohl RA: The nursing role in radiation oncology: symptom management of acute and chronic reactions, *Oncol Nurs Forum* 15:429, 1988.
93. Strohl RA: Radiation therapy: recent advances and nursing implications, *Nurs Clin North Am* 25:309, 1990.
94. Tighe MG and others: A study of the oncology nurse role in ambulatory care, *Oncol Nurs Forum* 12:23, 1985.
95. Van Drimmelen J, Rollins HF: Evaluation of a commonly used oral hygiene agent, *Nurs Res* 18:327, 1969.
96. Weiss JP and others: Treatment of radiation-induced cystitis with hyperbaric oxygen, *J Urol* 134:352, 1985.
97. Wescott WB: Dental management of patients being treated for oral cancer, *CDAJ* 13:42, 1985.
98. Wiley SB: Why glycerol and lemon juice? *Am J Nurs* 69:342, 1969.
99. Woodtli MA, Van Ort S: Nursing diagnoses and functional health patterns in patients receiving external radiation therapy: cancer of the head and neck, *Nurs Diagn* 2:171, 1991.
100. Yasko JM: *Care of the client receiving external radiation therapy,* Reston, Va, 1982, Reston.

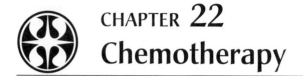

CHAPTER 22
Chemotherapy

MARTHA LANGHORNE

It is estimated that 1,359,150 people in the United States were newly diagnosed as having cancer in 1996. More than half of these people will receive systemic chemotherapy as a form of treatment because of disease recurrence, as secondary therapy after a local treatment, or for treatment of hematologic disease. The primary focus of chemotherapy is to prevent cancer cells from multiplying, invading adjacent tissue, or developing metastasis.[15,31,57,109]

DEFINITION

Chemotherapy is the use of cytotoxic drugs in the treatment of cancer. It is one of the four treatment modalities (the others being surgery, radiation therapy, and biotherapy) that provide cure, control, or palliation. Chemotherapy is a systemic treatment, rather than localized therapy, such as surgery and radiation therapy. Chemotherapy may be used in five ways[31]:

- *Adjuvant therapy*—a course of chemotherapy used in conjunction with another treatment modality (surgery, radiation therapy, or biotherapy) and aimed at treating micrometastases
- *Neoadjuvant chemotherapy*—administration of chemotherapy to shrink a tumor before it is removed surgically
- *Primary therapy*—the treatment of patients who have localized cancer for which an alternative but less than completely effective treatment is available
- *Induction chemotherapy*—drug therapy given as the primary treatment for patients who have cancer for which no alternative treatment exists
- *Combination chemotherapy*—administration of two or more chemotherapeutic agents to treat cancer; this allows each medication to enhance the action of the other or to act synergistically with it (an example of combination chemotherapy is the widely known MOPP regimen of nitrogen mustard, vincristine [Oncovin], procarbazine, and prednisone, which is used to treat patients with Hodgkin's disease)[5,37,42]

HISTORICAL PERSPECTIVE

Systemic therapy, in the form of metallic salts (arsenic, copper, lead), began with the Egyptian and Greek civilizations. This practice continued for centuries with limited success. Each generation had its own specific remedy for various illnesses. In the late 1880s some bacterial compounds were developed. However, none of these methods proved reliable and effective in treating these varied illnesses.[31]

Research for chemotherapy began in the early 1900s, when Paul Ehrlich used rodent models of infectious diseases to develop antibiotics. Further developments led to the use of rodents to test potential cancer chemotherapeutic agents. An additional discovery in drug development was made as the result of servicemen's exposure to mustard gas during World War I and World War II.[5,31,47] This exposure led to the observation that alkylating agents caused marrow and lymphoid suppression in humans. This experience resulted in the use of these agents to treat Hodgkin's and other lymphomas; the therapy was first attempted at Yale's New Haven Medical Center in 1940. Because of the secret nature of the gas warfare program, the work was not published until 1946. Chemotherapy as a treatment modality was introduced in the late 1950s and became established in medical practice in the 1970s.

Since the start of cytotoxic drug research, thousands of chemical agents have been tested for their ability to destroy cancer cells. More than 100 cytotoxic agents are available for commercial or experimental use with approval by the federal Food and Drug Administration.[31]

Research continues to contribute discoveries in the area of chemotherapy as a cancer treatment modality, and as a result of this intensive investigation, new areas have been tapped for further study, such as the use of chemotherapeutic agents as radiosensitizers and the strategy of chemoprevention.

PRINCIPLES OF CHEMOTHERAPY
Cell Generation Cycle

The cell cycle is the sequence of events that result in replication of deoxyribonucleic acid (DNA) and equal distribution into daughter cells, a process called *mitosis.* Normal cells and cancer cells go through the same division cycle, which is characterized by the following phases: G_0—resting or dormant phase; G_1—phase in which protein synthesis takes place in preparation for the S-phase–DNA synthesis; and G_2—phase for further protein synthesis in preparation for the M phase—mitosis and cell division. The generation time, or the time it takes a cell to complete the phase or cycle, varies from hours to days. Chemotherapeutic drugs are most active against frequently dividing cells, or in all the phases of the cell cycle except G_0. Normal cells with rapid growth changes that are most commonly affected by chemotherapeutic agents include bone marrow (platelets and red and white blood cells), hair follicles, the mucosal lining of the gastrointestinal (GI) tract, and skin and germinal cells (sperm and ova). Chemotherapy is given according to schedules that have proved most effective for tumor kill and that are planned to allow normal cells to recover.[15,31,36]

Tumor Growth

The regulatory mechanism that controls the growth of cancer cells differs from that of normal cells. Unlike normal cells, cancer cells grow by means of a pyramid effect; however, they grow at the same rate as the tissue from which they originated (e.g., breast cancer develops at the same rate of growth as normal breast tissue development). The time required for a tumor mass to reach a certain size is called *doubling time.* Tumors probably have undergone approximately 30 doublings from a single cell before they are clinically detected. Between the seventh and tenth doubling time, the possibility arises for the tumor to shed cells, a process called *micrometastasis.* During the early stages of tumor growth, doubling time is more rapid than at later stages; this pattern of growth is called *Gompertzian function.* Tumor cells are more sensitive than normal cells to chemotherapy agents that are toxic to rapidly dividing cells.[69]

Curative treatment for cancer focuses on killing the stem cells responsible for the neoplastic disease clone. In their attempts to understand the growth of tumor cells, investigators are trying to identify tumor-specific stem cells and then determine which cytotoxic drug is most effective against the tumor. Many investigators have tried to increase the efficiency of chemotherapy by using assays to evaluate the tumor clone's response to specific chemotherapy agents.[70,80]

The roles of tumor growth and cell kinetics are important in understanding the action of cytotoxic therapy. Hematologic diseases, such as leukemia and lymphoma, have many rapidly dividing cells. When chemotherapy is initiated, there is the potential for rapid, extensive cellular destruction because of the nature of the bone marrow stem cells and the rapidly dividing cancer cells. The treatment implications for these diseases and others are discussed later in the chapter.[57,58] (See Chapter 1 for a detailed discussion of the cell generation cycle and properties of tumor growth.)

Blood-Brain Barrier

An understanding of the blood-brain barrier is essential in comprehending the effects of some chemotherapeutic agents on brain and central nervous system (CNS) tumors. Brain tumors create greater obstacles for treatment by chemotherapy than do other tumors. This is partly because of the existence of the blood-brain barrier, the tumor's location inside the skull, and the lack of an adequate lymphatic drainage system.[23]

The blood-brain barrier is made up of cellular structures that can inhibit certain substances from entering the brain or cerebrospinal fluid (CSF). The barrier is formed by continuous supporting cells, particularly astrocytes, and the endothelial cells of brain capillaries, which form intertwining junctions. In many cases the blood-brain barrier acts as a screening device, protecting the brain and CSF from harmful particles or agents, although the exact nature of this mechanism is unknown. The permeability of the blood-brain barrier can be inconsistent throughout the tumor; it tends to be greater in or near the center of the tumor, where the blood supply usually is diminished. In addition, there frequently is a slowly dividing tumor core containing tumor cells that are not identical and therefore are prone to drug resistance (Figure 22-1).[77]

Certain metabolites, electrolytes, and chemicals have varying abilities to cross the barrier into the brain. This can have serious implications, because certain chemotherapeutic agents have a greater propensity than others for crossing the barrier. Neuwalt and others[86] have attempted to alter the integrity of the blood-brain barrier by infusing mannitol to "open" the barrier and administer greater concentrations of chemotherapy via a catheter in the carotid or vertebral artery. The concept is an interesting one that may offer a more favorable prognosis for these patients in the future.[23,77,86]

RADIOSENSITIZERS

The use of concomitant continuous infusion chemotherapy (CCIC) and radiation therapy in the treatment of a variety of tumors has produced substantial improvement in complete response and survival rates. The emphasis in chemotherapeutics has been directed toward treatment of systemic metastases, with seemingly less interest shown in improving the cure of local and local/

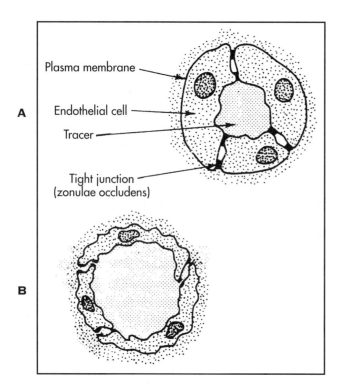

Figure 22-1 Schematic representation of the blood-brain barrier. **A,** Normal cerebral capillary showing tight junctions. **B,** Blood-brain barrier opening created by widening of the interendothelial tight junctions. When the endothelial cells shrink in a hypertonic environment, the permeability of the junctions increases. (From Groenwald SL and others: *Cancer nursing: principles and practice,* ed 3, Boston, 1993, Jones & Bartlett.)

regional disease. The goal of radiotherapy is to achieve maximum tumor-cell kill while minimizing injury to normal tissues; this is called the *therapeutic ratio.*[34] Efforts to improve the therapeutic ratio have led to the development of certain compounds called *radiosensitizers,* which are intended to be used to increase the radiosensitivity of tumor cells or to protect normal cells from the effects of radiation.[48,90]

Starting in the 1920s and for 30 years thereafter, radiosensitization was attempted with oxygen; in the 1950s, hyperbaric oxygen chambers were used. Well-oxygenated tumors are more responsive to radiation and more radiosensitive than poorly oxygenated tumors. The 1950s and 1960s brought systemic chemicals that changed the DNA structure and enhanced radiation response. The first hypoxic cell sensitizers were used in the 1970s and 1980s. It was thought that if radiation and chemotherapy were administered concurrently, treatment could be enhanced by the biochemical or molecular interactions that occur between them. This led to clinical use of the halogenated pyrimidines: iododeoxyuridine, bromodeoxyuridine, and fluorodeoxyuridine. The toxicities caused by combining these early drugs with irradia-

tion were so severe that interest turned to the use of chemotherapeutic agents as radiosensitizers.[90,96]

Today patients often receive combination treatment with radiation therapy and chemotherapy at some point in their management. The combination of radiation therapy and chemotherapy has potential benefit for patients. It may be part of a planned protocol, may be used when patients who have not responded to one modality are rescued by treatment with another, or may be used to reduce radioresistance.[24,95,96] Clinical trials are under way for various malignancies utilizing concomitant chemotherapy and radiation therapy.

Important principles and definitions in chemotherapy include the following:

1. *Spatial cooperation* is the ability of one agent to control disease spatially missed by the other, such as the practice of administering chemotherapy to eradicate micrometastases that are outside the radiation field.[90]
2. *Radiosensitizers* are compounds that apparently promote fixation of the free radicals produced by radiation damage at the molecular level.[48]
3. *Radioprotection* involves using drugs that may protect against radiation damage to normal tissue.[90]
4. It has been postulated that the drug and irradiation have a direct interaction within the tumor, producing greater cell kill than would be expected with either modality used alone.[90]

When a drug is selected to be used with radiation therapy, the drug's pharmacokinetics and the tumor cell kinetics are important considerations. Many chemotherapeutic agents are active in the cell during the phase of DNA synthesis. In some tumors this phase of the cell cycle is relatively short, and these chemotherapeutic agents usually have short half-lives; therefore bolus administration of the drug, with its rapid clearance, does not usually provide adequate exposure of the drug during this critical time in the cell cycle. The response to any chemotherapy is proportional to the serum concentration of the drug and the duration of exposure.[48,90,95,96]

If the tumor is one in which the DNA synthesis phase can vary from minutes to hours, prolonged drug exposure ensures that adequate amounts of the drug are present during the critical period. To achieve this, a continuous infusion is the route of choice, especially if the chemotherapeutic agent has a short half-life or is characterized by low cellular uptake or rapid cellular excretion. In addition, continuous infusion usually has low hematologic potential because no peak drug concentrations occur, as happens with a bolus administration.[90,95,96]

The mechanism of action that occurs with chemotherapy and radiation is not well known. One school of thought is that the separate effect of each modality may have an added therapeutic impact on the tumor. The drug may act as a sensitizer, causing a synergistic effect that leads to tumor cell kill.

Many classes of drugs have been found to interact with radiation; 5-fluorouracil (5-FU), cisplatin, and doxorubicin have been well documented and evaluated as radiosensitizers.

5-FU was developed in 1957 and has been widely used in the treatment of breast and gastrointestinal cancers. Various clinical studies have demonstrated that doses of radiotherapy that were growth inhibitory but not curative in rodents could be made curative by adding 5-FU. For more than 30 years, however, the drug's exact mechanism has remained unknown. The results report that combined treatment with 5-FU and radiotherapy leads to a dose- and time-dependent enhanced tumor kill.[78,83,95,96]

The exact mechanism of 5-FU and radiation therapy interaction is unknown. 5-FU is a pyrimidine analog that inhibits the synthesis of DNA. It also is taken up into the cell and combines with ribonucleic acid (RNA), which leads to defective RNA synthesis. Experimentation with a variety of cell types showed the need for CCIC anywhere from 8 hours to 5 days after irradiation.[78,96]

The infusion typically is begun 6 hours before the first radiation treatment and continues for 4 to 5 days. Complications with higher dosing primarily involve mucous membrane breakdown within the gastrointestinal tract, causing mucositis, stomatitis, or diarrhea. Myelosuppression is not usually a problem. With some of the low doses that are administered over a prolonged period, neurotoxicities (e.g., paresthesia of the hands and feet) can be a problem.[78,95,96]

Cisplatin is used as a radiation sensitizer, but its mechanism of action is also elusive. Covalent links are formed between cisplatin, DNA, and RNA. In the presence of radiation, these links break down.

Scheduling, concentration, and dosing vary. Drug studies have demonstrated that small doses of cisplatin and lower serum levels produce maximal effect. For increased tumor-cell kill, the cisplatin must be administered before and after irradiation; therefore continuous infusion of the drug is used. Nausea, vomiting, and renal toxicities are less problematic with a continuous infusion. The continuous infusion of cisplatin at 20 mg/m^2/day for 5 days produced a very low nephrotoxicity rate, with only 7% of patients experiencing grade 3 vomiting.[90,95]

Doxorubicin inhibits mitochondria and enzymatic repair of breaks in the DNA strands. The combination of doxorubicin and irradiation has been found to be synergistic at low doses. Despite many reports that the radiation-doxorubicin combination is well tolerated, its use has been avoided. Many believed that it was cardiotoxic and was associated with increased enteritis, esophagitis, and a recall reaction.

Several studies have been done to evaluate the efficacy of other chemotherapeutic agents as radiosensitizers, including paclitaxel[24,78,100,102] and ermustine.[113] The increasing use of CCIC with radiotherapy has provided clinicians with a wealth of information on the ability of radiosensitizers to improve the response rate in treating all but the most advanced carcinomas of the anus, rectum, esophagus, head and neck, and bladder. Gains also have been demonstrated with dose enhancement using CCIC in soft tissue sarcomas, suggesting in some instances that the amount of radiation needed could be reduced by 30% if it is administered concurrently with 5-FU. In certain gynecologic and colon malignancies, when liver metastasis is anticipated, it is not unreasonable to suggest the use of 5-FU infusion and radiation therapy not only for the primary tumor and lymph nodes, but also for the liver.[95]

CCIC and radiation therapy used in the treatment of a variety of tumors has produced substantial improvement in the complete response and survival rates. Current research is aimed at defining the required total dosing, fractionation of radiation, optimal concentration of drugs, and proper scheduling of the infusion. Randomized trials are needed to answer these and other questions about long-term toxicity. This form of therapy has had a major positive impact on survival and organ preservation and in reducing the need for radical surgery.[78,95]

DRUG CLASSIFICATION

Chemotherapeutic agents are classified according to their pharmacologic action and their interference with cellular reproduction. Following are the basic groups and their potential action.

- *Cell cycle phase-specific* drugs are active on cells undergoing division in the cell cycle; examples include antimetabolites, *Vinca* plant alkaloids, and miscellaneous agents such as asparaginase and dacarbazine. These drugs are most effective against actively growing tumors that have a greater proportion of cells cycling through the phase in which the drug attacks the cancer cell. Cell cycle phase-specific drugs are given in minimal concentration via continuous dosing methods.[15,37]
- *Cell cycle phase-nonspecific drugs* are active on cells in either a dividing or resting state; examples include alkylating agents, antitumor antibiotics, nitrosureas, hormone and steroid drugs, and miscellaneous agents such as procarbazine. These agents are active in all phases of the cell cycle and may be effective in large tumors that have few active cells dividing at the time of administration. Drugs of this nature are often given as single-bolus injections.

The mechanism of most chemotherapeutic drugs is targeting of the cell DNA in some manner. This action may result in direct interference with the DNA, inhibition of enzymes related to RNA or DNA synthesis or both, and/or destruction of the cells' necessary proteins.[15,31,37]

A general description of each drug classification follows,[38,41,57,59] and detailed information about the specific drugs in each class can be found in Appendix 22-1 at the end of this chapter.

- Alkylating agents are cell cycle phase-nonspecific. They act primarily to form a molecular bond with the nucleic acids, which interferes with nucleic acid duplication, preventing mitosis. This category of drugs has a phase activity similar to that observed in radiation therapy, with two peaks of maximum lethal activity, one in G_2 to M phase and one near the G_1–S phase boundary.
- *Antibiotics (antitumor agents)* are cell cycle phase-nonspecific. These drugs disrupt DNA transcription and inhibit DNA and RNA synthesis.
- *Antimetabolites* are cell cycle phase-specific. They exhibit their action by blocking essential enzymes necessary for DNA synthesis or by becoming incorporated into the DNA and RNA, so that a false message is transmitted.
- *Hormones* are cell cycle phase-nonspecific. These chemicals, which are secreted by the endocrine glands, alter the environment of the cell by affecting the cell membrane's permeability. By manipulating hormone levels, tumor growth can be suppressed. Hormone therapies are not cytotoxic and therefore not curative. Their purpose is to prevent cell division and further growth of hormone-dependent tumors.
- *Antihormonal agents* derive their antineoplastic effect from their ability to neutralize the effect of or inhibit the production of natural hormones used by hormone-dependent tumors.
- *Nitrosureas* are cell cycle phase-nonspecific. They have the ability to cross the blood-brain barrier. Their action is similar to that of the alkylating agents; synthesis of both DNA and RNA is inhibited.
- *Corticosteroids* exert an antiinflammatory effect on body tissues (e.g., they reduce intracranial or spinal cord compression and suppress lymphocytes). They may also promote a feeling of well-being and increase the appetite.
- *Vinca plant alkaloids* are cell cycle phase-specific. They exert a cytotoxic effect by binding to microtubular proteins during metaphase, causing mitotic arrest. The cell loses its ability to divide and so dies.
- *Miscellaneous agents* may be cell cycle phase-specific or nonspecific or both. These drugs act by a variety of mechanisms. For example, L-asparaginase is unique; it is an enzyme product that acts primarily by inhibiting protein synthesis.

Cell Kill Hypothesis

A single cancer cell is capable of multiplying and eventually killing the host. Every tumor cell must be killed to cure cancer. With each course of the drug therapy, a given dose of chemotherapeutic drug kills only a fraction, not all, of the cancer cells present (Figure 22-2).

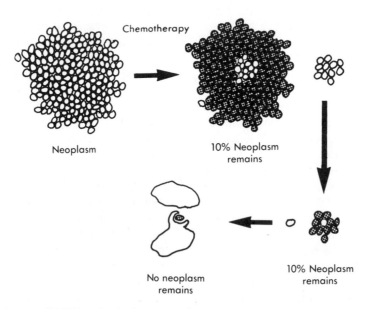

Figure 22-2 Cell kill hypothesis. (From Goodman MS: *Cancer: chemotherapy and care,* Bristol Laboratories, Evansville, Ind, Bristol-Myers Co.)

Repeated courses of chemotherapy must be used to reduce the total number of cancer cells. This cardinal rule of chemotherapy—the inverse relationship between cell number and curability—was established by Skipper and colleagues[15,32] in the early 1960s.

Factors Considered in Drug Selection[15,32]

- Patient's eligibility for chemotherapy (confirmed diagnosis; bone marrow, nutritional, hepatic, and renal status; expectation of longevity; history of chemotherapy and radiation therapy)
- Cancer cell type (e.g., squamous cell, adenocarcinoma)
- Rate of drug absorption (e.g., treatment interval and routes—oral, intravenous, intraperitoneal)[11]
- Tumor location (many drugs do not cross the blood-brain barrier)
- Tumor load (larger tumors are generally less responsive to chemotherapy)
- Tumor resistance to chemotherapy (tumor cells can mutate and produce variant cells distinct from the tumor stem cell of origin)[31,69,70,71]

Combination Chemotherapy

Chemotherapeutic drugs are most often given in combination because this enhances the effect of the drugs on the tumor cell kill. Considerations for drugs used in combination include verified effectiveness as a single agent, results in increased tumor cell kill, increased patient survival, presence of a synergistic action, varied toxicities, different mechanisms of action, and administration in repeated courses to minimize the immunosuppressive effects that might otherwise occur.[42,57,59] Combination chemotherapy provides additional benefits that are not possible with single-drug treatment, such as maximal cell kill within the range of toxicity tolerated by the host for each drug, a broader range of coverage of resistant cell lines in a heterogeneous tumor population, and prevention or slowing of the development of new resistant lines.[68,70,72,110]

Because numerous cellular variants exist within a metastasis by the time it is detected, therapy for metastatic disease often is directed toward characteristics of the secondary tumor rather than those of the primary tumor. Using combination chemotherapy rather than single sequential therapy maximizes the therapeutic response by addressing the diversity of cellular response.[42] See examples of commonly used combination therapies in the box at right.

CHEMOTHERAPY ADMINISTRATION
Calculation of Drug Dosage

The drug dosage for cancer chemotherapy is based on body surface area (BSA) in both adults and children.

Drug calculations should be verified by a second person to ensure accuracy of the dose. The dosage range of a drug may vary with different drug regimens.[16,32,79]

The dosages of some drugs are calculated proportionally to the patient's BSA. BSA is calculated in square meters (m^2). A nomogram is used to correlate height with weight to determine the BSA. The drug dose is ordered in milligrams per square meter.[16,93,108]

Drug Reconstitution

Pharmacy staff should reconstitute all drugs and pre-prime the intravenous tubings under a class II biologic safety cabinet. In certain conditions (the drug has short-term stability after mixing and the required administration time is unknown, as is the case with intrathecal injection of methotrexate using preservative-free diluent), nurses may be required to reconstitute medications. When the drugs are prepared and reconstituted, aseptic technique must be used in accordance with manufacturer's current recommendations. All syringes of reconstituted drugs are immediately labeled with the name of the drug.[32,79] Many chemotherapeutic agents are colorless and cannot be distinguished from one another after reconstitution[38] (see Safe Handling of Chemotherapeutic Agents, p. 537).

COMBINATION CHEMOTHERAPY REGIMENS

BREAST CANCER

CMF—cyclophosphamide, methotrexate, 5-fluorouracil
FUVAC—5-fluorouracil, vinblastine, Adriamycin, cyclophosphamide

LUNG CANCER

CAV—cisplatin, Adriamycin, vinblastine
CAMP—cyclophosphamide, Adriamycin, methotrexate, procarbazine

HODGKIN'S DISEASE

ABVD—Adriamycin, bleomycin, vinblastine, dacarbazine
MOPP—nitrogen mustard, Oncovin, prednisone, procarbazine

LYMPHOMA

CHOP-BLEO—cyclophosphamide, Adriamycin, Oncovin, prednisone, bleomycin
PROMACE-CytaBOM—prednisone, Oncovin, methotrexate, Adriamycin, cyclophosphamide, etoposide-cytarabine, bleomycin, leucovorin, dexamethasone, trimethoprim-sulfamethoxazole

TESTICULAR CANCER

VBP—vinblastine, bleomycin, cisplatin
VPV—VP-16 (etoposide), cisplatin, vinblastine

Administration Guidelines

Routes

Oral route. Emphasize the importance of the patient's complying with the prescribed schedule. Plan for drugs with emetic potential to be taken with meals; drugs that require hydration (e.g., Cytoxan) need to be taken early in the day.

Subcutaneous and intramuscular route. Demonstration with a return demonstration may be needed if the patient is giving self-injections. Be sure to rotate injection sites for each dose.[87]

Topical administration. Cover surface area with a thin film of medication; instruct the patient to wear loose-fitting cotton clothing. Wear gloves and be sure to wash hands thoroughly after procedure. Caution the patient not to touch ointment.[91]

Intraarterial route. This method requires catheter placement in an artery near the tumor; because of arterial pressure, administer the drug in a heparinized solution through an infusion pump. Throughout the infusion, monitor vital signs, color and temperature of extremity, and potential for bleeding at site. Instruct the patient and family in the care of the catheter and infusion pumps (e.g., routine filling and maintenance of the infusion pump) if chemotherapy is to be given at home.[38]

Intracavity route. Instill the drug into the bladder through a catheter or chest tube (or both) into the pleural cavity. Follow prescribed premedication dosage to minimize local irritation.

Intraperitoneal route. Deliver the drug into the abdominal cavity through the implantable port and/or external suprapubic catheter (e.g., Tenckhoff catheter). Use dry heat to warm the infusate solution to body temperature before administration. Monitor the patient for abdominal pressure, pain, fever, and electrolyte imbalance after the infusion; measure abdominal girth.[33]

Intrathecal route. Reconstitute all intrathecal medications with preservative-free sterile normal saline or sterile water. Medication may be infused through an Ommaya reservoir or implantable pump, if available, and/or through lumbar puncture. Usually the volume of medication given via an Ommaya reservoir or lumbar puncture is 15 ml or less. Maintain sterile technique throughout the procedure. The medication should be injected slowly. If chemotherapeutic drugs (cytarabine and/or methotrexate) are given in high doses, monitor the patient closely for potential neurotoxicity. Only a physician may administer intrathecal drugs via an Ommaya reservoir or lumbar puncture.[59]

Intravenous route. Drugs administered intravenously (IV) may be given through central venous catheters or peripheral venous access. Methods of administration include the following[88,89]:

- Push (bolus)—medication is administered through syringe directly into the vein.
- Piggyback (secondary setup)—drug is administered using a secondary bag (bottle) and tubing; primary infusion is concurrently maintained throughout drug administration.
- Side arm—drug is administered through a syringe and needle into the side port of a running (free-flowing) intravenous infusion.
- Infusion—drug is added to the prescribed volume of fluid in IV bag or bottle. Check for blood return before, during, and after infusion of chemotherapeutic drugs. Follow the agency's guidelines on how often continuous chemotherapeutic infusions are to be monitored. For continuous infusion of a vesicant drug, suggestions include validating blood return every 2 hours; for continuous infusion of a nonvesicant drug, validate blood return every 4 hours.[70,76]

Vein selection and venipuncture. Many chemotherapeutic agents irritate the veins and surrounding tissues. Venipuncture sites must be changed on a planned basis every 48 hours to reduce the possibility of phlebitis and infiltration. Peripheral sites should be changed daily before administration of vesicants. Veins suitable for venipuncture feel smooth and pliable, not hard or sclerotic. Select a vein that is large enough to allow adequate blood flow around the IV device.

Selection of the appropriate site and equipment is determined by the patient's age and vein status, the drugs to be infused, and the expected period of infusion. Observe and palpate the extremity. Use distal veins first, and choose a vein above areas of flexion. The distal veins of the hands and arms should be used first, and subsequent venipuncture should be done proximal to previous sites. Select the shortest catheter with the smallest gauge appropriate for the type and duration of the infusion. Veins commonly used include the basilic, cephalic, and metacarpal veins (Figure 22-3).

Large veins on the forearm are the preferred site. If a drug extravasates in this area, maximum soft tissue coverage is present to prevent functional impairment. Do not use the antecubital fossa and the wrist because extravasation in these areas can destroy nerves and tendons, resulting in loss of function.[88,89]

Procedure for administering chemotherapeutic drugs

- Verify the patient's identification, drug, dose, route, and time of administration with the physician's order.
- Review drug allergy history with the patient.
- Anticipate and plan for possible side effects or major system toxicity (Tables 22-1 and 22-2).
- Review appropriate laboratory data and other tests.
- Verify informed consent for treatment.
- Select appropriate equipment and supplies.
- Calculate the dose and reconstitute the drug using aseptic technique; follow safe handling guidelines.
- Explain the procedure to the patient and family.

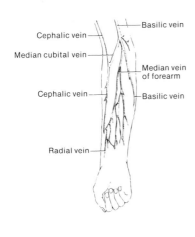

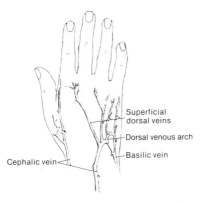

Figure 22-3 Venous anatomy. (From Perry A, Potter P: *Clinical nursing skills and techniques*, St Louis, 1986, Mosby.)

- Administer antiemetics or other prescribed medications.
- Initiate peripheral IV site and/or prepare central venous access site.
- Administer chemotherapeutic agents.
- Monitor the patient at scheduled intervals throughout the course of drug administration.
- Dispose of all used supplies and unused drugs in approved, puncture-proof, leak-proof containers outside of patient area.
- Document procedure according to agency policy and procedure.

Documentation recommendations
- Site assessment before and after infusion or injection of chemotherapeutic drug
- Establishment of blood return before, during, and after IV and intraarterial infusion of chemotherapy
- Establishment of catheter or device patency before, during, and after infusion of chemotherapy (e.g., intraperitoneal, intrathecal administration)
- Patient and family education about chemotherapy protocol: potential side effects and toxicities, self-

management of side effects, and schedule of follow-up blood counts, tests, and procedures
- Chemotherapeutic drug, dose, and route and time administered
- Premedications, postmedications, other infusions, and supplies used for chemotherapeutic regimen
- Any complaints by the patient of discomfort and symptoms experienced before, during, and after chemotherapeutic infusion[88,89]

SAFE HANDLING OF CHEMOTHERAPEUTIC AGENTS

The number of chemotherapeutic agents available and their use have increased considerably in recent years. Consequently, concern has emerged among health care workers about potential occupational hazards associated with the handling of these drugs. Clinical studies have indicated that many agents are carcinogenic, mutagenic, and teratogenic, or any combination of the three. Exposure to these chemotherapeutic agents can occur by inhalation, absorption, or digestion.[3,105,111] Safe handling guidelines should be followed when implementing policy and procedure within each agency that prepares, administers, stores, or disposes of supplies or unused chemotherapeutic agents.*[3,105]

Safe handling guidelines cover the following:
- Drug preparation
- Drug administration
- Disposal of supplies and unused drugs
- Management of spills
- Care of patients receiving chemotherapy (e.g., linen contamination, patient's excreta)
- Staff education
- Employment practice regarding reproductive health

Drug Preparation

To ensure safe handling, all chemotherapeutic drugs should be prepared according to the package insert in a class II biologic safety cabinet (BSC). Venting to the outside is desirable where feasible. Personal protective equipment includes disposable surgical latex gloves and a gown made of lint-free, low-permeability fabric with a closed front, long sleeves, and elastic or knit cuffs. Eye-protective splash goggles or a face shield must be worn when these drugs are prepared if BSC is not used.[3,105]

Gloves should be changed between preparation and administration of the drug and at least every 30 minutes

Text continued on p. 542.

---

*Recommendations for safe handling of chemotherapeutic drugs are available from the Occupational Safety and Health Administration (OSHA), the National Cytotoxic Study Commission, and the American Society of Hospital Pharmacists.

Table 22-1 Patient Teaching for Self-Management of Most Common Side Effects of Chemotherapeutic Drugs

Side effects	Points to cover
ACHES AND PAINS **Nursing action** Assess location, intensity, quality, and duration of pain	Pain medication should be taken on a regular schedule Side effects of pain medicine are constipation, dry mouth, and drowsiness Rest and relaxation strategies include music, progressive relaxation exercise, distraction, and positive imaging
ALOPECIA **Hair loss** Drugs associated with potential: cyclophosphamide, dacarbazine, dactinomycin, daunorubicin, doxorubicin, idarubicin, mechlorethamine, mitomycin, paclitaxel, topotecan, vinblastine, vinorelbine **Hair thinning** Drugs associated with potential: bleomycin, etoposide, 5-fluorouracil, floxuridine, vincristine	Hair loss occurs 10-21 days after drug treatment Hair loss is temporary, and hair will regrow when drug is discontinued Hair loss may occur suddenly and in large amounts; select wig, cap, scarf, or turban before hair loss occurs Avoid use of hair dryers, curling irons, and harsh or frequent shampoos Keep the head covered in summer to prevent a severe sunburn and in winter to prevent heat loss
ANOREXIA **Nursing action** Assess dietary history, monitor serum transferrin and weight loss	Eating is a social event; eat with others in a pleasant area with soft music and attractive settings Freshen up before meals, for example, with mouth care and exercise Small, frequent meals (five to six meals daily); avoid drinking fluids with meals to prevent feeling of fullness Concentrate on eating foods high in protein (e.g., eggs, milk products, peanut butter, tuna, beans, peas) Breakfast may be the most tolerable meal of the day; try to consume one third of daily calories at this time Monitor and record weight weekly; report weight loss
CONSTIPATION Drugs associated with potential: vinblastine, vincristine, vindesine, vinorelbine, narcotics **Nursing action** Determine normal bowel habits; advise patient not to strain with bowel evacuation and to respond immediately to urge to defecate	Increase intake of high-fiber foods (e.g., whole grain products, bran, fresh fruit, raw vegetables, popcorn) Increase fluid intake to 2-3 quarts of liquid daily; encourage fresh fruit juices, prunes, hot liquids on waking Follow prescribed schedule for use of stool softener; follow prescribed physician orders if patient has no bowel movement for 3 days or longer
CYSTITIS Drugs associated with potential: cyclophosphamide, ifosfamide **Nursing action** Observe urine for color and amount, and assess frequency of voiding; advise patient to take oral cyclophosphamide early in the day	Increase fluid intake to 3 quarts daily Empty bladder at least Q4hr especially at bedtime and at least once during the night Promptly report to physician increasing symptoms and frequency of bleeding, burning, pain, fever, chills
DEPRESSION **Nursing action** Assess for changes in mood, affect	Set small goals that are achievable daily Participate in enjoyable and diversionary activities (e.g., music, reading, outings) Share feelings and concerns with someone

From LaRocca JC, Otto SE, editors: *Pocket guide to intravenous therapy,* ed 3, St Louis, 1997, Mosby.

Table 22-1 Patient Teaching for Self-Management of Most Common Side Effects of Chemotherapeutic Drugs—cont'd

Side effects	Points to cover
DIARRHEA **Nursing action** Monitor serum fluid and electrolytes, as well as number, color, frequency, and consistency of diarrhea stools	Avoid eating high-roughage, greasy, and spicy foods; avoid using milk products or use boiled skim milk Avoid caffeine and alcoholic products and beverages Eat a bland diet Increase fluid intake to 3 quarts of liquid daily (weak, tepid tea; bouillon; grape juice) Record number and consistency of daily bowel movements; report information to physician Follow prescribed medication schedule if problem persists longer than 1 day Cleanse rectal area after each bowel movement
FATIGUE **Nursing action** Assess for possible causes (anemia, chronic pain, stress, depression, insufficient rest or nutritional intake)	Conserve energy, rest when tired, plan rest periods Plan for gradual accommodation of activities into life-style Monitor dietary and fluid intake daily
HEMATOPOIETIC CHANGES: LEUKOPENIA Most myelosuppressive agents produce white blood cell (WBC) nadir 7-14 days after drug administration; myelosuppression is severe and prolonged with increased dosages: for example, with cytarabine 3-6 g, busulfan 2-6 g, cyclophosphamide 2-3 g, methotrexate 6-8 g, etoposide 2-3 g **Nursing action** Monitor WBC and differential; change equipment as indicated—for example, oxygen (O_2) setup, denture cups, IV supplies; teach sexual hygiene	Avoid sources of infection, such as people with bacterial infections, colds, sore throats, flu, chickenpox, measles, or cold sores, or people recently vaccinated with live vaccines, such as measles-mumps-rubella (MMR) or diphtheria-pertussis-tetanus (DPT) Avoid having fresh fruit, plants, and flowers at or near bedside Avoid eating raw vegetables, fruits, and eggs Avoid cleaning animal litter boxes, since feces contain high levels of bacteria and fungi Maintain good personal hygiene—for example, bathe daily, wash hands before eating and preparing food, clean carefully after bowel movements, and keep nails clean and clipped short and straight across; maintain adequate fluid intake Conserve energy; get adequate rest and exercise Prevent trauma to skin and mucous membranes Avoid elective dental work or surgery Avoid enemas, use of rectal suppositories or thermometers, and catheterization Use toothettes or nonabrasive dental cleaning devices Report signs and symptoms of infection immediately to physician; for example, report fever of 100.4° F (38° C) or higher, cough, sore throat, shaking chill, painful or frequent urination, vaginal discharge
HEMATOPOIETIC CHANGES: THROMBOCYTOPENIA Drugs associated with delayed cumulative effect: mitomycin, nitrosureas **Nursing action** Monitor platelet counts; observe bleeding precautions; apply firm pressure to venipuncture site for 3-5 min; monitor pad count on menstruating girls and women; monitor environment for sharp objects	Avoid use of straight-edge razor, power tools, and physical activity that could cause injury Avoid use of drugs containing aspirin Humidify air; use lotion and lubricants on skin and lips; use soft bristle toothbrush Avoid invasive procedures: no intramuscular injections, rectal or vaginal examinations, enemas, suppositories, or use of rectal thermometers Discourage bare feet when ambulatory Use sanitary pads instead of tampons Immediately report these signs and symptoms to physician: bleeding gums, increased bruising, petechiae, purpura, hypermenorrhea, tarry stools, blood in urine, coffee ground emesis Check with physician before having any dental work

Continued.

Table 22-1 Patient Teaching for Self-Management of Most Common Side Effects of Chemotherapeutic Drugs—cont'd

Side effects	Points to cover
HEMATOPOIETIC CHANGES: ANEMIA **Nursing action** Monitor hematocrit and hemoglobin, especially during drug nadir	Adjust physical activity to accommodate rest periods Promptly report these signs and symptoms to physician: fatigue, dizziness, shortness of breath, palpitations
MUCOSITIS, RECTAL Symptoms occur 3-5 days after chemotherapy **Nursing action** Observe for electrolyte imbalance and monitor granulocyte count; monitor number, consistency, and amount of bowel movements and urine output; assess for rectal bleeding	Report weight loss to physician Eat low-residue, easily digestible foods Increase intake of liquids to replace fluid lost Follow prescribed medication schedule (e.g., antidiarrheal and pain-control drugs) Wash rectal area with soap and water after each bowel movement; pat or air dry
MUCOSITIS, VAGINAL Symptoms occur 3-5 days after chemotherapy and subside within 7-10 days after therapy	Report to physician any pain, ulceration, or bleeding of mucous membranes lining the perineum and vagina Sitz bath with warm saltwater may relieve vaginal itching and odor Use hydrogen peroxide (one quarter strength) with warm water after voiding to rinse perineal area Avoid commercial douches, tampons, and vaginal pads or liners containing deodorants
NAUSEA AND VOMITING Drugs with high emetic potential: cisplatin, dacarbazine, dactinomycin, daunorubicin, doxorubicin, mechlorethamine, paclitaxel; high-dose cytarabine, cyclophosphamide, and methotrexate **Nursing action** Premedicate with antiemetic before nausea begins, for example, 30 min before meals; patient may require routine antiemetics for 3-5 days after some chemotherapy protocols; monitor fluid and electrolyte status	Eat frequent, small meals Avoid greasy or fatty foods and very sweet foods or candies Avoid unpleasant sights, odors, and tastes Cold foods, salty foods, dry crackers, and dry toast may be more tolerable If vomiting is severe, restrict diet to clear liquids and notify physician Consider diversionary activities (e.g., music therapy, relaxation techniques) Recall strategies used successfully during pregnancy, illness, or other times of stress, such as, sipping on a flat cola drink
PHARYNGITIS AND ESOPHAGITIS Symptoms often are first noted by difficult or painful swallowing	Eat soft pureed or liquid diet Follow prescribed scheduled medication to relieve discomfort Report to physician any symptoms that persist longer than 3 days
SKIN CHANGES	Maintain good personal hygiene Use topical preparations to minimize itching (e.g., creams or lotions containing vitamins A, D, or E) Do not use perfume or perfumed lotion; avoid wearing fabrics such as wool or corduroy and tight-fitting clothing such as jeans or pantyhose
STOMATITIS, ORAL Symptoms occur 5-7 days after chemotherapy and persist up to 10 days	Continue brushing regularly; use soft toothbrush Use nonirritant mouthwash, such as a salt, soda, and water solution (¼ tsp salt, pinch of soda, 8 oz water) at least 4 times daily Avoid irritants to the mouth (e.g., tobacco, alcoholic beverages, spices, commercial mouthwashes) Avoid wearing dentures until mouth soreness abates Maintain good nutritional intake; eat soft or liquid foods high in protein; add sauces or gravies to foods to thin and moisten them Follow prescribed medication schedule, such as scheduled drugs for oral candidiasis Report persistent symptoms promptly to physician, and report any white patches on the tongue, back of the throat, or gums

Table 22-2 Major System Toxicity or Dysfunction and Nursing Management

Toxicity/dysfunction	Nursing management
CARDIAC TOXICITY Drugs associated with potential: chlorambucil, cyclophosphamide, daunorubicin, doxorubicin, mitoxantrone, high-dose ifosfamide	Verify baseline cardiac studies (e.g., electrocardiogram [ECG], ejection fraction, cardiac enzymes) before drug administration Monitor cardiac status and report symptoms such as tachycardia, shortness of breath, distended neck veins, gallop heart rhythm, ankle edema Monitor and record total cumulative dose of drug in patient's medical record; for example, the approximate maximum lifetime dose of doxorubicin is 500 mg/m^2
HEMATOPOIETIC TOXICITY (See Table 22-1) **HEPATIC TOXICITY** Drugs associated with potential: asparaginase, busulfan, carmustine, chlorambucil, cytarabine, doxorubicin, lomustine, mercaptopurine, methotrexate, mithramycin, streptozocin	Monitor liver function studies, such as lactate dehydrogenase (LDH), bilirubin, prothrombin time, and liver function tests (aspartate aminotransferase [SGOT] and alanine aminotransferase [SGPT]) Report to physician any signs of jaundice, tenderness over liver, and urine and stool color changes
HYPERSENSITIVITY REACTION Drugs associated with potential: asparaginase, bleomycin, docetaxel, doxorubicin (local erythema), etoposide, paclitaxel, teniposide	Review patient's allergy history Monitor for symptoms of hypersensitivity and anaphylaxis (e.g., agitation, urticaria, rash, chills, cyanosis, bronchospasm, abdominal cramping, hypotension); onset may be rapid or delayed; advise patient to report subjective symptoms promptly Make sure that proper medical equipment is nearby and in good working condition Drugs for emergency intervention should be readily available When administering a drug with potential for a reaction: give test dose, monitor vital signs, and observe for allergic response If allergic response occurs, stop drug administration and notify physician immediately
METABOLIC ALTERATIONS **Hypercalcemia**	Monitor serum calcium; observe for anorexia, constipation, nausea, vomiting, polyuria, mental status change
Hyperglycemia	Monitor serum and urine glucose; observe for symptoms of thirst, hunger, glucosuria, weight loss
Hyperkalemia	Monitor serum potassium; observe for symptoms of confusion, complaints of numbness or tingling, weakness, cardiac arrhythmias
Hypernatremia	Monitor serum sodium and weight loss; observe for symptoms of thirst; dry mucous membranes; poor skin turgor; rapid, thready pulse; restlessness, lethargy
Hyperuricemia Potential with treatment of highly proliferative tumors (e.g., leukemia, lymphoma)	Monitor serum and urine uric acid; as well as daily intake and output Initiate prescribed drug therapy (e.g., allopurinol) to inhibit formation of uric acid before administration of chemotherapeutic drug Provide vigorous hydration, such as oral and IV fluid intake (2000-3000 ml), beginning 12-24 hr after initiation of chemotherapy Alkalize urine to pH $\geq$ 7.0 by administering sodium bicarbonate (NaHCO$_3$) IV Report symptoms of pain, chills, fever, diminished urinary output

From LaRocca JC, Otto SE, editors: *Pocket guide to intravenous therapy,* ed 3, St Louis, 1997, Mosby.

Continued.

Table 22-2 Major System Toxicity or Dysfunction and Nursing Management—cont'd

Toxicity/dysfunction	Nursing management
Hypocalcemia	Monitor serum calcium; observe for symptoms of muscle cramping, tingling of extremities, depression, tetany
Hypomagnesemia	Monitor serum magnesium; observe for symptoms of personality change, anorexia, nausea, vomiting, lethargy, weakness, tetany
Hyponatremia	Monitor serum sodium; observe for symptoms of rales, shortness of breath, distended neck veins, weight gain, edema of sacrum or lower extremity, increasing changes in mental status
NEUROTOXICITY Drugs associated with potential: ifosfamide, vinblastine, vincristine, high peak plasma levels of etoposide, 5-fluorouracil; high-dose and/or intrathecal administration of cytarabine, cisplatin, and methotrexate	Monitor for and report symptoms of weakness and numbness and tingling in hands, arms, and feet; also hoarseness, jaw pain, hallucinations, mental depression, decreased or absent deep tendon reflexes, slapping gait or foot drop, severe constipation, paralytic ileus
OTOTOXICITY Drug associated with potential: cisplatin	Verify baseline audiogram Monitor for and report symptoms of tinnitus, hearing loss, vertigo
PULMONARY TOXICITY Drugs associated with potential: bleomycin, busulfan, carmustine	Verify baseline respiratory function Individuals over age 70 are at greater risk Monitor respiratory status and report to physician symptoms of dyspnea, dry cough, rales, tachypnea, fever
RENAL SYSTEM TOXICITY Drugs associated with potential: cisplatin, cyclophosphamide, ifosfamide, methotrexate, mithramycin, streptozocin, thioplex (thiotepa)	Assess 24-hr urine creatinine clearance before treatment Verify baseline renal function Encourage adequate fluid intake (e.g., 2-3 L for 24 hr before and after therapy) Monitor intake and output and weight changes Report diminished output to physician (e.g., less than 500 ml in 24 hr) Administer drug MESNA concomitantly with ifosfamide and with high-dose cyclophosphamide and thiotepa
REPRODUCTIVE SYSTEM DYSFUNCTION Drugs associated with potential: busulfan, chlorambucil, cyclophosphamide, mechlorethamine, thiotepa, vincristine Antihormonal agents: finasteride, flutamide, leuprolide, tamoxifen, goserelin	Assess for nature and frequency of sexual dysfunction Counsel patients about avoiding pregnancy and about sperm banking before administration of chemotherapy; provide information on contraceptives Most practitioners recommend that patients follow birth control practices for 2 yr after chemotherapy to allow for evaluation of disease response, to avoid possible teratogenic drug effects and, in men, to allow recovery of spermatogenesis Inform patient of potential for temporary or permanent infertility and loss of libido Women may experience symptoms such as amenorrhea, "hot flashes," insomnia, dyspareunia, and vaginal dryness; estrogen therapy may be helpful in managing these symptoms

during preparation and administration. Suggestions to minimize exposure include:
- Wash hands before and after drug handling.
- Limit access to drug preparation area.
- Keep labeled drug spill kit near preparation area.
- Put on gloves before handling drugs.

- Use aseptic technique when preparing drugs.
- Avoid eating, drinking, smoking, chewing gum, applying cosmetics, or storing food in or near drug preparation area.
- Place absorbent pad on work surface.
- Use Luer-Lok equipment.

- Open drug vials and ampules away from body.
- Vent vials with a hydrophobic filter needle or pin to prevent spraying of drug.
- Wrap alcohol wipe around neck of ampule before opening.
- Prime lines containing drugs inside BSC using original drug vial or a zip-close plastic bag.
- Cover tip of needle with sterile gauze or alcohol wipe when expelling air from syringe.
- Label all chemotherapeutic drugs.
- Clean up any spills immediately.
- Transport drugs to delivery area in a leak-proof container.

Drug Administration

- Wear protective equipment (gloves, gown, eyewear; Figure 22-4).[3,21,88,105]
- Explain to the patient that chemotherapeutic drugs are harmful to normal cells and that protective measures used by personnel minimize their exposure to these drugs.
- Administer drugs in a safe, unhurried environment.
- Place a plastic-backed absorbent pad under the tubing during administration to catch any leakage.
- Do not dispose of any supplies or unused drugs in patient care areas (see next section).

Disposal of Supplies and Unused Drugs

- Do not clip or recap needles or break syringes.
- Place all used supplies intact in a leak-proof, puncture-proof, appropriately labeled container.
- Place all unused drugs in containers in a leak-proof, closeable, puncture-proof, appropriately labeled container; keep these containers in every area where drugs are prepared or administered so that waste materials need not be moved from one area to another.[88,105]
- Dispose of containers filled with chemotherapeutic supplies and unused drugs in accordance with regulations of hazardous wastes (e.g., in a licensed sanitary landfill, or incinerate at 1832° F (1000° C).

Management of Chemotherapy Spills

Chemotherapy spills should be cleaned up immediately by properly protected personnel trained in the appropriate procedures. A spill should be identified with a warning sign so that other people will not be contaminated. The following are recommended supplies and procedures for managing a chemotherapy spill on hard surfaces, linens, personnel, and patients[5,88,105]:

Supplies[105]
- Chemotherapy spill kit (Figure 22-5)
  —Respirator mask for airborne powder spills
  —Plastic safety glasses or goggles
  —Heavy-duty rubber gloves
  —Absorbent pads to contain liquid spills

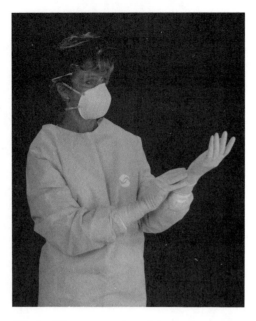

Figure 22-4 Woman wearing gloves, gown, eyewear, and mask. (Courtesy Biosafety Systems, Inc, San Diego, Calif.)

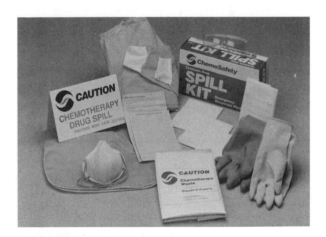

Figure 22-5 Chemotherapy spill kit. (Courtesy Biosafety Systems, Inc, San Diego, Calif.)

  —Absorbent towels for cleanup after spill
  —Small scoop to collect glass fragments
  —Two large waste disposal bags
- Protective disposable gown
- Containers of detergent solution and clear tapwater for postspill cleanup
- Puncture-proof, leak-proof closeable container approved for chemotherapy waste disposal
- Approved, specially labeled, impervious laundry bag
- Eyewash faucet adapters or fountain in or near work area[105]

Procedure for spill on hard surface[105]
- Restrict area of spill.
- Obtain drug spill kit.

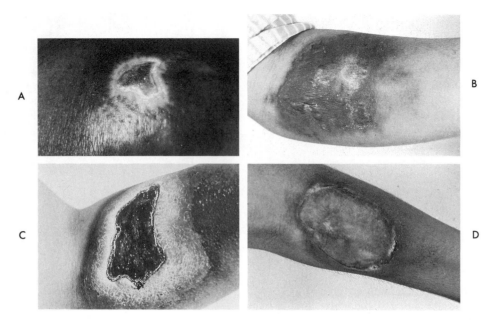

Figure 22-6 **A,** Cutaneous effects of vesicant extravasation; note central necrosis and surrounding erythema and induration. **B,** Lateral progression of initial cutaneous effects, which occurs over a period of weeks. **C,** Eschar requiring surgical debridement eventually develops. **D,** Wide surgical excision of involved area on forearm. (Courtesy Robert Dorr, University of Arizona, *Progressions* 2(4):4, 1990, Mosby.)

- Put on protective gown, gloves, and goggles and, if powder spill is involved, a respirator mask.
- Open waste disposal bags (double bag).
- Place absorbent pads gently on spill, being careful not to touch it.
- Place saturated absorbent pads in waste bag.
- Clean surface with absorbent towels using detergent solution and rinse clean with clean tapwater. Wipe dry.
- Place all contaminated materials (e.g., gown, gloves, saturated absorbent pads, towels) in double-bagged waste disposal bags.
- Discard waste bag and contents in approved container.
- Wash hands thoroughly with soap and water.
  Procedure for spill on linen[105]
- Restrict area of spill.
- Obtain drug spill kit.
- Obtain specially marked, approved laundry bag and labeled, impervious bag.
- Put on protective gown, gloves, and goggles.
- Remove soiled, contaminated linen from patient's bedside.
- Place linen in approved, specially marked, impervious laundry bag.
- Contaminated linen should be washed two times in the laundry; laundry personnel should wear surgical latex gloves and gown when handling this material.
- Clean contaminated area with absorbent towels and detergent solution.

- Place all contaminated supplies used for management of spill in waste disposal bag and discard in approved waste disposal container.
- Wash hands thoroughly with soap and water.
  Procedure for spill on personnel or patient[105]
- Restrict area of spill.
- Obtain drug spill kit.
- Immediately remove contaminated protective garments or linen.
- Wash affected area of skin with soap and water.
- *Eye exposure:* immediately flood affected eye with water for at least 5 minutes; obtain medical attention promptly.
- Follow procedures for contaminated linen.
- Notify physician if drug spills on patient.
  Documentation[105]
- Document in patient's medical record the management of the drug spill and notification of the patient's physician.
- Document on the agency's approved forms the management of the spill and whether it occurred on a hard surface, linen, or individual.

Caring for Patients Receiving Chemotherapeutic Drugs

Personnel handling blood, vomitus, or excreta from patients who have received chemotherapy within the previous 48 hours should wear disposable surgical latex gloves and gowns, which are discarded appropriately after use. Linen contaminated with chemotherapeutic drugs, blood, vomitus, or excreta from a patient who has received these drugs within 48 hours before should be placed in a specially marked, impervious laundry bag according to procedures for drug spills on linen.[21,105,111]

Staff Education

All personnel involved in any aspect of the handling of chemotherapeutic agents should receive an orientation to chemotherapeutic drugs, including their known risks, relevant techniques and procedures for handling, proper use of protective equipment and materials, spill procedures, and medical policies covering personnel handling chemotherapeutic agents who are pregnant or actively trying to conceive children (per OSHA requirements). Staff compliance can be evaluated through regular quality monitoring.[10,21,28,105]

Employment Practices Regarding Reproductive Issues

The handling of chemotherapeutic agents by women who either are pregnant or are actively trying to conceive and by those who are breast-feeding remains a sensitive and unsettled issue. Some suggest offering these employees the opportunity to transfer to areas that do not involve chemotherapeutic agents. All safe handling guidelines should be practiced with utmost care by all pregnant personnel.[6,15,21]

Extravasation Management

Vesicant extravasation is the accidental leakage of a drug that causes pain, necrosis, or sloughing of tissue into the subcutaneous tissue. A vesicant is an agent that can produce a blister or tissue destruction, or both. An irritant is an agent that can cause aching, tightness, and phlebitis at the injection site or along the vein line with or without an inflammatory reaction. A flare is a local allergic reaction without pain that usually is accompanied by red blotches along the vein line. Symptoms subside within 30 minutes with or without treatment.[13]

Injuries that may occur as the result of extravasation include tissue sloughing, infection, pain, and loss of mobility in an extremity. The degree of tissue damage is related to several factors, including drug vesicant potential, drug concentration, amount of drug extravasated, duration of tissue exposure,[2,9,52,76] veinpuncture site/device, and needle insertion technique and individual tissue responses (Figure 22-6). *Delayed extravasation* is an extravasation in which symptoms occur 48 hours after the drug is administered.[13]

Because of the harmful effect of vesicants on tissues, studies in human subjects are limited; thus controlled clinical trials demonstrating the effectiveness of treatment have been difficult to achieve. Most extravasation interventions have been based on preclinical studies using animal models, including mice, pigs, rabbits, and dogs. Treatment strategies for managing extravasation involve using specific antidotes and guidelines for immediate intervention to minimize tissue damage. Preventing extravasation and instituting prompt intervention are the key elements for successful management. Tissue destruction from drug extravasation may be subtle and progressive. Initial symptoms include pain or burning at the intravenous (IV) site, progressing to erythema, edema, and superficial skin loss (Figures 22-7 and 22-8). Tissue necrosis may not develop for 1 to 4 weeks after extravasation.* A list of nonvesicant chemotherapeutic drugs follows†:

Generic name	Trade name
Asparaginase	Elspar
Bleomycin	Blenoxane
Carboplatin	Paraplatin
Cisplatin	Platinol
Cladribine	Luestatin
Cyclophosphamide	Cytoxan
Cytarabine (ara-C)	Cytosar-u
Docetaxel‡	Taxotere
Floxuridine	FUDR
Fludarabine	Fludara
Fluorouracil	Efudex
Ifosfamide	IFEX
Methotrexate	Methotrexate
Mitoxantrone	Novantrone
Paclitaxel‡	Taxol
Pentostatin	Deoxycoformycin
Topotecan	
Thiotepa	Thioplex

Chemotherapeutic drugs with vesicant potential include†:

Generic name	Trade name
Dactinomycin	Actinomycin D, Cosmegen
Daunorubicin	Cerubidine, Daunomycin
Doxorubicin	Adriamycin
Epirubicin	Pharmorubin
Esorubicin	4-Deoxydrorubicin
Idarubicin	Idamycin
Mechlorethamine	Nitrogen Mustard, Mustargen
Mitomycin C	Mutamycin
Menogaril	Tomasar
Piroxantrone	Oxantrazole
Plicamycin	Mithracin
Vinblastine	Velban
Vincristine	Oncovin
Vindesine	Eldisine
Vinorelbine	Navelbine

---

*References 2, 9, 29, 34, 35, 76.

†From LaRocca JC, Otto SE, editors: *Pocket guide to intravenous therapy,* ed 3, St Louis, 1997, Mosby.

‡Recent documentation of vesicant potential (*Oncol Nurs Forum* 23[3]:541, 1996.)

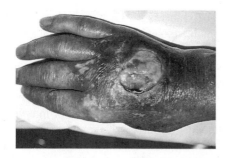

Figure 22-7 Doxorubicin extravasation in dorsum of right hand; note depth of wound. (From *Progressions* 2(4):4, 1990, Mosby.)

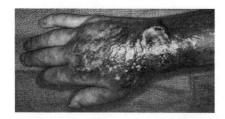

Figure 22-8 One month after doxorubicin extravasation in dorsum of right hand. (Courtesy Robert Dorr, University of Arizona, *Progressions* 2(4):4, 1990, Mosby.)

Chemotherapeutic drugs with irritant potential are*:

Generic name	Trade name
Carmustine (BCNU)	BiCNU
Dacarbazine	DITC-Dome
Etoposide	VePesid
Mitoguazone	Methyl-GAG, MGBG
Streptozocin	Zanosar
Teniposide	Vumon

Controversial Topics†[88,89]

Management of extravasation of chemotherapeutic drugs involves some controversial issues.

Use of antecubital fossa for drug administration
Favor antecubital fossa access
- Larger veins permit faster infusion of drug.
- Larger veins permit potentially irritating drugs to reach the general circulation sooner with less irritation.

Oppose antecubital fossa access
- Arm mobility is restricted.
- Infiltration may require extensive reconstructive efforts.

---

*From LaRocca JC, Otto SE, editors: *Pocket guide to intravenous therapy*, ed 3, St Louis, 1997, Mosby.
†Adapted from Oncology Nursing Society Task Force: *Cancer chemotherapy guidelines and recommendations for nursing education and practice: 1996 guidelines*, Pittsburgh, 1996, The Society.

- Early infiltration may be difficult to assess.
- Potential for venous fibrosis; blood drawing from antecubital fossa may be more difficult.

Methods of drug sequencing
Favor administering vesicants first
- Vascular integrity declines over time.
- Initial assessment of vein patency is most accurate.
- Possibility of diminishing patient awareness of symptoms related to drug infiltration.

Favor administering vesicants last
- Vesicants are irritating and may increase fragility of veins.
- Venous spasm may occur at onset of drug administration and alter assessment of venous access.

Needle or catheter size
Favor large gauge (18-19)
- Irritating chemotherapeutic agents can reach circulation sooner with less irritating effect on peripheral veins.

Favor small gauge (20-23)
- Smaller-gauge devices are less likely to puncture the wall of a small vein.
- Increased blood flow around a smaller gauge device increases dilution of chemotherapeutic agents.
- Phlebitis may be minimized with smaller gauge device.

Prevention of Extravasation[52,76,88,89]

Nursing staff responsibilities for preventing extravasation include the following:
- Acquiring a knowledge of drugs with vesicant potential (see list on p. 545).
- Explaining the vesicant potential to the patient before administering the drug, to obtain true informed consent for this treatment. This practice can significantly aid in identifying an early extravasation if one should occur.[13]
- Developing skill in drug administration.
- Identifying risk factors (e.g., multiple venipunctures, previous treatment).
- Anticipating extravasation and being knowledgeable about the approved management protocol.
- Obtaining a new venipuncture site daily if peripheral access is used.
- Considering central venous access if peripheral access is difficult.
- Being aware that most sources recommend 24-hour vesicant infusion via central venous access only.
- Administering the drug in a quiet, unhurried environment.
- Testing vein patency without using chemotherapeutic agents.
- Providing adequate drug dilution (e.g., side port infusion via free-flowing IV infusion)
- Carefully observing the access site and extremity throughout the procedure.

Table 22-3 Chemotherapeutic Vesicant Drugs with Recommended Antidotes

Drug	Antidote
ALKYLATING AGENTS Mechlorethamine (Mustargen, Nitrogen Mustard), Mitomycin C (Mutamycin)	Isotonic Sodium thiosulfate 1/6 molar, 4.4 g/10 ml Dilute 1.6 ml of sodium thiosulfate 25% with 8.4 ml of sterile water for injection; apply cold compresses
ANTIBIOTICS Daunorubicin (Daunomycin, Cerubidine) Doxorubicin (Adriamycin)	Apply *ice cold* compresses immediately for 30-60 min Alternate protocol: topical dimethyl sulfoxide (DMSO) 1-2 ml of 1 mmol DMSO 50%-100%; apply topically one time at site; apply *cold* compresses
BISANTRENE	Sodium bicarbonate 1 mEq/ml Mix equal parts of sodium bicarbonate with sterile normal saline (1:1 solution); resulting solution is 0.5 mEq/ml Inject 2-6 ml (1-3 mEq) IV through existing IV line and SQ into extravasated site; apply cold compresses
***VINCA* ALKALOIDS** Teniposide Vinblastine Vincristine Vindesine Vinorelbine	Hyaluronidase (Wydase) 150 U/ml Add 1 ml sterile sodium chloride Inject 1-6 ml (150-900 U) SQ into extravasated site with multiple injections; apply warm compresses; **do not** inject corticosteroids
DRUGS WITH NO KNOWN SPECIFIC ANTIDOTES Dactinomycin Epirubicin Esorubicin Idarubicin Menogaril Mitoxantrone Piroxantrone	
TAXANES Docetaxel (Taxotere) Paclitaxel (Taxol)	 Specific treatment for extravasation unknown at this time* Specific treatment for extravasation unknown at this time*

From LaRocca JC, Otto SE, editors: *Pocket guide to intravenous therapy,* ed 3, St Louis, 1997, Mosby.
*Recent documentation of vesicant potential (*Oncol Nurs Forum* 23[3]:541, 1996).

- Validating blood return from the intravenous site before, during, and after infusion of the vesicant drug.
- Educating patients about the symptoms of drug infiltration (e.g., pain, burning and stinging sensations at intravenous site).

Protocol for Extravasation Management at a Peripheral Site

Agency policy and procedure for management of extravasation with the responsible physician's prescription should be easily accessible to the staff. The approved antidotes should be readily available, and the following procedure should be initiated with a physician's prescription as soon as extravasation of a vesicant or irritant agent is suspected or occurs.[52,76,88,89]

- Stop the chemotherapeutic drug infusion.
- Leave the needle or catheter in place.
- Aspirate any residual drug and blood in the IV tubing,

needle, or catheter and suspected infiltration site.
- Instill the IV antidote (Table 22-3).
- Remove the needle.
- If unable to aspirate the residual drug from the IV tubing, remove the needle or catheter.
- Inject the antidote subcutaneously (SQ) clockwise into the infiltrated site using a 25-gauge needle; change the needle with each new infection.
- Avoid applying pressure to the suspected infiltration site.
- Photograph the suspected area of extravasation according to the agency's policy and procedure for documentation and follow-up.
- Apply a topical ointment if ordered.
- Cover lightly with an occlusive sterile dressing.
- Apply cold or warm compresses as indicated (see Table 22-3).
- Elevate the extremity.

- Observe regularly for pain, erythema, induration, and necrosis.
- Documentation of extravasation management:
  —Date
  —Time
  —Needle or catheter size and type
  —Insertion site
  —Drug sequence
  —Approximate amount of drug extravasated
  —Nursing management of extravasation
  —Photographic documentation
  —Patient's complaints and statements
  —Appearance of site
  —Notification of physician
  —Follow-up measures
  —Nurse's signature

Anaphylaxis

Nursing personnel administering chemotherapy in all settings should follow the listed guidelines for drug preparation, administration and disposal, vein selection, documentation of drug infusion, selection of venous access device and possible side effects, teaching of the patient about self-management of most common side effects, and management of chemotherapy spills and drug extravasation.[28,76] In addition to these guidelines, all

Table 22-4 Chemotherapeutic Drugs with Potential for Anaphylaxis

Drugs	Signs and symptoms	Precautions
Asparaginase (Elspar) *Test Dose Procedure:* Prepare 10,000 IU asparaginase with 5 ml NS; inject 0.1 ml of this solution (200 IU) into 9.9 ml NS; inject 0.1 ml of this concentration (2 IU) intradermally to make a wheal in inner aspect of arm; observe wheal for 60 minutes for erythema, swelling, and itching before doing infusion.	Respiratory distress, increased pulse, respirations, hypotension, facial edema, anxiety, flushed appearance, hives, itching; risk for anaphylaxis increases with each dose	Test dose before initial IV/IM dosing; monitor 30 min IM or 60 min IV after drug administration; keep vein open with IV normal saline before, during, and 30/60 min after IV administration of asparaginase. Initiate drug infusion slowly (mg/m^2/titrate infusion). Code Care; O_2, suction, drugs for anaphylaxis at or near patient's bedside
Bleomycin *Test Dose Procedure:* Inject 2 U of bleomycin intradermally to make a wheal in inner aspect of arm; observe for erythema or edema and itching before first 2 doses of bleomycin are infused	Dyspnea, hypotension, increased pulse and respiration, rash	Test dose before initial IV dosing; initiate drug infusion slowly (10-20 ml/15 min); monitor vital signs and auscultate breath sounds Q4hr during infusion and for 24 hours afterward, and/or on scheduled basis in outpatient setting
Etoposide (VP-16)	Hypotension, bronchospasm, chest pain, increased pulse and respirations, facial flush, fever, chills, diaphoresis	Initiate drug infusion slowly (10-20 ml/15 min). Infuse total volume over at least 60 min. Monitor vital signs Q15 min × 4; Q30 min × 2; and Q4hr during and for 24 hours after infusion
Teniposide (VM-26)	Severe hypotension, anxiety, increased pulse and respirations, fever	Initiate drug infusion *slowly* (10-20 ml/30 min). Total infusion time 60-120 min. Monitor vital signs Q15 min × 4; Q30 min × 2 during and after infusion; then monitor Q4hr × 24 hours
Paclitaxel (Taxol) Docetaxel (Taxotere)	Increased or decreased BP, increased temperature and pulse, restlessness, dyspnea, bronchospasm, facial flushing, hives *If any of these symptoms occur, stop drug infusion and notify physician immediately*	Premedicate with the following before Taxol or Taxotere infusion: dexamethasone 10-20 mg PO/IV 12-16 hr; diphenhydramine 50 mg IV push 30-60 min; cimetidine 300 mg IV over 30 min; infuse Taxol/Taxotere in a glass bottle with non-PVC tubing and a 0.22 μm filter; obtain baseline VS, then monitor Q15 min × 4, Q1 hr × 4, and Q4 hr × 4 during infusion. Ensure that emergency medications (Benadryl 50 mg, hydrocortisone 100 mg, adrenaline [epinephrine] 1:1000—all IV bolus), as well as O_2 and suction equipment are assembled and ready for use

From LaRocca JC, Otto SE, editors: *Pocket guide to intravenous therapy,* ed 3, St Louis, 1997, Mosby.
BP, Blood pressure; *IM,* intramuscular; *NS,* normal saline; *PO,* oral; *PVC,* polyvinyl chloride; *VS,* vital signs.

nursing personnel should be alert and prepared for the possible complications of anaphylaxis. The drugs and supplies needed to manage these complications must be readily available.[8,38] The nurse must be informed about and prepared for the specific drugs known to pose a risk of anaphylaxis. Test dosing before infusing the drug and following infusion precautions reduces the occurrence of anaphylaxis (Table 22-4).[57,59] Emergency medications and supplies for managing anaphylaxis include:

- Injectable aminophylline, diphenhydramine hydrochloride (Benadryl), dopamine, epinephrine, heparin, hydrocortisone
- Oxygen setup, tubing cannula, or mask and airway device
- Suction equipment
- IV fluids (isotonic solutions)
- IV tubings and supplies for venous access

Prompt, effective nursing intervention for anaphylaxis reduces complications. The nurse must be alert to the signs and symptoms of an anaphylactic response to a chemotherapeutic drug. All or some of these symptoms may be present: anxiety, hypotension, urticaria, cyanosis, respiratory distress, abdominal cramping, flushed appearance, and chills. The calm, reassuring presence of the nurse facilitates management of these symptoms, which proceeds as follows[88]:

- Immediately stop the drug infusion.
- Maintain an intravenous line with isotonic saline.
- Position the patient for comfort and to promote perfusion of the vital organs.
- Notify the physician, nursing agency and/or emergency medical services.
- Maintain the airway and anticipate the need for cardiopulmonary resuscitation.
- Monitor the vital signs according to agency policy.
- Administer the appropriate medications with an approved physician's order.
- Follow the nursing agency's protocol for follow-up care (e.g., evaluation of the patient by a physician).
- Document the incident in the patient's medical record.

An anaphylactic episode is very upsetting to the patient and family. Follow-up care is required to diminish their anxiety and to monitor for delayed side effects. Instruct the patient and family in the pertinent drug side effects, when and where to call for assistance, and what symptoms require immediate health care intervention (shortness of breath, rash on the body that increases in size and intensity, flushed appearance, fever, chills, abdominal cramping, feeling of anxiousness).[91,98]

ALTERNATIVE CARE SETTINGS

Improved drug delivery, cost containment, and consideration of the quality of life have affected trends in chemotherapy administration. Management of symptoms, such as controlling nausea and vomiting and innovative pain management, have reduced the need for hospitalization. Options for giving chemotherapy in outpatient settings include ambulatory care centers, physicians' offices, extended care facilities, and home health agencies. Certain principles of chemotherapy administration and standards of care for patients must be maintained by the staff regardless of the setting.[88,89,99,111]

Home health care will expand in the next decade. Oncology patients are now and will continue to be a major segment of this population of patients. Criteria specific to home administration of chemotherapy include (1) a caregiver is available who is able and willing to assist; (2) the patient's physical condition is stable and within the range of home care capabilities; (3) living conditions are stable and suitable, (cleanliness, plumbing, refrigeration, telephone); and (4) the patient has access to emergency assistance.[9,19,99]

Patients and family members involved in the infusion of chemotherapeutic drugs or the management of side effects, or both, require verbal, written, demonstration, and return demonstration procedural information. Following are suggested nursing interventions to facilitate education of the patient and family in drug administration in the home.[91,98]

Interventions

- Assess the patient's ability and willingness to learn, the availability of a caregiver, the home environment, the patient's ability to assume self-care, and compliance with the treatment regimen.
- Describe the purpose, schedule, and procedure of the chemotherapeutic regimen.
- Explain to the patient the possible side effects of chemotherapeutic drugs (nausea and vomiting, anorexia, stomatitis, constipation, diarrhea, alopecia, skin and hematopoietic changes).[37]
- Instruct the patient or caregiver in dealing with specific side effects.[25]
- Review symptoms, such as temperature elevation over 100.4° F (38° C), severe constipation or diarrhea, persistent bleeding from any site, sudden weight gain or loss, shortness of breath, pain that is not relieved by prescribed medications, and severe nausea and vomiting more than 24 hours after treatment. Emphasize the importance of promptly reporting these symptoms to the physician.[38]
- Instruct the patient or caregiver in the management of infusion devices.[91]
- Validate the aseptic technique and skills of the patient or caregiver for prescribed self-administration and discontinuation of chemotherapeutic drugs.
- Explain the safe handling precautions for administration and disposal of chemotherapeutic drugs.[19,28]
- Provide information and a list of resources for obtain-

ing, storing, and disposing of drugs and supplies. Also provide a schedule of follow-up tests and care.[49,82]

- Record the drug, dose, route, and time given in the home and provide this information to the agency responsible for care management.[82,87]
- Discard all unused drugs and used supplies in a recommended puncture-proof, leak-proof, closeable container. Return this container to the appropriate agency for disposal (Figure 22-9).[88,89]
- Use plastic sheeting to protect bedding or furniture if incontinence is possible.
- Carefully handle linen contaminated by chemotherapeutic drugs and excreta, and wash twice, separately from all other linen.[56,58]
- It is recommended that the patient receive the first chemotherapy dose in an acute care or outpatient setting.

FUTURE DIRECTIONS AND ADVANCES IN CHEMOTHERAPY

Future directions in chemotherapy offer many exciting opportunities. The use of effective adjuvant, neoadjuvant, and combination chemotherapies, as well as use of chemotherapy in combination with other treatment modalities, will increase. Continuing drug research will focus on new drug development and dose intensity schedules for most of the major cancer diseases, use of circadian chronotherapy, and chemoprevention. The emergence and ground swell of managed care packages, along with changes in insurance coverage, will demand an ambulatory/short-stay program for most chemotherapy administration. The "graying" of our population will create a larger population of oncology patients, whether for screening and detection, treatment, or palliative care.

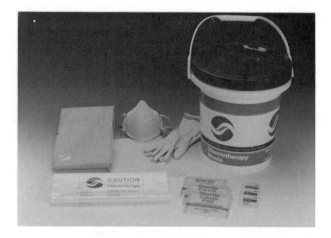

Figure 22-9 Home health care kit. (Courtesy Biosafety Systems, Inc, San Diego, Calif.)

This will evolve into the need for drugs that have greater efficacy, are administered in a timely fashion, and cause few or no side effects. The problem limiting the efficacy of chemotherapeutic drugs is the presence of drug resistance at the onset of therapy or the development of resistance during the course of therapy.

CANCER CARE FOR THE ELDERLY

A combination of recent factors, such as the increasing number of older people in the population and the increasing number of older people with cancer, has brought to the forefront the need to understand the special problems involved in treating older cancer patients. It is estimated that the number of Americans over age 85 will increase fourfold between 1980 and 2030. The incidence of cancer increases with age; the risk for a person over age 65 of developing cancer is 10 times that of a younger person.[26] Even though more than half of all cancers are diagnosed in people over age 67, studies rarely consistently enroll patients over age 70.[61]

The physiologic changes that occur with biologic aging are an important consideration in the treatment of cancer and chemotherapy pharmacokinetics. The hematopoietic system's inability to respond as readily as in a younger person partly determines the selection of chemotherapeutic agents and dose intensities and imposes an increased risk of infection. A gradual wasting of body muscle mass and an increase in fat can influence drug distribution, and decreased liver function and renal excretion affect drug metabolism and excretion. Cardiovascular changes must be taken into account when considering cardiotoxic chemotherapeutic agents or surgery as a cancer treatment modality.[107]

In the older age-group, perhaps more than any other, we have concern for the quality of life we are providing as well as the rate of cure. In caring for these individuals, any treatment of the tumor affects and is affected by the patient's previous experiences, behavior, and coping mechanisms and any support systems available.[4,22,61,107]

Likewise, it is important to remember that there can be wide degree of variability among older adults. Although many individuals in their 70s and 80s are physiologically challenged, others in the same age-group are running relays. Therefore while we recognize older adults as a group that has a greater vulnerability to cancer and the effects of treatment modalities, we also recognize a wide range of variability among individuals. Treatments should be selected based on the individual patient information, not age. Research should be conducted to determine the most appropriate use of current treatments and the efficacy of new treatments for this age-group, so that regimens are developed that address their needs.[61]

PREVENTION OF CANCER/CHEMOPREVENTION

Chemoprevention is the study of prevention of the development of cancer in humans. Currently there are three major approaches to cancer prevention. Primary prevention is the identification and elimination of agents that cause cancer. This usually refers to substances in the environment such as chemicals, radiation exposure, or viruses.

What immediately comes to mind are the risk factors of tobacco for lung cancer and sun exposure for skin cancer. It is estimated that 87% of lung cancers and 30% of all cancer deaths are attributable to cigarette smoking, and that 90% of the 700,000 skin cancers diagnosed in 1993 could have been prevented by using sunscreen, avoiding the midday sun, and wearing protective cover.[48]

Secondary prevention is the screening of individuals who are at increased risk for a particular malignancy in hopes of increasing their chances of survival with early detection and treatment. Recent advances in genetic testing soon will make it possible to determine an individual's inherited cancer susceptibility, and this information is valuable in determining the populations that would benefit from early preventive interventions.[97]

Chemoprevention refers to the concept of reducing cancer risk in individuals who are highly susceptible to certain cancers by prescribing certain natural or chemical synthetic products that may reduce or suppress the process of carcinogenesis. The development of cancer can be the result of a chemical, physical, or genetic insult to a cell. Carcinogenesis is a stepwise process that begins at the genetic level and progresses with cellular changes that initiate and promote the development of a malignancy. It is a widely held theory that there are many points in this chain of events where intervention can be beneficial.[46,48,97]

The third major chemoprevention approach is the use of biomarkers. A biomarker is a flag or signal that highlights specific stages in the initiation or progression of tumor development. A biomarker should provide the following benefits: (1) appear earlier in the process than the actual cancer and on a frequent basis, (2) be directly identified with tumor progression, (3) be reversible, (4) be used as a means of cancer detection that is cost saving, accurate, and convenient, and (5) be able to be validated. The biomarker of cholesterol indices has been used in the control and management of myocardial disease. Biomarkers are valuable tools in the detection, curtailing, and reversal of carcinogenesis and have provided a systemic pathway to chemoprevention studies.

Early work in the area of chemoprevention focused on the results of epidemiologic studies, which indicated that some substances that occur naturally in the diet were related to a decreased cancer incidence (vitamin A, selenium, vitamin E). Early work in the area of chemopre-

vention began in the 1980s, examining very few compounds. Originally the number of compounds thought to have an inhibitory effect on cancer was believed to be very large. Once thoroughly studied, however, the number that proceeded to clinical trials declined.

Today, under the National Cancer Institute's Chemoprevention Program, more than 400 possible chemoprevention agents are being studied, including 25 compounds in more than 60 clinical trials. Important points being reviewed are the drug's efficacy and safety and the overall potential of its chemoprevention properties. Studies for humans are staged as phase I, phase II, and phase III. A phase I clinical trial determines the drug's safety and pharmacokinetic profiles. Phase II develops biomarkers, which serve as surrogate endpoints for cancer. The compounds are then applied to assess their chemopreventive efficacy at these endpoints. The purpose of a phase III study is to demonstrate that the agent indeed reduces the cancer risk or that it will positively alter the surrogate endpoints in a large number of subjects over an extended period.[4,46,97]

Large-scale phase III trials are the next logical step in determining if these agents actually have chemopreventive properties. Phase III trials can last as long as 10 years and can involve thousands of subjects from many institutional settings. The population of trial subjects includes those at high risk for specific cancers as well as subjects from the general population. An added benefit of these large-scale trials is the time interval built in, which can confirm the efficacy, safety, and adverse effects of the agents, which may not have been determined in phase I and phase II.[97]

Trials in High-Risk Patients

Breast cancer prevention trial. A 10-year project begun in 1992, this study is attempting to determine whether tamoxifen will reduce the incidence of breast cancer in women at high risk for the disease. More than 16,000 women over age 35 are randomly selected to receive 20 mg of tamoxifen orally each day, versus a placebo, for a 5-year period. Previous studies estimate that tamoxifen may reduce the incidence in high-risk women by as much as 30%. It focuses on the high-risk breast cancer population because the potential benefits of using tamoxifen for this trial must outweigh the risk of endometrial cancers and other possible side effects.[12,39,46,62,85]

Linxian trials. The National Cancer Institute and The Cancer Institute of the Chinese Academy of Medical Sciences collaborated on two double-blind, randomized trials to determine whether daily ingestion of certain vitamins and minerals, multiple vitamins, or mineral supplements would reduce the incidence and mortality rates for esophageal and gastric cancer. In the Linxian area of China, roughly 20% of the population has esophageal dysplasia, which is considered a precancerous lesion. It was determined that certain substances (e.g., retinol, zinc, riboflavin, niacin, vitamin C, β-carotene, vitamin E, selenium) could have a chemopreventive effect. Beginning in 1986, in the General Population Trial, approximately 30,000 subjects were randomized. Each subject received one of four combinations of supplements for a period of 5½ years. The supplements contained doses equivalent to 1 to 2½ times the U.S. Recommended Daily Allowances.[4,46] The subjects who received the β-carotene/vitamin E/selenium combination had a 21% reduction in stomach cancer mortality, which contributed to a 13% reduction in the cancer death rate. The benefit of the β-carotene/vitamin E/selenium combination became evident approximately 2 years into the study and continued for its duration. An additional finding was an overall 9% drop in deaths from all causes for this group of subjects. The remaining three combinations did not affect the cancer risk.[46,50,67]

From this work a second study, the Dysplasia Trial, was conducted with 3,318 subjects who had cytologic evidence of esophageal dysphagia. In this randomized, 6-year study, participants received either a placebo or a daily supplement of 14 vitamins and 12 minerals, which were 2 to 3 times the U.S. Recommended Daily Allowances.

This study showed a 16% reduction in mortality from esophageal cancer.[46,48,97]

It is not possible to directly apply these results to Western cultures, however, because our well-nourished diet in the West tends to provide adequate multiple micronutrients.[46]

Prostate cancer prevention trial. Prostate cancer is the second most common cancer in men in the United States. It is estimated that 244,000 new cases were diagnosed and 40,400 deaths occurred from prostate cancer in 1995. Twenty-three percent of all men with cancer in the United States have prostate cancer, and it accounts for 12% of all cancer deaths. The Prostate Cancer Prevention Trial was designed to determine the ability of finasteride to prevent the development of prostate cancer in men age 55 or older. Because early development of prostate cancer is hormonally driven, this multicentered trial is aimed at determining whether inhibition of (DHT) by administration of finesteride may lead to a substantial reduction in the number of men who develop prostate cancer. Of the 18,000 men in this trial, half will receive a placebo and half will receive finasteride, 5 mg orally per day for 7 years.[30,46,64]

A-Tocopherol, B-Carotene Cancer Prevention Study (ATBC). The ATBC Trial, taking place in Finland, for the chemoprevention of lung cancer is being conducted by the National Cancer Institute and the National Public Health Institute of Finland. This study is examining whether daily oral supplementation with

α-tocopherol (vitamin E), β-carotene, or both would reduce the incidence of lung and other cancers. Nearly 30,000 men between the ages of 50 and 69 received either vitamin E alone, β-carotene alone, both vitamin E and β-carotene, or a placebo daily for 5 to 8 years. Results showed a 2% reduction in lung cancer for the men who received vitamin E, compared with an 18% higher incidence of lung cancer among those who took β-carotene. Those taking vitamin E and β-carotene together had an increase in the incidence of lung cancer relatively close to that of those taking β-carotene alone, which shows no significant interaction between these two supplements.[46,50,67,97]

When considering other cancers in regard to these supplements, it was found that vitamin E reduced prostate cancer by 34% and colorectal cancer by 16%, whereas β-carotene had little or no effect on the incidence of other cancers.

The results from the β-carotene group were surprising in light of the significant amount of evidence in the epidemiologic literature, suggesting that dietary β-carotene is associated with a low risk of lung cancer. Scientists speculate that perhaps the dietary supplement needed to be given over a longer interval to inhibit the development of lung cancer in long-term smokers. In addition, some of the men in the control group had higher blood levels of vitamin E or β-carotene before the start of the study. This could possibly indicate that there may be other constituents in foods high in vitamin E or β-carotene that could be responsible for the protective effect found in the epidemiologic studies.[46,50,67,97]

The role of chemoprevention in cancer care of the future is both exhilarating and challenging. There is now a significant interest in the biochemical and biologic mechanisms of cancer development. We will continue to see a concerted effort to develop new methods of identifying those who are at greatest risk and in turn to counsel those individuals in the areas of genetics, adjustment of life-styles, and avoidance of environmental factors. Chemoprevention as an area of study holds the promise of reducing cancer morbidity and mortality through early intervention, before carcinogenesis occurs or progresses to invasive disease.

CHRONOTHERAPY/CIRCADIAN RHYTHM

Circadian rhythm is a term used to describe a regular, repeated fluctuation in biologic functions during a 24-hour period. The term often is used in conjunction with the term *diurnal,* which refers to "events happening in the daytime." In the many ongoing physiologic mechanisms that take place in the human body, there are many variables that in part are affected by circadium rhythms. These *circadian variables* can influence drug absorption, metabolism, distribution and elimination.[1,43,55]

One of several possible examples is hepatic blood flow, which can be a major factor in the clearance of lipophilic, rapidly metabolized drugs. Age-related changes occur in hepatic function, such as a decrease in liver size, a decline in the number of functioning hepatocytes, less hepatic blood flow, and less ability to metabolize drugs.[1,43,55,56]

Early in the 18th century DeMairan described in detail the leaves of the mimosa plant, which opened during the day and closed during the night regardless of whether the plant was kept in total darkness. For the first time a scientist asserted the possibility that circadian rhythms arise internally and do not depend on an outside signal, making them endogenous to living organisms. Further work was done by Richter and by Johnson. Richter applied these findings to the diurnal activity of rats that were kept in constant darkness, whereas Johnson, who also studied animals housed in darkness, found that the "activity rhythms" of these animals did not fit into the normal 24-hour period. He believed that some other "internal physiologic clock" was at work that did not adhere to any stimulation or input from the environment.[1,43,55,83]

Interest in this phenomenon led investigators to examine cardiovascular disease, in which scientists observed a "morning increase" in the risk of acute cardiovascular disorders such as transient myocardial ischemia, myocardial infarction, sudden cardiac death, and stroke. These findings became a widely accepted tenet with both the public and the medical community. Later studies reported the occurrence of similar rhythmic patterns in numerous physiologic processes. For example, Panza and others[92] determined that "blood fibrinolytic activity is lower in the early morning hours, while platelet aggregability, plasma renin activity, and the rate of cortisol secretion are higher." Muller and Toffer[84] correlated the circadian rhythms in these findings in an epidemiologic manner to assert that "certain dynamic physiologic mechanisms contribute to, and even trigger, the onset of acute cardiovascular events." Biologic processes are often sequential, occurring in a specific, orderly fashion, and they usually depend on completion of one event before a second event can be initiated.[43,84,92]

Today, chronotherapy using antineoplastic agents is a relatively new strategy. Its purpose is to allow both dose intensification of the drug and reduction of cytotoxic side effects. Previous studies have revealed "time-dependent variations for both toxic side effects and therapeutic drug efficacy." Circadian variations are evident in several human parameters, such as DNA synthesis in the intestinal mucosal tissue, skin, bone marrow, spleen, testis, and thymus tissue. The numbers of circulating leukocytes, lymphocytes, erythrocytes, and platelets are not constant but are subject to diurnal fluctuations. Likewise, high-amplitude circadian rhythms in the epithelium of the human gut show the greatest DNA synthetic activity occurring each day at approximately 7 AM, fasting or non-fasting.[1,27,55]

Clinical trials conducted in this country and abroad thus far have sought to determine the benefit/risk ratio and efficacy of chemotherapeutic chronotherapy versus continuous infusion. Chronotherapy allows a subject to receive scheduled drug delivery at specific, predetermined time slots during a 24-hour period. Prior investigations determined that the therapeutic indices of these drugs can be affected by varying the timing of drug delivery, whereas a continuous, steady-rate infusion of antineoplastic agents can be a means of increasing antitumor activity with reduced toxicity. This is because a constant supply of the drug provides continuous exposure to the cancer cells and thus increases the probability of cytotoxic damage. An additional benefit is the avoidance of peak drug concentrations, which should minimize host cell injury.[1,27,43,55,83] For example, researchers have determined that nighttime administration of 5-FU in humans reduces toxic side effects. In a phase I study involving 34 patients who had advanced colorectal cancer, administration of the drug in a circadian-modulated delivery system allowed a mean dose of 7.5 g/m^2 for 5 consecutive days with relatively low toxicities. The 5-FU was administered via a curve, with the peak flow rate occurring at 4 AM. The dose was intensified to 1 g/m^2 per course for each patient. The normally anticipated side effects of stomatitis, diarrhea, leukopenia, and anemia were seen in fewer than 10%. A partial remission was attained by 10 patients, and the disease stabilized in 15 patients.[1]

An endometrial cancer trial using subjects with advanced or recurrent disease who had not received prior chemotherapy was conducted by the Gynecologic Oncology Group. The women were treated with doxorubicin and cisplatin. Doxorubicin, 60 mg/m^2, was infused over 30 minutes at 6 AM, whereas cisplatin, 60 mg/m^2, was given over 30 minutes at 6 PM, every 28 days. This study's overall response rate of 60% using both drugs was superior to the response attained with either drug as a single agent. There was also a 20% complete response rate, which is higher than that reported previously using both agents administered in a conventional manner. Toxicities were tolerable but not significantly reduced by the circadian-timed delivery.[7,102,103]

While we are familiar with the antitumor affect interferon-α, (IFN-α) has had on patients with hematologic malignancies, it also has been shown to be an effective tool in regression of solid tumors, such as renal cell carcinoma, malignant melanoma, bladder and carcinoid tumors, and Kaposi's sarcoma. However, questions remain about optimal dosing of IFN-α. A dose-response relationship exists for anticancer effects that suggests a benefit in dose intensification, but toxicities are a concern. Prior research points to evening administration of IFN-α as being better tolerated than morning treatment.[7,56]

A study was undertaken in which IFN-α was delivered as a 7-day continuous venous infusion at a circadian rhythm–modulated rate. The purpose was to determine the maximum tolerated dose (MTD) using this schedule in cancer patients who were resistant to conventional therapy, recording the therapeutic effect and measuring clinical toxicities. Clinical toxicities and treatment response were gauged by World Health Organization (WHO) criteria.[56]

IFN-α was administered via continuous infusion using an ambulatory pump (CADD Plus, Pharmacia, Sweden). The dose was increased by an amount equal to the starting dose six times, with a 1-week rest interval between each dose escalation. Participants received the drug on a daily, circadian-modulated schedule, with two thirds of the total dose delivered between 6 PM and 3 AM, and the remaining one third between 3 AM and 6 PM.[56,66]

Of the original 18 participants, two were removed from the study. Toxicities consisted of flu-like symptoms, which all patients experienced but which were limited for the most part to the first 2 to 3 days of treatment. Hematologic changes seen in 12 participants were mild and brief. One patient with anemia required blood transfusion. Ten patients had gastrointestinal symptoms, such as nausea and/or anorexia. All the subjects had transient elevations of alkaline phosphatase, which was asymptomatic. Toxicities appeared to increase with increasing doses of the drug but were rapidly reversed when the drug was discontinued. There was no significant reportable decline in performance status.[56]

Of the 16 participants, two who had been previously treated for renal cell carcinoma had partial response to IFN-α. One of these had a 75% reduction of the size of renal mass with resorption of all the pleural effusion and disappearance of all abdominal, mediastinal, and pulmonary lymph node enlargement, except for two small pulmonary lymph nodules. Both responses lasted longer than 3 months, and both patients lived longer than 1 year after therapy ended. Of the remaining 14 patients, 11 had progressive disease and 3 had stable disease at 6 weeks of therapy.[56]

Although the mechanism of diminished toxicity with evening infusion of IFN-α is unclear, it implies that the circadian rhythm of cortisol is involved. Therefore in this case, the circadian scheduling of IFN-α administration allowed an increase in dose intensity while reducing toxicities. Further clinical trials in the area of chronotherapy should investigate efficacy, toxicities, and dosing limits. This therapy's role in the treatment of cancer could allow maximum dosing for antitumor effect while limiting harmful toxicities.

Text continued on p. 559.

NURSING MANAGEMENT

Nursing management of the patient receiving chemotherapy requires multiple assessment and intervention strategies. Nursing care begins with a thorough understanding of five primary elements: the patient's condition; the goal of therapy; the treating drug or drugs dosage, route, and schedule; the principles of administration; and the potential side effects. Additional nursing management includes monitoring responses to therapy, reassessing and documenting signs and symptoms, and passing on pertinent information to other members of the health care team. Continual psychosocial evaluation and patient teaching components require astute nursing interventions. Many resources are available, both locally and nationally. The Oncology Nursing Society, the American Cancer Society, the National Cancer Institute, and the Leukemia Society all provide lay and professional educational materials.[19,81,88,105]

NURSING ASSESSMENT AND INTERVENTION

Chemotherapeutic drugs may cause adverse side effects and major system toxicity and dysfunction. Side effects and toxicity vary in severity according to the patient's individual response to the drug therapy. The most frequent side effects are myelosuppression, nausea, and vomiting. Myelosuppression can be a dose-limiting toxicity.[11] Myelosuppression, stomatitis, mucositis, and skin integrity are discussed extensively in Chapter 30. The chemotherapeutic drugs work by destroying and/or suppressing new leukocytes, platelets, and erythrocytes. These effects are monitored by evaluating the blood count at scheduled intervals. The time or level at which a blood count reaches its lowest point is the nadir. The nadir varies with individual drugs but usually occurs between 7 and 21 days after administration. Nausea and vomiting often are the most distressing side effects of chemotherapy[98]; they may be acute, anticipatory, delayed, or persistent. Acute nausea and vomiting occur within 1 to 2 hours of treatment and last approximately 24 hours. Anticipatory nausea and vomiting occur before the treatment. Nausea and vomiting after the initial 24 hours of treatment may be referred to as *delayed* or *persistent*. Cisplatin in particular is associated with this symptom. An estimated 60% of patients experience delayed emesis after receiving cisplatin, even if emesis is adequately controlled during the first 24 hours.[54]

Assessing and reporting the frequency, severity, patterns, and duration of symptoms aid in prevention and management. Prevention is best for nausea and vomiting. Behavioral interventions such as relaxation, distraction, and guided imagery may help with anticipatory nausea and vomiting. Allowing the patient to sleep through the peak hours of nausea and vomiting and/or chemotherapy may diminish these symptoms. Administering antiemetics 30 to 60 minutes before chemotherapy also alleviates the symptoms. Antiemetics should be continued at scheduled intervals throughout the expected duration of nausea and vomiting.[25,72]

In the past 10 to 15 years, antiemetic research has had a profound effect on the treatment of chemotherapy-induced nausea and vomiting. The incidence of these side effects is related to the emetic potential of the chemotherapy drug; the dose; the route, schedule, and duration; and combinations of administration (Table 22-5).[54,72] The combination of antiemetic drugs with different mechanisms, round-the-clock administration, and higher dosages have proved more effective than single-agent dosing and as-needed (PRN) schedules.[11] Several agents now used as single agents or in combination are metoclopramide, haloperidol, dexamethasone, lorazepam, and prochlorperazine (Tables 22-6 and 22-7). Many of these drugs act on the chemoreceptor trigger zone in the brain by blocking dopamine receptors.[17,25,74] Although these antiemetics have demonstrated their effectiveness, they are associated with undesirable side effects: sedation, extrapyramidal reactions, anxiety, mood changes, and diarrhea. Another major drawback is that most of these drugs are administered intravenously (IV), thus their use usually is not feasible for outpatients and children.[54,82]

With the development and use of the serotonin (5-HT3) antagonists (e.g., ondansetron [Zofran]), new strides have been made in effective antiemetic therapy. Although more costly than previous antiemetic drugs, the dosing schedule is less frequent (0.15 mg/kg 30 minutes before chemotherapy, then at 4 and 8 hours after the initial dose). Side effects thus far are mild: headache, constipation, and transient elevation of liver enzymes. Ondansetron has demonstrated its effectiveness as an oral agent and may be suitable for outpatient therapy and for children.[17,25,74]

The remaining side effects listed in Table 22-1 (e.g., aches and pains, alopecia, anorexia, constipation, cystitis, diarrhea, depression, fatigue, mucositis, pharyngitis, stomatitis) have listed nursing actions and points to cover for patient and family teaching. The nurse's responsibilities include evaluating the patient's response to the drugs, teaching the patient or caregiver self-management interventions, and monitoring laboratory data, as well as signs, and symptoms reported by the patient. This information is useful in developing the plan of care for the patient receiving chemotherapy.*

Pertinent information related to the major system toxicities (cardiac, hematopoietic, hepatic, hypersensitivity, neurologic, ototoxicity, pulmonary, reproductive, renal) and to metabolic alterations (see Table 22-1) imposes dose-limiting restrictions on many of the drugs. If symptoms occur and the chemotherapeutic drug dose or schedule (or both) is not altered or evaluated, the potential for irreversible side effects grows. All the toxicities listed in Table 22-1 require astute observation and intervention by all members of the health care team.[11,17,72,87] Selected nursing diagnoses and interventions appropriate for the patient receiving chemotherapy are listed below. Additional nursing diagnoses may be determined by assess-

---

*References 37, 41, 45, 49, 53, 57.

Table 22-5 Emetic Potential of Common Chemotherapeutic Drugs

Mild potential	Moderate potential	Severe potential
Bleomycin	Carboplatin	Cisplatin
Busulfan	Carmustine	Cyclophosamide
Chlorambucil	Cytarabine	Dacarbazine
Etoposide	Daunorubicin	Dactinomycin
5-Fluorouracil	Doxorubicin	Mechlorethamine
Hydroxyurea	Ifosfamide	Streptozotocin
Mercaptopurine	Lomustine	
Methotrexate (low dose)	Mitomycin C	
	Mitoxantrone	
Tamoxifen	Procarbazine	
Vinblastine	Taxol	

Table 22-6 Selected Parenteral Antiemetic Regimens

Drug	Dosage	Schedule
Metoclopramide (Reglan)	1-3 mg/kg IV	30 min before and 90 min after chemotherapy, then Q4hr PRN
Dexamethasone (Decadron)	20 mg IV	30-40 min before chemotherapy
Lorazepam (Ativan) *or*	1.5 mg/m^2 IV	30 min before chemotherapy
Diphenhydramine (Benadryl)	50 mg IV	30 min before chemotherapy
(The above drugs are used in varying doses and schedules depending upon severity of emetic episode.)		
Ondansetron (Zofran)	0.15 mg/kg in 30-50 ml; infused over 15-30 min	30 min before chemotherapy, then at 4 and 8 hr after initial dose

Data from American Society of Hospital Pharmacists, Inc, 1995, Bethesda, Md.

Continued.

Table 22-7 Selected Oral Antiemetic Regimens

Drugs	Dosage	Schedule
Chlorpromazine hydrochloride (Thorazine)	10, 25, 50, 100, 200 mg tablets; 75, 150, 200, 300 mg slow-release (SR) capsules	Give 30-75 mg in 2-4 hr in divided doses; give 1 hr before chemotherapy administration, then Q4-6hr PRN.
Dronabinol	2.5, 5, 10 mg SR capsules	Give 1-3 hr before chemotherapy administration; then 4-6 doses per day Q2-4hr (maximum 15 mg/m^2 per dose).
Ondansetron	8 mg (12 yr of age or older)	Give initial 8 mg dose 30 min before chemotherapy (maximum dose 3 times per day for 2-3 days).
	4 mg (4-11 yr of age)	Give initial 4 mg dose 30 min before chemotherapy (maximum dose 3 times per day for 2-3 days).
Prochlorperazine (Compazine)	5, 10, 25 mg tablets; 10, 15, 30 mg SR capsules	Give 10-25 mg 1 hr before chemotherapy administration, then 15-30 mg SR capsule Q12hr; repeat *one* of above doses Q3-4½hr.
Promethazine (Phenergan)	12.5, 25, 50 mg tablets	Give 25-50 mg 1 hr before chemotherapy administration, then 12.5-25 mg 4 times per day.
Trimethobenzamide hydrochloride (Tigan)	100, 250 mg capsules	Give 250 mg 1 hr before chemotherapy administration, then 250 mg 4 times per day.

Data from Physician Drug Reference, Medical Economics Data, Medical Economic Co, Montvale, NJ, 1995, and American Hospital Formulary Service, Bethesda, Md, 1995.

ing the patient's health and psychosocial issues and the specific side effects of the chemotherapeutic drugs. Additional circumstances that may affect the patient's response to a drug include the setting in which the drug is administered (acute care or home care), the needs posed by activities of daily living, and life-style changes.[11,16,25]

NURSING DIAGNOSIS

• *Knowledge deficit related to chemotherapeutic side effects*

OUTCOME GOAL

Patient will be able to:
• State drug side effects.

INTERVENTIONS

• Assess educational level, ability, desire to learn, and barriers to learning.
• Assess knowledge level relative to cancer, previous experience with diagnosis, and treatment of cancer.
• Evaluate understanding relative to the specific diagnosis, disease process, and potential treatment planned.
• Assess previous experience with chemotherapy.
• Determine availability of caregiver to participate in patient's care and treatment.
• Assess patient's and family's needs for consultation

with various resources (e.g., I can Cope Support Group, Reach to Recovery, Look Good–Feel Better, Ostomy, and Laryngectomy Support Groups[28,53,57]).

NURSING DIAGNOSIS

• *Oral mucous membrane, altered, related to side effects of drugs*[11,38,60]

OUTCOME GOALS

Patient will be able to:
• Exhibit signs of a healthy oral mucosa.
• Identify/demonstrate measures that promote good oral hygiene.

INTERVENTIONS

• Assess history of alcohol and/or tobacco use or other risk factors.
• Obtain history of current treatment: radiation therapy, chemotherapy, surgery, and biotherapy.
• Query patient about usual regimen for oral hygiene and date of last dental examination.
• Assess oral mucosa: palate, tongue, gums, teeth, lips, floor of mouth, and inner aspects of cheeks. Note redness, ulcerations, bleeding, and white patches, as well as color, amount, and consistency of saliva.

NURSING DIAGNOSIS

• *Injury, risk for, related to alteration in immune system; clotting factors*[37,41]

OUTCOME GOALS

Patient will be able to:
• Identify/report signs and symptoms of infection.
• Identify/demonstrate infection potential precautions.

INTERVENTIONS

• Monitor complete blood count (CBC), hemoglobin, prothrombin time (PT), partial thromboplastin time (PTT), and platelet count.
• Assess type of therapy (chemotherapy, radiation therapy) and current drugs (aspirin, anticoagulants) that may alter bleeding and clotting times.
• Assess factors (fever, sepsis, altered hepatic function, bone marrow function) that may alter clotting process.
• Identify potential date of nadir for platelets.
• Observe for and report symptoms: bruising; bleeding from venous access sites, nose, gums, vagina, rectum; hemoptysis, hematemesis; black, tarry, and/or gross blood in stools; increase in usual menstrual flow; change in vital signs; spontaneous petechiae or hematomas.

NURSING DIAGNOSIS

• *Nutrition, altered: less than body requirements, related to nausea and vomiting*[54,68,70]

OUTCOME GOALS

Patient will be able to:
• Maintain laboratory values within normal limits.
• Identify/demonstrate measures to minimize nausea and vomiting episodes.
• Consume sufficient calories to maintain weight goal.

INTERVENTIONS

• Assess nauseous episodes, including amount, color, consistency, and frequency of emesis.
• Determine what factors facilitate and/or prevent nausea and vomiting.
• Query patient about past strategies that were helpful in managing nausea and vomiting.
• Assess baseline weight before illness, onset of illness, changes since onset of treatment, and weight 1 month ago; note weight gains/losses.
• Monitor laboratory values: serum albumin, serum transferrin, CBC, electrolytes.
• Assess dietary history: food habits, food likes/dislikes, amount and type of food eaten at breakfast, lunch, supper, and snacks.
• Note altered bowel habits and presence of other related gastrointestinal (GI) distress (heartburn, feeling of fullness, cramping).

• Consult dietary services and/or plan with patient recommendations for nutritional intake that will stimulate appetite and facilitate calorie intake (e.g., cold foods, salads, cheeses, fruits, salty foods, colas).

NURSING DIAGNOSIS

• *Sensory/perceptual alterations, visual, related to photosensitivity and auditory related to ototoxicity*[70,72,91]

INTERVENTIONS

• Determine chemotherapy- and/or other treatment-related protocol that may affect sensory alterations.
• Assess severity of symptoms regarding compromises in activities in daily living.
• Assess environmental conditions (light, noise, room temperature).
• Assess sensory alteration: onset, severity, changes in duration, other discomforting symptoms.
• Instruct patient in precautions to follow: photosensitivity (wear sun glasses when outside, dim room lights, observe driving- and/or work-related restrictions), ototoxicity (limit or restrict environmental noise),
• Inform health care team about symptoms and restrictions affecting work, driving, and/or activities of daily living.

NURSING DIAGNOSIS

• *Body image disturbance related to alopecia*[8,10]

OUTCOME GOALS

Patient will be able to:
• Identify measures to protect/minimize scalp and hair damage.
• Utilize resources regarding changes in body image.

INTERVENTIONS

• Inform patient that hair loss is temporary and hair will regrow after treatment stops (hair growth usually returns in 2 to 6 months).
• Provide resources for purchase or loan of wigs, scarves, and caps.
• Inform patient about health care measures to protect scalp: use gentle shampoos, avoid hair dryers, curling irons, permanents, and hair drying; protect scalp in winter and summer (cold/heat loss); wear protective head covering when outdoors.
• Encourage sharing of feelings regarding body image changes. Inform patient about American Cancer Society support groups (e.g., I Can Cope, Look Good–Feel Better).

NURSING DIAGNOSIS[11,37,38]

• *Pain related to bone metastasis*
• *Oral mucous membrane, altered (mucositis)*

Continued.

OUTCOME GOALS

Patient will be able to:
- Achieve adequate control of pain.
- Identify/demonstrate measures to control or minimize pain episodes.

INTERVENTIONS

- Determine onset, location, duration, severity, intensity, and radiation of symptoms.
- Assess symptoms with patient's and family's suggestions: What makes the symptoms/discomfort better? What makes the symptoms/discomfort worse? For example: types and frequency of interventions; treatment-related interventions affecting hygiene, nutrition, and pain; time of intervention regarding food intake and mobility.
- Provide physician-prescribed medications and/or treatment interventions.
- Encourage relaxation/meditation/distraction strategies to facilitate coping with discomfort and enhance effects of medications and treatment interventions.
- Monitor electrolyte balance and granulocyte count.
- Assess skin, especially hidden areas (between toes, skin folds of breasts, buttocks, perineal area) on a scheduled basis; report changes and findings promptly.

NURSING DIAGNOSIS

- *Infection, risk for, resulting from immunosuppression, break in skin, or contamination of supplies*[11,49,53,81]

OUTCOME GOALS

Patient/caregiver will be able to:
- Identify and report signs and symptoms of infection.
- Identify/demonstrate appropriate hygiene measures.

INTERVENTIONS

- Monitor CBC and acute granulocyte count.
- Monitor expectation of nadir related to chemotherapy.
- Teach and monitor prudent handwashing technique: before any nursing intervention, before and after meals, after bathroom use, before any treatment-related activity for self-care.
- Restrict visitors with potential infections or those recently immunized with attenuated live vaccines, such as diphtheria-pertussis-tetanus (DPT) or measles-mumps-rubella (MMR).

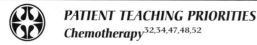

PATIENT TEACHING PRIORITIES
Chemotherapy[32,34,47,48,52]

Assess willingness, readiness to learn, and barriers to learning (acuity of illness, sensory deficits, pain, and/or fear and anxiety regarding diagnosis/treatment).

Inform patient/family about schedule of activities for chemotherapy administration and monitoring of laboratory and diagnostic tests.

Encourage practice and repetition of newly learned skill to enhance learner's performance for at-risk procedures.

Validate aseptic technique and skills of patient or caregiver for prescribed self-administration and discontinuation of chemotherapeutic drugs.

Provide written materials (e.g., those from the National Cancer Institute, "Chemotherapy and You." "What Are Clinical Trials All About"), 1-800-4-CANCER telephone number, and other materials as needed.

Teach and review specific drugs and related side effects patient may experience, and when, where, how, and whom to call if problems arise.

Provide information and list of resources for obtaining, storing, and disposing of drugs and supplies.[45,49]

GERIATRIC CONSIDERATIONS[52,54]
Chemotherapy

Consider potential for cardiac, renal, respiratory, and hepatic systems compromise: medication dosage and/or schedule of administration may be altered.

High-dose drug regimens have been associated with increased toxicity (e.g., neurotoxicity with high-dose cytarabine–patients over 50 years of age are particularly susceptible to this toxicity).

Consider neuromuscular and sensory deficits that may be present, such as visual and hearing losses and arthritic joints; plan individualized teaching sessions; use printed materials with large print for reading ease; return demonstration techniques may require more simplistic steps to facilitate patient/family ease in learning required technique.

Consider age-related changes in body function accommodations: bowel and bladder tonicity (unable to hold large-volume hydration, unable to retain large-volume bowel cleansing preparations); provide prompt and frequent elimination needs.

Premedications may cause drowsiness; encourage patient/family to utilize transportation resources (family, public, American Cancer Society) if receiving chemotherapy and/or undergoing required laboratory test monitoring.

Query patient/caregiver regarding over-the-counter and/or previous physician-prescribed medications; some of these medications may alter bleeding and clotting times and/or interfere with prescribed chemotherapy medications.

Assess abilities of patient and caregiver, and determine if additional resources are needed, such as a home-care agency, Meals on Wheels, and social services for financial assistance.[7,30,36]

- Monitor food intake: explain restrictions (no fresh vegetables or fruits) and emphasize that the nurse must be consulted before patient eats food brought into hospital.
- Ensure cleanliness of room and supplies used in routine care; change all supplies on a scheduled basis.

- Examine all sterile supplies before use; note expiration date for sterility, observe for any defect or interruption of product's integrity, and use sterile technique when opening and using product.

Patient teaching priorities and geriatric considerations are given in the boxes on p. 558.

CONCLUSION

Nurses have major responsibilities in caring for patients who receive chemotherapeutic agents. It is important that nurses know the treatment goals, drug classifications and modes of action, principles of tumor growth and cell kill, and administration protocols. Chemotherapeutic agents should be administered only by nurses who have been taught and are skilled in the various procedures. Patient and family education on the many aspects of chemotherapy (e.g., procedure, potential side effects and toxicities, follow-up care) requires competent nursing assessment and intervention. The nurse should encourage the patient and family to become an integral part of planning and implementing care. Keeping abreast of all the new drugs and their implications, along with the responsibilities just mentioned, offers many challenges for the nurse in the varied settings of oncology practice.

■ CHAPTER QUESTIONS

1. A patient experiencing chemotherapeutic drug anaphylaxis may have the following symptoms:
   a. Tachycardia, hypertension, dyspnea, back pain
   b. Bradycardia, hypotension, chest pain, fever
   c. Chills, constipation, diaphoresis, facial flushing
   d. Dyspnea, hypotension, hives, tachycardia
2. Chemotherapeutic vesicant drugs with extravasation potential include:
   a. Dactinomycin, daunorubicin, doxorubicin, Dilantin
   b. Carboplatin, cisplatin, cladribine, cyclophosphamide
   c. Methotrexate, menogaril, nitrogen mustard
   d. Vinblastine, vincristine, vindesine, vinorelbine
3. Nursing practice guidelines to prevent or diminish extravasation of chemotherapeutic drugs include:
   a. Knowledge of drugs with vesicant potential; testing vein with chemotherapeutic drug; validating blood return; monitoring drugs during bolus/continuous infusion
   b. Knowledge of drugs with vesicant potential; testing vein with normal saline; validating blood return after drug administration; monitoring drug during bolus/continuous infusion
   c. Knowledge of drugs with vesicant potential; testing vein with normal saline; validating blood return during drug administration; monitoring drug during bolus/continuous infusion
   d. Knowledge of drugs with vesicant potential; testing

vein with normal saline; validating blood return before, during, and after drug administration; monitoring drug during bolus/continuous infusion
4. Recommended nursing practice guidelines for safe handling of chemotherapy drugs include:
   a. Physician's order to use gown, gloves, goggles
   b. Gown and goggles only when administering intrathecal chemotherapeutic drugs
   c. Gown, gloves, goggles during preparation and administration only
   d. Gown, gloves, goggles during preparation, administration, and disposal; washing hands before and after handling drugs
5. Chemotherapeutic drugs that have potential for cardiac toxicity include:
   a. Chlorambucil, daunorubicin, doxorubicin, mitoxantrone
   b. Cyclophosphamide, etoposide, ifosfamide, teniposide
   c. Bleomycin, mitomycin, mithramycin, methotrexate
   d. Carboplatin, carmustine, cisplatin, cyclophosphamide
6. A visitor states to the nurse at the desk that "My mother's chemotherapy tubing came apart, and the drug is leaking." The nurse would:
   a. Obtain a chemotherapy spill kit and delegate the spill clean-up to housekeeping
   b. Obtain a chemotherapy spill kit; put on gloves; clean up the spill; and document the occurrence
   c. Obtain a chemotherapy spill kit; put on gown, gloves, and goggles; clean up the spill; and document the occurrence
   d. Obtain a chemotherapy spill kit; put on gown, gloves, and goggles; clean up the spill; wash hands; and document the occurrence
7. Chemotherapeutic drugs that have potential for neurotoxicity include:
   a. Cladribine, vinblastine, vincristine, vinorelbine
   b. Chlorambucil, cisplatin, cytarabine, lomustine
   c. Etoposide, ifosfamide, vinblastine, vincristine
   d. Vinblastine, vincristine, vinorelbine, prednisone
8. Patient/family education strategies for anorexia include:
   a. Eating alone; freshening up before meals; having small, frequent feedings; and concentrating on low-calorie foods
   b. Eating with others; freshening up before meals; having small, frequent feedings; and concentrating on high-calorie foods
   c. Eating with others; freshening up before meals; having large, frequent feedings; and concentrating on high-calorie foods

d. Eating alone; freshening up before meals; having small, frequent feedings; and concentrating on high-calorie foods

9. Myelosuppression from chemotherapeutic drugs increases the potential for infection; practices to diminish infection potential include:
   a. Avoiding sources of infection, maintaining good personal hygiene, getting adequate rest and exercise, and reporting signs and symptoms of infection immediately
   b. Avoiding sources of infection, maintaining good personal hygiene, omitting all exercise activity, and reporting signs and symptoms of infection immediately
   c. Avoiding sources of infection, maintaining good personal hygiene, getting adequate rest and exercise, and reporting signs and symptoms of infection at the next scheduled appointment
   d. Avoiding sources of infection, maintaining good personal hygiene, getting lots of exercise, and reporting signs and symptoms of infection immediately

10. The permeability of the blood-brain barrier tends to be greater in or near the center of the tumor, where the blood supply usually is diminished.
    a. True
    b. False

11. "Circadian variables" in the concept of circadian rhythm include:
    a. Drug absorption, distribution, dose intensification, metabolism
    b. Drug absorption, metabolism, drug administration, route, elimination
    c. Drug absorption, metabolism, distribution, elimination
    d. Drug absorption, distribution, dose intensification, elimination

12. The concept of chemoprevention involves reducing the risk of cancer in individuals highly susceptible to certain cancers by administering drugs that reduce or suppress carcinogenesis. The three major cancer diseases currently in chemoprevention trials are:
    a. Breast, cervical, and prostate cancer
    b. Cervical, lung, and prostate cancer
    c. Breast, lung, and prostate cancer
    d. Breast, lung, and testicular cancer

BIBLIOGRAPHY

1. Adler S and others: Chronotherapy with 5-fluorouracil folinic acid in advanced colorectal carcinoma: results of a chronopharmacolic phase I trial, *Cancer* 73(12):2905, 1994.
2. Alberts DS, Dorr RT: Case report: topical DMSO for mitomycin-C–induced skin ulceration, *Oncol Nurs Forum* 18(4):693, 1991.
3. American Society of Hospital Pharmacists: ASHP technical assistance bulletin on handling cytotoxic and hazardous drugs, *Am J Hosp Pharm* 47(5):1033, 1990.
4. Bailes J: Cost aspects of palliative cancer care, *Semin Oncol* 22(2)(2 suppl):64, 1995.
5. Baird SB and others: *Cancer nursing: a comprehensive textbook,* Philadelphia, 1991, Saunders.
6. Barnicle MM: Chemotherapy and pregnancy, *Semin Oncol Nurs* 8(2):124, 1992.
7. Barrett R and others: Circadian-timed combination doxorubicin-cisplatin chemotherapy for advanced endometrial carcinoma: a phase II study of the gynecologic oncology group, *Am J Clin Oncol* 16(6):494, 1993.
8. Barton-Burke MS: Potential toxicities and nursing management. In Barton-Burke MS and others: *Cancer chemotherapy: a nursing process approach,* Boston, 1991, Jones & Bartlett.
9. Beason R: Antineoplastic vesicant extravasation, *J Intravenous Nursing* 13(2):111, 1990.
10. Bender C: Implications of antineoplastic therapy for nursing. In Clark JC, McGee RF editors: *Core curriculum for oncology nursing,* ed 2, 1992, Philadelphia, Saunders.
11. Bjergaard J and others: Increased risk of myelodysplasia and leukaemia after etoposide, cisplatin, and bleomycin for germcell tumours, *Lancet* 338(8):359, 1991.
12. Boothe V, Pommier R, Vetto J: Tamoxifen in the treatment and chemoprevention of breast cancer, *Cancer Practice* 2(5):335, 1994.
13. Boyle D, Engelking C: Vesicant extravasation: myths and realities, *Oncol Nurs Forum* 22(1):57, 1995.
14. Brogen J, Nevidjon B: Vinorelbine tartrate (Navelbine): drug profile and nursing implications of a new vinca alkaloid, *Oncol Nurs Forum* 22(4):675, 1995.
15. Brown JK, Hogan CM: Chemotherapy. In Groenwald SL et al: *Cancer nursing principles and practice,* Boston, 1992, Jones & Bartlett.
16. Brown M, Mulholland JL: *Drug calculations: process and problems for clinical practice,* ed 4, St Louis, 1992, Mosby.
17. Button D: Recent developments in the management of emesis with the 5-HT3 antagonist granisetron, *Semin Oncol Nurs* 6(1 suppl):14, 1990.
18. Cain J, Bender C: Ifosfamide-induced neurotoxicity: associated symptoms and nursing implications, *Oncol Nurs Forum* 22(4):659, 1995.
19. Carey PJ and others: Appraisal and caregiving burdens in family members caring for patients receiving chemotherapy, *Oncol Nurs Forum* 18(8):1341, 1991.
20. Caruso CC and others: Cooling effects and comfort of four cooling blanket temperatures in humans with fever, *Nurs Res* 41(2):68, 1992.
21. Caudell KA and others: Quantification of urinary mutagens in nurses during potential antineoplastic agent exposure: a pilot study with concurrent environmental and dietary control, *Cancer Nurs* 11(1):41, 1988.
22. Cella D: Measuring quality of life in palliative care, *Semin Oncol* 22(2)(3 suppl):73, 1995.
23. Charette J: Contemporary approaches of chemotherapy, *Critical Care Nursing Clinics of North America* 7(1):135, 1995.
24. Choy and others: Investigation of Taxol as a potential radiation sensitizer, *Cancer* 71(11):3774, 1993.
25. Clark RA and others: Antiemetic therapy: management of chemotherapy-induced nausea and vomiting, *Semin Oncol* 5(2):53, 1989.
26. Cohen JH: Geriatric principles of treatment applied to medical oncology: an overview, *Semin Oncol* 22(1)(1 suppl):1, 1995.
27. Conroy T and others: Simplified chronomodulated continuous infusion of floxuridine in patients with metastatic renal cell carcinoma, *Cancer* 72(7):2190, 1993.

28. Creaton EM and others: A hospital-based chemotherapy education and training program, *Cancer Nurs* 14(2):79, 1991.

29. Dahlstrim KK and others: Fluorescence microscopic demonstration and demarcation of doxorubicin extravasation: experimental and clinical studies, *Cancer* 65(4):1722, 1990.

30. Davison B, Degner L, Morgan T: Information and decision-making preferences of men with prostate cancer, *Oncol Nurs Forum* 22(9):1401, 1995.

31. DeVita VT Jr.: Principles of chemotherapy. In DeVita VT Jr, Hellman S, Rosenberg SA, editors: *Cancer: principles and practice of oncology,* ed 4, Philadelphia, 1993, Lippincott.

32. Dison N: *Simplified drugs and solutions for nurses,* ed 10, St Louis, 1992, Mosby.

33. Doane LS, Fisher LM, McDonald TW: How to give intraperitoneal chemotherapy, *AJN* 90(4):58, 1990.

34. Dorr RT: Antidote vesicant chemotherapy extravasation, *Blood Rev* 4:41, 1990.

35. Dorr RT and others: High levels of doxorubicin in the tissues of a patient experiencing extravasation during a 4-day infusion, *Cancer* 64(12):2462, 1989.

36. Dudjak LA: Cancer metastasis, *Semin Oncol Nurs* 8(1):40, 1992.

37. Fields SM, Von Hoff DD: New anticancer agents, *Highlights on Antineoplastic Drugs* 10(2):16, 1992.

38. Finley RS: Drug interactions in the oncology patient, *Semin Oncol Nurs* 8(2):95, 1992.

39. Fisher B: Experimental and clinical justification for the use of tamoxifen in a breast cancer prevention trial: a description of the NSABP effort, *Proceedings Annual Meeting American Association of Cancer Researchers,* 40:A567, 1992.

40. Fumoleau P and others: Vinorelbine (Navelbine) in the treatment of breast cancer: the European experience, *Semin Oncol* 22(5):22, 1995.

41. Galassi A: The next generation: new chemotherapy agents for the 1990s, *Semin Oncol Nurs* 8(2):83, 1992.

42. Gatzemeier U and others: Combination chemotherapy with carboplatin, etoposide, and vincristine as first-line treatment in small cell lung cancer, *J Clin Oncol* 10(5):818, 1992.

43. Gibaldi M: Revisiting some factors contributing to variability, *Ann Pharmacother* 26:1002, 1992.

44. Gotaski G, Andreassi B: Paclitaxel: a new antimiotic chemotherapeutic agent, *Cancer Practice* 2(1):27, 1994.

45. Gosland MP, Lum BL: The 1991 ASCO and AACR meetings: a focus on drug resistance and dose intensification, *Highlights on Antineoplastic Drugs* 9(3):56, 1991.

46. Greenwald P and others: Chemoprevention, *CA Cancer J Clin* 45(1):31, 1995.

47. Groenwald SL and others: *Cancer nursing: principles and practice,* ed 2, Boston, 1990, Jones & Bartlett.

48. Groenwald S and others: Cancer nursing: principles and practice, ed 3, Boston, 1993, Jones & Bartlett.

49. Gullatte MM, Graves T: Advances in antineoplastic therapy, *Oncol Nurs Forum* 17(6):867, 1990.

50. Han J: Highlights of the cancer chemoprevention studies in China, *Prev Med* 22:712, 1993.

51. Hayes D, Henderson I, Shapiro C: Treatment of metastatic breast cancer: present and future prospects, *Semin Oncol Nurs* 22(5):5, 1995.

52. Hessen JA: Protocol for treatment of vesicant antineoplastic extravasation, *Hosp Pharm* 24(9):705, 1989.

53. Hiromoto BM, Dungan B: Contract learning for self-care activities: a protocol study among chemotherapy outpatients, *Cancer Nurs* 14(3):148, 1991.

54. Hogan CM: Advances in the management of nausea and vomiting, *Nurs Clin North Am* 25(2):475, 1990.

55. Hrushesky W, Bjarnason G: Circadian cancer therapy, *J Clin Oncol* 11(7):1403, 1993.

56. Iacobelli S and others: A phase I study of recombinant interferon-α administered as a seven-day continuous venous infusion at circadian rhythm–modulated rate in patients with cancer, *Am J Clin Oncol* 18(1):27, 1995.

57. Irani MA: Improving chemotherapy patient outcomes, *Highlights on Antineoplastic Drugs* 10(1):5, 1992.

58. Jenkins J: Biology of cancer: current issues and future prospects, *Semin Oncol Nurs* 8(1):63, 1992.

59. Kane B, Kuhn JG: Therapeutic drug monitoring in antineoplastic drug development, *Highlights on Antineoplastic Drugs* 10(2):21, 1992.

60. Kenny SA: Effect of two oral care protocols on the incidence of stomatitis in hematology patients, *Cancer Nurs* 13(6):345, 1990.

61. Kennedy B, Balducci L: Closing remarks, *Semin Oncol* 22(1)(1 suppl):35, 1995.

62. Kramer B, Brawley O, Johnson K: National Cancer Institute studies in primary prevention of breast cancer: tamoxifen and finasteride, *Cancer Research, Therapy and Control* 3:203, 1993.

63. Lavelle F and others: Preclinical evaluation of docetaxel (Taxotere), *Semin Oncol* 22(2)(4 suppl):3, 1995.

64. Lawrence T and others: The potential superiority of bromodeoxyuridine to iododeoxyuridine as a radiation sensitizer in the treatment of colorectal cancer, *Cancer Res* 52:3698, 1992.

65. Lebovics R, Delaney T: Sensitizers of photoradiation and ionizing radiation in the management of head and neck cancer, *Med Clin North Am* 77(3):583, 1993.

66. Levi F and others: Programmable in-time pumps for chronotherapy of patients with colorectal cancer with 5-day circadian-modulated venous infusion of 5-fluorouracil *Proceedings of the American Society of Clinical Oncology* 8:111, 1989 (abstract).

67. Li J and others: Nutrition intervention trials in Linxian, China: supplementation with specific vitamin/mineral combinations: cancer incidence and disease-specific mortality among adults with esophageal dysplasia, *J Natl Cancer Inst* 85:1492, 1993.

68. Lin EM: Nutrition support making the difficult decisions, *Cancer Nurs* 14(3):261, 1991.

69. Lind J: Tumor cell growth and cell kinetics, *Semin Oncol Nurs* 8(1):3, 1992.

70. Lobert S, Correia JJ: Antimiotics in cancer chemotherapy, *Cancer Nurs* 15(1):22, 1992.

71. Madeya ML, Pfab-Tokarsky JM: Flow cytometry: an overview, *Oncol Nurs Forum* 19(3):459, 1992.

72. Maher M: The conduct of clinical trials in the area of emesis control, *Semin Oncol Nurs* 6(1 suppl):10, 1990.

73. Mahon S and others: Safe handling practices of cytotoxic drugs: the results of a chapter survey, *Oncol Nurs Forum* 21(7):1157, 1994.

74. Marty M and others: Comparison of 5-hydroxytryptamine 3 (serotonin) antagonist ondansetron (GR38032F) with high-dose metoclopramide in the control of cisplatin-induced emesis, *N Engl J Med* 322(12):816, 1990.

75. Mayo D, Pearson D: Chemotherapy extravasation: a consequence of fibrin sheath formation around venous access devices, *Oncol Nurs Forum* 22(4):675, 1995.

76. McCaffrey D, Engelking C: Ten fallacies associated with the nature and management of chemotherapy extravasation, *Progressions* 2(4):3, 1990.

77. McCance K, Huether S: *Pathophysiology: the biologic basis for disease in adults and children,* ed 2, St Louis, 1994, Mosby.

78. McGinn C, Kinsella T: The experimental and clinical rationale for the use of S-phase–specific radiosensitizers to overcome tumor cell repopulation, *Semin Oncol* 19(4)(11 suppl):21, 1992.

79. McGovern K: 10 golden rules for administering drugs safely, *Nursing* 22(3):49, 1992.

80. McMillan SC: Carcinogenesis, *Semin Oncol Nurs* 8(1):10, 1992.

81. McNally JC and others: *Guidelines for oncology nursing practice,* ed 2, Philadelphia, 1991, Saunders.

82. Meade CD and others: Readability of American Cancer Society patient education literature, *Oncol Nurs Forum* 19(1):51, 1992.

83. Metzger G and others: Spontaneous or imposed circadian changes in plasma concentrations of 5-fluorouracil coadministered with folinic acid and oxaliplatin: relationship with mucousal toxicity in patients with cancer, *Clin Pharmacol Ther* 56(2):190, 1994.

84. Muller J, Tofler G: Circadian variations and cardiovascular disease, *N Engl J Med* 325:1038, 1991.

85. Nayfield S and others: Potential role of tamoxifen in prevention of breast cancer, *National Cancer Institute* 83:1450, 1991.

86. Neuwalt E, Howieson J, Frenkel J: Therapeutic efficacy of multiagent chemotherapy with drug delivery enhancement by blood-brain barrier modification in glioblastoma, *Neurosurgery* 19:573, 1986.

87. Newton M and others: Reviewing the "big three" injection routes, *Nursing* 22(2):34, 1992.

88. Oncology Nursing Society: *Cancer chemotherapy: guidelines and recommendations for nursing education and practice,* Pittsburgh, 1996, Oncology Nursing Press Inc.

89. Oncology Nursing Society: Clinical Practice Committee Module V of the cancer chemotherapy guidelines revised, *Oncol Nurs Forum* 16(2):275, 1989.

90. Ozols RF, editor: The clinical rationale for S-phase radiosensitization in human tumors, *Curr Probl Cancer* 17(5):277, 1993.

91. Padberg RM, Padberg LF: Strengthening the effectiveness of patient education: applying principles of adult education, *Oncol Nurs Forum* 17(1):65, 1990.

92. Panza J, Epstein S, Quyyyumi A: Circadian variation in vascular tone and its relation to α-sympathetic vasoconstrictor activity, *N Engl J Med* 325:986, 1991.

93. Richardson JK, Richardson LI: The mathematics of drugs and solutions with clinical application, St Louis, 1990, Mosby.

94. Rittenberg C, Gralla R, Rehmeyer T: Assessing and managing venous irritation associated with vinorelbine tartrate (Navelbine), *Oncol Nurs Forum* 22(4):707, 1995.

95. Rotman M: Chemoradiation: a new initiative in cancer treatment, 1991 RSNA Annual Oration in Radiation Oncology, *Radiation* 184(2):319, 1992.

96. Schilsky R: Biochemical pharmacology of chemotherapeutic drugs used as radiation enhancers, *Semin Oncol* 19(4)(11 suppl):2, 1992.

97. Szarka C, Grana G, Engstrom P: *Current problems in cancer,* vol 18, no 1, St Louis, 1994, Mosby.

98. Schulmeister L: Establishing a cancer patient education system for ambulatory patients, *Semin Oncol Nurs* 7(2):118, 1991.

99. Stevens KR: Safe handling of cytotoxic drugs in home chemotherapy, *Semin Oncol Nurs* 5(2):15, 1989.

100. Stromberg J and others: Lack of radiosensitization after paclitaxel treatment of three human carcinoma cell lines, *Cancer* 75(9):2262, 1995.

101. Tenenbaum L: *Cancer chemotherapy and biotherapy: a reference guide,* ed 2, Philadelphia, 1994, Saunders.

102. Tishler R and others: Taxol sensitizes human astrocytoma cells to radiation, *Cancer Res* 52:3495, 1992.

103. Trope C and others: Treatment of recurrent endometrial adenocarcinoma with doxorubicin and cisplatin, *Am J Obstet Gynecol* 149:379, 1984.

104. Tsavaris NB and others: Conservative approach to the treatment of chemotherapy-induced extravasation, *J Dermatol Surg Oncol* 16(6):519, 1990.

105. US Department of Labor, Office of Occupational Medicine, Occupational Safety and Health Administration: Work practice guidelines for personnel dealing with cytotoxic (antineoplastic) drugs, CPL 2-2.20B CH-4, Washington, DC, April 14, 1995, US Government Printing Office.

106. Viner CV and others: Ondansetron: a new safe and effective antiemetic in patients receiving high-dose melphalan, *Cancer Chemother Pharmacol* 25(6):449, 1990.

107. Wei J: Cardiovascular comorbidity in the older cancer patient, *Semin Oncol* 22(1)(1 suppl):9, 1995.

108. Weinstein SM: Math calculations for intravenous nurses, *J Intravenous Nursing* 13(4):231, 1990.

109. Wingo P, Tong T, Bolden S: Cancer statistics, 1995, *CA Cancer J Clin* 45(1):12, 1995.

110. Wujcik D: Current research in side effects of high-dose chemotherapy, *Semin Oncol Nurs* 8(2):102, 1992.

111. Xistris D, Schulmeister L: Complying with the new OSHA regulations: problem solving in office oncology, *Nursing* 6(4):1, 1992.

112. Yarbro JW: Oncogenes and cancer suppressor genes, *Semin Oncol Nurs* 8(1):30, 1992.

113. Yoshida D, Piepmeier J, Weinstein M: Estramustine sensitizes human glioblastoma cells to irradiation, *Cancer Res* 54:1415, 1994.

Appendix 22-1 Most Commonly Used Chemotherapeutic Drugs

Drug class	Disease	Route	Dose (mg/m²)	Nadir	Major side effects/toxicities	Nursing action
ALKYLATING AGENTS						
Busulfan (Myleran)	CML, BMT prep	PO	2-6 gm	12-30 days	Myelosuppression, nausea, vomiting, pulmonary fibrosis, alopecia, venoocclusive disease with high dose	Increased toxicity with high dose; promote compliance
Carboplatin (Paraplatin)	Ovarian, leukemia	IV, IP	250-600	21 days	Myelosuppression, nausea, vomiting, mild nephrotoxicity and neurotoxicity	Hydration; premedicate with antiemetics Drug decomposes if mixed with NS
Chlorambucil (Leukeran)	Lymphoma, CLL	PO IV	0.1-0.3 mg/kg 50-100	7-14 days	Myelosuppression, sterility, stomatitis, pulmonary infiltrates, hepatotoxicity	Promote compliance; inform patient about sexuality changes
Cisplatin (Cis-DDP)	Testicular, ovarian, lung, H&N, cervical, neuroblastoma, osteogenic sarcoma	IV, IP, IA	50-150	21 days	Nephrotoxicity, neurotoxicity, nausea and vomiting, ototoxicity, electrolyte imbalance (K⁺, Ca⁺⁺, Mg, P) Hypersensitivity reaction	Hydration; monitor I&O; premedicate with antiemetics, obtain 12-24 hr creatinine clearance
Cyclophosphamide (Cytoxan)	Leukemia, breast, pre-BMT, lymphoma, lung, ovarian, myeloma, neuroblastoma, Wilms', Ewing's sarcoma	IV, PO, IT	50-200 high dose: 2-6 g	7-14 days	Myelosuppression, alopecia, hemorrhagic cystitis, nausea and vomiting, cardiotoxicity, pulmonary fibrosis, temporary sterility Hypersensitivity reaction	Hydration; monitor I&O; encourage to void Q2-4 hr. EKG/MUGA scan with high doses; Preservative-free diluent for intrathecal injection
Estramustine	Metastatic prostate	PO	600	None	Nausea and vomiting, diarrhea, mild gynecomastia	May give drug in divided doses
Dacarbazine (DTIC)	Hodgkin's, soft tissue sarcoma, melanoma	IV	75-1500	7-21 days	Myelosuppression, nausea and vomiting, alopecia, diarrhea, anaphylaxis, extravasation, flu-like syndrome, hepatotoxic and renal impairment	Vesicant; administer drug via free-flowing IV; premedicate with antiemetics

ALL, Acute lymphocytic leukemia; *ADH,* antidiuretic hormone; *bid,* twice a day; *BMT,* bone marrow transplantation; Ca⁺⁺, calcium; *CI,* continuous infusion; *CLL,* chronic lymphocytic leukemia; *CML,* chronic myelogenous leukemia; *D₅W,* dextrose water 5%; *ECG,* electrocardiogram; *HD,* high dose; *HIV,* human immunodeficiency virus; *H&N,* head and neck; *I&O,* intake and output; *IA,* intraarterial; *IM,* intramuscular; *IP,* intraperitoneal; *IT,* intrathecal; *IV,* intravenous; *K⁺,* potassium; *Mg,* magnesium; *P,* phosphorus; *PO,* oral; *qd,* daily.

Continued.

Appendix 22–1 Most Commonly Used Chemotherapeutic Drugs—cont'd

Drug class	Disease	Route	Dose (mg/m²)	Nadir	Major side effects/toxicities	Nursing action
ALKYLATING AGENTS—cont'd						
Ifosfamide (Ifex)	Breast, lung, sarcoma, ovarian, lymphoma, testicular	IV	700-2 gm high dose:	7-21 days	Cardiotoxicity (high dose), alopecia, nephrotoxicity, nausea and vomiting, hemorrhagic cystitis, myelosuppression	Concurrent administration with Mesna; hydration; monitor I&O; premedicate with antiemetics
Melphalan (Alkeran)	Myeloma, ovarian, breast, multiple myeloma	PO	Varies	7-14 days	Myelosuppression (high dose), nausea and vomiting	Premedicate with antiemetics
Nitrogen mustard (Mechlorethamine HCl)	Hodgkin's, lymphoma, leukemia	IV, topical		7-21 days	Hypersensitivity reaction Severe nausea and vomiting, stomatitis, myelosuppression, alopecia, diarrhea, extravasation	Vesicant; premedicate with antiemetics; administer drug within 60 minutes after reconstitution
Thiotepa (Thioplex)	Preparation for BMT, breast, lymphoma, leukemia, bladder	PO, IV, instill bladder	6-10	7-28 days	Hypersensitivity reaction Myelosuppression, nausea and vomiting, menstrual and spermatogenesis dysfunction	Myelosuppression increases with high dose; monitor side effects
ANTITUMOR ANTIBIOTICS						
Bleomycin	Testicular, cervical, Hodgkin's lymphoma	IV, IM, SC	10-20 U/m²	7 days	Anaphylaxis Nausea and vomiting, rash, pneumonitis, pulmonary fibrosis, alopecia, stomatitis, hyperpigmentation, cystitis	Test dose before initial administration; auscultate breath sounds on a scheduled frequency
Dactinomycin (Actinomycin D, Cosmegen)	Choriocarcinoma, Ewing's and soft tissue sarcoma, rhabdomyosarcoma, Wilms' tumor	IV	1-2	7-14 days	Myelosuppression, extravasation, hepatotoxic, allergic reaction, alopecia, radiation recall, stomatitis	Vesicant; monitor skin irritation
Daunorubicin (Cerubidine, Daunomycin)	Leukemia (ALL, AML)	IV	30-60	7-14 days	Myelosuppression, cardiotoxicity, ECG changes, extravasation, nausea and vomiting, alopecia, stomatitis, anorexia, allergic reaction, red urine (24-48 hr) dermatitis in previously irradiated areas	Vesicant; cumulative dose ~500 mg/m²; monitor skin desquamation changes; inform patient about red urine status

Drug	Indications	Route	Dose	Nadir	Toxicity	Considerations
Doxorubicin (Adriamycin)	Breast, endometrial, H&N Ewing's, Kaposi's and osteogenic sarcomas, leukemia (ALL, AML), liver, Hodgkin's, myeloma lymphoma, Wilms', neuroblastomas and retinoblastomas	IV	Varies with protocol	7-14 days	Myelosuppression, cardiotoxicity, ECG changes, extravasation, nausea and vomiting, alopecia, stomatitis, anorexia, allergic reaction, red urine (24-48 hr) dermatitis in previously irradiated areas	Vesicant; cumulative dose ~550 mg/m²; monitor skin desquamation changes; inform patient about red urine status. Doxorubicin is incompatible with many drugs
Idarubicin (Idamycin)	Breast, leukemia	IV	18-25	7-14 days	Myelosuppression, myocardial toxicity, extravasation, nausea and vomiting, alopecia, stomatitis, diarrhea	Vesicant
Mitomycin C (Mutamycin)	Colorectal, gastric, esophageal, Ewing's and soft tissue sarcomas	IV	10-20	21 days	Myelosuppression, pulmonary toxicity, hepatotoxicity, renal toxicity, nausea and vomiting, extravasation, alopecia, urine color changes, stomatitis	Vesicant; inform patient about urine color changes
Plicamycin (Mithracin)	Testicular, hypercalcemia	IV	25-50	5 days	Hemorrhagic diathesis, nausea and vomiting, hepatic and renal damage, hypocalcemia	Vesicant; irritant
ANTIMETABOLITES						
Cytarabine (Cytosar, Ara-C)	Leukemia (ALL, AML), lymphoma	IV, IT, IP, SC	Varies with protocol	7-10 days	Myelosuppression, neurotoxicity, sudden respiratory distress with high doses, rash, nausea and vomiting, stomatitis, diarrhea, conjunctivitis, hepatotoxicity, alopecia Anaphylaxis	Monitor neurotoxicity via scheduled neurologic assessments; premedicate with antiemetics; use Decadron eye drops as prophylaxis for conjunctivitis Preservative-free diluent intrathecal injection
Floxuridine (FUDR)	Colorectal, hepatic metastasis, liver	IA	5-20	7-14 days	Myelosuppression, nausea and vomiting, oral and GI ulceration, alopecia, dermatitis, hepatic dysfunction	Requires placement of temporary arterial catheter and/or implantable pump for drug infusion; monitor catheter and extremity on a scheduled basis
Fludarabine (Fludara)	Leukemia (CLL, hairy cell), low-grade lymphoma	IV	30	7-14 days	Myelosuppression, CNS toxicity, visual disturbance, nausea and vomiting, renal damage with HD, tumor lysis syndrome	Hydration; premedicate with antiemetics; monitor CNS toxicities on a scheduled basis

Continued.

Appendix 22-1 Most Commonly Used Chemotherapeutic Drugs—cont'd

Drug class	Disease	Route	Dose (mg/m^2)	Nadir	Major side effects/toxicities	Nursing action
ANTIMETABOLITES—cont'd						
Fluorouracil (5-FU)	Breast, colorectal, liver, endometrial, esophageal, pancreatic, bladder	IV	400-600	7-14 days	Myelosuppression, diarrhea, oral and GI ulcerations, alopecia, hyperpigmentation, nausea and vomiting	Diarrhea and ulcerations are more severe when 5-FU is given in combination with leucovorin. Incompatible with anthracyclines
Hydroxyurea (Hydrea)	CML chronic phase	IV, PO	1000-1500 1000	7-21 days	Myelosuppression, nausea and vomiting, stomatitis, dysuria, alopecia, allergic reaction	Premedicate with antiemetics; administer in divided doses; monitor for allergic reaction
Gemcitabine (Gemzar)	Pancreatic, lung cancer	IV	Varies	7-14 days	Myelosuppression, fatigue	Monitor myelosuppression
Mercaptopurine (6-MP)	Leukemia (ALL, CML)	PO	100	7-14 days	Myelosuppression, nausea and vomiting, diarrhea, oral and GI ulcerations, pancreatitis	Monitor oral dosing compliance
Methotrexate (MTX, Folex)	Breast, lymphoma, leukemia (ALL), bladder, choriocarcinoma, H&N, esophageal, mycosis fungoides	IV, IT, PO, IM	Varies with protocol	7-14 days	Myelosuppression, diarrhea, oral and GI ulcerations, pulmonary infiltrates and fibrosis, nausea and vomiting, stomatitis, renal toxicity, hepatotoxicity, CNS toxicity with IT infusion, alopecia. Hypersensitivity reaction	Dosage: 1 gm/m^2 or more requires hydration and alkalinization of urine and leucovorin rescue; diarrhea and ulcerations are more severe when drug given in high-dose. Preservative-free diluent with intrathecal administration
Thioguanine (6-TG)	Leukemia (ALL)	PO	100	7-21 days	Myelosuppression, diarrhea, stomatitis, hepatic damage	Monitor oral dosing compliance
Trimetrexate (Neutrexin)	*Pneumocystitis carinii*, H&N, non-small-cell lung, urothelial cancer	IV	8-12 × 5 days	7-14 days	Myelosuppression, mucositis, fever, chills, nausea and vomiting, rash, pruritus, hyperpigmentation, nephrotoxicity, diarrhea	Monitor toxicities; administer antiemetics and antidiarrheal drugs
HORMONAL AGENTS			Dosage *not* in mg/m^2			
Aminoglutethimide (Cytadren)	Breast, prostate	PO	500-1000 mg	None	Nausea, rash, drowsiness, hypotension, masculinization, fever	Caution patient about concomitant prescriptions with aminoglutethimide

Drug	Use	Route	Dose		Side effects	Nursing considerations
Corticosteroids (Dexamethasone, Decadron, Solu-Cortef, Solu-Medrol, Prednisone)	Used in many chemotherapy disease protocols	PO, IV, IM	Varies with protocol	None	Fluid and electrolyte disturbances, neuromuscular imbalances, changes in appetite and energy, requires glucose/insulin adjustments, potential weight gain	Decadron IV rapid bolus results in severe rectal itching; Corticosteroids long-term use requires dose tapering principles
Diethylstilbestrol (DES)	Breast, prostate	PO	Varies	None	Nausea and vomiting, gynecomastia in men, breast tenderness, loss of libido, hypertension, changes in menstrual flow	Inform patient about sexuality changes
Finasteride (Proscar)	Prostate	PO	5 mg	None	Impotence, decreased libido, teratogenicity	Inform patient about sexuality changes
Flutamide (Eulexin)	Prostate	PO	250-750 mg	None	Nausea, diarrhea, gynecomastia, hepatotoxicity	Inform patient about sexuality changes
Leuprolide (Leupron)	Prostate	IM, SC	Varies	None	Impotence, testicular atrophy, hot flashes, gynecomastia, CNS effects, peripheral edema, transient increase in bone pain	Inform patient about sexuality changes
Megestrol (Megace)	Breast, prostate	PO	Varies	None	Menstrual changes, hot flashes, nausea and vomiting, headache, fluid retention, weight gain, edema	Inform patient about sexuality changes
Tamoxifen (Nolvadex)	Breast	PO	Varies	None	Vaginal bleeding and discharge, hot flashes, rash, nausea and vomiting, hypercalcemia, peripheral edema, transient increased bone or tumor pain, thrombocytopenia	Inform patient about sexuality changes
Goserelin (Zoladex)	Breast, prostate	IM, SC	Varies	None	Postmenopausal symptoms, impotence, testicular atrophy, gynecomastia, hot flashes, transient increased bone pain	Inform patient about sexuality changes

Continued.

Appendix 22-1 Most Commonly Used Chemotherapeutic Drugs—cont'd

Drug class	Disease	Route	Dose (mg/m²)	Nadir	Major side effects/toxicities	Nursing action
NITROSOUREAS						
Carmustine (BCNU)	Glioblastoma, myeloma, lymphoma, pre-BMT	IV	200-225	3-4 wk	Myelosuppression, nausea and vomiting, pulmonary fibrosis, renal and liver damage, seizures, myocardial ischemia, leukemia, phlebitis	Irritant; administer slowly, contains alcohol, patient may feel inebriated; myelosuppression is increased with high-dose administration
Chlorozotocin (DCNU)	Brain	IV		2-4 wk	Myelosuppression, nausea and vomiting, phlebitis, renal and liver damage, diarrhea, hyperglycemia, fever	Irritant; monitor glucose/insulin levels
Lomustine (CCNU)	Brain, leukemia, Hodgkin's lymphoma, melanoma, myeloma, bladder	PO	100-150	4-6 wk	Myelosuppression, nausea and vomiting, pulmonary fibrosis, neurologic reactions, renal damage, leukemia, transient elevated liver enzymes	Administer at bedtime with antiemetics
Semustine (Methyl-CCNU)	Brain, colorectal, gastric	PO	150-200	4-6 wk	Myelosuppression, nausea and vomiting, renal and hepatic toxicities	Administer on an empty stomach with antiemetics
Streptozocin (Zanosar)	Colorectal, liver, pancreas	IV	Varies	2-4 wk	Myelosuppression, CNS effects, renal and liver damage, hypoglycemia/hyperglycemia, diarrhea, nausea and vomiting, phlebitis	Irritant; monitor glucose/insulin levels
VINCA ALKALOIDS						
Etoposide (VP-16)	Lung, testicular, Kaposi's and osteogenic sarcomas, leukemia, neuroblastoma, prep-BMT, lymphoma	IV, PO	50-100 200	7-10 days	Myelosuppression, nausea and vomiting, diarrhea, fever, hypotension, phlebitis, anaphylaxis, rash, alopecia, peripheral neuropathy, mucositis, hepatic damage with high doses	Test dose and/or administer drug slowly IV; increased severity of side effects with high doses
Teniposide (VM-26)	Leukemia (childhood ALL)	IV	165	7-14 days	Myelosuppression, extravasation, alopecia, constipation, neuropathy	Vesicant; monitor neurotoxicities and bowel function; promote hydration

Drug	Cancer	Route	Dose	Nadir	Side effects	Nursing considerations
Vinblastine (Velban)	Testicular, Hodgkin's, lung, lymphoma, bladder, Kaposi's sarcoma, renal	IV	2-6	5-10 days	Myelosuppression, extravasation, nausea and vomiting, alopecia, stomatitis, loss of deep tendon reflexes, jaw pain, paralytic ileus	Vesicant; monitor neurotoxicity; promote hydration and high-fiber diet; administer oral stool softener
Vindesine (Eldisine)	Squamous cell (esophagus)	IV	2-4	7-14 days	Myelosuppression, peripheral neuropathy, constipation, extravasation, skin changes	Vesicant; monitor neuropathy and constipation; promote hydration
Vincristine (Oncovin)	Leukemia (ALL, CML), lymphoma, myeloma, retinoblastoma, Wilms' brain, Ewing's and Kaposi's sarcomas, rhabdomyosarcoma	IV	0.5-2 mg	5-7 days	Extravasation, alopecia, stomatitis, constipation, paralytic ileus, peripheral neuropathy, jaw pain, inappropriate ADH secretion, mild myelosuppression, optic atrophy	Vesicant; monitor bowel function and promote hydration and high-fiber diet; administer oral stool softener; monitor neurotoxicity changes
Vinorelbine (Navelbine)	Breast, lung, Hodgkin's, H&N	IV	30 dilute concentration > 3 ml	7-10 days	Myelosuppression, alopecia, injection site reactions (erythema, discoloration, phlebitis, pain), nausea and vomiting, anorexia, stomatitis, peripheral neuropathy, constipation, weakness, fatigue	Vesicant; monitor neurotoxicity and bowel function; follow manufacturer's reconstitution guidelines; prehydrate patient with 100 ml NS or D_5W to flush the vein; administer drug over 10 min via free-flow IV

MISCELLANEOUS CHEMOTHERAPEUTIC DRUGS

Drug	Cancer	Route	Dose	Nadir	Side effects	Nursing considerations
Altretamine (Hexamethylmelamine)	Lymphoma, lung, H&N, breast, ovarian	PO	150-400 in 4 divided doses	21 days	Myelosuppression, nausea and vomiting, CNS depression, peripheral neuropathy, ataxia, tremors, alopecia, rash	Premedicate with antiemetics; ensure medication is taken qid; (PC & HS)
L-asparaginase (Elspar)	Leukemia (ALL)	IV, IM	1000-6000 IU/kg	None	Nausea and vomiting, chills, headache, CNS depression, abdominal pain, coagulation defects, hyperglycemia, hepatic and renal damage, fever; Anaphylaxis	Maintain IV access; follow anaphylaxis protocol; monitor for 2-4 hr after drug infusion

Continued.

Appendix 22-1 Most Commonly Used Chemotherapeutic Drugs—cont'd

MISCELLANEOUS CHEMOTHERAPEUTIC DRUGS—cont'd

Drug class	Disease	Route	Dose (mg/m²)	Nadir	Major side effects/toxicities	Nursing action
(Leustatin) Cladribine, 2-CdA (Leustatin)	Hairy cell leukemia, low-grade lymphoma	IV CI × 7 days	0.09 mg/kg	7-14 days	Myelosuppression, peripheral neuropathy with high doses, fever, fatigue	Incompatible with D_5W; calculate dose by multiplying patient's weight in kg by 0.09 mg (50 kg × 0.09 mg = 4.5 mg/day); administer via central venous access/ambulatory pump
Mitoxantrone (Novantrone)	Leukemia, breast, lymphoma, childhood T-cell ALL and lymphoma	IV	15	7-14 days	Myelosuppression, cardiotoxicity, alopecia, nausea and vomiting, stomatitis, phlebitis, hepatic and renal damage, temporary blue-green pigment in urine and sclera	Inform patient about urine and sclera blue-green pigment changes 24-48 hr after drug infusion
Pentostatin (2'-deoxycoformycin)	Hairy cell leukemia, chronic lymphocytic leukemia, lymphoma	IV, SC	2-4	7-14 days	Myelosuppression, nephrotoxicity, CNS depression, nausea and vomiting, myalgia, rash, photophobia, conjunctivitis	Monitor toxicities; teach patient to recognize and report symptoms
Procarbazine (Matulane)	Lymphoma, lung, brain, Hodgkin's	PO	100-150	3-5 wk	Myelosuppression, CNS depression, nausea and vomiting, stomatitis Avoid alcohol, antidepressants, antihistamines, foods rich in tyramine (yeast)	Teach patient diet (e.g., bananas, yogurt), medication, and ethanol restrictions
Suramin	Prostate, breast, multiple myeloma	IV	350-1400	7-14 days	Myelosuppression, proteinuria, tearing, photophobia, elevated liver enzymes and serum creatinine, blurred vision	Inform patient about visual changes
Taxol (Paclitaxel)	Breast, lung, ovarian	IV	200	7-14 days	Myelosuppression, angioedema, dyspnea, hypotension, alopecia, urticaria, cardiotoxicity, peripheral neuropathy Anaphylaxis	Maintain IV access; follow anaphylaxis protocol; use non-PVC tubing/glass bottle for drug administration; *vesicant properties*
Taxotere (Docetaxel)	Breast, lung, ovarian	IV	100	7-14 days	Myelosuppression, fluid retention, skin desquamation, mucositis, phlebitis, vomiting, diarrhea Anaphylaxis	Maintain IV access; follow anaphylaxis protocol; irritant; use non-PVC tubing/glass bottle for drug administration; *vesicant properties*

Drug	Indication	Route	Dose	Nadir	Side effects	Nursing considerations
Topotecan	Lung, breast, esophagus, tumors, lymphoma, myelodysplastic syndrome	IV	2 mg CI × 5 days	7-14 days	Myelosuppression, nausea and vomiting, diarrhea, fever, fatigue, alopecia, rash, elevated liver enzymes	Premedicate with antiemetics
Tretinoin (Vesanoid)	Skin cancers	Topical	Daily	None	Rash, stinging, erythema, blistering, hypersensitivity, contact dermatitis	Provide prudent skin care

INVESTIGATIONAL CHEMOTHERAPEUTIC DRUGS

Drug	Indication	Route	Dose	Nadir	Side effects	Nursing considerations
Amonafide	Leukemia, esophagus	IV, PO	75-450	7-14 days	Myelosuppression, alopecia, rash, temporary orange urine, myalgia, nausea and vomiting	Inform patient about urine color change 24-48 hr after drug infusion
Amsacrine (m-AMSA)	Leukemia, breast	IV	120	7-14 days	Myelosuppression, phlebitis, nausea and vomiting, alopecia, cardiotoxicity, hepatic and renal dysfunction	Irritant; monitor for anaphylaxis and cardiotoxicity
Azacitidine (Ladakamycin, 5-Azacytidine)	Leukemia (refractory AML)	IV	200	7-14 days	Myelosuppression, fever, rash, diarrhea, nausea and vomiting, drowsiness, hepatic toxicity and cardiotoxicity. Anaphylaxis	Premedicate with antiemetics
Didemnin B	Lung, breast, ovarian, sarcoma, kidney	IV	5	7-14 days	Nausea and vomiting, diarrhea, elevated liver enzymes. Anaphylaxis	Follow anaphylaxis protocol; premedicate with antiemetics
Edatrexate (10-EDAM)	H&N, colorectal, breast, lymphoma, lung, soft tissue sarcomas	IV	80-100	7-14 days	Myelosuppression, mucositis, fatigue, diarrhea, alopecia, nausea and vomiting, elevated liver enzymes	Premedicate with antiemetics
Fazarabine	Lung	IV	2	7-14 days	Myelosuppression, elevated liver enzymes, nausea and vomiting	Reconstitute with D_5W and/or lactated Ringer's solutions
Irinotecan	Metastatic colorectal, pancreatic, gastric	IV	Varies	7-10 days	Myelosuppression, severe diarrhea, nausea and vomiting, abdominal cramping, diaphoresis, flushing	Administer antidiarrheal medications
Isotretinoin (Accutane)	Cervical	PO	1 mg/kg	7-14 days	Fatigue, headache, nausea and vomiting, xerostomia, rash, conjunctivitis, anorexia, pruritus, bone and joint pain, nose bleeds	Provide prudent mouth care and offer medications for dry eyes/conjunctivitis

Continued.

Appendix 22-1   Most Commonly Used Chemotherapeutic Drugs—cont'd

Drug class	Disease	Route	Dose (mg/m²)	Nadir	Major side effects/toxicities	Nursing action
INVESTIGATIONAL CHEMOTHERAPEUTIC DRUGS—cont'd						
Merbarone	Pancreatic, gastric, melanoma	IV	1 g CI × 5 days	7-14 days	Alopecia, elevated liver enzymes, nausea and vomiting, diarrhea, phlebitis, anorexia	Irritant; premedicate with antiemetics; monitor liver enzymes
Mitotane (Lysodren)	Adrenocortical carcinoma	PO	9-10 g/day divided doses	None	CNS depression, nausea and vomiting, diarrhea, visual disturbance, rash, pulmonary infiltrates, hypertension	Provide hydration; monitor CNS effects
Octreotide (Sandostatin)	Carcinoid cancers	SC	100-600 µg	None	Nausea and vomiting, diarrhea, gallstones, increased secretion of sebaceous glands	Promote prudent hygiene
Pala	Colorectal	IV	250	7-14 days	Nausea and vomiting, diarrhea, stomatitis	Premedicate with antiemetics
Piritrexim	Melanoma, urothelial cancers, H&N	PO	75-150 mg bid	7-14 days	Myelosuppression, mucositis, stomatitis, nausea and vomiting, anorexia, skin rash	Premedicate with antiemetics
Piroxantrone (Oxantrazale)	Breast, prostate, H&N, melanoma	IV	150	7-14 days	Myelosuppression, nausea and vomiting, alopecia, mucositis, diarrhea, lethargy, extravasation	Vesicant; premedicate with antiemetics
MISCELLANEOUS DRUGS USED IN CHEMOTHERAPY PROTOCOLS						
Allopurinol	Leukemia, Hodgkin's, lymphoma	PO	200-600 mg/qd	None	Myelosuppression, headache, drowsiness, anorexia, nausea and vomiting, alopecia	Promote hydration; administer before chemotherapy drug initiation
Leucovorin	Used in multiple chemotherapy regimens (e.g., 5-Fluorouracil)	PO, IV	Varies	7-14 days	Hypersensitivity, pruritus, erythema, urticaria, wheezing	Promote hydration and compliance in self-administration regimens
Levamisole	Used in multiple chemotherapy regimens	PO	1-5 mg/kg	None	Mild GI complaints	Observe
Mesna	Used most often with ifosfamide and Cytoxan regimens	IV	Varies	None	Nausea and vomiting, diarrhea, altered taste, rash, headache, fatigue, joint pain, hypotension	Always administer concurrently with and/or before ifosfamide and high-dose cyclophosphamide

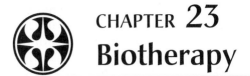

CHAPTER 23
Biotherapy

PAULA TRAHAN RIEGER

The rapid introduction of novel agents and approaches and an improved understanding of the biology of cancer have opened an exciting era in cancer therapy. Traditionally, surgery, radiation therapy, and chemotherapy, either singly or in combination, have been the mainstays of cancer therapy. Since the 1980s, biotherapy, or biologic therapy, has emerged as an important fourth modality for treating cancer.[49,63,74,102,156]

Oncology nurses whose patients receive biotherapy need a basic understanding of the immune system, the rationale for this therapy, and its primary clinical agents (see Chapter 30 for a review of the immune system). This chapter reviews the history of immunotherapy and other biotherapy approaches, scientific advances that led to clinical trials with biologic agents, the rationale for the use of these agents, their clinical indications, and the associated nursing care for patients receiving them.

THEORY OF IMMUNE SURVEILLANCE

Host defense mechanisms protect the body by detecting and eliminating substances recognized as "foreign" or "nonself." The theory of immune surveillance, refined and expanded by McFarlane Burnet,[28,90,111] states that certain cells undergo neoplastic transformation but are recognized by the immune system as foreign and subsequently destroyed. At first T cells were thought to be primarily responsible for this reaction, but it is now known that other immune cells such as natural killer (NK) cells and macrophages are also involved.[111] If an atypical cell somehow escapes detection or destruction, a clinically detectable tumor eventually develops.

Although this theory remains controversial, many clinical phenomena and laboratory observations support it. Spontaneous tumor regression has been observed in patients with solid tumors such as melanoma and renal cancer and with acute leukemia[193]; that is, tumors shrank or patients entered remission without treatment. Some of these regressions have been associated with infectious complications, which may suggest an immunologic mechanism.[90,153,193]

Immunologic defense mechanisms are relatively weak in the young and the aged, and the incidence of malignancy in humans peaks correspondingly during early childhood and old age. In these periods, impaired or immature defense mechanisms may allow abnormal cells to escape immune surveillance and proliferate.

An increased incidence of cancer is also seen in patients with immune deficiencies resulting from immunosuppressive therapy or other causes; for example, individuals undergoing chronic immunosuppressive therapy for the maintenance of organ allografts. Patients with immunodeficiencies exhibit a higher incidence of malignancies, especially of the lymphoid type, than does the general population.[111,163]

The fact that immune cells infiltrate tumors also supports this theory. Pathologic examination of surgical specimens shows infiltration by lymphocytes, macrophages, and plasma cells, and it has been suggested that immune mechanisms may be responsible for reducing the growth rate of tumors.[170]

A variety of experiments lend further support to the theory of immune surveillance. Neonatal thymectomy causes mice to accept tumor transplants, whereas mice possessing normal thymic function reject the transplants.[3] The use of antilymphocyte serum and immunosuppressive therapy in animals can increase the incidence and development of both spontaneous tumors and those induced by viruses and chemical carcinogens. Lymphocytes appear to be essential to the recognition and destruction of aberrant cells.[90]

If, as this evidence suggests, immune surveillance is an important part of antitumor host defense, how do transformed cells escape detection by the immune system? Krueger[111] proposes four basic mechanisms: (1) a basic defect in function of effector cells responsible for immune surveillance; (2) an imbalance of the immune response to the tumor; (3) malignant cells not sufficiently immunogenic to elicit an immune response; and (4) production of blocking factors that interfere with the immune response to tumors.

Although skepticism remains regarding the theory of

immune surveillance, it is an attractive explanation for the occurrence of cancer. Further experimentation will continue to clarify the relationship between the immune system and malignant cells.

HISTORICAL PERSPECTIVE

The observation of interactions between the immune system and malignant cells led to the development of therapies that could manipulate this natural process. Traditionally, this field has been known as *immunotherapy*.[90,193] The immunotherapy of cancer can be divided into two approaches, active and passive. *Active immunotherapy* consists of giving a tumor-bearing host agents that are designed to elicit an immune response capable of retarding or eliminating tumor growth. The two types of active immunotherapy are specific and nonspecific. *Active specific* immunotherapy is immunization with tumor cells or tumor-cell extracts, either alone or in vaccines. The use of monoclonal antibodies as vaccines is an area of active investigation. *Active nonspecific* immunotherapy is an attempt to boost overall immunity through the use of adjuvants such as bacterial extracts. The latter approach was based on the observation that adjuvants administered in animal systems could cause tumor regression. It was also based on the idea that those with tumors have diminished defense mechanisms.[90,193]

Passive immunotherapy is the administration or transfer of previously sensitized immunologic reagents such as antisera (which contain sensitized antibodies) or immune-reactive cells to a tumor-bearing host. These reagents directly or indirectly mediate antitumor responses. The term *adoptive immunotherapy* is still used to refer to the passive transfer of sensitized cells such as lymphocytes or macrophages.[90,191,193]

Principles for immunotherapy of human cancer are based mainly on knowledge gained from animal experiments. First, immunotherapeutic approaches appeared most successful for small tumor burdens. Therefore tumor burden was to be reduced by conventional treatment, followed by immunotherapy. Second, the host had to be immunocompetent, or immunocompetence had to be restored, for immunotherapy to be maximally effective. Third, the timing of immunotherapy was crucial. How long after conventional treatment immunotherapy should be started to allow for restoration of immunosuppressive effects was a concern. Fourth, the site of immunization for active immunotherapy, especially active specific immunotherapy, was extremely important. Active specific immunotherapy was often given in tumor-free lymphatic drainage areas.[90]

Initial attempts at boosting the immune systems of cancer patients to destroy tumors used a variety of microorganisms, fractions of microbial products, or other immunomodulators. Since the 1960s many clinical studies have attempted nonspecific stimulation of the immune system by using such products as bacille Calmette-Guérin (BCG) or its methanol extraction residue (MER), *Corynebacterium parvum,* and levamisole. Although initial trials seemed positive, well-controlled, prospective, randomized trials did not show significant overall survival gains in the arm utilizing immunotherapy.[156]

These early trials failed to establish immunotherapy as a major modality most likely for a variety of reasons, such as the lack of purity and definition of immunotherapeutic agents, lack of analogy between animal model systems and humans, variability of experimental procedures, and inadequate administration of immunotherapeutic agents.[156,193]

TECHNOLOGIC ADVANCES

During the 1970s and 1980s, several scientific and technologic developments led biologic therapy to emerge as a major modality in the treatment of cancer. Our overall understanding of the relationship between host defense mechanisms and cancer and of the basic biology of cancer has improved. Recombinant deoxyribonucleic acid (DNA) technology (see Figure 23-1) has allowed the production of large quantities of highly purified products from the human genome, as hybridoma technology has done for highly purified, highly specific immunoglobulin reagents. Methods of growing large volumes of effector cells in culture have been developed, and advances in computer hardware and software have led to the isolation and purification of biologic molecules.[73,156]

These discoveries have led to the modern era of biotherapy. The use of this term is more appropriate than heretofore because this field encompasses a much broader basis than only the immune system. Although the use of agents affecting the immune system remains a subcategory, biotherapy includes treatments affecting other biologic responses such as growth and differentiation factors, chimeric molecules (genetically engineered molecules that may have some parts added or removed to tailor them for a particular use, as when a chimeric monoclonal antibody has part human and part murine fragments), and agents that may affect tumor cells' ability to metastasize.

BIOTHERAPY DEFINED

Biotherapy may be defined as treatment with agents derived from biologic sources and/or affecting biologic responses. Most of its agents are derived from the mammalian genome.[156] The Subcommittee on Biologic Response Modifiers (BRMs) of the National Cancer Institute's Division of Cancer Treatment defines BRMs as "agents or approaches that modify the relationship between tumor and host by modifying the host's biologic

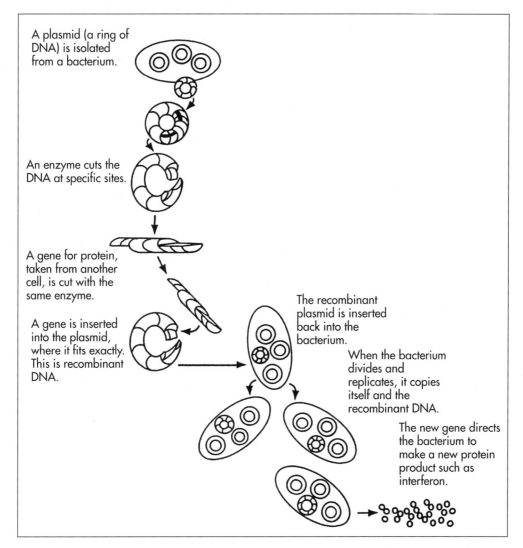

A plasmid (a ring of DNA) is isolated from a bacterium.

An enzyme cuts the DNA at specific sites.

A gene for protein, taken from another cell, is cut with the same enzyme.

A gene is inserted into the plasmid, where it fits exactly. This is recombinant DNA.

The recombinant plasmid is inserted back into the bacterium.

When the bacterium divides and replicates, it copies itself and the recombinant DNA.

The new gene directs the bacterium to make a new protein product such as interferon.

Figure 23-1   Recombinant DNA technology. Genetic engineering, known as recombinant DNA technology, allows scientists to pluck genes from one type of organism and combine them with genes of a second organism, inducing cells to make large quantities of human protein, such as interferon and interleukins. Microorganisms also can be made to manufacture proteins from infectious agents, such as the hepatitis virus and the acquired immunodeficiency syndrome (AIDS) virus, for use in vaccines. (From Schindler LW: *Understanding the immune system*, NIH Pub No 88-529, Bethesda, Md, 1988, US Department of Health and Human Services.)

response to tumor cells, with a resultant therapeutic effect."[138]

The explosion of biotherapy research, coupled with the aforementioned technologic advances, has led to the use of numerous agents, both commercially and in clinical trials. Although nonspecific immunomodulating agents such as BCG and *C. parvum* are still used, a variety of newer agents, such as interferons, interleukins, monoclonal antibodies, and hematopoietic growth factors, are now undergoing clinical investigation (Tables 23-1 and 23-2). Many of these are naturally occurring body sub-

stances that act as messengers between cells. A generic term for these messengers is *cytokine*, which refers to protein products from cells that serve as cell regulators. More specifically, lymphokines are products of lymphocytes, and monokines are products of monocytes. The name *interleukin* refers to proteins that act as messengers between cells.[46,170,193]

A system of classification is often useful for looking at the agents' mechanisms of action. However, the way many BRMs work against tumors is not fully understood. Many agents may have more than one antitumor mode

Table 23-1   Biologic Activity of Cytokines

Cytokine	Abbreviation	Primary cellular source	Biologic activity
INTERFERONS			
Interferon-alpha	IFN-α	Leukocytes	Antiviral activity
Interferon-beta	IFN-β	Fibroblasts	Antiproliferative effects; augments NK cell activity; induces MHC class I antigens
Interferon-gamma	IFN-γ	T cells, NK cells, monocytes/macrophages	Antiviral activity; induces MHC class I, II antigens; potent immunomodulatory effects; interacts with other cytokines
HEMATOPOIETIC GROWTH FACTORS			
Granulocyte colony-stimulating factor	G-CSF	Stromal cells, endothelial cells, monocytes/ macrophages	Stimulates growth of granulocyte colonies; activates mature granulocytes; augments ADCC
Granulocyte/macrophage colony-stimulating factor	GM-CSF	Fibroblasts, endothelial cells, T cells, stromal cells	Stimulates growth of monocyte, granulocyte, and early erythroid progenitors; activates mature granulocytes and monocytes; enhances ADCC and cell-mediated cytotoxicity
Macrophage colony-stimulating factor	M-CSF	Fibroblasts, stromal cells, monocytes/macrophages	Stimulates growth of monocyte colonies; activates mature monocytes
Erythropoietin	Epo	Peritubular cells in the kidney	Stimulates erythrocyte progenitors; primary regulator of erythropoiesis
Thrombopoietin	Tpo	Hepatic cells, endothelial cells, fibroblasts	Primary regulator of platelet production
Stem cell factor	SCF	Stromal-derived cells	Stimulates multiple and committed stem cells, mast cells, megakaryocytes; potent costimulatory factor
INTERLEUKINS			
Interleukin-1	IL-1	Monocytes/macrophages; B, T, and NK cells; fibroblasts; endothelial cells	Hematopoietic effects; induces acute-phase responses (e.g., fever, sleep, ACTH release); mediates inflammation; activates resting T cells
Interleukin-2	IL-2	T cells	Primary T-cell growth factor; cofactor for growth and differentiation of B cells; induction/release of cytokines
Interleukin-3	IL-3	T cells	Stimulates early progenitor cell growth; supports mast cell growth; supports growth of pre-B cell lines
Interleukin-4	IL-4	T cells, mast cells, macrophages	Growth factor for activated B cells; growth factor for resting T cells; supports mast cell growth; enhances cytolytic activity of cytotoxic T cells
Interleukin-5	IL-5	T cells, mast cells	Induces differentiation and proliferation of eosinophil progenitors; cofactor for induction of cytotoxic T cells
Interleukin-6	IL-6	T cells, monocytes/ macrophages, fibroblasts, endothelial cells	Costimulates T cells; induces IL-2 production; induces acute-phase response; hematopoietic effects; augments NK and LAK cytotoxicity
Interleukin-7	IL-7	Bone marrow stromal cells	Induces LAK activity; supports growth of B-cell precursors; induces cytokine secretion by monocytes
Interleukin-8	IL-8	Monocytes/macrophages	Strongly chemotactic for neutrophils, T and B cells, and monocytes; depending on cofactor, enhances or inhibits growth of hematopoietic progenitors
Interleukin-9	IL-9	T-helper cells	Stimulates antigen-specific T-helper cell clones; stimulates mast cell growth; supports erythroid colony formation

Data from Tushinski RJ, Mulé JJ: Biology of cytokines: the interleukins. In DeVita VT, Hellman S, Rosenberg SA, editors: *The biologic therapy of cancer,* ed 2, Philadelphia, 1995, Lippincott; and Rosenberg SA: Principles and applications of biologic therapy. In DeVita VT, Hellman S, Rosenberg SA, editors: *Cancer principles and practice of oncology,* ed 4, Philadelphia, 1993, Lippincott.
ACTH, Adrenocorticotropic hormone; *ADCC,* antibody-dependent cellular cytotoxicity; *LAK,* lymphokine-activated killer; *MHC,* major histocompatibility complex; *NK,* natural killer.

Table 23-1   Biologic Activity of Cytokines—cont'd

Cytokine	Abbreviation	Primary cellular source	Biologic activity
INTERLEUKINS—cont'd			
Interleukin-10	IL-10	T cells, B cells, macrophages	Costimulator to enhance growth of mast cell lines; costimulator for proliferation of activated T cells; inhibits macrophage activity; stimulates B-cell proliferation
Interleukin-11	IL-11	Stromal fibroblasts	Synergizes with IL-3 to support megakaryocyte colonies; stimulates proliferation of $CD34^+$ cells
Interleukin-12	IL-12	B lymphoblastoid cell lines	Enhances NK activity; stimulates antigen-activated $CD4^+$ and $CD8^+$ cells; induces production of IFN-γ; hematopoietic effects
Interleukin-13	IL-13	T cells	Induces IgE synthesis; enhances class II MHC antigen expression on resting B cells
Interleukin-14	IL-14	T cells	Induces B-cell proliferation; inhibits immunoglobulin secretion
Interleukin-15	IL-15	Activated monocytes/ macrophages	T-cell growth factor (some functions overlap with those of IL-2); stimulates NK cells

Table 23-2   Clinical Status of Major Biologic Response Modifiers

Agent	Status/indication
INTERFERONS	
Interferon-α	
Interferon alfa-2a (Roferon-A, Roche Laboratories)	FDA approved for hairy cell leukemia, AIDS-related Kaposi's sarcoma, chronic myelogenous leukemia
Interferon alfa-2b (Intron-A, Schering Corp.)	FDA approved for hairy cell leukemia, AIDS-related Kaposi's sarcoma, adjuvant therapy for high-risk melanoma, condyloma acuminata, chronic hepatitis non-A, non-B/C, and chronic hepatitis B
Interferon-α leukocyte (Alferon, Purdue Fredrick)	Condyloma acuminata
Interferon-β	
Interferon-β (Betaseron, Berlex Laboratories)	FDA approved for multiple sclerosis
Interferon-γ	
Interferon γ-1b (Actimmune, Genentech)	FDA approved for chronic granulomatous disease
INTERLEUKINS	
IL-1-α	In clinical trials
IL-1-β	In clinical trials
IL-2 (Proleukin, Chiron)	FDA approved for renal cell cancer
IL-4	In clinical trials
IL-6	In clinical trials
IL-12	In clinical trials
HEMATOPOIETIC GROWTH FACTORS	
GM-CSF	FDA approved for acceleration of myeloid recovery in patients with
Sargramostim	non-Hodgkin's lymphoma, acute lymphoblastic leukemia, and Hodgkin's
(Leukine, Immunex)	disease undergoing autologous BMT, treatment of delayed engraftment, support of elderly patients with acute myelogenous leukemia (AML) receiving high-dose chemotherapy
G-CSF	FDA approved to reduce incidence of infection in patients with nonmyeloid
Filgrastim	malignancies receiving myelosuppressive anticancer drugs, autologous bone
(Neupogen, Amgen)	marrow transplantation, cyclic neutropenias
M-CSF	In clinical trials
IL-3	In clinical trials

Continued.

Table 23-2   Clinical Status of Major Biologic Response Modifiers—cont'd

Agent	Status/indication
HEMATOPOIETIC GROWTH FACTORS—cont'd	
Erythropoietin	
Epoetin alfa	Indicated for treatment of anemia in patients with chronic renal failure
Epogen (Amgen)	
Procrit (Ortho Biotech)	Indicated for treatment of: anemia in patients with chronic renal failure; anemia related to therapy with zidovudine (AZT) in patients infected with the human immunodeficiency virus (HIV); and anemia in cancer patients undergoing chemotherapy
IL-11	In clinical trials
Thrombopoietin	In clinical trials
Stem cell factor	In clinical trials
MONOKINES	
Tumor necrosis factor (TNF)	In clinical trials
MONOCLONAL ANTIBODIES (MAbs)	
Oncoscint, Cytogen	FDA approved for diagnostic imaging of colon and ovarian cancer
RETINOIDS	
all-*trans*-retinoic acid	
Tretinoin (Vesanoid, Roche Laboratories)	FDA approved for the induction of remission in patients with acute promyelocytic leukemia.
13-*cis*-retinoic acid (13-cRA)	In clinical trials
Isotretinoin	
Fenretinide	In clinical trials
Etretinate	In clinical trials
EFFECTOR CELLS	
Lymphokine-activated killer cells (LAK)	In clinical trials
Tumor-infiltrating lymphocytes (TILs)	In clinical trials
Gene-altered TILs	In clinical trials

of action, and with certain agents it is often difficult to determine which mode of action is most important to the antitumor effect. It may be one action or the combination of several. In addition, many agents have both immunologic actions and other biologic effects.

Although several classification schemes exist, in general, BRMs can be classified into three major divisions: agents that augment, modulate, or restore the host's immunologic mechanisms; agents that have direct antitumor activity (cytotoxic or antiproliferative mechanisms); and agents that exert other biologic effects (those that affect differentiation or maturation of cells, that interfere with the ability of a tumor cell to metastasize, or that affect initiation or maintenance of neoplastic transformation).[37,110]

MAJOR AGENTS IN USE

INTERFERONS

Interferon (IFN) was first characterized in 1957 by virologists Isaacs and Lindemann.[97] They found that this newly discovered protein was produced by virally infected cells and was capable of protecting other cells from viral infection. A great deal has been learned since about the IFN system and its biologic effects. Interferon has proved effective in the treatment of several malignancies and viral diseases.

Interferons are divided into three major classes, according to antigenic type: alpha, beta, and gamma. IFN-α and IFN-β are produced primarily by leukocytes and fibroblasts respectively; IFN-γ is made primarily by T lymphocytes. The interferons may be called a family of glycoprotein hormones possessing pleiotropic biologic effects.[14,61]

Biologic Effects

All IFNs mediate their cellular effects after binding to a specific receptor. IFN-α and IFN-β share a receptor, whereas IFN-γ uses a different one. The interferons have a wide range of biologic effects, including antiviral, antiproliferative, and immunomodulatory. Exactly how they exert their antitumor effects is unknown. It is unclear which of their many biologic effects may be most important in obtaining tumor responses (e.g., direct effects versus immune stimulation). This is further complicated by the likely diversity of patients' responses to the agents and the differing effects of IFN on different diseases. In addition, there are differences in biologic effects between different classes of interferon.[14,61]

The antiviral activity of IFN renders uninfected cells resistant to attack by the offending virus as well as by a variety of other viruses. Internalization of the IFN-receptor complex causes a sequence of events that results in the production of antiviral proteins and enzymes. Both in vitro and in vivo experimentation have demonstrated the antiproliferative effects of IFN. Although the exact mechanism is unknown, IFN extends all phases of the cell cycle and lengthens overall cell generation time. The proteins also may inhibit DNA and protein synthesis to block the growth of tumor cells. Cellular protooncogenes play an important role in the regulation of cell growth, and IFNs are known to inhibit expression of protooncogenes.

A variety of immunomodulatory effects have been described for the IFNs; these differ for the different classes of IFN. In vitro, IFN increases the killing potential of NK cells by recruiting pre-NK cells and enhancing the cytotoxic activity of activated cells. Low doses of IFN appear to stimulate antibody production, but higher doses have a suppressive effect. IFN-γ appears to be a more potent activator of macrophage function than IFN-α or IFN-β; however, all three are capable of inducing tumoricidal activity and increasing phagocytosis. Interferons also are capable of affecting the production of other lymphokines that regulate immune responses. Little is known about the positive and negative feedback regulation between IFNs and other lymphokines. Current investigations will continue to define the immunomodulatory effects on IFNs and their interactions with other cytokines.[14,61]

Phenotypic Effects

Interferon is also capable of affecting the phenotypic properties of neoplastic cells. In vitro studies have shown that IFN can enhance differentiation of certain cell lines. IFN can also induce or enhance expression of human leukocyte antigens (HLAs) and increases tumor-associated antigens in melanoma and other cell lines. This may improve endogenous host antitumor activity.[14,61]

Clinical Indications

Initial clinical trials with IFN were carried out in the early 1970s using the Cantell preparation of leukocyte IFN (IFN-α), which was manufactured by Kari Cantell and coworkers at the Finnish blood bank.[30] Although supplies of leukocyte IFN were scarce, expensive, and very impure, a few important pharmacologic studies were done. The National Cancer Institute (NCI) in 1975 and the American Cancer Society in 1978 expanded this

work. Although initial trials showed responses in patients with breast cancer and lymphoma, large-scale clinical trials have not supported widespread efficacy in these two diseases. Large-scale clinical trials with IFN became possible during the 1980s with the advent of recombinant DNA technology. Large quantities of very pure IFNs of all types are now available because of these industrial-scale production methods.[164]

The U.S. Food and Drug Administration (FDA) approved two recombinant IFN-α products for the treatment of hairy cell leukemia (HCL) in 1986: IFN alfa-2b (Intron A) and IFN alfa-2a (Roferon A). Use of these IFNs in high doses has also been approved for the treatment of AIDS-related Kaposi's sarcoma.[188,199] Since then, Intron A has received additional approval for the treatment of condyloma acuminata, chronic hepatitis non-A, non-B/C, and chronic hepatitis B, and as adjuvant therapy in patients with melanoma at high risk for recurrence.[199] In late 1995, Roferon A received regulatory approval for the treatment of patients with chronic myelogenous leukemia in the chronic phase.[199]

The treatment of HCL with IFN-α has shown dramatic antitumor effects. Doses as low as 3 million U/m^2/day have been shown to be of benefit in as many as 95% of patients.[172,173] The median time to response is 4 to 6 months, with most patients achieving normalization of peripheral blood values, resulting in a decrease in transfusion requirements and the incidence of infection. Once therapy is stopped, patients ultimately relapse. Today, newer therapies, such as cladribine, have replaced IFN-α as frontline therapy for HCL. Chronic myelogenous leukemia (CML), a more common leukemia, is characterized by the presence of the Philadelphia chromosome in most patients. The use of IFN in this population, at doses of 2 to 5 million U/m^2/day results in normalization of peripheral blood counts. In approximately 15% of patients with chronic-phase CML, IFN therapy has been shown to eliminate the malignant clone of cells (those bearing the Philadelphia chromosome).[77,220-222] Other hematologic diseases against which IFN-α has shown efficacy include low-grade lymphomas[210,226] and multiple myeloma.[127] In these diseases several studies have shown the use of IFN as maintenance therapy after chemotherapy to result in an improved rate of failure-free survival and median survival. In solid tumors, such as melanoma, renal cell cancer, ovarian carcinoma (using the intraperitoneal route), and superficial bladder carcinoma, IFN has also demonstrated efficacy[2] (Tables 23-3 and 23-4). In patients with melanoma, no adjuvant therapy has traditionally been effective in extending relapse-free or overall survival. In late 1995, based on a study by the Eastern Cooperative Oncology Group, Intron A was approved as an adjuvant to surgical treatment of melanoma in patients who are free of disease but at a high risk for recurrence. These are patients with a deep primary lesion (greater than 4 mm thickness) or any

Table 23-3 Response of Various Hematologic Malignancies to IFN-α

Tumor type	Response rate*
Hairy cell leukemia	80%-90%
Chronic myelogenous leukemia	
Newly diagnosed	70%-80%
Advanced	10%-25%
Philadelphia-negative myeloproliferative disorders	
Essential thrombocythemia and polycythemia vera	75%
Cutaneous T-cell lymphomas	
No prior therapy	80%
Previously treated	55%
Non-Hodgkin's lymphomas (relapsed)	
Low grade	40%-50%
Intermediate and high grade	15%
Hodgkin's disease (relapsed)	20%
Multiple myeloma	
No previous therapy	50%
Previously treated	15%-25%
Chronic lymphocytic leukemia	10%-15%
Acute leukemia	10%-20%

From Kurzrock R, Talpaz M, Gutterman JU: Other tumors. In DeVita VT, Hellman S, Rosenberg SA, editors: *The biologic therapy of cancer*, Philadelphia, 1991, Lippincott.
*Responses signify a partial or complete regression of tumor.

Table 23-4 Response of Various Solid Tumors to IFN-α

Tumor type	Response rate*
Cervical intraepithelial neoplasia	80%-90%
Basal cell cancer	90%
Superficial bladder cancer	60%-70%
Malignant neuroendocrine tumors	30%-80%
Kaposi's sarcoma (AIDS related)	35%
Ovarian cancer	
Parenteral administration	10%-15%
Intraperitoneal administration	40%
Gliomas	30%
Renal cell cancer	15%-20%
Nasopharyngeal cancer	20%
Melanoma	10%-15%
Colorectal cancer	<10%
Osteogenic sarcoma	<10%
Lung (small and non-small cell)	<10%
Breast cancer	<10%

From Kurzrock R, Talpaz M, Gutterman JU: Other tumors. In DeVita VT, Hellman S, Rosenberg SA, editors: *The biologic therapy of cancer*, Philadelphia, 1991, Lippincott.
*Responses signify partial or complete tumor regression.

patient with primary or recurrent nodal involvement. Median disease-free survival was extended from 1 to 1.7 years and overall survival from 2.8 to 3.8 years.[106] (For a comprehensive review of IFN therapy, see DeVita and others,[49] Estrov and others,[61] Parkinson,[161] Rieger,[185] Rosenberg,[193] Skalla,[207] and Yarbro and others[246].) IFN-β remains under clinical investigation in patients with cancer but has received regulatory approval for the treatment of multiple sclerosis.[18] Although IFN-γ remains under investigation for the treatment of cancer,[175] it is commercially available for the treatment of chronic granulomatous disease.[72,75]

Interferon continues to be explored as a single agent and in combination with other BRMs and chemotherapeutic agents.[147,185] Initial clinical trials evaluating the combination of IFN and fluorouracil (5-FU) for the treatment of colon cancer yielded exciting results. A pilot study conducted by Wadler and coworkers[236] in 1989 reported a response rate of 81% with 13 of 16 previously untreated patients with advanced colon carcinoma. These results led other investigators to attempt to duplicate Wadler's regimen and to evaluate this combination in other cancers. However, several recent large-scale randomized studies have not demonstrated any clear superiority for the combination, compared with 5-FU alone.[42] An additional area of investigation is the combination of IFN-α

and 13-*cis*-retinoic acid for the treatment of squamous cell carcinomas of the skin and cervix.[121] Although responses have been demonstrated, randomized trials are required to clarify the ultimate role of the combination in these diseases. Randomized trials have demonstrated no additional benefit for the addition of IFN-α to high-dose therapy with interleukin-2 (IL-2) in patients with melanoma or renal cell carcinoma.[54]

An occasional problem in patients receiving chronic treatment with IFN-α is development of neutralizing antibodies. Although the clinical significance of this phenomenon is uncertain, in a number of clinical trials the development of neutralizing antibodies has been associated with resistance to therapy. Factors that may contribute to formation of antibodies are immunogenicity, underlying disease, routes of administration, dosing regimens, and duration of treatment. It has been difficult to determine the true incidence of antibody formation. Additional factors that may be important are blood sampling time and assay methodology. Until comparative studies are well controlled for these variables, the formation of antibodies and their effect will remain controversial.[11]

Administration

Although numerous clinical trials have been conducted, the optimal dose, route, and frequency of administration for interferon have yet to be determined. The most common routes of administration are intramuscular and subcutaneous, although IFN is also given intravenously, intralesionally, intraperitoneally, intravesically, intraarteri-

Table 23-5   Interferon Dosage

Interferon protocol	Dose (million U/m²)
Low dose	0-3
Intermediate dose	3-10
High dose	>10

ally, and intrathecally.[41,193] Pharmacokinetics differ by types of IFN and route of administration. Intravenous administration results in rapid clearance with a half-life of 4 to 8 hours. With subcutaneous or intramuscular administration, peak serum levels occur at about 6 to 8 hours and complete clearance occurs by 16 to 24 hours.[83] IFN is metabolized in the kidneys, and most metabolites are completely reabsorbed. Although at first IFN was given by a predetermined standard dosage, it is now more commonly prescribed by body surface area (million U/m²). Dosage requirements for IFN-α vary among patients and diseases. A rough classification for dosage is given in Table 23-5. In general, the higher the dose, the more severe the side effects and the inhibition of the patient's performance status.

IFN-α is supplied commercially as a sterile, lyophilized powder with accompanying diluent or as a sterile solution. It must be stored in a refrigerator at 35.6° to 46.4° F (2° to 8° C). The vial should not be shaken when the powder is reconstituted, because this will make the medication foam. For further information, such as the availability of differing vial strengths and shelf-life stability, see the manufacturer's product literature.[188,199]

Handling issues are a concern to all oncology nurses. To date there has been no formal research on the safest way to handle IFNs or other BRMs. Many institutions place BRMs in the same classification as chemotherapy, instructing staff to follow institutional policy on the handling and disposal of cytotoxic drugs. Patients taught to self-administer interferon are advised to dispose of vials, needles, and syringes in a puncture-resistant container. Guidelines for disposal of used equipment in the home setting are available from the U.S. Environmental Protection Agency (EPA). In some clinical trials, patients are requested to return unused vials to the dispensing institution.[41,86,183]

Side Effects

The toxicity of interferon has been well established. In general, side effects are similar for all classes of interferon, with slight variations according to dosage, schedule, and type. Although at higher doses the effects of IFN can be quite debilitating, side effects are generally reversible upon cessation of therapy. Because interferon is generally given as long-term therapy, side effects can be divided into those occurring early (acute) and those oc-

curring as therapy progresses (late or chronic). Some side effects occur only occasionally or rarely.

Nearly all patients beginning therapy with IFN have flu-like symptoms. Although the symptoms may be severe at first, tachyphylaxis (adjustment to symptoms over time) prevents them from becoming dose limiting. Symptoms include chills 2 to 4 hours after injection followed by fever spikes up to 104° F (40° C). Patients may have headaches, myalgia, arthralgia, and malaise. High-risk patients (e.g., those with a history of cardiac problems, debilitated patients) should be premedicated, monitored closely, and kept well hydrated.[84]

Chronic side effects tend to increase in intensity and maintain their level of intensity after patients have been undergoing therapy for several weeks. Of prime concern are fatigue and anorexia with resultant weight loss; these can become dose limiting. The patient's interferon therapy may have to be halted or the dosage reduced if these side effects become too severe. Patients also experience lethargy, lack of concentration,[137] neutropenia, mild thrombocytopenia, elevated transaminase levels, proteinuria, and asymptomatic hypotension.

A number of side effects are less widespread; they vary in frequency between individual patients and in intensity depending on the dose. These include gastrointestinal effects such as nausea, vomiting, diarrhea, and altered taste (patients complain of foods tasting metallic or bitter). Nausea, in particular, is more commonly seen in patients with malignant melanoma who are receiving higher doses of IFN-α by the intravenous route during the induction phase. Patients may exhibit central nervous system (CNS) or neurologic changes such as depression, mood alterations, decreased libido, memory problems, electroencephalographic (EEG) abnormalities, and peripheral neuropathies.[137] Inflammation at the injection site, reactivation of herpes simplex, rash, exacerbation of psoriasis, and mild alopecia (thinning of hair as opposed to full-scale hair loss) have all been reported. Laboratory values should be watched for changes indicating anemia, hypercalcemia, hyperkalemia, elevated blood urea nitrogen (BUN), and elevated lactate dehydrogenase.[174,193,234]

In general, patients receiving low doses tolerate side effects well. Although not proved by research, a frequent recommendation is that IFN be given at bedtime so that patients will sleep through the worst of the side effects. The most common life-threatening toxicity is acute cardiac failure, which is extremely rare. It is generally recommended that patients with a strong history of cardiovascular disease should not undergo IFN therapy.

INTERLEUKINS

The term *interleukin* literally means "between leukocytes." Traditionally, when biologic proteins were characterized, they were given acronyms based on their functional properties (e.g., T-cell growth factor). When genes for these cytokines were ultimately cloned, it was found that a number of these substances were in fact the same molecule. At international symposia, the terminology interleukins was agreed on to name these biologic proteins. Hence, as more of these cytokines are discovered and their amino acid sequences established, they are named numerically (e.g., IL-5, IL-6) (see Table 23-1).*

As of December 1995, research has progressed through the discovery of IL-15.[118] This section will concentrate on interleukin-2 (IL-2), which received FDA approval in 1992, and will briefly cover other interleukins that are currently in clinical trials. Interleukin-3 will be covered under the discussion of hematopoietic growth factors.

Interleukin-1

Interleukin-1 (IL-1) was originally described as an endogenous pyrogen and lymphocyte-activating factor.[55] It is a complex and heterogeneous molecule now known to be produced by a variety of cells. Its biologic activities include serving as an endogenous pyrogen; inducing the release of lymphokines from activated T cells and fibroblasts; enhancing antibody responsiveness through synergism with other lymphokines that affect B-cell function; inducing the proliferation of fibroblasts; serving as a chemotactic factor for neutrophils, macrophages, and lymphocytes; and serving as a mediator of the inflammatory response.[55,214] Two genes coding for proteins with IL-1 properties have been discovered. These have been called *interleukin-1-alpha (IL-1-α)* and *interleukin-1-beta (IL-1-β)*. They share the same cell surface receptor and various biologic activities.

Several phase I trials have evaluated IL-1 in patients.[104,214,231] In general, these studies demonstrated a delayed increase in leukocytes and platelets. In patients receiving IL-1-β after treatment with 5-FU, it appeared to exert a myeloprotective effect (fewer days of neutropenia).[44] However, the difference between those patients receiving IL-1-β and those receiving 5-FU alone was not statistically significant. A study by Vadhan-Raj and coworkers[231] demonstrated that IL-1-α increased circulating platelet counts and enhanced platelet recovery after treatment with carboplatin (CBDCA) in patients with ovarian cancer. Common toxicities experienced in these phase I trials were chills and fever, constitutional symptoms (headache, myalgia, arthralgia, fatigue, nausea), hypotension at higher doses, tachycardia, and inflammation at injection sites. Occasional toxicities, especially at doses above 300 ng/kg, were cardiac dysrhythmias, reversible renal insufficiency, abdominal pain, and transient CNS changes. Further studies evaluating IL-1 in a

variety of settings, as well as IL-1 in combination with IL-2, are in progress. Future trials will continue to evaluate the role of IL-1 in the pathology of septic shock, inflammatory bowel disease, and autoimmune diseases such as rheumatoid arthritis.[202,214] Clinical studies are now investigating the role of IL-1 receptor antagonist (IL-1RA), a molecule capable of blocking the biologic effects of IL-1. This agent may have efficacy in the treatment of septic shock or as a means of selectively suppressing the toxic effects of other cytokines such as IL-2.

Interleukin-2

Interleukin-2 is a glycoprotein mainly produced by activated T-helper cells. First discovered in 1976 by Morgan and coworkers,[141] it was originally named T-cell growth factor. Since then, intensive research has proved IL-2 to be a potent modulator of immune responses. The release of IL-2 in vivo occurs in response to two signals presented to T lymphocytes. The first is activation of T cells by antigen or mitogen, and the second is through interactions with IL-1. Like many polypeptide hormones, IL-2 exerts its biologic effects by binding to membrane-bound receptors on certain immune cells. It is now known that the IL-2 receptor has low-, intermediate-, and high-affinity forms. Hence, a resting cell may display very few IL-2 receptors. Once activated, it may display thousands of receptors and respond to activation by IL-2.[8,14,46,208,237]

Biologic effects. The biologic effects of IL-2 are numerous and have been well documented.[8,14,46,208,237] IL-2 supports the growth and maturation of subpopulations of T cells both in vitro and in vivo, stimulates cytotoxic T cells, stimulates the proliferation and activity of NK cells, and develops the capacity in lymphoid cells incubated with IL-2 to lyse fresh tumor cells. These cells, known as lymphokine-activated killer (LAK) cells, have served as the basis for adoptive immunotherapy regimens. IL-2 also enhances antibody responses by activating other lymphocytes to produce lymphokines important to B-cell function (IL-4 and IL-6), stimulates the expression of its own cell surface receptor, and induces the release of other lymphokines, such as IFN-γ and granulocyte/macrophage colony-stimulating factor (GM-CSF), that can mediate physiologic effects. Both in vitro and in vivo studies have demonstrated that IL-2 can reverse immune deficiencies in mice and humans. It appears that there are no differences in activity between naturally occurring IL-2 and the recombinant forms available.

Clinical indications. In 1992, IL-2 (aldesleukin) was approved by the FDA for the treatment of renal cell cancer.[35] The approved regimen uses high doses of IL-2: 600,000 or 720,000 IU/kg by intravenous bolus every 8 hours, up to 15 doses. This approval was based on a multicenter study of more than 200 patients, who had an overall response rate of 14%. (For a complete chronology on the clinical investigation of IL-2, see Atkins,[8]

---

*References 12, 46, 56, 202, 225, 240.

Dillman,[54] Fisher,[66] Kolitz,[109] Parkinson,[162] Rosenberg,[191,193,194] Sharp,[202] Sznol,[218] Wagstaff,[237] and Wheeler.[240]) The first phase I clinical evaluations of IL-2 began in 1983 with IL-2 obtained from a human lymphoma tumor cell line. Although production methods limited supplies, a few clinical trials were conducted for patients with malignant tumors or acquired immunodeficiency syndrome (AIDS). Therapy was given intravenously and produced minimal side effects. However, no therapeutic responses were seen.[123,124]

When the DNA sequence coding for IL-2 was elucidated, recombinant DNA technology made possible the production of large quantities of purified IL-2. As a result, phase I trials using recombinant IL-2 (rIL-2) were initiated in 1984.[124] Concurrently, studies conducted by Rosenberg[193] showed that adoptive immunotherapy with LAK cells was well tolerated by patients. These LAK cells were generated from fresh peripheral blood lymphocytes obtained through lymphocytapheresis and then incubated with IL-2.

In 1984 studies of the combination of IL-2 and LAK cells began. Results reported by Rosenberg and associates[193] in December 1985 showed that of 25 patients, 11 exhibited tumor responses. These responses were seen in patients with melanoma, renal cancer, and colorectal and pulmonary adenocarcinoma.

The excitement over these results generated an explosion of clinical trials with IL-2. Numerous clinical trials have evaluated a variety of doses, routes of administration, and schedules for IL-2. Trials have been conducted using IL-2 alone and in combination with LAK cells. Although patients with a variety of cancers have been treated, most trials have focused on patients with renal cell cancer and melanoma because of the successes seen in these solid tumors. Randomized trials have now demonstrated that the addition of LAK cells does not offer an advantage over the use of high-dose IL-2 alone.[54,66]

Research efforts continued to find cells with more potent antitumor activity. A different subpopulation of lymphocytes, denoted *tumor-infiltrating lymphocytes (TILs)*, appeared to have greater efficacy in the treatment of experimental tumors than did LAK cells. TILs are obtained by removing tumor specimens from the host. Human TILs are T cells and can be isolated by growth in single-cell suspensions. They appear to be less dependent on adjunctive systemically administered IL-2 than are LAK cells. Early clinical trials using IL-2 plus TILs by Rosenberg and coworkers reported remissions in 11 of 20 patients with metastatic melanoma treated with this combination. A recent report on his 5-year experience with this combination showed an overall response rate of 34% in patients with advanced melanoma. Work continues on how to achieve the optimal therapeutic benefit and to find predictors of response.[193]

The combination of IL-2 with other cytokines, mono-clonal antibodies, and chemotherapy is another active area of focus. Preclinical studies in animal models have shown antitumor activity to be enhanced by use of the combinations just mentioned.* Phase I and II trials evaluating the efficacy of these combinations continue. One promising area appears to be the use of IL-2 in combination with chemotherapy in patients with melanoma. Several clinical trials across the country are evaluating multidrug chemotherapy, using cisplatin, dacarbazine, carmustine, and tamoxifen (Dartmouth regimen) or cisplatin, vinblastine, and dacarbazine (CVD), in combination with IL-2 and IFN-α. Reported response rates to these combinations have been 53% or higher, although toxic effects are severe. Randomized studies are in progress to determine whether biochemotherapy is truly superior to chemotherapy alone.[29,66] Also of important consideration in these regimens is whether biotherapy is given before, during, or after chemotherapy.

Evaluation of chimeric molecules is an active area of pursuit. One such example is the use of an IL-2 molecule with diphtheria toxin attached that is administered to patients whose malignancies express the IL-2 receptor. Phase I and II trials with this molecule continue,[160] as does its evaluation for the treatment of rheumatoid arthritis. In patients who have received both autologous and allogeneic bone marrow transplantation, administration of low-dose IL-2 to reduce the incidence of relapse by stimulating a graft-versus-leukemia effect and to restore immune function is under investigation. A current area of focus, especially in patients with renal cell cancer, is the use of low-dose regimens administered in the ambulatory setting that maintain efficacy yet reduce toxicity.[213] Over the next several years, increased use of IL-2 will be seen in the clinical setting as research defines optimal dosing and schedules and its concomitant use with effector cells and other biologic or chemotherapeutic agents.[66,202,240]

Administration. As with other BRMs, the optimal therapeutic dosage, route, and schedule for IL-2 have yet to be determined. The most common route of administration is intravenous, using either bolus or continuous infusion.[35] Investigations continue to evaluate other routes such as subcutaneous, intraperitoneal, and intraarterial, with most ambulatory regimens using the subcutaneous route. The trend in dosing is toward expression of the dose in common international units. The recommended dose for aldesleukin (Proleukin) is 600,000 IU/kg every 8 hours by a 15-minute IV infusion, for a total of 15 doses.[35] Pharmacokinetic studies show rapid initial plasma clearance (6 to 7 minutes) after bolus administration. With longer infusions, however, a more prolonged clearance is seen (half-life of approximately 30 minutes). These observations suggest a multicompart-

---

*References 8, 9, 54, 65, 66, 126, 147, 148, 162.

mental model of pharmacokinetics.[7,123,124] Inactivation appears to occur in the kidneys, with inactive metabolites excreted in the urine.

Other concerns about drug administration that are important to nurses include handling procedures, which are determined by hospital policy; manufacturer's instructions for administration; how long the drug is stable in solution; whether the drug can pass through a micropore filter; and evaluation of compatibility with concomitant medications such as antiemetics and vasopressors.[41,183]

Side effects. Although responses to therapy with IL-2 are seen, severe systemic toxicities associated with high-dose IL-2 therapy make it difficult to tolerate. The range and severity of toxicity seen with IL-2 are related to and influenced by dose, schedule, and concomitant use of adoptive immunotherapy, other BRMs, and chemotherapy.[204]

How many side effects arise from IL-2 remains a mystery. Although IL-2 may directly cause some side effects, the induction of other cytokines by IL-2 may also play a role. One encouraging note is that most IL-2–related side effects disappear once therapy is completed. IL-2 is often administered on a cyclic basis similar to that of chemotherapy. This gives patients an opportunity to recuperate between cycles or courses, although cumulative toxicity does occur with repeated cycles. Patients have exhibited a marked decline in performance status over time, and more severe toxicity and impairment have been observed as the dose increases. Because the toxicity of existing IL-2 regimens can be severe enough to require hospitalization, ongoing trials continue to search for dosage schedules that can maximize therapeutic responses with a more acceptable level of toxicity.[66,202,240] See the box, p. 585, for an overall summary of IL-2 side effects by system.

As with other BRMs, patients receiving IL-2 have constitutional or flu-like symptoms, including chills followed by fever of up to 104° F (40° C), headache, myalgia, arthralgia, and general malaise. Pretreatment with acetaminophen and indomethacin or another nonsteroidal antiinflammatory drug (NSAID) helps control these side effects. With continuous infusions of IL-2, the medications just mentioned are often necessary around the clock to control fevers. The major cardiovascular and pulmonary toxicity associated with IL-2 administration stems from cumulative, dose-related fluid imbalances caused by a capillary leak syndrome. Shortly after administration, a rapid decrease in systemic vascular resistance occurs and fluids shift from the vascular bed to the interstitium. This causes a drop in mean arterial blood pressure, increased cardiac output, and increased heart rate.[193]

Weight gains of as much as 10% of baseline weight have been observed in high-dose trials.[193] Fluid retention is usually manifested as peripheral edema and abdominal ascites. These effects may progress to interstitial pulmonary edema, with subsequent dyspnea and decreased partial oxygen pressure (P_{O2}) in some patients. In extreme cases of respiratory distress, patients require intubation.[62]

Although clinically patients appear fluid overloaded, in reality they are hypovolemic. This hypovolemia leads to hypotension, decreased central venous pressure (CVP), and renal hypoperfusion. These physiologic changes increase the demand on the heart, and transient dysrhythmias may be observed. Because of this, patients usually undergo rigorous pretherapy screening for underlying cardiac problems before beginning treatment with IL-2. Medical treatment includes administration of colloid solutions (5% albumin), judicious use of fluids to avoid pulmonary edema, and the use of vasopressors.[183,244]

The multiple hemodynamic abnormalities associated with IL-2 therapy often lead to the development of renal hypoperfusion and prerenal azotemia. Renal toxicity is evidenced by oliguria, proteinuria, azotemia, and increases in BUN and creatinine levels. These effects, seen at various doses, usually return to baseline after therapy. Medical treatment includes fluids, diuretics (if blood pressure and CVP are within normal limits), and pressors such as low-dose dopamine to stimulate renal blood flow.

Acute gastrointestinal effects are common with IL-2. Nausea and vomiting closely parallel chemotherapy-associated nausea and vomiting. Patients often complain that food odors increase nausea. Unfortunately, for some patients, IL-2–associated nausea and vomiting have proved resistant to pharmacologic treatment. Often, aggressive use of multiple antiemetics around the clock is required. In addition, patients lose their appetite; therefore weight loss over time becomes a major concern. Diarrhea may be acute or chronic and is often watery and profuse. Mucositis, glossitis, and xerostomia can further damage nutritional status.

Baseline assessment of mental status is important in patients receiving IL-2. CNS toxicity may be manifested as confusion, lethargy, decreased concentration, extreme somnolence, depression, hallucination, paranoia, combativeness, agitation, and nightmares.[16,48,98,137,211] Occasionally these toxicities are severe enough to cause the delay or discontinuation of therapy.

Skin changes occurring with IL-2 therapy are profound and cumulative; they are a major source of discomfort for patients. Varying degrees of erythema, erythematous rash, pruritus, dryness, and occasionally dry desquamation all may be seen, either alone or in combination. Skin biopsies have not elucidated the etiology of these skin changes. Aggravation of underlying dermatologic conditions, as well as recall phenomena, may also be seen.[71]

Patients may develop neutropenia, thrombocytopenia, or anemia. In programs using lymphocytapheresis, ane-

INTERLEUKIN-2 TOXICITIES

CONSTITUTIONAL SYMPTOMS

Chills, fever
Headaches
Malaise
Myalgia, arthralgia
Fatigue
Nasal congestion

CARDIOVASCULAR SYSTEM

Hypotension
Decreased systemic vascular resistance
Tachycardia
Atrial arrhythmias
Edema
Weight gain
Ascites

PULMONARY SYSTEM

Pulmonary edema
Dyspnea
Decreased Po_2

RENAL FUNCTION

Oliguria
Increased BUN, creatinine
Proteinuria
Azotemia

GASTROINTESTINAL SYSTEM

Nausea, vomiting
Diarrhea
Decreased appetite
Mucositis
Glossitis
Xerostomia

ENDOCRINE SYSTEM

Hypothyroidism

INTEGUMENTARY SYSTEM

Erythema
Erythematous rash
Dry skin
Pruritus
Dry desquamation

CENTRAL NERVOUS SYSTEM

Confusion, disorientation
Somnolence
Lethargy
Combativeness
Psychoses
Anxiety
Depression

HEMATOLOGIC FUNCTION

Anemia
Thrombocytopenia
Eosinophilia
Lymphopenia

HEPATIC FUNCTION

Increased bilirubin
Elevated aspartate aminotransferase (AST, formerly SGOT), alanine aminotransferase (ALT, formerly SGPT), and lactate dehydrogenase (LDH)

RELATED LABORATORY VALUES

Hypophosphatemia
Hypocalcemia
Hypomagnesemia
Decreased serum albumin

OTHER

Potential for catheter-related sepsis

From Rieger PT, Weatherly B: *Dimens Oncol Nurs* 3(3):9, 1989.

mia is often exacerbated. With prolonged IL-2 administration, marked eosinophilia often occurs. The clinical significance of this is uncertain, although it may be responsible for the fluid shifts observed.[179] Significant lymphopenia occurs within minutes of IL-2 administration. However, rebound lymphocytosis occurs within 24 hours after discontinuation of a treatment. As with other IL-2 side effects, these changes are usually reversible upon cessation of therapy.

Patients receiving IL-2 often have several abnormal laboratory values. Patients should be monitored for increased bilirubin, elevated hepatic enzymes (AST, ALT, LDH), hypomagnesemia, hypophosphatemia, hypocalcemia, decreased serum albumin, and respiratory alkalosis.

Replacement therapy should be instituted as appropriate.

The incidence of catheter-related sepsis appears higher in patients receiving high doses of IL-2. Trials have evaluated the use of prophylactic antibiotics in this patient population. In patients with indwelling catheters, antibiotics are often administered prophylactically. It is often difficult to differentiate signs of infection from those associated with IL-2; therefore patients must be monitored closely.[244]

In patients receiving adoptive immunotherapy with either LAK or TILs, most side effects are attributable to IL-2. Chills and fever are the major side effects noted with cell infusions. These are readily treatable with meperidine. A further risk is that of infection, because lym-

MEDICATIONS COMMONLY USED IN THE MANAGEMENT OF IL-2 TOXICITY

ANTIPYRETIC ANALGESIC AGENTS

Acetaminophen

ANTIINFLAMMATORY AGENTS

Indomethacin
Naproxen
Sulindac

HISTAMINE H$_2$-ANTAGONIST AGENTS

Cimetidine
Ranitidine

ANTIEMETIC AGENTS

Lorazepam
Prochlorperazine maleate
Promethazine HCl
Droperidol
Ondansetron
ABH (lorazepam, diphenhydramine, haloperidol)
Scopolamine patches

ANTIDIARRHEAL AGENTS

Codeine phosphate
Kaolin and pectin
Opium tincture
Diphenoxylate HCl with atropine So$_4$

ANTIANXIETY, ANTIHALLUCINOGEN, AND HYPNOTIC AGENTS

Diphenhydramine
Diazepam
Fentanyl
Flurazepam
Haloperidol

DIURETIC AGENTS

Furosemide
Metolazone

AGENTS TO CONTROL CHILLS

Meperidine HCl
Indomethacin
Dilaudid SL

VASOPRESSORS AND ANTIARRHYTHMIC AGENTS

Dopamine HCl
Verapamil HCl
Atropine So$_4$

ANTIHYPOTENSIVE MEASURES

0.9% Sodium chloride boluses
5% N serum albumin

ANTIPRURITIC AGENTS

Hydroxyzine hydrochloride
Diphenhydramine
Colloidal oatmeal

From Rieger PT: Patient management. In Rieger PT, editor: *Biotherapy: a comprehensive overview,* Boston, 1995, Jones & Bartlett. Adapted and revised from original source: Padavic-Shaller K: *Semin Oncol Nurs* 4(2):142, 1988.

phocytes incubated in culture medium for 3 to 4 days may be contaminated with viruses or bacteria[193] (see the box above for medications commonly used during IL-2 therapy).

Interleukin-4

Primarily produced by activated T cells, IL-4 has a number of biologic effects. It stimulates the growth of resting B cells in vitro; it increases production of immunoglobulin in vitro; it may stimulate certain T-cell lines in vitro; it produces CSF-like activity in vitro; and it may stimulate growth and maturation of mast cells in vitro. In addition, IL-4 has a variety of effects on cytotoxic cells such as LAK or TIL cells; these effects depend on the type of cell, the presence of other cytokines such as IL-2, and the state of activation of the cytotoxic cells.*

Several phase I trials have evaluated tolerance of IL-4

*References 46, 99, 113, 171, 202, 224.

in patients, utilizing several routes of administration: intravenous (IV) bolus, short-term IV infusion, and subcutaneous (SC) injection. Toxicities experienced were low-grade delayed fevers, nausea, reversible elevation in liver enzymes, and nasal congestion. Occasional toxicities, especially at higher doses, were chills, hypotension, and edema with weight gain. Rare instances of therapy complicated by gastroduodenal erosion or ulceration have been reported.[195] A phase II outpatient dose and schedule have been established at 5 μg/kg/day by the SC route. Phase II trials are in progress, with greatest interest in hematologic malignancies (multiple myeloma, indolent lymphoma, B-cell chronic lymphocytic leukemia [BCLL], intermediate-grade lymphoma, Hodgkin's disease, and chronic myelogenous leukemia [CML]). Several clinical trials have evaluated the combination of IL-2 and IL-4, with both high-dose and low-dose regimens for each of these agents. As yet the few responses documented have been in patients with either renal cell cancer or melanoma.[202,224,240]

Interleukin-6

Interleukin-6 (IL-6) is a cytokine produced by many cells in the body and induced by other cytokines such as tumor necrosis factor (TNF) and IL-1. As with other cytokines, it has pleiotropic effects and plays an important role in coordinating systemic host defense responses to injury. Its expression has been noted in several disease states, and it may be involved in certain aspects of the pathogenesis of infection, autoimmunity, and malignancy. Multiple myeloma has been linked to autocrine growth stimulation by IL-6. IL-6 has an important role in promoting differentiation of B lymphocytes into antibody-secreting cells; is involved in the activation of T cells and promotion of T-cell differentiation; induces production of acute-phase proteins by the liver; increases the proliferation of multilineage progenitor cells and increases the number of megakaryocytes; and serves as a messenger between the nervous and immune systems. It works synergistically with many other cytokines in vivo.[21,46,113,224]

Phase I/II trials are currently in progress evaluating the use of IL-6 in patients with cancer as both an antitumor and as a myeloprotective agent. In a study published by Weber and colleagues at the National Cancer Institute, IL-6 given by the SC route resulted in no clinical responses. Elevations in platelet counts were seen at higher doses. The most common toxic effects included constitutional symptoms, transient anemia, and hyperglycemia.[238] Other investigators have administered IL-6 by the IV route in patients with melanoma or renal cell cancer; minor clinical responses were documented. Further study is necessary to determine this agent's utility as an anticancer agent, as well as its optimal dose, route, and schedule. Its value as a marker of disease activity is also under investigation.[113,240]

HEMATOPOIETIC GROWTH FACTORS

Hematopoietic growth factors (HGFs) are a family of glycoprotein hormones responsible for the proliferation, differentiation, and maturation of hematopoietic cells in vitro. They also stimulate functions of certain mature leukocytes.[38] The four classic growth factors, known as colony-stimulating factors (CSFs), are granulocyte/macrophage colony-stimulating factor (GM-CSF), granulocyte colony-stimulating factor (G-CSF), macrophage colony-stimulating factor (M-CSF), and IL-3 (multi-CSF). All are now produced in recombinant form. GM-CSF (sargramostim) and G-CSF (filgrastim) have both received regulatory approval, whereas clinical trials with IL-3 and M-CSF continue. The characterization of other hematopoietic growth factors is also being pursued. After in vitro studies elucidate their biology, the next step will be assessment of their clinical efficacy in vivo.[70] For the four classic CSFs, current investigations attempt to

further define appropriate dosages, schedules, and routes of administration, as well as the diseases and conditions for which these agents are best used.[133-135,235]

The HGFs were discovered through research into the process and regulation of hematopoiesis. These glycoproteins were detected because of their mandatory and unique role in stimulating hematopoietic cells to proliferate[57] (Figure 23-2). The use of semisolid colony assay systems to culture hematopoietic cells revealed that specific regulatory molecules (CSFs) were necessary to sustain progenitor cells and to form colonies. The ability to clone these agents greatly enhanced the ability to study them.

There appear to be overlapping functions, as well as synergism, between different HGFs. Because these are all receptor-mediated molecules, differences in effects on different hematopoietic lineages may be related to the distribution of receptors.[133-135]

To understand the HGFs, one needs a basic understanding of hematopoiesis, or the production and development of blood cells. This process normally occurs in the bone marrow, where cells of various lineages proliferate, differentiate, and mature. Most blood cells have a relatively short life span; therefore they must be constantly produced to offset continual turnover. For example, baseline levels of granulocytes and macrophages are maintained within a narrow range. However, the body has a remarkable ability to increase production in response to stresses such as infection and inflammation. Factors thought to be important in the control of hematopoiesis are the bone marrow microenvironment, cell-to-cell interaction, and humoral substances.[122]

The process starts with a multipotent or pluripotent stem cell. These cells have the capacity for self-renewal and the ability to form multilineage colonies, although they are relatively quiescent under normal circumstances. Cells become successively more proliferative during differentiation, and their capacities to renew themselves and to form multilineage colonies become more restricted. The factors controlling hematopoiesis have not been entirely delineated. Constitutive substances that may affect the lineage commitment status of a cell are being investigated. CSFs appear more important in the stress response, and they seem to help control the number of effector cells in the immune response.[85,122]

Biology and Clinical Applications

The biologic activity of the HGFs is summarized in Table 23-1. In vitro studies suggested that the CSFs may have clinical value in a variety of settings. CSF clinical trials continue to evaluate (1) reducing cancer treatment morbidity by decreasing myelosuppression (both intensity and duration) and the incidence of febrile neutropenia; (2) improving survival by allowing patients to receive chemotherapy treatments on schedule; (3) speeding mar-

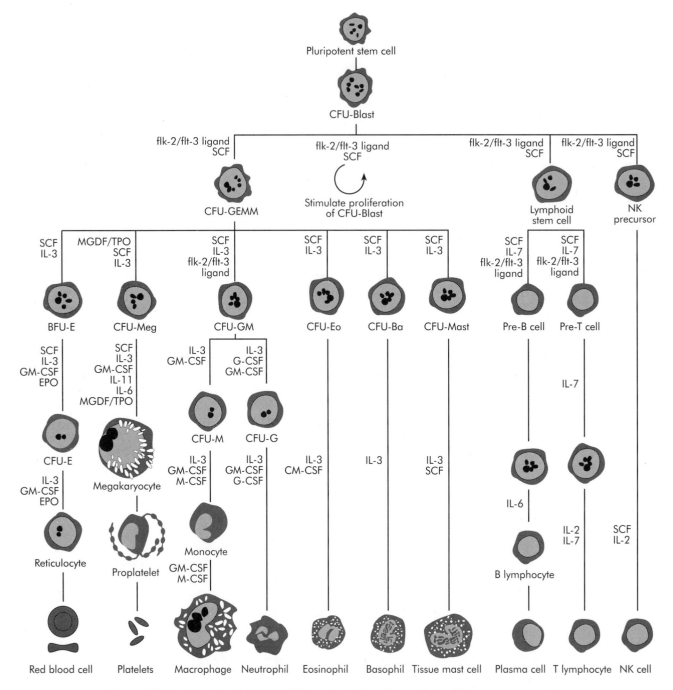

Figure 23-2 Hematopoietic tree. All hematopoietic cells are derived from a common stem cell under the influence of various growth factors or combinations of growth factors. *BFU-E,* Erythrocyte burst-forming units; *CFU,* colony-forming units; *CFU-Ba,* basophil CFU; *CFU-Eo,* eosinophil CFU; *CFU-g,* granulocyte CFU; *CFU-GEMM,* granulocyte/erythroid/macrophage/ megakaryocyte CFU; *CFU-GM,* granulocyte/macrophage CFU; *CFU-M,* macrophage CFU; *CFU-mast,* mast cell CFU; *CFU-Meg,* megakaryocyte CFU; *NK,* natural killer; *SCF,* stem cell factor; *IL-3,* interleukin-3; *GM-CSF,* granulocyte-macrophage colony-stimulating factor; *Epo,* erythropoietin; *IL-11,* interleukin-11; *IL-6,* interleukin-6; *MGDF,* megakaryocyte growth and development factor; *Tpo,* thrombopoietin; *M-CSF,* macrophage colony-stimulating factor; *G-CSF,* granulocyte colony-stimulating factor; *IL-7,* interleukin-7; *IL-2,* interleukin-2. (From Hunt P, Foote MA: *Curr Opin Biotech* 6:692, 1995.)

row recovery after bone marrow transplantation; (4) supporting the harvest of peripheral blood stem cells; (5) restoring bone marrow function in aplastic anemia, myelodysplastic syndrome, myelomas, leukemias, and acquired and congenital neutropenias; (6) combining CSFs with other BRMs to further enhance effector cell functions; (7) treating leukemia by promoting terminal cell maturation; and (8) treating burns, overwhelming sepsis-related infections, and parasitic infections.* Although the use of HGFs has had a significant impact as supportive therapy in patients receiving chemotherapy and after bone marrow transplantation,[152] issues of cost effectiveness are a continuing concern. Because a major issue in the changing health care environment is controlling cost, the American Society of Clinical Oncology (ASCO) published guidelines and recommendations for the use of these factors in 1995.[139]

Granulocyte/Macrophage Colony-Stimulating Factor (GM-CSF)

Of the multilineage CSFs, GM-CSF has received the most extensive clinical evaluation. Early clinical trials evaluated its application in patients with AIDS,[82] myelodysplastic syndromes, and aplastic anemia,[227,228] and in cancer patients after chemotherapy[10] and autologous bone marrow transplantation.[22] All studies showed dose-dependent increases in leukocytes, especially neutrophils, eosinophils, and monocytes. The duration of neutropenia appeared shorter after chemotherapy, and leukocyte recovery was enhanced after transplantation, compared with controls. Overall, no significant effects on platelet recovery were seen. Counts rose during therapy in a dose-dependent manner but fell rapidly once therapy was discontinued. In general, courses were well tolerated, and side effects were dose dependent. Recombinant human GM-CSF, sargramostim (Leukine), received regulatory approval in 1991 for the acceleration of myeloid recovery in patients with non-Hodgkin's lymphoma (NHL), acute lymphoblastic leukemia (ALL), and those with Hodgkin's disease who were undergoing autologous bone marrow transplantation (BMT).[95] Patients receiving GM-CSF had neutrophil recovery 7 days earlier than the group receiving placebo, fewer infections, fewer days taking antibiotics, and fewer days of hospitalization. Subsequent approvals include use in BMT graft failure and engraftment delay and as supportive therapy for elderly patients with acute myelogenous leukemia receiving high-dose chemotherapy. Issues to be addressed in future trials include evaluation of GM-CSF's effects on the incidence and seriousness of neutropenic infections after chemotherapy or transplantation, the timing of therapy in relation to administration of che-

motherapy,[133,140,169,229,243] long-term toxicity, its antitumor effect in both solid tumors and leukemias, and its use in infectious disease.

Administration. GM-CSF is manufactured by several pharmaceutical companies; however, only one brand is commercially available in the United States. Nurses should consult pharmacy resource personnel or the package insert about issues related to reconstitution, filterability, and stability. Pharmacology studies show GM-CSF has a relatively short half-life, with the second phase lasting 1 to 3 hours.[31] In early trials GM-CSF was given by IV infusion (continuous infusion, bolus); however, SC administration is also used.

In general, doses of 125 to 250 $\mu g/m^2$ (3 to 5 $\mu g/kg$) are fairly well tolerated. The recommended dose for sargramostim is 250 $\mu g/m^2$/day for 21 days as a 2-hour IV infusion beginning 2 to 4 hours after the autologous bone marrow infusion.[95] Toxicity is dose related, and the dose-limiting side effects are myalgia, arthralgia, capillary leak syndrome with edema, and pericardial and pleural effusions, which develop at doses above 16 to 32 $\mu g/kg$.[10]

Side effects. Side effects are affected by the dosage, route of administration, patient population, and setting used (postchemotherapy, post-BMT). Common side effects are constitutional symptoms (low-grade fever), bone pain, fatigue, and anorexia. Other reported side effects, generally seen at higher doses, are rashes, flushing, phlebitis,[82] gastrointestinal disturbances, erythema at the injection site, hypotension, fluid retention, pericarditis, pleural and pericardial effusion, thrombocytopenia, and thrombus formation at the catheter tip.[10] These effects are generally reversible when therapy stops.*

Granulocyte Colony-Stimulating Factor (G-CSF)

The early clinical trials investigating G-CSF focused on its use after chemotherapy.[144] Trials with combination chemotherapy for urothelial carcinoma[69] and high-dose chemotherapy for small-cell lung cancer[23] demonstrated a shorter duration of severe neutropenia after G-CSF therapy. Gabrilove's study showed that patients who received G-CSF had fewer days of antibiotic therapy and a reduced incidence and severity of mucositis and were more likely to be able to stay on their chemotherapy schedules than other patients. Patients exhibited a dose-dependent increase in leukocyte counts, mainly because of an increase in the absolute number of neutrophils. Counts fell rapidly once therapy was stopped. G-CSF has also been investigated in neutropenia arising from other causes.[64] In patients with HCL, for example, G-CSF dramatically increased the absolute neutrophil count.[78] In patients with myelodysplastic syndrome, patients have

*References 70, 133, 145, 169, 235, 243.

*References 10, 22, 85, 126, 227, 228.

increased their neutrophil counts over baseline levels fivefold to fortyfold.[145]

Recombinant human G-CSF, filgrastim (Neupogen) received FDA approval in 1991. Its initial indication was to reduce the incidence of infection in patients with non-myeloid malignancies receiving myelosuppressive anti-cancer drugs associated with a significant incidence of severe neutropenia with fever. In 1994 filgrastim received regulatory approval for use in BMT in nonmyeloid malignancies. An additional indication is the use of filgrastim to treat patients with severe chronic neutropenia.[4] Current clinical trials continue to study its use in a variety of bone marrow failure states, infections, in dose-intensified chemotherapy, mobilization of peripheral blood stem cells, radiotherapy, and in combination with other HGFs.[145,169,243]

Administration and side effects. The recommended starting dose of filgrastim is 5 μg/kg/day, administered subcutaneously or intravenously as a single daily injection[4] 24 hours after chemotherapy (for complete dosing instructions, consult the package insert). Nurses should consult pharmacy resource personnel or the package insert about issues related to reconstitution, filterability, and stability. Therapy is generally well tolerated, with medullary bone pain as the only consistent toxicity reported. This pain is usually mild to moderate in severity and is generally well controlled with nonnarcotic analgesics. Erythema is occasionally seen at the site of subcutaneous injections (see the box at right for a review of potential clinical uses of GM-CSF and G-CSF).

Erythropoietin

Physiologically, erythropoietin is a natural body glycoprotein essential for the growth of erythroid progenitor cells. Erythropoiesis is regulated by erythropoietin in response to changes in tissue oxygenation. Secreted primarily by the kidneys, erythropoietin acts on specific target cells in the bone marrow to increase the rate of production and release of red blood cells.[212] Recombinant human erythropoietin, epoetin alfa (Epogen and Procrit) was approved by the FDA in 1989 as a treatment for chronic anemia in end-stage renal disease after phase I and II trials demonstrated clinical efficacy.[60] The recombinant form is produced in cultured mammalian cells. When receiving it intravenously three times a week, virtually all patients achieved normalization of hematocrit (Hct) and were transfusion independent. Therapy is well tolerated in general, and most side effects (hypertension, seizures, increased clotting of venous access grafts) appear to be related to increased Hct.[6] Patients are generally started at a dosage of 50 to 100 U/kg three times a week intravenously or subcutaneously. Maintenance doses are generally titrated in 25-unit increments to keep the Hct in a chosen target range (e.g., 36% to 38%).

CLINICAL POTENTIAL OF GM-CSF AND G-CSF

Adjunct to standard chemotherapy
• Reduce morbidity
• Allow full doses to be delivered on time
Permit dose intensification of chemotherapy
• Reduce the morbidity of autologous or allogeneic marrow or peripheral stem-cell transplantation
• Allow larger doses of drugs to be administered
• Increase the frequency of chemotherapy cycles
Reversal of marrow failure
• Malignancies with marrow infiltration, chronic lymphatic leukemia, hairy cell leukemia, lymphoma
Differentiation-inducing agents
• Myelodysplastic syndromes
• Myeloid leukemia
Recruitment of malignant cells before chemotherapy
• Myeloid leukemia
Direct anticancer effects

From Metcalf D, Morstyn G: Colony-stimulating factors: general biology. In DeVita VT, Hellman S, Rosenberg SA, editors: *Biologic therapy of cancer,* Philadelphia, 1991, Lippincott.

Anemia is one of the major side effects of treatment with zidovudine, an antiviral drug used in the treatment of patients infected with the human immunodeficiency virus (HIV). Double-blind, placebo-controlled trials led to regulatory approval of epoetin alfa in this population for patients with an endogenous serum erythropoietin level below 500 U/L. Doses of epoetin alfa at 100 U/kg by intravenous infusion three times a week resulted in an increase in Hct and a decrease in transfusion requirements. In 1993 Procrit received regulatory approval for the treatment of anemia in cancer patients undergoing chemotherapy.[1,158,184,212,247] At doses of 150 U/kg given by subcutaneous injection three times weekly, patients experienced an increase in Hct values from baseline and a decrease in transfusion requirements. Quality of life indices in responding patients showed improvement in energy levels, ability to engage in daily activities, and improvement in overall quality of life. Epoetin alfa is being studied for its use in autologous blood donation, acute blood loss and surgery, and treatment of myelodysplastic syndrome, as well as in combination with other HGFs.

Macrophage Colony-Stimulating Factor

The inherent biologic activity of M-CSF has aroused considerable interest in its use, alone or in combination with other biologic agents, in the treatment of malignancy.[13,149,151] Early phase I/II trials are in the process of evaluating dosage and toxicity for both the subcutaneous and intravenous routes. In trials evaluating subcutaneous administration, doses up to 12,800 $\mu g/m^2$ have been administered. In general, toxicity has been mild, consisting of local reaction, arthralgia, and fatigue. At the highest dose levels, thrombocytopenia and monocytosis have been observed.[28] A dose-dependent decrease in cholesterol and lipoproteins has also been observed. Future trials will further define dosage and evaluate the efficacy of M-CSF in treating cancer. It is also being studied as a treatment for fungal infections in patients undergoing BMT.[235]

Interleukin-3

The ability of IL-3 to target multipotential committed progenitor cells provides a strong rationale for its evaluation in the treatment of bone marrow failure states. Phase I/II clinical trials continue to evaluate the use of IL-3 alone and in combination with other HGFs for patients with bone marrow failure, normal hematopoiesis but advanced malignancy, or prolonged cytopenia after radiotherapy or chemotherapy.[89,111] In trials with IL-3 alone, all studies showed a delayed increase in leukocytes (granulocytes, eosinophils, and basophils), and occasional increases in platelets and reticulocytes. Both subcutaneous and intravenous routes were used, with doses up to 1000 $\mu g/m^2$/day being fairly well tolerated.[76,112,235] The most common toxicities experienced were low-grade fever and headaches with occasional flushing, erythema at injection sites, bone pain, lethargy, and nausea and vomiting. Future trials will further refine dosage and the application of IL-3 in bone marrow failure states and its ability to provide a myeloprotective effect after chemotherapy or radiotherapy.[169,235,243] In vivo simian studies with IL-3 have shown marked stimulation when it is given in combination with GM-CSF.[57] Preliminary clinical results suggest that this combination may have a synergistic effect on hematopoietic progenitor cells and may be of value in reducing chemotherapy-induced neutropenia.

PIXY321

PIXY321 is a recombinantly engineered fusion molecule. It consist of GM-CSF and IL-3, fused together with a linker protein. It has demonstrated biologic effects consistent with both of these growth factors and is thought to have a greater multilineage effect than either alone. PIXY321 is being evaluated both (1) alone in a variety of bone marrow failure states or after chemotherapy and (2) in combination with other HGFs. Doses range from 50 to 750 $\mu g/m^2$/day as an intravenous or subcutaneous injection for up to 14 days. Studies have shown a dose-dependent increase in white blood cell counts (mainly neutrophils) and platelets. Common toxic effects include erythema at the injection site, flu-like symptoms, bone pain, and fatigue. Phase III confirmatory trials of PIXY321 are in progress at several centers, evaluating

its use in the areas of chemotherapy-induced cytopenias and high-dose chemotherapy and BMT.[169,230,232,235,243]

Other Growth Factors

Several new growth factors are being investigated in early phase I/II clinical trials. Stem cell factor (SCF) is thought to exert its effects on the pluripotent stem cell. It is a potent costimulatory factor when given in combination with other HGFs, causing increases in the size and number of hematopoietic progenitor cells. In fact, it has little clinical activity when given alone at low doses.[125,146,235] Interleukin-11, known to have hematopoietic effects, is being evaluated in phase III trials for its ability to abrogate chemotherapy-related thrombocytopenia.[107,235] Thrombopoietin, a platelet-specific growth factor, has recently been identified. It is characterized as the primary regulator of platelet production. Its most likely clinical use will be in concert with other HGFs.[105,136] Several interleukins (IL-1, IL-3, and IL-6) are being evaluated as myeloprotective agents, both alone and in combination with other HGFs.[169,224]

TUMOR NECROSIS FACTOR

Discovered in 1975 in the serum of animals treated with injections of BCG or *C. parvum* followed by endotoxins, tumor necrosis factor (TNF) is a protein that selectively targets transformed cells.[14] Normal human fibroblasts appeared insensitive to TNF. These findings generated considerable interest in the use of TNF in the treatment of cancer. The gene for TNF has been isolated, identified, and cloned to produce recombinant TNF (rTNF). Further investigations have analyzed TNF's relationships with other cytotoxic factors produced by immune effector cells. Cachectin was isolated by Beutler and colleagues,[19] who believed it to be important in the pathogenesis of cachexia. Amino acid sequencing and cloning techniques proved human cachectin and TNF to be the same molecule.[19,223] This TNF, primarily produced by activated macrophages, is called *TNF-α*. Another cytokine, lymphotoxin, which shares biologic activity with TNF-α, has been called TNF-β. It is produced primarily by lymphocytes. This section focuses on TNF-α.

Biologic Effects

Although primarily synthesized in vivo by activated macrophages, TNF is also produced by lymphocytes, NK cells, astrocytes, and microglial cells of the brain. This polypeptide hormone, pivotal in the pathogenesis of infection, inflammation, and injury, participates in the beneficial processes of host defense and tissue homeostasis. TNF interacts with high-affinity receptors on normal tissue cells, with resultant internalization of the receptor-ligand complex. Details of this process remain unclear.

Several biologic activities of TNF may be responsible for its antitumor effects: it is cytotoxic or cytostatic to some human tumor cells; it promotes the induction of other mediators (IL-2 and GM-CSF)[68,223]; it enhances chemotactic, phagocytic, and cytotoxic activity of macrophages and neutrophils; and it causes the induction of several cell-surface antigens. It also serves as the primary mediator of endotoxic shock[128] and as a growth factor by stimulating fibroblasts and mesenchymal cell proliferation.[14,26,223]

Clinical Indications

Both preclinical studies in animal models and human clinical trials have evaluated the effectiveness of TNF as an antitumor agent. An overview of phase I experience with TNF in the United States indicates that more than 200 patients with a variety of malignancies have undergone therapy with TNF. However, to date, therapeutic responses are unimpressive.[20,33,68,205] An editorial by Frei[68] concludes that until the cellular mechanisms of TNF cytotoxicity and tumor cell resistance are understood, clinical trials will not be able to exploit the full potential of this agent. Current efforts are focused on phase II investigations and on evaluating combination therapy of TNF with other cytokines,[147,148] isolated limb perfusions in combination with IFN-γ and in the transfer of the gene coding for TNF into TIL (a form of gene therapy).[191]

Administration

TNF has been administered by intramuscular, subcutaneous, intravenous[20,205] (via both bolus and continuous infusion), and intraperitoneal routes. The maximum tolerated dose as defined in phase I trials varies with route and schedule. TNF has not received FDA approval and therefore is administered only in investigational settings.

Pharmacy resource personnel should be consulted about stability, filterability, and other administration concerns (e.g., intravenous lines are often preprimed with albumin and normal saline before TNF administration). Handling procedures should follow hospital policy.

Side Effects

Toxicity associated with TNF has been well documented in early clinical trials.[26] The side effects are similar to those seen with other biologic agents, are dose dependent, and in general resolve upon discontinuation of therapy. Dose-limiting toxicities with IV administration have been constitutional symptoms and shocklike manifestations, including fever and hypotension.[26] As with IFN, patients may exhibit tachyphylaxis to many of the side effects.

Common side effects include fever, severe chills or rigors, fatigue, myalgia, headache, soreness at the injection site (erythema and tenderness), nausea and/or vomiting, and loss of appetite, with resultant weight loss. Pretreatment with meperidine is often helpful in controlling chills and rigors. Depending on the dose and schedule, these side effects may lessen or disappear with subsequent doses.

Occasional side effects include hematologic changes (leukopenia, thrombocytopenia), cardiovascular changes (hypotension, dizziness), hepatic changes (elevated transaminases, hyperbilirubinemia), elevated triglycerides, and decreased serum cholesterol. These changes are usually reversible with cessation of therapy. Hypotension can generally be managed with fluid administration, with prehydration used at higher IV doses of TNF (≥ 100 μg/m^2).

Although rare, more severe toxicity associated with changes in the central nervous or respiratory systems has occurred.[137] Neurologic deficits observed include transient ischemic attacks and strokelike symptoms. Patients who develop these symptoms should be removed from the study and evaluated to determine the etiology of the symptoms. Respiratory insufficiency, evidenced primarily by dyspnea, has also been observed. Morice and associates[142] monitored 19 patients receiving subcutaneous or intravenous TNF. All but two demonstrated impairment of gas exchange as measured by diffusion lung capacity (DLCO), a measurement of alveolar gas exchange. This toxicity appeared to be dose related but resolved in most patients with the cessation of therapy.

MONOCLONAL ANTIBODIES

Monoclonal antibodies (MAbs), produced by the fusion of antibody-producing cells and myeloma tumor cells (hybridomas), have been shown to be highly specific for a single target antigen. With the development of hybridoma technology in 1975,[108] large amounts of pure antibodies with a predetermined specificity could be produced. This rekindled interest in the use of antibodies for the diagnosis and treatment of cancer. Their potential was implicated in the early 1900s, when Paul Ehrlich observed that antiserum from tumor-bearing mice, when injected into tumor-bearing animals of the same strain, was capable of causing tumor rejection. He called these antibodies magic bullets and proposed using them as carriers to deliver drugs and toxins to tumor cells.[58]

An antigen is any substance that the body recognizes as foreign and attacks with an immune response. The humoral immune response produces immunoglobulins against the invading antigen from B cell–derived plasma cells. These immunoglobulins, or antibodies, react specifically with the antigenic determinants or epitopes of the inducing antigen. The antigenic determinants are parts of the antigen recognized by the antibodies. Each antigen has any number of epitopes, depending on the complexity of its structure. Individual B cells produce an antibody specific for a single antigenic determinant; therefore when an antigen invades the body, a variety of antibodies against it are produced.[170]

Hybridoma technology begins with immunizing a mouse with a chosen antigen (Figure 23-3). After the mouse mounts an immune response, its spleen is removed to obtain B lymphocyte–producing antibodies. Because lymphocytes cannot grow indefinitely in culture, they are fused with mouse myeloma cells (plasma cells) to immortalize the antibody-producing B lymphocytes. These new cells, *hybridomas,* can grow indefinitely in culture and produce antibodies with predetermined specificity—MAbs. The next step is to select and clone for the desired antibody. Once the desired hybridoma is obtained, it can be frozen for future use, grown in culture to produce continuous quantities of MAbs, or reinjected into mice and grown as tumors to produce MAbs in ascites fluid.[50]

As previously discussed, when the body encounters a foreign substance, an immune response is mounted. It has long been hypothesized that tumor cells express cell-surface molecules (antigens) different from those expressed on normal cells. Antigens found only on malignant cells are called *tumor-specific antigens (TSAs),* whereas antigens found also on normal tissues but to a greater degree in malignant cells are called *tumor-associated antigens (TAAs).*[15,50,53,200] Most malignant cells express TAA. One example is oncofetal antigens, which are normally expressed on embryonic cells and later reexpressed on malignant cells. Whereas most current therapies are toxic for both malignant and normal cells, MAbs can be used to attack the tumor cell directly. Theoretically, antibody therapy is the most tumor-specific approach to cancer treatment.[50,53]

Unconjugated Antibody

Biology and clinical applications. Numerous clinical trials have been conducted with native MAbs—those not bound to drugs, toxins, or isotopes—for a large number of malignancies. An unconjugated antibody may demonstrate an anticancer effect in several ways. One is to mediate an antitumor cytotoxic effect through complement-dependent cytotoxicity or antibody-dependent cellular cytotoxicity. The constant region (F_c) of the immunoglobulin reacts with either the first component of the complement system or with immune effector cells; the end result is tumor cell lysis.[15] Tumor cells express a variety of receptors important for growth and proliferation advantages. A second approach employs MAbs directed against cell-surface receptors involved in proliferation, such as the epidermal growth factor (EGF) receptor. The intent is to block or downgrade the number of available receptors, thereby inducing an antiproliferative effect.[15,53,200] An extensively studied approach is the use of antiidiotype antibodies. Idiotypes are the variable regions of the immunoglobulin molecule that contain the antigen-combining region. A malignant B-cell clone produces cells that express and occasionally secrete a specific antibody. Infusions of antibodies directed against a B-cell lymphoma idiotype may suppress that clone back to its baseline.[50,53,200]

Another approach, actually a method of passive immunization, uses antibodies as surrogate tumor antigens to stimulate an immune response against the tumor. For example, suppose a murine antibody (AB1) is selected to recognize a certain TAA. A second antibody (AB2) is raised against the idiotype of AB1. This second antibody, AB2, is an antiidiotype antibody. The patient is immunized with this antibody. An antiidiotype response to AB2 produces a third antibody, AB3. This third antibody has the same capacity to react with the desired TAA as AB1 because its idiotype is the mirror image of this antigen. In essence, by receiving AB2, the patient becomes self-immunized, developing his or her own human antibodies against the tumor. This technique is also used to immunize against invading organisms such as viruses be-

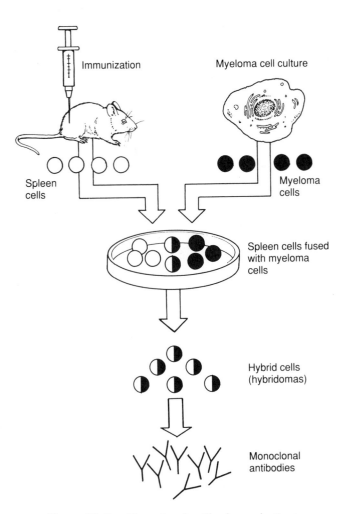

Figure 23-3 Monoclonal antibody production.

cause it avoids vaccination with whole virus or viral antigens. In the treatment of cancer, the use of MAbs as vaccines is an active area of clinical investigation[15] (see Figure 23-4).

The first MAb clinical trials were conducted in patients with hematologic malignancies—leukemias and lymphomas. Trials soon followed evaluating MAbs in solid tumors such as melanoma, colorectal cancer, prostate cancer, breast cancer, and lung cancer.* To date this approach has led only to transient clinical responses.

Several problems can affect the therapeutic efficacy or toxicity (or both) of MAbs. A major concern is the development of human antimouse antibodies (HAMA) after murine MAbs are administered.[15,50,176] HAMA may trigger immune complex formation, which mediates tissue damage, neutralization of MAbs (preventing them from binding to tumor cells), and alteration of MAb clearance and organ distribution. Strategies being evaluated to abrogate the development of HAMA include infusion of antibody fragments, infusion of large doses of MAb to induce tolerance, immunosuppressive therapy, and use of human or chimeric (part murine/part human)[15,50] antibodies.

*References 15, 50, 53, 79, 115, 193, 200.

Another concern is antigenic modulation. Surface antigens decline during this process, being either internalized and later reexpressed or shed from the cell surface. Antigenic modulation is especially problematic in hematologic malignancies. Within minutes of exposure to MAbs, modulation can occur. Once circulating levels of MAb decrease, antigen is reexpressed. Obviously, once modulation occurs, MAbs cannot effectively bind to malignant cells. Strategies for circumventing this problem include administration of mixed MAbs (a cocktail) to recognize different antigens and choosing MAbs specific for nonmodulating antigens.[50,53,200]

Other problems include poor tumor vascularity (poor circulation inhibits delivery of MAbs to the tumor site); cross-reactivity of MAbs with normal tissues; tumor heterogeneity (expression of more than one TAA); lack of sufficient antigen expression on the tumor cell surface; and lack of in vivo cytotoxicity of the antibody alone. Clinical trials are evaluating strategies to overcome these obstacles so that the full therapeutic benefit of MAbs can be realized.[15,50,176] For example, one area of focus is the combination of native MAbs and other BRMs. An example is the use of an HGF such as GM-CSF to increase the number of immune cells capable of interacting with MAbs to destroy tumor cells.[15]

Immunoconjugates. An active area of investigation

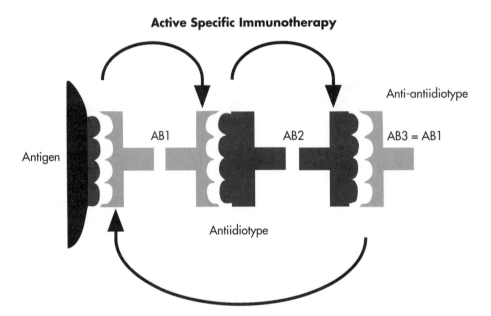

Active Specific Immunotherapy

Figure 23-4 Production of monoclonal antibodies to be used as vaccines. A murine antibody (AB1) is chosen to recognize a certain tumor-associated antigen, such as a melanoma-associated antigen. A second antibody (AB2) is made to recognize the idiotype of AB1; this second antibody is an antiidiotype antibody, which is used as the vaccine. The patient is immunized with AB2 and responds by producing an antiidiotype antibody against AB2; this third antibody, designated AB3, has the same ability to react with the desired tumor-associated antigen as AB1, because its idiotype is the mirror image of AB1. Thus the patient becomes self-immunized, developing his or her own human antibodies against the tumor.

is the conjugation of MAbs to toxins (immunotoxins),[160] chemotherapy (chemoimmunotoxins),[165] radioisotopes (radioimmunotherapy),[80] and BRMs (immunobiologics).[15] The ricin A chain, a toxin, has been conjugated to several antitumor murine MAbs, and clinical trials are progressing.[157,160] Although most responses are transient, patients with hematopoietic tumors tend to respond better than those with solid tumors. The most significant complications have included a capillary leak type of syndrome exhibited clinically by hypoalbuminemia, proteinuria, weight gain, and pulmonary edema. Clinical trials are investigating immunoconjugates of chemotherapeutic agents such as methotrexate, doxorubicin, and cisplatin, to MAbs. By selectively delivering these drugs to the tumor, investigators hope to increase tumor cell kill while avoiding systemic toxicity. Problems include acquired drug resistance and the need to deliver large amounts of drug (as opposed to small amounts with toxins) to the tumor.

Another exciting area is conjugation of radioisotopes to MAbs. Two important advantages to this approach are the ability to kill antigen-negative bystander cells and elimination of the need for internalization by the tumor cell to exhibit their cytotoxic effect. Clinical trials are in progress in this area, with most successes seen in the hematologic malignancies.[50,80]

Major problems with all types of conjugates include damage to normal tissue as a result of cross-reactivity and systemic toxicity should the MAb and the conjugate dissociate. Toxicity is related primarily to the effects of the radioisotope on the bone marrow, with platelets being the most sensitive.

Diagnostic imaging with radiolabeled antibodies. The use of radiolabeled MAbs in diagnostic imaging has received intense study.[116,193] When low doses of radioisotopes such as indium-111 and iodine-131 are conjugated with MAbs that react to specific tumor antigens, MAbs can be used to locate both primary and metastatic tumors. The ability of radiolabeled MAbs to detect tumors is being compared with conventional x-rays and isotope scans. In some instances, antibodies are more sensitive than conventional scans. Currently, Oncoscint CR/OV is the only MAb with regulatory approval for the detection of cancer in patients with colorectal and ovarian cancer. Problems that are associated with radioimmunoimaging include tumor size (lesions less than 1 cm in size do not image well), tumor heterogeneity, nonspecific uptake of MAbs by other organs (especially the liver and spleen), tumor vascularity, toxicities, and the HAMA response, which may limit administration to a single course. A current area of investigation is the use of a hand-held probe during surgery to detect radiolabeled areas of tumor foci within the abdomen. This approach might be used to rule out metastasis in the lymph nodes and to determine tumor-free margins for resection.[15]

Other clinical applications. For diagnosis, MAbs may be used in serologic detection of clinically unapparent tumors or to aid in the differential diagnosis of tumors that look alike on routinely processed light microscopy specimens. The latter field, *immunohistochemistry,* has been used increasingly over the past several years. MAbs have been used extensively to classify leukemias and lymphomas.[200]

MAbs have also been used in BMT. One of the more severe complications of allogeneic transplantation is the development of graft-versus-host disease (GVHD). In an attempt to prevent the development of GVHD, MAbs reactive with immunocompetent T cells are incubated in vitro with donor marrow before the marrow is infused into the recipient. An attractive therapeutic option in this area is the use of MAbs to purge autologous marrow of lingering malignant cells before transplantation.

The use of monoclonal antibodies and antibody conjugates continues to progress (see box below). The future holds further exploration and refinement in this area and investigation into the use of human monoclonal antibodies, chimeric monoclonal antibodies, and bifunctional antibodies. Also, a considerable number of clinical trials are investigating the use of MAb-based therapies in other disease states, such as bacterial and viral infections, the treatment of septic shock, and autoimmune disease.*

Administration. Most MAbs remain investigational. Administration of MAbs involves intravenous, intraarterial, intraperitoneal, and intralymphatic routes.[50,193] Dosage depends on investigational protocols and whether the MAb is being used for diagnostic or therapeutic purposes. Antibodies are generally diluted in normal saline and administered over several hours via an infusion

*References 15, 50, 53, 79, 115, 200.

ANTIBODIES IN CANCER THERAPY

Antibodies
  Cytotoxic
  Regulatory
  Immunization
Immunoconjugates
  Radiolabeled antibodies
  Chemoimmunoconjugates
  Immunotoxins
  Immunobiologics
Bone marrow transplantation
  Allogeneic
  Autologous

From Dillman RO: Antibody therapy. In Oldham RK, editor: *Principles of cancer biotherapy,* ed 2, New York, 1991, Dekker.

pump to prevent accidental bolus infusion.[41,183,196] Handling procedures may vary among institutions; however, appropriate cytotoxic handling procedures should be used with chemoimmunoconjugates and immunotoxins. Radiation safety procedures should be employed whenever radiolabeled MAbs are used. Pharmacy resource personnel should be consulted about filterability, solution compatibility, stability, and other pertinent issues.[183,196]

Side effects. Allergic reaction to mouse protein is a major concern for patients receiving murine MAbs. The major acute toxicity is anaphylaxis, manifested as generalized flushing and/or urticaria, followed by pallor and/or cyanosis. Respiratory distress may also occur. If left untreated, anaphylaxis can progress to systemic vascular collapse, unconsciousness, and death. Fortunately, its occurrence is rare. Treatment involves immediately stopping the antibody infusion and administering fluids and emergency drugs such as epinephrine, diphenhydramine, and hydrocortisone sodium succinate.

Subacute toxicity includes fever, chills, and rigors, diaphoresis, malaise, urticaria, pruritus, nausea, vomiting, dyspnea, and hypotension. Fevers, chills, diaphoresis, and shaking rigors are often seen when MAbs bind to circulating leukemic cells.[51,52] These toxicities can occur in the first 24 hours to 1 week after the infusion. They are usually easily treated before or during the infusion with acetaminophen, antihistamines, meperidine, or antiemetics.[50-52,183,196]

Serum sickness, the major delayed toxicity seen with MAb therapy, can occur 2 to 4 weeks after infusion. It results when circulating immune complexes are deposited in the tissues and produces symptoms such as urticaria, pruritus, arthralgia, generalized adenopathy, and flu-like symptoms. Treatment includes aspirin, acetaminophen, and occasionally corticosteroids. Symptoms usually resolve as the complexes are cleared from the body.[50-52]

On occasion, when MAbs cross-react with normal tissues, other types of toxic effects may be seen. For example, antibodies targeted against the GD_2 ganglioside in melanoma cause intense pain during infusion. This is hypothesized to be a result of cross-reactivity with nerve tissue.[15]

RETINOIDS

The retinoids are a class of agents consisting of vitamin A (retinol) and related derivatives (all-trans-retinoic acid [tretinoin] and 13-cis-retinoic acid [13-cRA] isotretinoin) that are involved in growth, reproduction, epithelial cell differentiation, and immune function. Specific effects of the retinoids on the immune system include enhancement of humoral antibody responses and certain cell-mediated immune responses, and improved phagocytosis by macrophages. The biologic effects of retinoids appear to oc-

cur from changes in gene expression that occur via specific nuclear receptors. Retinol and retinoic acid (RA) are known to bind to cellular retinol or RA-binding proteins. These proteins facilitate the transfer of RA and retinol from the cytoplasm to the nucleus, where they bind to one of several nuclear RA receptors. This ultimately leads to the transcription of appropriate target genes through binding to specific DNA sequences.[92,121,209]

Preclinical studies with RA have demonstrated several potentially beneficial effects: induction of cell differentiation in both normal epithelial cells and certain tumor cell lines, and direct growth inhibition with or without differentiation. Because of the unique biology of the retinoids, a number of clinical trials are evaluating their use in the treatment of cancer patients. Toxicity in these trials can be classified according to mucocutaneous, visual, skeletal, lipid, liver, and teratogenic side effects. Mucocutaneous toxicities are generally the most troublesome and include dryness of the mucosal tissues, erythema and desquamation of the skin, and cheilitis. Because of the strong teratogenic effect of the retinoids, extreme caution should be exercised to avoid their use during pregnancy.[92,121,209]

A series of clinical studies with oral RA has demonstrated high complete remission rates (CR) in patients with acute promyelocytic leukemia (APL). Although many responses are not lasting despite continued therapy, the role of RA alone and in combination with conventional therapy for APL continues to be evaluated.[219] In November 1995 tretinoin (Vesanoid) received regulatory approval for the treatment of APL for induction of remission in patients who are refractory to or who have relapsed from anthracycline chemotherapy, or for whom anthracycline-based therapy is contraindicated. Because optimal consolidation or maintenance regimens have not been determined, all patients should receive a standard consolidation and/or maintenance chemotherapy regimen for APL after induction therapy with Vesanoid unless otherwise contraindicated.[189] Additional clinical trials, both phase I and phase II, are evaluating the use of RA alone and in combination with other agents such as IFN in myelodysplastic syndrome, other hematologic malignancies (multiple myeloma, mycosis fungoides), and solid tumors (cervical, squamous cell cancer of the head and neck, breast, and prostate carcinoma).[92,121,209]

Another exciting area is the use of retinoids in the chemoprevention of upper aerodigestive tract carcinomas.[17,119,120] Clinical trials have evaluated the effectiveness of both natural agents and synthetic retinoids in reversing oral premalignant lesions. A randomized, placebo-controlled trial of 13-cRA has been reported by Hong and associates.[92] Reversal of dysplasia occurred in 54% of the retinoid group and in only 10% of the placebo group. Two significant problems were encountered in this study: toxicity from 13-cRA and a relapse rate of over 50% within 3 months of stopping therapy. A second trial evaluated an induction phase with higher doses (1.5 mg/kg/day) followed by a 9-month maintenance program with either low-dose 13-cRA (0.5 mg/kg/day) or β-carotene (30 mg/day). Preliminary data demonstrate that the relapse rate after 9 months is 8% in the low-dose 13-cRA group and 55% in the β-carotene group. Other trials include evaluation of high-dose 13-cRA to prevent second primary tumors (SPT) in patients with squamous cell cancer of the head and neck. With a median follow-up of 42 months, only 6% of the 13-cRA group developed SPT, compared with 28% of the placebo group. Two important directions for future chemoprevention trials will be establishing effective doses that reduce toxicity and evaluating other retinoids, such as fenretinide or etretinate.[43] A phase III trial comparing tretinoin with β-carotene in the treatment of oral premalignant lesions is in progress.

OTHER IMMUNOMODULATORS

This section briefly reviews agents that either boost immunologic responses (specifically or nonspecifically) or cause the induction of cytokines. Although many of these agents were more actively investigated in the 1960s and 1970s, they may still be encountered today. For example, they may now be used alone via different routes (intraperitoneal, intrapleural), or smaller subunits may be used in an attempt to elicit an immune response. Further possible uses include combining these agents with newer BRMs.

Bacillus Calmette-Guérin

Bacillus Calmette-Guérin (BCG) was used in first-generation immunotherapy trials.[90] Developed in the early 1900s, it is an attenuated form of the living bovine tubercle bacillus. It is believed to have a nonspecific immunostimulating effect. The initial work with BCG in animal models was done by Old and co-workers,[155] who demonstrated that BCG could stimulate the reticuloendothelial system and the immune response. Clinical trials reported by Mathé[129] in 1969 demonstrated positive therapeutic results of BCG therapy for children with acute lymphocytic leukemia (ALL). Although early trials with BCG in a multitude of settings appeared promising, further investigations did not support these results.[90,193] Trials with BCG continue. When comparing the results of different clinical trials of BCG, it is of prime importance to note the variability in the strains of BCG used (Pasteur, Glaxo, Phipps, and so on), as well as the route of administration, dosage, and schedule. BCG is approved for the treatment of bladder cancer by intravesical instillation.[198]

BCG can be administered intralesionally; intradermally by scarification, the tine technique, or the Heaf-

gun; or intracavitarily (to the pleura, peritoneum, or bladder). Side effects can include local inflammatory reactions, flu-like symptoms, hypersensitivity, and the serious complication of disseminated BCG infection.

Levamisole

Levamisole is an orally active synthetic agent that is an isomer of tetramisole, a broad-spectrum antihelminthic agent. Ergamisol[100] has been approved by the FDA for use with 5-FU as an adjuvant treatment for colon cancer (Duke's stage C). A randomized study showed that patients in Duke's stage C disease who were treated with levamisole and 5-FU had a higher 5-year survival rate than untreated patients.[117] Toxicity has been minimal with levamisole alone, and no more severe than expected for 5-FU alone, when the two drugs were combined.

Tumor Antigens

This form of therapy rests on the premise that tumor cells express immunogenic determinants that are not associated, or are associated to a lesser degree, with normal cells. The immune system will theoretically recognize these cells as foreign and mount an immunologic response. Tumor vaccines employ tumor cells or purified components of tumor cell membrane. To increase the immunogenicity of the cells, the surface is often treated with viruses, irradiation, or neuramidase. Tumor vaccines are also given in combination with other immunostimulants such as BCG or *C. parvum*. Vaccines are usually administered by multiple intradermal injections, with patients receiving vaccines prepared from their own tumor cells. Although historically this approach has been unsuccessful, recent randomized, phase II trials to evaluate active specific immunotherapy in colorectal cancer have proved efficacy. One hindrance has been the technical limitations of such individualized vaccines. The process is technologically complex, labor intensive, and expensive. Research with MAbs may lead to characterization and purification of reactive antigenic molecules that could be mass produced as a generic vaccine.[15,87]

GENE THERAPY

An exciting area of current focus is gene therapy, defined as the insertion of a functioning gene into the cells of a patient to correct an inborn genetic error or to provide a new function to the cell. Somatic cell gene therapy, which does not have the potential of passing changes on to future generations, is currently the only technique approved for use in humans. To ensure the patient's safety, the approval process is quite lengthy and rigorous, necessitating institutional, FDA, and National Institutes of Health authorization.[103,187] Work in this area has been pioneered by Rosenberg and associates at the National Cancer Institute. Trials are in progress evaluating the insertion of the gene for TNF into TIL cells. Theoretically, TILs would secrete large amounts of TNF locally at the tumor site.[190,191] Other studies include administration of fibroblasts, transduced with the gene coding for IL-4, and tumor vaccines in patients with advanced melanoma or renal cell, breast, or colon cancer. Another approach under investigation is insertion of the multidrug resistance gene into bone marrow progenitor cells in an attempt to prevent dose-limiting myelosuppression while using higher doses of chemotherapy.[94]

To date, the most common approach for insertion of genes into somatic cells is through the use of a retroviral vector. A retrovirus, incapable of replicating, is used as a carrier to enter the cell and insert the desired gene into the cell's genome. Safety concerns include the fear of replication-competent viruses arising from vector cell lines or the disruption of normal cell growth when the retroviral vector randomly inserts the gene into the target cell. To address these issues, alternative delivery systems such as the use of the gene gun or antibody-coated liposomes are under evaluation. At this point, minimal toxic effects have been noted with gene therapy. However, it is important to remember that this therapy is still in its infancy. Ethical concerns over the manipulation of genes is also an area of importance. As genetic tests are developed to identify patients at risk for developing certain types of cancer, the use of gene therapy to inactivate or replace defective genes will become more prevalent.[187]

FUTURE DIRECTIONS AND ADVANCES IN BIOTHERAPY

Treatment with biologic agents is becoming more and more widespread, and new agents and novel combinations of agents will continue to make their way into the clinical setting.* For example, interleukin-12, a potent cytokine with effects on NK and T cells, is now in phase I/II trials.[27,89] It is imperative that oncology nurses be knowledgeable about biotherapy in order to care for patients receiving it. In their roles as educator, advocate, and caregiver, nurses are key figures in facilitating management of patients receiving biologic agents. Over the next few years BRMs will continue to receive FDA approval, which will increase their availability. Clinical trials will continue to define appropriate dosage, route, and clinical indications for many agents and combinations.[9,147,148] In addition, research efforts are now focusing on delineating the pathophysiology of BRM-associated side effects. It is hoped that these efforts will lead to improved tolerance of the more severe side effects.[179,201]

For years, determination of the maximum tolerated dose has been the standard in chemotherapy trials. However, this approach may not be appropriate for biotherapy. Recent attention has focused on determining the optimal immunomodulatory dose. Lower doses may be more effective than the maximum tolerated dose in boosting an immune response. In addition, determining the full range of biologic effects in vivo will assist in determining dosage. Investigators are also faced with the challenge of developing therapeutic regimens that maximize response yet are tolerable to patients, cost effective, and realistically managed.[181,193]

Clinical investigations evaluating combinations of cytokines and of cytokines and chemotherapy continue to be an area of active focus. The availability of recombinant cytokines has led to evaluation of their efficacy in vivo as single-modality cancer therapy. Although clinical benefits have been achieved, few patients have been cured. An additional problem is the toxicity of cytokines when given at high doses. Is there a way to maximize response while achieving acceptable toxicity? Studies in animal models using combinations of cytokines have demonstrated synergism and a resultant increase in antitumor effect. Combining agents may make it possible to use smaller doses while maintaining therapeutic benefit. This has provided a rationale for the use of combinations of cytokines such as IFN-α and IL-2, TNF, and IL-2, and monoclonal antibodies and IL-2. It is hoped that effective combinations of BRMs with or without chemotherapy will result in improved therapeutic benefits and decreased toxicity.[9,147,148] Randomized trials will ultimately be necessary to prove any benefit for combination therapies.[53]

Progress in the basic sciences will continue to explore the mystery of cancer on a cellular level. This new understanding will serve as the foundation for future cancer therapies.[114,186,245] Key regulatory molecules and signaling pathways in the cells will provide important targets for future diagnostic, therapeutic, and preventive strategies. Therapies will become increasingly selective and targeted toward repairing or blocking the negative effects of the underlying cellular defect. Depending on the existing mutation, strategies might be designed either to block or to stimulate transcription of a gene. Examples of this approach currently under clinical investigation include the use of "antisense" therapy, synthetic strands of DNA that bind to specific sites on the nucleic acids and inhibit the synthesis of disease-related proteins.[215] Numerous current and future clinical trials are aimed at restoring normal function to the mutated *p53* gene.[32] This gene, classified as a tumor-suppressor gene, is important in controlling abnormal cell growth.[239] As basic research begins to describe the metastatic process, new avenues for therapeutic intervention will be opened. One example under clinical investigation is the use of

---

*References 40, 59, 113, 114, 156, 186, 192, 225.

Text continued on p. 606.

Nursing Management

Caring for patients receiving biotherapy is both challenging and exciting. Because many biologic response modifiers are now available for commercial use, many oncology nurses have become more familiar with this once new form of therapy. As research continues, biotherapy advances over the next few years will be exponential. Nurses working in this area will be compelled to remain up-to-date and will have an opportunity to be on the cutting edge in developing standards of care for patients receiving biotherapy.[63,102] Although the mode of action and pattern of toxicity for biotherapy differ from those for chemotherapy, nurses can draw on their expertise in managing chemotherapy-related side effects to meet the challenge of dealing with side effects unique to biotherapy.

Nursing Diagnoses: Neurologic Function

- *Sensory/perceptual alterations (visual, auditory)*
- *Sleep pattern disturbance*
- *Social interaction, impaired*
- *Thought processes, altered*

Nursing Diagnosis: Renal Function

- *Urinary elimination, altered*

Nursing Diagnoses: Hematologic Function

- *Injury, risk for, related to weakness or bleeding*
- *Infection, risk for, related to decreased WBC*
- *Activity intolerance related to anemia*

Nursing Diagnosis: Skin

- *Skin integrity, impaired*

Nursing Diagnoses: Gastrointestinal System

- *Nutrition, altered: less than body requirements*
- *Diarrhea*
- *Oral mucous membrane, altered*
- *Skin integrity, impaired, risk for, related to diarrhea*

Nursing Diagnoses: Cardiovascular System

- *Tissue perfusion, altered cardiopulmonary, peripheral*
- *Fluid volume deficit*

Nursing Diagnoses: Pulmonary System

- *Gas exchange, impaired*
- *Anxiety related to respiratory distress*

Nursing Diagnoses: Miscellaneous

- *Fatigue*
- *Activity intolerance*
- *Body temperature, altered, risk for*
- *Pain*

- *Self-care deficit (hygiene, grooming, feeding)*
- *Knowledge deficit (biotherapy treatment side effects)*

Nursing Diagnoses: Psychosocial Adjustment

- *Coping, ineffective, individual or family*
- *Decisional conflict (treatment regimen)*
- *Hopelessness*
- *Sexuality patterns, altered*

Outcome Goals

Patient/significant other/caregiver will be able to:
- Discuss their disease and the rationale for the use of biotherapy in their disease (e.g., as treatment, for detection or diagnosis, as a supportive measure).
- Describe their treatment regimen and associated laboratory and diagnostic tests, clinic visits, hospitalizations, and other special requirements.
- State the side effects common to the agent they are receiving and specific management strategies.
- Verbalize reportable signs and symptoms.
- Demonstrate proper skills for self-administration of medications.
- Lists resources available to assist them in coping with their disease and treatment (e.g., financial and reimbursement issues, community resources).

ASSESSMENT AND PLANNING

From the first encounter, nurses play a key role in managing patients undergoing biotherapy. (For the purposes of this chapter, the word *patient* includes the patient and family or significant other as applicable.) The physician generally obtains a detailed history and physical examination before starting a patient on therapy. The physician explains the purpose of therapy, the treatment schedule, associated side effects, and financial concerns as appropriate. The physician also obtains informed consent for patients in a clinical trial. It is important that nurses understand the ethical and legal foundations of informed consent, for they serve as both educator and advocate for the patient.* The nurse may have to answer many questions that the patient is either afraid or embarrassed to ask the physician. Within the scope of independent nursing practice, the nurse can do much to reinforce information and clarify misconceptions. Assessing whether patients understand their therapeutic plan is crucial, and this information should be relayed to other members of the health care team as appropriate.

The nurse should perform a baseline assessment using a body systems approach, including psychosocial concerns, before the patient starts therapy. This should

---

*References 100, 118, 169, 188, 220, 233, 242.

Continued.

include current symptoms related to disease or previous treatment, level of functional status, and hopes, fears, and expectations related to therapy. Documentation of other intercurrent medical illnesses (e.g., cardiovascular disease) that may place the patient at risk for more severe toxic effects is essential. A medication profile should also be obtained, because many medications are contraindicated with certain biologic agents or can contribute to side effects. The initial assessment should also include evaluation of the patient's support systems. When biotherapy trials are investigational, the patient often receives therapy away from home and his or her usual support systems. Patients may be concerned about finances; appropriate housing; family, friends, and job while they are away; loneliness; and fear of the unknown. It is especially helpful to allow patients to voice their concerns and resolve problems through appropriate referrals.

The nurse plays a crucial role in assessing and facilitating the patient's tolerance of side effects while undergoing therapy. A basic understanding of the biology, mode of action, and side effects (acute and chronic) of the agent administered is a must. This knowledge can be applied through regular, systematic assessment of the patient. It is necessary to evaluate symptoms for duration, frequency, and severity in order to plan the appropriate care. Information and care plans should be documented in the patient's medical record.

The nurse must also assess the therapeutic plan in order to develop a plan of care and intervene appropriately. Questions would include the following:
- Will the therapy be given in the hospital, an ambulatory care setting, or both? In the ambulatory care setting, assessment of the patient's compliance with the therapeutic plan is especially important.
- What types of laboratory tests (routine laboratory work, special laboratory work, and pharmacology) and diagnostic procedures will be required?
- What agent or agents will the patient receive, and what are the associated side effects?
- Is the agent under investigation or FDA approved?
- If under investigation, has informed consent been secured?
- What is the nature of the agent? Are there special handling precautions or storage requirements? Is any special equipment or are any emergency supplies needed?
- What type of teaching will the patient need (e.g., self-administration techniques, side effects, and management)?
- What type of monitoring will be required? Are special vital signs necessary (e.g., orthostatic blood pressures)?

A thorough assessment both before and during therapy helps in formulating and updating the patient's plan of care.*

---

*References 24, 25, 41, 93, 101, 130, 183, 196.

HANDLING ISSUES

As previously mentioned, handling issues are a matter of concern to all oncology nurses. Policies and procedures governing safe handling of cytotoxic agents during preparation, administration, and disposal have been well established nationwide. However, there has been no formal research to date regarding the safest way to handle biologic agents. The nurse is advised to check institutional policy regarding handling of BRMs at the place of employment. Most BRMs do not directly affect DNA and are therefore not considered genotoxic substances; however, many institutions place them in the category of cytotoxic products requiring special handling. In the future, new generation BRMs may require special handling. The addition of chemotherapeutic agents or toxins to BRMs would necessitate special handling, and the addition of radioisotopes would require appropriate radiation safety procedures.[41,183]

MANAGEMENT OF SIDE EFFECTS

The oncology nurse plays a key role in the management of side effects associated with biologic therapy. This is especially true because many of these effects are not "life threatening" but have a tremendous impact on the patient's quality of life. A sound foundation in symptom management can guide the nurse in developing strategies to manage biotherapy-related side effects.[177]

Neurologic Side Effects

To ensure prompt recognition of CNS toxicity, patients should be assessed before therapy for baseline data and regularly during therapy for changes in level of consciousness, orientation, and mental status. Changes should be reported to the physician. The nurse should also evaluate the patient's medication profile for other drugs that can contribute to CNS toxicity. The patient should be taught which signs and symptoms to report. Family members are often the first to recognize subtle changes and should be encouraged to report them to the health care team. Often the nurse and the patient together can creatively deal with minor CNS changes, such as slowed thinking, decreased concentration, and memory problems.[16,36,98,137,211]

For more serious problems, such as confusion, disorientation, and somnolence, safety concerns arise. Patients should be protected from injury when appropriate with fall precautions or bed sensors and should be reoriented as needed. Especially in the intensive care unit, the nurse should allow normal periods of sleep and rest. Patients receiving BRMs may experience depression. Allowing patients to verbalize their feelings is often helpful. However, a psychiatric consultation should be sought when appropriate.

For a review of BRM-related side effects and their frequency of occurrence, see Table 23-6.

Table 23-6   Side Effects of Biologic Response Modifiers

System	Interferons	Interleukin-2	Hematopoietic growth factors	Monoclonal antibodies	Tumor necrosis factor	Retinoids
Central nervous system	Impaired concentration, headache, lethargy, confusion, depression	Impaired concentration, headache, lethargy, confusion, anxiety, psychoses, depression	Rare	Rare	Confusion, seizures (rare)	Headache,* visual disturbances, changed visual acuity, anxiety, insomnia, depression
General	Constitutional symptoms,* fatigue*	Constitutional symptoms,* fatigue,* weight gain during therapy, followed by weight loss*	Mild constitutional symptoms, fatigue (mostly with GM-CSF)	Constitutional symptoms, allergic reactions, anaphylaxis (rare)	Constitutional symptoms,* rigors,* fatigue*	Fever,* malaise
Cardiovascular system	Hypotension, tachycardia, arrhythmias, myocardial ischemia (rare)	Hypotension* edema,* ascites, arrhythmias, decreased systemic vascular resistance*	Hypertension (rare) with epoetin alfa	Hypotension, chest pain	Hypotension,* arrhythmias	Hypotension, hypertension, flushing
Pulmonary system	Rare	Dyspnea, pulmonary edema	Rare occurrence of dyspnea with first dose of GM-CSF	Dyspnea, wheezing	Dyspnea	Dyspnea, pleural effusion in patients with APL experiencing RA-APL syndrome
Renal/hepatic systems	Proteinuria, elevated liver enzymes*	Oliguria,* increased BUN, creatinine* proteinuria, azotemia, increased bilirubin, SGOT, SGPT, LDH	Elevation of LDH (rare), alkaline phosphatase with G-CSF	Rare	Increased bilirubin, liver enzymes	Elevation of triglycerides and cholesterol*; elevation of liver function tests*
Gastrointestinal system	Nausea, vomiting, diarrhea, anorexia*	Nausea, vomiting,* diarrhea,* anorexia,* mucositis	Rare	Nausea, vomiting	Nausea, vomiting, anorexia, diarrhea	Nausea, vomiting,* mucositis,* diarrhea
Genitourinary system	Impotence, decreased libido	Decreased libido	Rare	Rare	Decreased libido	Rare

Modified from Rieger PT: Biotherapy: the fourth modality of therapy. In Barton-Burke M, editor: *Cancer chemotherapy: a nursing process approach,* Boston, 1996, Jones & Bartlett.
*Common side effect.
APL, Acute premyelocytic anemia; *BUN,* blood urea nitrogen; *G-CSF,* granulocyte colony-stimulating factor; *GM-CSF,* granulocyte/macrophage colony-stimulating factor; *LDH,* lactate dehydrogenase; *SGOT,* aspartate aminotransferase (AST); *SGPT,* alanine aminotransferase (ALT).

Continued.

Table 23-6 Side Effects of Biologic Response Modifiers—cont'd

System	Interferons	Interleukin-2	Hematopoietic growth factors	Monoclonal antibodies	Tumor necrosis factor	Retinoids
Integument	Alopecia, rash	Rash,* dry desquamation,* erythema,* pruritus,* inflammatory reaction at injection sites*	GM-CSF/G-CSF: inflammation at injection site; rash (rare)	Urticaria, rash, pruritus	Inflammatory reaction at injection sites	Dryness of skin and mucous membranes,* pruritis, increased sweating
Hematologic system	Leukopenia,* anemia, thrombocytopenia	Anemia,* thrombocytopenia, lymphopenia,* eosinophilia*	Leukocytosis (expected biologic effect of HGF use); eosinophilia (GM-CSF)	Leukopenia in hematologic malignancies	Thrombocytopenia, granulocytopenia	Leukocytosis in patients with APL
Musculoskeletal system	Myalgia,* arthralgias*	Myalgia, arthralgia	Bone pain* with GM-CSF and G-CSF	Arthralgia (rare)	Myalgia, arthralgia	Bone pain,* myalgias,* arthralgia*

Renal Side Effects

In all treatment settings, patients should be evaluated for renal toxicity through assessment of blood urea nitrogen (BUN) and creatinine levels, and changes should be reported to the physician. With IL-2 therapy, renal toxicity is more problematic. Patients should be placed on strict intake and output and weighed regularly. Because urine output is often decreased, intake and output usually will not balance. The physician usually sets a minimum output per shift that can be used as a guideline for reporting changes. Nursing includes administration of fluids, diuretics, and pressors as ordered.[41,178,183,244]

Hematologic Side Effects

Patients are monitored for changes in complete blood count, including differential and platelet counts. When ordered, the coagulation profile should also be assessed. The patient should be taught signs and symptoms to report, along with appropriate precautions (e.g., bleeding precautions for thrombocytopenia, measures to guard against infection should white counts decrease, conservation of energy for anemia), in case a problem develops. Replacement therapy with blood and platelets should be administered as ordered. With biologic therapy, counts generally recover very quickly after therapy stops.

Hepatic Side Effects

Nursing includes assessing the patient for changes in serum transaminases and bilirubin and for jaundice or hepatomegaly. Nursing diagnoses should be formulated as

appropriate. If significant changes occur in laboratory values, therapy may need to be withheld and reinstituted at a lower dose after laboratory measurements recovery and the patient's status improves.

Skin Changes

Skin changes are most commonly seen with IL-2 and retinoid therapy, although rashes have been reported with IFN and GM-CSF. The baseline assessment of skin condition should include a history of underlying skin conditions such as psoriasis. Patients should be taught signs and symptoms to be expected as well as an appropriate skin care routine. Skin should be observed daily for signs of infection and breakdown. Therapeutic measures for dry skin include gentle cleansing (avoid scrubbing the skin), tepid rather than hot baths, frequent use of water-based lotions and creams, soft cotton clothing, and bath oils.* Patients should be taught to avoid the use of perfumed lotion, because it can further irritate already sensitive skin. Pruritus can also be a major problem. Helpful measures include antipruritic medications (often with around-the-clock administration), soft clothing, and the use of colloidal oatmeal baths. In some cases a room humidifier is helpful.[178] It is important to caution patients against the use of topical steroids, since this is contraindicated in many IL-2 protocols.

Irritation, with resultant erythema and swelling, may

---

*References 41, 45, 71, 93, 101, 183, 196.

occur at subcutaneous injection sites. Patients should be reassured that this inflammatory reaction usually resolves within several days. In patients receiving IL-2 by subcutaneous injection, "knots" may persist under the skin for several months. Although not generally painful, they reduce the number of sites available for subsequent injections.[240] For inflammatory reactions, no treatment is generally necessary; however, if applications of cold or heat are considered, they should be verified with the physician.

Gastrointestinal Side Effects

Teaching the patient to maintain nutritional status is of prime importance, because anorexia and weight loss over time are common side effects of many BRMs. Baseline nutritional status and dietary intake should be assessed and documented. Measures commonly used with other oncology patients (e.g., small, frequent meals and calorie supplements) are appropriate here. A dietary consultant should be used as necessary. If weight loss becomes significant, tube feedings or hyperalimentation may have to be considered. Antiemetics usually abate nausea and vomiting; however, with IL-2, more aggressive around-the-clock therapy is usually necessary. Prophylactic antiemetic administration and an odor-free environment are often necessary with IL-2. Diarrhea is controlled through the use of antidiarrheal medications. Special consideration should also be given to the skin integrity in the perianal area through assessment, hygienic measures, and use of barrier creams as indicated.[41,93,101,183,196]

Mucositis may also occur, especially with IL-2 therapy. The oral cavity should be assessed and its condition documented. A pretreatment oral assessment by a dental oncologist to identify and treat preexisting oral disease may be recommended. Patients should be taught meticulous oral hygiene using saline and baking soda mouth rinses, soft toothbrushes, alterations in diet for comfort, and avoidance of solutions such as commercial mouthwashes, which can exacerbate oral dryness. If dryness of oral mucous membranes is extreme, artificial saliva may be helpful.[178]

Cardiovascular/Pulmonary Side Effects

A thorough assessment of cardiopulmonary parameters is important with all biologic agents, but it is extremely important with IL-2 therapy or in patients receiving ricin-based immunotoxins, because of capillary leak syndrome. Nursing specific for this syndrome includes evaluation of cardiovascular status by monitoring heart rate, blood pressure (including orthostatic checks), central venous pressure as indicated, and other cardiac indices. Accurate daily weight and strict intake and output measures are necessary to evaluate fluid imbalances.*

*References 41, 93, 101, 183, 196, 244.

Patients should be assessed for edema and abdominal ascites. They should be taught signs and symptoms to report, as well as to rise from a lying to a sitting position slowly to prevent dizziness that may result from sudden drops in blood pressure. Because of edema, the use of tight clothing or restrictive jewelry should be avoided. Bed rest may be indicated if the systolic blood pressure consistently runs below 80 mm Hg and the patient is symptomatic. Nursing assessment of pulmonary status includes monitoring the respiratory rate, ausculating breath sounds, monitoring laboratory values of oxygenation, and heeding complaints of shortness of breath or altered breathing patterns. Patients should be taught which signs and symptoms to report and should be reassured that toxicity is dose related and reversible. Nurses should position patients for maximum respiratory effort.

Constitutional Symptoms

Chills followed by fever are seen with almost all biologic agents.[84] Patients should be told to expect this reaction and that tachyphylaxis will occur. Because chills are usually transient and self-limiting, nursing focuses primarily on comfort measures. Patients are often premedicated with acetaminophen or other NSAIDs. They should be kept warm with blankets and warm clothing during chills and should be instructed to avoid cold beverages. For severe chills, intravenous meperidine or sublingual morphine may be necessary. Fevers are usually controlled with regular administration of acetaminophen. However, for prolonged or extreme temperature elevations, cool sponging or hypothermia blankets may be necessary. When therapy is initiated, vital signs, including temperature, are usually monitored for the first day or so; patients with cardiovascular or pulmonary problems require more intensive monitoring. Patients should monitor their temperature several times a day so that fever patterns can be established. It should never be assumed that all fevers in a patient receiving a BRM are related to the therapy. Variables such as length of time the patient has been receiving the agent, comparison of the fever with the patient's usual fever patterns, spiking fevers despite administration of antipyretics, and other signs and symptoms of infection should all be considered. Appropriate interventions can then be instituted. An adequate fluid intake should be encouraged during high fevers to prevent dehydration. Acetaminophen, massage, and heating pads can be used as appropriate to control headache, myalgia, arthralgia, and bone pain.

Fatigue

Fatigue is common with many biologic agents, is usually chronic, and in some instances can be the dose-limiting side effect.[206] Because its etiology is unknown, nursing interventions are aimed at helping patients cope with this often distressing side effect. Although few tools

Continued.

can objectively measure fatigue, nurses can document the patient's fatigue by gathering data on contributing factors (e.g., anemia, stressors, depression, other treatment regimens); diagnosis, disease stage, and prognosis; degree of immobility; manifestations of fatigue; and patterns of fatigue. Which factors alleviate fatigue and which exacerbate it? When is fatigue the greatest? How long does it persist? Interventions focus on four areas: conservation of energy, nutritional management, stress management, and management of contributing factors.* When teaching patients about this side effect and its management, nurses should stress that this fatigue is chronic, not acute, and that more sleep often exacerbates the problem instead of alleviating it. Many patients fear that increased fatigue signals progression of disease. The nurse should reassure such patients that fatigue is an expected side effect of the medication. If fatigue becomes so severe that the patient's functional status is acutely impaired, therapy may have to be stopped or the dosage

---

*References 36, 47, 81, 150, 166-168, 206, 241.

reduced. Nursing research is beginning to evaluate the use of exercise programs as an intervention for managing cancer-related fatigue.

Allergic Reactions

Allergic reactions are most commonly associated with MAb infusions.[51,52,183] The patient's vital signs should be monitored regularly, in many cases as often as every 15 minutes, and observed closely. Emergency drugs must be kept at the bedside, and a crash cart must be on hand. Nursing may include medication of the patient before or during therapy to prevent chills, fever, and urticaria. Fever is common with certain MAbs, and should be evaluated for its relationship to the course of therapy (early versus late).

Psychosocial Difficulties

When investigational biotherapy is used, patients often are extremely optimistic that therapy is going to help them, especially if there is no effective therapy for their particular disease or if they have failed several courses

---

EDUCATIONAL RESOURCES AVAILABLE FROM PHARMACEUTICAL COMPANIES

Amgen, Inc.
Analogy Book
Calendar with laboratory data
Chemotherapy and Neupogen
Neupogen (Filgrastim) Patient Fact Sheet
Neupogen Reimbursement Guide for the Patient
Patient Guide to Therapy with Neupogen (video, handout)
Pediatric Package (includes Sammy Syringe, Marvin's Marvelous Medicine, Your Body and G-CSF—pamphlets)
Questions and Answers About Therapy with Neupogen (Filgrastim)
Self-Injection Chart (step-by-step guide)
Self-Injection Video (English and Spanish)
Your Personal Daily Journal

Cetus Corp.
Hospital Based Therapy
Understanding Proleukin (Aldesleukin) for Injection

Immunex Corp.
The Cells of the Hematopoietic Cascade (video, monograph)
Hematopoiesis Chart
A Patient Guide to Self-Injection (video)
A Patient Guide to Self-Injection (instruction and site recording chart)
Understanding Your Bone Marrow Transplant: A Videotape for Patients
Understanding Your Bone Marrow Transplant: A Patient Guide (written accompanying BMT videotape)

Ortho Biotech, Inc.
Anemia in Cancer: Getting Your Energy Back
Coping with Fatigue Videotape
Dimensions of Caring: Understanding and Overcoming Fatigue
Patient Diary
Resource Catalogue
r-HuEpo and the Anemia of Cancer and Chemotherapy: Two Sides of an Inpatient Story (book and audiocassette)
Self-Injection Starter Kit
Subcutaneous Injection: A Patient Guide to Correct Injection Technique (video, flipchart)
Understanding and Overcoming Fatigue (audiotape)
Understanding and Overcoming Fatigue (brochure)

Roche Laboratories
Complete home administration kit
Medication travel cooler
Patient Guide
Refrigerator magnet for expiration date
Self-Administration (video)
Syringe disposal container

Schering-Plough Corp.
Patient Information Card
Patient kit: home supplies plus brochures on self-administration and side effect management
Self-Injection (video)
Taking Control of Your Therapy (booklet)

Modified from Rumsey KA: Patient education. In Rieger PT, editor: *Biotherapy: a comprehensive overview*, Boston, 1995, Jones & Bartlett.

PATIENT TEACHING PRIORITIES
Biotherapy

Assessment

Time available
Learning needs
People available to teach
Barriers to learning
Resources needed

Teaching content

Treatment plan
  Goals of therapy
  Commercial versus investigational agent
  Treatment regimen
  Associated laboratory and diagnostic tests
  Special requirements
Side effects
  Expected side effects
  Management of symptoms experienced
  Reportable signs and symptoms
Self-administration of BRMs
  Aseptic technique
  Reconstitution of powdered medications
  Drawing up the proper dose
  Proper site selection and rotation
  Administration of the injection
  Storage of the drug
  Proper disposal of equipment at home
Psychosocial/economic concerns
  Coping skills/resources
  Reimbursement resources

Documentation

Time frame for teaching
Patient/significant others taught
Tasks/information disseminated
Resources utilized
Evaluation/need for referrals

GERIATRIC CONSIDERATIONS
Biotherapy

Factors affecting medication dosage and administration

Alterations in hepatic and renal function may necessitate adjustment of dosage and/or schedule.

Decreases in cardiovascular function may require lower doses of BRMs such as interferon and interleukin-2, which have side effects that may stress the cardiovascular system.

Alterations in neurosensory/perceptual protective mechanisms may place elderly patients at higher risk for problems with CNS-associated side effects of BRMs such as confusion, depression, memory loss, or slowed thinking.

Decreased functional status may place patients at a higher risk for intolerance of fatigue associated with many BRMs.

Altered nutritional intake (less than body requirements) may be increased due to anorexia associated with some BRMs.

Decreased tissue, skin, and mucous membrane integrity may place patients at higher risk for IL-2–related skin toxicity.

The patient's current medication profile should be evaluated to detect drugs that may be contraindicated with BRMs and/or may cause additive toxicity.

Factors affecting patient teaching

Assess for neuromuscular and sensory deficits (e.g., vision problems, hearing losses, arthritic joints) that may inhibit teaching/learning. Utilize appropriate teaching tools for deficits present (e.g., large print, minimal illustrations for patient with vision problems).

Assess for reading level and comprehension, since many people 65 or older have completed 8 or fewer years of formal schooling. Utilize reading materials targeted for the appropriate reading level and/or audiovisual aids. Frequently reinforce information presented.

Factors affecting social support systems

Approximately 30% of patients 65 or older live alone, the majority being women. The difficulties of living alone are often intensified by poverty, having few relatives or other social supports, and decreased functional status.

Many BRMs are given on an outpatient basis; hence patients are required to learn self-care. Evaluation of formal and informal support networks, functional capacity, and economic status should be incorporated into the nursing assessment and referrals made to community resources as needed.

Spouses should be evaluated for early indicators of caregiver role strain and appropriate interventions initiated.

Modified from Boyle DM, and others: *Oncol Nurs Forum* 19(6):913, 1992.

---

of therapy. Although hope is important, expectations should be realistic. The nurse can be instrumental in helping patients voice their hopes and fears, answering questions, and discussing the patient's expectations. Depression is common, either as a side effect of BRMs, related to fatigue, or as a result of failing therapy. The failure of therapy can be extremely difficult for patients, and the nurse's most effective tool is often his or her presence. Even when a cure is not possible, the nurse can foster hope that something can be done for the patient and can reassure the patient that he or she will not be abandoned.

As previously mentioned, patients are often away from their usual support systems. Family dynamics are often

Continued.

disrupted, and therapy may be more difficult to tolerate than anticipated. Support groups, individual counseling, and simple ventilation of feelings to the nurse all can be helpful. Serving as an advocate for the patient, the nurse can make appropriate referrals to help resolve problems.[91]

Patient Instructions

The nurse is responsible for teaching patients about the particular biologic agent or agents they are to receive, for preparing them for participation in experimental trials, for describing side effects and how to cope with them, and for teaching self-administration of the medication.[143,180,197,203,217] The keys are early assessment of the patient for learning needs and barriers (physical, psychologic, and verbal deficiencies and dysfunctions) and use of appropriate written and audiovisual materials that reinforce teaching. The box, p. 604, outlines patient education materials specific to biologic agents produced by pharmaceutical companies. A teaching plan specific for the patient can be formulated and documented in the medical record.

Sufficient time should be allotted to teach patients to administer their medication. This should always be anticipated with interferon therapy and CSFs. Patients need to learn how to reconstitute the medications (if applicable), how to draw up the proper dose, the proper technique for intramuscular or subcutaneous injection, the proper technique for site selection and rotation, storage requirements for the medication, and proper disposal of needles and syringes at home. A variety of vital concentrations are available for IFN. The nurse can exercise considerable latitude in selecting a concentrations that is cost effective and easy for the patient to use. The nurse also should accommodate dose escalations if applicable without the need to reteach the patient continually. Because many biologic agents require refrigeration or freezing, special arrangements for transport must be made. Patients are also instructed in reportable signs and symptoms.

With CNS side effects, changes are often subtle. Family members are usually the first to recognize changes and can report them to the health care team. Many patients are asked to keep a daily log or diary of associated side effects, time and location of injections, and other medications used. If the patient is not self-sufficient, appropriate referrals should be made before discharge. Priorities for patient teaching in biotherapy and geriatric considerations are given in the boxes, p. 605.

Nursing Research

Biotherapy follows a pattern different from that of standard chemotherapy, often lasting months to years. The associated toxicities are complex, chronic, usually subjective, and prone to having a major effect on the quality of life.[25] The etiology of many side effects is unknown, which makes treating them difficult or empirical. A clearer understanding of the nature of these side effects is essential to the development of effective strategies for dealing with them. Biologic therapy is ripe with opportunities for research, including nursing research in conjunction with clinical trials.[216]

One difficulty with research in this area is accurately measuring symptoms.[67,132] Although observer-rated toxicity scales used in clinical trials have been adapted to accommodate symptoms associated with BRMs, often they are not sensitive enough for research purposes.[154] The subjective nature of most BRM-associated symptoms makes their measurement a challenge. Nursing research efforts require a means to quantify side effects before interventions to prevent and control them can be studied.[183] These research efforts might be focused on the development of tools to measure side effects, determination of the most effective time of drug administration to alleviate side effects, interventions to control or prevent toxicity, evaluation of teaching methods, evaluation of quality of life and symptom distress, and drug handling issues. Such studies have begun; however, a great deal of work remains to be completed.[47,98,183,206]

antiangiogenesis factors that ultimately would deprive a tumor of its blood supply.[88]

A final area of concern is reimbursement. Because of recent economic trends in health care, funding agencies and third-party payors often are unwilling to underwrite the cost of phase I and II investigations for drugs not approved by the FDA.[39] In the case of approved agents, they may be unwilling to pay for indications not included in the original FDA approval. Treatment with many BRMs can be costly in both the inpatient and ambulatory care setting; therefore this problem is of major importance to both patients and health care profession-

als.[171,248] Patients who receive investigational drugs as part of an approved clinical trial receive the drug at no cost; however, they are responsible for all other associated costs. In the case of an FDA-approved drug, patients must pay for the drug. Because extended therapy can be quite expensive, some pharmaceutical companies have programs to assist patients in receiving drugs if they are no longer able to pay or have reached a yearly maximum (cost assistance programs).[5,34,96,159] In addition, most pharmaceutical companies sponsor reimbursement hotlines that will assist patients and health care professionals with reimbursement concerns.

CONCLUSION

Oncology nurses who care for patients receiving biotherapy are on the cutting edge of cancer therapy. They must stay abreast of continual changes, be knowledgeable about therapeutic agents and modalities, and develop standards of care and nursing interventions to manage toxicity. The possibilities for nurses to participate in this exciting new therapeutic modality are limitless.

■ CHAPTER QUESTIONS

1. Biotherapy is best defined as the use of agents that:
   a. Suppress the immune system
   b. Are cytotoxic
   c. Are derived from biologic sources and/or affect biologic responses
   d. Potentiate the effects of chemotherapy
2. The theory of immune surveillance proposes that:
   a. Cancer cells arise in the body continuously, are recognized as foreign, and are then destroyed by the individual's immune system.
   b. Cancer cells arise in the body, appear similar to normal cells, and therefore are allowed to grow into tumors.
   c. The development of cancer is not related to the immune system in any way.
   d. Cancer cells arise in the body only when the immune system is depressed or deficient.
3. Which of the following is true about biotherapy?
   a. Biologic response modifiers currently used clinically are given only in combination with chemotherapy.
   b. All classes of biologic response modifiers have received at least one regulatory (FDA) approval.
   c. Biotherapy is a new mode of therapy in which no clinical success has been seen.
   d. Biotherapy is not an accepted form of therapy.
4. The following have contributed to the development of biotherapy:
   a. Increased knowledge of the immune system, increased knowledge of the biology of cancer, and improved third-party payment for investigational trials
   b. Increased knowledge of the immune system, the advent of recombinant DNA technology and hybridoma technology, and increased knowledge of the biology of cancer
   c. The advent of recombinant DNA technology and hybridoma technology, increased acceptance by physicians, and encouragement from managed care consortiums for the use of biotherapy over chemotherapy
   d. Increased knowledge of the immune system, improved third-party payment for investigational trials, and increased acceptance by physicians
5. Biotherapy differs from chemotherapy in that:
   a. There is no classification system for biologic agents.
   b. It is given only by the subcutaneous route.
   c. Special handling procedures are never required.
   d. It utilizes natural body proteins as therapeutic agents.
6. For which of the following diseases has interferon-alfa *not* received FDA approval in the United States?
   a. Renal cancer
   b. Melanoma
   c. Hairy cell leukemia
   d. Chronic myelogenous leukemia
7. Ms. Brewer is admitted to the outpatient area for her first dose of interferon-alfa. She is very nervous, and not sure about what side effects to expect. The nurse's best response would be:
   a. "Relax, it has the same side effects as chemotherapy."
   b. "You'll probably have nausea and vomiting, but we can treat you for that."
   c. "Most patients experience flu-like symptoms that gradually lessen over time."
   d. "You'll be fine; interferon has very few side effects because it's a natural body protein."
8. Which of the following side effects is a common chronic side effect for patients receiving interferon or interleukin-2?
   a. Neutropenia
   b. Skin changes
   c. Fatigue
   d. Alopecia
9. Mr. Roberts is on his fourth day of a 4-day course of continuous infusion interleukin-2 (IL-2). Your morning assessment finds a weight gain of 5 kg since he started therapy, a blood pressure of 90/60 mm Hg, and a urine output of 200 ml for the previous shift. Which of the following IL-2 toxicities is the most likely cause of these changes?
   a. Excessive nausea and vomiting
   b. Capillary leak syndrome
   c. Cardiac dysrhythmias
   d. Eosinophilia
10. A major clinical application for the hematopoietic growth factors might be:
    a. The treatment of bleeding disorders, such as hemophilia
    b. The treatment of primary and secondary bone marrow failure
    c. The treatment of stomatitis
    d. The treatment of chronic myelogenous leukemia
11. Which of the following is not a hematopoietic growth factor?
    a. M-CSF
    b. TPO
    c. CDDP
    d. PIXY321
12. It is important to monitor fever in a patient receiving GM-CSF because:
    a. Fevers caused by sepsis are often difficult to differentiate from normal side effects.
    b. Excessively high fevers are common and can compromise the patient's cardiac status.
    c. GM-CSF is an investigational agent and therefore monitoring of fever is a protocol requirement.
    d. Fever is an untoward side effect, and the drug should be stopped immediately.

13. Which of the following is true about monoclonal antibody therapy?
    a. The only clinical success has been seen in patients with solid tumors.
    b. It should never be given by the intravenous route, because this type of administration increases the potential for an allergic reaction.
    c. Monoclonal antibodies are obtained primarily from goat serum.
    d. Monoclonal antibodies can be used for both diagnostic and therapeutic purposes.

BIBLIOGRAPHY

1. Abels RI: Use of recombinant human erythropoietin in the treatment of anemia in patients who have cancer, *Semin Oncol* 19(3)(suppl 8):29, 1992.
2. Aggarwala SS, Kirkwood JM: Interferons in the therapy of solid tumors, *Oncology* 51(2):129, 1994.
3. Allison AC, Taylor RB: Observations on thymectomy and carcinogenesis, *Cancer Res* 27:703, 1967.
4. Amgen, Inc: Neupogen (filgrastim) (package insert), Thousand Oaks, Calif, 1995, Amgen.
5. Amgen, Inc: Neupogen reimbursement hotline: (1-800-272-9376), Thousand Oaks, Calif, 1990, Amgen.
6. Amgen: Epogen (epoetin alfa) (package insert), Thousand Oaks, Calif, 1989, Amgen.
7. Atkins MB and others: Phase I evaluation of recombinant interleukin-2 in patients with advanced malignant disease, *J Clin Oncol* 4(9):1380, 1986.
8. Atkins M, Mier JW, editors: *Therapeutic applications of interleukin-2,* New York, 1993, Dekker.
9. Atkins MB, Mier JW, Trehu EG: Combination cytokine therapy. In DeVita VT, Hellman S, Rosenberg SA, editors: *Biologic therapy of cancer,* ed 2, Philadelphia, 1995, Lippincott.
10. Antman KS and others: Effect of recombinant human granulocyte-macrophage colony-stimulating factor on chemotherapy-induced myelosuppression, *N Engl J Med* 319(10):593, 1988.
11. Antonelli G: Development of neutralizing and binding antibodies to interferon (IFN) in patients undergoing IFN therapy, *Antiviral Res* 24:235, 1994.
12. Aulitzky WE and others: Interleukins: clinical pharmacology and therapeutic use, *Drugs* 48(5):667, 1994.
13. Bajorin DF, Cheung NV, Houghton AN: Macrophage colony-stimulating factor: biological effects and potential applications for cancer therapy, *Semin Hematol* 28(2)(suppl)2:42, 1991.
14. Balkwill FR, editor: *Cytokines in cancer therapy,* Oxford, 1989, Oxford University.
15. Baquiran DC, Dantis L, McKerrow J: Monoclonal antibodies: innovations in diagnosis and therapy, *Semin Oncol Nurs* 12(2):130, 1996.
16. Bender CM: Cognitive dysfunction associated with biological response modifier therapy, *Oncol Nurs Forum* 21(3):515, 1995.
17. Benner SE, Lippman SM, Hong WK: Chemoprevention strategies for a lung and upper aerodigestive tract cancer, *Cancer Res* 52(9)(suppl):2758, 1992.
18. Berlex Laboratories: Betaseron (interferon-beta 1B) package insert, Richmond, Calif, 1993, Berlex Laboratories.
19. Beutler B, Cerami A: Cachectin: more than a tumor necrosis factor, *N Engl J Med* 316(7):379, 1987.
20. Blick M and others: Phase I study of recombinant tumor necrosis factor in cancer patients, *Cancer Res* 47:2986, 1987.
21. Borden EC, Chin P: Interleukin-6: a cytokine with potential diagnostic and therapeutic roles, *J Lab Clin Med* 123(6):824, 1994.
22. Brandt SJ and others: Effects of recombinant human granulocyte-macrophage colony-stimulating factor on hematopoietic reconstitution after high-dose chemotherapy and autologous bone marrow transplantation, *N Engl J Med* 318(14):869, 1988.
23. Bronchud MH and others: Phase I/II study of recombinant human granulocyte colony-stimulating factor in patients receiving intensive chemotherapy for small cell lung cancer, *Br J Cancer* 56:809, 1987.
24. Brophy LR, Rieger PT: Biotherapy. In Clark JC, McGee RF, editors: *Core curriculum for oncology nursing,* ed 2, Philadelphia, 1992, Saunders.
25. Brophy LR, Sharp EJ: Physical symptoms of combination biotherapy: a quality-of-life issue, *Oncol Nurs Forum* 18(1)(suppl):25, 1991.
26. Brophy LR: Tumor necrosis factor. In Rieger PT, editor: *Biotherapy: a comprehensive overview,* Boston, 1995, Jones & Bartlett.
27. Brunda MJ, Gately MK: Interleukin-12: potential role in cancer therapy. In DeVita VT, Hellman S, Rosenberg SA, editors: *Important advances in oncology,* Philadelphia, 1995, Lippincott.
28. Burnet FM: The concept of immunological surveillance, *Prog Exp Tumor Res* 13:1, 1970.
29. Buzaid AC, Legha SS: Combination of chemotherapy with interleukin-2 and interferon-alfa for the treatment of advanced melanoma, *Semin Oncol* 6:23, 1994.
30. Cantell K, Hirvonen S: Preparation of human leukocyte interferon for clinical use, *Tex Rep Biol Med* 35:138, 1977.
31. Cebon J and others: Pharmacokinetics of human granulocyte-macrophage colony-stimulating factor using a sensitive immunoassay, *Blood* 72:1093, 1988.
32. Chang F, Syrjanen S, Syrjanen K: Implications of the p53 tumor-suppressor gene in clinical oncology, *J Clin Oncol* 13:1009, 1995.
33. Chapman P and others: Clinical pharmacology of recombinant human tumor necrosis factor in patients with advanced cancer, *J Clin Oncol* 5:1942, 1987.
34. Chiron Corp: Proleukin reimbursement line (1-800-775-7533), San Francisco, Calif, 1992, Chiron.
35. Chiron Therapeutics: Proleukin (aldesleukin) for injection (package insert), Emeryville, Calif, 1994, Chiron Corp.
36. Cimprich B: Symptom management: loss of concentration, *Semin Oncol Nurs* 11(4):279, 1995.
37. Clark J, Longo D: Biological response modifiers, *Mediguide Oncol* 6(2):1, 1986.
38. Clark SC, Kamen R: The human hematopoietic colony-stimulating factors, *Science* 236:1229, 1987.
39. Coleman T: Health system reform and clinical research, *Oncology* 9:118, 1995.

40. Cohen JS, Hogan ME: The new genetic medicines, *Sci Am* 271:76, 1994.

41. Conrad KJ, Horrell CJ, editors: *Biotherapy: recommendations for nursing course content and clinical practicum,* Pittsburgh, 1995, Oncology Nursing Press.

42. Corfu-A Study Group: Phase III randomized study of two fluorouracil combinations with either interferon alfa-2a or leucovorin for advanced colorectal cancer, *J Clin Oncol* 13:921, 1995.

43. Costa A and others: Prospects of chemoprevention of human cancers with the synthetic retinoid fenretinide, *Cancer Res* 54(suppl 7):2032, 1994.

44. Crown J and others: A phase I trial of recombinant human interleukin-1 alone and in combination with myelosuppressive doses of 5-fluorouracil in patients with gastrointestinal cancer, *Blood* 78(6):1420, 1991.

45. Dangel RB: Pruritus and cancer, *Oncol Nurs Forum* 13(1):17, 1986.

46. Dawson MM, editor: *Lymphokines and interleukins,* Boca Raton, Fla, 1991, CRC Press.

47. Dean GE and others: Fatigue in patients with cancer receiving interferon-alpha, *Cancer Practice* 3:164, 1995.

48. Denicoff KD and others: The neuropsychiatric effects of interleukin-2/lymphokine–activated killer cell therapy, *Ann Intern Med* 107:293, 1987.

49. DeVita VT, Hellman S, Rosenberg SA, editors: *Biologic therapy of cancer,* ed 2, Philadelphia, 1995, Lippincott.

50. DiJulio JE, Liles TM: Monoclonal antibodies. In Rieger PT, editor: *Biotherapy: a comprehensive overview,* Boston, 1995, Jones & Bartlett.

51. Dillman JB: Toxicity of monoclonal antibodies in the treatment of cancer, *Semin Oncol Nurs* 4(2):107, 1988.

52. Dillman RO and others: Toxicities and side effects associated with intravenous infusions of monoclonal antibodies, *J Biol Response Mod* 5:73, 1986.

53. Dillman RO: Antibodies as cytotoxic therapy, *J Clin Oncol* 12(7):1497, 1994.

54. Dillman RO: The clinical experience with interleukin-2 in cancer therapy, *Cancer Biother* 9(3):183, 1994.

55. Dinarello CA: Interleukin-1 and interleukin-1 antagonism, *Blood* 77(8):1627, 1991.

56. Dinarello CA, Mier JW: Lymphokines, *N Engl J Med* 317(15):940, 1987.

57. Donahue RE and others: Stimulation of hematopoiesis in primates by continuous infusion of recombinant human GM-CSF, *Nature* 321:872, 1986.

58. Ehrlich P: *Studies in immunity,* ed 2, New York, 1910, Wiley & Sons.

59. Engelking C: New approaches: innovations in cancer prevention, diagnosis, treatment and support, *Oncol Nurs Forum* 21:62, 1994.

60. Eschbach JW and others: Correction of the anemia of end-stage renal disease with recombinant human erythropoietin, *N Engl J Med* 316(2):73, 1987.

61. Estrov Z, Kurzrock R, Talpaz M, editors: *Interferons: basic principles and clinical applications,* Austin, Texas, 1993, Landis.

62. Farrell MM: The challenge of adult respiratory distress syndrome during interleukin-2 therapy, *Oncol Nurs Forum* 19(3):475, 1992.

63. Farrell MM: Biotherapy and the oncology nurse, *Semin Oncol Nurs* 12(2):82, 1996.

64. Fazio MT, Glaspy JA: The impact of granulocyte colony-stimulating factor on quality of life in patients with severe chronic neutropenia, *Oncol Nurs Forum* 18(8):1411, 1991.

65. Figlin RA and others: Concomitant administration of recombinant human interleukin-2 and recombinant interferon alfa-2a: an active outpatient regimen in metastatic renal cell carcinoma, *J Clin Oncol* 10(3):414, 1992.

66. Fisher R, editor: Interleukin-2: advances in clinical research and treatment, *Semin Oncol* 20(6)(suppl 9):1, 1993.

67. Frank-Stromborg M, editor: *Instruments for clinical nursing research,* Boston, 1992, Jones & Bartlett.

68. Frei E, Spriggs D: Tumor necrosis factor: still a promising agent, *J Clin Oncol* 7(3):291, 1989.

69. Gabrilove JL and others: Effect of granulocyte colony-stimulating factor on neutropenia and associated morbidity due to chemotherapy for transitional-cell carcinoma of the urothelium, *N Engl J Med* 318(22):1414, 1988.

70. Gabrilove JL, Golde D: Hematopoietic growth factors. In DeVita VT, Hellman S, Rosenberg SA, editors: *Cancer: principles and practice of oncology,* ed 4, Philadelphia, 1993, Lippincott.

71. Gallagher J: Management of cutaneous symptoms, *Semin Oncol Nurs* 11(4):239, 1995.

72. Gallin JI and others: Interferon-gamma in the management of infectious diseases, *Ann Intern Med* 123(3):216, 1995.

73. Gallucci B: The immune system and cancer, *Oncol Nurs Forum* 14(suppl 6):3, 1987.

74. Galvani DW, Cawley JC, editors: *Cytokine therapy,* New York, 1992, Cambridge University Press.

75. Genentech, Inc: Actimmune (Interferon gamma 1 b) (package insert), San Francisco, Calif, 1991, Genentech, Inc.

76. Gianella-Borradori A: Present and future clinical relevance of interleukin-3, *Stem Cells* 12 (suppl) 1:21, 1994.

77. Giralt S and others: The natural history of chronic myelogenous leukemia in the interferon era, *Semin Hematol* 32(2):152, 1995.

78. Glaspy JA and others: Therapy for neutropenia in hairy cell leukemia with recombinant granulocyte colony-stimulating factor, *Ann Intern Med* 109(10):789, 1988.

79. Goldenberg D: New developments in monoclonal antibody for cancer detection and therapy, *CA Cancer J Clin* 44(1):43, 1994.

80. Goldenberg DM, editor: *Cancer therapy with radiolabeled antibodies,* Boca Raton, Fla, 1995, CRC Press.

81. Graydon JE and others: Fatigue-reducing strategies used by patients receiving treatment for cancer, *Cancer Nurs* 18:23, 1995.

82. Groopman JE and others: Effect of recombinant human granulocyte-macrophage colony-stimulating factor on myelopoiesis in the acquired immunodeficiency syndrome, *N Engl J Med* 317(10):593, 1987.

83. Gutterman JU and others: Recombinant leukocyte α-IFN: pharmacokinetics, single-dose tolerance, and biologic effects in cancer patients, *Ann Intern Med* 96(5):549, 1982.

84. Haeuber D: The flu-like syndrome. In Rieger PT, editor: *Biotherapy: a comprehensive overview,* Boston, 1995, Jones & Bartlett.

85. Haeuber D, DiJulio JE: Hematopoietic colony-stimulating factors: an overview, *Oncol Nurs Forum* 16(2):247, 1989.

86. Hahn MB, Jassak PF: Nursing management of patients receiving interferon, *Semin Oncol Nurs* 4(2):95, 1988.

87. Hanna MG and others: Fundamental and applied aspects of successful active specific immunotherapy of cancer. In Oldham RK, editor: *Principles of cancer biotherapy,* New York, 1991, Dekker.

88. Hawkins MJ: Clinical trials of antiangiogenic agents, *Curr Opin Oncol* 7(1):90, 1995.

89. Hendrzak JA, Brunda MJ: Interleukin-12: biologic activity, therapeutic utility, and role in disease, *Lab Invest* 72(6):619, 1995.

90. Hersh EM, Gutterman JU, Mavligit G, editors: *Immunotherapy of cancer in man: scientific basis and current status,* Springfield, Ill, 1973, Thomas.

91. Hogan CM: Coping with biotherapy: physiological and psychosocial concerns, *Oncol Nurs Forum* 18(1)(suppl)1:19, 1991.

92. Hong WK, Lotan R, editors: *Retinoids in oncology,* New York, 1993, Dekker.

93. Hood LE, Abemathy E: Biological response modifiers. In Baird SB, McCorckle R, Grant M, editors: *Cancer nursing: comprehensive textbook,* Philadelphia, 1991, Saunders.

94. Hwu P: Gene therapy of cancer, *Principles and practice of oncology updates,* Philadelphia, 1995, Lippincott.

95. Immunex Corp: Leukine (Sargramostim) (package insert), Seattle, 1995, Immunex.

96. Immunex Corp: A reimbursement support program for Leukine (1-800-321-4669), Seattle, 1990, Immunex.

97. Isaacs A, Lindemann J: Virus interference, *Proc Soc Biol* 147:257, 1957.

98. Jackson BS and others: Long-term biopsychosocial effects of interleukin-2 therapy, *Oncol Nurs Forum* 18(4):683, 1991.

99. Jansen JH and others: Interleukin-4: a regulatory protein, *Blut* 60:269, 1990.

100. Janssen Pharmaceutica: Ergamisol (levamisole hydrochloride) (package insert), Piscataway, NJ, 1990, Janssen Pharmaceutica.

101. Jassak PF: Biotherapy. In Groenwald SL and others, editors: *Cancer nursing: principles and practice,* ed 3, Boston, 1993, Jones & Bartlett.

102. Jassak P: An overview of biotherapy. In Rieger PT, editor: *Biotherapy: a comprehensive overview,* Boston, 1995, Jones & Bartlett.

103. Jenkins J, Wheeler V, Albright L: Gene therapy for cancer, *Cancer Nurs* 17:447, 1994.

104. Johnson C: Interleukin-1: therapeutic potential for solid tumors, *Cancer Invest* 11(5):600, 1993.

105. Kaushansky K: Thrombopoietin: primary regulator of platelet function, *Blood* 86(2):419, 1995.

106. Kirkwood JM and others: Interferon alfa-2b adjuvant therapy of high-risk resected cutaneous melanoma: the Eastern Cooperative Oncology Group Trial EST 1684, *J Clin Oncol* 14(1):7, 1996.

107. Kobayashi S and others: Interleukin-11, *Leuk Lymphoma* 15(1-2):45, 1994.

108. Köhler G, Milstein C: Continuous cultures of fused cells secreting antibody of predefined specificity, *Nature* 256:495, 1975.

109. Kolitz JE, Mertelsmann R: The immunotherapy of human cancer with interleukin-2: present status and future directions, *Cancer Invest* 9(5):529, 1991.

110. Krown SE, Jacubowski A, Houghton A: Biologic response modifiers. In Wittes RE, editor: *Manual of oncologic therapeutics 1991/1992,* Philadelphia, 1991, Lippincott.

111. Krueger GRF: Abnormal variation of the immune system as related to cancer. In Herberman RB, editor: *Influence of the host on tumor development,* Dordrecht, 1989, Kluwer.

112. Kurzrock R and others: Phase I study of recombinant human interleukin-3 in patients with bone marrow failure, *J Clin Oncol* 9(7):1241, 1991.

113. Kurzrock R, Talpaz M, editors: *Cytokines: interleukins and their receptors,* Boston, 1995, Kluwer.

114. Kurzrock R, Talpaz M, editors: *Molecular biology in cancer medicine,* New York, 1995, Oxford University Press.

115. Kuzel TM, Rosen ST: Antibodies in the treatment of human cancer, *Curr Opin Oncol* 6(6):622, 1994.

116. Larson SM and others: Overview of clinical radioimmunodetection of human tumors, *Cancer* 73(suppl 3):832, 1994.

117. Laurie JA and others: Surgical adjuvant therapy of large-bowel carcinoma: an evaluation of levamisole and the combination of levamisole and fluorouracil, *J Clin Oncol* 7(10):1447, 1989.

118. Leuko WM and others: Interleukin-15 and the growth of tumor-derived activated cells, *Cancer Biother* 10(1):13, 1995.

119. Lippman SM, Benner SE, Hong WK: Cancer chemoprevention, *J Clin Oncol* 12:851, 1994.

120. Lippman SM and others: Strategies for chemoprevention study of premalignancy and second primary tumors in the head and neck, *Curr Opin Oncol* 7(3):234, 1995.

121. Livera MA, Vidali G, editors: *Retinoids: from basic science to clinical application,* Boston, 1994, Birkhausen Verlag.

122. Long MW, Wicha MS, editors: *The hematopoietic microenvironment: the functional and structural basis of blood cell development,* Baltimore, 1993, John Hopkins University Press.

123. Lotze MT and others: In vivo administration of purified human interleukin-2. I. Half-life and immunologic effects of the Jurkat cell line–derived IL-2, *J Immunol* 134:157, 1985.

124. Lotze MT and others: In vivo administration of purified human interleukin-2. II. Half-life, immunologic effects and expansion of peripheral lymphoid cells in vivo with recombinant IL-2, *J Immunol* 135:2865, 1985.

125. Lyman AD, Williams DE: Biological activities and potential therapeutic uses of steel factor, *Am J Pediatr Hematol Oncol* 14(1):1, 1992.

126. Lynch M, Yanes L, Todd R: Nursing care of AIDS patients participating in a phase I/II trial of recombinant human granulocyte-macrophage colony-stimulating factor, *Oncol Nurs Forum* 15(4):463, 1988.

127. Mandelli F and others: Maintenance treatment with recombinant interferon alfa-2b in patients with multiple myeloma responding to conventional induction chemotherapy, *N Engl J Med* 322:1430, 1990.

128. Marincola FM and others: Combination therapy with interferon alfa-2a and interleukin-2 for the treatment of metastatic cancer, *J Clin Oncol* 13:1110, 1995.

129. Mathé G and others: Active immunotherapy for acute lymphoblastic leukemia, *Lancet* 1:697, 1969.

130. Mayer DK: Biotherapy: recent advances and nursing implications, *Nurs Clin North Am* 25(2):291, 1990.

131. McCabe MS: Reimbursement for biotherapy. In Rieger PT, editor: *Biotherapy: a comprehensive overview,* Boston, 1995, Jones & Bartlett.

132. McCorkle R, Young K: Development of a symptom distress scale, *Cancer Nurs* 1(3):373, 1978.

133. Mertelsmann R, Herrmann F, editors: *Hematopoietic growth factors in clinical applications,* ed 2, New York, 1995, Dekker.

134. Metcalf D: The granulocyte-macrophage colony-stimulating factors, *Science* 229:16, 1985.

135. Metcalf D: The colony-stimulating factors: discovery, development and clinical applications, *Cancer* 65(10):2185, 1990.

136. Metcalf D: Thrombopoietin: at last, *Nature* 369:519, 1994.

137. Meyers C: Mental status changes. In Rieger PT, editor: *Biotherapy: a comprehensive overview,* Boston, 1995, Jones & Bartlett.

138. Mihich E, Fefer A, editors: Biological response modifiers: subcommittee report, National Cancer Institute Monograph, p 63, 1983.

139. Miller L, editor: American Society of Clinical Oncology recommendations for the use of hematopoietic colony-stimulating factors: evidence-based, clinical practice guidelines, *J Clin Oncol* 12:2471, 1994.

140. Moore MAS: Does stem cell exhaustion result from combining hematopoietic growth factors with chemotherapy? If so, how do we prevent it? *Blood* 80(1):3, 1992.

141. Morgan DA, Ruscetti FW, Gallo RC: Selective in vitro growth of T lymphocytes from normal human bone marrows, *Science* 193:1007, 1976.

142. Morice RC and others: Pulmonary toxicity of recombinant tumor necrosis factor (rTNF), *Proc Am Soc Clin Oncol* 6:29, 1987 (abstract).

143. Morra ME, Grant M, editors: Cancer patient education, *Semin Oncol Nurs* 7(2):79, 1991.

144. Morstyn G and others: Treatment of chemotherapy-induced neutropenia by subcutaneously administered granulocyte colony-stimulating factor with optimization of dose and duration of therapy, *J Clin Oncol* 1(10):1554, 1989.

145. Morstyn G, Dexter TM, editors: *Filgrastim (r-metHuG-Csf) in clinical practice,* New York, 1994, Dekker.

146. Morstyn G and others: Stem cell factor is a potent synergistic factor in hematopoiesis, *Oncology* 51(2):205, 1994.

147. Mulé JJ, Rosenberg SA: Combination cytokine therapy: experimental and clinical trials. In DeVita VT Jr, Hellman S, Rosenberg SA, editors: *Biologic therapy of cancer,* Philadelphia, 1991, Lippincott.

148. Mulé JJ, Rosenberg SA: Immunotherapy with lymphokine combinations. In DeVita VT, Hellman S, Rosenberg SA, editors: *Important advances in oncology,* Philadelphia, 1991, Lippincott.

149. Munn DH, Cheung N-KV: Preclinical and clinical studies of macrophage colony-stimulating factor, *Semin Oncol* 19:395, 1992.

150. Nail LM, Winningham ML: Fatigue and weakness in cancer patients: the symptom experience, *Semin Oncol Nurs* 11(4):272, 1995.

151. Nemunaitis J: Macrophage function–activating cytokines: potential clinical application, *Crit Rev Oncol Hematol* 14:153, 1993.

152. Nemunaitis J: Overview of the role of hematopoietic growth factors in bone marrow transplant recovery and bone marrow transplant failure, *Support Care Cancer* 2(6):374, 1994.

153. Oettgen HF, Old LJ: The history of cancer immunotherapy. In DeVita VT Jr, Hellman S, Rosenberg SA, editors: *Biologic therapy of cancer,* Philadelphia, 1991, Lippincott.

154. Oken MM and others: Toxicity and response criteria of the Eastern Cooperative Oncology Group, *Am J Clin Oncol* 5(6):649, 1982.

155. Old LJ and others: The role of the reticuloendothelial system in the host reaction to neoplasia, *Cancer Res* 21:1281, 1961.

156. Oldham RK: Biotherapy: general principles. In Oldham RK, editor: *Principles of cancer biotherapy,* ed 2, New York, 1991, Dekker.

157. Oratz R and others: Antimelanoma monoclonal antibody—ricin A chain immunoconjugate (XMMME-001-RTA) plus cyclophosphamide in the treatment of metastatic malignant melanoma: results of a phase II trial, *J Biol Response Mod* 9(4):345, 1990.

158. Ortho Biotech: Procrit (epoetin alfa) (package insert), Raritan, NJ, 1993, Ortho Pharmaceutical.

159. Ortho Biotech: PROCRIT line (reimbursement hotline 1-800-553-3851), Raritan, NJ, 1991, Ortho Pharmaceutical.

160. Pai LH: Immunotoxins and recombinant toxins. In DeVita V, Hellman S, Rosenberg S, editors: *Biologic therapy of cancer,* ed 2, Philadelphia, 1995, Lippincott.

161. Parkinson DR (guest editor): The expanding role of interferon-alfa in the treatment of cancer, *Semin Oncol* 21 (6 suppl 14):1, 1994.

162. Parkinson DR, Sznol M: High-dose interleukin-2 in the therapy of metastatic renal cell carcinoma, *Semin Oncol* 22:61, 1995.

163. Penn I: Principles of tumor immunity: Immunocompetence and cancer. In DeVita VT Jr, Hellman S, Rosenberg SA, editors: *Biologic therapy of cancer,* Philadelphia, 1991, Lippincott.

164. Pestka S: The purification and manufacture of human interferons, *Sci Am* 249:37, 1983.

165. Pietersz GA and others: Chemoimmunoconjugates for the treatment of cancer, *Adv Immunol* 56:301, 1994.

166. Piper BF, Lindsey AM, Dodd MJ: Fatigue mechanisms in cancer patients: developing a nursing theory, *Oncol Nurs Forum* 14(6):17, 1987.

167. Piper BF and others: Recent advances in the management of biotherapy-related side effects: fatigue, *Oncol Nurs Forum* 16(6)(suppl)6:27, 1989.

168. Piper BF: Alteration in comfort: fatigue. In McNally JC and others, editors: *Guidelines for oncology nursing practice,* ed 2, Philadelphia, 1991, Saunders.

169. Pitler LR: Hematopoietic growth factors, *Semin Oncol Nurs* 12(2):115, 1996.

170. Post-White J: The immune system, *Semin Oncol Nurs* 12(2):89, 1996.

171. Puri R, Siegel J: Interleukin-4 and cancer therapy, *Cancer Invest* 11(4):473, 1993.

172. Quesada JR and others: Interferon for induction of remission in hairy cell leukemia, *N Engl J Med* 310(1):15, 1984.

173. Quesada JR, Gutterman JU, Hersh EV: Treatment of hairy cell leukemia with alpha interferons, *Cancer* 57:1678, 1986.

174. Quesada JR and others: Clinical toxicity of interferons in cancer patients: a review, *J Clin Oncol* 4:234, 1986.

175. Quesada JR: Biologic therapy with interferon-gamma. In DeVita VT, Hellman S, Rosenberg SA, editors: *Biologic therapy of cancer,* ed 2, Philadelphia, 1995, Lippincott.

176. Reilly RM and others: Problems of delivery of monoclonal antibodies: pharmaceutical and pharmacokinetic solutions, *Clin Pharmacol Ther* 28(2):126, 1995.

177. Rhodes VA, McDaniel RW, editors: Cancer symptom management, *Semin Oncol Nurs* 11(4):231, 1995.

178. Rieger PT, Weatherly B: Can your nursing skills meet the challenge of a patient receiving IL-27? *Dimens Oncol Nurs* 3(3):9, 1989.

179. Rieger PT: The pathophysiology of selected symptoms associated with BRM therapy, Emeryville, Calif, 1992, Cetus Corp (monograph).

180. Rieger PT, Rumsey KA: Responding to the educational needs of patients receiving biotherapy. In Carroll-Johnson RM, editor: *The biotherapy of cancer.* V, Pittsburgh, 1992, Oncology Nursing Press (monograph).

181. Rieger PT: Dosing and scheduling of biological response modifiers. In Rieger PT, editor: *Biotherapy: a comprehensive overview,* Boston, 1995, Jones & Bartlett.

182. Rieger PT, editor: *Biotherapy: a comprehensive overview,* Boston, 1995, Jones & Bartlett.

183. Rieger PT: Patient management. In Rieger PT, editor: *Biotherapy: a comprehensive overview,* Boston, 1995, Jones & Bartlett.

184. Rieger PT, Haeuber D: A new approach to managing chemotherapy-related anemia: nursing implications of epoetin alfa, *Oncol Nurs Forum* 22:71, 1995.

185. Rieger PT: Interferon-alpha: a clinical update, *Cancer Practice* 3(6):356, 1995.

186. Rieger PT: Future projections in biotherapy, *Semin Oncol Nurs* 12(2):163, 1996.

187. Robinson KD, Abernathy E, Conrad KJ: Gene therapy of cancer, *Semin Oncol Nurs* 12(2):142, 1996.

188. Roche Laboratories: Roferon-A (package insert), Nutley, NJ, 1995, Hoffman-LaRoche.

189. Roche Laboratories: Vesanoid (package insert), Nutley, NJ, 1995, Hoffman-LaRoche.

190. Rosenberg SA: Gene therapy of cancer. In DeVita VT Jr, Hellman S, Rosenberg SA, editors: *Important advances in oncology,* Philadelphia, 1991, Lippincott.

191. Rosenberg SA: The immunotherapy and gene therapy of cancer, *J Clin Oncol* 10(2):180, 1992.

192. Rosenberg SA, Barry JM, editors: *The transformed cell: unlocking the mysteries of cancer,* New York, 1992, Putnam.

193. Rosenberg SA: Principles and applications of biologic therapy. In DeVita VT, Hellman S, Rosenberg SA, editors: *Cancer principles and practice of oncology,* ed 4, Philadelphia, 1993, Lippincott.

194. Rosenberg SA and others: Treatment of 283 consecutive patients with metastatic melanoma or renal cell cancer using high-dose bolus interleukin-2, *JAMA* 271:907, 1994.

195. Rubin JT, Lotze MT: Acute gastric mucosal injury associated with the systemic administration of interleukin-4, *Surgery* 111(3):274, 1992.

196. Rumsey KA, Rieger PT, editors: *Biological response modifiers: a self-instructional manual for health professionals,* Chicago, Ill, 1992, Precept.

197. Rumsey KA: Patient education. In Rieger PT, editor: *Biotherapy: a comprehensive overview,* Boston, 1995, Jones & Bartlett.

198. Schellhammer PF, Ladaga LE, Fillion MB: Bacillus Calmette-Guérin for superficial transitional cell carcinoma of the bladder, *J Urol* 135:261, 1986.

199. Schering Corp: Intron A: interferon alfa-2b recombinant for injection, Kenilworth, NJ, 1995, Schering.

200. Schlom J: Monoclonal antibodies in cancer therapy. In DeVita VT, Hellman S, Rosenberg SA, editors: *Biologic therapy of cancer,* ed 2, Philadelphia, 1995, Lippincott.

201. Sergi JS: The physiology of the flu-like syndrome and the cardiopulmonary and renal symptoms associated with BRM therapy, Emeryville, Calif, 1991, Cetus Corp, (monograph).

202. Sharp E: The interleukins. In Rieger PT, editor: *Biotherapy: a comprehensive overview,* Boston, 1995, Jones & Bartlett.

203. Sharp E and others: A teaching tool for patients receiving continuous IV infusion recombinant interleukin-2 therapy, *Oncol Nurs Forum* 21(5):911, 1994.

204. Siegel JP, Puri RK: Interleukin-2 toxicity, *J Clin Oncol* 9(4):694, 1991.

205. Silverman P, Berger NA: Recent clinical experience with tumor necrosis factor and advances in understanding its physiologic function and cellular activities, *Curr Opinion Oncol* 2:1133, 1990.

206. Skalla KA, Rieger PT: Fatigue. In Rieger PT, editor: *Biotherapy: a comprehensive overview,* Boston, 1995, Jones & Bartlett.

207. Skalla KA: The interferons, *Semin Oncol Nurs* 12(2):97, 1996.

208. Smith KA: Interleukin-2, *Sci Am* 262(3):50, 1990.

209. Smith MA and others: Retinoids in cancer therapy, *J Clin Oncol* 10(5):839, 1992.

210. Solal-Celigny P and others: Recombinant interferon alfa-2b combined with a regimen containing doxorubicin in patient with advanced follicular lymphoma, *N Engl J Med* 329:1608, 1993.

211. Sparber A, Biller-Sparber K: Immunotherapy and neuropsychiatric toxicity, *Cancer Nurs* 16(3):188, 1993.

212. Spivak JL, editor: Erythropoietin: basic and clinical aspects, *Hematol Oncol Clin North Am* 8(5):863, 1994.

213. Stadler WM, Vogelzang NJ: Low-dose interleukin-2 in the treatment of metastatic renal cell carcinoma, *Semin Oncol* 22:67, 1995.

214. Stames HF: Biological effects and possible clinical applications of interleukin 1, *Semin Hematol* 28(2)(suppl)2:34, 1991.

215. Stein CA, Narayanan R: Antisense oligodeoxynucleotides, *Curr Opin Oncol* 6:587, 1994.

216. Stetz KM and others: 1994 Oncology Nursing Society research priorities survey, *Oncol Nurs Forum* 22(5):785, 1995.

217. Straw LJ, Conrad KJ: Patient education resources related to biotherapy and the immune system, *Oncol Nurs Forum* 212:1223, 1994.

218. Sznol M, Parkinson DR: Clinical applications of IL-2, *Oncology* 8:61, 1994.

219. Tallman MS: All-*trans*-retinoic acid in acute promyelocytic leukemia and its potential in other hematologic malignancies, *Semin Hematol* 31(4 suppl 5):38, 1994.

220. Talpaz M and others: Hematologic remissions and cytogenic improvement induced by recombinant human interferon A in chronic myelogenous leukemia, *N Engl J Med* 314(17):1065, 1986.

221. Talpaz M and others: Interferon alpha in the therapy of CML, *Br J Haematol* 79(suppl)1:38, 1991.

222. Talpaz M: Use of interferon in the treatment of chronic myelogenous leukemia, *Semin Oncol* 6:3, 1994.

223. Tracey KJ, Vlassara H, Cerami A: Cachectin tumor necrosis factor, *Lancet* 1:1122, 1989.

224. Truitt RL and others: Role of IL-4, IL-6 and IL-12 in cancer therapy. In DeVita VT, Hellman S, Rosenberg SA, editors: *Biologic therapy of cancer,* ed 2, Philadelphia, 1995, Lippincott.

225. Tushinski RJ and Mulé JJ: Biology of cytokines: the interleukins. In DeVita VT, Hellman S, Rosenberg SA, editors: *Biologic therapy of cancer,* ed 2, Philadelphia, 1995, Lippincott.

226. Urabe A: Interferons for the treatment of hematological malignancies, *Oncology* 51(2):137, 1994.

227. Vadhan-Raj S and others: Effects of recombinant human granulocyte-macrophage colony-stimulating factor in patients with myelodysplastic syndromes, *N Engl J Med* 317(25):1545, 1987.

228. Vadhan-Raj S and others: Stimulation of myelopoiesis in patients with aplastic anemia by recombinant human granulocyte-macrophage colony-stimulating factor, *N Engl J Med* 319(25):1628, 1988.

229. Vadhan-Raj S and others: Abrogating chemotherapy-induced myelosuppression by recombinant granulocyte-macrophage colony-stimulating factor in patients with sarcoma: protection at the progenitor cell level, *J Clin Oncol* 10(8):1266, 1992.

230. Vadhan-Raj S and others: Effects of PIXY321, a granulocyte-macrophage colony-stimulating factor/interleukin-3 fusion protein, on chemotherapy-induced multilineage myelosuppression in patient with sarcoma, *J Clin Oncol* 12:715, 1994.

231. Vadhan-Raj S and others: Effects of interleukin-1α on carboplatin-induced thrombocytopenia in patients with recurrent ovarian cancer, *J Clin Oncol* 12(4):707, 1994.

232. Vadhan-Raj S: PIXY321 (GM-CSF/IL-3 fusion protein): biology and early clinical development, *Stem Cells (Dayt)* 12(3):253, 1994.

233. Varrichio CG, Jassak PF: Informed consent: an overview, *Semin Oncol Nurs* 5(2):95, 1989.

234. Vial T, Descotes J: Clinical toxicity of the interferons, *Drug Safety* 10(2):115, 1994.

235. Vose JM, Armitage JO: Clinical applications of hematopoietic growth factors, *J Clin Oncol* 4:1023, 1995.

236. Wadler S and others: Fluorouracil and recombinant alfa-2a-interferon: an active regimen against advanced colorectal carcinoma, *J Clin Oncol* 7(12):1769, 1989.

237. Wagstaff J, editor: *The role of interleukin-2 in the treatment of cancer patients,* Boston, 1993, Kluwer.

238. Weber J and others: Phase I trial of subcutaneous interleukin-6 in patients with advanced malignancies, *J Clin Oncol* 11:499, 1993.

239. Weinberg R: Oncogenes and cancer suppressor genes, *CA Cancer J Clin* 44:160, 1994.

240. Wheeler V: Interleukins: the search for an anticancer therapy, *Semin Oncol Nurs* 12(2):106, 1996.

241. Winningham ML and others: Fatigue and the cancer experience: the state of the knowledge, *Oncol Nurs Forum* 21:23, 1994.

242. Winters W, Glass E, Sakurai C: Ethical issues in oncology nursing practice: an overview of topics and strategies, *Oncol Nurs Forum* 20(suppl):21, 1993.

243. Wujcik D: Hematopoietic growth factors. In Rieger PT, editor: *Biotherapy: a comprehensive overview,* Boston, 1995, Jones & Bartlett.

244. Yarbro CH, editor: Management of patients receiving interleukin-2 therapy, *Semin Oncol Nurs* 9(suppl 3):1, 1993.

245. Yarbro JW: The new biology of cancer: future clinical applications, *Semin Oncol* 16(3):254, 1989.

246. Yarbro JW, Bornstein RS, Mastrangelo MJ: Interferon: advances in biotherapy, *Semin Oncol* 18(5)(suppl)7:1, 1991.

247. Yarbro JW, Bornstein RS, Mastrangelo MJ: Management of anemia in oncology, *Semin Oncol* 19(3)(suppl)8:1, 1992.

248. Yasko JM, Ver Furth M: Closing comments: economic trends, *Semin Oncol Nurs* 8(2):156, 1992

CHAPTER 24
Bone Marrow Transplantation

CLAIRE KELLER

Bone marrow is a spongy tissue found in the inner cavities of bone. Normal functioning marrow is rich in progenitor or stem cells, which eventually proliferate into mature erythrocytes, leukocytes, and platelets (see Chapters 13 and 30 for further information). Bone marrow transplantation (BMT) is the process of replacing diseased or damaged bone marrow with normal-functioning bone marrow. Bone marrow transplants (BMTs) are used in the treatment of a variety of diseases and offer a chance for long-term survival.

HISTORICAL PERSPECTIVE

The first known documented cases of human BMT occurred as early as the 19th century. Medical practitioners experimented with bone marrow as a treatment modality for poorly understood diseases for which there was no existing treatment. Bone marrow was injected into or sometimes even fed to patients. Some positive results occurred; however, these benefits were sporadic, and the reasons for improvement were poorly understood. These primitive attempts were for the most part abandoned.

Later in the 20th century an interest in BMT again arose as an experimental approach for the treatment of some hematologic diseases. A variety of approaches were used, and many important discoveries were made. Developments in antibacterial, fungal, and viral therapies; blood-banking techniques; chemotherapeutic regimens; growth factors; graft-versus-host disease (GVHD) prophylaxis and treatment; and tissue typing have made BMT a more effective, viable treatment option. Table 24-1 summarizes the highlights of these significant developments.

TYPES OF BONE MARROW TRANSPLANTATION

There are two major types of BMT: autologous and allogeneic. The type of transplant is identified by the recipient's relationship to the donor. An *autologous BMT* is a transplant in which the patient's own bone marrow

is collected (harvested), placed in frozen storage (cryopreserved), and reinfused into the patient after the conditioning regimen. Therefore the patient is his or her own donor. An *allogeneic BMT* is a transplant in which the patient receives someone else's bone marrow. There are several types of allogeneic BMT, with each type named according to the donor: *syngeneic*—the donor is the patient's identical twin; *related*—the donor is related to the recipient and is usually a sibling; *unrelated*—the donor is no relation to the recipient.

Peripheral Blood Stem Cells

Although stem cells have been traditionally harvested from bone marrow cavities, functional hematopoietic stem cells can be found circulating in peripheral blood as well. These peripheral blood stem cells (PBSCs) can be effectively transplanted, as evidenced in 1986 when the first successful PBSC transplants were reported.* Today the collection of PBSCs for hematopoietic support after high-dose chemotherapy (HDCT) has become common practice in the treatment of a variety of diseases (Table 24-2). Despite increased use of PBSCs for transplantation, debate continues over the advantages and disadvantages of PBSC transplant versus autologous BMT (Table 24-3). It is difficult to determine if one approach is more cost-effective than the other. Advocates of PBSC transplant cite early engraftment as a cost-saving measure because of shortened length of stay and the need for fewer blood products and antibiotics. Others argue that PBSC transplants appear less costly because many centers are providing a major portion of the post-BMT care in their outpatient facilities. PBSC collection may be less costly than traditional marrow harvest, but if multiple apheresis sessions are required, the cost can easily exceed the cost of a bone marrow harvest. There is no clear-cut cost advantage to either approach.[36]

The process of PBSC transplantation involves several phases: mobilization, apheresis, HDCT, reinfusion, and engraftment.

*References 9, 16, 34, 39, 50, 63.

Table 24-1 Significant Historical Events in Bone Marrow Transplantation (BMT)

Year	Researcher	Significant finding
1896	Quine	Attempted BMT by injecting or feeding bone marrow to patients; poor results.
1939	Osgood et al.	Attempted to cure aplastic anemia by massive intravenous (IV) injections of marrow cells.
1950	Relders et al.	Attempted BMT in dogs. Adequate doses of bone marrow, but inadequate radiation exposure did not allow for sufficient immunosuppression for engraftment.
1951	Lorenzo et al.	Demonstrated that guinea pigs and mice exposed to lethal radiation could be protected by infusion of bone marrow.
1955	Lindsley et al.	Radiation protection described earlier was result of growth of donor bone marrow.
1956	Ford et al.	Cytogenetic techniques used to show that radiation protection resulted from transfer and survival of donor marrow cells.
1957	Thomas et al.	Large quantities of bone marrow could be safely infused IV; one patient showed transient engraftment. Estimated necessary dose of marrow cells and warned against graft-versus-host disease reactions.
1959	Thomas et al.	Demonstrated that IV infusion of marrow from identical twin could protect against lethal radiation doses in patients with refractory leukemia.
1964	Mathe	First to achieve enduring bone marrow graft in patient with leukemia.
1968	Epstein et al.	Detected DL-A antigen in dogs and showed that marrow grafts between litter mates were almost always successful.
1968	Gatti et al.	Performed first marrow transplant from a matched sibling for an infant with immunodeficiency.
1975	Thomas et al.	Performed series of successful transplants using HLA-A–identical siblings.

Mobilization. Peripheral blood in its steady state does not contain adequate numbers of stem cells to allow for efficient collection. Bone marrow contains up to 100 times the number of stem cells found in peripheral blood.[36,71] To collect an adequate number of stem cells in the least number of apheresis sessions, it is necessary to stimulate the production of PBSCs through a process called *mobilization*. There are two techniques typically used to mobilize PBSCs, using hematopoietic growth factors (G-CSF or GM-CSF) alone or in combination with chemotherapy.

When growth factors are used alone, they are generally given for a set number of days and followed by a preset number of apheresis sessions. The main advantage to this approach is that the apheresis sessions can be scheduled in advance.[31] Cyclophosphamide is the most frequently used chemotherapeutic agent in PBSC mobilization, although other agents have been used. Chemotherapy is used to treat the disease and to take advantage of the accelerated hematopoiesis that occurs during the recovery period that follows myelosuppressive treatment.[59] When chemotherapy and growth factors are used together, there is an increase in the number of stem cells in the blood and a lengthening in the time they are present.[71] There are two primary disadvantages to chemotherapy-induced mobilization: it can result in neutropenic fever and infection, and it is difficult to predict when the patient will be ready to begin apheresis. However, the most significant mobilization seems to occur when chemotherapy and growth factors are used together rather than when either is used alone.[59,71] It has been reported that the combined use of chemotherapy and growth factors for mobilization also enhances engraftment.[71]

Apheresis. PBSCs are collected by a process called *apheresis*, using standard commercially available cell separators. The cell separators are programmed to collect either lymphocytes or low-density leukocytes.[36] The remaining blood components are returned to the patient. Apheresis is performed for 3 to 10 days. Each session is 3 to 4 hours long, but the duration is based on the rate of blood flow through the central venous catheter. A flow rate of 50 to 70 ml/minute is considered optimal.[59,71]

To collect PBSCs, a large-bore, double-lumen central venous catheter is required. This is necessary to provide adequate blood flow through the cell separator. A variety of catheters are in use; generally at least a 12 French is needed to maintain blood flow. Catheters that have narrower lumens or those constructed of soft material such as silicone may not be able to provide adequate flow rates.[15,72] Complications related to the central venous catheters have been reported, including thrombosis, occlusion, malpositioning, and infection. These complications contribute to the morbidity and cost of the procedure. The "ideal" apheresis catheter has not yet been found. Current technology does not allow one to identify the circulating stem cells. Several techniques are in development to help determine if an adequate number of stem cells has been collected to ensure engraftment. The easiest and most accessible is to measure the number of mononuclear cells in the apheresis product. Mononuclear cell counts of 4 to 5×10^8 per kilogram of patient body weight routinely contain adequate stem cells for engraftment. Another method is to measure the population of

Table 24-2 Diseases Treated with Bone Marrow Transplant (BMT) or Peripheral Blood Stem Cell (PBSC) Transplant

Type	Disease
BMT	
Malignant	Acute myelogenous leukemia
	Acute lymphocytic leukemia
	Chronic myelogenous leukemia
	Myelodysplastic syndrome
	Hodgkin's disease
	Non-Hodgkin's lymphoma
	Multiple myeloma*
	Breast cancer*
	Neuroblastoma
	Testicular cancer*
	Ewing's sarcoma*
	Rhabdomyosarcoma*
	Wilms' tumor*
	Malignant melanoma*
	Lung cancer*
Nonmalignant	Aplastic anemia
	Myelofibrosis
	Wiskott-Aldrich syndrome
	Severe combined immunodeficiency syndrome
	Mucopolysacharoidosis
	Osteopetrosis
	Lipid storage diseases*
	Thalassemia*
	Paroxysmal nocturnal hemoglobinuria*
PBSC TRANSPLANTATION[12]	
	Acute leukemia
	Brain tumors
	Breast cancer
	Hodgkin's disease
	Multiple myeloma
	Neuroblastoma
	Non-Hodgkin's lymphoma
	Ovarian cancer
	Small cell lung cancer
	Testicular cancer
	Ewing's sarcoma
	Chronic myelogenous leukemia

*Role of BMT is still under investigation.

Table 24-3 Advantages and Disadvantages of Peripheral Blood Stem Cell (PBSC) Transplant and Autologous Bone Marrow Transplant (ABMT)

Advantages	Disadvantages
PBSC TRANSPLANT	
Outpatient procedure	Processing and cryopreservation of PBSCs labor intensive
No general anesthesia needed for PBSC collection	Low cell yield requires multiple pheresis sessions
No harvest-related pain	Malignant cells may be present
Can be done when bone marrow is fibrotic, hypocellular, or diseased	Requires large-bore double-lumen central venous catheter
Possibility of less tumor contamination than in bone marrow	
Tumor cells in peripheral blood may have less ability to proliferate	
More rapid hematopoietic recovery; may result in lower costs from increased need for blood products and antibiotics, increased risk of infection, and shorter length of stay	
Faster reconstitution of immune function from increase in number of committed lymphocytes	
Potential for serial transplants	
ABMT	
Offers treatment options for older adults	Longer period of neutropenia
	Harvest requires general anesthesia and hospitalization
	Pain from multiple aspirations

cells that express CD34+ using flow cytometry. It is believed that stem cells are found within the group of cells carrying the CD34+ antigen. Currently this is one of the most widely used methods to estimate the number of stem cells in the apheresis product.[59]

Side effects of apheresis are minimal but include transient hypocalcemia from the anticoagulant used in the apheresis process, fatigue, anemia, and thrombocytopenia. After each collection the stem cells are placed in a blood bag and cryopreserved using dimethylsulfide (DMSO) as a cryoprotectant. The cells are kept frozen at $-196°$ C.

High-dose chemotherapy. HDCT for PBSC transplant requires hospital admission. It is administered in much the same way as the conditioning regimens for other types of transplants and varies based on the patient's disease and the treatment protocol of the transplant center.

Reinfusion. Transplantation of PBSC is performed in the same way as an autologous BMT. The side effects include hemoglobinuria, red urine, hypertension, fever, chills, vomiting, tachypnea, elevated serum bilirubin, cough, diarrhea, elevated serum creatinine, flushing, and headache. Studies have suggested that these side effects may occur more frequently in patients who receive a large volume of PBSCs or in patients whose dose of PBSCs contain a large volume of red blood cells (RBCs).[35]

Engraftment. Acute complications seen in the neutropenic period are similar to those of patients receiving an autologous BMT. Patients receiving PBSCs engraft as early as day 5 after stem cell infusion, on average 11 to 16 days after stem cell infusion.[36]

Unrelated Donors

Another option for donor availability is the attainment of an unrelated donor. The National Marrow Donor Program (NMDP) was established in 1987 for this purpose. The registry contains more than 2 million available bone marrow donors, all of whom have had tissue typing completed and have expressed a desire to donate bone marrow. Ethnic minorities are underrepresented in the registry. The NMDP is placing major emphasis on the recruitment of minority donors. The registry search determines which listed donors have compatible typing with the recipient patient. Several other donor registries also contain approximately 1 million donors located throughout the world who are available for searches. It is not inconceivable that a patient in the United States could receive bone marrow from a donor located somewhere in Europe, Asia, Africa, or anywhere else in the world. The system is an anonymous one. When chosen, the donor does not know who is receiving the marrow, and the recipient does not know from which donor the marrow came or where that donor is located. More than 4200 unrelated BMTs have been made possible as a result of efforts of the NMDP.

Cord Blood Transplantation

As with bone marrow, umbilical cord blood is rich in PBSCs. It is now possible to collect and store cord blood for use in place of bone marrow or PBSCs. As of January 1996, 150 cord blood transplants have been performed worldwide.[13] Cord blood transplants have been successfully performed in patients with leukemia, aplastic anemia, Fanconi's anemia, immunodeficiency, and genetic and metabolic disorders.

Most early cord blood transplants were from siblings, but 90 transplants from unrelated donors have been performed.[13,47] The New York Blood Bank Center has banked more than 5000 cord blood samples. So far, cord blood has been used primarily in children because of the low number of PBCs in the cord blood. It is not yet known how many PBSCs are required to ensure engraftment, but at least four patients weighing more than 70 kg have been successfully transplanted.[13]

Collecting cord blood is a simple procedure and poses no risk to the donor. After delivery, the umbilical cord is clamped and the blood withdrawn from the umbilical vein using a needle and syringe. It is then cryopreserved in much the same way as PBSCs or bone marrow.[24,53] A national cord blood bank, standards for collecting and storing cord blood, and data collection related to cord blood transplantation are expected in the near future.

	Mother		Father	
	M-1	M-2	F-1	F-2
A	1	2	3	9
B	5	7	12	13
DR	1	2	4	5

	Child #1		Child #2		Child #3		Child #4	
	M-1	F-1	M-1	F-2	M-2	F-1	M-2	F-2
A	1	3	1	9	2	3	2	9
B	5	12	5	13	7	12	7	13
DR	1	4	1	5	2	4	2	5

Figure 24-1 Human leukocyte antigen (HLA) inheritance.

Cord blood transplantation will have an increasing impact on transplant medicine in the near future.

Human Leukocyte Antigen Typing

Tissue typing of the patient and potential donors is the first step in identifying whether a patient has a compatible donor. To determine a person's tissue type, a small amount of peripheral blood is drawn, and antigens on the surface of the leukocytes are analyzed. These antigens make up the human leukocyte antigen (HLA) system, which plays a role in immune surveillance by constantly identifying "self" from "nonself."[74] There are a pair of antigens at several sites on the white blood cells (WBCs) called *loci*. Three of these loci, the HLA-A, HLA-B, and HLA-DR, are important in determining whether a patient and potential donor are compatible. The best match is one in which the antigens of the patient and potential donor match at all three loci. Matching at the A, B, and DR loci minimizes the risk of graft-versus-host disease (GVHD) and graft rejection.

The antigens that make up the HLA system are inherited from one's parents. Each offspring receives a set of antigens, referred to as a *haplotype,* from each parent (Figure 24-1). Thus the best chance of finding a matched donor occurs among full siblings. Statistically, each sibling has a one in four (25%) chance of receiving the same haplotypes from the same parents. It is possible but unlikely that parents or children of a patient will match, since they are usually only a one-haplotype (half) match. In general, relatives outside the immediate family have approximately the same chance of matching as someone from the general population. Overall, the chances of matching someone in the general population are approximately 1 in 20,000, depending on how common the individual's haplotypes are.

HLA-A and HLA-B (class I) antigens are identified by serologic testing using a small blood sample and a typing tray containing known antisera.[73] HLA-DR antigens are identified using deoxyribonucleic acid (DNA) technology. DNA technology identifies genes that specify the DR and DQ antigens; this allows for more accurate DR typing and therefore the identification of better matches. DNA technology has become the standard method used by many transplant centers and is now required by the NMDP.[74]

Mixed-lymphocyte culture (MLC) testing, in which donor and recipient lymphocytes are grown in culture together to assess their reaction, was considered important in determining HLA-DR antigen compatibility, but the results are often difficult to analyze or reproduce. The advent of DNA technology has caused many centers to consider MLC testing obsolete.[74]

Mismatched donors are used in allogeneic transplants, for which no true match exists. Mismatches currently considered for transplant are either one or two antigen mismatches. The mismatch can occur at either the A, B, or DR loci. The higher the number of mismatches, the higher the incidence is of GVHD or graft rejection and the poorer the chances are of the patient's survival.[3]

Mismatching does not refer to ABO incompatibility. Corrections can be made to overcome ABO incompatibility so that, for example, a patient with blood type O can receive a BMT from a donor with blood type A. When ABO incompatibility occurs, the donor's erythrocytes can be removed from the bone marrow before transplant. Therefore the donor's erythrocytes are not infused and side effects from the ABO incompatibility are minimized. The recipient will eventually seroconvert to the donor's blood type.

INDICATIONS FOR BONE MARROW TRANSPLANTATION

BMT is a treatment modality for a variety of malignant and nonmalignant diseases (see Table 24-2). Most BMTs are performed for malignancies. The type and stage of the disease, the patient's age and performance status, and donor availability determine the type of transplant that can be done and the chances of survival. Table 24-4 identifies approximate 5-year disease-free survival (DFS) for autologous and allogeneic transplants. Allogeneic BMT is used for the treatment of patients with hematologic malignancies, marrow failure, severe combined immunodeficiency syndrome (SCIDS), and some inherited metabolic disorders. Currently, most allogeneic transplants are performed for acute myelocytic leukemia (AML), acute lymphocytic leukemia (ALL), and chronic myelogenous leukemia (CML).[28,29] Autologous BMT is used primarily for the treatment of diseases in which the patient's own bone marrow contains adequate PBSCs that can eventually generate functioning erythrocytes, leukocytes, and platelets. For example, autologous BMT is not a viable option for the treatment of aplastic anemia, since the patient's own bone marrow is lacking PBSCs; however, it can be a treatment option for patients with limited disease in their bone marrow.

Table 24-4 Survival Rates: Approximate 5-Year Disease-Free Survival (DFS) of Patients Receiving Autologous or Matched-Sibling BMT

Disease	DFS
AUTOLOGOUS TRANSPLANTS	
AML (1st CR)	40%-50%
AML (2nd CR)	30%-40%
ALL (1st CR)	40%-50%
ALL (2nd CR)	30%
CML (chronic)*	10%
Hodgkin's disease	20%-60%
Non-Hodgkin's	40%-60%
Breast cancer	Stage II and III: 75%
	Stage IV: 20%
ALLOGENEIC TRANSPLANTS	
AML (1st CR)	50%-65%
AML (>1st CR)	25%-35%
ALL (1st CR)	40%-60%
ALL (2nd CR)	30%-60%
CML (chronic)	65%
CML (accelerated)	30%-45%
CML (blastic)	15%
Hodgkin's disease	25%-55%
Non-Hodgkin's	20%-65%
Multiple myeloma*	30%
Aplastic anemia	60%-80%
MDS	30%-60%

See text for abbreviations.
*Limited number of patients and follow-up.

Autologous BMT is being used increasingly for the treatment of hematologic malignancies. Since 1990 the number of autologous BMTs has outpaced the number of allogeneic BMTs.[65]

A variety of approaches are being used to improve the efficacy of autologous transplant. The most promising is the use of dose-intensity therapy. BMT allows for the use of much higher doses of chemotherapy and or radiation than would otherwise be possible. By increasing the dose intensity of the treatment, one can increase the likelihood of curing patients of their disease.[14,58,65] A second approach is the use of sequential autologous BMTs. Often, using PBSCs this approach allows for several courses of dose-intensive therapy with PBSC rescue in the hope of curing the patient's disease.

A concern associated with autologous transplant and PBSC transplant is the potential for contamination with tumor cells. A variety of purging techniques have been developed. A lack of prospective clinical trials, a lack of sensitive and specific assays to measure residual tumor, and the concern that stem cells can be damaged during the purging process have kept marrow purging controversial.[20]

Hematologic Malignancies

Leukemia

Acute lymphocytic leukemia (ALL). Allogeneic BMT has been performed on patients with ALL in remission and in relapse. Survival for patients transplanted in first remission is comparable to survival with conventional chemotherapy.[28,29] However, performing an allogeneic BMT in first remission is beneficial for patients who present with a high WBC count at diagnosis, the Philadelphia chromosome, or other chromosomal abnormalities. Allogeneic BMT for ALL in second or subsequent remission has shown a survival advantage over conventional chemotherapy.

Autologous BMT and PBSC transplant may also be done if no suitable donor is available. ALL is the most common leukemia among children; 60% to 70% of these children are cured with conventional chemotherapy. For most children with ALL, BMT is not considered unless the child relapses with treatment. BMT in first remission is indicated only if the Philadelphia chromosome or other chromosomal abnormality is present.[50,56] For those patients who do not have a suitable donor, autologous BMT has been done, but these patients have a relapse rate of 70% to 75%.[56]

Acute myelocytic leukemia (AML). Survival rates of AML patients with allogeneic BMT are 35% to 60%, compared with conventional chemotherapy survival rates of 20% to 50%. Timing of transplant remains controversial, but survival is best when the patient is transplanted in first remission. For patients without suitable donors, autologous and PBSC transplants done during first remission offer survival rates of 40% to 50%. The relapse rate is higher after autologous BMT, but complications of allogeneic BMT (e.g., GVHD) result in similar DFS rates.

Chronic myelogenous leukemia (CML). For patients with CML, allogeneic BMT is the only treatment option that is curative.[41,42] The disease phase at the time of transplantation is the factor most strongly associated with treatment success.[42] Patients who have a BMT in the chronic phase have higher rates of success. The best results are seen in young patients, transplanted in chronic phase within a year of the diagnosis.[2]

For patients without a suitable donor, autologous BMTs for CML have been done. Marrow or PBSCs must be collected while the patient is in chronic phase. Patients are transplanted when they progress to accelerated phase. Although this treatment is not curative, patients with chronic-phase CML have been successfully restored for 4 months to 1 year.[65]

Five percent of the leukemias in children are chronic. There are two types, adult type CML and juvenile chronic myelogenous leukemia (JCML). Adult type CML is more common and is characterized by high WBC count and the presence of the Philadelphia chromosome.

Allogeneic BMT is the only hope of cure and should be performed early after diagnosis. JCML occurs in very young children, usually less than 5 years of age. JCML frequently presents like acute leukemia but cannot be effectively treated with chemotherapy. Allogeneic BMT provides a 30% to 50% chance of survival and the only hope of cure.[50,56]

Lymphoma. BMT in the malignant lymphomas, Hodgkin's and non-Hodgkin's, is very widely used as a salvage treatment. Because of the high chemotherapy and radiation sensitivity of these tumors, patients with lymphoma are optimal candidates for BMT.[70]

Autologous, allogeneic, and recent PBSC transplants are used, although autologous BMTs are done most frequently because of better donor availability and decreased complications. Autologous BMT also allows for treatment of older patients, which is especially important in non-Hodgkin's lymphoma.[70]

Patients with lymphoma who have good performance status, have had less than two prior chemotherapy regimens, and have a low tumor burden at the time of transplant have the best survival rates.[70] In Hodgkin's disease, BMT is usually indicated for patients who fail to achieve a complete response to three or four courses of chemotherapy or who are in early relapse after initial complete response.[27,32,43] In non-Hodgkin's lymphoma, BMT is usually indicated for patients who have relapsed after an initial complete response or who remain responsive to chemotherapy but have residual disease.[27,32,70] For patients with residual disease or highly aggressive non-Hodgkin's lymphoma, BMT should be carried out as a consolidation procedure.[27]

Other hematologic malignancies

Myelodysplastic syndrome (MDS). MDS consists of a number of disorders characterized by peripheral cytopenias. Allogeneic BMT is the only curative treatment for patients with MDS. Results are better in patients without excess blasts; cure rates of 60% to 70% have been reported in this population. Patients with excess blasts have a survival rate of 25% to 40%.[3]

Multiple myeloma (MM). Allogeneic BMT is being used more frequently for patients with MM. Overall survival rates for patients who fail first-line chemotherapy average 30% to 35%.[3] Allogeneic BMT is not an option for many MM patients because of their advanced age and lack of suitable donors. Autologous BMT can be tolerated by patients up to age 65. Favorable results reported with autologous BMT showed that patients most likely to benefit have primary resistant or responding disease with low β-microglobulin and lactate dehydrogenase (LDH) levels.[67]

Solid Tumors

Autologous BMT is most often done for patients with solid tumors. Solid tumors are the malignancies most frequently treated with dose-intensive strategies. For BMT to be effective, the disease must be responsive to treatment. Although BMTs are currently being performed on a variety of solid tumors, many are still considered investigational. The diseases currently receiving the most attention and study are breast cancer and neuroblastoma. Other tumors for which BMT has shown some positive responses are Ewing's sarcoma, malignant melanoma, rhabdomyosarcoma, testicular cancer, Wilms' tumor, ovarian cancer, and small cell lung cancer.

Breast cancer. Breast cancer now represents the most common disease treated by autologous BMT.[65] Conventional chemotherapy shows a dose-response effect, providing the rationale for the use of HDCT.[11] Studies show that HDCT with PBSC or marrow transplant in patients with chemotherapy-responsive metastatic disease has a 50% rate of complete remission, with a 5-year DFS rate of 20%. For patients with high-risk stage II (10 nodes or more) and stage III disease, the 5-year DFS rate with conventional treatment is 25% to 57%. With HDCT and PBSC transplant, this increases to 70%. Indicators of favorable prognosis for these patients are chemotherapy-responsive disease, limited tumor bulk, limited number of disease sites, absence of liver involvement, and good performance status. HDCT and autologous BMT alone are not curative; dose-intensive therapies must be integrated with other treatment modalities into the overall treatment of breast cancer.[11,65]

Neuroblastoma. Neuroblastoma is the most frequent pediatric solid tumor treated with BMT. Approximately 60% of patients have advanced disease and only a 10% chance of cure with conventional therapy.[45,57] Recent studies of autologous BMT in these patients suggests an overall 5-year DFS of 20% to 40%. Again, the small number of patients and the brief follow-up make these results encouraging but inconclusive. Further clinical trials are needed to determine if autologous BMT provides optimal treatment.[25,57]

Nonmalignant Diseases

Aplastic anemia. Allogeneic BMT is responsible for approximately an 80% overall survival rate in patients with aplastic anemia.[1] Patients who have had blood product transfusions before BMT have a higher rate of graft rejection. Therefore, at the time of diagnosis, HLA typing is done on the entire family. All patients younger than age 45 should be considered for BMT. Although patients are immunosuppressed because of the disease, a conditioning regimen is usually administered.[74] This is especially important for patients who have received transfusions because of the increased possibility of rejection.[2]

Severe combined immunodeficiency syndrome (SCIDS). The earliest successful BMTs were in patients with SCIDS.[1] Most patients with SCIDS die within 1 year of diagnosis, and since this disease occurs so early

in life, a matched-sibling donor may be unavailable.[1,74] Therefore the use of a haplo-identical parent and, in some patients, matched unrelated donors is considered.[1] Approximately 70% of patients receiving a matched BMT will be cured.[1,74] The survival rate is slightly lower for patients receiving a haplo-identical parent match because of the increased incidence of graft rejection and GVHD.[1] Because the disease has already immunosuppressed the patient, no conditioning regimen is usually given.

BONE MARROW TRANSPLANTATION PROCEDURE
Pretreatment Work-up

An extensive evaluation is performed on the BMT recipient before transplant. This is done to establish the recipient's physical and psychosocial status. For allogeneic transplants, the donor is also thoroughly assessed. The assessment is done on an outpatient basis and includes a variety of tests, procedures, and consultations (see box, p. 621). A team approach is usually used and typically includes psychology, social work, surgery, chaplaincy, and radiology in addition to nursing and medicine.

The patient's family and significant others are also included in this process. These evaluations alert the BMT team to potential problems that can occur, such as physical hindrances, negative coping mechanisms, or financial difficulties. This assessment also ensures that the patient has adequate support systems to help him or her throughout the rigorous BMT process.

Marrow Harvest

Harvesting is the process of obtaining bone marrow for transplantation. This procedure occurs in the operating room, typically with the patient under general anesthesia. Bone marrow is obtained by performing multiple punctures with a large-bore needle into the patient's posterior and occasionally anterior iliac crests. Usually two physicians work simultaneously, one on either side of the patient. Multiple punctures are necessary because each aspiration obtains only 2 to 5 ml of bone marrow.

The amount of bone marrow collected depends on the size of the recipient and donor as well as the type of BMT (autologous or allogeneic). Usually, 10 to 15 ml per kilogram of body weight will yield the amount of needed stem cells. Therefore a 50 kg patient would contribute approximately 500 to 750 ml of bone marrow, and if obtaining about 5 ml per aspiration, approximately 100 to 150 aspirations are required to obtain the desired 500 to 750 ml of marrow. This is only about 5% of the bodies total marrow volume. Ideally, this amount of marrow should contain 1 to 4×10^8 nucleated cells.[2]

Once collected, the marrow is mixed with a heparinized solution, filtered to remove bone fragments and fat, and placed in a blood bag. At this point the marrow can be treated or purged. *Purging* is the process of removing residual malignant cells from the marrow for autologous transplant. It is performed using monoclonal antibodies or chemotherapeutic agents. Marrow collected for allogeneic BMT may also be treated. One such treatment is that of T-cell depletion, which is the process of removing T lymphocytes from the marrow to prevent acute GVHD. If an ABO incompatibility exists, the RBCs may also be removed from the allogeneic marrow.

When an allogeneic BMT is to be done, the marrow is immediately transfused into the recipient. The marrow is usually brought directly to the recipient's room from the operating room. For an autologous BMT, the collected marrow is mixed with the preservative DMSO,

placed in a blood bag, and cryopreserved. It is thawed and transplanted at a later date.

After bone marrow harvest, postoperative recovery time is minimal. A large pressure dressing will have been applied to the iliac crests. Nursing responsibilities after bone marrow harvest include routine postoperative care such as maintaining comfort and mobility, providing care of the dressing, and monitoring vital signs and blood counts. Postoperatively, patients can expect discomfort at the sites for approximately 1 week. This discomfort can typically be relieved with acetaminophen. With an allogeneic BMT, the donor's psychologic and emotional needs must not be overlooked. Many donors experience anxiety over whether the BMT will be a success or a failure. Nursing must allow for the ventilation of donor feelings and offer support.

Conditioning Regimens

The conditioning regimen is the process of preparing the patient to receive bone marrow. It accomplishes three vital functions: obliterate the malignant disease, destroy the patient's preexisting immunologic state, and create space in the marrow cavity for the proliferation of the transplanted stem cells.[68] In effect, conditioning regimens destroy the patient's own bone marrow. The proliferation of new erythrocytes, leukocytes, and platelets cannot occur unless new functioning bone marrow is given to the patient. On completion of the conditioning regimen, the patient must receive a BMT or die. The conditioning regimen consists of HDCT with or without total body irradiation. There are several regimens using various combinations of chemotherapy and/or radiation that last 4 to 10 days (Table 24-5). Cyclophosphamide, carmustine, etoposide, busulfan, and cytarabine are all common chemotherapeutic agents used in conditioning regimens. The regimen chosen depends on the type of disease and the amount and response to previous radiation or chemotherapy.[40]

In addition to severe myelosuppression, the patient may experience many other side effects (Table 24-6). Most of these are immediate responses to the chemotherapy and radiation and can continue for several weeks after BMT. Management of these side effects focuses on control of the symptoms, prevention of further complications, and maintenance of patient comfort. Long-term effects, such as cataracts and gonadal dysfunction, also can occur and are discussed in the section on complications.

Transplantation of Marrow

After completion of the conditioning regimen, the bone marrow must be infused. If the regimen was one in which chemotherapy was the last treatment given, there is a rest period of 24 to 72 hours before transplant. This rest period is necessary because of the drug's half-life. Com-

Table 24-5   Common Conditioning Regimens for BMT

Regimen	Description									
Busulfan/cyclophosphamide										
Day	−7	−6	−5	−4	−3	−2	−1	0		
Busulfan 1 mg/kg every 6 hours	X	X	X	X						
Cyclophosphamide 60 mg/kg/day					X	X				
Rest day							X			
Transplant day								X		
Busulfan/cytarabine/cyclophosphamide										
Day	−9	−8	−7	−6	−5	−4	−3	−2	−1	0
Busulfan 1 mg/kg every 6 hours	X	X	X	X						
Cytarabine 2 gm/m² every 12 hours					X	X				
Cyclophosphamide 60 mg/kg/day							X	X		
Rest day									X	
Transplant day										X
Cyclophosphamide/total body irradiation (TBI)										
Day	−6	−5	−4	−3	−2	−1	0			
Cyclophosphamide 60 mg/kg/day	X	X								
Rest day			X							
TBI 200 Gy twice daily				X	X	X				
Transplant day						X				
Cyclophosphamide/etoposide/carmustine										
Day	−7	−6	−5	−4	−3	−2	−1	0		
Cyclophosphamide 1.8 g/m²/day	X	X	X	X						
Etoposide 200 mg/m² every 12 hours	X	X	X	X						
Carmustine 600 mg/m²/day					X					
Rest day						X	X			
Transplant day								X		
Cyclophosphamide/TBI										
Day	−8	−7	−6	−5	−4	−3	−2	−1	0	
Cyclophosphamide 50 mg/kg/day	X	X	X	X						
TBI 300 Gy every day					X	X	X*	X		
Transplant day									X	
Cyclophosphamide										
Day	−5	−4	−3	−2	−1	0				
Cyclophosphamide 50 mg/kg/day	X	X	X	X						
Rest day					X					
Transplant day						X				

*Lungs shielded for this dose.

pared with the donor search, extensive pretransplant work-up, and toxic conditioning regimen, most patients describe the actual transplantation of marrow as quite anticlimactic.

For autologous BMTs, the frozen marrow is brought to the recipient's room for transplant. The bag of marrow is thawed in a normal saline bath, drawn up in large syringes, and given through a rapid intravenous (IV) push via central venous catheter. The entire process takes approximately 20 to 30 minutes depending on the volume of bone marrow being transplanted. Patients often experience minimal shortness of breath, because of the rapid infusion of bone marrow, and nausea and vomiting from the preservative DMSO. DMSO also gives off a strange garliclike odor as it is excreted through the patient's respiratory system for 24 to 48 hours after autologous BMT.

For allogeneic transplants the marrow is infused on the same day as it is collected. This procedure resembles an RBC transfusion in that the bag of marrow is hung and transfused via the patient's central venous catheter. Unfiltered tubing must be used to prevent precious stem cells from becoming trapped and not being infused. The total time of infusion depends on the amount of marrow but usually lasts between 1 and 5 hours. Possible side effects from an allogeneic BMT are similar to those that can occur with a blood transfusion: shortness of breath, chills, fever, rash, chest pain, and hypotension. These reactions are more likely to occur if the marrow is ABO incompatible. If reactions do occur, the patient is treated with diphenhydramine, hydrocortisone, epinephrine, and/or oxygen therapy as necessary.

Patients may be premedicated with diphenhydramine and/or hydrocortisone to prevent or minimize these re-

Table 24-6 Side Effects of Conditioning Regimens for BMT

Regimen	Major side effects	Management
Busulfan	Nausea, vomiting, diarrhea, seizures (possible during administration and up to 48 hours after last dose)	Administer antiemetic at scheduled intervals. Check emesis for busulfan tablets and replace 1 for 1. Establish seizure precautions and monitor for seizure activity. Administer anticonvulsant at scheduled intervals as ordered. See Chapter 22.
Carmustine (BCNU)	Nausea, vomiting, diarrhea Hypotension Alcohol intoxication (drug is reconstituted in an alcohol base) Stomatitis Venoocclusive disease (hepatic failure occurs in first 4 weeks)	Administer antiemetic at scheduled intervals. Monitor blood pressure (BP) throughout administration. Maintain adequate hydration. Monitor for possible intoxication, maintain safe environment, and keep patient in bed during administration and several hours afterward. Monitor for ascites, edema, and elevated liver function. Administer diuretics, lactulose, and albumin and restrict fluids as ordered. See Chapter 22.
Cyclophosphamide (Cytoxan)	Nausea, vomiting, diarrhea Hemorrhagic cystitis Alopecia Cardiac toxicity	Administer antiemetic at scheduled intervals. Maintain adequate hydration. Monitor for blood in urine. Maintain continuous bladder irrigation as ordered and provide catheter care. Administer MESNA and pain medications as ordered. Ensure that electrocardiogram is done and checked before administration of each dose. See Chapter 22.
Cytarabine (ARA-C)	Nausea, vomiting, diarrhea Erythema Neurotoxicity Hemorrhagic conjunctivitis Alopecia	Administer antiemetics at scheduled intervals. Monitor palms and soles for erythema; provide creams and assistance with activities of daily living as needed. Monitor for cerebellar toxicity (ataxia). Administer steroid eye drops at scheduled intervals up to 48 hours after last dose. See Chapter 22.
Etoposide (VP-16)	Nausea, vomiting, diarrhea Hypotension Alopecia	Administer antiemetics at scheduled intervals. Monitor BP throughout administration. Maintain adequate hydration. See Chapter 22.
Total body irradiation (TBI)	Nausea, vomiting, diarrhea Stomatitis Alopecia Venoocclusive disease Fever Parotitis Erythema	Administer antiemetics 30 minutes before and immediately after treatment. Monitor for ascites, edema, and elevated liver function. Administer diuretics, lactulose, albumin, and fluid restriction as ordered. Monitor temperature every 2 to 4 hours and observe fever pattern. Assess for signs and symptoms of infection. Administer antipyretics as ordered. Apply hot/cold packs to affected areas. Administer pain medications as ordered. Monitor skin integrity and keep skin clean and dry. Avoid harsh soaps and irritants. If desquamation occurs, use dressings, ointments only as ordered. See Chapter 21.

Table 24-7   Common Antibiotics, Antifungals, and Antivirals Administered after BMT

Medication	Route/dose	Indications/precautions
ANTIBIOTICS		
Cefoperazone	IV 2 g every 8 hours	Suspected gram-negative sepsis. Infuse over 30 minutes. Not approved for pediatric patients. Monitor prothrombin time and for diarrhea. Administer vitamin K as ordered.
Ceftazidime	IV 150 mg/kg/day every 8 hours	Suspected gram-negative sepsis. Infuse over 30 minutes. Maximum dose 2 g every 8 hours. Monotherapy for pediatric patients, second-line therapy for adults. Monitor for diarrhea and development of drug resistance.
Norfloxacin	PO 400 mg BID	Reduction of bowel flora, anaerobes. Administer on empty stomach. Do not administer with antacids or carafate. Monitor for rash, nausea, vomiting, and diarrhea. Discontinue when granulocyte recovery is maintained.
Penicillin VK	PO 250 mg BID	Prophylaxis of gram-positive infections after BMT. Check for allergy to penicillin. Monitor for rash.
Tobramycin	IV 5 mg/kg/day	Suspected gram-negative sepsis. Infuse over 20 to 30 minutes. Do not administer at same time as ceftazidime or cefoperozone. Monitor peak and trough blood levels. Monitor for nephrotoxicity (elevated BUN and creatinine) and ototoxicity (ataxia, diminished hearing).
Trimethoprim-sulfamethoxazole	PO 1 DS tablet BID IV 15-20 mg/kg/day	Prophylaxis of *Pneumocystis carinii* pneumonia after BMT. Avoid with sulfa allergy. Administer per transplant center protocol. Monitor for rash, decreasing WBC, and increasing BUN and creatinine.
Vancomycin	IV 1 g every 12 hours (adult patients) IV 40 mg/kg/day (pediatric patients) PO 125 mg every 6 hours	Suspected or proven gram-positive infections. Infuse over 60 minutes. PO is used for *Clostridium difficile* enterocolitis only (not absorbed orally). Monitor peak and trough blood levels. Monitor for nephrotoxicity (elevated BUN and creatinine) and ototoxicity (ataxia, diminished hearing).
ANTIFUNGALS		
Amphotericin B	IV 0.5-1 mg/kg/day	Treatment of fungal infections resistant to fluconazole. Infuse through D_5W only over 3 to 6 hours. Administer test dose at initiation of therapy (1 mg in 100 ml D_5W). Monitor for increased temperature and chilling rigor during infusion. Premedicate with diphenhydramine, acetaminophen, or hydrocortisone as ordered. Monitor electrolytes and for nephrotoxicity.
Fluconazole	PO 500 mg BID IV 100-200 mg/day	PO for reduction of bowel flora (used with norfloxacin). IV for treatment of fungemia. Monitor for overgrowth of resistant strains of fungus—surveillance cultures. Monitor for elevated liver function tests and nephrotoxicity. Discontinue PO when granulocyte recovery is maintained.

IV, Intravenous; *PO*, oral; *BID*, twice a day; *BUN*, blood urea nitrogen; *WBC*, white blood cell count.

Table 24-7 Common Antibiotics, Antifungals, and Antivirals Administered after BMT—cont'd

Medication	Route/dose	Indications/precautions
ANTIVIRALS		
Acyclovir	PO or IV 250-500 mg/m² every 8 hours	Prophylaxis and treatment of herpes simplex virus (HSV) or cytomegalovirus (CMV). Infuse over 2 hours (doses >500 mg must be diluted in 500 ml of fluid). Monitor for increased BUN and creatinine.
Ganciclovir	IV 2.5 mg/kg every 8 hours IV 5 mg/kg every 12 hours	Prophylaxis and treatment of CMV. Infuse over 1 hour; handle administration and disposal using chemotherapy precautions. Administer with immunoglobulin for cases of CMV pneumonitis. Monitor for decreased WBC and increased BUN and creatinine. Colony-stimulating factors may be given to maintain WBC.
Foscarnet	IV 40-60 mg/kg every 8 hours	Second-line therapy for HSV or CMV infections. Monitor for electrolyte disturbances, nephrotoxicity, and decreased WBC. Monitor for seizure activity.
Immunoglobulin	IV 0.4 g/kg every week for 6 weeks PO 50 mg/kg/day every 6 hours	IV prophylaxis for HSV and CMV. IV treatment for CMV pneumonitis in conjunction with ganciclovir. PO treatment of rotavirus. Administer IV slowly 20 to 30 ml/hour. Monitor for chills, hypotension, and increased temperature during infusion.

actions. In both transplant procedures, emergency equipment is always available at the patient's bedside. The physician is also available throughout the entire transplant. The nursing staff is responsible for closely monitoring vital signs and for signs and symptoms of reaction. Teaching is also an important aspect of nursing care. The patient and family/significant others will have been exposed to much information about this procedure before its occurrence; however, several questions always arise, along with patient and family anxiety, on this eventful day. Some patients view their transplant day as a "birthday" of sorts, since in their eyes they are given a new chance at life.

Engraftment Period

The engraftment period is the time immediately after BMT when the transfused stem cells migrate, by some unknown phenomenon, to the recipient's bone marrow space and begin to regenerate. This usually takes 2 to 3 weeks and is evidenced by increasing blood counts. During this period the patient experiences severe pancytopenia and immunosuppression. Immediate complications that can occur include infection and bleeding. The patient's care during this time focuses on prevention of and early treatment of infection and bleeding. Patients typically receive numerous antibiotics and blood components during this time (Tables 24-7 and 24-8).

Because infections and bleeding can be major com-

plications immediately after BMT, one goal is to shorten the length of the pancytopenic period. Hematopoietic growth factors aid in this process (see Chapter 23). These include, but are not limited to, granulocyte-macrophage colony stimulating factor (GM-CSF), granulocyte colony-stimulating factor (G-CSF), and interleukin 3 (IL-3). These factors affect the function of mature myeloid cells and the ability to stimulate the proliferation of myeloid precursor cells at various stages of differentiation.[48]

GM-CSF and G-CSF are both myeloid-stimulating factors. GM-CSF (sargramostin) activates mature granulocytes and macrophages and has a multilineage factor. GM-CSF is indicated for the acceleration of myeloid recovery in patients with NHL, ALL, and Hodgkin's disease undergoing autologous BMT. G-CSF (filgrastim) is lineage specific and regulates the production of neutrophils within the bone marrow. It reduces the incidence of infection, as manifested by febrile neutropenia in patients with nonmyeloid malignancies who are receiving myelosuppressive anticancer drugs associated with severe neutropenia and fever.

IL-3 has the additional potential of assisting even earlier multilineage progenitor cells to maturation and therefore may also have an impact on hastening platelet and RBC recovery after BMT.[49] This could lead to decreased bleeding problems for the patient, who therefore requires less blood transfusion therapy. The administration of IL-3 with or without GM-CSF or G-CSF may have an

Table 24-8   Blood Component Therapy

Component	Indications	Special considerations
PACKED RED BLOOD CELLS (PRBCS)	Hemoglobin is <8.0 g. Patient is symptomatic. Active bleeding occurs.	Type and cross-match procedure is necessary. Infuse over 2 to 4 hours. Monitor for transfusion reaction (fever, chills, urticaria).
Leukocyte-poor PRBCs: leukocytes are removed during transfusion.	Patient has experienced febrile transfusion reactions. Patient is at risk for alloimmunization.	Infuse through a special filter (Pall).
Washed PRBCs: blood is washed with 1000 ml normal saline and repacked before transfusion.	Patient has known severe allergic reaction to plasma and leukocytes.	Infuse at 20-30 gt/minute until completion of unit. Unit expires within 24 hours of washing.
PLATELET CONCENTRATES	Platelet count is <20,000. Active bleeding occurs. Platelets are given before minor procedures or surgery.	ABO compatibility is preferred but not necessary. 1-hour or 24-hour posttransfusion increments are monitored to determine effectiveness. Splenomegaly, disseminated intravascular coagulation, fever, and sepsis may increase demand. Monitor for transfusion reactions. Prophylaxis is done with diphenhydramine, acetaminophen, and hydrocortisone.
Random-donor platelets (RDPs): several units (6-10) harvested from whole blood are pooled into one bag.	Patient has had no prior transfusions. Patient has had no reactions or alloimmunization.	Units expires about 4 hours after pooling.
Leukocyte-poor RDPs: leukocytes are removed before or during transfusion.	Patient is at risk for alloimmunization. Patient has experienced febrile transfusion reactions.	Unit is either centrifuged and leukocytes mechanically trapped (Leukotrap) or a special filter (Pall) is used for infusion.
Single-donor platelets (SDPs): platelets are collected by pheresis from one donor.	Patient is refractory to RDPs. Patient is at risk for alloimmunization.	Try to match ABO/Rh of patient. Usually transfuse with special filter (Pall). Unit expires within 24 hours of collection.
HLA-matched platelets: platelets are collected by pheresis from a donor whose HLA typing closely matches patient's type.	Patient is refractory to RDPs and SDPs. Patient is at risk for alloimmunization.	Patient must have been HLA typed. Unit expires within 24 hours of collection.
Resuspended platelets: plasma is removed from pooled units, and an equivalent amount of normal saline is added.	Patient has experienced severe reaction to platelet concentrates despite prophylaxis.	Prophylaxis is usually needed.
FRESH FROZEN PLASMA	Patient has had multiple PRBC transfusions. Abnormal coagulation factors are evident.	Provide ABO-compatible component. Transfuse immediately after thawing.
IRRADIATED COMPONENTS Gamma radiation delivered to blood components inactivates lymphocytes within product.	Severely immunocompromised patients are at risk for graft-versus-host disease.	Component is not radioactive. Component should be labeled as being irradiated. RBCs and platelets are not affected.

even greater impact on granulocyte recovery than the use of single agents.[22,66]

Erythropoietin is being studied to see if it decreases the need for RBC transfusions. Early studies are inconclusive. The efficacy of erythropoietin remains to be seen. It will also be important to balance the benefit compared with the cost of erythropoietin therapy.[44]

COMPLICATIONS OF MARROW TRANSPLANTATION

BMT recipients experience toxic complications associated with the conditioning regimen. The major complications characteristic of BMT are graft failure, infections, pneumonitis, venoocclusive disease, graft-versus-host disease (GVHD), and recurrence of original disease (Table 24-9).

Graft Failure

Graft failure or rejection after BMT is a relatively rare occurrence, but an incidence of 5% to 15% has been reported.[2] Graft failure is defined as failure of marrow recovery to return or the loss of marrow function after an initial period of recovery.[2,3] An increased risk of graft failure is seen in patients who receive T-cell-depleted marrow, a low marrow cell dose, or HLA-mismatched marrow or who have extensive marrow fibrosis before BMT. Patients with aplastic anemia who have been previously transfused or receive only cyclophosphamide for their conditioning regimen are at an increased risk for graft failure.[3]

Infection

Alterations in the integrity of physical barriers and severe granulocytopenia from the pretransplant regimen set up an environment for serious bacterial and fungal infections during the first 6 weeks after BMT.[64] Usually the causative agents are from the patient's own microflora, particularly from the gastrointestinal (GI) tract and integumentary system. Common agents are gram-positive and gram-negative bacteria, such as *Staphylococcus, Escherichia coli,* and *Pseudomonas.*[1] Fungal infections are less common than bacterial infections, accounting for only 10% to 15% of systemic infections.[64,78]

Viral infections occur at varying times after BMT. Herpes simplex virus (HSV) and cytomegalovirus (CMV) are causative agents generally in the first 3 to 6 months after BMT. Varicella-zoster virus is usually not seen until later in the first year after the transplant. Viral infections are also typically associated with the incidence of chronic GVHD and can occur at any time during the course of chronic GVHD.[1,4]

During the first 6 weeks after BMT, prevention of infections is the most important step in counteracting infections. Maintaining protective environments, providing good hygiene, frequently monitoring vital signs, and performing head-to-toe assessments are very important. The greater the speed of marrow recovery, the less is the incidence of bacterial and fungal complications.[64] For this reason, there is a strong interest in the benefits of growth factors to stimulate engraftment.

Pneumonitis

Interstitial pneumonia is the most common cause of death in the first 100 days after BMT. Greater than 50% of interstitial pneumonitis is caused by CMV.[1] Interstitial pneumonitis peaks in incidence around 2 to 3 months after BMT and carries a 60% mortality rate.[1,64,69] The risk factors for interstitial pneumonitis are total body irradiation, presence of GVHD, advanced age of patient (more than 45 years), prior lung injury, and CMV serologic status of recipient and/or donor.[1,64]

Because CMV infection is a significant complication, screening for CMV during the pretransplant work-up is routine. This screening is valuable to identify patients at risk, evaluate the need for prophylaxis, and guide clinical steps if an infection is suspected. Screening consists of serologic testing of the recipient and donor for CMV. The incidence of recipient seropositivity before BMT is 40% to 70%.[75] In an allogeneic transplant a seropositive donor may transmit CMV to a seronegative recipient. In autologous transplants a seronegative patient may convert to seropositive because of blood product transfusion.

Prevention, early detection, prompt treatment, and immune restoration are important to a successful outcome.[69] One means of preventing CMV transmission is to provide seronegative blood products to BMT recipients who are seronegative and have a seronegative marrow source. Because this can put a great strain on the blood bank, an alternative is to provide leukocyte-depleted blood components.[75] This is usually accomplished by the use of special filters during the transfusion of the blood product. Prophylaxis with acyclovir or ganciclovir in seropositive recipients with CMV has also been used to decrease the chance of CMV infections. However, the use of these drugs in this manner must be weighed against the risk of bone marrow toxicity as a side effect.[75] The most successful treatment of CMV is ganciclovir and intravenous immunoglobulins (IVIGs).

Venoocclusive Disease

Venoocclusive disease (VOD) of the liver occurs in approximately 20% of patients undergoing allogeneic BMT and 10% of patients undergoing autologous BMT. Mortality rates of up to 50% have been reported. VOD is a complication of the conditioning regimen; the risk is greater for those patients receiving total body irradiation.

Table 24-9 Major Complications after BMT

Complication	Appearance	Signs/symptoms	Management
GRAFT REJECTION	1-4 weeks	Absent/prolonged neutropenia Partial marrow recovery Hypoplasia Hemolysis	Administer blood component therapy. Consider retransplantation.
INFECTION			
Bacterial	1-5 weeks	Fever	Maintain protective environment.
Fungal	1-5 weeks	Dry, nonproductive cough	
Viral		Change in breath sounds	Provide good hygiene.
Herpes virus	1-3 months	Erythema—oropharynx/catheter site	Monitor vital signs frequently.
Cytomegalovirus (CMV)	3 months	Diarrhea	Perform frequent head-to-toe systems
Varicella-zoster virus	1st year	Lesions—skin or mucous membranes	assessments.
		Hypotension	Administer colony-stimulating factors. Ensure CMV-negative blood products. Administer broad-spectrum antibiotics. Administer acyclovir and/or ganciclovir. Administer IV immunoglobulins.
VENOOCLUSIVE DISEASE			

(VOD)	1-3 weeks	Weight gain
		Ascites
		Hepatomegaly
		Right upper quadrant pain
		Bilirubin level above 2 mg/dl
			Maintain intravascular volume.
			Administer RBCs and IV fluids.
			Frequent physical assessments.
			Weigh twice daily.
			Measure abdominal girth daily.
			Administer low-dose dopamine, heparin,
			  and/or recombinant tissue
			  plasminogen activator (rTPA).

PNEUMONITIS			
Interstitial	1-4 months	Fever	Ensure CMV-negative blood products.
Toxic	1-6 months	Dry, nonproductive cough Shortness of breath Tachypnea Interstitial changes on x-ray film	Ensure leukocyte-poor blood products. Administer colony-stimulating factors. Administer ganciclovir. Administer IV immunoglobulins.

ACUTE GRAFT-VERSUS-HOST DISEASE (GVHD)	3-14 weeks	Maculopapular skin rash
		Nausea, vomiting, uncontrollable
		  diarrhea
		Jaundice
		Elevated liver function tests
		Hepatomegaly
			Provide immunosuppression with
			  cyclosporine-A, steroids,
			  methotrexate, and/or tacrolimus
			  (Prograf).
			Provide symptomatic treatment of skin,
			  gastrointestinal tract, and/or liver.

CHRONIC GVHD			

Skin	Months-years	Hyperpigmentation or
		  hypopigmentation, patchy
		  erythematous scaling,
		  thickening/hardening resembling
		  scleroderma, hair loss in involved
		  areas
			Provide immunosuppression with
			  cyclosporine-A, steroids, azathioprine
			  (Imuran), and/or thalidomide
			  (investigational).

Mouth		White striae and erythema on mucosa,
		  decreased salivary flow with dryness
		  of mouth
			Manage symptoms of affected organ or
			  system.

Eyes		Dryness, redness, itching/burning; corneal thickening	
Sinuses		Chronic sinusitis, predisposition to gram-positive infections	

Table 24-9 Major Complications after BMT—cont'd

Complication	Appearance	Signs/symptoms	Management
CHRONIC GVHD—cont'd			
Gastrointestinal tract		Difficulty swallowing, retrosternal pain, abdominal discomfort, diarrhea	
Pulmonary		Productive cough, progressive dyspnea, wheezing, pneumothorax	
Vagina		Inflammation, dryness, stenosis	
Muscle		Occasional polymyositis, proximal weakness	
Genitourinary tract		Cystitis, mild nephrotic syndrome	
Hematopoietic		Eosinophilia, thrombocytopenia, hypoplastic marrow, marrow fibrosis	
Lymphoid		Hypocellularity and atrophy of lymph tissues, functional asplenia	
Endocrine		Decreased growth rates, delayed pubertal development, autoimmune hyperthyroidism	
Nervous system		Entrapment neuropathy, peripheral neuropathy, myasthenia gravis	
LATE EFFECTS			
Cataracts	1-6 years	Loss of vision Dryness	Consider surgical intervention.
Gonad dysfunction	Variable	Infertility Menopause	Administer replacement sex hormones. Refer for psychosexual counseling.
Growth failure	Variable	Impaired growth of facial skeleton and dentition (<6 years old) Absent growth spurts No height changes	Administer supplemental growth hormone. Administer replacement sex hormones.
Hypothyroidism	1-15 years	Dry skin Hoarse speech Lethargy/apathy Weight gain with appetite loss Increased susceptibility to cold	Administer replacement hormones.
Secondary malignancy	Months-years	Specific to disease	Determine by type and extent of disease and patient's physical and psychologic status.
RECURRENCE	Months-years	Signs/symptoms of original disease	Determine by extent of disease and patient's physical and psychologic status.

VOD is the occlusion of the central veins of the liver resulting in venous congestion and stasis; this results in damage to the hepatic cells. The onset of VOD is usually early after BMT, in the first 3 weeks, but has been seen later. VOD is usually diagnosed by its classic symptoms of weight gain greater than 5% over baseline, hepatomegaly, right upper quadrant pain, total serum bilirubin level above 2 mg/dl, and ascites. Risk factors include a history of hepatitis, elevated transaminase at the time of transplant, mismatched or unrelated transplant, and the use of methotrexate as GVHD prophylaxis.

Treatment is aimed at maintaining intravascular volume to minimize further liver damage and maintain renal perfusion. Other treatment approaches remain controversial. Low-dose dopamine infusions have been used to increase renal perfusion, but this practice has been questioned. Low-dose heparin infusions also have been used for prophylaxis and treatment; some studies show favorable results in decreasing the incidence of VOD but results are inconclusive. Prostaglandin has vasodilatory, antithrombotic, and thrombolytic effects. Early studies in the use of prostaglandins for treating VOD have shown efficacy but have also shown significant toxicity. Recombinant tissue plasminogen activator (rTPA), a thrombo-

Table 24-10   Acute Graft-Versus-Host Disease (GVHD) Severity Grading

Stage	Skin	Liver	Gastrointestinal tract
+	Maculopapular rash over <25% of body surface	Bilirubin 2-3 mg/dl	Diarrhea >500 ml/day
++	Maculopapular rash over 25%-30% of body surface	Bilirubin 3-6 mg/dl	Diarrhea >1000 ml/day
+++	Generalized erythroderma	Bilirubin 6-15 mg/dl	Diarrhea >1500 ml/day
++++	Generalized erythroderma with bullous formation (>2 cm vesicle) and desquamation	Bilirubin >15 mg/dl	Severe abdominal pain with or without ileus

lytic agent, has been used to treat VOD, and early studies show it to be safe and effective in about 50% of patients.[5,55,79]

Graft-Versus-Host Disease

GVHD is a complication that can occur after allogeneic BMT. It is an immune-mediated reaction of the newly grafted marrow to the body of the recipient. Two types of GVHD have been identified: acute and chronic. They are distinguished from each other by the target organs, pathology, and timing after BMT. Chronic GVHD may occur after acute GVHD, but not always. A patient may also develop chronic GVHD without ever having had acute GVHD.

Acute GVHD. Acute GVHD is typically defined as occurring before 100 days after BMT. There is a 45% incidence in HLA-matched sibling donor transplants and greater than 75% incidence in HLA-mismatched related donor transplants.[17] The risk factors related to the incidence of acute GVHD are advanced patient age (more than 45 years), HLA mismatch, and donor-recipient gender mismatch.[41] The skin, GI tract, and liver are the primary target organs of acute GVHD. The occurrence of acute GVHD also prolongs immunodeficiency.

Skin involvement is characterized by a maculopapular rash that can proceed to a desquamating dermatitis. A biopsy of the skin is necessary to confirm the diagnosis and rule out other causes for the rash. In the first 20 days after BMT, this can be difficult because of changes in the skin related to the conditioning regimen.[1] The GI involvement is typically characterized by nausea, vomiting, and diarrhea. Again, a biopsy of the GI mucosa is the only definitive way to make a diagnosis. The pathologic changes seen in the GI tract are similar to those seen in the skin. In both the skin and the GI mucosa, secondary infections can occur because the acute GVHD has altered their integrity. Liver involvement is characterized by jaundice, elevated liver function studies, and hepatomegaly.

Acute GVHD can range from mild to life-threatening and is graded to distinguish its severity (Table 24-10). In its mildest form, acute GVHD typically can be con-

Table 24-11   Example of Immunosuppression Schedule

Day of BMT	Cyclosporine-A	Methylprednisolone
−2	IV 5 mg/kg/day continuous infusion	
+4	IV 3 mg/kg/day continuous infusion	
+8		IVP 0.5 mg/kg BID
+15	IV 3.75 mg/kg/day continuous infusion	IVP 0.375 mg/kg BID
+23		IVP 0.25 mg/kg BID
+29	PO 7.5 mg/kg BID	
+31		PO 0.125 mg/kg BID
+36	PO 5 mg/kg BID	
+38		PO 0.25 mg/kg × 1
+40		PO 0.25 mg/kg × 1
+42		PO 0.25 mg/kg × 1
+84	PO 4 mg/kg BID	
+98	PO 3 mg/kg BID	
+120	PO 2 mg/kg BID	
+181	Discontinue	

IV, Intravenous; *IVP,* IV push, *PO,* orally.

trolled and actually benefits those patients receiving transplants for malignancies. Patients with acute GVHD have a decreased incidence of disease recurrence.[17]

Because acute GVHD can be a life-threatening complication, means of preventing its occurrence are routinely administered. One of the most common means of preventing GVHD is the use of cyclosporine-A (CSA), steroids, and/or methotrexate (MTX). Tacrolimus (Prograf) is an immunosuppressant similar pharmacologically to cyclosporine but about 100 times more potent. Early studies show a lower incidence of GVHD using tacrolimus instead of CSA, but randomized clinical trials are ongoing.[2] All these agents provide immunosuppression after BMT and are given according to a scheduled regimen (Table 24-11). Because GVHD is immune mediated, suppressing immune reactions after BMT should prevent its occurrence. The T cells have been identified as the primary culprit in GVHD. Depleting the marrow of T cells before infusion into the recipient has greatly reduced the incidence and severity of acute GVHD.[17] However, the incidence of graft rejection and/or relapse is also significantly increased.[17]

Treatment for acute GVHD centers around increasing immune suppression. Often first-line therapy for GVHD is prednisone. Antithymocyte globulin (ATG) is often used as second-line therapy. Increasing the doses of CSA or tacrolimus may also be beneficial, but serum drug levels must be closely monitored. About 50% of patients with grade II or III GVHD respond to treatment. The mortality rate can be as high as 50%.[2,3]

Chronic GVHD. The onset of chronic GVHD is typically 100 days after transplant; however, it can occur at 70 days or up to years after transplant. It affects as many as 50% of matched sibling transplants and is life-threatening in about 5% of cases. It is characterized by scleroderma-like features and persistent immunodeficiency. It is a systemic multiorgan syndrome that resembles collagen-vascular diseases.[1,4] Chronic GVHD can be a continuation of acute GVHD, can occur after acute GVHD has resolved, or it can occur without any acute GVHD preceding it. The risk factors related to incidence are advanced age of recipient (more than 45 years), occurrence of preceding acute GVHD, T-cell-replete marrow, and female donor to male recipient.[4]

Almost every organ in the body can be affected by chronic GVHD (see Table 24-9). The basic effect is that of dermal thickening, fibrosis, and dryness. Bacterial, fungal, and viral infections are common in patients with chronic GVHD and are the most frequent cause of death.[4] Late interstitial pneumonitis occurs frequently. Mortality is highest in patients with progressive acute to chronic GVHD and those with multiorgan involvement.[62] Currently, standard treatment for chronic GVHD is prednisone; it is effective in 50% to 70% of cases.[3] Other agents have been used such as CSA, tacrolimus, azathioprine, and thalidomide.

Recurrence

Disease recurrence remains the most significant problem after BMT. It is the major factor related to patient mortality longer than 3 months after BMT.[1,49,64] Relapse is more frequent after autologous BMT because of hidden malignant cells in the transplanted marrow.[1,49] In allogeneic BMT the presence of GVHD is associated with decreased incidence of recurrence.[17] Some patients have been successfully retransplanted. Factors associated with better survival after a second transplant are a diagnosis of CML, AML in remission, good performance status, and duration of posttransplant remission of longer than 1 year. Patients with CML who relapse have been successfully treated with interferon.[2,3]

Late Effects

Long-term effects of BMT can occur several months to several years after transplant. Late effects are a common concern as more patients survive disease-free for as long as 20 years after-BMT.[21,37] The more common effects are cataracts, hypothyroidism, growth failure, gonadal dysfunction, and secondary malignancies. The late effects of BMT are of particular concern in the pediatric population and for patients with the possibility of cure with less intensive treatment.[37]

Cataracts. Cataracts are of concern primarily in patients who receive total body irradiation (TBI). Since radiation is more commonly being given in fractionated doses, the incidence of cataracts has decreased. Patients receiving TBI in a single dose have an 80% incidence of cataracts versus a 20% incidence when TBI is given in fractionated doses.[21,37] Patients receiving conditioning regimens of chemotherapy only do not have significant risk of developing cataracts.

Gonadal dysfunction. Sexual development is impaired in both males and females. Older patients (more than 40 years) are less likely to recover their reproductive functioning.[21] After TBI most females (90%) experience ovarian failure and require hormone replacement.[21,37] After TBI, males will recover production of testosterone but have absent or abnormal spermatogenesis.[21,37] If TBI is not used as part of the conditioning regimen, both males and females have a better chance of recovering gonadal functioning. There are several reports of patients having children after transplant.[21]

Growth failure. Impairment of growth is a common problem in children after BMT. Again, the incidence is high in those children who received TBI.[37] Of children who received TBI, 40% to 55% have decreased growth hormone, causing a retardation of spinal growth and the pubertal growth spurt.[21,37] Administration of growth hormone has shown some effect on growth velocity, and some catch up in growth can occur.

Hypothyroidism. The incidence of hypothyroidism is also related to preparation with TBI. Thyroid function is affected in as many as 60% of patients receiving single-dose TBI and as many as 25% of those receiving fractionated TBI.[21] Patients who have received conditioning regimens of chemotherapy only usually have normal thyroid function.[21]

Secondary malignancy. New malignancies may develop 6 months to years after BMT. A 4% to 6% incidence of secondary malignancies has been reported in long-term survivors of allogeneic BMT.[2] TBI, immunosuppression, immunodeficiency, viral infection, chronic immune stimulation, and genetic predisposition are factors that have been identified with increased risk of second malignancy after-BMT.[21] Radiation appears to be the most important risk factor. Non-Hodgkin's lymphoma is the most frequently reported new malignancy and develops more often in donor cells.[37] The incidence of leukemia and solid tumors as secondary malignancies is rare. Most often the appearance of leukemia is a recurrence of the original disease.[37] Overall, BMT recipients have a sixfold to sevenfold higher tumor incidence than nontransplanted individuals.[21]

Quality of life/survivorship. Interest on the part of researchers in quality of life after BMT has increased in recent years. A number of studies have been done to assess quality of life at various intervals after transplant. A number of tools have been used to collect this information. Some examples are Profile of Mood States, Psychological Adjustment to Illness Scale, Functional Living Index—Cancer, and the Cancer Rehabilitation Evaluation System. There is a need for more research in this area to develop better tools and determine the best times to measure quality of life throughout the transplant process.[76,77]

FUTURE DIRECTIONS AND ADVANCES IN BONE MARROW TRANSPLANTATION

According to data from the International Bone Marrow Transplant Registry, the number of patients undergoing BMT continues to increase annually. Future advances will include the use of cord blood stem cells for gene therapy because they are more efficient at taking up genes than are stem cells from other sources; fetal therapy; transplanting stem cells in utero for patients with congenital diseases such as SCIDS; and expansion of stem cells in the laboratory so fewer stem cell will be needed. Collection of PBSC is already expanding to include allogeneic donors; we can expect this to increase. The donor pool will continue to expand with an increase in the number of donors in the NMDP and the creation of a national cord blood bank.

Outpatient resources and transplantation via the outpatient mode will continue to expand. Third-party reimbursement, length of hospital stay, and financial resources for medications used in transplant recovery will have ongoing scrutiny.

Ongoing research will continue to look for better conditioning regimens and more effective treatments for infection and GVHD. Biologic response modifiers, cytokines, and colony-stimulating factors used to reduce relapse and enhance hematologic function will have continued exploration.

CONCLUSION

Bone marrow transplantation, regardless of the source of stem cells, offers cure and new hope for the future to many patients with life-threatening diseases. Continued expansion of the donor pool and ongoing research ex-

ploring better conditioning regimens, hematopoietic growth factors, and antibiotic/antifungal/antiviral drugs will be ongoing challenges. Financial reimbursement issues will continue to be a challenge: managed care is already having an impact. Many insurance companies are already expecting transplant centers to negotiate a fixed price; this will increase competition among transplant centers, because the lowest bidder will get the contracts and therefore the patients. Patients will no longer be able to choose a transplant center. There will be ongoing debate about which indications for transplantation are experimental. Transplantation is constantly changing but this challenging practice environment will continue to provide opportunities for skilled nurses.

The following is a list of resources and support services for patients and families undergoing bone marrow transplantation:

1. American Cancer Society
   Atlanta, Georgia
2. Aplastic Anemia Foundation of America
   Baltimore, Maryland
3. BMT Family Support Network
   Avon, Connecticut
4. BMT Link
   Southfield, Michigan
5. BMT Newsletter
   Highland Park, Illinois
6. Cancer Information Service
   Bethesda, Maryland
7. Candlelighters Childhood Cancer Foundation
   Bethesda, Maryland
8. Children's Tranplant Association
   Dallas, Texas
9. Corporate Angel Network
   White Plains, New York
10. Immune Deficiency Foundation
    Bethesda, Maryland
11. Leukemia Society of America
    New York, New York
12. LIFE-SAVERS Foundation of America
    Covina, California
13. National Marrow Donor Program
    Minneapolis, Minnesota
14. National Cancer Institute
    Bethesda, Maryland
15. National Children's Cancer Society
    St. Louis, Missouri
16. National Coalition of Cancer Survivorship
    Silver Springs, Maryland
17. Oncology Nursing Society Bone Marrow Transplant Special Interest Group
    Pittsburgh, Pennsylvania
18. Ronald McDonald Houses and Children's Charities
    Chicago, Illinois

Text continued on p. 638.

NURSING MANAGEMENT

Bone marrow transplantation is a strenuous medical treatment that in and of itself can be life threatening. As with any major medical treatment and life-threatening situation faced by patients and families, the general stresses that affect the patient and family must be addressed. These stresses are not necessarily unique to transplant; however, throughout the transplant process there are periods of transition when these general stresses increase in occurrence and/or intensity.

Prior experiences affect a patient/family examination of the risks and benefits of transplant. For some patients, the decision to have a transplant comes on the heels of being informed that they have a life-threatening illness and transplant must be done as soon as possible and is the only chance of cure. For other patients, the decision for transplant comes after a course or more of chemotherapy and living with their disease for a period of time pretransplant. Still other patients are informed at the time of diagnosis that a transplant is the only curative option and needs to be done within a certain time frame. Also affecting the patient's reaction to transplant is the ability to locate a donor if they cannot be their own donor and do not have a match within their family.

The idea of transplantation as a treatment option generally creates a wide spectrum of emotional reactions. Patients may experience anxiety, fear, depression, denial, grieving, and hopefulness all at different times. Coping styles that the patient and family have relied on in the past will be those they most likely fall back on at this time. Dysfunctional or disruptive coping behaviors, such as substance abuse, may resurface. Past or current psychiatric problems may also become intensified.

Everyday life for these patients and their families will be disrupted by transplantation. There will be changes in patients' roles within the family. When the transplant center is a distance from home, the family may be separated for several months. The relocation of the patient and a family member may be necessary. Child care as well as elder care can be affected by changes in the roles of family members. New routines also have to be incorporated into family life. Life-style changes after transplant may be permanent or temporary and can be a major disruption on family life.

The financial impacts of transplant can be devastating to families. Transplantation is a costly treatment. This is because of the numerous resources necessary to care for the patient. The cost of housing, food, dependent care, and transportation can seriously affect the financial status of any family. Reimbursement continues to vary based on the third-party payor and the disease being treated. Third-party payors may detail which diseases they accept as being treatable by transplantation and which are experimental. Very rarely are the costs of searching for an unrelated donor covered by third parties. They may cover the cost of the patient's care throughout the transplant, but the cost of searching for an unrelated donor is not covered.

Donors for allogeneic transplants also have special considerations that need to be addressed. The most important is the one of choice. Potential donors need to be adequately educated as to their role in a transplant if they are a match. It is the donor's choice to donate. In families with less than ideal relationships, this can be a challenge. Donors also need to be aware that agreeing to donate carries some amount of responsibility for the recipient's health. However, they must also understand that once they have donated, they have no control over what happens to the recipient. This is especially important in cases where patients develop GVHD.

Caring for patients undergoing BMT requires comprehensive and consistent nursing management. Patient/family teaching is key to providing assistance to patients and family members throughout the transplant process. Table 24-12 outlines the teaching priorities by stage of transplantation. Examples of nursing diagnoses and interventions for patients undergoing BMT follow.

NURSING DIAGNOSIS

Body image disturbance, risk for, related to treatment process

OUTCOME GOALS

Patient will be able to:
- Verbalize and demonstrate acceptance of appearance.
- Demonstrate a willingness and ability to resume self-care roles and responsibilities.

INTERVENTIONS

- Encourage patient to verbalize feelings about appearance and perceptions of life-style changes.
- Validate perceptions and assure that responses are appropriate.
- Promote acceptance of positive, realistic body image.
- Explore ways that the patient can cope with body image changes within their cultural expression.

NURSING DIAGNOSIS

Pain, risk for, related to side effects of treatment regimens

OUTCOME GOALS

Patient will be able to:
- Identify activities that increase or decrease pain
- Relate pain relief

Continued.

Table 24-12 Patient/Family Teaching Priorities

Topic	Before transplant	During transplant	After transplant
TRANSPLANT PROCESS			
Donor identification	X		
Tissue typing	X		
Recipient workup	X		
Donor workup	X		
Goal of transplant	X	X	
Duration of process	X	X	
Conditioning regimen	X	X	
Bone marrow harvest	X	X	
Immunosuppression	X	X	X
Unit environment	X	X	
CENTRAL VENOUS CATHETER			
Insertion	X	X	
Catheter care		X	X
ROUTINE CARE			
Hygiene/skin care	X	X	
Oral care	X	X	
Nutrition	X	X	
Infection precautions	X	X	
Bleeding precautions	X	X	
SIDE EFFECTS			
Nausea/vomiting	X	X	
Diarrhea	X	X	
Alopecia	X	X	
Stomatitis	X	X	
Seizures	X	X	
Hypotension	X	X	
Cystitis	X	X	
Acral erythema	X	X	
Conjunctivitis	X	X	
Fever	X	X	
Parotitis	X	X	
COMPLICATIONS			
Graft rejection	X	X	X
Infections	X	X	X
Pneumonitis	X	X	X
GVHD	X	X	X
Late effects	X	X	X
Recurrence	X	X	X
SUPPORTIVE CARE			
Blood components	X	X	X
Antibiotics	X	X	X
Antifungals	X	X	X
Antivirals	X	X	X
Parenteral nutrition	X	X	X
PSYCHOSOCIAL			
Coping strategies	X	X	X
Sexuality	X	X	X
Socialization	X	X	X
Resources	X	X	X

GVHD, Graft-versus-host disease.

Table 24-12 Patient/Family Teaching Priorities—cont'd

Topic	Before transplant	During transplant	After transplant
DISCHARGE			
Follow-up schedule		X	X
Medications		X	X
Diet		X	X
Activity	X	X	X
Precautions	X	X	X
Work/school	X	X	X
Emergency contact	X	X	X

INTERVENTIONS

- Assess patient's pain:
  —Location
  —Onset
  —Frequency
  —Intensity
  —Quality
- Identify effective pain control measures.
- Administer medications as ordered and needed.
- Assess for effectiveness of pain control measures.
- Intervene at onset of pain.
- Instruct patient in relaxation techniques (see Chapter 29).

NURSING DIAGNOSIS

- *Coping, ineffective individual, related to transplant process and potential life-style changes*

OUTCOME GOALS

Patient will be able to:
- Identify coping patterns and the consequences of the behavior that results
- Identify personal strengths and accept support

INTERVENTIONS

- Assess patient's level of distress and anxiety related to:
  —Uncertainty of future
  —Bothersome symptoms
  —Changes in self-concept
- Assess for signs of maladaptive or risky behaviors that interfere with responsible health practices.
- Identify patient's support system, resources, and communication patterns.
- Assess patient's ability to problem solve.
- Listen attentively and provide support.
- Encourage verbalization of fears.
- Assist patient with problem solving as needed.
- Provide reassurance that anxiety or distress are common feelings among transplant patients.
- Initiate referrals to social work, psychology, or community resources as appropriate (see Chapters 27 and 31).

NURSING DIAGNOSIS

- *Coping, ineffective family, compromised, related to transplant process* and *role changes*

OUTCOME GOALS

Patient/family will be able to:
- Identify responses that are neglectful or harmful
- Verbalize the need for assistance
- Access available community resources

INTERVENTIONS

- Assess past family relationships and coping patterns.
- Provide opportunities for family to express feelings.
- Assist family members in adapting to changes in roles and activities as appropriate.
- Listen attentively and provide support.
- Encourage communication and positive interaction between patient and family.
- Assess cultural issues that are unfamiliar.
- Initiate referrals to social work, psychology, or community resources as appropriate.

NURSING DIAGNOSIS

Fluid volume deficit or excess, risk for, related to compromised regulatory mechanisms, as evidenced by altered electrolytes

OUTCOME GOALS

Patient will be able to:
- Maintain normal fluid volume and electrolyte balance as evidenced by:
  —Normal blood and urinary laboratory values
  —Maintaining baseline weight
  —Normal skin turgor
  —Moist mucous membranes
  —Normal mentation

INTERVENTIONS

- Monitor patient's:
  —Intake and output
  —Weight
  —Abdominal girth

Continued.

—Edema
—Serum electrolytes
—Blood urea nitrogen
—Hemoglobin and hematocrit
• Assess patient for signs of fluid overload or dehydration.
• Administer diuretics as ordered.
• Maintain fluid restrictions as needed.

NURSING DIAGNOSIS

Growth and development, altered, related to late effects of treatment

OUTCOME GOALS

Patient will be able to:
• Demonstrate an increase in behaviors in personal, social, language, and cognition or motor activities appropriate for age-group

INTERVENTIONS

• Monitor patient's growth according to standard growth charts.
• Assess for accomplishments of normal growth and developmental tasks.
• Monitor for learning disabilities.
• Provide referrals for educational and emotional support as needed.
• Administer growth hormone as ordered and assess for response.

NURSING DIAGNOSIS

• *Infection, risk for, related to myelosuppression and immunosuppression*

OUTCOME GOAL

Patient will be able to:
• Be free of infection as evidenced by absence of fever (<38.5° C) and chills, pulse within normal limits, absence of adventitious breath sounds, absence of burning on urination, absence of redness or swelling at central line site, negative cultures

INTERVENTIONS

• Assess for signs and symptoms of infection:
—Fever
—Cough
—Erythema
• Institute measures to prevent exposure to potential sources of infection:
—Meticulous handwashing
—Meticulous hygiene
—Good oral hygiene after meals
• Monitor white blood count and differential.
• Monitor vital signs and head-to-toe systems assessments frequently.

• Obtain cultures of blood, urine, stool, sputum as ordered and appropriate.
• Administer antibiotics, antifungals, antivirals, and antipyretics as ordered.
• Instruct patient and family in prevention of infections.
• Monitor culture results and serum antibiotic levels as needed.
• Implement protective isolation precautions per hospital policy.
• Minimize invasive procedures.

NURSING DIAGNOSIS

• *Injury, risk for related to thrombocytopenia*

OUTCOME GOALS

Patient will be able to:
• Be aware of and report signs and symptoms of bleeding
• Demonstrate measures to prevent bleeding
• Demonstrate absence of bleeding

INTERVENTIONS

• Monitor platelet count and anticipate nadir.
• Assess for signs and symptoms of bleeding:
—Petechiae
—Ecchymosis
—Epistaxis
—Vaginal or rectal bleeding
• Administer platelet transfusions as ordered.
• Observe patient for signs of transfusion reaction and response to transfusions.
• Teach patient to avoid:
—Shaving with razor
—Flossing teeth
—Picking nose or scabs
—Forceful nose-blowing

NURSING DIAGNOSIS

• *Knowledge deficit related to transplant process*

OUTCOME GOALS

Patient/family will be able to:
• Discuss knowledge or experience related to BMT
• Discuss rationale for BMT
• Acknowledge potential therapeutic and adverse effects of BMT
• Describe medical and nursing interventions available and required during treatment

INTERVENTIONS

• Evaluate patient and family readiness to learn.
• Identify barriers to learning such as language, physical deficiencies, psychological deficiencies, intellectual development.

- Determine patient and family knowledge of the transplant process.
- Review information patient and family have already been given.
- Provide written or audiovisual education materials and review with patient and family; consider culture-sensitive materials.
- Allow adequate time for verbalization of questions, concerns, and fears.
- Reinforce and clairfy information as needed.

NURSING DIAGNOSIS

- *Nutrition, altered: less than body requirements, related to effects of treatment process*

OUTCOME GOALS

Patient will be able to:
- Report/maintain adequate nutritional status during periods of decreased oral intake
- Report strategies to manage altered taste
- Experience minimal or no nausea and vomiting

INTERVENTIONS

- Assess nutritional intake and monitor calorie counts.
- Assess for causes of decreased nutritional intake:
  —Nausea and vomiting
  —Xerostomia
  —Taste changes
- Provide small, frequent meals.
- Determine cultural preferences and meanings of foods.
- Initiate referral to dietician for assessment of food preferences and appropriateness of diet (see Chapter 27).

NURSING DIAGNOSIS

- *Sexuality patterns, altered, related to treatment process and to late effects*

OUTCOME GOALS

Patient/significant other will be able to:
- Share concerns regarding sexual function
- Express satisfaction with sexual patterns

INTERVENTIONS

- Assess for physical symptoms that may affect libido.
- Assess for fear, anxiety, depression, and diminished self-concept.
- Consider culture/sensitive interventions.
- Promote open communication about sexual issues by bringing up the subject.
- Instruct patient on appropriate hygiene and contraceptive measures (see Chapter 32).

NURSING DIAGNOSIS

- *Skin integrity, impaired, risk for, related to treatment process and to GVHD*

OUTCOME GOAL

Patient will be able to:
- Have intact skin and be free of infection

INTERVENTIONS

- Assess impaired area every shift for:
  —Color
  —Scaling
  —Bleeding
  —Drainage
  —Tenderness
- Avoid use of harsh soaps, hot water, perfume, deodorant, and oil-based creams.
- Maintain meticulous hygiene with antibacterial soap.
- Instruct patient to avoid activities and clothing that irritate affected areas.
- Instruct patient to avoid exposure to the sun and to use sun screen when outdoors.
- Use therapeutic beds and pain medications as needed for severe skin GVHD (see Chapters 29 and 30).

NURSING DIAGNOSIS

- *Management of therapeutic regimen, ineffective, risk for, related to posthospitalization follow-up*

OUTCOME GOALS

Patient/family will be able to:
- Explain and discuss treatment regimen, rationale of regimen, expectations of regimen, side effects of regimen, life-style changes needed, follow-up care needed, resources support available
- Relate an intent to practice health behaviors needed for recovery and prevention of complications

INTERVENTIONS

- Identify factors that influence learning.
- Explain the need for close follow-up after BMT.
- Explain the need to remain close to the BMT center for 100 days or as appropriate.
- Explain the expectations of family and caregiver.
- Explain home alterations needed.
- Provide written material.
- Consider culture-sensitive materials and interventions.

■ CHAPTER QUESTIONS

1. Side effects of the apheresis procedure include:
   a. Hypocalcemia, fatigue, anemia, thrombocytopenia
   b. Hypernatremia, fatigue, anemia, thrombocytopenia
   c. Hyponatremia, fatigue, anemia, leukopenia
   d. Hypocalcemia, fatigue, anemia, leukopenia
2. The purpose of mobilization in peripheral stem cell transplantation is:
   a. To stimulate the production of PBSCs to collect an adequate number in the least number of pheresis sessions
   b. To move as many PBSCs as possible through the cell collector in as short a time as possible
   c. To ensure that there are no tumor cells in the stem cell product
   d. To prevent occlusion of the central venous catheter during apheresis
3. Autologous bone marrow transplants are performed for all of the following diseases *except:*
   a. Breast cancer
   b. Ovarian cancer
   c. Aplastic anemia
   d. Leukemia
4. The following are all symptoms of VOD *except:*
   a. Weight gain
   b. Ascites
   c. Hepatomegaly
   d. Fever
5. Acute GVHD targets primarily which organs:
   a. Skin, liver, GI tract
   b. Skin, lungs, GI tract
   c. Skin, liver, lungs
   d. Liver, lungs, GI tract
6. Potential long-term side effects after BMT include all of the following *except:*
   a. Cataracts
   b. Infertility
   c. Secondary malignancy
   d. Acute GVHD
7. Measures to prevent GVHD include all of the following *except:*
   a. T-cell depletion
   b. Cyclosporin
   c. Tacrolimus
   d. Ganciclovir
8. Neutropenia, breakdown of physical barriers, and posttransplant immunosuppression increase the risk for:
   a. GVHD
   b. Infection
   c. VOD
   d. Graft failure

BIBLIOGRAPHY

1. Abramowsky CR, Coccia PF: Bone marrow transplantation in pediatrics. In Abramowsky CR, Colvin RB, editors: *Organ transplantation in children,* Basel, 1989, Karger.
2. Anderlini P, Przepiorka D: Allogeneic marrow transplantation. In Pazdur R, editor: *Medical oncology: a comprehensive review,* Huntington, NY, 1995, PRR.
3. Applebaum FR: Allogeneic bone marrow transplantation for treatment of malignancy. In Macdonald JS, Haller DG, Mayer RJ, editor: *Manual of oncologic therapeutics,* Philadelphia, 1995, Lippincott.
4. Atkinson K: Chronic graft-versus-host disease following marrow transplantation, *Marrow Transplant Rev* 2:1, 1992.
5. Ayash LJ and others: Hepatic venoocclusive disease in autologous bone marrow transplantation of solid tumors and lymphomas, *J Clin Oncol* 8:1699, 1990.
6. Ballester OF: Allogeneic bone marrow transplantation for multiple myeloma, *Semin Oncol* 20(suppl 6):5, 1993.
7. Barlogie B, Gahrton G: Bone marrow transplantation in multiple myeloma, *Bone Marrow Transplant* 7:71, 1991.
8. Belec RH: Quality of life: perceptions of long-term survivors of bone marrow transplantation, *Oncol Nurs Forum* 19:31, 1992.
9. Bell AJ and others: Peripheral blood stem cell autografting, *Lancet* 1:1027, 1986.
10. Benisinger WI, Berenson RJ: Peripheral blood and positive selection of marrow as a source of stem cells for transplantation, *Prog Clin Biol Res* 337:93, 1990.
11. Bierman PJ, Armitage JO: Autologous bone marrow transplantation. In Macdonald JS, Haller DG, Mayer RS, editors: *Manual of oncologic therapeutics,* Philadelphia, 1995, Lippincott.
12. *BMT Newsletter:* Peripheral stem cell transplants, 11:1, 1992.
13. *BMT Newsletter:* Cord blood transplants, 7:1, 1996.
14. Bolwell BJ: Autologous bone marrow transplantation for Hodgkin's disease and non-Hodgkin's lymphoma, *Semin Oncol* 21(suppl 7):4, 1994.
15. Buchsel PC, Kapustay PM: Peripheral stem cell transplantation, *Oncol Nurs* 2:2, 1995.
16. Castaigne S and others: Successful haematopoietic reconstitution using autologous peripheral blood mononucleated cells in a patient with acute promyelocytic leukemia, *Br J Haematol* 62:209, 1986.
17. Champlin RE: T-cell depletion for bone marrow transplantation: effects on graft rejection, graft-versus-host disease, graft-versus-leukemia, and survival, *Cancer Treat Res* 50:99, 1990.
18. Chielens D, Herrick E: Recipients of bone marrow transplants: making a smooth transition to an ambulatory care setting, *Oncol Nurs Forum* 17:857, 1990.
19. Crouch MA, Risse C: Post-induction autologous bone marrow transplantation. In Wujcik D, editor: *Nursing care issues in adult leukemia,* Huntington, NY, 1995, PRR.
20. Crouch MA, Ross JA: Current concepts in autologous bone marrow transplantation, *Semin Oncol Nurs* 10:1, 1994.
21. Deeg HJ: Delayed complications of marrow transplantation, *Marrow Transplant Rev* 2:10, 1992.
22. Donahue RE and others: Human IL-3 and GM-CSF act synergistically in stimulating hematopoiesis in primates, *Science* 241:1820, 1988.
23. Ersek M: The process of maintaining hope in adults undergoing bone marrow transplantation for leukemia, *Oncol Nurs Forum* 19:883, 1992.
24. Gale RP: Cord-blood-cell transplantation: a real sleeper, *N Engl J Med* 332:6, 1995.
25. Gale RP, Armitage JO, Dicke KA: Autotransplants: now and in the future, *Bone Marrow Transplant* 7:153, 1991.

26. Gaston-Johansson F, Franco T, Zimmerman L: Pain and psychological distress in patients undergoing autologous bone marrow transplantation, *Oncol Nurs Forum* 19:41, 1992.

27. Gorin NC: Autologous bone marrow transplantation in hematological malignancies, *Am J Clin Oncol* 14(suppl 1):S5, 1991.

28. Gould DA, Franco T: Allogeneic bone marrow transplantation, *Semin Oncol Nurs* 10:1, 1994.

29. Gould DA, Franco T: Allogeneic bone marrow transplantation. In Wujcik D, editor: *Nursing care issues in adult acute leukemia,* Huntington, NY, 1995, PRR.

30. Haas R and others: Successful autologous transplantation of blood stem cells mobilized with recombinant human granulocyte/macrophage colony-stimulating factor, *Exp Hematol* 18:94, 1990.

31. Janssen WE: Peripheral blood and bone marrow hematopoietic stem cells: are they the same? *Semin Oncol* 20(suppl 6):5, 1993.

32. Jones RJ: Autologous bone marrow transplantation in hematologic malignancies, *Curr Opin Oncol* 3:234, 1991.

33. Kessinger A: Autologous peripheral stem cell transplantation, *Marrow Transplant Rev* 2:5, 1992.

34. Kessinger A and others: Reconstitution of human hematopoietic function with autologous cryopreserved circulating stem cells, *Exp Hematol* 14:192, 1986.

35. Kessinger A and others: Cryopreservation and infusion of autologous peripheral stem cells, *Bone Marrow Transplant* 5:25, 1990.

36. King CR: Peripheral stem cell transplantation: past, present, and future. In Buchsel PC, Whedon MB editors: *Bone marrow transplantation: administrative and clinical strategies,* Boston, 1995, Jones and Bartlett.

37. Klob HJ, Bender-Gotze CH: Late complications after allogeneic bone marrow transplantation for leukaemia, *Bone Marrow Transplant* 6:61, 1990.

38. Klumpp TR: Complications of peripheral blood stem cell transplantation, *Semin Oncol* 22:3, 1995.

39. Korbling M and others: Autologous transplantation of blood-derived hematopoietic stem cells after myeloablative therapy in a patient with Burkitt's lymphoma, *Blood* 67:529, 1986.

40. Lum LG, Storb R: Bone marrow transplantation. In Flye MW, editor: *Principles of organ transplantation,* Philadelphia, 1989, Saunders.

41. Marks DI, Goldman JM: Bone marrow transplantation in chronic myelogenous leukemia, *Marrow Transplant Rev* 2:17, 1992.

42. McGlave P: Bone marrow transplants in chronic myelogenous leukemia: an overview of determinants of survival, *Semin Hematol* 27:23, 1990.

43. McMillan A, Goldstone A: What is the value of autologous bone marrow transplantation in the treatment of relapsed or resistant Hodgkin's disease? *Leuk Res* 15:237, 1991.

44. Miller AM: Hematopoietic growth factors in autologous bone marrow transplantation, *Semin Oncol* 20(suppl 6):5, 1993.

45. Moss TJ: Bone marrow transplantation for solid tumors in pediatrics, *Cancer Treat Res* 50:279, 1990.

46. Nemunaitis J: Growth factors in allogeneic transplantation, *Semin Oncol* 20(suppl 6):5, 1993.

47. *Oncology News International:* Cord blood is used as a source of stem cells for pediatric transplantation, 4:7, 1995.

48. Peters WP: The myeloid colony stimulating factors: introduction and overview, *Semin Hematol* 28(suppl 2):1, 1991.

49. Rabinowe SN and others: The impact of myeloid growth factors on engraftment following autologous bone marrow transplantation for malignant lymphoma, *Semin Hematol* 28(suppl 2):6, 1991.

50. Ramsey NK: Bone marrow transplantation in pediatric oncology. In Pizzo PA, Poplack DG editors: *Principles and practice of pediatric oncology,* Philadelphia, 1993, Lippincott.

51. Reiffers J and others: Successful autologous transplantation with peripheral blood hematopoietic cells in a patient with acute leukemia, *Exp Hematol* 14:312, 1986.

52. Rowe JM and others: Recommended guidelines for the management of autologous and allogeneic bone marrow transplantation, *Ann Intern Med* 120:2, 1994.

53. Rubenstein P and others: Stored placental blood for unrelated bone marrow reconstitution, *Blood* 81:7, 1993.

54. Sable CA, Donowitz GR: Infections in bone marrow transplant recipients, *Clin Infect Dis* 18(3):273, 1994.

55. Safah HF, Weiner RS: Veno-occlusive diseases following bone marrow transplantation, *Mediguide Oncol* 14:4, 1994.

56. Sanders JE: Bone marrow transplantation for pediatric leukemia, *Pediatr Ann* 20:12, 1991.

57. Seeger RC, Reynolds CP: Treatment of high-risk solid tumors of childhood with intensive therapy and autologous bone marrow transplantation, *Pediatr Clin North Am* 38:393, 1991.

58. Simone JV: Autologous bone marrow transplantation in childhood cancer, *J Clin Oncol* 11:8, 1993.

59. Stadtmauer EA, Schneider CJ, Silberstein LE: Peripheral blood progenitor cell generation and harvesting, *Semin Oncol* 22:3, 1995.

60. Steeves RH: Patients who have undergone bone marrow transplantation: their quest for meaning, *Oncol Nurs Forum* 19:899, 1992.

61. Stuart RK: Autologous bone marrow transplantation for leukemia, *Semin Oncol* 20(suppl 6):5, 1994.

62. Sullivan KM: Prevention and treatment of chronic graft-versus-host disease, *Marrow Transplant Rev* 2:8, 1992.

63. Tilly H and others: Haemopoietic reconstitution after autologous peripheral blood stem cell transplantation in acute leukemia, *Lancet* 11:154, 1986.

64. Tutschka PJ: Early complications of bone marrow transplantation in children and adults, *Bone Marrow Transplant* 4(suppl 4):22, 1989.

65. Ueno NT, Champlin RE: Autologous transplantation: basic concepts and controversies. In Pazdur R, editor: *Medical oncology: a comprehensive review,* Huntington, NY, 1995, PRR.

66. Ulich TR and others: Acute and subacute hematologic effects of multi-colony stimulating factor in combination with granulocyte colony stimulating factor in vivo, *Blood* 75:48, 1990.

67. Varterasian ML: Biologic and clinical advances in multiple myeloma, *Oncology* 9:5, 1995.

68. Vitale V, Barra S, Frazone P: Total body irradiation in the conditioning regimen for hematological malignancies, *Bone Marrow Transplant* 8(suppl 1):28, 1991.

69. Volker DL: Clinical characteristics of cytomegalovirus infection, *Nurs Acumen* 3:1, 1992.

70. Vose JM, Armitage JO, Bierman PJ: Bone marrow transplantation for Hodgkin's disease, non-Hodgkin's lymphoma, and multiple myeloma, *Cancer Treat Res* 50:259, 1990.

71. Vose JM, Armitage JO, Kessinger A: High-dose chemotherapy and autologous transplant with peripheral-blood stem cells, *Oncology* 7:8, 1993.

72. Walker F, Roethke SK, Martin G: An overview of the rationale, process, and nursing implications of peripheral blood stem cell transplantation, *Cancer Nurs* 17:2, 1994.

73. Welte K: Matched unrelated transplants, *Semin Oncol Nurs* 10:1, 1994.

74. Whedon MB, editor: *Bone marrow transplantation: principles, practice and nursing insights,* Boston, 1991, Jones and Bartlett.

75. Whedon MB: Cytomegalovirus-seronegative autologous bone marrow transplant patient, *Nurs Acumen* 3:4, 1992.

76. Whedon MB, Ferrell BR: Quality of life in adult bone marrow transplant patients: beyond the first year, *Semin Oncol Nurs* 10:1, 1994.

77. Winer EP, Sutton LM: Quality of life after bone marrow transplant, *Oncology* 8:1, 1994.

78. Wingard JR: Infections in allogeneic bone marrow transplant recipients, *Semin Oncol* 20(suppl 6):5, 1993.

79. Wujcik D, Ballard B, Camp-Sorrell D: Selected complications of allogeneic bone marrow transplantation, *Semin Oncol Nurs* 10:1, 1994.

CHAPTER 25
Cancer Clinical Trials

SUSAN BRENNAN GIACALONE

As a medical and nursing specialty, oncology has grown rapidly over the past 20 years. The efforts of a nationwide network of physicians and nurses performing clinical trials have resulted in improved surgical outcomes, new chemotherapeutic agents, less toxic radiation therapy, and the testing of numerous biologic agents and growth hormones. Many cancers that were once fatal are now curable, and many other cancers now are considered chronic diseases, with many long-term survivors. Nurses are at the forefront of this battle against cancer. Oncology nurses now administer first-time treatments to patients. In clinical trials, nurses ensure that treatments are given safely and that patients are monitored closely for known and unknown side effects. Nurses perform numerous expanded roles in all phases of clinical trials, but they are much more than mere participants. Nurses are independent clinical researchers who study the human response to diseases and treatments. Clinical trial patients present nurses with the opportunity to identify and study the effects, responses, and sequelae of new medical therapies and to define appropriate nursing interventions.

This chapter provides the framework for understanding the history, purpose, and implementation of clinical trials. The roles of the oncology nurse as direct caregiver, educator, advocate, coordinator, administrator, and researcher are discussed.

HISTORICAL PERSPECTIVE

The U.S. federal government founded the National Institutes of Health (NIH) in 1887. The purpose of the NIH is to support research into the causes, diagnosis, prevention, and cure of human disease.[55] As one of the largest biomedical research facilities in the world, the NIH is part of the U.S. Department of Health and Human Services (DHHS).

Many of the early clinical trials in the United States focused on the prophylaxis and treatment of infectious diseases.[54] By the 1930s, cancer was identified as a major health problem requiring a large-scale national plan of action. In 1937 Congress unanimously passed the *National Cancer Institute Act,* which appropriated $700,000 to establish the National Cancer Institute (NCI), now the largest of the 12 NIH institutes. The NCI expected to break new theoretic ground by conducting its own research, promoting research in other institutions, and coordinating cancer-related activities throughout the United States.[14] The NCI underwent numerous reorganizations and expansions over the next decades.

The Warren Grant Magnuson Clinical Center was established in 1953 on the NIH campus. The center is shared by the NIH institutes that are conducting combined laboratory and clinical studies. Both inpatients and ambulatory care patients from all over the world participate in cancer clinical trials at this facility. Travel, nursing care, and medical care are provided to these patients at no cost.[55]

The trials performed within the NIH clinical center are called *intramural research studies. Extramural research studies* trials are those NCI-sponsored studies conducted at universities, medical schools, and hospitals across the United States. Extramural trials are supported by grants, contracts, or cooperative agreements and use about 80% of the funds appropriated to the NIH by the U.S. Congress.[55]

The post–World War II years brought successes in cancer treatment with the development of new chemotherapeutic agents. The *National Chemotherapy Program,* funded through congressional appropriations in 1955, was devoted to testing new chemicals that might prove to be effective antineoplastic agents. The Cancer Chemotherapy National Service Center at the NCI functioned as a pharmaceutical house to move new drugs into both the intramural and the extramural trials. In 1965 the program expanded to include international drugs.

The motivated efforts of a public and private campaign ultimately resulted in the signing of the *National Cancer Act* in 1971. This created a national cancer program administered by the NCI, with its director appointed by and reporting to the president of the United States. This legislation was a landmark in the history of cancer treatment and research. Increased power and funding created new opportunities for physicians, improving the quality and increasing the accessibility of cancer care for patients across the United States.

In 1991, on the twentieth anniversary of the National Cancer Act, Harold Freeman, chairman of the President's Cancer Panel, testified before a house panel and listed the following accomplishments in cancer treatment[10]:

- Fewer amputations for osteosarcoma patients
- A 50% survival rate for patients with acute lymphocytic leukemia, improved from 28%
- Improvement in 5-year survival rate of women with breast cancer from 85% to 91%
- Prostate cancer 5-year survival rate of 71%, up from 50%

The following programs, initiated by the NCI since 1971, increased the number of cancer specialists and organized a structure to coordinate national research and to translate research advances into clinical practice.

Oncology Training Programs

The NCI funded fellowship programs in medical oncology and radiotherapy. There were 100 medical oncologists in the 1960s; now there are more than 4000.[14] The first certifying examinations for medical oncologists were in 1974. The increased numbers of radiation therapists and medical oncologists allowed movement of this specialty from predominantly university settings into community hospitals and into many less urban settings.

Comprehensive Cancer Centers

The National Cancer Act of 1971 formally authorized the *Cancer Centers Program*.[14] The NCI was challenged to develop a network of specialized and comprehensive cancer centers to serve as a national resource for research and a multidisciplinary treatment approach, as well as a community resource through outreach programs and cancer control.[13] Designation as a comprehensive cancer center requires meeting eight criteria established by the NCI: (1) basic research, (2) mechanisms for technology transfer, (3) clinical research, (4) program of high-priority clinical trials, (5) cancer prevention and control research, (6) research training and continuing education programs, (7) cancer information services, and (8) community service and outreach activities.[13] In 1995 there were 27 comprehensive cancer centers, a tremendous increase since the year of the National Cancer Act, when there were only three.

Cooperative Research Groups

Cooperative research groups consist of researchers who jointly develop and conduct cancer treatment clinical trials in a multiinstitutional setting.[13] These groups are funded by the NCI through cooperative agreements. The cooperative group program started with the National

Chemotherapy Service Center funding in 1955. The original purpose of the groups was to test the new chemotherapeutic agents developed at the NCI. The scope of the program has broadened through the years, and current areas of research include evaluation of multimodality therapies, basic science, supportive care, quality of life, and chemoprevention trials.[13] The results of cooperative group research are reported through group-wide meetings and published in scientific journals.

The goals of cooperative group research are the following[14]:

- To improve survival and quality of life for cancer patients
- To conduct basic scientific research into cancer biology, pathology, epidemiology, and supportive care
- To serve as a research base for the implementation of cancer control research
- To conduct oncology nursing research

Cooperative groups share common goals but may differ in their clinical focus. The focus may be the multimodality treatment of all adult cancers or all pediatric cancers. Other groups focus on a specific type of cancer or specific type of treatment. Currently, 13 cooperative groups are funded by the NCI (see box below). The names of certain groups may imply a geographic focus (Southwest Oncology Group), but they include members from across the United States and from some international locations as well.

Cooperative groups are generally similar in structure. They are composed of an operations office, statistical center, and various standing committees. The *operations office* manages the administrative affairs of the group and houses the group chairman. The *statistical center*, which

---

NCI-FUNDED COOPERATIVE RESEARCH GROUPS

Brain Tumor Cooperative Group (BTCG)
Cancer and Leukemia Group B (CALGB)
Children's Cancer Study Group (CCSG)
Eastern Cooperative Oncology Group (ECOG)
European Organization for Research and Treatment of Cancer (EORTC)
Gynecological Oncology Group (GOG)
Intergroup Rhabdomyosarcoma Study (IRS)
National Surgical Adjuvant Project for Breast and Bowel Cancers (NSABP)
National Wilms' Tumor Study (NWTS)
North Central Cancer Treatment Group (NCCTG)
Pediatric Oncology Group (POG)
Radiation Therapy Oncology Group (RTOG)
Southwest Oncology Group (SWOG)

may be in a different location, houses the group biostatistician and protocol data coordinators. This office handles protocol registration, quality control of data, and ongoing statistical analysis of protocols. Each cooperative group has *standing disease and discipline committees* that represent the group's focus.[85]

The role of oncology nurses in cooperative research groups has strengthened over the past decade. Most cooperative groups have a standing nurse oncologist committee, with the chairperson being a member of the board of governors. Nurses review protocols before activation to assess the impact of the proposed treatment on the nursing unit. Nurses also are principal investigators or co-investigators on companion studies and cancer control studies. The issue of nursing research in clinical trials is addressed later in this chapter. Nurses may be involved in the research process as independent researchers, co-investigators, protocol coordinators, or clinical research associates (historically referred to as *data managers*).

Community-Based Research Programs

Cooperative Group Outreach Program. The Cooperative Group Outreach Program (CGOP), implemented in 1976, was the NCI's first comprehensive effort to extend participation in clinical trials to community physicians. The objectives of the program are to make state-of-the-art cancer treatment available to patients in the community setting, adding to the pool of patients available for clinical trials. The program consists of individual community oncologists, surgeons, or radiation therapists contracting with a member institution of a cooperative group to register patients for research protocols. The amount of funding the CGOPs receive is based on the number of eligible patients they enter into studies.[13]

Community Clinical Oncology Program. The Community Clinical Oncology Program (CCOP) was initiated by the NCI in 1983 to disseminate state-of-the-art cancer research to patients in community settings. CCOP institutions are groups of community-based physicians who are linked to cooperative groups and cancer centers that serve as their research bases.[13]

This mechanism is beneficial to the patients, the community, and the NCI. Patients now have access to investigational therapies without traveling to a geographically distant treatment center. The local medical community benefits through opportunities for education and exchange of information. The NCI benefits by having available more patients potentially eligible for registration on clinical trials.

All studies available for CCOP participation through the 17 research bases are assigned a "credit" value by the NCI. Generally, treatment studies are assigned one to two credits per patient depending on the complexity of the study. CCOPs are required to accrue at least 50 treatment credits each year.

Minority-based CCOPs. The CCOP model was expanded in 1993 when the NCI funded 13 minority-based CCOPs. These are located in areas that serve ethnic minorities and poor populations. Minority-based CCOPs accrue patients for both treatment studies and cancer control studies.

Cancer control. Cancer control is the reduction of cancer incidence, morbidity, and mortality through an orderly sequence from research or interventions (including their impact on populations) to the broad, systematic appreciation of the research results.[35] With the National Cancer Act in 1971, cancer control activities were formalized as part of the National Cancer Program and recognized as a distinct program entity. With the creation of the Division of Cancer Control and Rehabilitation (DCPC) at the NCI in 1974, a national effort for effective intervention was made possible for the first time.[37] DCPC research priorities include tobacco-use control; diet, nutrition, and cancer prevention; chemoprevention; early detection; and access to state-of-the-art diagnosis and treatment.

Because of the relatively large number of participants required to complete cancer control research, it is frequently implemented through the cooperative group mechanism. Each cooperative group has a standing cancer control committee composed of interested oncology nurses, physicians, epidemiologists, and statisticians. Cancer control concepts are developed and submitted to the DCPC for review. Once the concept is approved, a protocol is developed and resubmitted to the NCI for final review, approval, and eventual activation by the research group. In 1986 the NCI mandated CCOP participation in cancer control research. CCOPs are required to accrue 50 cancer control credits per year. Cancer control studies are usually assigned a portion of credit (0.1, 0.3, 0.5) per patient registered.[13]

Oncology nurses, well versed in the mechanisms of clinical trials, are primarily responsible for the implementation, data collection, and conduct of the study.[40] Oncology nurses may evolve into independent prevention investigators in trials that treat well populations with essentially toxic agents.[88] Table 25-1 lists examples of current NCI-approved cancer control trials.[85]

Non-NCI-Supported Research

Although the NCI supports a large network of cancer centers, cooperative research groups, and community programs, most cancer clinical trials are not NCI sponsored. Comprehensive cancer centers and university hospitals contribute patients to NCI studies, but they also conduct their own cancer research activities. These research studies are developed by physician investigators

Table 25-1 Examples of Current NCI-Approved Cancer Control Trials

Trial*	Description
SWOG-9041	Phase III pilot study on chemoprevention of recurrent adenomas and second primary colorectal carcinoma†
NSABP P1	Clinical trial to determine efficacy of tamoxifen in preventing breast cancer†
SWOG-9201 RTOG 91-11	Phase II trial to preserve larynx: induction chemotherapy and radiation therapy versus concomitant chemotherapy and radiation therapy
SWOG-9221 RTOG-9113	Phase III double-blind trial of 13-*cis*-retinoic acid (13-CRA) to prevent second primary tumors (SPTs) in stage 1 non–small cell lung cancer†
RTOG-9115	Chemoprevention trial to prevent SPTs with 13-CRA in head and neck cancer†

*See box, p. 642, for group names represented by acronyms.
†High priority.

in their own institution. Studies include early trials with new chemotherapeutic or biologic agents and comparative randomized trials to identify new or more effective drug combinations. Cancer clinical trials are also conducted by radiation therapists in these institutions.

The pharmaceutical industry sponsors many clinical trials to evaluate new agents. The pharmaceutical company contracts with institutions or individual investigators to register patients in their studies. In recent years there has been a striking increase in clinical trials conducted by private pharmaceutical firms, largely related to a marked expansion in the field of biotherapeutics.[13]

DRUG DEVELOPMENT

The NCI is the largest single sponsor of studies using antineoplastic agents. More than 100 such agents are currently in clinical testing, and even more are in preclinical testing.[13] New drugs are also developed by pharmaceutical companies. Agents at the NCI are developed through the Investigational Drug Branch (IDB), a division of the Cancer Therapy and Evaluation Program (CTEP). The development of new agents, whether through IDB or industry, is extremely costly in terms of labor, time, and financial resources.

Identification

The first and most obvious step is the discovery of the new agent. Two basic approaches exist for the selection of chemicals to be tested: the empiric and the rational. The *empiric approach* is a systematic screening of chemicals from a wide variety of plant, animal, and min-

eral sources. For example, bryostatin 1, an agent currently under study, is derived from marine animals,[76] and vincristine, an effective commercially available drug, was extracted from the *Vinca* alkaloid plant. Natural products are emphasized because of the observation that many human diseases are successfully treated by these substances.[17]

Drawbacks of the traditional discovery process are that thousands of substances must be screened to find one that has activity in human cancer. After investing large amounts of time and money, it is still unknown why the response is produced or how it may be improved. *Rational drug design* addresses these shortcomings by attempting to identify the cell receptor site responsible for a given effect and, through a systematic process, specifically design compounds to stimulate or inhibit the receptor. Techniques of molecular biology refined in the biotechnology industry and computer technology aid in this process. The Division of Cancer Treatment at the NCI has established a grant program, the National Cooperative Drug Discovery Groups. These groups promote collaboration among scientists from academia, government, and industry in developing new cancer agents.[27,53,54]

Drug Screening

Identified compounds are entered into the NCI's Division of Cancer Treatment's drug testing program. Computer analysis and application of specific criteria for selection reduce the chance of duplicating drugs already under evaluation. The NCI selects approximately 10,000 of the 40,000 available substances for further testing.[39] These 10,000 compounds then undergo a screening process that uses both animal and human tumor systems. The tumor system most frequently used from 1955 to 1975 was the murine L1210 leukemia system. Tumors of uniform and predictable behavior were transplanted into mice, and the new drugs were given to the mice to evaluate tumor shrinkage and prolonged survival. This screening system was eventually found to be effective in selecting drugs active against leukemias and lymphomas but ineffective against solid tumors.[17] Now the initial screening is performed in a system called the *P388 mouse leukemia*. Approximately 250 agents will demonstrate antitumor effect in this system and advance to a tumor panel consisting of human tumors transplanted into immunodeprived ("nude") mice. The current panel includes L1210 leukemia, B16 melanoma, M5076 mouse tumor, and MX-1, a human mammary xenograft.[39] The agent must show efficacy against at least one of the tumors to advance to further testing. The human tumor cloning system developed in 1980 can grow human cancer cells in culture for the purpose of anticancer drug screening. This system has identified effective drugs that showed no activity in the P388 screening system.[17]

Formulation and Production

Ten of the compounds that successfully pass through the screening system will be selected for identification, purification, and definition of chemical structure. Large amounts of the drug must be produced so that there is sufficient quantity for further testing. The agent Taxol (paclitaxel) is a recent example of a drug production problem. This agent, known to be effective against ovarian cancer and possibly lung and breast cancer, is found in the bark of the Pacific yew tree. A huge volume of yew bark must be harvested to produce even small quantities of Taxol. Because a particular type of owl, an endangered species, inhabits these trees, debate erupted among the scientific community, conservationists, and the government. Currently, clinical trials are in progress using an agent known as docetaxel. This agent is produced from the leaves of the Pacific yew rather than the bark, thereby preserving the tree and the dependent wildlife.

Toxicity Testing

Preclinical testing for drug toxicity is required once formulation and production problems are solved. Usually, seven to nine compounds are tested per year. The goals of toxicology studies are to predict the safest starting dose for clinical trials and to determine if and when organ system toxicity occurs.[27] Toxicity testing is done in mice. Testing formerly was done in a number of larger animals, but this was expensive and did not increase the safety of the drugs.[17] The mice are used to develop a dose-response curve. The lethal dose in 10%, 50%, and 90% of the animals is determined. The dose that is lethal in 10% of the mice, called the *LD10,* is used to establish an initial dose for human trials. To maximize safety, if an unknown compound is being given in humans, only 10% of the LD10 is used at first.

Investigational New Drug Application

Before a drug can be studied in humans, its sponsor, either the NCI or a pharmaceutical company, submits an Investigational New Drug Application (IND) to the Food and Drug Administration (FDA) to request permission to evaluate the agent in human cancer.[88] The sponsor may begin to investigate the drug 30 days after the FDA has received the application.[58] The development process for a new drug is lengthy and costly, taking approximately 12 years and 50 to 70 million dollars from screening to commercial availability.[39]

Physician Approval

Physicians participating in the human clinical trials of investigational drugs must first be approved by the FDA. The FDA requires that these physicians, through medical training and experience, can assume responsibility for compliance with the protocol requirements for drug ad-

ministration, data monitoring, and toxicity reporting. The physicians sign an agreement that outlines their responsibilities in clinical research—Form FDA 1573.[50]

Clinical trials are carefully controlled experiments aimed at using the smallest number of subjects to determine with statistical confidence the effectiveness of treatments while maintaining patient safety.[53] The primary goal of clinical cancer research is to identify treatments that ultimately translate into improved quality of life and improved survival.[66]

Two major steps must occur before a clinical trial is implemented: (1) the design and writing of the cancer treatment protocol and (2) the approval of regulatory boards.

CANCER PROTOCOLS

A protocol is a formal document written to clearly describe the proposed experiment.[66] Both cancer treatment and cancer control experiments are written as protocol documents. *Protocols* provide the rationale for the proposed study, the study objectives or questions to be answered, and a concise description of the treatment involved. Protocols are written in a similar format and contain the same basic elements regardless of whether the study originates in a cancer center, cooperative group, or pharmaceutical company. The protocol is written by the principal investigator and must be approved by the study sponsor before distribution to participating investigators. The protocol is then followed by everyone involved in the study: physicians, nurses, data managers, pharmacists, study sponsor, and statisticians. The protocol document may be revised or amended as needed by the study sponsor throughout the course of the clinical trial. It is helpful to have a set of protocol notebooks with all the active studies near the area (hospital oncology unit or clinic setting) where protocol patients are evaluated and treated.

Table 25-2 lists the basic elements of a protocol, describes the purpose of each element, and presents nursing actions to be taken in evaluating and treating protocol patients.

ETHICAL ISSUES AND REGULATIONS

Before a clinical trial can be initiated in an institution, certain ethical and regulatory conditions must be met. First, the study must be approved for human use by the institutional review board, and the patient must voluntarily give his or her consent to participate.

Historical Perspective

These conditions, aimed at the protection of human subjects, developed over the past 50 years. The Nuremberg

Table 25-2 Protocol Elements, Purpose, and Nursing Interventions

Protocol element	Purpose	Nursing interventions
Objectives Background	Defines intent of study Describes previous studies and justification for current study	Understand objectives and background of study and incorporate them in patient/family teaching plan to ensure adequacy of informed consent process and to enhance patient's understanding and compliance.
Drug information	Describes animal toxicology studies, human toxicity previously observed, mechanisms of drug action, drug storage, preparation, administration, supplier	Have adequate knowledge of drugs, especially investigational drugs, before drug administration. Demonstrate knowledge of safe dose range, expected side effects, correct preparation, administration, and organs of drug excretion and metabolism.
Patient eligibility	Defines parameters of patient participation: Disease confirmation Major organ function Performance status Medical history	Accurately assess patient's cancer history and previous treatments applicable to eligibility. Evaluate patient's performance status. Evaluate required hematologic and chemistry results. Assess radiologic tests for bidimensionally measurable disease. Ensure all prestudy tests are performed within required time frame.
Treatment plan	Details initial and subsequent doses, administration guidelines and schedule, duration of treatment	Verify body surface area (BSA) for all doses and initial and subsequent dose calculations. Validate method of drug administration. Ensure correct dose modifications for subsequent courses based on criteria defined by protocol. Provide patient/family teaching regarding side effects, self-care, and administration schedule for drugs. Administer additional medications as needed, including antiemetics, laxatives, and antidiarrheal agents.
Study parameters	Schedule of required evaluations and treatment	Provide patient/family teaching about follow-up blood counts, office visits, hospitalizations, and appointments for scans and x-ray films. Ensure required tests are performed, with results available before ordering the next treatment. Provide patient/family with phone numbers of appropriate contacts for questions.
Criteria for response	Defines response: Complete remission Partial remission Stable disease Increasing disease	Demonstrate knowledge of current disease status. Assess patient's response at required intervals per protocol, incorporating physical examination findings and radiologic and biochemical results. Give emotional support to patient during response evaluation. Note any change in response requiring change in treatment plan.
Discipline review	Verification of correct pathologic diagnosis and radiation therapy by a designated review panel	Ensure required slides, blood samples, films, etc., are submitted to correct address within required time. Coordinate these activities with other departments (laboratory, pathology, radiation therapy).
Data submission	Defines required data forms and submission intervals	Complete data forms, ensuring all submitted information is found in patient's medical record. Verify accurate documentation of treatment, required laboratory and radiology parameters, toxicity and response evaluations. Submit within time constraints of research group.

Table 25-2 Protocol Elements, Purpose, and Nursing Interventions—cont'd

Protocol element	Purpose	Nursing interventions
Statistical considerations	Defines accrual goals, study design, statistical analysis	Know expected number of patients to be accrued and expected length of study.
Toxicity criteria	Grading of treatment-related toxicities according to standardized scale	Ensure use of correct scale.
		Accurately assess and document toxicities in patient chart.
		Record toxicity grade on flow sheets at required intervals.
		Distinguish between side effects of disease and treatment.
		Provide patient/family teaching regarding symptom management.
		Implement appropriate medical and nursing interventions to lessen morbidity of disease process or treatment or both.
Informed consent	Sample form that must be modified to meet institutional guidelines	Verify institutional review board (IRB) approval date before patient registration; all protocols must be initially approved, followed by annual full board review.
		Verify patient has given informed consent before telephone registration. Provide patient with copy of consent.
Adverse drug reaction (ADR) reporting	Defines ADR and reporting responsibilities	Demonstrate knowledge of previously reported drug toxicities.
		Inform physician of possible observed ADR.
		Do thorough clinical investigation to determine whether adverse effect is caused by study drug.
		Notify appropriate authorities, and submit required reporting forms according to time frame.

trials of 1947 exposed the horrors of human experimentation performed on Nazi concentration camp prisoners during World War II. In 1949 the *Nuremberg Code* set forth standards for physicians and scientists conducting biomedical experiments on human subjects.[86] These codes set forth the absolute requirement of "voluntary consent of the human subject."[74] Unfortunately, several examples of subject abuse in medical research occurred in the United States. There was no regulation on clinical research in the United States before 1960. The Tuskegee Study, begun in Macon County, Alabama, in 1932 under the auspices of the U.S. Public Health Service, left hundreds of black men with syphilis untreated so that long-range effects of the disease could be studied. This study, intended to last 6 months, continued until 1973, when the Department of Health, Education, and Welfare halted it only after the national media reported the story the year before.[33,52,76] Another example of failure to disclose research information was the Willowbrook experiment, conducted between 1956 and 1970 on 700 to 800 retarded children. Consent was given by parents to enroll their children in this study to better understand hepatitis and to possibly develop more effective vaccines. Incentives were used to gain parental consent, including

earlier admission of their child to the hospital and better hospitalization conditions for children in the study.[52,87]

The *Helsinki Declaration,* passed by the World Health Organization (WHO) in 1964 and revised in 1975, provided recommendations to guide physicians in biomedical research.[54] In the United States in 1966 the first research regulations were issued by the surgeon general's office requiring internal review for all research protocols.[33,59] The Congress strengthened this regulation in 1974 by passing the *National Research Act* (Public Law 98-348), which required review of all research with human subjects by an institutional review board (IRB) before any grants or contracts could be funded.[33,59] The National Commission for the Protection of Human Subjects of Biomedical and Behavioral Research ("the commission") was created by the 1974 National Research Act. The commission published a series of reports and recommendations on human research. This information, known as the *Belmont Report,* was published in 1979.[5] The three ethical principles stated in the Belmont report are as follows:

1. Respect for persons *(autonomy)*
2. Minimization of risk and maximization of benefits to the subjects *(beneficence)*

3. Fairness in the distribution of research burdens and benefits *(justice)*

These three principles are the foundation of the IRB and informed consent.

Institutional Review Boards

To protect human subjects from research abuses, the DHHS requires all federally funded institutions to have IRBs. The Office for Protection from Research Risks (OPRR) is the administrative subdivision of DHHS that negotiates assurances of compliance with individual institutions.

The *assurance program* requires that all investigational clinical protocols are subjected to full board review before human research subjects can be recruited and at least annually thereafter. Each institution must send IRB certification information to the cooperative group's operations office.

The IRB is composed of at least five members with professional competence, experience, and qualifications. The board should include both men and women and should represent a variety of backgrounds, races, and cultural considerations. At least one member should be a nonmedical professional, and one person must have no direct affiliation with the institution performing the research.

The protocol review process provides the investigator, the institution, and the patient with the assurance that the research is medically and ethically sound.[54]

Informed Consent

Before a research subject can be registered on an IRB-approved research study, the DHHS requires that informed consent must be given by the subject. *Informed consent* is defined as "the knowing consent of an individual or his legally authorized representative so situated as to be able to exercise free power of choice without inducement or any element of force, fraud, deceit, distress, or any other form of constraint or coercion."[16]

Information must be provided in a language understandable to the subject. It is not complete unless the patient understands what he or she has been told and is able to use the information to decide whether to participate in the study. The physician must verify that the patient understood what was read and heard. Patients must be allowed to ask questions, and the physician should question the patient to determine the patient's level of understanding.

The required elements of informed consent include the following[55]:

• Statement of research, purpose of the research, expected duration of participation, and description of procedures, including identification of any experimental procedures
• Description of risks and benefits of the study treatment

• Disclosure of alternative procedures or treatments that may be advantageous to the subject
• Description of confidentiality; disclosure of possibility of FDA inspection
• Explanation as to whether compensation and medical treatments are available if injury occurs
• Whom to contact about research, patient's rights, and research-related injury
• Instruction that participation is voluntary and results in no penalty or loss of benefits to which the subject is otherwise entitled

Inclusion of Women and Minorities in Clinical Trials

To date, the cancer clinical trials that have been conducted nationally have included relatively few poor and minority participants. This can be explained partly by a lack of access to health care of such populations, as well as the failure of researchers to accommodate cultural and economic variables when planning and conducting clinical trials.[26]

When such populations were represented in adequate numbers in clinical trials, it has been noted that by controlling for socioeconomic status, one can greatly reduce and in some instances nearly eliminate the apparent mortality and disparity of occurrence of cancer among and between ethnic groups and economic levels.[27] This finding has provided the impetus for additional mandates from the NIH for the development of active recruitment procedures at designated comprehensive cancer centers to ensure adequate representation of women and minorities, or these centers may risk losing funding and comprehensive cancer center designation. In addition, the American Cancer Society (ACS), the American Society of Cancer Institutes, and the Association of Community Cancer Centers have come forth in recent years to endorse appropriate representation of women and minorities in clinical trials and to encourage the public and health care professionals alike to consider protocol therapy when and where it exists.[65] The challenge to health care providers in dealing with those patients who may not have adequate insurance or access to care is to avoid segregating them from cancer clinical trial participation based on barriers that could be broken down with a committed effort by providers and administrators within health care centers.[26]

PHASES OF CLINICAL RESEARCH

There are four phases of clinical trials in humans: I, II, III, and IV.

Phase I

The purpose of a phase I trial is to determine the maximum tolerated dose (MTD) in humans, to determine the most effective schedule of administration, and to identify and quantify toxic effects in normal organ systems. Studying the pharmacokinetics of the agent, including drug absorption, distribution, metabolism, and excretion, is a primary aim of these trials. The previous animal testing helps predict human toxicities, but careful and frequent monitoring of all human organ systems is required to define the dose-limiting toxicities.

Patients eligible for phase I trials have often been heavily pretreated with available standard therapies before having entered the study. Major organ function must meet the study eligibility criteria; life expectancy is required to be at least 1 to 2 months; and toxicity from previous treatments must be resolved. Objectively measurable disease is usually not a requirement in these trials, since therapeutic response is not an endpoint of the study.

The initial drug dose in a phase I trial is one tenth of the dose that was lethal to 10% of the mice in toxicity testing. Three patients are entered at this dose, each about a week apart. Patients are then observed for toxicity for a specified period. When no irreversible, life-threatening, or fatal toxicities have occurred, three more patients are entered at the next higher dose level. The MTD is usually defined within five dose escalations; thus a phase I trial requires 15 to 20 subjects.[39] The escalation of doses in tiers of patients is called the *Fibonacci search method*.[17] Efforts are underway to attempt to expedite dose escalation by using pharmacologic data to determine the starting dose, to guide dose escalation, and to define the MTD using fewer subjects.[53]

Antitumor response or lack of response does not contribute directly to moving the agent into phase II trials. Drugs are selected based on suggestion of therapeutic benefit. An effective agent may not produce responses in phase I trials because the optimal dose and schedule is unknown at the initiation of phase I studies.[54]

Phase I trials are usually performed in single institutions so that the data can be monitored very closely by the study sponsor. Data are submitted biweekly, and study summaries are required every 6 months to comply with FDA regulations. The first occurrence of any toxic reaction is reported by telephone to the Cancer Therapy and Evaluation Program for NCI-sponsored drugs to allow rapid information dissemination to other investigators using the agent.[17]

Not all cancer trials involve the use of chemotherapeutic agents. Trials may also investigate biologics, radiation therapies, surgical interventions, mechanical devices, or psychometric tools.[10] Cancer control studies all progress through the three phases of clinical trials.

Phase II

Phase II evaluation of a new anticancer drug is designed to determine whether the compound has objective anti-tumor activity in a variety of cancers. Attention is focused on the types of tumors that respond and the dose-response relationship. Unlike phase I studies, these trials are disease oriented. It is impossible to test the new drug for all types of cancer to determine which ones respond, so the Drug Development Program of the NCI's Division of Cancer Treatment evolved the concept of signal tumors. These *signal tumors* include breast cancer, colorectal cancer, lung cancer, melanoma, acute leukemia, and lymphoma. These represent the minimum number of cancers against which the new drug must be evaluated. This panel includes tumors that are at opposite extremes in sensitivity to chemotherapy and those that are leading causes of cancer deaths.[39] If a drug is inactive in these patients, it is likely to be inactive in other tumors.

Eligibility for a phase II study does require measurable or evaluable lesions, since these areas are followed for tumor response. Depending on the drug and disease under study, previous treatment with chemotherapy and other treatment modalities may or may not be allowed. Adequate hematologic, hepatic, renal, and cardiac parameters are specified by the protocol. Life expectancy of at least 8 weeks is required, and patients must be capable of partial self-care to be eligible for most phase II trials.

The phase II study is a plan to ensure that adequate numbers of patients with the greatest probability of benefit are treated with the optimal dose and schedule of the drug. The recommended dose and schedule from phase I are tested in a variety of tumor types. The main problem in phase II trials is maintaining uniformity in treatment and study population. A phase II study will require 15 to 30 patients; each phase II drug is assigned by the NCI to two different cooperative groups.

The endpoints of a phase II trial may vary with the type of disease under study. For example, an endpoint of complete remission would not be realistic for a typically treatment-resistant disease such as metastatic melanoma. Because minimal effective treatment exists for this disease, the sole endpoints may be identifying the response rate and toxicity of the new agent.[66]

Phase III

A phase III trial establishes the value of the new treatment relative to standard treatments by a randomized or comparative study. The best role for the new drug must be defined. Different study methods that may be used to define this role are comparing the new drug with the best standard drug; using the new agent in a current, effective drug combination; and comparing combined-modality treatment with the previous best single modality. There must be reasonable evidence to suggest that the new drug or combination of drugs is equivalent to or more effective than the currently accepted standard therapy.

Eligibility for a phase III trial is similar to that for phase II in that patients must have histologically confirmed disease that is bidimensionally measurable, have adequate major organ function, and be capable of performing at least partial self-care. Patients in phase III trials have received little or no previous therapy.

Phase III trials are large studies that involve hundreds of patients and generally multiple institutions. More phase III trials are being performed through the intergroup mechanism of the NCI, whereby several cooperative groups cosponsor the study. This allows patients to be accrued from a wider geographic segment, thus allowing a more rapid completion and analysis of the study. Community-based programs contribute significant numbers of patients to phase III trials.

These trials are often randomized, meaning that the patient is arbitrarily assigned to one of two or more possible treatments. Neither the physician nor the patient knows which treatment will be assigned until after informed consent is given and registration completed. The purpose of *randomization* is to remove potential biases in allocating patients to each treatment so that similar numbers of "like" patients receive each treatment.[66] Another advantage of randomized trials is that treatment

groups can be "balanced" according to prognostic factors by means of stratification.[62] The *stratification process* may involve such variables as age, performance status, extent of disease, or prior therapy. This method ensures that patients with a good prognosis and those with a poor prognosis are distributed equally among all treatment arms so that valid conclusions may be drawn when the study is completed.

The primary endpoint of a phase III trial is to improve on existing treatment. Investigators measure for higher complete response rates, increased disease-free survival, and longer overall survival. As treatment results improve, long-term toxicities become an important endpoint. Recently, more attention has focused on quality of life as a study endpoint.[71]

Phase IV

Briefly, a phase IV clinical trial is designed to determine the optimal use of a treatment as a standard therapy. In this design study a large number of subjects are recruited. Phase IV studies build on the endpoints of successful phase III trials to enhance scientific findings. As mentioned, the primary endpoint of these "refining" protocols is the determination of optimal treatment use.

Text continued on p. 654.

NURSING MANAGEMENT

Historically, nurses only provided physical care to the patients in clinical trials. Chemotherapy research was one of the first areas that emphasized active collaboration of nurses in research. The need for skilled chemotherapy nurses stimulated the development of role expansion. Nurses provided patient education regarding the various aspects of clinical trials. More recently, the role of nurses in clinical trials has expanded from the nurse as a participant in medical research to the nurse as principal investigator for independent research.

The roles of nursing in clinical trials include the areas of direct patient care, education, advocate coordination, administration, and independent research. These roles are accomplished by a variety of individuals, who may include hospital staff nurse, ambulatory care nurse, research nurse, clinical research associate, clinical nurse specialist, and unit manager. Maintaining coordinated efforts among these individuals requires skill in both organization and communication. Successful implementation and conduct of clinical trials results in safe patient care and generalizable research results.

Greater numbers of nurses than ever are actively involved in clinical trials because of the extension of these trials into the community. Nurses practicing in institutions that do not perform clinical trials still need a work-

ing knowledge of these studies because they may refer patients to centers for possible entry into a trial. In addition, in this era of managed care, clinical trial participants who are not receiving investigational medications are frequently referred back to the community setting for treatment and follow-up. The education and support an informed nurse can lend in this stressful situation are invaluable.

Nursing diagnoses and interventions for patients participating in phases I, II, III, and IV clinical trials follow.

NURSING DIAGNOSES

- *Knowledge deficit related to disease pathology, new diagnosis*
- *Knowledge deficit related to clinical trials process, randomization process, informed consent process*
- *Knowledge deficit related to experimental chemotherapy, side effects*
- *Decisional conflict related to involvement in clinical trial versus standard therapy*
- *Anxiety related to new diagnosis or disease progression*
- *Anxiety related to treatment with experimental agent or procedure*
- *Anxiety related to completion of quality of life tools*

- *Coping, ineffective individual, related to new diagnosis or change in prognosis and new treatment*
- *Powerlessness related to involvement in a large clinical trial*

INTERVENTIONS: Phase I Clinical Trials

- Assess adequacy of informed consent, and notify physician if patient does not fully understand risk-benefit relationship.
- Know mechanism of drug action, route of administration, absorption, metabolism, and excretion.
- Know results of animal toxicology studies to anticipate human toxicities.
- Assess for, evaluate, and document unexpected adverse drug reactions (ADRs).
- Provide nursing care to minimize disease-related and treatment-related morbidity.
- Understand disease process to distinguish between disease-related and treatment-related effects.
- Carefully document objective and subjective responses to treatment.
- Document acute, chronic, delayed, and cumulative side effects.
- Perform and document results of pharmacokinetic studies.
- Participate in decisions concerning dose escalation, schedule manipulation, and determination of optimal dose.

INTERVENTIONS: Phase II Clinical Trials

- Know results of phase I drug studies:
  —Side effects
  —Dose-limiting toxicities
  —Method of administration
  —Drug metabolism and excretion
- Provide patient education and support:
  —Treatment plan
  —Expected side effects
  —Symptom management
  —Disease process

INTERVENTIONS: Phase III and Phase IV Clinical Trials

- Ensure drug doses are calculated correctly.
- Document toxicities and grade correctly
- Modify doses correctly and consistently.
- Evaluate tumor measurements appropriately for response determination.
- Ensure patient's understanding of randomization process.
- Assess for new and unexpected side effects of drug.
- Assess performance status.
- Administer quality of life assessment tools.

Follow-up after treatment completion:

- Teach patient importance of follow-up visits even years after treatment is completed.

- Report data on survival and late effects until patient dies.
- Develop systems to maintain contact with patients who have moved or changed physicians.
- Encourage patients to return to a healthful life-style in light of knowing cancer may recur.
- Teach recommendations for screening and early detection appropriate to patient's age.
- Counsel other family members of patients at high risk for developing cancer.

PATIENT CARE

The area of patient care includes the informed consent process, treatment administration, toxicity assessment, and documentation.

Informed Consent

In the past the nursing responsibility in the informed consent process consisted mainly of verifying that the signature on the consent document was that of the patient. Responsibility for disclosure rested entirely with the physician. Nurses answered questions to reinforce the physician's explanation.[15]

The changing role of the nurse and the autonomy of expanded roles, especially in ambulatory and clinical trials, bring new professional and legal responsibilities for informed consent to the nurse. Establishing the diagnosis and choosing a treatment plan are independent functions of the physician, but administering medical and nursing treatments and diagnosing and managing human responses to health problems are independent functions of the nurse. Clinical trials are an area of collaboration. The physician may introduce the idea of participation in a clinical trial and give an overview of the treatment, but often the protocol nurse must explain the details of the consent form and obtain the signature. In doing so, the protocol nurse accepts the delegated responsibility of providing information to aid the decision.[12,57] In this role the nurse assumes greater responsibility than that of "witness." For this reason, and to prevent future potential conflicts, a third party should be called in to witness the patient's signature when the protocol nurse accepts the responsibility of participating in the informed consent process. The following factors assist in the process of informing the patient:

- Allow patient to take the consent form home to read before making a decision.
- Write down treatment information.
- Draw a diagram of randomization and treatment schedule.
- Provide *What Are Clinical Trials All About* pamphlet from the NCI.
- Encourage patient to call the NCI hotline (1-800-4-CANCER) for information regarding disease and treatment.

Continued.

PATIENT TEACHING PRIORITIES
Cancer Clinical Trials

Cancer control

Review American Cancer Society Guidelines on prevention strategies for diet, smoking cessation, and sun protection measures.

Teach early detection measures (breast, skin, and testicular self-examinations).

Review Cancer Control Study Guidelines (purpose, treatment/drug schedule, side effects of drugs), preparation and schedule for diagnostic examinations, and follow-up plan.

Clinical trials

Assess and clarify issues related to the informed consent, clinical trial, and randomization process.

Review the purpose and treatment schedule; drugs and their related side effects; symptom management (e.g., fever, pain); appointments for diagnostic tests/x-ray films; monitoring of blood counts; return office/clinic visits and/or hospitalization; resources to contact for emergent care; and questions about clinical trials.

Ineffective therapies

Use nonjudgmental approach in providing and clarifying information on ineffective therapies; offer reliable information from NCI, NIH, FDA, and American Medical Association (e.g., pamphlets, resources to contact, referrals for second opinions).

GERIATRIC CONSIDERATIONS
Cancer Clinical Trials

Cancer clinical trials and cancer control research have established eligibility criteria for patient accrual; refer to age-related guidelines.

Consider sensory and neuromuscular deficits (e.g., visual, hearing, mobility) in selection of educational materials.

Review current prescription and over-the-counter medication guidelines that may interact with scheduled drugs/treatments.

Initiate assessment and intervention strategies for additional limitations, such as fixed income, transportation, caregiver resources, and age-related functional status.

- Show audiovisual information about chemotherapy and side effects.
- Provide telephone numbers for patient to call if questions arise.
- Assess patient's anxiety level and integration of new information.
- Question patient to determine whether he or she understands the treatment.
- Continue to review and reinforce information throughout treatment.

See the boxes above for patient teaching priorities and geriatric considerations.

Treatment Administration

Protocol guidelines must be strictly followed so that results from a group of patients treated in precisely the same manner can be analyzed and the study repeated and validated.[11] The treatment nurse should always verify the body surface area (BSA) calculation, protocol dose calculations and modifications, pretreatment laboratory values, and method of administration. Treatment nurses should be provided with protocol abstracts in the patient chart or a set of protocols in the treatment area to facilitate these activities. Experimental drugs may be administered by a staff nurse, clinic nurse, research nurse, or chemotherapy nurse.

Toxicity Assessment

The observation skills of oncology nurses are crucial to assess treatment-related toxicities in clinical trials. The nurse's observation of the patient after treatment identifies the side effect profile and ultimately is the basis for the care plan of patients receiving experimental treatment in the future.[55] The nurse may be the first person to recognize a side effect, perhaps even before the patient is aware of the experience.

Documentation

Accurate nursing documentation is the foundation of good clinical research. All data that are reported on flow sheets or case report forms must be verifiable in the patient's medical record. Nurses must document treatments and assessments accurately. Study investigators can extrapolate hematologic toxicity from laboratory work but cannot document other, more subjective toxicities unless nursing documentation is objective. Areas requiring precise nursing assessment and documentation include patient's level of activity, oral assessment, nausea, vomiting, anorexia, diarrhea, constipation, skin condition, weight loss, changes in sexual capability, and psychologic changes. Inaccurate assessment or documentation of toxicities may result in patients receiving ineffective low doses or toxicity-producing high doses during the subsequent course of therapy. The previous Interventions section lists specific nursing responsibilities for phases I, II, III, and IV clinical trials.

Miaskowski and Nielsen[67] have published excellent documentation forms that could be used to document nursing care for clinical trial patients. All observations must be recorded in the medical record. Information recorded directly onto protocol specific forms are not considered valid source documents.

EDUCATOR
Patient Education

One of the vital roles in clinical trials is that of patient educator. The beginning of a clinical trial is a time of unique stress for the patient. The patient feels hopeful that the experimental therapy will work but also fears that it will not be successful and is anxious about unknown side effects. Nursing diagnoses for the clinical trial patient are listed on pp. 650-651.

The nurse can help the patient cope by describing the concept of clinical trials to the patient and family. Written information about the treatment schedule, side effects, and follow-up plan give some structure for the patient. The patient should have the telephone number of the protocol nurse or assigned clinic nurse and should be instructed to call with any questions. A telephone call from the protocol or clinic nurse the day after an outpatient treatment allows assessment of immediate side effects and gives assurance to the patient.

Nursing Education

Staff nurses are an integral component of the research team and must be knowledgeable about research protocols in which they are participating. Areas of education include the purpose and history of the protocol treatment, design of the study, previously observed toxicity, treatment administration, and management of side effects.

A clinical nurse specialist (CNS), when available in an institution, educates the staff about cancer treatment protocols and patient care. More frequently, however, the role of educator is found in a variety of other expanded nursing roles.[88] When available, research nurses are expert resources for information about the research process and details of particular protocols. Both the CNS and research nurse provide education and consultation about the research study. The primary focus of the CNS is nursing management of the patient and nursing skill development, whereas the priority of the research nurse is the successful implementation of the study.[88]

ADVOCATE

The nurse is an important advocate for the patient. Because the nurse is more accessible than the physician, the patient may feel more comfortable expressing fears or concerns to the nurse. The nurse advocates for the patient by ensuring that adequate information is given, that the patient has a clear understanding of the risk-benefit

relationship, and that adequate time is available for questions. The nurse must support the patient who refuses treatment or who wants to withdraw from the study.

The nurse largely determines the quality of the informed consent. Oncology nurses have the competence, the rapport with clients, and the tradition of collaboration with colleagues to safeguard the right to informed consent.[16]

COORDINATOR

Cancer treatment protocols require the coordination of numerous hospital-based and outpatient services, including hematology, chemistry, blood bank, pathology, pharmacy, hospital patient units, radiation therapy, and outpatient clinics. The research nurse is responsible for organizing and coordinating such activities as specimen collection for phase I pharmacokinetic studies; mailing blood, marrow, or tissue specimens to reference laboratories; and ensuring that radiation therapy materials are submitted for review. Good communication and interpersonal skills are required to accomplish these tasks. Without clear communication among departments, the patient may receive confusing or contradictory information and health care can become fragmented.[64] In addition, the protocol nurse is responsible for coordinating patient appointments. To promote patient compliance and avoid protocol violations, the nurse must be cognizant of potential scheduling conflicts when maneuvering the patient through the health care maze.

ADMINISTRATOR

McEvoy and colleagues[64] state that the role of the administrative nurse includes coordinating both the patients' care and the research project. The administrator is responsible for analyzing the impact of the research study, the resources available, and the existing organizational structure within which the trial will take place.[23] Administrators work with study sponsors to coordinate the implementation of studies and to negotiate funding for new studies. They may serve as liaison among hospital administrators, physician investigators, the research staff, and the institutional review board (IRB). Information must be disseminated to many individuals within the research program. Characteristics of the nurse performing the administrative role of a clinical trial include the ability to interact comfortably with a variety of professionals and to organize and implement group meetings.[64]

RESEARCHER

The role of nurses as merely data collectors for medical research has changed and expanded over the past decades of clinical trials. Nurses are independent investigators for nursing research studies. One purpose of nursing research in clinical trials is to evaluate patients' responses

Continued.

to treatment or disease.[64] Another is to evaluate the impact of specific nursing interventions on management of symptoms associated with cancer therapy. One method of implementing nursing research through the clinical trials mechanism is by companion studies. *Companion studies* include nurse-sponsored studies "piggybacked" on an existing medical study or as complementary, parallel studies. The latter studies are initiated in response to a nursing concern that may have been generated by observation of patients in an ongoing study. Some nursing studies are implemented through the cooperative group mechanism after being developed within the group's nursing committee. Funding for these studies is available through the cooperative group mechanism, the Division of Cancer Prevention and Control, and the NIH's Center for Nursing Research.[13]

Nurses may be involved with the generation of knowledge through identifying trends in patient experiences, the dissemination of knowledge through presenting research results, and the utilization of knowledge through incorporating research results into their daily nursing practice.[24,64]

ACCRUAL ON CLINICAL TRIALS

More than 1 million Americans are diagnosed with cancer annually; one half of these individuals will eventually succumb to the disease.[25,43] Historical data verify that fewer than 3% of patients receiving cancer therapy are treated through clinical trials.[43] More than 1 million people were diagnosed with cancer in 1994. Only 0.5% to 2.5% of these patients were entered on a cancer clinical trial. Some patients are not eligible for studies, but fewer than 10% of patients eligible for NCI-sponsored studies will be registered.[25,91] In 1987 Friedman[29] reported that in NCI-sponsored cooperative group trials, only 1% to 1.5% of potentially eligible breast cancer patients, 0.5% of rectal cancer patients, and 1% of colon cancer patients were actually registered as participating in a study by their physicians. This slow accession of patients is a contributing factor to three major cooperative group studies taking 32%, 113%, and 119% longer to complete than projected. For studies in which the endpoint is reduction in mortality, 18 to 24 months should be sufficient to accrue the needed number of patients. Given the present accrual rates, however, 3 to 8 years or longer may be necessary to provide sample sizes of acceptable magnitude.[91] In addition to the expense of keeping a trial open for an extended period, slow accrual also delays analysis of the study and therefore dissemination of new information into standard practice.[85]

Strategies to Increase Accrual

Community Clinical Oncology Program. The CCOP, as discussed previously, was implemented by the NCI in 1983. A primary goal was to increase the available numbers of potentially eligible patients for clinical trials, thus improving accrual rates. Southwest Oncology Group (SWOG) figures attest to the community contribution: in 1983, the year CCOP accrual began, 209 CCOP patients were registered on SWOG studies. The following year the CCOP contribution increased to 1230 patients.[21]

Recent data indicate that 60% of patients entered in cancer clinical trials are from the community setting.[25] Even in the community setting, however, only approximately 30% of patients are eligible for participation, and only 10% of these are registered.[45] This number may continue to decrease in the face of managed care. In a study published by the Association for Community Cancer Centers, 484 medical oncologists were surveyed regarding patient participation in clinical trials. Results indicated that 670 patients in a 1-year period were not entered in clinical trials because of third-party payor denial.[2]

High-priority trials. In 1988 the NCI implemented the High-Priority Clinical Trials Program to enhance accrual to important cooperative group phase III trials. These studies are selected from existing cooperative group protocols because they require large numbers of patients, involve common malignancies, and answer important questions, the results of which will likely lead to improved patient survival.[13] Physicians who are not participating in clinical trials through the other available mechanisms may affiliate with a group as high-priority investigator. These physicians are reimbursed for the number of eligible patients they register into study. Table 25-3 lists the most recent set of studies, Series IV High-Priority Trials. The High-Priority Trials program has been successful in increasing patient accrual. Historically, these trials account for only 6% of currently active phase II studies but accrue 27% of current phase III patients.[85]

Obstacles to Accrual

Various reasons and explanations are cited for poor patient accrual on clinical trials. Johansen and co-workers[56] group these obstacles into patient-related, nurse-related, and physician-related obstacles.

Patient-related obstacles. These authors identify potential patient-related barriers as financial costs (transportation, lodging, meals, loss of income); concerns of privacy and confidentiality; lack of interest in, disapproval of, or low opinions of clinical research; fear; anxiety; denial; and family influences.[56]

Table 25-3 Examples of NCI High–Priority Clinical Trials

Protocol ID	Title
INT-0080, SWOG-8710, CLB-8891, EST-1887	Phase III Randomized Comparison of Cystectomy Alone vs Neoadjuvant MVAC (MTX/VBL/DOX/CDDP) plus Cystectomy in Patients with Locally Advanced Transitional Cell Carcinoma of the Bladder
INT-0163, CLB-9082, CAN-NCIC-MA13, SWOG-9114	Phase III Randomized Comparison of High-Dose CTX/CDDP/BCNU with Autologous Marrow and Peripheral Stem Cell Support vs Standard-Dose CTX/CDDP/BCNU Following Adjuvant CTX/DOX/5-FU in Women with Stage II/IIIA Breast Cancer with at Least 10 Positive Axillary Nodes
INT-0116, SWOG-9008, CLB-9195, EST-6290, NCCTG-904151, RTOG-9018	Phase III Randomized Study of Adjuvant Chemoradiotherapy with 5-FU/CF in Patients with Resected Gastric Cancer
RTOG-9111, EST-R9111, SWOG-9201	Phase III Randomized Trial of Laryngeal Preservation with CDDP/5-FU Followed by Radiotherapy vs Concomitant Radiotherapy and CDDP vs Radiotherapy Alone in Patients with Stage III/IV Squamous Cell Cancer of the Glottic and Supraglottic Larynx
VA-CSP-407, PIVOT-1, NCI-T94-0131O, CLB-9492, SWOG-9450, E-VA407	Phase III Randomized Study of Prostatectomy vs Expectant Observation with Palliative Therapy for Stage I/II Prostate Cancer (PIVOT)

Nurse-related obstacles. Numerous nursing barriers to accruing patients on clinical trials also exist. Treating research patients increases the job responsibilities of nurses, and conflicts in responsibility may arise. Many nurses do not have the opportunity for education regarding clinical research and feel poorly prepared to assume these responsibilities. Lack of rewards and recognition for members of the research team and a lack of investigator/nurse and nurse/nurse collaboration may produce frustration.[56]

Physician-related obstacles. Numerous authors discuss physician obstacles to registering patients on research studies.* An early trial conducted by the National Surgical Adjuvant Breast and Bowel Project (NSABP) studied reasons surgical principal investigators chose not to enter patients in a large, multicenter, cooperative group trial. The clinical trial compared segmental mastectomy with postoperative radiation therapy, segmental mastectomy alone, and total mastectomy. Patient accrual was so far below expected accrual that it threatened the successful completion of the trial.[80] Of the 94 surveyed principal investigators, 91 responded to the survey. These physicians identified the following reasons for not entering eligible patients:

- Concern that the physician-patient relationship would be affected by a randomized clinical trial
- Difficulty with informed consent
- Dislike of open discussion involving uncertainty
- Perceived conflict between the roles of scientist and clinician

- Practical difficulties in following procedures
- Feelings of personal responsibilities
- Feelings of personal responsibility if the treatments were found to be unequal

Additional factors that inhibit participation in clinical trials were identified in a 1989 American Medical Association (AMA) survey. These factors include lack of time, bureaucratic administration of research, professional liability concerns, ethics of patient care, lack of interest, and reimbursement.[1] However, three fourths of these physicians had a positive view of clinical trials.

Financial barriers. Financial barriers have become increasingly problematic over the past decade. There are three major areas of expense in cancer clinical trials. The first is for the actual implementation and conduct of the trial and includes research personnel, data collection and analysis, and study monitoring.

The second major area of expense is direct patient care, including the cost of drugs, tests, and hospitalization. Historically, these costs were shared by the treating institution, the NCI, the pharmaceutical companies, insurance companies, and the patient.[3] With a recessionary economy, spiraling health care costs, and increased competition for fewer government dollars, the burden of covering costs is shifting. The result of these changing economic conditions is that institutions and health professionals may be less able to participate in clinical trials without adequate reimbursement.

The third area of financial barriers relates to expenses incurred by the patient and his or her family. These expenses can be defined as reimbursable and nonreimbursable or "out-of-pocket" expenses associated with treat-

*References 1, 3, 29, 31, 56, 83, 92.

ment.[7] For patients, decisions about participation in a clinical trial may be affected by the insurer's willingness to reimburse expenses.[56]

One specific problem in reimbursement is the third-party coverage for *off-label use* of chemotherapeutic agents. When the FDA approves the commercial use of an agent, it is for the specific condition listed on the package insert. Clinical trials and years of experience, however, often indicate that these agents are effective in conditions other than those listed on the label. These drugs become "standard care" and are prescribed for many patients. The General Accounting Office conducted a 1991 survey to determine the extent of off-label drug use in the practice of medical oncology; 680 respondents reported the recommendations they made to their last three patients and also designated agents they often use to treat specific malignancies.[31] The survey found that one third of all prescribed drugs were for off-label indications, and 44% of all combination drug treatments were off-label. Half the respondents reported insurance reimbursement problems. The problem is that some insurers have considered off-label use of the drug to be "investigational" and therefore a nonreimbursable expense. This interpretation of off-label use has not been supported by the FDA, Health Care Financing Administration (HCFA), or current state legislation and is actively being addressed in the cancer care arena.[3]

Out-of-pocket expenses are the other, often overlooked, financial barrier faced by patients. A number of categories of out-of-pocket expenses have been identified in the general health care literature and in the cancer literature. These expense categories have also been referred to in literature specific to cancer clinical trials. Specifically, such expenses as loss of work, income, and leisure time by patients and caregivers associated with frequent attendance at treatment facilities have been noted.[33] Transportation costs, food and nutritional supplements, over-the-counter medications, cosmetics, clothing, additional household expenses, child care, and home health care are all examples of nonreimbursed expenses associated with cancer treatment.[7,25]

Other published works have linked these economic distresses with cancer patients' refusal to enter into a clinical trial and with treatment noncompliance. Along with unmet emotional needs, patients cite unmet financial and transportation needs as creating a significant burden for themselves and their families. Personal reports of unmet needs by cancer patients and their selected family members are positively associated with increased financial obligations.[25,33]

A noteworthy point discovered in this review of literature regarding out-of-pocket expenses is the apparent significant financial impact of health care on women. In almost all instances, women encounter greater out-of-pocket costs than men. This factor also is addressed in recent NCI mandates for strategic imperatives designed to enhance the accrual of women and minorities in cancer clinical trials.[25,33]

Strategies to Overcome Obstacles

Presently, clinical research in cancer is being threatened by inadequacies in the accrual of patients for clinical trials. A concerted effort by physicians, nurses, their respective professional organizations, and the NCI can identify solutions to this accrual crises.

Education is an effective tool in overcoming many barriers. The NCI, through its *Patient to Patient* campaign, is attempting to increase public knowledge about and acceptance of clinical trials. Products of this campaign include press releases, the brochures *What are Clinical Trials All About?* and *Cancer Treatments: Consider the Possibilities,* and a videotape, *Patient to Patient: Cancer Clinical Trials and You.* Patients can also be encouraged to call the NCI Hotline (1-800-4-CANCER) to obtain information about the disease, treatment centers, and available clinical trials. The Physicians Data Query (PDQ) data base now has treatment-related information available by fax. This program is called CancerFax and is accessed by dialing 301-402-5874 from the telephone on the fax machine. Anecdotal experience even at this early stage suggests that enhancing public awareness of and demand for access to clinical trials may be one of the most effective means of increasing accrual rates.[91]

Nurses are at the core of this patient education task. Patient education about clinical trials focuses on defining the purpose and relevance of cancer research, including the significance of control groups and randomization.[56] Teaching is accomplished either in an individual setting with the patient and significant others or in a group setting. Participating in an ACS speakers' bureau provides opportunities to educate the public about the benefits of clinical trials. To overcome the obstacle of increased job responsibilities for nurses in clinical trials, Johansen and co-workers[56] propose two strategies: adjusting the nurse/patient ratio when additional duties are required for clinical trial patients and demonstration of support of clinical research nurses by primary nurses and administrators. The authors also suggest the following as forms of recognition for the nurses' research involvement: coauthorships, attending educational conferences, and educational material for the nursing unit. Physicians may reciprocate support by cooperating with associated nursing research. It is also suggested that recognition is influenced by the type and amount of research involvement and should be negotiated before trial implementation.[56]

Nurses can help increase patient accrual in several ways. Physicians can be better informed of available studies and eligibility requirements through improved verbal or written communications. Tumor registries and medical records departments can provide information on newly diagnosed patients, whose charts are then evaluated by the research nurse for protocol eligibility. Nurses can coordinate prestudy testing, evaluation of results, planning, and troubleshooting of potential barriers. These mechanisms decrease the amount of physician time required to prepare patients for registration. Because one of the main physician obstacles to registration is lack of time, these measures may increase physician enthusiasm regarding participation in clinical research.

To reduce both time involvement and costs of clinical trials, most trial sponsors have review mechanisms to ensure that studies are cost-conscious but maintain the scientific integrity necessary to fulfill the clinical objectives.[40] This action results in decreasing the frequency of expensive tests such as computed tomography (CT) scans and eliminating interesting but nonessential testing. Chemotherapy is often administered in the outpatient setting. Study sponsors are simplifying and standardizing data collection forms to decrease the amount of time required for record keeping. The Pediatric Oncology Group (POG) implemented electronic data transmission of protocol information from the participating institution to their statistical center. This started as a pilot project in 1991 and is being expanded to other institutions.

INEFFECTIVE CANCER THERAPIES

The ACS defines unproven cancer therapies as "those diagnostic tests or therapeutic modalities which are promoted for cancer prevention, diagnosis, or treatment and which are on the basis of careful review by scientists and/or clinicians not deemed proven or recommended for current use."[44] Furthermore, the American Society of Clinical Oncology's Subcommittee on Unorthodox Therapies states that the term *quackery* implies a knowing intent to misrepresent, whereas belief based on inadequate knowledge may be the underlying promotional incentive rather than the deliberate intent to defraud.[41] The important common feature to all these treatments is *ineffectiveness*.

The impact of ineffective therapies in today's society is tremendous. The number of patients subjected to ineffective therapies may never be known, but it is known that more than $2 billion is spent annually by people with cancer and those desiring an easy method to prevent cancer. Promoters of ineffective therapies accumulate millions every year, and the cancer patient, who may be curable through conventional treatment, bears the financial burden of the promoter's financial gain.

The medical professional may perceive the cancer pa-

tient who seeks unproven therapy as naive. However, although patients discuss the latest "cure" through the extensive and accessible "underground" of patients sitting in clinic waiting rooms, it may be the health care professionals who are naive. Fear of discontinuation of medical treatment often precludes the verbalization of these ideas to physicians and nurses.

Historical Perspective

Ineffective cancer treatments have been documented as early as 1748, when George Washington and James Madison of the Virginia General Assembly appointed a committee to evaluate Mary Johnson's recipe for curing cancer. The cure, containing sorrel, black celandine, and spring water, was so well defended by testimonials from the "cured" that Mary Johnson was indeed awarded 100 pounds by the assembly.[36] Numerous unproven treatments flourished, and advertisements by promoters abounded.

In 1906 the U.S. Congress passed the *Food and Drug Act.* In 1910, the first time it was challenged, the U.S. Supreme Court ruled that it applied only to truthful labeling of ingredients in a product.[51] The court concluded that individuals could not be prosecuted for what was termed "mistaken praise" for their treatments.[63] In 1912 President Taft urged Congress to pass tougher legislation. This produced the *Sherley Amendment,* which made it a crime to make false or fraudulent claims of therapeutic efficacy. However, it was the prosecution's responsibility to prove intent to defraud. An important piece of legislation, passed by Congress in 1938, finally required scientific proof of drug safety before marketing. A Supreme Court ruling in 1943 determined that the responsibility for establishing safety lies with the drug manufacturer. In 1962 Congress further clarified the Food and Drug Act and added the essential element of *proof of drug efficacy.* This represents research in its current form: data are collected from animal studies evaluating safety and efficacy, an investigational new drug application is filed with the FDA, and on approval of that application the drug enters human clinical trials. When all phases of clinical trials are complete, the company can market the drug if it is indeed safe and effective. The problem is that patients can still choose to use an ineffective and unproven therapy. The FDA is responsible for enforcement of the Food and Drug Act, which is difficult at best. The FDA's legal base is interstate commerce, so promoters operating entirely within a state can totally avoid FDA laws. The U.S. government has no control over ineffective therapies outside the United States.

It is apparent that the health care profession cannot rely solely on governmental legislation and enforcement to protect patients from unproven and possibly dangerous treatments. The health care provider must help patients recognize these methods for what they are and make informed decisions regarding their cancer treatment.

Recognizing Ineffective Cancer Therapy

The American Society of Clinical Oncologists' Subcommittee on Unorthodox Therapies published its paper *Ineffective Cancer Therapy: A Guide for the Layperson* in 1983.[81] The committee identified the following 10 ways to recognize ineffective therapy:

1. *Is the treatment based on an unproven theory?* Promoters of ineffective cancer therapy are experts at using confusing scientific language in brochures. However, these claims are not backed with peer-reviewed publication in scientific journals. Encourage patients to use the National Library of Medicine Medlars Computer through their local reference library to determine whether the claims are published in scientific literature.

2. *Is there a need for special nutritional support when the remedy is used?* People have believed in the medicinal power of certain foods for centuries, and proper nutrition is essential for good health. However, promoters may capitalize on the notion that certain natural foods can cure or prevent cancer. Many ineffective therapies claim that special food preparation or nutritional supplements are required to achieve the treatment's full effect.

3. *Is there a claim made for harmless, painless, non-toxic treatment?* These claims may be especially difficult to resist, particularly when the promoter reinforces this with such phrases as "burning radiation," "poisonous chemotherapy," and "mutilating surgery."

4. *Are claims published frequently in the mass media?* Although promoters' claims are not published in scientific literature, they have an attentive audience in the media, often quick to publicize a "new cure" without full investigation. Because the FDA can enforce misleading drug labels but not media claims, the belief that "they couldn't say it if it weren't true" is simply not the case.

5. *Are claims of benefit the result of the power of suggestion?* Promoters rely heavily on testimonials of their "cured" clients. This can overwhelm the cancer patient, who does not know that some of these people never had cancer and that others who gave testimonials succumbed to cancer a short time later. Predictably, the placebo effect of any treatment, when backed with faith and expectation, can result in subjective improvements for short periods. The only scientifically valid evidence, however, is objective tumor response.

6. *Are the major promoters recognized experts in cancer treatment?* Many ineffective therapy promoters

look like experts; they wear white coats and have framed degrees hanging in the office. Some are physicians but lack expertise in cancer research and care. The patient should check the Directory of Medical Specialists, which lists individuals who have recognition, special training, and experience in cancer research and treatment.

7. *Do promoters back up their claims with controlled studies?* Promoters claim excellent results from their treatment. However, the demonstration may be from patients' testimonials rather than from controlled trials. Promoters may claim they do not have the staff or money to conduct such investigations. This claim is difficult to believe when they collect millions of dollars in profits every year.

8. *Is there a claim that only specially trained physicians can produce results with their drug, or is the formula a secret?* Formulations of reputable cancer drugs are published in scientific journals, and the information is available to all physicians.

9. *Do the promoters attack the medical and scientific establishment?* Claims of a conspiracy in the medical community to prevent a cancer cure, thus securing the incomes of its members, are often voiced by promoters. However, members of the establishment also die of cancer, as do their loved ones. Ineffective promoters segregate themselves from the medical community, often performing their cures in hotel rooms and discouraging consultation with medical experts.

10. *Is there a demand for "freedom of choice" regarding drugs?* Americans revere the word "freedom," and so promoters claim the patient's freedom of choice would be limited if promoters were not allowed to sell their products. The freedom to misrepresent facts in drug labeling and selling is no freedom at all, but simply a license to steal from the public.

A pamphlet discussing these 10 points, available from Upjohn Pharmacia Inc., is helpful for patients who want to evaluate an option for treatment.

Types of Ineffective Therapy

More than 100 types of ineffective therapy have been or are available. Table 25-4 lists some of the more common treatments and their rationale. The ACS and FDA have files on unproven treatments accessible to both professionals and lay persons.

PATIENT MOTIVATIONS FOR THE USE OF INEFFECTIVE THERAPY
Fear

The psychologic factors that influence a patient to seek ineffective therapies are multiple and complex, but the

Table 25-4   Common Ineffective Cancer Treatments

Treatment	Rationale/mechanism of action	Comments
MACHINES/DEVICES		
Oscilloclast (Hubbard E meter, Drown radio therapeutic instrument, Orgon energy devices, Dotto electronic reactor)	Detect disharmonious disease-causing oscillations of body's electrons and adjust back to harmonious state.[70] Normalize bad vibrations or counteract harmful currents that cause cancer.[68]	Devices more often used at turn of century. FDA proved oscilloclast worthless and made it illegal.
DRUGS		
Koch antitoxin therapy	Developed reagent useful as oxidation catalyst and body stimulant antagonist to cancer cells. Process built on normal cell metabolism and retarded functioning of anaerobic cancer cell.[19]	Developed in 1919 by W.F. Koch, MD, PhD. Popular in 1940s and 1950s. Treatment was extremely pure distilled water with one part per trillion of "reagent" glyoxylide.[63] Koch indicted in 1943 after FDA hearings; ended in mistrial after defense produced 104 witnesses offering testimonials. Koch moved to Brazil in 1948. Treatment is illegal in United States but can be obtained through underground medical community or in Mexico.[63]
Hoxsey method	"Restore body to physiologic normalcy."[47] Proposed that as a result of chemical imbalance, body cells matured and became cancerous.	Internal and external therapy: "pink medicine" and "black medicine." External treatment was paste applied to tumor. Federal court injunction stopped sales in 1960 after 10 years of litigation. FDA estimates patients spent more than $50 million on treatment. Available at Biomedical Center in Tijuana, Mexico.
Krebiozen (carcalon)	Stimulates body's inherent anticancer substances and thus slows or arrests growth of cancer.[44]	Endorsed by Andrew Ivy, MD, PhD, vice-president of University of Illinois in 1951. Tested by NCI in 1961; substance identified as an amino acid found in all animal tissue. Later investigations showed samples contained mineral oil alone or with small amount of amyl alcohol and methylhydantoin.[36] Prescribed by thousands of U.S. physicians. Many unsuccessful legal battles; FDA unable to outlaw because of intense pressure by supporters.[44] Continued to be dispensed until Ivy's death in 1977.
Laetrile	Cyanogenic glucoside, derived from variety of fruit and plant sources, was found too toxic in cancer treatment in 1920s. Purified in 1950s—β-glucoronic analogue of amygdalin.[20] Theory: cancer cells contain enzyme β-glucosidase, which releases cyanide after drug administration. Normal cells low in enzyme so they are spared toxic effect while cancer cells are killed.[61] In 1970, transformed cyanogenic glycosides into substance dubbed B$_{17}$—labeled as vitamin ("vitamin theory").	Biggest success among unproven treatments in 1970s despite opposition by FDA and cancer research groups. NCI-sponsored clinical trial proved laetrile ineffective (1957-1977). Toxicity: fever, rash, headache, hypotension, vomiting, diarrhea, motor disturbances, agranulocytosis.

Continued.

Table 25-4 Common Ineffective Cancer Treatments—cont'd

Treatment	Rationale/mechanism of action	Comments
DRUGS—cont'd		
DMSO (dimethylsulfoxide)	Combination therapy with DMSO allegedly yields decreased side effects of chemotherapy while potentiating its therapeutic effects. Theoretic basis suggests that the immune system of cancer patients forms a shell around cancer cells, and DMSO can penetrate the shell and enter the cell, carrying with it any other drugs patient is receiving.	ACS review of literature found no data supporting DMSO's antineoplastic activity.[84] FDA in 1978 approved use of 50% aqueous solution of DMSO (RIMSO-50) for relief of interstitial cystitis by bladder instillation. In 1983 ACS published statement that DMSO lacks scientific evidence of efficacy and declared it an unproven method.[84]
BIOLOGIC PRODUCTS		
Rand vaccine	Made from animal blood injected with material from human cancer collected from operating rooms.[4]	IND application failed. Production halted in 1967.[35]
Lewis method	Injections of coupled tumor protein antigen (CPTA).	
Helt cancer serum	Contains *Escherichia coli* and *Streptococcus faecalis*.[35]	
METABOLIC THERAPIES		
Gerson diet	Cancer causes generalized tissue damage, especially in liver. With tumor lysis, toxic degradation products appear in bloodstream, which leads to coma and death as a result of liver failure.[32] Theory: cancer is caused by constipation or inadequate elimination of waste. Cure can be achieved through dietary manipulation. Basis for dietary recommendations: • Detoxifying of whole body • Providing essential contents of potassium • Adding oxidizing enzymes continuously (green leaf juice, fresh calf's liver juice)	Developed in 1920s by German physician. Currently more than 20 modifications of original program. Diet demands no foodstuffs other than fresh fruits and vegetables (chopped by Gerson-sold chopper) and oatmeal. No escape of steam during food preparation. No tobacco, alcohol, sodium, spices. Protein allowed only after sixth week of diet. Multiple additional iodine and niacin supplements used as well as coffee enemas.
Macrobiotic diet	Origins of cancer "rooted in the quality of the external factors that we are selecting and consuming."[60] Factors crucial to cancer prevention and control: overall blood quality, mental orientation, way of life. Specific causes of cancer result from excess of yin and yang foods. Health and happiness only result with proper balance of yin and yang, the two major world forces.[68]	Ten macrobiotic diets exist: diet no. −3 to diet no. 7, which is 100% brown rice. Foods eliminated gradually in progressing from diet no. −3 to no. 7. No scientific basis for this diet in cancer therapy. Nutritional value inadequate in vitamins, minerals, protein, calories.[60]
SPIRITUAL/MYSTICAL TECHNIQUES		
Psychic surgery	Cancer can be removed from any part of body without incisions by use of prayers, "psychic surgeries," massage. "Operation" done in hotel room. Body area covered with salve, then cotton-soaked square. Blood is splattered over site and a bloody piece of tissue held up. "Operative site" is wiped clean and diseased area is "whole" again.[77]	Patient's faith in method is major promotional factor. Arguments of simple faith used to counter scientific arguments. Psychic surgery done mostly in Philippines. Opposition believes done by sleight of hand using animal tissues and blood-filled capsules hidden by "psychic surgeon."
Spiritualists	Claim to have special healing abilities given by God. Rely on laying on of hands on the cancer site.	Patient must admit sinfulness and guilt to be cured.

Table 25-4 Common Ineffective Cancer Treatments—cont'd

Treatment	Rationale/mechanism of action	Comments
SPIRITUAL/MYSTICAL TECHNIQUES—cont'd		
Seances/trances/incantations	Invoke "mystical universal powers" to cure cancer. "Miracle injections" may be administered after trance is over.[75]	
PSYCHOLOGIC METHODS		
Simonton method	Attitude and stress may be crucial factors in the causation and cure of cancer. Uses relaxation and mental imagery to visualize cancer cells as weak and body as strong army attacking cancer cells.[79] Advocate that patients continue to receive conventional treatment in conjunction with their counseling sessions.	Founded by Carl and Stephanie Simonton. Established cancer counseling and research center in Ft. Worth, Texas. Entire program is described in their book *Getting Well Again.* Although medical/scientific community supports notion that positive attitude promotes an optimal therapeutic response, no controlled studies demonstrate objective response with this method. Individuals may feel guilty, believe their personality type caused cancer. Also may be encouraged to forego standard treatment if they become overdependent on this method. Positive aspects of treatment include increased feelings of well-being, promotion of relaxation, decreased feelings of helplessness, adaptation to situation.
IMMUNOLOGIC THERAPY		
Immuno-augmentative therapy (IAT)	Immune stimulation enables body's normal defenses to destroy cancer cells. Treatment program consists of daily immunocompetence tests and IAT. Length of treatment ranges from 4 weeks to several months.[22]	Therapeutic approach based on reasonable scientific theory; scientific documentation of treatment results are lacking.[22] Lawrence Burton, PhD, a zoologist, founded treatment and uses it at the Immunology Researching Center in the Bahamas. He has publicized therapy widely but has not reported findings in scientific literature. Withdrew IND application after FDA requested further information. Some states have passed law protecting physicians who prescribe IAT from malpractice suits.[37]

strongest motivator may be fear.[49] A Gallup poll in 1976 surveyed 1548 men and women about their fear of disease; 58% of those interviewed stated cancer was the disease they feared most.[72] Many people see cancer as a frightening, painful process ending in death. In addition to fear of death, fears of an uncertain future, pain, mutilation, loss of family, dependence, costly medical care, and alienation dominate.[80]

Family Pressure

Pressures from family and friends may add to these psychologic fears. In a sincere and well-meaning attempt to help, they look for a cure, determined to leave no stone unturned in their search. When cancer is diagnosed,

people immediately relate success stories of others they know who may have been cured by conventional means, but they also tell stories of those cured by mystical and "innovative" means. Fear and pressure may lessen objectivity and increase vulnerability to the claims of ineffective therapy promoters. The family, as the patient's strongest support system, feels a responsibility to help decide on treatment, and the patient, fearing alienation from family, may succumb to their wishes.

Recurrence and Progression

Many people resort to unproven therapies when the initial diagnosis is made; others who start with conventional therapy make that same decision when they find their disease has recurred or metastasized. A period of searching for a second opinion or reason for error in diagnosis is followed by anxiety, sometimes bordering on panic, and depression. Depression changes sleeping and eating patterns and impairs the ability to work and concentrate. The patient may reach a point of hopelessness and helplessness, knowing a cure may now be out of reach. At this time of emotional turmoil, thoughts may turn to pursuing unproven methods as a last resort.[46]

Mistrust of Medical System

Medical professionals would like to believe they are held in high regard by lay people, but this is not always true. Today's society has a medical sophistication unknown to previous generations. Health maintenance and prevention and treatment of disease are common topics in the national and local news. News from the latest *New England Journal of Medicine* may be heard on the nightly news before the issue arrives in the mail. While people are assuming more responsibility for their own health, they are actively assimilating new information. Some of this information includes knowledge of the side effects of conventional cancer treatments. They associate alopecia, nausea, vomiting, lack of energy, and loss of appetite with chemotherapy. They see surgery that may cure but may result in disfigurement. The concept of radiation therapy is particularly frightening, since it cannot be seen or felt. The disillusionment some people feel with science and technology may carry over into the physician's office, where this authority figure speaks in a medical language not easily understood and can easily rebuff patients who are already understandably apprehensive.

Promoters of ineffective therapies understand well the anxieties of patients in the conventional medical system. They deal with the apprehension, loss of control, and feelings of isolation very effectively by making the patient an active part of the treatment program. Coupled with a promise for cure without discomfort, a close camaraderie soon develops between the provider and patient, both of whom are outside the medical system.

Nursing Role

Patients may perceive their physicians as too busy to answer questions about unproven methods, and so they frequently direct these queries to the nurse. Angry memories of curable patients who opted for laetrile may make the nurse's first emotional reaction to lecture the patient and tell him or her that these people have nothing to offer and only want money. This approach may quickly confirm the distrust for the medical community and encourage the patient to seek other treatment options. Patients need factual information delivered in a calm, objective, and nonjudgmental manner. This is the appropriate time to evaluate what the patient has read or heard about the alternative therapy and what the perceived benefits are. What is the level of interest in the unproven method? What is the level of understanding about current therapy and treatment goals?

This is an important opportunity to provide accurate information about unproven methods. All currently accepted treatments were unproved at one time. The FDA and NCI protect patients by requiring proof of safety and efficacy before generalized use of a drug. The following interventions may help the patient evaluate unproved methods and improve nurse-patient relationships:

1. Explain how to access the Medlars system to determine scientific testing of treatment.
2. Check resources to verify promoter's cancer expertise:
   - Directory of Medical Specialists
   - American Federation of Clinical Oncologic Societies
   - American Association for Cancer Research
   - American Society of Clinical Oncology
   - National Cancer Institute Hotline (1-800-4-CANCER)
3. Offer reliable information:
   - *Ineffective Cancer Therapies* (Adria Laboratories)
   - *What Are Clinical Trials All About?* (NCI)
4. Examine the patient's expectation of current treatment plan.
5. Offer quality-of-life versus quantity-of-life information.
6. Help reestablish hope.
7. Identify ways to make the patient and family more involved in treatment.
8. Consider referrals for a second opinion, which may increase confidence in current treatment or identify additional therapeutic alternatives.

If unproven methods or promotional techniques seem to the nurse or physician to warrant further legal investigation, the following organizations should be notified: local health department, consumer protection office, and appropriate medical society. The federal agencies and national organizations involved in the investigation, regulation, or reporting of such practices include the FDA, Federal Trade Commission (FTC), U.S. Postal Service, Consumer Product Safety Commission, and AMA.[33]

FUTURE DIRECTIONS AND ADVANCES

Through clinical research and the clinical trials network, progress has been made in cancer treatment over the past 20 years. Combinations of surgery, radiation therapy, and chemotherapy have made a number of cancers curable. Even more cancers may become curable in the next two decades with the addition of biologic response modifiers to the therapeutic armamentarium. Curable cancers include acute lymphoblastic leukemia (ALL) in both children and adults, acute myeloblastic leukemia, Hodgkin's lymphoma, diffuse histiocytic and Burkitt's lymphoma, testicular tumors, Wilms' tumor, osteogenic sarcoma, and rhabdomyosarcoma.

Clinical trials also supply blood and tissue specimens for clinical research. This has greatly increased the knowledge of disease biology. Childhood ALL can now be subclassified into a variety of prognostic groups and the treatment tailor-made to yield the best outcome. Human tumor tissue can be cloned for testing with a variety of drugs to determine the most effective treatment. Polyglycoprotein, identified on the cell surfaces of some patients with multiple myeloma, ovarian cancer, and acute multiple myeloma, indicates a high risk for drug resistance. New tumor markers are being studied for prognostic significance. The study of oncogenes sheds further light on the biology of cancer. Advances in cytogenetic studies may identify high-risk subsets of patients requiring more aggressive therapy. Finally, the identification and mapping of the human genome will direct cancer research in this century and the next.

In 1986 the NCI presented its highly publicized *Year 2000* goal: to reduce the mortality of cancer 50% by the year 2000. Since the National Cancer Program was established in 1971, much has been learned about the causes and cures of many forms of cancer. The source of the progress in understanding cancer has been a vigorous basic, clinical, and cancer research program. The knowledge gained about cancer can be used now to control a significant portion of the disease.[27,85]

One of the main emphases of the cancer control objectives is the prevention of cancer. According to Hennekens and Buring,[41] 68% of cancer deaths are attributed to preventable causes: alcohol (3%), tobacco (30%), and nutrition (35%). Therefore health professionals are faced with the potential to impact more than one half of all cancers with prevention techniques. The NCI identified the priority areas of research as chemoprevention, diet and nutrition, occupational cancer control, and screening and early detection.

These studies present new challenges and opportunities for oncology nurses. Rather than treatment of the patient with cancer, the health population will be the focus. Cancer control studies will take nurses into the community for many of the studies. New physician networks will be identified. From the NCI perspective of funding, cancer control trials will be as important as clinical trials.

In recent years, gene-transfer therapy has emerged as a promising cancer treatment. Currently in various stages of phase I and II trials, this treatment technique involves the manipulation of the genetic production of enzymes, which control every chemical process in the body. Studies are underway involving oncogenes and tumor suppressor genes.[43]

Innovative therapeutic treatment trials are rapidly becoming an integral part of this era of health care reform

evaluations of the economic impact of novel and conventional treatment regimes. As issues of reimbursement become greater obstacles to the development of innovative treatment options, health care providers will be forced to investigate the financial as well as the physical outcomes of cancer treatment.

CONCLUSION

These are exciting times for nurses involved in cancer research. New chemotherapeutic agents are being identified, the role of the biologic response modifier is being determined, technology is rapidly changing the world of diagnostics, and cancer control requires a new flexibility in health care systems. The challenges of cancer clinical trials are many, but the rewards justify the efforts.

■ CHAPTER QUESTIONS

1. Cancer control clinical trials are designed to:
   a. Detail initial and subsequent doses of new antineoplastic agents
   b. Establish the value of a new treatment relative to the standard treatment for a disease entity
   c. Examine approaches to reduce cancer incidence, morbidity, and mortality through an orderly sequence
   d. Determine cancer incidence rates in a given population
2. Standard elements of a research protocol include all the following *except:*
   a. Nursing interventions
   b. Criteria for response
   c. Data submission
   d. Treatment plan
3. Required elements of informed consent for participants in clinical trials include:
   (1) Statement of researcher or institutional compensation by the research sponsor
   (2) Description of confidentiality and disclosure of possibility of FDA inspection
   (3) Purpose of the research
   (4) Whom to contact about research, patient's rights, and research-related injury
   (5) Description of patient's risks/benefits and any experimental procedures to be performed
   a. (2), (3), (4), and (5)
   b. (1), (4), and (5)
   c. All the above
   d. (1), (3), (4), and (5)
4. How many phases are there in human clinical trials?
   a. 1
   b. 2
   c. 3
   d. 4
5. Cooperative groups that perform clinical trials include all the following *except:*
   a. Eastern Cooperative Oncology Group
   b. North American Cancer Research Group
   c. Intergroup Rhabdomyosarcoma Group
   d. Gynecologic Oncology Group

BIBLIOGRAPHY

1. AMA Council on Scientific Affairs: Viability of cancer clinical research: patient accrual, coverage, and reimbursement, *J Natl Cancer Inst* 83(4):254, 1991.
2. Antman K: Reimbursement issues facing patients, providers, and payers, *Cancer* 72:2842, 1993.
3. Antman KH and others: Cost-effectiveness and reimbursement in patients' care, *Semin Hematol* 26(suppl):32, 1989.
4. Arje SL, Smith LV: The cruelest killers. In Barrett S, Knight G, editors: *The health robbers,* Philadelphia, 1976, Stickley.
5. *Belmont Report: Ethical principles and guidelines for the protection of human subjects of research,* DHEW Pub No (05)-78-0012, Washington DC, 1978, US Government Printing Office.
6. Berlin NI: Unorthodox therapy. In Moosa AR, Robson C, Schimpff SC, editors: *Comprehensive textbook of oncology,* Baltimore, 1986, Williams & Wilkins.
7. Birenbaum LK, Clarke-Steffen L: Terminal care costs in childhood cancer, *Pediatr Nurs* 18(3):285, 1991.
8. Bohigian G: *Reliability of cancer research patient accrual,* Paper presented at the American Medical Association Home of Delegates, Chicago, 1989.
9. Bujorian GA: Clinical trials: patient issues in the decision-making process, *Oncol Nurs Forum* 15(6):779, 1988.
10. *The Cancer Letter* 17(40):6, 1991.
11. Cassidy J, Macfarlane DK: The role of the research nurse in clinical cancer research, *Cancer Nurs* 14(3):124, 1991.
12. Chamorro T, Applebaum J: Informed consent: nursing issues and ethical dilemmas, *Oncol Nurs Form* 15(6):803, 1988.
13. Cheson BD: Clinical trials programs, *Semin Oncol Nurs* 7(4):235, 1991.
14. *Closing in on a cure: solving a 5000 year old mystery,* Washington, DC, 1987, US Department of Health and Human Services.
15. Creighton H: Informed consent, *Nurs Manage* 17(10):11, 1986.
16. Department of Health and Human Services: Protection of human subjects: informed consent, Washington DC, *Federal Register,* Jan 27, 1981, Part IX.
17. DeVita VT: Principles of chemotherapy. In DeVita VT Jr, Hellman S, Rosenberg SA, editors: *Cancer: principles and practice of oncology,* ed 4, Philadelphia, 1993, Lippincott.
18. Donovan CT: Ethics in cancer nursing practice. In Groenwald S and others, editors: *Cancer nursing: practice and principles,* ed 2, Boston, 1991, Jones and Bartlett.
19. Donsbach KW, Walker M: *Metabolic cancer therapies,* Huntington Beach, Calif, 1981, International Institute of National Health Sciences.
20. Dorr R, Pazxinos J: The current status of laetrile, *Ann Intern Med* 89(3):389, 1978.
21. Durant J: Current status of clinical trials, *Cancer* 65(suppl):2371, 1990.
22. Easy cures for cancer still find support, *JAMA* 246(7):714, 1981.
23. Engelking C: Clinical trials: impact evaluation and implementation considerations, *Semin Oncol Nurs* 8(2):148, 1992.
24. Fawcett J: A typology of nursing research activities according to educational preparation, *J Prof Nurs* 1:75, 1985.
25. Fleming ID: Barriers to clinical trials, *Cancer* 74:2662, 1994.
26. Freeman HP: Poverty, race, racism and survival, *Ann Epidemiol* 3:145, 1993.
27. Freeman HP: The impact of clinical trial protocols on patient care in a large city hospital, *Cancer* 3:2834-2839, 1993.
28. Freireich EJ: The design and planning of clinical trials. In Moosa AR, Robson MC, Schimpff SC, editors: *Comprehensive textbook of oncology,* Baltimore, 1986, Williams & Wilkins.
29. Friedman MA: Patient accrual to clinical trials, *Cancer Treat Rep* 71:557, 1987.
30. Galassi A: New antineoplastic agents. In Hubbard SM, Greene PE, Knobf MT, editors: *Current issues in cancer nursing practice,* Philadelphia, 1991, Lippincott.
31. General Accounting Office: *Off label drugs: initial results of a national survey,* GAO/PEDM-91-12BR, Washington, DC, 1991, US General Accounting Office.
32. Gerson M: The cure of advanced cancer by diet therapy: a summary of 30 years clinical experimentation, *Physiol Chem Physics* 10:449, 1978.
33. Given CW, Given BA, Stommel M: Family and out-of-pocket costs for women with breast cancer, *Cancer Pract* 2:187, 1994.
34. Grady C: Ethical issues in clinical trials, *Semin Oncol Nurs* 7(4):288, 1991.
35. *Grant guidelines for cancer control: areas of programmatic interest,* Washington, DC, 1992, US Department of Health and Human Services.
36. Grant RN, Bartlett I: Unproven cancer remedies—a primer. In *Unproven methods of cancer management,* New York, 1971, American Cancer Society.
37. Green S: Let's stop driving cancer patients to unproven treatments, *Med Work News* 23(12):188, 1982.
38. Greenwald P, Cullen JW, Weed D: Cancer prevention and control, *Semin Oncol* 17(4):383, 1990.
39. Gross J: Clinical research in cancer chemotherapy, *Oncol Nurs Forum* 13(1):59, 1986.
40. Guy JL: New challenges for nurses in clinical trials, *Semin Oncol Nurs* 7(4):297, 1991.
41. Hennekens CH, Buring JE: Contributions of observational evidence and clinical trials in cancer, *Cancer* 74:2625, 1994.
42. Henney JE: Unproven methods of cancer treatment. In DeVita VT Jr, Hellman S, Rosenberg SA, editors: *Cancer: principles and practice of oncology,* ed 2, Philadelphia, 1985, Lippincott.
43. Ho RCS: The future direction of clinical trials, *Cancer* 74:2739, 1994.
44. Holland J: The krebiozen story, *JAMA* 200:125, 1967.
45. Holland J: Why patients seek unproven cancer remedies: a psychological perspective, *CA Cancer J Clin* 32(1):10, 1982.
46. Houts PS and others: Nonmedical costs to patients and their families associated with outpatient chemotherapy, *Cancer* 53:2388, 1984.
47. Hoxsey HM: *You don't have to die,* New York, 1956, Milestone.
48. Hunter CP and others: Selection factors in clinical trials: results from the community clinical oncology physicians' patient log, *Cancer Treat Rep* 71:559, 1987.
49. Ingelfinger FJ: Cancer! Alarm! Cancer! *N Engl J Med* 293:1329, 1975.
50. *Investigators' handbook, Cancer Therapy Evaluation Program,* Bethesda, Md, 1986, Division of Cancer Treatment, National Cancer Institute.

51. Jannsen WF: Cancer quackery: the past in the present, *Semin Oncol* 6:526, 1979.

52. Jassak PF, Ryan MP: Ethical issues in clinical research, *Semin Oncol Nurs* 5(2):102, 1989.

53. Jenkins J, Curt G: Implementation of clinical trials. In Baird SB, McCorkle R, Grant M: *Cancer nursing: a comprehensive textbook,* Philadelphia, 1991, Saunders.

54. Jenkins J, Hubbard S: History of clinical trials, *Semin Oncol Nurs* 7(4):228, 1991.

55. Jenkins JF, Lake PC: Celebration of an era of public service at the National Institutes of Health and the National Cancer Institute, *Cancer Nurs* 11(1):58, 1988.

56. Johansen MA, Mayer DK, Hoover HC: Obstacles to implementing cancer clinical trials, *Semin Oncol Nurs* 7(4):260, 1991.

57. Kelly ME: Informed consent. In Northrup CE, Kelly ME, editors: *Legal issues in nursing,* St Louis, 1987, Mosby.

58. Kessler DA: The regulation of investigational agents, *N Engl J Med* 320(5):281, 1989.

59. Kreuger J: Safeguarding the rights of human subjects. In Davis A, Kreuger J, editors: *Patients, nurses, and ethics,* New York, 1980, AJN.

60. Kushi M: *Macrobiotic approach to cancer,* Wayne, NJ, 1982, Avery.

61. Laetrile: the political success of a scientific failure, *Consumer Rep,* August 1977.

62. Leventhal BG: An overview of clinical trials in oncology, *Semin Oncol* 15(5):414, 1988.

63. Luursk J: Unproven methods of treatment. In Groenwald S, editor: *Cancer nursing: practice and principles,* Boston, 1987, Jones and Bartlett.

64. McEvoy MD, Cannon L, MacDermot ML: The professional role for nurses in clinical trials, *Semin Oncol Nurs* 7(4):268, 1991.

65. McKenna RJ: Reimbursement issues in cancer clinical trials, *Cancer* 65:2405, 1990.

66. Melink TJ, Whitacre MY: Planning and implementing clinical trials, *Semin Oncol Nurs* 7(4):243, 1991.

67. Miaskowski C, Nielsen B: Documentation of the nursing process in cancer nursing. In Baird SB, McCorkle R, Grant M, editors: *Cancer nursing: a comprehensive textbook,* Philadelphia, 1991, Saunders.

68. Miller NJ, Ruben JH: Unproven methods of cancer management. Part I. Background and historical perspectives, *Oncol Nurs Forum* 10(4):46, 1983.

69. Miller NJ, Ruben JH: Unproven methods of cancer management. Part II. Current trends and implications for patient care, *Oncol Nurs Forum* 10(4):52, 1983.

70. Milstead JC, Davis JB, Dobelle M: Quackery in the medical device field. In *Proceedings from the Second National Congress on Medical Quackery,* 1963.

71. Monipour CM and others: Quality of life endpoints in cancer clinical trials: review and recommendations, *J Natl Cancer Inst* 81:485, 1989.

72. Mor V and others: The changing needs of patients with cancer at home, *Cancer* 69:829, 1992.

73. Most feared diseases, *Parade,* Feb 6, 1977.

74. The Nuremburg Code, 1949. In Beauchamp T, Childress J, editors: *Principles of biomedical ethics,* ed 2, St Louis, 1981, Mosby.

75. Patrick PKS: Cancer quackery: information, issues, responsibility, action. In Marino LB, editor: *Cancer nursing,* St Louis, 1981, Mosby.

76. Pettit GR: The bryostatins. In Herz W and others, editors: *Progress in the chemistry of organic natural products,* Vienna, 1991, Springer-Verlag.

77. Psychic surgery can mean fiscal excision with tumor retention, *JAMA* 228:278, 1974.

78. Reiser J, Dyck AJ, Curran WJ, editors: *Ethics in medicine: historical perspectives and contemporary concerns,* Cambridge, Mass, 1977, MIT.

79. Simonton OC: Unproven methods of cancer management, *CA Cancer J Clin* 32(1):58, 1982.

80. Spike J, Holland JC: The care of the patient with potentially fatal disease. In Strain J, Grossman S, editors: *Principles of liaison psychiatry,* New York, 1975, Appleton-Century-Crofts.

81. Subcommittee on Unorthodox Therapies, American Society of Clinical Oncology: Ineffective cancer therapy—a guide for the layperson, *J Clin Oncol* 1:154, 1983.

82. Taylor A, Bantham J: Changes in out-of-pocket expenditures for personal health services, 1977 and 1987, AHCPR Pub No 94-0065, *National Medical Expenditure Survey Research Findings* 21, Rockville, Md, 1994, Agency for Health Care Policy and Research, Public Health Service.

83. Taylor KM, Margolese RG, Soskolne CL: Physicians' reasons for not entering eligible patients in a randomized clinical trial of surgery for breast cancer, *N Engl J Med* 310(21):1363, 1984.

84. Unproven methods: DMSO, *CA Cancer J Clin* 33(2):122, 1983.

85. *Update,* October 1996, Bethesda, Md, National Cancer Institute.

86. Varricchio CG, Jassak PF: Informed consent: an overview, *Semin Oncol Nurs* 5(2):95, 1989.

87. Veatch RM: *Case studies in medical ethics,* Cambridge, Mass, 1977, Harvard University Press.

88. Wheeler V: Preparing nurses for clinical trials: the cancer center approach, *Semin Oncol Nurs* 7(4):275, 1991.

89. Winn R: From opera to chemoprevention, *Oncol Issues* 7(2):13, 1992.

90. Wittes RE: Cancer emphasis in the clinical drug development program of the NCI. In DeVita VT Jr, Rosenberg SA, Hellman S, editors: *Cancer: principles and practice of oncology,* Update 1(12):1, Philadelphia, 1987, Lippincott.

91. Wittes RE: Paying for patient care in treatment research—who is responsible? *Cancer Treat Rep* 71:107, 1987.

92. Wittes RE, Friedman MA: Accrual to clinical trials, *J Natl Cancer Inst* 80:884, 1988.

93. Young F and others: The FDA's new procedures for use of investigational drug in treatment, *JAMA* 259(15):2267, 1988.

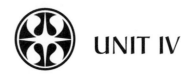

UNIT IV

CANCER CARE SUPPORTIVE THERAPIES

CHAPTER 26
Fatigue

MARGARET L. BARNETT

"Whether the disease is cured, in remission, under control, or progressing, we have the privilege of watching our patients do everyday things heroically; we gain an appreciation of them and how they get the most out of living."

Maryl L. Winningham, 1995

Fatigue is the most frequently experienced symptom of cancer and cancer treatment.[1,4,6,11] It can alter functional status, sense of well-being, and relationships. Cancer-related fatigue often influences patient decisions about treatment and physician decisions about chemotherapy or biologic response modifier doses.[8,13,18] Patients find the symptom of fatigue very distressing. Lack of energy, as many patients refer to fatigue, also negatively affects quality of life.[15,18,19] Morbidity of cancer and cancer treatment may be increased with fatigue as a result of adverse effects on appetite, impairment of role, and diminished quality of life.[18] Fatigue is difficult to measure, and little is understood about its mechanisms.[4,25] The purpose of this chapter is to highlight what are presently identified as factors that relate to fatigue. By understanding these factors that relate to cancer and cancer treatment fatigue, the nurse can plan interventions to assist patients in managing fatigue more effectively, resulting in an improved quality of life.

The Oncology Nursing Society sponsored the Fatigue Initiative Through Research and Education (FIRE^SM) seminar in 1995. The program's primary focus was research and education regarding fatigue in the oncology patient. The FIRE program will advance the education of health care professionals, consumers, patients, and the general public in understanding the magnitude of the fatigue problem.

DEFINITION

No universal definition of fatigue exists. Fatigue has been viewed in terms of both objective performance and subjective experience.[9,15] An objective indicator would identify a point at which performance declined either physically or mentally. Exercise endurance and accuracy of completion of a mental task are examples of the use of objective indicators. In the subjective state, the patient's self-report—perception of fatigue and how it relates to that individual's functioning—is the most important indicator of fatigue.[10,15,17,19] As nurses care for the patient with cancer fatigue, the subjective view is most relevant to the assessment and development of a plan of care that will help the patient deal with the experience.[15] Fatigue is described as a human response to cancer and its treatment that may be characterized by subjective feelings of weakness, exhaustion, and lack of energy resulting from prolonged exertion or stress.[1,3,12,14] The outcome is an impaired functional status including mental and physical activities, which ultimately has an impact on quality of life. Fatigue also has the quality of overwhelmingly sustained exhaustion, which remains in spite of rest.[21]

Fatigue, from a nursing perspective, is defined as a subjective feeling of physical or mental tiredness that is influenced by physical, psychosocial, and spiritual domains.[6,8,30] Fatigue can be classified as acute or chronic. Acute fatigue is an expected occurrence after energy has been expended; it has a short duration of hours, days, or weeks.[2,20] Acute fatigue serves as a protective mechanism. In contrast, chronic fatigue is regarded as abnormal or excessive and may be described as involving the whole body. Multiple domains of life are affected such as the physical, psychosocial, and spiritual. Chronic fatigue is not relieved by rest and is overwhelming.[2,20,21] It may also involve multiple and additive causes such as cancer treatments and their related side effects. Chronic overwhelming fatigue results in decreased activity and may eventually lead to disability.[31,33]

Pathophysiology

Because fatigue is multidimensional and multicausal, no clear support for any of the major hypotheses or models has emerged.[2,15,33] Each of the theories, frameworks, or models in Table 26-1 represent aspects of fatigue experienced by individuals with cancer. These potential causes of fatigue assist nurses in planning interventions. Most hypotheses relating to fatigue in cancer patients remain untested. Winningham suggests that fatigue has a unique relationship to other symptoms based on how the symptoms affect the individual's level of activity (Figure 26-1). Cancer patients who become less active as a result of disease or treatment-related symptoms lose energizing metabolic resources such as oxygen and nutrients.[31] Winningham has listed ten propositions describing the theoretic relationships among activity level, perception of fatigue, symptom management, and functional status (box below). These propositions emphasize a need for balance between restorative activity and restorative rest.

TEN PROPOSITIONS EXPLAINING FATIGUE IN CANCER

The relationship between activity, fatigue, symptom management, and functional status in people with cancer can be summarized in the following propositions:

- Too much rest as well as too little rest contributes to increased feelings of fatigue.
- Too little activity as well as too much activity contributes to increased feelings of fatigue.
- A relative balance between activity and rest promotes restoration; an imbalance promotes fatigue and deconditioning.
- Deconditioning is the adaptive energetic response whereby an organism's biological work potential is decreased over time.
- Everyday energy expenditure in activity is the most potent known regulator of the body's energy systems. ("Use it or lose it.")
- Any symptom/condition that contributes to decreased activity will lead to deconditioning, increased fatigue, and decreased functional status.
- Any intervention that provides relief of a symptom/condition that contributes to decreased activity may simultaneously serve to mitigate fatigue and promote functioning providing that intervention does not have a sedating or catabolic effect.
- The experience of fatigue potentiates distress associated with other symptoms/conditions.
- The experience of other symptoms/conditions potentiates feelings of fatigue.
- Deconditioning and perceived fatigue interact to make every aspect of life more stressful and negatively impact quality of life, thus contributing to increased suffering.

From Maryl L. Winningham. Copyrights 1992, 1995.

Table 26-1 Nursing Theories, Models, and Frameworks[1,8,14,20,32]

Theory/model/framework	Description
Accumulation hypothesis	Suggests that accumulation of waste products in the body results in fatigue.
Depletion hypothesis	Suggests that muscular activity is impaired when the supply of substances such as carbohydrate, fat, protein, adenosine triphosphate (ATP), and protein is not available to the muscle. Anemia can also be considered a depletion mechanism.
Biochemical and physiochemical phenomena	Proposes that production, distribution, use, equalization, and movement of substances such as muscle proteins, glucose, electrolytes, and hormones may influence the experience of fatigue.
Central nervous system control	Grandjean proposes that the central control of fatigue is placed in the balance between two opposing systems: the reticular activating system (RAS) and the inhibitory system, which is believed to involve the reticular formation, the cerebral cortex, and the brain stem.
Adaptation and energy reserves	Selye suggests that each person has a certain amount of energy reserve for adaptation, and that fatigue occurs when energy is depleted. Selye's hypothesis incorporates ideas from the other hypotheses but focuses on the person's response to stressors.
Psychobiologic entropy	Proposes to associate activity, fatigue, symptoms, and functional status based on clinical observations that persons who become less active as a result of disease or treatment-related symptoms lose energizing metabolic resources.
Aistars' organizing framework	This framework is based on energy and stress theory and implicates physiologic, psychologic, and situational stressors as contributing to fatigue. Aistars attempts to explain the difference between tiredness and fatigue within Selye's general adaptation syndrome.
Piper's integrated fatigue model	Piper suggests that fatigue mechanisms influence signs and symptoms of fatigue. Changes in biologic patterns such as host factors, metabolites, energy substrates, disease, and treatment, along with psychosocial patterns, impact a person's perception and leads to fatigue manifestations. The fatigue manifestations are expressed through the person's behavior.
Attentional fatigue model	Use of attentional theory linked to attentional fatigue. When increased requirements or demands for directed attention exceed available capacity, the person is at risk for attentional fatigue.

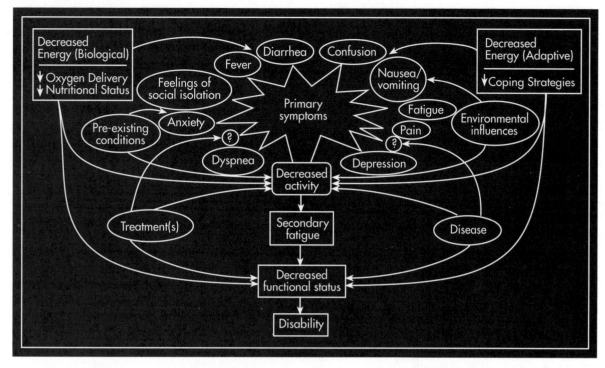

Figure 26-1   The psychobiological–entropy model of functioning. (Redrawn from Maryl L. Winningham. Copyright 1995. All rights reserved.)

An individual's spiritual orientation (values and meaning) determines direction and amount of energy needed for day-to-day functioning. Quality of life in the physical, psychologic, and social domains is affected by the distribution of energy among those domains.[31] Others, however, suggest that spirituality is one of the four domains that affects fatigue.[6,8]

Persons with cancer require energy to successfully manage symptoms and side effects. They may also have to deal with disruption in their usual reenergizing activities when nausea, pain, or other symptoms interfere with sleep, rest, and exercise.[15] Factors that contribute to fatigue and strategies that allay fatigue are listed in the first box, p. 672.[15,31-33]

CANCER AND FATIGUE

Most patients with cancer experience some level of fatigue. Patients with lung cancer rate fatigue as severe and as the most problematic symptom.[7] Many factors contribute to an individual's feeling of fatigue. It is not clear how all these factors interact physically and mentally to produce the symptom of fatigue (see first box, p. 672). Patients with cancer are commonly advised to slow their pace and get plenty of rest.[1,15,16,33] However, decreased activity may be a contributing factor to their fatigue instead of a benefit. This decrease in activity may cause an increase in energy loss resulting in decreased function of organ systems.[33] Organ systems affected often in-

clude the cardiorespiratory, musculoskeletal, and central nervous systems.[11,16,33] Clinical signs and symptoms of these physiologic changes are listed in the middle box, first column, p. 672. It is a nursing responsibility to recognize those patients who are at risk for fatigue and implement appropriate nursing interventions before quality of life deteriorates.[16]

CANCER TREATMENTS
Surgery

Most patients with cancer usually have at least one surgery to obtain a diagnosis of cancer.[16] Patients with cancer recovering from surgery consistently report fatigue, which may persist as long as 6 months.[16,17,19] Some patients have multiple surgeries related to their cancer and may experience cumulative fatigue.[16] Several physiologic mechanisms are proposed for surgery-related fatigue (third box, first column, p. 672).[16,33] It is known that surgery-related fatigue does improve with time unless other cancer treatment interventions are implemented or the cancer itself progresses.[33] The relationship between fatigue and anxiety in surgical patients was examined.[5] The researchers concluded that preoperative anxiety was not a significant factor in the development of postoperative fatigue and that postoperative fatigue may be caused by physiologic rather than psychologic factors.[5] Attentional fatigue, or the decreased capacity to direct attention, was present postoperatively in women

PROPOSITIONS RELATING FATIGUE, ENERGY, QUALITY OF LIFE, AND SPIRITUALITY

• The cancer experience is often characterized by decreases in energy capacity and by increases in perceived fatigue.
• The cancer experience usually requires an increase in adaptive energy expenditure in responding to disease- and treatment-related exigencies, as well as an alteration of activities related to quality-of-life domains.
• Fatigue becomes a critical factor in the cancer experience when less energy is available to address everyday life challenges.
• Conflicts reflect the stress caused by energy demands of life in contrast to the individual's inability to meet those demands and contribute to increased perception of fatigue.
• An individual's spiritual orientation (values and meaning) determines direction and amount of energy focused on everyday functioning in the separate domains of quality of life.
• Coping techniques reflect appraisal of energy resources versus demands to resolve conflicts and thus reduce energy waste.
• Quality of life at any stage in the cancer experience depends on the satisfactory resolution of energy conflicts consistent with an individual's spiritual system.

From Maryl L. Winningham. Copyright 1994.

CLINICAL SIGNS AND SYMPTOMS OF PHYSIOLOGIC CHANGES RELATED TO FATIGUE IN CANCER[11,16,33]

• Decreased strength
• Increased dyspnea
• Tachycardia with exertion accompanied by frequent need to slow down or stop and rest
• Difficulty concentrating

POTENTIAL CAUSES OF POSTOPERATIVE FATIGUE

• Increased cardiac effort
• Use of anesthetics
• Route of administration of analgesics
• Alteration in nutrition
• Decreased physical activity
• Use of variety of treatment methods

FACTORS ASSOCIATED WITH CHEMOTHERAPY FATIGUE

• Pathologic
• Environmental
• Psychologic
• Nutritional
• Duration of illness
• Concurrent medical condition
• Drug interactions
• Age of subject

who had either mastectomy or breast conservation surgery.[11] The attentional deficits in the postsurgical period were present regardless of the extent of the surgery.[11]

Chemotherapy

The most commonly reported side effect of chemotherapy is fatigue.* Investigators have reported that 80% to 99% of patients receiving cytotoxic agents experience fatigue.[5] After pain, fatigue was the second most distressing symptom reported by patients receiving investigative chemotherapy.[15] There are many cytotoxic agents with variability in administered dose and schedule, and fatigue seems to be cumulative with repeated chemotherapy courses.[4,33]

The symptom of fatigue is an important problem. Patients with cancer have skipped doses or withdrawn from potentially curative chemotherapy treatment because of fatigue.[33] Fatigue levels peak about 7 to 10 days after chemotherapy and then return to baseline levels before the next cycle.[18,33] At this time patients state that they are just beginning to feel better and get their energy back. Nursing knowledge of potential fatigue patterns is essential to develop a plan of care and interventions for the patient with chemotherapy-related fatigue.

Multiple factors associated with chemotherapy-related fatigue (box above) have been investigated, but no single responsible cause has been cited. Some researchers have found that a correlation exists between the presence of fatigue and the number of other symptoms experienced, such as pain, nausea, vomiting, or cachexia.[15,23,33] The duration of illness also impacts the fatigue experience.

It is unknown how drowsiness from antiemetics, analgesics, antianxiety agents, and antidepressants impact fatigue in the person receiving chemotherapy. The patterns of fatigue in individual chemotherapy regimens are not well documented because of the variability of onset, duration, pattern, and severity of the fatigue associated with particular drugs.

---

*References 4, 13, 15, 16, 18, 20, 33.

FACTORS THAT INCREASE THE RISK FOR FATIGUE WITH RADIATION THERAPY

- Age >34 years
- Weight loss
- Mood disturbance
- Pain
- Symptom distress
- Length of treatment
- Advanced disease

Radiation Therapy

Skin problems and fatigue are the most frequently reported side effects of radiation therapy.[33] Most radiation side effects are local and predictable based on the site of the treatment field. Patients who have radiation and chemotherapy are at increased risk for fatigue. Causes of fatigue in radiation therapy patients are not clear, but some research suggests that the risk for fatigue increases with the factors listed in the box above.[4,13,19,33] The incidence of fatigue is 65% to 100% in patients receiving radiation treatment.[16] Patients receiving radiation therapy have multiple disease sites and receive different doses for different cancers. Because of these factors, it has been suggested that a central mechanism may be responsible for the symptom of fatigue (see first box, p. 672).[16]

Fatigue associated with radiation therapy is an important clinical problem for patients receiving treatment.[13] It is the only common systemic side effect of local radiation therapy; it is also the most severe, especially during the last week of radiation treatment.[15]

Over the course of radiation therapy, the prevalence of fatigue can vary. Fatigue is usually intermittent at the beginning of treatment and then gradually increases as the treatment progresses. The exception to this is the patient with lung cancer, whose fatigue is more severe at the beginning of radiation treatment and gradually decreases as the tumor responds to therapy. The improved energy level may be related to newly opened airways resulting in less effort to breathe.[16] Fatigue may decline over the weekend when patients are not receiving radiation therapy treatment.[15,16,33] Early afternoon and evening are the most common times for patients to feel fatigued.[16] Usually within 3 months after radiation therapy is completed, fatigue decreases to pretreatment levels.[13,14,16]

Biotherapy

Biologic response modifiers (BRMs) are a category of biologic agents that alter the immune system by stimulating or suppressing it.[16] Types of BRMs include interferon, interleukin-2, tumor necrosis factor, and colony-stimulating factors. Each of these agents may affect the type and pattern of fatigue experienced by the individual

Table 26-2 Biologic Response Modifier Agents and Common Side Effects[6,20,24]

BRM agent	Comments
Interferons	Physical and mental fatigue are common dose-limiting side effects. Fatigue may be worse in older patients and those receiving other BRMs concurrently. Flu-like syndrome occurs.
Interleukin-2	Greater fatigue occurs than from other BRMs and is dose-limiting toxicity. Fatigue increases with length of treatment and flu-like syndrome. Cognition and orientation decline.
Tumor necrosis factor (TNF)	Muscle wasting may be mediated by TNF. Flu-like syndrome occurs.
Colony-stimulating factors (CSF)	Difficult to assess—fatigue is already present when most CSFs are started. Erythropoietin could reverse fatigue related to anemia. Cumulative fatigue occurs with GM-CSF, especially in the AIDS population.

GM, Granulocyte-macrophage; *AIDS,* acquired immunodeficiency syndrome.

(Table 26-2).[15,20,24,27,33] The pattern or duration of fatigue is affected by the BRM agent, dose, and route of administration. Fatigue associated with interferon is most severe in the afternoon and evening.

Toxicity from the biotherapy agents are dose limiting, requiring reduction in dosages, postponement of treatment, or termination of treatment.[16] Biotherapy is responsible for fatigue that is more severe than the fatigue related to surgery, radiation therapy, or chemotherapy.[15,24] Fatigue related to biotherapy is only a part of a group of symptoms, e.g., fever, chills, myalgia, headache, and malaise. Additional side effects include mental fatigue and cognitive deficits. Because fatigue is so pervasive and severe in patients receiving BRMs, preventing and relieving the fatigue becomes a high priority in the plan of care.

FACTORS INFLUENCING FATIGUE

Initially, patients may not notice how fatigue has changed some of their activities. But over time, they eventually reach a values-determined balance between their energy at hand and their desire to do what they want.[31] Quality of life as it relates to fatigue is a nebulous concept. What one patient deems to be quality is not the same for another. Nurses must help patients discover their own balance between fatigue, energy, quality of life, and spirituality.

FACTORS THAT INFLUENCE FATIGUE*

PHYSICAL	PSYCHOSOCIAL
Pain	Depression isolation
Sleep/rest patterns	Anxiety
Nutrition	Appearance
Gastrointestinal problems	Control
Bone marrow suppression	Roles/isolation
Multiple medications	Relationships/affection/
Overall physical condition	' sexual function
	Finances

*References 1, 2, 4, 10, 15, 16, 33.

In addition to cancer and cancer treatment, patients experience a variety of problems that may elicit mental, physical, and emotional fatigue. Physical, psychosocial, functional, and spiritual factors influence fatigue. Physical factors such as symptom distress and psychologic factors contribute to fatigue and its impact on the life of the patient with cancer (box above).*

The value and meaning that individuals give to the changes in their life that have been caused by fatigue will influence their level of functioning and their contentment with the overall situation.[16] Some patients find a week or two of fatigue acceptable in light of their personal goals for a cure, remission, or relief of a symptom such as pain. Other patients may find that fatigue for any length of time is an unacceptable experience.[16] Being able to carry out the functions of everyday living are important considerations for patients, whether it be their activities at home, at work, or socializing. Attentional fatigue (decreased capacity to concentrate) affects functioning as well.[5] Patients often keep books at their hospital bedside but never seem to find the energy to read them. Mental demands are routinely placed on patients to digest complex information regarding diagnosis, tests, treatments, prognosis, and other information. Attentional fatigue may be common during and after cancer treatment.[11,33] More research is needed in this area.

Spirituality is another aspect of personhood that affects how fatigue is managed. Winningham[31] describes spirituality as "expanding boundaries inward, outward, and upward." In trying to make sense of what has happened in their lives, patients attempt to attach some value or meaning to their diagnosis, treatment, suffering, recovery period, and possible impending death. By searching for value or meaning in their experiences, patients consider the meaning and consequences of their diagnosis. Patients also review their life and look for ways to cope by being hopeful, changing their priorities, and learning to live with their diagnosis.[8]

All these spiritual and emotional activities take energy in an already fatigued individual. In some instances patients are thought to be "depressed" but in reality they may be demonstrating an energy-saving behavior—withdrawal.[31] Patients are attempting to balance an interrelationship of fatigue, spirituality, and quality of life by their own value system. Nurses must assess where patients *are* in that process and not where nurses *expect them* (or their families) *to be*. Winningham's model (see Fig. 26-1) illustrates the interrelationships between energy available, energy expenditure, and quality-of-life domains. The amount of energy that healthy individuals commit to role expectations and daily activities in each domain is fairly consistent over time.[31] However, a diagnosis of cancer and the demands of cancer treatment require reallocation of the amount of energy spent on each activity. Conflict or coping will influence the energy available to the person. A patient's spiritual focus determines the direction and amount of energy used on daily activities in the separate domains of quality of life.[31] The first box, p. 672, identifies relationships among fatigue, energy, quality of life, and spirituality.[31]

Fatigue in Advanced Cancer

Fatigue in patients with advanced cancer is chronic and continues without relief. This unrelenting fatigue promotes an aversion to activity with a desire to escape.[22] Significant factors that relate to fatigue in patients with advanced cancer are length of illness, intensity of pain experience, and mood disturbance.[4] Patients with lung cancer have more severely limited physical functions than other cancer patients regardless of age.[4] Women seem to experience greater fatigue than men.[7] Research has demonstrated that age and morbidity are significantly correlated; however, age plays less of a role in physical function than does symptom distress associated with the cancer. Symptom distress is the amount or intensity of physical or mental distress or suffering experienced from a specific symptom. It is reflective of the individual's response to his or her physical, psychosocial, spiritual, familial, and cultural background experience along the cancer continuum. For example, a patient with a sedentary life-style before his or her illness may not be very upset at the changes fatigue might bring to an already quiet life-style. However, a young man who is married with children and active in seasonal sports would tend to be more upset in his life-style changes related to fatigue.

Hope or the "fighting spirit" plays a therapeutic role in the coping process of patients with cancer.[22] Hope instills an expectation of a future good that is realistically possible and significant to the patient. It may be possible to decrease fatigue and increase quality of life in the patient with advanced cancer by using nursing strategies that attempt to decrease stress, anxiety, depression, and fear.[22]

*References 1, 6-8, 15, 22, 33.

NURSING MANAGEMENT

Fatigue is the most common symptom of cancer and cancer treatment and is the least understood or researched. Because fatigue is not life threatening, health care providers often minimize the impact that it has on patients' level of functioning and quality of life.[8] At present, practice guidelines are based on clinical judgement rather than research.[16] Despite limitations in the knowledge about prevention and treatment of fatigue, nursing has much to offer in helping patients manage fatigue. Careful nursing assessment, collaboration, planning the interventions, evaluation, and modification of the nursing plan are key elements in the management of fatigue. The nursing diagnosis of *Fatigue* should focus on the patient's response to the occurrence of symptoms in the physical, psychosocial, functional, and spiritual areas. The nurse should also explore the meaning that the patient assigns to these symptoms. The goal for nursing care for the patient with cancer or treatment-related fatigue is to maintain the highest possible level of functioning and quality of life by helping the patient balance energy requirements with the energy on hand.

Patients underestimate the occurrence and severity of fatigue related to cancer and cancer treatment. Patients' perceived ability to deal with symptom distress correlates with fatigue distress.[16,18,33] Less symptom distress will be experienced by education of patients and families about the effects of fatigue as it relates to their cancer or cancer treatment.

NURSING DIAGNOSES: Cancer and Cancer Treatment–Related Fatigue[16,20,23,24]

- *Fatigue*
- *Pain*
- *Mobility, impaired physical*
- *Nutrition, altered: less than body requirements*
- *Coping, ineffective individual*
- *Knowledge deficit (affects of fatigue after chemotherapy, radiation therapy, or BRM)*
- *Social isolation (changes in roles/relationships, activity level)*
- *Anxiety*
- *Spiritual distress (distress of the human spirit)*
- *Hopelessness*

OUTCOME GOALS

The patient, caregiver, and/or significant other will be able to:
- Identify and discuss the causes of fatigue.
- Share feelings regarding the effects of fatigue on lifestyle.
- Establish priorities for daily and weekly activities.
- Participate in activities that stimulate and balance physical, cognitive, affective, and social domains.

ASSESSMENT

Factors to consider in assessment of the patient with fatigue[11,12,15,33]
- Assessment should not be a burden to an already fatigued patient.
- Timing of the assessment is important to gain pertinent information.
- If fatigue does not gradually decrease once the treatment had been completed, an evaluation should be done to rule out other potential medical problems.

Qualitative assessment of the cancer patient's level of fatigue[10,12,15,33]
- Assess changes in functional ability by using theoretic models such as Piper or Winningham (see Table 26-1).
- Ask the patient to describe a typical day now and before the illness.
- What has the patient stopped doing because of fatigue?
- Which of these things are most important for the patient to continue and which of these could be done by someone else?
- What time of day is the fatigue lowest and most severe?
- How does the feeling of fatigue relate to the patient's cancer treatment?
- What does the patient do to lessen the fatigue and is it beneficial?
- Ask the patient how he views the fatigue and what it means to him?
- What does the patient identify as a strength, ability, or interest?
- How is the patient/family coping with fatigue, and how has the patient coped in the past?
- Review present medical history and data for present or suspected presence of other medical conditions that might cause fatigue, e.g., pulmonary disease, sleep disruption, dehydration, anemia.

Factors to consider in measurement
- Method of measurement should not be a burden to an already fatigued patient.
- Measurement methods should match the developmental stage of the patient.
- Culture and primary language will influence measurement options.
- Various self-report tools that range from a simple yes-no question to a multiple adjective checklist are used for fatigue measurement. The Rhoten fatigue scale is a linear 0-10 scale, with *0* being not tired, full of energy, or peppy and *10* representing total exhaustion.
- Measurement should be done at multiple points in time (e.g., baseline, pretreatment, nadir).
- Fatigue measurement is not well developed; however, consider the criteria just listed and find a consistent, helpful measure.

Continued.

INTERVENTIONS

- Facilitate rest or sleep by the following[9,10,26]:
  - —Provide environmental comforts (e.g., room temperature, light/dark, noise/interruptions).
  - —Minimize symptoms that interfere with sleep such as pain, nausea/vomiting, or anxiety.
  - —Administer prescribed medication PRN or on schedule as indicated.
  - —Encourage patients to use strategies that relieve fatigue (e.g., conversation, hobbies, regular light exercise).
  - —Sleep just long enough. Curtailing time in bed helps patient feel refreshed and avoids fragmented and shallow sleep.
  - —Strengthen circadian cycling by regular arousal time and bedtime.
  - —Offer bedtime snack to prevent hunger from disturbing sleep.
  - —Explore how naps affect the patient (e.g., feel refreshed, feel more tired and listless, sleep better at night, sleep poorly).
  - —Avoid stimulants such as cola, caffeine, and chocolate, especially after lunch.
  - —Avoid alcohol ingestion near bedtime because it may fragment sleep.
- Prioritize activities by encouraging the patient to[15,16,23,33]:
  - —Save energy for most important or enjoyed activities.
  - —Set limits (it is alright to say "no").
  - —Pace activities to save energy.
  - —Keep a log of activities (e.g., daily routines and accompanying energy levels to assist in setting priorities and planning ahead).
  - —Plan daily activities in advance to manage physical and emotional stressors. (See box on right.)
- Exercise[15,16,29,30,32]
  - —Teach self-care techniques for exercising such as walking diary, pulse monitoring, and avoiding temperature extremes.
  - —Contraindications to exercise include unusual fatigability, unusual muscle weakness, irregular pulse, leg pain or cramps, chest pain, nausea, vomiting within previous 24-36 hours, dyspnea, or IV chemotherapy within the past 24 hours.
  - —Facilitate hospitalized patients by scheduling light activity periods and referring to occupational or physical therapy department for assistance in activity planning.
  - —Exercise is helpful in providing stimulation opportunities to prevent boredom-related fatigue.
- Other interventions[23,33]
  - —Assist patient with personal hygiene to save energy for priority activities.
  - —Encourage small meals—less energy is needed for digestion.
  - —Provide nutritious, high-protein meals and snacks throughout the day.
  - —Administer prescribed agents that alter metabolism, for example, Megace®
  - —As fatigue decreases, gradually reintroduce normal activities into the daily routine and monitor fatigue status.
  - —Use assistive devices (e.g., walkers, wheelchairs) to conserve energy.
  - —Suggest attention-restoring activities for those patients with mental fatigue, such as walking or sitting in a natural environment, tending plants or gardening, or bird watching.
  - —If a patient's fatigue does not gradually decrease within a few months of completing the treatment, a medical evaluation should be done.

EVALUATION

- Evaluate response to interventions by using the patient's subjective response and activity log.
- Determine if patient/family are satisfied; if so, continue nursing care plan.
- If patient/family are not satisfied; look first at the goals and goal attainment.
  - —Are the goals reasonable?

 PATIENT/FAMILY TEACHING PRIORITIES*
Fatigue

Think of energy as a bank account; deposits and withdrawals must be planned on a daily to weekly basis.

Rest when tired; sit or lie down frequently.

Avoid physical and emotional stress.

Pace daily activities according to energy level.

Plan workload around your best times of the day.

If fatigue increases, set priorities and reduce activities.

Solicit help for household chores, child care, errands.

Food will help energy levels; eat nutritious snacks.

Mild to moderate exercise (walking, golfing or swimming) increase energy levels; avoid heavy exercise.

Do whatever you can while sitting (use shower bench or lawn chair while in shower and to dry off).

Loose fitting clothes allow easier breathing.

Organize work space to save energy.

Use cookwear you can serve from.

To relieve mental fatigue, reading, sitting outdoors, gardening, and talking with friends are helpful.

Try to keep a balance between the activities you must do and those that make you happy.

*References 10, 16, 20, 21, 24, 26, 33.

—Ask the patient/family if the importance of the intervention is understood and if the interventions are practical for them.
—If goals and the patient/family understanding are adequate, repeat the nursing process starting with as-

sessment (a different measurement tool may be helpful).
—If interventions are not practical or applicable for the patient/family, modify the nursing plan and then reevaluate.

CONCLUSION

Present research documents a high incidence of fatigue in patients with cancer and those receiving cancer treatment. The patient's self-report is the most satisfactory measure of fatigue. Care of the person with fatigue is based on clinical judgement rather than on research. Further research is needed to improve the care of patients with fatigue, including the measurement, interventions, economic cost, and development of education strategies.[15,16,33]

With the present knowledge and future research data, it is hoped that outcomes in patients with fatigue will continue to improve. This will have a positive impact on quality of life for many individuals.

■ CHAPTER QUESTIONS

1. Patients with lung cancer generally have more fatigue at the beginning of radiation than after the treatment is completed. Which response best explains this improvement in the patient?
   a. The patient has stopped smoking recently.
   b. The tumor is decreasing in size, allowing improved breathing, which consequently decreases fatigue.
   c. Radiation therapy always decreases fatigue in patients with any type of cancer.
   d. Patients eat better while receiving radiation and consequently have more energy.
2. What cancer therapy seems to produce the most severe fatigue that may result in the patient stopping therapy?
   a. Surgery
   b. Chemotherapy
   c. Biologic response modifiers
   d. Radiation therapy
3. What interventions are most helpful in alleviating fatigue?
   a. Avoid going out of the house, and limit contact with friends.
   b. Rest in bed more, and limit activity.
   c. Continue normal level of activity except limit social activities.
   d. Rest periods, napping, mild exercise, and a good night's sleep.
4. Which of the following types of cancer results in severe fatigue?
   a. Breast cancer
   b. Ovarian cancer
   c. Lung cancer
   d. Prostate cancer

5. In assessing fatigue, the most reliable information comes from:
   a. Assessment of the behavior of the person
   b. The self-report of the person
   c. Muscle function testing
   d. Report of the nurse or family of the person with fatigue
6. The patient keeping an activity log will assist in the nursing care plan by providing information in what area(s)?
   a. Prioritizing activities
   b. Setting realistic goals with the patient
   c. Identifying rest/sleep patterns
   d. All the above
7. Benefits of mild to moderate exercise in the patient with fatigue include:
   a. Increased energy
   b. Increased sense of well-being, improved functional capacity and energy
   c. Improved functional capacity
   d. All the above
8. Patient education information should include:
   a. Encouraging patient to rest when feeling tired; avoid physical and emotional stress—it uses a lot of energy.
   b. Preparing patient and family for fatigue through education about its occurrence and causes.
   c. Teaching the patient to think of his or her energy as a bank account; deposits and withdrawals must be planned on a daily and weekly basis to be able to enjoy priority activities.
   d. All the above.

BIBLIOGRAPHY

1. Aistars J: Fatigue in the cancer patient: a conceptual approach to a clinical problem, *Oncol Nurs Forum* 14(6):25, 1987.
2. Baird SB, McCorkle R, Grant M: *Cancer nursing,* Philadelphia, 1991, Saunders.
3. Billings JA: *Outpatient management of advanced cancer,* Philadelphia, 1985, Lippincott.
4. Blesch KS: Correlates of fatigue in people with breast or lung cancer, *Oncol Nurs Forum* 18(1):81, 1991.
5. Cimprich BE: Attentional fatigue following breast cancer surgery, *Res Nurs Health* 1:199, 1992.
6. Dean GE, Spears L, Ferrell BR: Fatigue in patients with cancer receiving interferon alpha, *Cancer Pract* 3(3):164, 1995.
7. Degner LF, Sloan JA: Symptom distress in newly diagnosed ambulatory cancer patients and as a predictor of survival in lung cancer, *J Pain Symptom Manage* 10(6):423, 1995.
8. Ferrell BR and others: Quality of life in long-term cancer survivors, *Oncol Nurs Forum* 22(6):915, 1995.

9. Graydon JE and others: Fatigue-reducing strategies used by patients receiving treatment for cancer, *Cancer Nurs* 18(1):23, 1995.

10. Groenwald M and others: *Cancer nursing principles and practice,* Boston, 1993, Jones & Bartlett.

11. Hansen M, Kehlet H: Fatigue and anxiety in surgical patients, *BR J Surg* 79:165, 1992.

12. Held JL: Cancer care: managing fatigue—help your patients cope with persistent fatigue during their cancer treatments, *Nursing* 24(2):26, 1994.

13. Irvine D, and others: A critical appraisal of the research literature investigating fatigue in the individual with cancer, *Cancer Nurs* 14(4):188, 1991.

14. Irvine D and others: The prevalence and correlates of fatigue in patients receiving treatment with chemotherapy and radiotherapy, *Cancer Nurs* 17(5):367, 1994.

15. Love RR and others: Side effects and emotional distress during cancer chemotherapy, *Cancer* 63:604, 1989.

16. Nail L, Jones L: Fatigue side effects and treatment and quality of life, *Qual Life Res* 4(1):8, 1995.

17. Nail L, King K: Fatigue, *Semin Oncol Nurs* 3(4):257, 1987.

18. Pickard-Holley S: Fatigue in cancer patients: a descriptive study, *Cancer Nurs* 14(1):13, 1991.

19. Piper B, Lindsey A, Dodd M: Fatigue mechanisms in cancer patients: developing nursing theory, *Oncol Nurs Forum* 14(6):17, 1987.

20. Piper BF and others: Recent advances in the management of biotherapy-related side effects: fatigue, *Oncol Nurs Forum* 16(6):27, 1989.

21. Potempa KM: Chronic fatigue, *Annu Rev Nurs Res* 11:57, 1993.

22. Rhodes VA, McDaniel RW: Fatigue and advanced illness, *Qual Life Res* 4(1):14, 1995.

23. Rhodes V, Watson P, Hanson B: Patients' descriptions of the influence of tiredness and weakness on self-care abilities, *Cancer Nurs* 11:186, 1988.

24. Robinson KD, Posner JD: Patterns of self-care needs and interventions related to biologic response modifier therapy: fatigue as a model, *Semin Oncol Nurs* 8(1):17, 1992.

25. Ryden M.: Energy: a crucial consideration in the nursing process, *Oncol Nurs Forum* 16:71, 1977.

26. Skalla KA, Lacasse C: Patient education for fatigue, *Oncol Nurs Forum* 19(10):1537, 1992.

27. St. Pierre B, Kasper C, Lindsey A: Fatigue mechanisms in patients with cancer: effects of tumor necrosis factor and exercise on skeletal muscle, *Oncol Nurs Forum* 19(3):419, 1992.

28. Varricchio C: Selecting a tool for measuring fatigue, *Oncol Nurs Forum* 12(4):122, 1985.

29. Winningham M: Walking program for people with cancer, *Cancer Nurs* 14:270, 1991.

30. Winningham M: How exercise mitigates fatigue: implications for people receiving cancer therapy, *Biotherapy Cancer* 16, 1991.

31. Winningham M: Fatigue: the missing link to quality of life, *Qual Life Res* 4(1):2, 1995.

32. Winningham M, MacVicar M, Burke C: Exercise for cancer patients: guidelines and precautions, *Physician Sportsmed* 14:125, 1986.

33. Winningham M and others: Fatigue and the cancer experience: the state of the knowledge, *Oncol Nurs Forum* 21(1):23, 1994.

CHAPTER 27

Home Care, Alternative Care Settings, and Cancer Resources

FRANCES H. CORNELIUS

The advent of rising health care costs and efforts to contain these costs, such as diagnosis-related groups (DRGs), have resulted in increased emphasis on home care and alternative care settings. A major contributing factor to the exponential growth experienced in home health care is the belief that it can prevent rehospitalization, avoid nursing home placement, and save health care dollars. Other factors include demographic changes in America, technologic advances, and consumerism. Most Americans, 71%, prefer receiving health care in the comfort of their home instead of some form of institutional care.[25,33] The number of patients receiving home care under Medicare benefits in 1995 was 3.5 million, nearly doubling in the past 5 years. Conservative estimates projected that this number rose to more than 4 million in 1996.[7,16] Home care has become increasingly "high tech," providing intravenous (IV) infusions, parenteral nutrition, supplemental oxygen, and respirators in the home setting. Consequently, patients are discharged after only a short hospital stay, whereas in the past, they would have remained hospitalized for ongoing assessment and evaluation of their status and response to treatment. Many cancer therapies that were previously administered only in acute care settings are now given routinely in an outpatient or home care setting. To date, approximately 10% to 20% of cancer care is given in the traditional acute care hospital setting, and the remainder is given in alternative settings for care, such as home care and outpatient clinics. The advances in cancer treatments and the availability of improved technology have made outpatient and home cancer treatment both safe and effective. It is expected that more than 110,000 cancer patients will receive chemotherapy in the home in 1997.[77]

It is important to note that accompanying the decreased hospital stay, emergency department use and subsequent rehospitalization have increased. According to Smith, "Patients who are frequent Emergency Room visitors or who have frequent readmissions to the hospital due to exacerbations of chronic illnesses are often patients who could or should have received home health care at an earlier time."[84] As the trend for earlier discharge continues, nurses are expected to facilitate the transition between the acute care and community or convalescent setting. This transition is a complex and challenging task that requires comprehensive data-gathering and decision-making skills.[1] The health care professional must be able to collect and analyze pertinent information to develop an appropriate discharge plan. Leiby and Shupe[49] have identified elderly patients as more at risk for hospitalization and recurrent hospitalizations and note that home health care does reduce the number of hospital readmissions. The authors further state that early discharge:

. . . results in less time during hospitalization for health professionals to instruct the patient in the self-care practices necessary to further their recovery within the home. This health teaching, therefore, needs to be continued after hospital discharge to lessen the chance of illness exacerbation and rehospitalization. And of course early discharge may mean that the patient remains acutely ill. Thus, nursing care is needed for the facilitation of the patient's self-care practices, health teaching, continuation of skilled assessments, and communication of changes in condition to the physician.[49]

The trend for more economical, home-based, family-supported cancer care and treatment is on the increase. However, it is important to note that demographic changes in U.S. society and the decline of traditional extended family support systems necessitate (1) utilization of additional community-based support services to maintain the patient in the home setting or (2) consideration of alternative settings for care that are now more frequently available through managed care systems. It is essential that the health care professional accurately assess and identify the specific needs of the client and, if the family is available, their ability to take on the care-

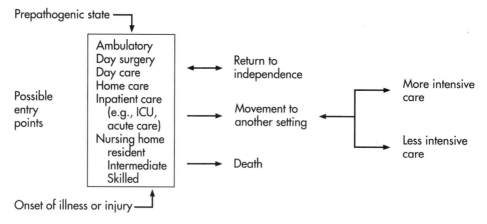

Figure 27-1   Illness-wellness continuum through discharge planning. (From Kelly K, Mc-Clelland E: Discharge planning: home care considerations. In Martinson IM, Widmer A, editors: *Home health nursing,* 1989, Philadelphia, Saunders.)

giving role. Identification of the presence or absence of adequate caregiving supports is central to determining if home care or an alternative care setting is appropriate.

It is also imperative that health care providers, especially the oncology nurse, be cognizant of all the variables that will affect the patient's response to treatment when he or she is at home or in an alternative care setting. The goal is to ensure the patient's safety and facilitate the transition throughout a coordinated system of health care delivery. This system includes various settings within a continuum of care in which comprehensive assessment of patient/family needs are communicated consistently to health care providers involved in the patient's care. To accomplish this, the oncology nurse must thoroughly assess and accurately identify the patient's/family's abilities and learning needs, as well as the environmental factors in the home that may interfere with the patient's safety and well-being.

Researchers have determined that supporting the caregiver in the caregiving role, particularly with the day-to-day management of care, is of paramount importance.[38,55,73] It has been determined "that the intervention most needed is the provision of assistance to family members caring for cancer patients. This intervention should be tailored to meet individual needs but must include information and skills relative to physical care, emotional support, and respite when possible."[73]

The discharge planning process is an organized, systematic approach used primarily in the acute care setting to facilitate the transition from the hospital to home. As health care delivery systems attempt to control costs and avoid duplication of services while maintaining high-quality care, the oncology nurse must be aware that the assessment and planning process characteristic of discharge planning should not be limited to the acute care setting. Patients seen in the outpatient oncology clinic

have discharge planning needs as well. This process is ongoing and should continue as the patient moves through a variety of health care settings during the course of the illness. A patient-centered approach to provide continuity of care facilitates the delivery of holistic health services that serve the patient's best interests while assisting providers to plan services that are based on needs.[32,46]

Discharge planning, an essential component of quality patient-centered care, is supported by a federal law passed in December 1994. The law requires that standards and guidelines for discharge planning contain the following seven components[18]:

1. The hospital must identify, at an early stage of hospitalization, patients who are likely to experience adverse health consequences if discharged without adequate discharge planning.
2. Hospitals must provide a discharge planning evaluation for patients identified under the requirement listed above and for other patients at the request of the patient or his or her representative or physician.
3. Any discharge planning evaluation must be made on a timely basis to ensure that appropriate arrangements for posthospital care will be made before discharge and to avoid unnecessary delays in discharge.
4. This evaluation must include the patient's likely need for and availability of appropriate posthospital services.
5. The discharge planning evaluation must be included in the patient's medical record for use in establishing an appropriate discharge plan, and the results of the evaluation must be discussed with the patient or his or her representative.
6. At the request of the patient's physician, the hospital must arrange for the development and initial implementation of a discharge plan for the patient.

7. A registered professional nurse, social worker, or other appropriately qualified staff member must develop or supervise any discharge planning or discharge plan required under this act.

In the literature, discussions regarding discharge planning focus primarily on the transition from the acute care setting. On examination, the process used in the hospital setting can be directly applied to the outpatient setting or any other health care setting in which a health care professional identifies unmet needs.

A model developed by Kelly and McClelland[46] achieves the balance between the realities of health care delivery today and the ideals of continuity of care (Figure 27-1). This model addresses the following key points:

1. Discharge planning can begin at any entry point in the health care system—not just as the client prepares to leave a 24-hour acute care setting.
2. Any point on the health continuum can serve as a basis for entry into the health care system. This may range from enrollment in a fitness clinic to a hospice program.
3. Movement through the care continuum may be multidirectional.
4. The intensity of care may be increased or decreased as the setting changes.

DISCHARGE PLANNING PROCESS

Discharge planning is a process that involves assessment, identification of continuing care needs, planning, and implementation of a plan to meet those needs. The trend to expedite patient transfers to more cost-effective levels of care at the earliest possible time necessitates not only the development of an effective tool to facilitate the process, but also professional standards of practice for discharge planning. Discharge planning is performed by a variety of health care professionals, including nurses, social workers, and others who, regardless of their background, must have the basic skills necessary to assess, develop, and implement individualized continuing care plans. Hamilton[32] acknowledges the importance of standards for discharge planning. She identifies the following seven essential components that should be included in the standards of practice for discharge planning and has developed a flow chart to demonstrate the process (Figure 27-2 and box, pp. 682-683):

- Assessment
- Needs identification
- Planning
- Documentation and communication
- Implementation
- Patient/family education
- Program evaluation

Adherence to standards of discharge planning and utilization of a systematic approach such as this example is

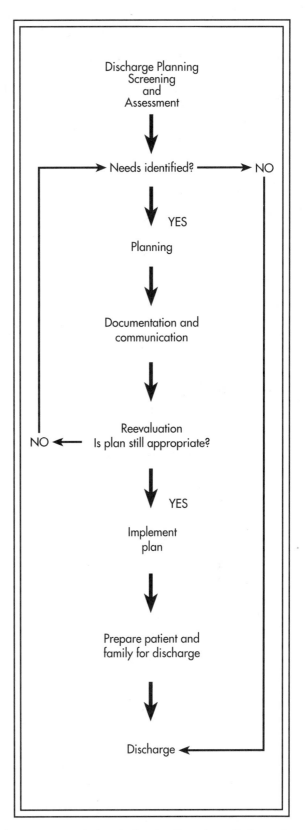

Figure 27-2 Discharge planning flow sheet. (Redrawn from Hamilton M: *Contin Care,* September 1995, p 34.)

STANDARDS OF PRACTICE FOR DISCHARGE PLANNING

STANDARD ONE: ASSESSMENT

Expected outcome: all patients will be screened as soon as possible after admission to identify continuing care needs. Accurate assessments are essential to development of appropriate discharge plans.

A. Assessment/screening triggers
 1. Admission review
 2. Case-finding criteria
 3. Continued-stay review
 4. Receipt of order/referral
B. Data collection sources
 1. Patient/family interviews
 2. Clinical/medical record
 3. Physicians, nurses
 4. Other health care professionals
C. Patient components
 1. Physical
  a. Age (high risk: over age 65, pediatric cases)
  b. Admitting diagnoses (high risk: HIV/AIDS, cancer, cerebrovascular accident (stoke), substance abuse, psychiatric diagnoses, chronic illnesses)
  c. Medical history, prognosis
  d. Response to treatments
  e. Functional capacity and ability to perform activities of daily living (ADLs) safely (e.g., feeding, bathing, mobilizing, ambulating, vision, hearing, communicating, toileting, shopping, housekeeping, using the telephone, sleeping)
  f. Medications
  g. Nursing care/therapy needs
  h. Nutritional status
  i. Skin integrity
  j. Pain
  k. Exercise, activity tolerance
 2. Emotional/cognitive/behavioral
  a. Level of consciousness, orientation, memory, competence, judgment
  b. Motivation and readiness for self-care
  c. Learning ability
  d. Personal goals, preferences
  e. Self-perception, health perception
  f. Presence of confusion, dementia, depression, anxiety
  g. Communication
  h. Coping mechanisms
 3. Psychosocial
  a. Adequacy of living arrangements/caregivers
  b. Familial/social support systems
  c. Availability of community resources
  d. Roles, relationships, ability to socialize
  e. Values, beliefs, cultural/spiritual preferences
  f. Designated party for health care decisions
  g. Advance directives
 4. Financial
  a. Insurance/benefits, contractual considerations
  b. Income, occupation, employment
  c. High-risk: homeless, indigent, Medicare, Medicaid, and nonfunded patients

STANDARD TWO: NEEDS IDENTIFICATION

Expected outcome: assessment data will provide a basis for indentification of actual or potential continuing care needs or problems that may affect discharge planning decisions.

A. Home with no aftercare needs identified
B. Home health care
 1. Nursing services/attendant care
 2. Home medical equipment
 3. Therapy services (e.g., occupational/physical/speech therapies)
 4. Social services
 5. Nutritional support
 6. Clinical laboratory, radiology
C. Transportation needs
 1. Frequency
 2. Distance
 3. Public assistance
D. Financial assistance
 1. Availability of third-party coverage
 2. Family resources
 3. Public assistance
E. Board and care/assisted living
F. Rehabilitation services
 1. Inpatient
 2. Outpatient
G. Nursing facility
 1. Extended care facility (ECF)
 2. Transitional care unit (TCU)
 3. Subacute care facility
 4. Convalescent/long-term care facility
H. Transfer to another acute care facility
 1. Acute care hospital
 2. Long-term acute care hospital (LTAC)
I. Hospice care/palliative care program

STANDARD THREE: PLANNING

Expected outcome: individualized plan of care will be developed from the information obtained in the assessment and needs identification processes. This plan will include input from the multidisciplinary health care team, patient, and family.

A. Prioritize identified discharge planning needs
B. Identify available resources
 1. Equipment
 2. Personnel
 3. Facilities
 4. Supportive services/agencies
C. Select actions/interventions to achieve desired goals

STANDARD FOUR: DOCUMENTATION AND COMMUNICATION

Expected outcome: all aspects of discharge planning process will be documented and communicated in a timely manner.

A. Multidisciplinary care plan/discharge record (if available)
 1. Name of discharge planner
 2. Date of patient contacts

STANDARDS OF PRACTICE FOR DISCHARGE PLANNING—cont'd

    3. Identified needs
    4. Expected outcomes
    5. Interventions
  B. Progress notes
    1. Date of consultation/referral
    2. Referral source
    3. Assessment (physical, emotional, psychosocial, financial, and personal data)
    4. Updates, reassessments
    5. Needs identified
    6. Requirements to meet continuing care needs
    7. Referrals to outside agencies/services
    8. Anticipated disposition/date
  C. Communicate/collaborate on plans
    1. Patient and family
    2. Attending physicians
    3. Nursing/ancillary services
    4. Community resources
    5. Insurance/utilization review (UR)/case management

STANDARD FIVE: IMPLEMENTATION

Expected outcome: individualized patient's plan of care will be implemented in a timely, effective manner to ensure postdischarge needs are met.
  A. Contact appropriate and available resources
  B. Coordinate placement
    1. Initiate patient transfer and referral record
    2. Initiate chart/copies process
  C. Order needed equipment, supplies, transportation, services
  D. Assist with referrals
    1. Social services
    2. Agencies
    3. Legal counsel
    4. Support groups
    5. Medicaid, Medicare, etc.
  E. Obtain consent for authorization to release medical records (as appropriate)

STANDARD SIX: PATIENT EDUCATION

Expected outcome: health care team, patient, and family will be knowledgeable about the discharge plan and the responsibilities to meet patient's ongoing health care needs.
  A. Multidisciplinary team
    1. Nursing
    2. Physical/occupational/speech therapies
    3. Pharmacy
    4. Nutritional services
    5. Social services
    6. Respiratory therapy
    7. Physicians
  B. Patient/family teaching
    1. Identify learning needs/barriers
    2. Assess readiness to learn
    3. Identify resources available
    4. Verbal/written discharge instructions

STANDARD SEVEN: PROGRAM EVALUATION

Expected outcome: to meet and exceed customer expectations through an ongoing performance improvement program.
  A. Periodic program evaluation
    1. Assess timeliness of screening
    2. Ensure appropriateness/accuracy of assessments
    3. Determine effectiveness of interventions
    4. Assess for preventable readmissions
  B. Monitor outcome through feedback
    1. Community resources/facilities
    2. Patients/families
    3. Physicians, nursing
    4. Multidisciplinary health care team
  C. Communicate outcomes through appropriate channels
    1. Financial
    2. Clinical
    3. Satisfaction indicators

Modified from Hamilton M: *Contin Care,* September 1995, pp. 33, 34, 36.

---

beneficial because it not only helps to develop a comprehensive plan of care, but also provides a built-in mechanism for ongoing reevaluation and modification of the plan.

ASSESSMENT

The oncology nurse in the acute care setting has a unique opportunity to perform a comprehensive assessment of the patient's strengths and limitations over days and sometimes weeks. This allows for the establishment of rapport between the nurse and patient. Frequently, when care is given over days, the nurse's keen eye may note a patient care need that may not have been previously assessed. The inpatient setting is extremely hectic, and frequently nurses do not have the luxury of spending extended periods with patients exploring their discharge needs when they, as well as the other patients in the nurse's care, have many needs that must be addressed immediately. Often it becomes a matter of prioritization: what needs to be done now and what can wait? It is important to understand that discharge planning *cannot* wait until the day the patient is going home or to an alternative setting for care.

Similarly, the oncology nurse in the outpatient clinic or alternative setting also has the opportunity to assess for and identify the patient's specific health care needs. A skilled practitioner can perform this task. The experienced oncology nurse can quickly and effectively assess, identify, and respond to newly identified patient/family needs as these needs surface if the nurse is continuously cognizant of the importance of planning for continued care and has a workable tool to facilitate the process.

A more detailed tool that facilitates the assessment and needs identification process was developed by Slevin and Roberts[83] at St. Francis Medical Center, Peoria, Ill, in 1987. It is a good example for discussion, although many other tools are available in the literature that are equally useful.[82] Many factors must be considered before discharge, and advance planning is imperative. Slevin and Roberts provide a helpful detailed approach to effective discharge planning transition from the acute care setting to the home setting. This process necessitates not only thorough assessment and evaluation, but also extensive planning, communication, and coordination. The authors identify the patient admission data form and the chart as the initial sources of data for the discharge planner to screen and identify patients that may have continuing care planning needs.[83] The experienced oncology nurse, while using secondary sources of data such as the patient's record, also relies on his or her first-hand observations and assessment of the patient. Hamilton[32] identifies specific patient components that identify patients who are in particular need for continuing care planning, including the following:

- Age (over age 65 or pediatric cases)
- Admitting diagnoses (human immunodeficiency virus/ acquired immunodeficiency syndrome [HIV/AIDS], cancer, cerebrovascular accident (CVA, stroke), substance abuse, psychiatric diagnoses, chronic illnesses)
- Medical history and prognosis
- Response to treatment
- Functional capacity and ability to perform activities of daily living (ADLs) safely
- Medications
- Nursing care and therapy needs
- Nutritional status
- Pain
- Exercise and activity tolerance

No matter how the patient with continuing care needs is identified, this screening process should be followed by (1) the patient interview, (2) identification of the specific problems or needs, and (3) development of a plan for solving client problems or needs. These three major components of the discharge planning process have specific subcomponents that, when addressed, both clarify and simplify the continuing planning process. These are discussed next.

Patient Interview[83]

1. Make introduction (if necessary).
2. Establish the relationship of the patient to (a) spouse, (b) family, including children, (c) neighbors, (d) church, and (e) senior-citizen support activities (if applicable).
3. Establish how the patient's illness has affected his or her role and function in the family, with special attention to (a) financial support, (b) shopping, (c) meal preparation, (d) transportation, and (e) living arrangements.
4. Determine the patient's prehospital daily routine.
5. Assess the patient's learning and comprehension ability.
6. Assess the patient's interest in discharge planning services.

In addition to Slevin and Robert's six steps in the patient interview, it is important also to determine the patient's goals and expectations of treatment and rehabilitation. This important factor is frequently overlooked by health care providers and is critical to the planning process.

Identification of Continuing Care Problems and Needs

After the patient interview is completed and it is determined that some needs or potential problem areas exist and the patient is interested in having continuing care planning services, the next step is to clearly identify the specific needs. Slevin and Roberts[83] identify the following factors warranting consideration at this stage of the planning process:

1. Inadequate or no support system
2. Inadequate financial resources
3. Poor environmental conditions
4. Inability to carry out treatment and medication regimen
5. Inability to carry out ADLs
6. Poor socialization
7. Potential problems (i.e., related to disease progression or treatment)

These seven cues help clarify the patient's specific and individual needs or problems and give direction to the development of an individualized plan of care to address these concerns.

PLANNING

Development of Plan for Solving Patient's Problems and Addressing Needs

After the patient's problems or needs are identified, a collaborative process involving the patient, family or significant others, and health care professionals should occur. At this time the oncology nurse should assist the patient, family, and significant others to look realistically at their goals and expectations and subsequently develop a plan for care. This may entail placement in an extended care facility or linkage with community-based agencies providing service in the home setting. With the diverse services available, it is necessary to address the following factors when assisting the patient and family in this decision-making process[83]:

1. Assist patient or family to identify the specific problem(s).
2. Assist patient or family to set priorities among the problems.
3. Assist patient or family to identify the services or resources needed.
4. Interpret services of the available resources to patient or family.
5. Establish patient's financial status.
6. Work out details of selected plan with patient or family.
7. Obtain patient or family consent to contact the resources in their behalf.
8. Establish criteria for evaluation of the effectiveness of the plan (usually a follow-up telephone call—discussed later in the chapter).

At this point, it should be apparent that the transition to home or alternative settings for care is complex and that it is necessary to consider many factors. It is important to keep in mind that health care is provided on a continuum and is a multidisciplinary effort. The nurse should utilize the resources available in his or her practice setting and establish a collaborative relationship with the continuing care team to facilitate the process for the benefit of the patient. If this is not possible, the nurse should network with colleagues and professionals in the community.

Often, because of early discharge, there is not sufficient time to initiate all the appropriate referrals to community support services. In such cases the referrals may be made after the patient is home. Since it has been well documented that the caregiving role is stressful, it is preferable that the professional doing the discharge planning make the initial contacts with the support services. A responsible family member may be willing to follow up on a referral made by the professional. The nurse should give this individual the name of the referred agency, the phone number, and the agency contact person.

If the patient needs skilled nursing care in the home setting, a referral to a skilled home care agency should be made. Most hospitals have continuing patient care forms that must be completed when a referral is initiated. The nurse should include information about other identified needs and request that the home care agency's personnel assist the patient with the referral process. It is essential that all relevant patient information is communicated and documented clearly, concisely, and in a timely manner. In addition to information about identified support needs, the referral for continuing patient care in the home care setting should also include information about significant factors related to this hospitalization, relevant past medical history, current medications and treatment orders, identified nursing problems, and results

of recent diagnostic tests or blood work. Concise and comprehensive referrals are essential to facilitate the transition from one setting of care to another and to promote continuity of care. It should be remembered that while nurses in the institutional settings have ready access to the patient's extensive medical record, the home care nurse frequently has only the continuing patient care referral form. The information on the referral form is often not comprehensive, thus making the home care nurse's job even more difficult. A list of national community resources is given in the Appendix at the end of this chapter. These organizations help identify available local community resources.

According to Magilvy and Lakomy[53]:

In summary, the transfer of information about a patient is essential to initiating prompt, effective care tailored to the specific needs of the patient. When accurate, timely information is available, the nurse who opens the case can accomplish the initial assessment more efficiently to facilitate continuity of care and assist the patient and family with the transition into home care.

Assessment of Caregiver and Informal Supports

In most institutions, assessment of supports of family, friends, and available organized institutions is routinely done if it is determined that the patient needs assistance in the home setting. Frequently, a primary caregiver, usually the spouse, has been identified, and some in-hospital teaching has been initiated by the nurses before discharge. However, this is not enough. A caregiver assessment must also be done. As the trend for early discharge continues, "the family support system must assume greater responsibility for maintaining what is often a very aggressive post-hospitalization treatment plan."[46] The stress and anxieties associated with the caregiving responsibilities can be overwhelming. Often, unasked questions and feelings of inadequacy in their ability to care for their loved one properly and safely add to the caregiving burden. "Probably their greatest challenge is developing the confidence to do what is right for the patient. 'Have I changed the dressing correctly?' 'Have I suctioned the patient in the proper manner?' One question often leads to a hundred more! Teaching them not only the 'what to do's' but also the 'what to expect' is one of the best stress reducers."[46]

Family members or friends provide approximately 80% of in-home care in the United States. Often these individuals do not have the option of quitting this role because of a sense of responsibility and duty and as an expression of love and devotion to the patient.[10,63,70] Most frequently, women over 55 years of age are the caregivers of the patient. Often these women receive assistance from other family members. Older males with cancer are usually cared for by their spouse. Elderly women with cancer, because of their longevity, are cared for by their adult children. Middle-aged cancer patients are cared for primarily by their spouse. The level of depression among caregivers is highest for wives, followed by daughters and then other female caregivers. Spousal caregivers are at particular risk for caregiver burden and illnesses associated with caregiver stress, since they maintain the caregiving role for longer periods and provide more extensive and comprehensive care. In addition, they believe that they are obligated to do so, with or without formal or informal assistance. More people enter nursing homes because of caregiver burnout than because of a significant change in their condition.[36,63,97]

Feuer[22] recommends that an extensive assessment of the caregiver also be conducted as part of the discharge planning process. He identifies 24 key issues and questions that should be addressed as part of this process:

1. Has the caregiver's age been considered as well as the patient's?
2. Does the caregiver's mental and physical condition allow that person to assume this responsibility?
3. Will the caregiver live in the patient's home?
4. If the caregiver is not in the home, how accessible will that person be?
5. Who can provide some relief or free time for the caregiver?
6. Is the caregiver aware of the patient's medical condition?
7. Has the caregiver received instructions on administering medications, observing for possible side effects, and managing them?
8. Is the caregiver aware of the expected course of treatment?
9. If there is to be a change in the patient's condition, does the caregiver know what problems to watch for?
10. If the patient's condition changes, does the caregiver know whom to call?
11. Does the caregiver know the name of the physician directing the home care plan?
12. If a home care agency will provide care at home, has the caregiver received the name and phone number of the company?
13. If the patient will be using medical equipment in the home, has the caregiver been given the name of the company that supplies it?
14. Has the caregiver been helped to develop a list of emergency phone numbers: (a) community emergency numbers, (b) rescue emergency numbers, (c) physician, (d) home care agency, (e) equipment supplier, and (f) other family members?
15. Does the caregiver know about any follow-up medical appointments scheduled for the patient?
16. Has the caregiver been instructed in what *not* to do for the patient as well as what to allow the patient to do for himself or herself?
17. If prescriptions must be filled, are there immediate funds available to do this? Also, if a prescription is difficult to obtain at local pharmacies, advise the caregiver where it is available.
18. Have questions regarding financial matters related to the patient's home care needs been arranged before discharge? Is the caregiver attending to financial matters?
19. If the caregiver can no longer assume responsibility, whom should he or she notify?
20. Does the caregiver have medications for the patient's first 24 hours home? If not, is there a plan developed to obtain these medications?
21. Has the caregiver been made aware of any appropriate support groups available in the community?
22. Have you supplied the caregiver with suitable educational materials regarding the patient's diagnosis?
23. Does the caregiver have the name and phone number of the person who arranged for home care services and who can be called to clarify issues or further explain services to be expected?
24. Has the discharge planner asked the caregiver if he or she has any questions or problems concerning the discharge, date, time, transportation home, or the services the caregiver and patient will be receiving?

Value of Humor

Humor as a preventive therapy for family caregivers is one type of respite that has been underused in primary

Table 27-1 Holistic Effects of Humor

Human dimension	Effects of humor
Musculoskeletal system	Upward movement of cheeks and upper lip; vocal cords function to produce laughter sounds; movement of arms, hands, torso, head
Respiratory system	Rapid, shallow breathing; ratio of expirations to inspirations increased; ventilation increased
Cardiovascular system	Circulation stimulated; cardiac muscle stimulated; production of thrombosis-preventing plasminogen activator stimulated
Immune system	T-lymphocyte production stimulated
Endocrine system	Catecholamine production stimulated, especially epinephrine (Adrenalin); endorphin release stimulated
Behavioral system	Stress-worry cycle interrupted; effects of stress, tension, anxiety decreased; expression of emotion facilitated; learning and memory enhanced; self-concept and/or self-acceptance reflected and reinforced; consensual validation, bonding, social cohesiveness facilitated; negative feelings, attitudes, and ideas expressed in socially acceptable manner
Spiritual system	Existential paradox of God-mortal and death paradox of sad-glad played with; absurdities of life and human condition held up to jest; human spirit rescued from despair

Modified from Pasquali EA: *Home Healthc Nurse* 9(3):34, 1991.

prevention of caregiver burnout.[72] Humor is not just the telling of jokes. It is a concept that includes wit, laughter, joking, comedy, kidding, teasing, mimicking, and satire. What is seen as humorous varies with different personalities, culture, and background as well as with levels of stress and pain.[15] The uses and beneficial effects of humor have been well documented (Table 27-1).[15,72,95] Humor can help "recharge" family caregivers physically and psychologically and can improve the quality of their lives. Humor can also facilitate communication and promote positive interpersonal relationships among health care providers, patients, and their families. To use humor therapeutically, oncology nurses must first understand the family's and caregivers' coping patterns, level of anxiety, and sense of humor.[15,71,94]

SETTINGS FOR CARE

In the past the hospital was the primary setting for care. In recent years, hospitals, as well as other health care providers and payors, have created innovative alternative care sites that reduce the cost but not the income while maintaining quality care.

Extended Care

Usually in the outpatient setting, extended care placement is not an identified need; however, it is wise to have a working knowledge about these resources. At times, family members may find the caregiving burden too overwhelming and request information on and assistance with extended care placement. If it is determined that the patient's care needs necessitate placement in an extended care facility, the facility that will most effectively meet the patient's needs must then be identified. The following six basic types of extended care facilities vary according to the amount and type of care needed by the patient:

1. Subacute care facilities
2. Skilled care facilities
3. Intermediate care facilities
4. Adult foster or sheltered care facilities
5. Residential care facilities
6. Adult day-care facilities

Subacute care facilities, also known as long-term care hospitals, are a recent development in the health care system. These are cost-efficient settings that provide a variety of medical-surgical, oncologic, rehabilitation, and additional specialty care services in an alternative setting for those patients who no longer need acute care services but are too ill to send home. This alternative care setting is preferred by case managers and managed care organizations because it offers outcome-focused care as well as cost efficiency.[86,88] Many hospitals have begun to add subacute facilities to enhance revenues while still providing appropriate care to patients with specialized needs such as highly skilled nursing and therapy services.[67] An

added benefit to providing such a facility for care is that it separates the chronically ill patients from others. This enables health care providers to consider the underlying assumptions of care and the appropriateness of aggressive care measures while still providing care for chronically critically ill patients in specialized "low-tech" units without compromising prospects for recovery.[43,59]

Skilled care facilities provide around-the-clock skilled nursing care and observation. In addition, there is frequent medical supervision. *Intermediate care facilities* provide around-the-clock basic nursing care for patients who are medically stable but unable to care for themselves. *Adult foster care* or *sheltered care facilities* are for individuals who require a protective living arrangement that provides general supervision and assistance with bathing, dressing, meals, and other personal needs.[83]

Adult foster care, also known as sheltered care, is a reasonable option for adults needing care regardless of income or age. Usually, adult foster care is less expensive than nursing home care. Although some overlap occurs between the populations served by nursing and foster care homes, residents in foster care tend to be less functionally and cognitively impaired than those in nursing homes.[64]

Residential care facilities are for individuals who no longer want to live alone or have no place to live. In general, these facilities also provide similar services as a sheltered care facility and occasionally, in times of illness, may provide intermediate care for their residents.[83] These facilities often have various levels of living arrangements, ranging from independent to assisted living.

Adult day-care facilities can provide various levels of care for cancer patients and much needed respite for family caregivers. Adult day-care programs serve as a bridge between traditional care services and the home where there otherwise might be a gap in service delivery. Some adult day-care programs also provide services for the caregiver, ranging from counseling to caregiver support groups.[93]

Since many extended care facilities are available, it becomes an overwhelming task to select the best one. The long-term care ombudsman office in each state will provide lists of certified extended care facilities that offer the various levels of care. This state office will also provide information regarding reimbursement of these facilities by Medicare or Medicaid. This is a helpful starting point for patients and their family members. It is recommended that the patient or significant other tour the facilities before making a selection.

Home Care

Home care has seen an increase in utilization in the past 14 years because of the implementation of DRGs and subsequent earlier discharges. Increased momentum of consumerism and the desire to exercise more control over personal health care have also been influencing factors.

Home care is on the cutting edge of change in nursing and health care. In a time of increasing concern over federal health care expenditures, home care represents a humane, sensible alternative to institutionalized care for an increasing number of Americans. It also offers other benefits, including eliminating the risk of nosocomial infection, maintaining patients' and families' social and cultural patterns, and promoting patients' self-esteem, independence, and personal involvement in care.[20]

The option of home care services is understandably attractive to cancer patients and their families, who face an illness that often strips away much of their sense of personal control. Remaining in the comfort of their own home and receiving care is preferred over institutionalization by 71% of Americans.[16,33]

Two types of home care services are available to health care consumers: traditional home care and high-technology home care. Traditional home care services generally provide skilled nursing care, including patient assessment and intervention, patient and family education; rehabilitative services such as physical, occupational, and speech and language therapies; social work intervention; and home health aide support.

Recent improvements in and the increasing availability of high technology in the home setting have made home care a viable option for cancer patients at all stages of treatment and illness. High-technology home care for patients with cancer generally refers to the home management of infusional therapies such as the following[54]:
1. Antifungal therapy
2. Antibiotic therapy
3. Chemotherapy
4. Hemotherapy
5. Hydration therapy
6. Venous access device maintenance
7. Pain management
8. Total parenteral and enteral nutrition

Home IV therapy is one of the most rapidly growing trends in the home care industry. Cost containment and the growing threat of communicable disease transmission in hospitals are the two major factors contributing to this trend.[45,56] Not all patients with cancer are good candidates for home infusion therapy. These patients and their families must be properly screened before initiating such therapies in the home setting to ensure that the treatment is both safe and efficacious (see box on right). In addition, physician support and accessibility for clear, open communications must be present to ensure continuity of care and safe infusion therapy in the home setting.[65]

Patients who receive infusional therapy in the home must have a venous access device to ensure a reliable, safe, and patent access site. A variety of infusion pumps

that are compact, reliable, and easy to manage are available for the home setting and ensure that the prescribed medication is administered as ordered. A variety of types of central venous catheters are available. Tables 27-2, 27-3, and 27-4 present a general overview of tunneled central venous catheters and peripherally inserted central venous catheters (PICC lines), as well as guidelines for care and management. Table 27-5 provides a general overview of infusion pumps.

Total parenteral therapy (TPN) and enteral therapy for cancer patients have been controversial issues from medical, ethical, and financial perspectives. Nevertheless, this form of treatment is frequently provided in the home setting. It is generally believed that improved nutritional status improves the quality of life but does not necessarily prolong life. During the end stage of illness, however, when vital organs begin to shut down, infusional therapies are not advised. This is particularly dif-

---

CRITERIA FOR PATIENT SCREENING FOR HOME INFUSION THERAPY

1. Patient must want to receive therapy at home.
2. Patient must be medically stable for home treatment.
3. Patient should have a venous access device in place or adequate venous access via peripheral route (or a plan must exist should peripheral access become exhausted).
4. Patient or caregiver must be able to care for central line and demonstrate proficiency and competency in maintaining access device.
5. Patient or caregiver must be knowledgeable about therapy, including:
   a. Name of drug(s)—both infusional and adjunct medications
   b. Dosage(s)
   c. Potential side effects
   d. Actions to take to prevent or minimize side effects
   e. Potential adverse reactions to medication
   f. Storage of drug(s)
6. Patient or caregiver must be knowledgeable and proficient in functioning of infusion pump as follows:
   a. Operation of pump
   b. Using alarm system
   c. How to check if pump is working
   d. Troubleshooting pump
7. Patient's home environment must be conducive to home care (e.g., physical layout, telephone access, support person[s], running water, electricity).
8. Patient must have the financial means to pay for home treatment (e.g., insurance, private pay).
9. Patient or caregiver must have an emergency 24-hour number to call for problems (e.g., clinic RN, physician's office, homecare agency).

Modified from Maloney CH, Preston F: *Oncol Nurs Forum* 19(1):77, 1992.

ficult for families to accept and understand because they frequently believe that since the patient is not eating or drinking, IV lines are necessary. If the rationale for withholding, discontinuing, or decreasing fluids to keep vein open (KVO) is not clearly explained to families at this time, they may be concerned that the patient is being denied vital treatment. More information regarding home care for the terminally ill and symptom management can be obtained from several helpful handbooks listed in the Appendix at the end of this chapter.

As many as 70% of patients with cancer experience pain during their illness, and at least 90% of this cancer-related pain can be effectively relieved with existing pain management techniques. Although the oral route of pain medication is the preferred method by pain experts, high-technology pain management is a reasonable option to patients whose pain can not be effectively controlled otherwise. The American Pain Society, a national chapter of the International Association for the Study of Pain, publishes a helpful booklet, *Principles of Analgesic Use in the Treatment of Acute Pain and Chronic Cancer Pain,* which can be obtained for a small fee. In addition, the American Pain Society may be contacted to obtain addi-

tional information regarding pain management and consult with another health care professional experienced in pain management techniques (see Appendix and Chapter 29).

With the advances in anticancer therapies and the availability of portable infusion pumps, chemotherapy administration in the home setting has become both safe and effective. Lokich[51] cites many advantages of continuous infusional chemotherapy: "(1) increased exposure to chemotherapeutic agents with continuous infusion, thereby increasing the tumorcidal effect, (2) an increased cumulative dose delivered to the tumor, and (3) a decrease in occurrence and severity of toxicities." As a result, this has become an increasingly common practice in the home setting. It is important that patients receive their first dose of chemotherapy in an inpatient or outpatient setting to facilitate expedient and proper treatment if any untoward reactions occur. In addition, a plan for properly disposing of all biohazardous waste should be in place (see Chapter 22).

It is also important that antibiotic and antifungal therapies be initiated in the inpatient or outpatient setting because side effects typically occur with these medications.

Text continued on p. 696.

Table 27-2 Examples of Tunneled Central Venous Catheters Currently Marketed in the United States

Model/material (manufacturer)	French size	Inner diameter	Total lumen volume (priming volume)
SINGLE-LUMEN DEVICES			
Hickman Single Lumen Catheter/silicone (Bard)	9	1.6 mm	1.8 ml
Groshong Single Lumen Catheter/silicone (Bard)	7 and 8	1.3-1.5 mm	0.7-1.2 ml
Quinton Single Lumen Central Venous Access Catheter/silicone (Quinton)	3.9-9.7*	0.75-1.5 mm	0.9-2.0 ml
Harborin Single Lumen Central Venous Catheter/polyurethane (Harbor Medical Devices)	7	1.5 mm	0.9 ml
DOUBLE-LUMEN DEVICES			
Hickman Dual Lumen Catheters/silicone (Bard)	7	0.8 mm/1.0 mm	0.6 ml/0.8 ml
	9	0.7 mm/1.3 mm	0.6 ml/1.3 ml
	12	1.6 mm/lumen	1.8 ml (each lumen)
Leonard Dual Lumen Catheter/silicone (Bard)	10	1.3 mm/lumen	1.3 ml/lumen
Groshong Dual Lumen Catheter/silicone (Bard)	9.5	1.1 mm/1.33 mm	0.5 ml/0.8 ml
Cook TPN Double Lumen Central Venous	5	0.5 mm/lumen	0.2 ml/lumen
Catheters/silicone (Cook Critical Care)	7	0.7 mm/1.0 mm	0.4 ml/0.6 ml
	9	1.0 mm/1.3 mm	0.6 ml/1.0 ml
	12	1.0 mm/1.6 mm	1.6 ml/2.3 ml
Quinton RAAF Dual Lumen Central	9	1.1 mm/lumen	1.2 ml/lumen
Venous Catheters/silicone	12	1.5 mm/lumen	2.2 ml/lumen
	13.5	2.0 mm/lumen	2.5 ml/lumen
TRIPLE-LUMEN DEVICES			
Nutritional Support Catheter/polyurethane (Arrow International)	7		0.7 ml/0.5 ml/0.5 ml
Hickman Triple Lumen Catheter/silicone (Bard)	12.5	1.0 mm/1.0/mm/1.5 mm	0.7 ml/0.7 ml/1.6 ml
Quinton Triple Lumen Central Venous Access Catheter/silicone	11.7	1.0 mm/1.0 mm/1.25 mm	1.0 ml/1.1 ml/1.2 ml

Modified from Finley RS: *Highlights Antineoplast Drugs* 13(2):15, 1995.
*Size depends on model.

Table 27-3 Examples of Peripherally Inserted Central Venous Catheters (PICCs) Currently Marketed in the United States

Model or trade name/material (manufacturer)	French size	Lumen diameter	Length	Priming volume
SINGLE-LUMEN DEVICES				
Groshong PICC/silicone (Bard)	4	0.8 mm	56 cm	0.3 ml
C-PICS/silicone (Cook Critical Care)	5	0.91 mm	60 cm	0.6 ml
V-Cath/silicone (HDC Corporation)	2	0.3 mm	40 cm	0.1 ml
	4	0.9 mm	60 cm	0.4 ml
L-Cath PICCs/polyurethane	5	1.2 mm	56 cm	0.9 ml
(Luther Medical Products)	3.5	0.7 mm	56 cm	0.4 ml
	2.6	0.5 mm	56 cm	0.2 ml
DOUBLE-LUMEN DEVICES				
D/L PICC/silicone (Bard)	5	0.8 mm/0.6 mm	55.9 cm	0.4 ml/0.3 ml
Double-Lumen Per-q-cath/silicone (Bard)	4	0.5 mm/0.3 mm	60 cm	0.1 ml/0.6 ml
	5	0.8 mm/0.4 mm	60 cm	0.3 ml/0.1 ml

Modified from Finley RS: *Highlights Antineoplast Drugs* 13(2):15, 1995.

Table 27-4 Central Venous Catheters: Recommended Nursing Management

Type	Heparinization*	Dressing	Blood sampling
ADULT			
Central venous catheters, short-term use, subclavian Single/dual/triple lumen	After each use, flush *each* lumen with 5 ml normal saline (N/S), then heparinized saline 2 ml (100 U/ml). For catheter *not* in use, flush *each* lumen with heparinized saline 2 ml (100 U/ml) *every 12 hours.*	Daily sterile dressing change at the site for duration of catheter placement. Gauze dressing change every 24 hours. Change Luer-Lok injection caps *every 72 hours.*	Shut off all IV lines for *1 full minute.* Withdraw 5 ml blood. Discard. Withdraw blood sample. Flush lumen with 5 ml N/S, then heparinize or resume IV line. *Total parenteral nutrition (TPN): shut off IV line 10 minutes.*
Peripherally inserted central venous catheters Long-line PICC† Single/dual lumen Use gentle pressure on syringe plunger for PICCs.)	After each use, flush lumen with 2 ml N/S, then heparinized saline 1 ml (100 U/ml). For catheter *not* in use, flush lumen with heparinized saline 1 ml (100 U/ml) every 12 hours.	Sterile dressing change after first 24 hours, then every 72 hours. Change Luer-Lok injection caps every 72 hours.	Shut off all IV lines for *1 full minute.* Withdraw 1.5 ml blood. Discard. Withdraw blood sample. Flush lumen with 2.5 ml N/S, then heparinize or resume IV line. *TPN: shut off IV line 10 minutes.*
Tunneled catheters, long-term use Hickman Quinton/Raaf Single/dual/triple lumen	After each use, flush *each* lumen with 5 ml N/S, then heparinized saline 2 ml (100 U/ml). For catheter *not* in use, flush *each* lumen with heparinized saline 2 to 5 ml (100 U/ml) daily/biweekly.	Daily sterile dressing change at exit site for initial 14 days. Gauze dressing change every 24 hours. Thereafter, cleanse exit site daily (Betadine/alcohol). Optional daily clean dressing. Change Luer-Lok injection caps *weekly.*	Shut off all IV lines for *1 full minute.* Withdraw 5 ml blood. Discard. Withdraw blood sample. Flush lumen with 5 ml N/S, then heparinize or resume IV line. *TPN: shut off IV lines 10 minutes.*

From LaRocca JC, Otto SE, editors: Pocket Guide to Intravenous Therapy, ed 3, St Louis, 1997, Mosby.

*Heparinization of central venous catheters varies in frequency, volume of solution, concentration of the heparin dilution, type of device, and patient's age and weight. Confirm with physician managing patient's care and agency/institution for nursing management protocol regarding heparinization of central venous catheters/implantable ports.

Consider patient with an alteration in coagulation factors and/or heparin allergy/intolerance with frequency of use of intermittent device. Potentially these patients may require low-concentration (e.g., 10 U/heparin/ml) and/or alternative flushing solution (e.g., sodium citrate, 1.4% solution).

†Use 5 ml or larger syringes when flushing and/or blood sampling from PICC.

‡Selected oncologists use 2 to 5 ml heparinized saline (100 U/ml).

§Check manufacturer's specific recommendations regarding volume. Oncologists use heparin, 10 ml (100 U/ml).

‖Assess patient, disease, platelet count with frequency/volume/concentration of heparinization schedule.

Table 27-4 Central Venous Catheters: Recommended Nursing Management—cont'd

Type	Heparinization*	Dressing	Blood sampling
Groshong Single/dual lumen	Does not require heparin to maintain catheter patency. *Use force when flushing.* Flush *each* lumen with 5 ml N/S after each use, except for TPN, then flush with 30 ml N/S. For catheter *not* in use, flush with 5 ml N/S weekly.‡	Daily sterile dressing change at exit site for initial 14 days. Gauze dressing change every 24 hours. Thereafter, cleanse exit site daily (Betadine/alcohol). Optional daily clean dressing. Change Luer-Lok injection caps *weekly.*	Shut off all IV lines for *1 full minute.* Withdraw 5 ml blood. Discard. Withdraw blood sample. Flush lumen with 30 ml N/S vigorously, then resume IV line or apply injection cap.‡ *TPN: shutoff IV line 10 minutes.*
Implantable vascular access devices Davol Port Infuse-A-Port Life Port Port-A-Cath	After each use, flush *each* port with Huber needle: 10ml N/S, followed by heparinized saline (100 U/ml).§ For port *not* in use, flush each port with 3 to 10 ml heparinized saline (100 U/ml) *every 30 days* (venous placement). Intermittent flush >1/day use N/S and/or low-dose/low-volume heparin.‖	Sterile bio-occlusive dressing when port accessed. Steri-strips at new incision site for 3 days. When incision site healed and port not accessed, no dressing required. When port is accessed for continuous infusion, change needle and extension tubing every 5-7 days.	Shut off all IV lines for *1 full minute.* Withdraw 5 ml blood. Discard. Withdraw blood sample. Flush with 20 ml N/S, followed by 3 to 10 ml heparinized saline (100 U/ml)‡ or resume IV line. *TPN: shut off IV line 10 minutes.*
PEDIATRIC			
Short-term use, subclavian Single lumen/or multilumen	After each use, flush *each* lumen with 2 ml N/S, followed by 1 ml heparinized saline solution, 10 U/ml, after each use or at least twice a day.	Daily sterile dressing change at site for duration of catheter placement. Gauze dressing change every 24 hours. Change Luer-Lok injection caps every 24 hours.	Shut off all IV lines for *1 full minute.* Withdraw 3 ml blood. Discard. Withdraw blood sample. Flush lumen with 2 ml N/S, then heparinize or resume IV line. *TPN: shut off IV line 10 minutes.*
Peripherally inserted catheters Long-line PICC† Single/dual lumen (Use gentle pressure on syringe plunger for PICCs.)	After each use, flush lumen: *Pediatrics:* 2 ml N/S in 5 ml syringe or larger, followed by 1ml heparinized saline (10 U/ml) after each use or at least twice a day. *Special care nursery (neonates):* 0.5 ml N/S, preservative free, in 5 ml syringe or larger, followed by 0.5 ml heparinized saline (4 U/ml). Intermittent flush schedule every 4 to 8 hours: consult with physician orders.	Sterile dressing change after first 24 hours, then every 72 hours. Change Luer-Lok injection caps every 72 hours.	Shut off all IV lines for *1 full minute.* Withdraw 1.5 ml blood. Discard. Withdraw blood sample. Flush lumen with 2.5 ml N/S, then heparinize or resume IV line. *TPN: shut off IV line 10 minutes.*
Tunneled catheters, long-term use Broviac	After each use, flush lumen with 2 ml N/S, then heparinized saline 1 ml (10 U/ml). For catheter *not* in use, flush lumen with heparinized saline 1 ml (10 U/ml) daily.	Daily sterile dressing change at exit site for initial 14 days. Gauze dressing change every 24 hours. Thereafter, cleanse exit site daily with Betadine. Apply sterile 2 × 2 Change Luer-Lok injection caps *weekly.*	Shut off all IV lines for *1 full minute.* Withdraw 3 ml blood. Discard. Withdraw blood sample. Flush lumen with 2 ml N/S, then heparinize or resume IV line. *TPN: shut off IV line 10 minutes.*
Implantable vascular access devices Port-A-Cath	After each use, flush the port with Huber needle, 5 ml N/S, followed by 2 ml heparinized saline (100 U/ml). For port *not* in use, flush port with 2 ml heparinized saline (100 U/ml) *every 30 days* (venous placement).	Sterile bio-occlusive dressing when port accessed. Steri-strips at new incision site for 3 days. When incision site healed and port not accessed, no dressing required. When port is accessed for continuous infusion, change needle and extension tubing every 5-7 days.	Shut off all IV lines for *1 full minute.* Withdraw 3-5 ml blood (depending on size of child). Discard. Withdraw blood sample. Flush with 5 ml N/S, then heparinize or resume IV line. *TPN: shut off IV line 10 minutes.*

Table 27-5 Features of Ambulatory Infusion Devices

Name/model (manufacturer)	Pumping mechanism	Drug reservoir/ accessories	Battery/power source	Range of infusion rates	Alarms/safety features	Keep open rate	Program modes	Weight	Size
AMBULATORY, SINGLE CHANNEL									
WalkMed 440 PIC (Medex, Division of Ivion)	Linear peristaltic	Disposable 65, 150, 250 ml bags; dedicated pump sets	9 V disposable battery (450-650 ml/battery)	1-30 ml/hr (can also be programmed as mg/hr)	Near end of program; volume limit; occlusion; system malfunction; low battery; depleted battery; end of infusion; door open; programming error; lockout levels	0-9.9 ml/hr	PCA; intermittent; continuous	360 g	1.6 × 11.2 × 10.2 cm
WalkMed 350 (Medex Ambulatory Infusion Systems, Division of Ivion)	Linear peristaltic	Disposable 65, 150, 250 ml bags; dedicated pump sets	9 V alkaline battery (3-21 days)	0.1-19.99 ml/hr (increments of 0.01 ml)	Occlusion; system malfunction; low battery; depleted battery; prime; door open		Continuous	360 g	4.6 × 11.2 × 10.2 cm
WalkMed PCA (Medex Ambulatory Infusion Systems, Division of Ivion)	Linear peristaltic	Disposable 65, 150, 250 ml bags; dedicated pump sets	9 V alkaline battery (1-21 days depending on infusion rate)	0.1-19.99 ml/hr (increments of 0.01) or 0.1-30 ml/hr (increments of 0.1 ml)	Near end; volume limit; occlusion; system malfunction; low battery; depleted battery; end of infusion; total volume delivered; programming error		Continuous; continuous with patient-activated bolus; bolus only	360 g	4.6 × 11.2 × 10.2 cm
Provider One (Abbott)	Rotary peristaltic	Any collapsible IV bag; dedicated tubing	Two disposable 9 V lithium batteries (4800 ml); or 12 V rechargeable batteries (4,000 ml)	1-400 ml/hr	Occlusion; cartridge improperly inserted; programming error; computer error; air in line; low battery; low reservoir; end of infusion	1 ml/hr	Continuous; tapering	400 g	132 × 86 × 33 cm
Provider 5500 (Pancretec/Abbott)	Rotary peristaltic	Any collapsible IV bag	9 V alkaline battery	0.1-250 ml/hr	Occlusion; air in line; low reservoir; low battery; ending infusion; system problem; latch open	0.1 ml/hr	Continuous; PCA	400 g	

Pain Management Provider (Abbott)	Rotary peristaltic	Any collapsible IV bag		0.1-25 ml/hr in 0.1-ml increments	Security lock box available		Continuous; loading dose; PCA (suitable for epidural injection)		
CADD-Plus (Pharmacia Deltec)	Linear peristaltic	50, 100, 250 ml custom cassettes or any collapsible IV bag with custom adapter	9 V disposable alkaline or lithium battery	0.1-75 ml/hr	High pressure; low reservoir; low battery; power-up failure; pump in stop mode; programmed volume depleted; high pressure; system error	0-10 ml/hr	Continuous; intermittent; delay start	425 g	2.8 × 8.9 × 16 cm
CADD-I (Pharmacia Deltec)	Linear peristaltic	50, 100, 250 ml custom cassettes or any collapsible IV bag with custom adapter	9 V disposable alkaline or lithium battery	0-299 ml every 24 hours or 90 ml/hr in fixed high-flow mode	Power-up fault; pump in stop mode; low battery; low reservoir; low volume; programmed volume depleted; high pressure; system error		Continuous	425 g	2.8 × 8.9 × 16 cm
CADD-PCA Ambulatory Infusion Pump Model 5800	Linear peristaltic	50, 100, 250 ml custom reservoir or any IV bag with remote adapter	9 V alkaline or lithium battery	0-20 ml/hr (may also be programmed in mg/hr)	Power-up failure; low battery; depleted battery; low reservoir; programmed volume depleted; high pressure; system error		Continuous; patient-activated bolus; continuous plus patient-activated bolus	425 g	2.8 × 3.5 × 6.4 cm
CADD-TPN Ambulatory Infusion System Model 5700 (Pharmacia Deltec)	Linear peristaltic	Collapsible IV bag with dedicated adapter tubing	9 V alkaline (6 hour) or lithium (18 hour) battery, rechargeable battery pack (11 hour), or AC adapter	10-250 ml/hr with 9 V battery or 10-400 ml/hr with AC adapter	Low reservoir; programmed volume depleted; infusion period completed; low battery; depleted battery; invalid rate; high pressure; power-up fault; system error	5 ml/hr	Continuous; continuous with tapering up or down	369 g	2.8 × 8.9 × 13.3 cm
EZ Flow Model 80-2 (Creative Medical Development)	Displacement chamber	Disposable 100 and 250 ml cassettes or large-volume adapter	Rechargeable NiCad battery or AC power adapter	0.6-250 ml/hr (16 incremental rates)	Infusion complete; occlusion; low battery	0.2 or 1 ml/hr	Continuous; intermittent	14 oz	6.75 × 3.5 × 1.27 inches

Modified from Finley RS: *Highlights Antineoplast Drugs* 13(2):15, 1995.

Continued.

Table 27-5 Features of Ambulatory Infusion Devices—cont'd

Name/model (manufacturer)	Pumping mechanism	Drug reservoir/ accessories	Battery/power source	Range of infusion rates	Alarms/safety features	Keep open rate	Program modes	Weight	Size
AMBULATORY, SINGLE CHANNEL—cont'd									
MedMate 1100 (Patient Solutions)	Peristaltic	Custom cassettes or any IV bag	Two disposable 9 V alkaline or lithium batteries or external recharger	0.1-500 ml/hr	Programming error; system fault; low battery; dose due; air in line; door open; dose complete; low bag; bag end	0.1-9.9 ml/hr	Continuous; tapering; patient-controlled anesthesia (PSA); intermittent; delay start	17 oz	4.4 × 3.3 × 1.4 inches
Vector MTI (Infusion Technology)		Any collapsible IV bag	Two 9 V alkaline batteries or AC power	0.1-400 ml/hr	Reservoir empty; infusion complete; over pressure; check cassette; dead battery; system malfunction; air in line; low battery; low reservoir	0-5 ml/hr	Continuous; intermittent; PCA; taper	14.5 oz	5.6 × 3.5 × 1.4 inches
MAXX 100 (Medication Delivery Devices)	Controlled-pressure technology	100 ml custom bag	9 V alkaline battery	50, 100, or 200 ml/hr	Pump malfunction; low battery; occlusion; end of infusion; overflow		Continuous	10.5 oz	6.7 × 4.7 × 1.4 inches
SideKick (I-Flow)	Spring-driven infusion	50 and 100 ml minibags; custom IV sets that determine flow rate	Self-contained spring	50, 100, or 200 ml/hr	None		Continuous		
MEDFLO II (Secure Medical Products)	Elastomeric	Unit is disposable balloon reservoir: 100, 200, and 300 ml	None	50, 100, 175, and 200 ml/hr	None	NA	Continuous		2.75 × 4.25 to 7.0 inches
ReadyMed (McGaw)	Elastomeric	50, 100, 250 ml reservoirs	None	50, 100, 167, and 200 ml/hr	None	NA	Continuous		
Intermate LV System (Baxter)	Elastomeric	Unit is disposable balloon reservoir: 105, 275 ml	None	50, 100, 200, and 250 ml/hr	None	NA	Continuous		

						PCA			
Infusor (Baxter)	Elastomeric	Unit is disposable balloon reservoir: 65-275 ml	None	0.5-10 ml/hr or 12-240 ml/day		With patient-controlled module attachment, lockout of 15 or 60 minutes	Continuous;		
AMBULATORY, MULTICHANNEL									
The VIVUS 4000 Infuser (I-Flow Corporation), four channel	Positive displacement	Any IV bag; dedicated tubing; manifold line to connect up to four tubings to single IV line; programmer required for operation; communicator unit for remote programming	5 (5000 ml delivery) or 10 (10,000 ml delivery) AA disposable alkaline batteries; 1.5 V DC or external 110/120 V AC adapter	0.1-200 ml/hr	Low battery; dead battery; occlusion; empty reservoir; internal malfunction; runaway infusion; open door	0.1-200 ml/hr	Continuous; sequential; continuous bolus; intermittent	1.05 kg	19.7 × 11.43 × 5.1 cm
Intelliject (Ivion), four channel	Rack and pinion drive (syringe driver)	Dedicated 30 ml syringes and manifold	Two 9 V disposable batteries	5.4-40 ml/hr/channel	Occlusion; low battery; low reservoir; program error; electronic fault	Any preset rate	Continuous; bolus; continuous plus bolus; sequential; alternating	1.54 kg	25.4 × 16.5 × 7.1 cm
Verifuse (Block Medical)	Linear peristaltic	Any IV container	Two 9 V alkaline batteries; rechargeable NiCad battery, or AC power adapter	0.1-300 ml/hr	Door open; barcode fault; change batteries; low batteries; pump interrupted; air in line; low reservoir; occlusion; bad batteries; pumping complete; overvoltage; end of program; malfunction	Any preset rate	Continuous; tapering up or down; loading dose; delay start; PCA; intermittent	17 oz	6.4 × 3.1 × 1.1 inches

Once the patient's tolerance to the medication has been established, this treatment modality in the home setting is preferable to extended hospitalization if the patient is medically stable.

The patient is generally more comfortable at home, and the health care cost savings are considerable when such high-technology services are provided in the home setting. In addition, patient hospitalizations are reduced, there is increased quality of life for patients and their families, and patients have a sense of control and active participation in their treatment plan.

Geriatric Considerations

Ill older adults generally want to be home among family and familiar surroundings. Family members often feel inadequate in their abilities to care properly for their parent/spouse and may be reluctant to bring them home. This in turn may result in feelings of guilt and fears that they may be judged as uncaring. In addition, family members have feelings of guilt and helplessness associated with their parent's/spouse's illness. The nurse must provide an opportunity for family members to discuss their fears, feelings, and concerns. Consideration should be given also to how this illness is affecting the family's ability to meet their continuing needs.[6,17,53]

McAnear[58] developed the following set of questions that enable the nurse to gain a more thorough awareness of the family's needs and coping abilities:

Needs
1. What difficulties is the family experiencing with the medical treatment? (This would include management and changes in course of illness.)
2. What are the sources of financial strain from direct and indirect costs related to the illness?
3. What changes are required in ADLs for the family?
4. In what manner has the illness fostered social isolation?
5. How have relationships within the family been affected?
6. What impact has the illness or its management had on the ability to meet their continuing needs?

Coping strategies
1. What is the level of knowledge and technical skill the family has gained concerning the illness and its treatment?
2. What strategies does the family employ to help maintain a sense of normalcy in family life?
3. Who are identified supportive people or groups, and what do they provide for the family?
4. What activities do the family members use to enhance positive coping strategies?
5. Does this illness have any positive aspects or results as perceived by this family?

These questions are a good starting point for gathering assessment data. After the establishment of rapport with the family, it is expected that each of these areas can be explored in more depth. Then the nurse and the family can work together to identify and implement mutually acceptable interventions that will promote optimal family functioning.[53]

It is important to provide the family with education to enable them to care adequately for their parent/spouse and to provide the necessary resources to support their primary caregiving role and to foster optimal family functioning. Refer to the following teaching section for more discussion regarding this topic.

Many community resources are available to aid and support families experiencing difficulties associated with caring for an elderly person who has cancer. These resources are listed in the Appendix at the end of this chapter.

Hospice

Any discussion of home care for patients with cancer would not be complete without considering hospice and the vital care provided by health care professionals within this domain of practice. Hospice offers the health care community an approach to dealing with death and dying from a familial framework.[31] The advent of consumerism and the desire for increased control over the delivery and quality of care, particularly when all other treatment options have been exhausted or judged to be ineffective, have contributed to the increased public awareness of and interest in the hospice concept. Even though the term *hospice* is familiar to most, many do not understand the type of services provided under hospice.

A common misconception of the public and health care professionals is that hospice is a specific type of extended care facility. *It is not.* Hospice is a philosophy of care that provides high-quality, comprehensive care to persons with a terminal disease and their families. Hospice care is not exclusively terminal care. It is sensitive and skilled care that addresses the physical, psychologic, and spiritual needs of the patient and family and is provided by an interdisciplinary team of professionals and volunteers. The setting for this care is usually in the home; however, hospitalization is available during acute medical crisis, impending death, or to give the family a short respite (2 to 5 days). Medical crises may include uncontrolled pain, nausea and vomiting, or other situations that may warrant a brief hospitalization until the client's symptoms are controlled.

In home care, an assessment of the family and their ability to provide care and support the patient is essential. Gulla[31] provides a family assessment tool that addresses this area (see box, p. 697). In the early 1980s, hospice treatment was formally acknowledged through reimbursement by Medicare and private insurance companies. This official recognition has made it easier for people to die at home by providing them with some fi-

---

PERTINENT TOPICS INVOLVED IN FAMILY SYSTEM ASSESSMENT

1. Which family members are present during the initial evaluation?
2. Which members appear to be the decision makers?
3. Which family member is the hospice intake worker addressing the most during the intake process?
4. Does there appear to be consent (harmony) or discontent (disharmony) among various family members? If so, which ones?
5. What position does terminal member maintain within family structure: e.g., leader/follower, contributor/ bystander, hero/scapegoat (hero: family member whose role is designed to save or protect the family from internal or external conflict; scapegoat: family member whose role is designed to take the blame for families' mishaps and problems)?
6. Are there any family members who are emotionally attached to terminal member but who are not present at the meeting and/or may not be seen as part of decision-making process? This may especially focus on children, grandchildren, and siblings of terminal member who are emotionally involved and will clearly be part of bereavement process but may be overlooked by immediate family members.
7. Do family members appear to accept the terminal diagnosis? Are they open in speaking with terminal member concerning diagnosis, or do they want to protect/conceal medical data?
8. Are any of the immediate family members, including the terminal member, affected by substance abuse, gambling, or other addictive disorders?
9. Is there a history of any mental illness within the family system?
10. Is there a history of any antisocial behavior (e.g., criminal behavior) with any family members?
11. Have there been other losses experienced by family members? What was the nature of these losses? When did they occur? How did family members cope and adjust to them?
12. What impressions does family give concerning their experiences with attending physicians? This may indicate families who have difficulty in dealing with the medical community or with authority figures.

Modified from Gulla JP: *Am J Hospice Palliative Care* 7:32, 1990.

---

nancial and professional support, by setting standards to regulate the professional care they receive, and by educating physicians, nurses, and the public about the home death alternative. In slightly more than a decade, the grass-roots, volunteer-based reform movement became an integral part of the mainstream health system in America.[7,34,51,66]

The goal of hospice is to enhance the quality of life for the patient who is dying and for the surviving family members. Hospice care makes it possible for dying patients to live their last days in their own homes.[62,74] Hospice programs enable terminally ill patients to remain comfortable in their own homes by providing the necessary support services. Some hospice programs have expanded the range of services available to hospice patients and their families by establishing hospice day-care centers. These centers increase the continuity of care, provide additional support services such as individual counseling and/or support groups, and increase the patient's and family's sense of connectedness with others. These centers are cost efficient, since care is provided in a congregate setting and is staffed primarily by volunteers.[94]

Recently, in many areas of the United States, several hospice programs have been particularly innovative in reaching out to the community at large by developing educational and bereavement programs that teach others not in hospice programs how to confront and ultimately cope with loss and grief. These programs target school-age children (kindergarten to grade 12), individuals who have lost loved ones to AIDS/HIV, and the general population. These hospices also provide training programs and manuals to health care providers and teachers to enable them to form support groups in their community. Many hospice programs provide consultation services to other health care providers and institutions.[2,94]

The hospice team is truly a multidisciplinary team of professionals, consisting of physicians, nurses, social workers, spiritual care advisors, pharmacists, nutritionists, and volunteers. Often, attorneys are available to provide legal aid to patients and their families. Most hospice programs provide ongoing bereavement services to families after the patient's death. For additional information about hospice, support resources, innovative programs, and training opportunities, see the Appendix at the end of this chapter.

Private Duty

Many home care organizations provide supplemental home care services on a fee-for-service basis. These additional services, such as nursing, nursing aides, companions, and housekeepers, can supplement available caregiving resources or provide care when there is no available caregiver, thereby preventing or delaying institutionalization. Private-duty home care is often not included in most health insurance policies as a benefit; therefore the patient or family is responsible to pay for this service. This can be a significant financial burden, but when one considers the alternative of institutionalization, it can be well worth the expense. Agencies that provide these services are required by law to be licensed and can be found in the local Yellow Pages.

If the cost of such services through an agency is prohibitive for the patient and family, the nurse may suggest that they make arrangements with a friend or neighbor for light housekeeping, meal preparation, or sitter/companion services for nominal compensation.

As the trend for managed care continues, some supplemental home care services probably will be included in the patient's health insurance plan. Third-party payors have long noted that paying for additional support services to maintain the patient in the home or in nonhospital settings reduces the overall cost of long-term care.

Cultural Issues

In the complex American health care system, multiculturality is a pressing, mainstream issue. For the individual with cancer, one's native language and treasured traditions can become an obstacle, especially if the skills of the health care professionals are not tempered with cultural sensitivity.[98] One result of the absence of culturally sensitive care is the breakdown of communication and trust, often leading to the reluctance of minorities to utilize available health resources. Issues related to access and acceptability of care and services have also contributed to cultural barriers to cancer care in America.[14,34,60,68,98] Many organizations have made significant efforts to reduce cultural barriers to cancer care. Innovations include the following[14,61,69]:

- Establishing a minority/cultural group: task force composed of members of the target group to identify specific barriers and a plan to reduce these obstacles
- Establishing a community speakers bureau that utilizes members of the targeted minority or cultural group
- Involving culturally specific minority media
- Involving culturally specific spiritual and religious institutions
- Forming culturally specific minority support groups
- Recruiting diverse health care workers through employment advertising in publications aimed at ethnic groups
- Forming an informal "language bank" of bilingual employees
- Utilizing available technology, such as the AT&T Language Line, to facilitate communication through an over-the-phone interpretation service

As community-based and home-based health care continue to grow, health care providers will encounter individuals from diverse cultures and ethnic groups. Although an important first step is to improve communication with these groups, it is imperative that health care providers be knowledgeable in issues related to cultural diversity and conceptual differences between cultures. These providers must be proficient in modifying cancer care accordingly to provide culturally sensitive care.[14]

Reimbursement Issues

In the United States, most health care is provided through third-party payors, that is, private health insurance companies or government health care assistance at state or federal levels. It is estimated that more than 37 million people are without health care insurance and that 30 to 60 million people are underinsured.[25,42] This inequity among U.S. citizens is a major component of discussions regarding health care reform on all levels.

Another problem area included in these discussions is the present manner in which long-term care for elderly patients is being financed. About 1 million nursing home residents currently rely on Medicaid to pay for nursing home expenses. According to Townsend[95]:

Something is wrong when a society forces so many of its citizens onto welfare simply for growing old and needing care. . . . Long-term care needs should not be viewed as welfare needs. . . . We owe it to the nation's elderly to create a comprehensive, coordinated long-term care system.

Economic assessments, analysis, and outcome measures are being increasingly used to provide health care providers, payors, and policy decision makers with the meaningful data regarding oncology studies, innovative treatments, and alternative care settings to facilitate identification of optimal treatment and care strategies. As third-party payors and health care institutions are attempting to control spiralling health care costs and implement health care reform proactively, such data will guide and direct the allocation of health care service and resource funding.[80] Currently, in an effort to supervise more closely the delivery of health care, a variety of health care models are being considered. Among these, *managed care* is likely to be the predominant health care delivery system in the future. More and more people are receiving care in a managed care system. In 1994 approximately 51.1 million members were in a managed care system. Government health programs are also shifting to managed care. At the end of 1996 the membership in managed care systems was estimated to exceed 62 million, an increase of approximately 10% per year.[87,89]

As a result of this shift, a dramatic increase probably will occur in the number of subacute care facilities and a variety of alternative care facilities to provide the necessary services to avoid high-cost nursing home placements. Currently the cost of subacute care is 20% to 60% less than in an acute care setting. Subacute care facilities provide care that is outcome focused, which is also a factor contributing to cost efficiency. Unlike acute care facilities, subacute care facilities are not bound by the prospective payment system (PPS) because long-term facilities generally have patients whose stay exceeds 25 days and have few short-stay, low-cost cases. Subacute care facilities can either be free-standing long-term care institutions or housed within an existing acute care hospital as long as the federal guidelines and criteria for such facilities are met.

Although managed care has been highly praised for

its efficient management of health care dollars, concerns have been raised by some health care providers and the public that high-quality, individualized care and access to some treatment modalities have been sacrificed. This dimension in the discussion concerning health care reform and resource allocation cannot be ignored. Nurses, as patient advocates, can and should play an important role in clinical and community-based research that includes quality measures, patient outcomes, and access to care in addition to economic assessments and analysis. Nurses should also take an active part in provider negotiations and in establishing new standards of care as part of their patient advocacy role.[43,75]

Currently, most health care insurance policies cover home care and hospice services. All require that the service is ordered by a physician and that a medical plan of care is signed by the physician. The care provided must be intermittent, and the patient must also need skilled professional care provided by a nurse, physical therapist, or speech therapist and have a medical condition that warrants ongoing assessment and evaluation. Patients must also be *homebound,* that is, unable to leave home without assistance of others and assistive devices. If the patient or caregiver requires no additional instruction regarding the disease process or its management and the patient is medically stable for more than 2 weeks, he or she is no longer considered in need of ongoing skilled nursing service unless specific treatments are ordered, such as monthly catheter changes or vitamin B_{12} injections.

Insurance coverage for home care services and alternative care settings varies from policy to policy. In most cases, insurance benefits are negotiated individually for group policies and benefit packages. More frequently now, health insurance providers are becoming more flexible regarding the services and benefits available to individuals because the cost-saving benefits have been well documented. Prior approval usually is necessary. The medical plan of care must be reviewed and updated periodically and again signed by the physician. The certification periods—the specified time frame the plan of care is valid—is usually 30 or 60 days, depending on the payor (Table 27-6; see box, p. 700).

PATIENT AND FAMILY TEACHING

Nurses play a major role in educating individuals about cancer detection methods, life-style risks, disease process, and treatment options.[30,63] Given the importance of this role, the oncology nurse must be proficient in patient and family education.

The trend of consumerism and the complex nature of cancer and current, often aggressive treatment modalities necessitate improved, comprehensive patient and family education. "The goal of patient education is more than information giving; the intent is to provide individuals and their families support, with control, and knowledge to empower them to manage self-care deficits more effectively."[39] It is well documented that patients and families with increased knowledge of their illness and treatment plan experience significantly less anxiety and stress.[73] Researchers have also noted that different pa-

Table 27-6   Payor Source Guidelines

Medical insurance	Prior authorization	Services covered	Certification period	Durable medical equipment
Medicare	No	SN, PT, ST, OT, MSS, HHA	2 months, 60-62 days	Yes, need medical order
Medicaid	Yes	SN, PT, ST, HHA, no MSS*	2 months	Yes, need medical order
Blue Cross Basic	Yes	SN, PT, OT, ST, MSS, HHA	30 days	No, coverage only with major medical
Blue Cross: Blue Care Network or Personal Choice	Yes	SN, PT, OT, ST, MSS, HHA, nutrition (if agency certified for this)	30 days	Yes, with approval
Federal Blue Cross: Hi-option	Yes	SN, PT, OT, ST, MSS, HHA	30 days	Yes
Federal Blue Cross: Lo-option	No, all visits reimbursed 75%	25 SN/yr; 50 PT/yr; no HHA, OT, or ST	30 days	Yes, coverage at 75%
Commercial: Aetna, Prudential, etc.	Yes	Varies with benefit plan	60 days	Yes, varies with benefit plan
Managed care: health maintenance organizations, (HMOs), Group Health Plans, Health Alliance Plans, etc.	Yes	SN, PT, OT (MSS, HHA with authorization*)	60-62 days	Yes, varies with benefit plan

SN, Staff nurse; *PT,* physical therapy; *ST,* speech therapy; *OT,* occupational therapy; *MSS,* medical social service; *HHA,* home health aide.
*Refer to the box, p. 700, for list of services that are often provided through managed care.

HOME CARE SERVICES PROVIDED BY MANAGED CARE ORGANIZATIONS

HIGH-TECHNOLOGY SERVICES

Infusion therapy
Parenteral therapy
Enteral nutrition
Home dialysis
Home monitoring
Customized equipment

SKILLED SERVICES

Medical
Nursing (RN)
Physical therapy
Speech therapy
Occupational therapy
Vocational services
Respiratory therapy

SEMISKILLED SERVICES

Nursing (LPN)
Home health aides
Therapy assistants
Personal response systems

PHARMACY

Antibiotics
Nutrition
Infusion solutions
Chemotherapy
Other

HOME MEDICAL EQUIPMENT

Basic mobility aids
Daily living assistive devices
Extensive mobility aids
Advanced high-technology equipment
Oxygen therapies
Medical supplies

REHABILITATION/ASSISTIVE TECHNOLOGY

Mobility aids
Adaptive equipment
Custom seating and positioning
Orthotics and prosthetics
Aids for daily living

HOSPICE SERVICES

Bereavement counseling
Social work services
Palliative services

CUSTODIAL SERVICES

Companions
Personal aides
Housekeeping
Shopping
Cooking
Transportation

From Hammill CT, Parver CP: *J Home Health Pract* 7(4):18, 1995.

tients have individual learning and informational needs. The oncology nurse must consider individual differences as well as cultural differences when beginning patient or family teaching. Important areas to evaluate are readiness, motivation, past experiences, physical and intellectual abilities, and physical and psychologic comfort.[25,29] As in the nursing process, a thorough assessment must take place. Determining what the patient or family member already knows is imperative to avoid boredom and "tuning out." Simply asking the individual if he or she is interested in obtaining additional information is a good first step. The nurse should remember that often the individual may not know what specific learning opportunities are available. It is helpful to have a list from which the individual may select appropriate topics (see box on right). Hileman and colleagues[36] researched and identified the unmet needs of home caregivers of patients with cancer (see box, p. 701) and concluded that most caregivers' unmet needs were psychologic and informational. Oncology nurses in acute, community, clinic, and outpatient settings need to emphasize more the psychosocial and informational needs of family home caregivers. Because of shorter hospitalizations, nurses must begin this

SAMPLE TOPICS FOR PATIENTS AND FAMILIES

Specifics related to illness
Specifics related to treatment and effects
Exercise/activity and rest
Safety
Financial issues
Insurance issues
Social interactions
Emotional concerns
Support groups/resources
Family concerns
Rehabilitation
Adaptive techniques
Returning to work
Long-term planning
Others: _____
_____
_____
_____

From Hileman JW, Lackey NR, Hassanein RS: *Oncol Nurs Forum* 19(5):771, 1992.

TOP 25 UNMET NEEDS OF HOME CAREGIVERS

1. Information about the underlying reasons for symptoms
2. Information about what symptoms to expect
3. Information about what to expect in the future
4. Information about treatment of side effects
5. Information about community resources
6. Honest and updated information
7. Ways to reassure patient
8. Ways to deal with patient's decreased energy
9. Ways to deal with unpredictability of the future
10. Information about medications (side effects, scheduling)
11. Ways to encourage patient
12. Information about patient's psychologic needs
13. Methods to decrease caregiver's stress
14. Ways of coping with patient's diagnosis of cancer
15. Information about type and extent of patient's illness
16. Ways to cope with role changes
17. Information about physical needs of patient
18. Activities that will make patient feel purposeful
19. Ways to be more patient and tolerant
20. Ways to deal with caregiver's depression
21. Ways to maintain a normal family life
22. Ways to discuss death with patient
23. Ways to deal with caregiver's fears
24. Ways to combat fatigue
25. Ways to provide patient with adequate nutrition

From Hileman JW, Lackey NR, Hassanein RS: *Oncol Nurs Forum* 19(5):775, 1992.

educational process early and continue the counseling process, especially on psychologic and informational needs, after discharge. This could be done directly or by linking families to volunteer and professional community agencies with appropriate services.

In a study of educational wants of family caregivers, Mathis[56] determined that adults perceive that they need information about how to deal with real-life situations and, if given such information, they will be motivated to learn. If such educational opportunities are not afforded, caregivers might reject the caregiving role. It is also important to use the principles of adult learning. These include encouraging immediate application of learned material, providing adequate practice time and materials, and giving specific feedback promptly.[29] Often, teaching materials and supplies are not readily available because of the lack of an organized storage system. If the practice site is in an ambulatory, acute care, or similar setting, the nurse might consider using movable carts, setting up one cart per teaching topic, and putting appropriate supplies and teaching materials in each.[47] If the practice site is in home care or similarly transient, the nurse might consider using carrying cases instead.

Educational reading material is usually written at a sixth- to eighth-grade reading level, but even this may be too high. Glazer-Waldman and others[28] determined that 60% of their research sample of 101 hospital inpatients and outpatients could not read and understand material written at a sixth-grade level. Literacy is a problem in the United States today, with more than 20% of the general population functionally illiterate. Twenty million adults can read at an eighth-grade level, and another 20 million can read at or below the fourth-grade level. Results of other studies indicate that reported reading levels are significantly higher than the actual reading levels of patients.[12,29,30] Illiteracy is more endemic among the elderly and poor persons. Keeping this in mind, the oncology nurse should determine the patient's reading capabilities. This is not easily done. Many adults are embarrassed about the inability to read and over the years become very skillful in covering up this deficit. Excuses such as "I don't have my glasses with me now; can you read it to me?" or "I'll read it later" may serve as cues on which the nurse should follow up. Other indicators identified by Meade and co-workers[63] include lack of interest in the material, expressions of frustration, lack of reading speed, and inability to answer questions about the content of the text.

In addition to these informal methods of assessing reading ability, the Wide-Range Achievement Test (WRAT) II developed by Janstak and Wilkinson[44] is a helpful tool. To assess the readability of written material or when developing written material, the Cloze procedure developed by Taylor[92] may be used to make certain that the material is not written at too high a level. Other readability formulas, such as the Flesch Formula and the Forcast, may also be used.[63]

Meade and colleagues[63] conducted an analysis of the readability of American Cancer Society (ACS) patient education literature in 1991 and determined that ACS publications written before 1985 had a mean reading level of grade 12.7, whereas those written during and after 1985 had a mean reading level of grade 10.9. Of the 51 booklets analyzed in this study, only six booklets were written at an 8.9-grade level or below, whereas 45 were written at ninth-grade level or above. In view of these results, it is important that the oncology nurse realize the importance of a multifaceted, creative approach to patient and family education. The findings of Meade and co-workers do not negate the value of the written material available currently from ACS and institutions. The oncology nurse be aware of the limitations of these materials, individualizing the teaching plan to meet the unique needs of each patient. The nurse must also assess for the appropriate instructional method for the individual, using *all* available educational resources and modalities, such as audiovisual, pictorial, and didactic as well as written material. These can only enhance and facilitate the learning process. It is well documented that

Name _____ Date _____ Age _____

Diagnosis _____ Sex [ ] F [ ] M

Highest level of education [ ] Elementary

[ ] Intermediate [ ] High School [ ] College/University

[ ] Other _____

Patient's interest in learning is:

1	2	3	4
Total disinterest or defers to significant other	Minimal information desired	Moderate information desired	Desires all there is to know

Preferred learning method: [ ] Books [ ] Pictorial

[ ] Audiovisual [ ] Other _____

Any reading or visual problems? [ ] no [ ] yes _____

Any neurosensory impairments? [ ] no [ ] yes _____

Questions related to:

Universal self-care requisites
[ ] Nutrition   [ ] Safety
[ ] Elimination   [ ] Financial
[ ] Activity & Rest   [ ] Social Interactions

[ ] Others _____

Developmental self-care requisites
[ ] Emotional Concerns   [ ] Family Concerns

[ ] Support Groups/Resources [ ] Others _____

Health deviation self-care requisites
[ ] Illness   [ ] Treatment and Effects

[ ] Others _____

Are there any other questions? _____

I hereby acknowledge the above information to be an assessment of my current learning needs. I understand I am encouraged to participate in my health care utilizing self-care measures. I will have opportunities during my outpatient visits to seek further knowledge as questions or problems develop.

Client's signature _____ Date _____

Figure 27-3 Learning needs assessment tool. (From Hiromoto BM, Dungan J: *Cancer Nurs* 14(3):148, 1991.)

Learning Interest #1
Chemotherapy: A Guide for patients with cancer (Adria pamphlet) (given to significant other)
Taking time (NIH booklet) (given to significant other)
Living with cancer (American Cancer Society—support group)

Other resources: _____

Learning Interest #2
We care (American Cancer Society brochure)
Chemotherapy: A guide for patients with cancer (Adria pamphlet)
Living with cancer (American Cancer Society—support group)

Other resources: _____

Learning Interest #3
Chemotherapy & you: A guide to self-help during treatment (NIH booklet)
Taking time (NIH booklet)
Nausea/vomiting (hospital's handout)
Symptom alert sheet for chemotherapy (hospital's handout)
Living with cancer (American Cancer Society—support group)
Chemotherapy slide show (OPTIONAL)   OR
Chemotherapy & you (Adria Laboratories picture book)
                                 (OPTIONAL)

Other resources: _____

Learning Interest #4
Chemotherapy & you: A guide to self-help during treatment (NIH booklet)
Taking time (NIH booklet)
Nausea/vomiting (hospital's handout)
Symptom alert sheet for chemotherapy (hospital's handout)
Cancer terms: A guide for patients with cancer (Adria pamphlet)
Eating hints: Recipes and tips for better nutrition during cancer treatment
Living with cancer (American Cancer Society—support group)
Chemotherapy slide show (OPTIONAL)   OR
Chemotherapy & you—(Adria Laboratories picture book)
                                 (OPTIONAL)

Other resources: _____

Figure 27-4 Teaching materials provided according to level of learning interests. (From Hiromoto BM, Dungan J: *Cancer Nurs* 14(3):148, 1991.)

the use of multiple instructive modalities greatly improves the amount of learning. Thus it is advisable to use a variety of teaching techniques. An extensive list of written educational materials is available in the Appendix at the end of this chapter.

Hiromoto and Dungan[39] recommend a contract learning protocol to provide a systematic, comprehensive approach to the individual's learning needs. The researchers have found that contract learning has had good results when used with adult learners, since it includes concepts of independent, individualized, and self-directed learning. They developed a useful learning needs assessment tool designed specifically for chemotherapy learning needs (Figure 27-3) and a form documenting the instructional material provided based on the assessment (Figure 27-4). This example can assist development of an appropriate tool for one's own particular practice setting.[15,39]

The education process, as with the nursing process, includes the steps of assessing, planning, implementing, and evaluating. The primary learner in the family must be identified and his or her learning needs assessed. After this assessment, a mutually acceptable plan to meet the identified educational needs is developed by the nurse/teacher and patient/learner. Appropriate teaching strategies are used to implement the plan and are mutually evaluated, with the evaluation serving as a basis for further decision making.[81] Addressing the educational wants and needs of the family caregiver is a top priority if the patient is to receive proper care and be able to remain in the home.[56]

ADVANCE DIRECTIVES

Since 1991, when the Patient Self-Determination Act (PSDA) became law, hospitals have responded to the mandate by creating pamphlets and educational materials regarding advance directives. These are usually presented to patients on admission to the acute care facility, which is not ideal because at that time patients are usually either ill, anxious, or under great stress. This lack of timing does not facilitate a well-reasoned health care decision. It is preferable that patients and their families collaborate with their primary health care provider well before hospitalization. Many people have misconceptions regarding advance directives, believing that these are only for elderly or terminally ill patients and that if one does have an advance directive, it will result in limited or denied care in the future.[68] The oncology nurse must address these misconceptions. Keeping in mind the barriers to education created by illiteracy and cultural differences, the information regarding advance directives must be provided in an easily readable and clear manner. Neumark[68] developed a patient teaching tool that does an excellent job of presenting the concept of advance directives (see box, pp. 704-705).

DISCHARGE INSTRUCTIONS

To help facilitate the transition to the home or alternative care setting and ensure continuity of care and medical follow-up, it is important to clearly convey specific discharge instructions to the patient and family members at discharge. The time of discharge is particularly hec-

tic, and often instructions given at this time may not be remembered accurately or at all. Consequently, it is advisable to have specific written instructions to review with and give the patient and family at discharge.

Accessing the Health Care System

Many institutions have discharge instruction sheets that are completed by the nurse and include instructions regarding follow-up appointments and medications. However, this is not enough. Patients and their families need to know how to access the health care system after discharge. They need to know the answers to such questions as the following:

- Whom should I call when questions arise that cannot wait until the next appointment?
- What should I expect?
- When do I worry?
- When should I call?
- How can I reach these professionals?
- What about after hours? Who is the contact person then?

As can be seen, the list of questions can be endless. However, questions can be anticipated by the experienced health care professional. An individualized discharge instruction sheet (Figure 27-5) can be helpful in reducing stress and anxiety.

In addition, the experienced oncology nurse, in either the inpatient or the outpatient setting, can anticipate any potential problems that may arise as a result of treatment or disease progression. In this case it is appropriate for the nurse to provide the patient or responsible caregiver with information regarding anticipated problems (e.g., stomatitis associated with chemotherapy) and measures to manage these problems. If the institution does not have patient instruction sheets and pamphlets about common side effects or problems, a considerable amount of literature for both professionals and patients is available from the ACS, The U.S. Department of Health and Human Services, and other organizations. Often, pharmaceutical companies provide informational pamphlets for patients as well as health care professionals (see Appendix at end of chapter).

Again, it is important to consider the patient's reading ability and assess the readability of the written material provided. If the reading skills of the patient or family member are limited, it may be more appropriate and more effective to write out very simple instructions or information specifically tailored for the individual. Alternative teaching modalities such as audio or video tapes may also be effective teaching tools to augment any teaching plan (see Appendix for resources). Nurses may even consider making their own audio tapes for patients, giving step-by-step instructions that patients and families would be able to follow more easily.

MAKING YOUR OWN CHOICES: A GUIDE TO HELP YOU DECIDE ABOUT ADVANCE DIRECTIVES

This guide is to help you learn how you can make your own choices about health care. You have the right to make choices about your health care.

There is a law called the Patient Self-Determination Act. This law states that most hospitals have to tell you about something called "advance directives."

This guide gives you some facts about advance directives. It will explain:
• What advance directives are
• How you make advance directives
• Why advance directives are important
• What to include in your advance directive

WHAT ARE ADVANCE DIRECTIVES?

If you are ever unable to make your own health care choices or to communicate what you want to do, other people will have to make choices for you. *Advance directives* are a way to let your family, friends, and health care providers know your wishes to receive—or not to receive—medical care and treatment. An advance directive protects your right to make your own choices. It gives you the power to control your own care.

MAKING YOUR ADVANCE DIRECTIVE

To make sure that your family, friends, and health care providers understand your choices, it is important to have your advance directive in writing.

There are two common types of advance directives. One type is called a *living will*. The second type is called a *durable power of attorney for health care*. Both are legal pieces of paper that allow you to state your wishes in writing.
• *Living will:* this explains your wishes about health care and treatments. It is used only if you become terminally ill, if you are in an accident and have permanent brain damage, or if you are in a permanent coma.
• *Durable power of attorney for health care:* this names another person to make choices for you if you cannot make choices for yourself. This person is called your *agent* or your *proxy.* It is a good idea to name a second person to make decisions for you in case your first choice is not available for some reason.

Your agent should be someone whom you know and trust. It is very important to talk about your feelings and choices about health care and treatment with your agent.

To make sure your choices are clearly known, it is best to write them down. It is helpful to be as clear as possible so that your agents understand what you would want. Any advance directive can be changed or cancelled by you at any time.
• Sign your name and put the date on the advance directive. It is best to do this in front of a notary public.
• Give a copy of your advance directive to your doctor to put in your medical file.
• Give a copy of your advance directive to each of the people you have asked to be your agents.

• Put a card in your wallet that says you have an advance directive (and where to find it).
• *Review your advance directive often. Make sure it expresses your wishes clearly.*

WHY ADVANCE DIRECTIVES ARE IMPORTANT

The purpose of an advance directive is to help other people make choices for you if you cannot make your own choices. *You want them to make the same choices that you would make.* Your advance directive guides other people to follow your wishes.

PREPARE ADVANCE DIRECTIVES WHILE YOU ARE ABLE TO MAKE YOUR OWN CHOICES

You are never too young or too healthy to have an advance directive. A time may come when an accident or illness will keep you from being able to make or communicate your own health care choices.

Some times when you may not be able to decide for yourself would be if you are:
• *Permanently unconscious:* this means there is no chance to become conscious (in a permanent coma).
• *Irreversibly brain damaged:* this can affect your ability to think or communicate.
• *Brain dead:* this means all brain function has stopped permanently and will not return.

WHAT TO INCLUDE IN YOUR ADVANCE DIRECTIVE

What you choose to write in your advance directive depends on things that are most important to you.

These things are your beliefs and values. The beliefs and values that may influence your health care choices may include what you think or feel about:
• Being independent and having control
• Making your own decisions
• Pain or suffering
• Being with your loved ones at death
• What makes you happy and sad
• Where you live
• Your religious background and beliefs
• Your finances
• Your health care providers
• Your health care relationships
• Prolonging life
• Donating parts of your body

WHAT ARE YOUR CHOICES?

Before you make an advance directive, it is important to think about what you might feel if you were near death. It is helpful to express your feelings about having or not having certain forms of medical treatment. *Often having these treatments will keep you alive longer.*

Some of the medical treatments that you may have to make choices about:
• *Life-sustaining treatment/extraordinary care:* this is any treatment that keeps you alive longer and delays death.

From Neumark DE: *Oncol Nurs Forum* 21(4):771, 1994.

MAKING YOUR OWN CHOICES: A GUIDE TO HELP YOU DECIDE ABOUT ADVANCE DIRECTIVES—cont'd

- *Cardiopulmonary resuscitation (CPR):* this is a method that will attempt to restore stopped breathing and/or heartbeat.
- *Code:* this means calling a special team of doctors and nurses to start CPR when your heart stops beating or you stop breathing.
- *Do not resuscitate (DNR)/no code:* this is a doctor's order that lets other staff know that you do not want to receive CPR.
- *Intravenous (IV) therapy:* this is when thin tubes are put in your vein to give you food, water, and/or medicine.
- *Feeding tubes:* this is when tubes are put in your mouth, nose, or stomach to give you liquid food if you cannot eat normally.
- *Respirator or ventilator:* this is a machine that breathes for you or helps you breathe. A tube is put in through your mouth, nose, or a hole in your neck. The tube goes into your lungs and is attached to the machine.
- *Dialysis:* This means using a machine to remove waste products from your blood if your kidneys do not work the right way.

An advance directive lets you make choices about future medical care and treatments under various circumstances. You can ask your doctor or nurse to help explain the pros and cons of the different types of medical treatments.

If you make choices while you are able, your wishes about the end of your life will be honored.

SHARING YOUR BELIEFS

Talk about your beliefs and values with the people who may have to make choices for you in the future. It is hard to think about many of these issues. But, if you talk about your wishes when you are able, the people who will have to make difficult choices for you will feel relieved that they know what you would have chosen.

Even if you do not know exactly how you feel about certain types of treatments, share your feelings with your family, friends, doctor, nurse, or spiritual leader.

Remember, advance directives let you *make your own choices.*

For more information

Laws for advance directives are different in each state. Sample forms and more information may be available from a hospital, home health service, hospice, lawyer, or your state medical society. Other good sources to learn more about advance directives:

Legal Hotline for Older Americans
PO Box 23810
Pittsburgh, PA 15222
1-800-262-5297

Choice in Dying
200 Varick St.
New York, NY 10014
212-366-5540

Legal Counsel for the Elderly (Associated with American Association for Retired Persons)
1331 H Street NW
Washington, DC 20005
202-434-2120

Follow-up Appointments

Central to an effective treatment of any cancer is consistent medical follow-up. Ongoing assessment and evaluation and subsequent modification of the treatment plan are critical as the trend for more aggressive posthospital treatment continues. Follow-up appointments are important but are often difficult endeavors for patients and their families. The nurse can implement several actions to facilitate keeping follow-up appointments.

First and foremost is the almost universal concern about transportation. Patients may not have transportation resources available to them, and frequently this issue is not addressed when they are given the follow-up appointment. It is important to ask the patient or family member if transportation is a problem. If so, they may be referred to local agencies that provide such services. The ACS and the American Red Cross are national organizations that have local offices that provide transportation to and from medical facilities at no charge or minimal cost. Many private companies provide transportation services for disabled persons for a fee.

In addition to information about transportation resources, patients need to know what assistance is available when they arrive for their follow-up appointment. If a wheelchair is needed, how do they arrange to have one available? Most hospitals and clinics have wheelchairs available for such purposes. This should be determined before the appointment. If a wheelchair is not available, the patient should be advised to arrange for one's use.

At busy oncology clinics, follow-up appointments can become an all-day endeavor. Patients frequently are scheduled for blood work before their appointment with the physician and later may receive chemotherapy or be scheduled for other tests. Patients and their families should be advised to bring the medications that they may need to take while still at the clinic, especially PRN pain medications. Patients and their families should be told

NAME: _____

MEDICATIONS:

_____
(name, dose, route, frequency, and common
_____ side effects) _____

_____

_____

TREATMENTS:

_____
(specify tx, procedure, frequency)
_____ or refer to attached handout of hospital _____
_____ treatment protocol _____

WHEN TO CALL NURSE/DOCTOR:
IF TEMPERATURE IS 100° OR HIGHER
IF YOU HAVE PAIN THAT WON'T GO AWAY
IF YOU CAN'T KEEP FOOD OR LIQUIDS DOWN FOR 24 HOURS
   OR MORE
IF YOU HAVE NO BOWEL MOVEMENT FOR 3 OR MORE DAYS
IF YOU HAVE DIARRHEA FOR 24 HOURS OR MORE
IF YOU HAVE URINARY DIFFICULTIES
   PAIN OR BURNING
   BLEEDING
OTHER: _____

_____

_____

IMPORTANT PHONE NUMBERS:
DR. _____   _____ (phone)
NURSES' STATION   _____ (phone)
DISCHARGE PLANNER   _____ (phone)
HOME CARE AGENCY   _____ (name)

_____   _____
   (contact person)   (phone)
DURABLE MEDICAL EQUIP. SUPPLIER_____ (name)

_____   _____
   (contact person)   (phone)
   Items to be delivered: w/c, commode, cane, walker, shower
   chair, hospital bed,_____ (other) ____ on ____ (date)

_____
   (please list)

YOUR NEXT APPOINTMENT WITH _____
IS ON _____ AT _____ AM/PM AT
THE ONCOLOGY OUT PATIENT CLINIC (include specific location).
   PLEASE CALL (clinic phone #) IF YOU ARE UNABLE TO KEEP
   THIS APPOINTMENT TO RESCHEDULE.

Figure 27–5 Discharge instruction sheet. (From Slevin JB, Roberts AS: *Nurs Manage* 18(12):47, 1987.)

what to expect at the follow-up appointment, especially if the patient is going to receive a treatment or particular diagnostic test for the first time. Knowing what to expect greatly reduces fears and anxieties associated with the unknown.

In many health care settings, minimal interaction occurs among the various departments that provide cancer treatment. This often results in a breakdown in continu-

ity of care and greatly diminishes interdepartmental, interdisciplinary collaboration and collegiality.

Some institutions make interdepartmental experiences available as part of the orientation process. Such opportunities have direct benefits for both the patient and the health care professional. Drummand and Hagenstad[21] have developed a program to provide inpatient oncology nursing staff with the opportunity to spend one-half or a full day in a full-service oncology office. The authors found that this not only improved morale, but also "improved communication between the oncology unit nurses and the oncology office staff and physicians."[21] In addition, this program fostered greater cohesiveness and collaboration among members of the oncology team. An added benefit was the increased awareness of the outpatient diagnostic procedures, prehospital admission process, and postdischarge care, all of which constitute important information that the nurse can, in turn, share with patients.[21]

Follow-up Phone Call

A follow-up phone call to patients and their families should be made within 24 to 48 hours after discharge. It is helpful for the nurse to have a copy of the continuing patient care form and discharge instruction sheets to enable him or her to ask appropriate questions to facilitate obtaining accurate information about the patient's status. A helpful starting point is to ask the patient or family the following questions:
1. How are things going since you came home?
2. Have any problems occurred?
3. Do you have any questions that I can answer for you? These questions can open communication, but the nurse must ask specific questions related to the patient's illness and treatment plan to ensure an accurate assessment of the home situation. If it becomes apparent that activities are not going well in the home, the nurse may recommend that the patient be brought in to see the physician.

Often, home care needs are not easily identified before discharge, but once the patient is at home, this need becomes apparent. If a home care referral has not been made, the nurse may determine at this time that a referral is warranted and initiate this process.

Durable Medical and Adaptive Equipment

Durable medical equipment (DME) includes hospital beds, wheelchairs, and much more. Many assistive devices are available to patients and their families that can simplify home care management and also promote home safety. Essential equipment such as hospital beds, wheelchairs, and bedside commodes should be in the home at discharge, but some equipment and adaptive devices should not be ordered until a home evaluation can be done. Although an experienced nurse can assess and

NURSING MANAGEMENT

As previously discussed, many essential steps are necessary to facilitate transition to the home setting and ensure continuity of care. Assessment with planned interventions and an evaluation of the outcomes will enhance a smooth transition for the patient and family members. Following is an example of a nursing diagnosis with multiple assessment and intervention strategies that can be adapted to meet the varied individual patient needs.

NURSING DIAGNOSIS

• *Home maintenance management, impaired, related to:*
Patient
—Inability to perform household activities secondary to side effects of chemotherapy
—Inability to perform household activities secondary to disease progression
—Inability to engage in self-care activities secondary to chronic debilitating disease
Caregiver
—Inability to maintain self and patient secondary to unavailable support system
—Inability to maintain caregiver role secondary to lack of knowledge, inadequate supports/resources

OUTCOME GOALS

Patient/caregiver will be able to:
• Identify factors that restrict self-care and home management.
• Demonstrate the ability to perform skills necessary for care of patient or home.
• Express satisfaction with home situation.
• Experience less anxiety and stress related to caregiving role.
• Identify personal strengths and receive support through nursing relationship and community resources.

INTERVENTIONS

The following interventions apply to many individuals with impaired home maintenance management, regardless of etiology:
• Assess for causative or contributing factors:
—Lack of knowledge
—Insufficient funds
—Lack of necessary equipment or aids
—Inability to perform household activities (illness, sensory deficits, motor deficits)
—Impaired cognitive functioning
—Impaired emotional functioning
—Factors affecting learning
• Reduce or eliminate causative or contributing factors if possible.

• Determine with patient and family the information needed to be taught and learned:
—Monitoring skills needed (pulse, circulation, urine)
—Medication administration (procedure, side effects, precautions)
—Treatment procedures
—Equipment use/maintenance
—Safety issues (e.g., environmental)
—Community resources
—Follow-up care
—Anticipatory guidance (e.g., emotional and social needs of family, alternatives to home care)
• Be sensitive to patient's and families' time schedules.
• Reduce or eliminate barriers for learning (e.g., delay teaching until person ready, cultural barriers, health beliefs, past experiences).
• Promote patient/family learning (e.g., reduce anxiety; provide quiet, nonstressful environment; promote positive attitude and active participation in learning process).
• Initiate teaching and give detailed written instructions. Refer to a community nursing (home care) agency for follow-up.
• Determine type of equipment or aids needed, considering availability, cost, and durability:
—Seek assistance from agencies that rent or loan supplies.
—Teach care and maintenance of supplies that increase length of use.
—Consider adapting equipment to reduce cost.
• If patient/family has insufficient funds, consult with social service department and service organizations for assistance, such as American Heart Association, The Lung Association, and American Cancer Society (see Appendix).
• Determine type of assistance needed to perform household activities (e.g., meals, housework, transportation) and assist patient to obtain them.
• Discuss with family the possibility of freezing complete meals that require only heating (e.g., small containers of soup, stew, casseroles).
• Determine availability of meal services for ill persons (e.g., Meals on Wheels, church groups).
• Teach patient/family about foods that are easily prepared and nutritious (e.g., hard-boiled eggs).
• Contract with an adolescent for light housekeeping, or refer to community agency for assistance with housework.
• Determine availability of transportation for shopping and health care:
—Request rides with neighbors to places they drive routinely.

Continued.

—Consult transportation resources in community.
- If patient has impaired mental processes, assess ability to maintain household safely:
  —Reduce/eliminate causative or contributing factors, if possible.
  —Initiate health teaching regarding impairment, and make appropriate referrals.
- Determine if patient has impaired emotional functioning:
  —Assess severity of dysfunction.
  —Assess causative or contributing factors.
  —Assess patient's present coping strategies.
  —Teach constructive problem-solving techniques and coping skills.
  —Assist patient to develop appropriate strategies based on his or her personal strengths and previous experience.
  —Find outlets that foster feelings of personal achievement and self-esteem.
  —Correct lack of support systems.
  —Reduce or eliminate social isolation caused by lessened contact with others.
  —Initiate health teaching.
  —Assist with managing new roles/responsibilities.
  —Initiate appropriate referrals.
- Provide anticipatory guidance for caregivers.
- Discuss implications of caring for a chronically ill family member:
  —Amount of time involved

—Effects on other role responsibilities (spouse, children, job)
—Physical requirements (lifting)
- Share alternatives to reduce strain and fatigue of caregiving responsibilities:
  —Acquire relief from responsibilities at least twice a week for at least 3 hours (sitter, neighbors, relatives).
  —Enlist aid of others to meet some of patient's needs (e.g., hairdresser, transporting to physician's office).
  —Plan to set aside at least 1 hour a day as leisure time (after patient asleep).
  —Maintain contacts with friends and relatives even if only by phone. Caregivers should inform friends that they do use sitters so friends can include them in some social activities.
  —Give caregivers the opportunity to share problems and feelings.
  —Include humor therapy strategies to help patient/caregiver relieve stress and anxiety and enhance feelings of well-being.
- Commend caregivers for their concern, diligence, and perseverance in caring for patient at home.
- Initiate health teaching and referrals as indicated:
  —Refer to support groups (e.g., American Cancer Society, Encore, Y-Me).
  —Refer to community nursing agency.
  —Refer to community agencies (e.g., volunteer visitors, meal programs, homemakers, adult day care).

evaluate home equipment needs, a physical or occupational therapist should be consulted. These therapists have an extensive knowledge of available equipment and may be able to meet the patient's equipment needs more effectively.

Most insurance policies provide coverage for some DME; however, a physician's order and an accompanying related neuromusculoskeletal diagnosis is usually required. Some insurance companies require prior approval before the equipment can be delivered to the patient. DME companies can help with this process. See Table 27-6 for a general overview of insurance coverage and the Appendix for national durable medical and adaptive equipment resources. Also, DME companies can be found in the local Yellow Pages.

COMMUNITY RESOURCES

Utilization of available community resources is low even when these services are needed. The reasons are not clear, but contributing factors may include the following[26]:
- Service cost
- Access/availability

- Lack of awareness of available resources
- Lack of flexibility in services
- Inappropriate use of limited resources
- Consumer dissatisfaction
- Labeling of services

Further investigation into these factors is warranted to provide appropriate, well-coordinated community resources in a cost-efficient manner. In some U.S. areas, health care providers have attempted to fill the gap in support services for cancer patients and their families through innovative, comprehensive programs. Good examples of these efforts include The Santa Monica Wellness Community, The R.H. Bloch Support House, The Cancer Support Foundation, The Cancer Wellness Center, and The Cancer Support Network (see Appendix at end of chapter). These programs have proved that significant support services can have a major impact on the lives of cancer patients and their families.[40]

Many national and local community resources are available to cancer patients and their families, ranging from personal services, informational services, social services, and support services. A phone call to the Cancer Information Service (1-800-4-CANCER) and the local ACS chapter is a good starting point when first attempting to identify resources available in the community. Local community services often include agencies that provide and/or assist with the following:

1. Chore or housekeeping services
2. Adult day care
3. Socialization services (e.g., Friendly Visitor, In-Home Companion)
4. Nutritional services (e.g., Meals on Wheels, nutrition sites, food supplements, food banks/cupboards)
5. Financial savings and grant program
6. Transportation services
7. Support groups and counseling services

A list of national organizations that provide assistance to cancer patients and their families is included in the Appendix. These organizations will help nurses identify local community support services, obtain educational materials, and facilitate networking within the community.

CONCLUSION

Patients with cancer move through a number of health care settings during the course of their illnesses. Inherent within this movement are encounters with many health care professionals. A successful transition through these settings depends on the collaborative efforts of the health care providers. Ongoing communication is the key to the effectiveness of these efforts.[51]

In addition to collaboration, a thorough assessment and evaluation of the unique and specific care requirements of the patient must be performed to identify the appropriate community support services to facilitate this transition along the continuum. Subsequent reevaluation and modification of the continuing care plan must be done periodically to ensure attainment of expected outcomes and to avoid inappropriate use of limited services. It is a challenge to meet the increasingly complex, multidimensional needs of patients with cancer and their families. Nurses must be prepared and knowledgeable to meet these needs successfully. They must also remember that what most people want is *not* the power of hospital technology in their homes or alternative settings for care, but the *security* of care that a multidisciplinary team can provide.[7]

■ CHAPTER QUESTIONS

1. Factors that have influenced increased emphasis on home care and alternative care settings include all the following *except:*
   a. Implementation of diagnosis-related groups (DRGs)
   b. Demographic changes in American society
   c. Limited available extended care facilities
   d. Efforts to contain rising health care costs

2. Of the following patient characteristics, which would *not* indicate high risk or need for discharge planning?
   a. Newly diagnosed cancer
   b. Pediatric patient
   c. Diminished functional capacity
   d. Diabetes

3. In the United States, family members and friends provide approximately what percentage of in-home care?
   a. 50%
   b. 65%
   c. 70%
   d. 80%

4. The primary reason more people do *not* have an advance directive is:
   a. Poor timing of health care provider in offering information to patient
   b. Fear that having an advance directive will limit care in the future
   c. Belief that advance directives are only for elderly and terminally ill patients
   d. Poor literacy level among patient population

5. Subacute care is becoming an increasingly common setting for care primarily because of cost efficiency, costing 20% to 60% less than acute care settings. Factors that directly influence the cost efficiency include all the following *except:*
   a. Delivery of outcome-focused care
   b. Short-term, low-cost patient stays
   c. Independence from prospective payment systems
   d. Ability to provide highly skilled, specialized care

6. Which of the following statements regarding hospice goals and objectives is *false?*
   a. Hospice strives to enhance the quality of life for the patient who is dying.
   b. Hospice enhances the quality of life for the surviving family through ongoing bereavement services.
   c. Hospice provides a setting for care that is supportive of both the terminally ill individual and the family.
   d. Hospice provides a comprehensive, well-coordinated, multidisciplinary approach to terminal and palliative care.

7. The primary goal of patient education is to:
   a. Provide information and knowledge to empower individuals to manage self-care deficits
   b. Provide individuals and their families with support and control
   c. Provide a competent alternative for care delivered by a health care worker
   d. Decrease anxiety and stress experienced by patients and their families

8. Utilization of available community resources is low even when these resources or services are needed. Factors that contribute this include all the following *except:*
   a. Consumer dissatisfaction with services provided
   b. Flexibility of services
   c. Lack of access or availability of services
   d. Lack of awareness of available services

BIBLIOGRAPHY

1. Aitken MJ: Matching models to environments: a planning guide to the selection of pediatric home care models, *Home Healthc Nurse* 7(2):13, 1989.
2. Amenta MO, Lippert C: Hospice is a concept, not a place, *Home Healthc Nurse* 12(3):71, 1994.
3. Baldwin PD: Resources for indigent patients, *Semin Oncol Nurs* 10(2):130, 1994.
4. Broydo L: Sometimes doctors don't present all the options, *Mother Jones Magazine,* March/April 1996, p 18.
5. Bates IV: A secret shared, *Hospice* 1(4):20, 1990.
6. Beach DL: Caregiver discourse: perceptions of illness-related dialogue, *Hospice J* 10(3):13, 1995.
7. Campion EW: New hope for homecare? *N Engl J Med* 333(18):1213, 1995.
8. Cancer resources in the United States, *Oncol Nurs Forum* 22(9):1421, 1995.
9. Carpenito LJ: *Nursing diagnosis: application to clinical practice,* Philadelphia, 1983, Lippincott.
10. Carter R, Golant S: *Helping yourself help others: a book for caregivers,* New York, 1996, Times Books.
11. Cohen MH, Pinnick NP: Home care of children. In Martinson IM, Widmer A, editors: *Home health care nursing,* Philadelphia, 1989, Saunders.
12. Cooley ME and others: Patient literacy and the readability of written cancer educational materials, *Oncol Nurs Forum* 22(9):1345, 1995.
13. *Coping Magazine's* guide to educational information and support services, *Cope* 11(3):32, 33, 1995.
14. Cuthbert-Allman C, Conti PA: VNA of Boston addresses: cultural barriers in home-based care, *Caring Magazine,* 14(12):22, 1995.
15. Davidhizer R, Giger JN: Humor-care for the caregiver, *Caring Magazine* 14(10):64, 1995.
16. Deets H: Home care in the 21st century, *Caring Magazine* 14(9):50, 1995.
17. de Menses MR, Perry GRB: The plight of the caregiver, *Home Healthc Nurse* 11(4):10, 1993.
18. *Discharge planning: conditions of participation,* Fed Register 59(238), December 1994, *Rules and regulations,* final rule, Health Care Financing Administration, 42 CER, Pts 405 and 482, Medicare and Medicaid Programs; *Revisions to conditions of participation for hospitals,* p 64141.
19. Dixon E, Park R: Do patients understand written health information? *Nurs Outlook* 38(6):278, 1990.
20. Dolan MB: *Community and home health care plans,* Springhouse, Pa, 1990, Springhouse.
21. Drummand PA, Hagenstad RR: Oncology outpatient experience: a unique approach to staff development, *Nurs Manage* 18(9):88, 1987.
22. Feuer LC: Discharge planning: home caregivers need your support, too, *Nurs Manage* 18(4):58, 1987.
23. Finley RS: Drug-delivery systems: infusion and access devices, *Highlights Antineoplast Drugs* 13(2):15, 1995.
24. Folden SL: Caring for older homebound adults: a chronic illness perspective, *J Home Health Care Pract* 2(1):57, 1989.
25. Ginsberg JA, Prout DM: Access to health care, *Ann Intern Med* 112(9):641, 1990.
26. Given BA: Believing and dreaming to improve cancer care, *Oncol Nurs Forum* 22(6):929, 1995.
27. Given BA, Stommel M, Given CW: Depression as an overriding variable in explaining caregiver burdens, *J Aging Health* 2(1):81, 1990.
28. Glazer-Waldman H, Hall K, Weiner MF: Patient education in a public hospital, *Nurs Res* 34:184, 1985.
29. Gorski LA: Patient education in high-tech home care, *Caring Magazine* 14(5):22, 1995.
30. Griffiths M, Leek C: Patient education needs: opinions of oncology nurses and their patients, *Oncol Nurs Forum* 22(1):16, 1995.
31. Gulla JP: Family assessment and its relation to hospice care, *Am J Hospice Palliative Care,* 7:32, 1990.
32. Hamilton M: Standards of practice for discharge planning, *Contin Care,* September 1995, p. 33.
33. Hammill CT, Parver CP: Home health care services: a vital component of managed care, *J Home Health Care Pract* 7(4):16, 1995.
34. Harper BC: Report from the National Task Force on Access to Hospice Care by Minorities, *Hospice J* 10(2):1, 1995.
35. Health beat, *Contin Care magazine* 28, May 1995.
36. Hileman JW, Lackey NR, Hassanein RS: Identifying the needs of home caregivers of patients with cancer, *Oncol Nurs Forum* 19(5):771, 1992.
37. Hillner BE: The Schulman/Yabroff article reviewed, *Oncology* 9(6):528, 1995.
38. Hinds C: The needs of families who care for patients at home: are we meeting them? *Adv Nurs Pract* 10:575, 1985.
39. Hiromoto BM, Dungan J: Contract learning for self-care activities, *Cancer Nurs* 14(3):148, 1991.
40. Horton JR, Gosey M, Fay A: Cancer support services: a working prototype, *J Oncol Manage* 3(4):10, 1994
41. Hyatt L: Subacute services solve the managed care puzzle, *Contin Care* 13(8):20, 1994.
42. Jacobs P: *The economics of health and medical care,* ed 3, Gaithersburg, Md, 1996, Aspen.
43. Jaime AJ: Putting the pieces together: effective case management in long-term rehabilitation essential for positive outcomes, *Contin Care,* 15(1):5, 1996.
44. Jastak S, Wilkinson GS: *Wide-Range Achievement Test: revised administration manual,* Washington, DC, 1984, Janstak.
45. Johnston J, Clark B: Orientation to home care: maximizing Medicare reimbursement, *Home Healthc Nurse* 8:45, 1990.
46. Kelly K, McClelland E: Discharge planning: home care considerations. In Martinson IM, Widmer A, editors: *Home health care nursing,* Philadelphia, 1989, Saunders.
47. Kennis N: Maximizing your patient teaching potential, *RN,* February 1996, p 21.
48. Kinsey R, Doty T: Cancer resources in the United States, *Oncol Nurs Forum* 22(9):1421, 1995.
49. Leiby SA, Shupe DR: Does home care lessen hospital readmissions for the elderly? *Home Healthc Nurse* 10(1):37, 1992.
50. Loescher LJ: Genetics in cancer prediction, screening and counseling. Part II. The nurse's role in genetic counseling, *Oncol Nurs Forum* 22(2 suppl):16, 1995.
51. Lokich J: The delivery of cancer chemotherapy by continuous venous infusion, *Cancer* 50:2731, 1982.
52. MacDonald D: Hospice entropy and the 1990's: towards a hospice world view, *Am J Hospice Palliative Care,* 8(4):35, 1991.

53. Magilvy JK, Lakomy JM: Transitions of older adults to home care, *Home Health Care Serv Q* 12(4):59, 1991.

54. Maloney CH, Preston F: An overview of home care for patients with cancer, *Oncol Nurs Forum* 19(1):75, 1992.

55. Mathis EJ: Top 20 educational wants of current family caregivers of disabled adults, *Home Healthc Nurse* 10(3):23, 1992.

56. Mathis EJ: Family caregivers want education for their caregiving roles, *Home Healthc Nurse* 10(4):19, 1992.

57. McAbee RR, Grupp K, Horn B: Home intravenous therapy. Part I. Issues, *Home Health Care Serv Q* 12(3):59, 1991.

58. McAnear S: Parental reaction to a chronically ill child, *Home Healthcare Nurse* 8(3):35, 1990.

59. McClinton DH: Subacute care, *Contin Care* 14(9), 1995.

60. McClinton DH: Oncology care management, *Contin Care* 15(1):8, 1996.

61. McDonald R: Caring enough to reach out: a hospice considers its minority services, *Hospice,* Summer 1990.

62. McMillan SC, Mahon M: The impact of hospice services on the quality of life of primary caregivers, *Oncol Nurs Forum* 21(7):1189, 1994.

63. Meade CD, Diekmann J, Thornhill DG: Readability of American Cancer Society patient education literature, *Oncol Nurs Forum* 19(1):51, 1992.

64. Mehrotra CMN, Kosloski K: Foster care for older adults: issues and evaluations, *Home Health Care Serv Q* 12(1):115, 1991.

65. Meredith D: Patient selection criteria for home IV therapies from A to Z, *Caring Magazine* 14(5):18, 1995.

66. Moore V: *Hospice care systems,* New York, 1987, Springer.

67. Murer CG, Brick LL: Long-term hospitals add revenues, *Contin Care* 14(4):25, 1995.

68. Neumark DE: Providing information about advance directives to patients in ambulatory care and their families, *Oncol Nurs Forum* 21(4):771, 1994.

69. Noggle BJ: Identifying and meeting needs of ethnic minority patients, *Hospice J* 10(2):85, 1995.

70. Nottingham JA: Navigating the seas of caregiving: allies and ideas for success, *Caring Magazine* 14(4), 1995.

71. O'Hare PA, Terry MA: Community-based care management: a framework for delivery of services, *Home Healthc Nurse* 9(3):26, 1991.

72. Pasquali EA: Humor: preventive therapy for family caregivers, *Home Healthc Nurse* 9(3):13, 1991.

73. Perry G, Rhoades de Meneses M: Cancer patients at home: needs and coping styles of primary caregivers, *Home Healthc Nurse* 7(6):27, 1989.

74. Phillips K: Pediatric hospice: home care for the terminally ill child, *J Home Health Care Pract* 1(3):37, 1989.

75. Powell SK, Dalton ME: Shifting roles, *Contin Care,* 15(1):10, 1996.

76. Reimbursement assistance programs, *Cope* 11(5):34, 1995.

76a. Resources: educational information and support services, *Cope* 11(3):18, 1995.

77. Sandrick K: Oncology: who's managing out-patient programs? *Hospitals* 64(3):32, 1990.

78. Sankar A: *Dying at home: a family guide for caregiving,* Baltimore, 1992, The Johns Hopkins University Press.

79. Schonwetter RS, Walker RM, Robinson BE: The lack of advance directives among hospice patients, *Hospice J* 10(3):1, 1995.

80. Schulman KA, Yabroff: Measuring the cost-effectiveness of cancer care, *Oncology* 9(6):523, 1995.

81. Shannon M: Skills in family teaching. In Martinson IM, Widmer A, editors: *Home health care nursing,* Philadelphia, 1989, Saunders.

82. Sherry D: Cost effectiveness and home care: myth or reality? *Home Healthc Nurse* 10(1):27, 1992.

83. Slevin AP, Roberts AS: Discharge planning: a tool for decision making, *Nurs Manage* 18(12):47, 1987.

84. Smith JB: Competition and continuity of care in home health nursing, *Home Healthc Nurse* 9(1):9, 1992.

85. Straw LJ, Conrad KJ: Patient education resources related to biotherapy and the immune system, *Oncol Nurs Forum* 21(7):1223, 1994.

86. Stahl DA: Managed care and subacute care: a partnership of choice, *Nurs Manage* 26(1):16, 1995.

87. Stahl DA: 1995 leadership challenges for SNF's, *Nurs Manage* 26(3):17, 1995.

88. Stahl DA: Maximizing reimbursement for subacute care, *Nurs Manage* 26(4):16, 1995.

89. Stahl DA: Merger mania, alliances and subacute care, *Nurs Manage* 26(11):16, 1995.

90. Stahl DA: Competition in the subacute care market: who will prevail? *Nurs Manage* 26(12):14, 1995.

91. Stahl DA: Accreditation, managed care and subacute care, *Nurs Manage* 27(2):16, 1996.

92. Taylor WI: Cloze procedure: a new tool for measuring readability, *Read J Q* 30:415, 1953.

93. Tompson B: Hospice day care, *Am J Hospice Care* 7(1):28, 1990.

94. Tong KL: Vancouver General Hospital palliative care unit utilization review, *J Palliative Care* 9(1), 1993.

95. Townsend CH: Humor and elderly caregivers, *Home Healthc Nurse* 12(6):35, 1994.

96. Weeks JC: The Schulman/Yabroff article reviewed, *Oncology* 9(6):529, 1995.

97. Woodward W, Thobaben M: Special home healthcare nursing challenges: patients with cancer, *Home Healthc Nurse* 12(3):33, 1994.

98. Zanca J: The challenge of multi-culturality or, how do you say cancer care in American? *Cancer News* 48(1):8, 1994.

APPENDIX CANCER RESOURCES

NATIONAL RESOURCES

About Face
Suite 1405
123 Elm St.
Toronto, Ontario, Canada M5G-1E2
416-593-1448
A support organization for patients who are facially disfigured, their families, and their friends. Membership is $10 annually, and benefits include a variety of publications, a video library, a reference library, and linkage through a computer network.

AIDS Action Council
1875 Connecticut Ave. NW, Suite 700
Washington, DC 20009
202-986-1300
202-986-1345 (fax)
This organization advocates at the federal level for more effective AIDS policy, legislation, and funding, representing more than 1000 community-based AIDS service organizations in the United States. A good referral source for local support services.

AIDS Hotline
800-342-AIDS

Airport Owners and Pilots Association
Medical Department
412 Aviation Way
Frederick, MD 21701-4798
301-695-2139
This organization maintains a directory of U.S. medical transportation firms. Contact to obtain a free copy of the directory.

American Brain Tumor Association
2720 River Rd., Suite 146
Des Plaines, IL 60018
708-827-9910
800-886-2282 (patient line)
708-827-9918 (fax)
This organization provides written information about brain tumors and treatment options, patient education materials, support group referrals, CONNECTIONS Pen-Pal program, and information about nationwide treatment facilities. Also available is a triannual newsletter, *Message Line.*

American Cancer Society
1599 Clifton Rd. NE
Atlanta, GA 30329
404-320-3333 (general information)
404-329-7616 (department of nursing)
800-ACS-2345 (for cancer information)
Local facilities are listed in the telephone directory. The ACS provides a wide range of services encompassing the following:
• Information to the public on all sites of cancer, community resources, rehabilitation programs

• Home care items for use by patients
• Transportation to assist cancer patients to and from medical appointments
• Patient and family education programs to provide a better understanding of the disease and its management
• *Cancer Nursing News:* newsletter mailed to nurses, free on request
• Housing: local divisions near cancer treatment centers, providing housing for patients with cancer and a family member at a Hope Lodge or local hotel/motel.
The following programs are offered by the American Cancer Society:
• *CanSurmount:* short-term visitor program for patients with many types of cancer and for families of patients. The one-on-one visit by a person who has experienced the same type of cancer offers functional, emotional, and social support.
• *I Can Cope:* structured educational program provides information and supportive materials to persons with cancer and their families.
• *International Association of Laryngectomees:* program provides information and supportive materials to laryngectomy patients. Laryngectomy visitors provide preoperative and postoperative support to patients who have recently undergone laryngectomy surgery.
• *Look Good, Feel Better:* joint venture of ACS Society and the Cosmetic, Toiletry and Fragrance Association assists those recovering from cancer by improving their quality of life through personal appearance and body image.
• *Reach to Recovery:* program provides emotional support and practical information to women with breast cancer. especially those who have had a mastectomy. Postoperative visits are provided by women who have had a mastectomy, and literature and a temporary prosthesis are provided.
• Ostomy rehabilitation program
• Cancer prevention and early detection programs for general public
• Resources, information, and guidance for general public and health care professionals

American Foundation for Urologic Disease, Inc.
300 West Pratt St., Suite 401
Baltimore, MD 21201-2463
410-727-2908
410-528-0550 (fax)
This national nonprofit organization focuses on prevention and cure for urologic diseases, offering material for men, women, and children; national awareness programs; research funding; and prostate cancer support groups for patients and their families.

American Liver Foundation
1425 Tompton Ave.
Cedar Grove, NJ 07009
800-223-0179
This nonprofit organization distributes educational materials, assists with transplant availability information, offers grants for research, and on the local level, conducts support groups and other activities.

American Lung Association

1740 Broadway
New York, NY 10019
212-315-8700
This nonprofit organization is dedicated to eliminating lung disease and promoting lung health. It conducts programs to inform the public of air conservation, occupational health, smoking and health hazards, lung disease, and community health. It also provides professional educational programs, publications, films, fellowships, and research grants.

American Red Cross

PO Box 37243
Washington, DC 20013
202-639-3250
This nonprofit organization provides a wide range of support services to the community. Contact the branch in your area for specific information.

Appearance Concepts Consulting Group

Appearance Concepts Foundation
12543 Totem Lake, Suite 142
Kirkland, WA 98033
800-227-7730
This group specializes in needs of women with cancer by providing professional beauty consultation and information about hair alternatives, makeup, skin care, and clothing. It offers training seminars for health care professionals, beauty and fashion professionals, and people with cancer or other cosmetic disabilities. It also provides direct assistance to women who have limited financial resources, using goods and services that have been donated by product manufacturers and professionals and cosmetologists. The founder of this organization has written a book, *Beauty and Cancer,* and conducts a series of seminars and workshops on the topic. *Man to Man* offers group education, discussion, and support to men with prostate cancer and their wives.

Association for Applied Psychophysiology and Biofeedback

BF Training and Treatment Center
Suite 158, Southdale Medical Building
6545 France Ave. South
Edina, MN 55435
612-920-5700
This organization provides information on biofeedback as a technique to help patients cope with pain. For more information and/or a referral to a trained specialist in your area, write to AAPB, 10200 W 44th Ave., Suite 304, Wheatridge, CO 80033; include a stamped, self-addressed envelope.

Better Together Club

c/o ConvaTec
PO Box 4291
Syosset, NY 11791-9706
800-422-8811
This is a nationwide club for ostomates created and funded by ConvaTec, an ostomy supply company. It provides members with such benefits as discounts on food, travel, entertainment, and a quarterly newsletter containing information on the latest medical and product news, travel hints, athletic tips, contests, and personal accounts of the emotional and practical aspects of living with an ostomy.

Bone Marrow Transplant Family Support Network

PO Box 845a
Avon, CT 06001
800-826-9376
This network provides support to families who are coping with the decision to undergo a transplant and describes daily routines before and after the transplant and follow-up medical care.

Cancer Care, Inc.

1180 Avenue of the Americas
New York, NY 10036
212-221-3300
A nonprofit social service agency founded to help cancer patients and their families cope with the impact of cancer. Psychologic and financial support is provided. Counseling is available on both a group and an individual basis.

Cancer Federation, Inc.

21250 Box Springs Rd. #204
Moreno Valley, CA 92557
909-849-HEAL
909-849-0156 (fax)
This organization provides referral information to cancer patients and their families, supports and funds cancer immunology research, provides scholarships, and supports various hospices. A 24-hour hotline is also available.

Cancer Hot-Line

800-525-3777
800-638-6070 (in Alaska)
800-636-5700 (in Washington, DC)
808-524-1234 (in Hawaii, neighboring islands, call collect)

CDC National AIDS Clearinghouse

800-458-5231
This resource provides centralized information regarding HIV/AIDS-related groups, programs, services, testing centers, support groups, and educational materials.

Concern for Dying

250 W. 57th St.
New York, NY 10107
212-246-6962
This nonprofit educational organization provides information regarding the living will, durable power of attorney, death and dying, and euthanasia. Psychologic and legal counseling regarding terminal care decision making is provided.

Corporate Angel Network

Westchester County Airport
Building 1
White Plains, NY 10604
914-328-1313
This network helps cancer patients by providing air transportation to and from cancer treatment centers.

Disabilities Resources, Inc.

516-585-0290

This organization offers a revised and expanded edition of a guide to toll-free telephone services for people with disabilities.

Encore^plus

YWCA of the USA Encore^plus Program
Office of Women's Health Initiatives
624 9th St., 3rd Floor
Washington, DC 20001
202-628-3636
202-723-7123 (fax)

Encore, the national YWCA, offers a systematic approach to women's health promotion, especially related to breast and cervical cancer education and control. Program is designed to meet the needs of all women, including minorities, those with limited incomes, and elderly women who do not use appropriate health care and preventive services. Also included are health education programs, support groups, and exercise programs for women who have had breast cancer surgery. The exercise program consists of floor and pool exercises and group discussion sessions that provide opportunities for sharing common concerns.

Gynecological Cancer Foundation

401 N. Michigan Ave.
Chicago, IL 60611
312-644-6610
312-527-6640 (fax)

This organization's primary focus is an aggressive campaign to disseminate information to the medical community and the public about current trends and techniques in gynecologic cancer.

Help for Incontinent People

PO Box 8310
Spartanburg, SC 29305
803-579-7900
803-579-7902 (fax)
800-BLADDER

This nonprofit organization provides advocacy, education, and support to the public and health professionals regarding causes, prevention, diagnosis, treatments, and management alternatives for incontinence. Send a long, stamped, self-addressed envelope for an introductory packet about incontinence and a list of HIP publications and member services.

In Path

800-296-1217

This volunteer organization provides air ambulance service to patients.

International Association of Cancer Victors and Friends, Inc.

7740 W. Manchester Ave., No. 110
Playa Del Rey, CA 90293
213-822-5032

This organization supports independent research for cancer treatments, disseminates information on chemotherapies, and provides education on nutrition, cancer, and carcinogens in air, food, and water. A quarterly publication, *Cancer Victors Journal,* is available, as well as books, pamphlets, reprints of speeches, tapes, and referral lists.

International Myeloma Foundation

2120 Stanley Hills Dr.
Los Angeles, CA 90046
800-452-CURE

This organization provides information about myeloma and its treatment and management to physicians and patients.

Johanna's On Call to Mend Esteem

Cancer Rehabilitation Nurse Consultants
199 New Scotland Ave.
Albany NY 12208
518-482-4178

This nonprofit cancer rehabilitation nursing service provides a wide range of preventive, restorative, supportive, and palliative nursing interventions for individuals with cancer. It also publishes audiovisual and written material for public and professional education.

Legal Counsel for the Elderly (in association with American Association for Retired Persons, AARP)

1331 H Street NW
Washington, DC 20005
202-434-2120

Legal Hotline for Older Americans

PO Box 23810
Pittsburgh, PA 15222
800-262-5297

Leukemia Society of America

600 Third Ave.
New York, NY 10016
212-573-8484
800-955-4LSA

National and local organization for support of patients and families with leukemia and related disorders. Services include financial counseling, assistance with payment for outpatient drugs, laboratory costs, transportation, radiation therapy, and patient/family support groups.

Look Good, Feel Better

The Cosmetic, Toiletry, and Fragrance Association Foundation
1101 17th Street NW, Suite 300
Washington, DC 20036
202-331-1770
800-395-LOOK

This is a free, national, public service program focusing on teaching women with cancer (through hands-on experience) beauty techniques that will help them restore their appearance and self-image during chemotherapy and radiation treatment. This organization provides a trained and certified cosmetologist for individual or group sessions. Also available are complimentary makeup kits, pamphlets, and videotapes. This is a joint venture of the ACS, the Foundation, and the National Cosmetology Association. Contact your local ACS office or call the toll-free number.

LymphEdema Foundation

PO Box 834
San Diego, CA 92014-0834
800-LYMPH-DX/800-596-7439
This large, nonprofit, all-volunteer, educational organization provides information and resources to patients with lymphedema and health care professionals who treat them. Membership and quarterly publication, *LymphEdema Digest,* are free.

Make Today Count

1235 East Cherokee
Springfield, MO 65804-2263
417-885-2273
800-432-2273
An international organization for persons with cancer or other life-threatening illnesses. Support groups and educational programs are provided, and brochures and handouts are available.

Medical Insurance Claims, Inc.

Kinnelon Professional Complex
170 Kennelon Rd., Suite 10
Kinnelon, NJ 07405
This organization was established in response to the perceived need by the public for assistance in handling insurance claims. These services can be used by senior citizens and family members too involved with the patient's illness to deal with paperwork. It has a full range of services for a fee, including filing claims and pursuing any missing information from health care providers to complete a claim.

National Association of Meal Programs

204 E. Street NE
Washington, DC 20002
202-547-6157
This organization provides referrals to the public regarding the nearest available meal preparation and delivery service in your area.

National Black Leadership Initiative on Cancer

Executive Plaza North
Room 240-D
Bethesda, MD 20892
301-496-8589
301-496-8675 (fax)
This community-based cancer prevention and control outreach program of the National Cancer Institute targets black Americans. Its focus is to address the barriers that limit or prevent access to quality health care that prevents, controls, and treats cancer.

National Brain Tumor Foundation

785 Market St., Suite 1600
San Francisco, CA 94103
415-284-0208
415-284-0209 (fax)
800-934-CURE
This organization supports research into causes and treatments of brain tumors and offers information and support-group re-ferrals for patients and their families. An informational publication for brain tumor patients, *The Resource Guide,* and a newsletter, *Search,* are available through the foundation. A telephone consultation with a brain tumor survivor, nurse, or family member of a brain tumor patient can be arranged by calling this organization.

National Breast Cancer Coalition (NBCC)

1707 L St. NW, Suite 1060
Washington, DC 20036
202-296-7477
202-265-6854 (fax)
A grass-roots advocacy group, whose members consist of women and concerned others, is a leader in the national movement to bring changes in public policy that benefit breast cancer patients and their survivors. This organization also has a National Alert Network that provides up-to-date information regarding breast cancer and related issues.

National Cancer Institute (NCI)

Cancer Information Service
301-496-8664
1-800-4-CANCER/800-422-6237
The Cancer Information Service is available to answer questions by telephone from the general public, patients and their families, and health professionals. Also available are referrals to local resources and printed materials on many topics related to cancer. Callers can also be connected to the NCI's PDQ clinical trial data base for health professionals, which is a comprehensive service providing state-of-the-art cancer treatment. See Professional Organizations and Resources for more about PDQ.

National Coalition for Cancer Research

426 C Street NE
Washington, DC 20002
202-544-1880
202-543-2565 (fax)
This organization's primary focus is to provide education to the public, health professionals, and elected officials in an effort to promote research and public education in order to eradicate cancer and facilitate implementation of the National Cancer Act.

National Coalition for Cancer Survivorship (NCCS)

1010 Wayne Ave., Fifth Floor
Silver Spring, MD 20910
301-650-8868
301-565-9670 (fax)
A network of independent organizations and individuals working in the area of cancer support and survivorship. The primary goal is to generate a nationwide awareness of cancer survivorship. NCCS facilitates communication between persons involved with cancer survivorship, promotes the development of cancer support activities, serves as a clearinghouse for information and materials on survivorship, advocates the interest of cancer survivors, and encourages the study of survivorship.

National Hispanic Leadership Initiative on Cancer

En Accion Coordinating Center
South Texas Health Research Center
University of Texas Health Sciences Center at San Antonio
7703 Floyd Curl Dr.
San Antonio, TX 78284-7791
210-614-4496
210-615-0661 (fax)

This national network of experts in public health and medicine, in collaboration with grass-roots community-based organizations, has conducted a comprehensive assessment of cancer risk factors for all Hispanic/Latino populations. The goal is to provide these targeted populations with the knowledge and the resources to prevent and control cancer among their own people.

National Hospice Organization

1910 North Fort Meyer Dr., Suite 307
Arlington, VA 22209
703-243-5900

This nonprofit organization provides literature and information about hospice to patients and their families and makes referrals to local, regional, and national resources.

National Lymphedema Network

2211 Post St., Suite 404
San Francisco, CA 94115
414-421-2911
800-541-3259

This organization provides educational information, exercise programs, a quarterly newsletter, Internet service, a computer data bank, a resource guide of lymphedema support groups, and health care list and U.S. treatment centers.

National Neurofibromatosis Foundation, Inc.

141 Fifth Ave., Suite 7-S
New York, NY 10010
800-323-7938
212-460-8980

This organization sponsors research, publishes educational materials, and assists in the development of clinical centers and diagnostic protocols. Information packets about neurofibromatosis and support groups are available.

Oley Foundation

214 Hun Memorial, A 23
Albany Medical Center
Albany, NY 12208
518-445-5079
800-776-OLEY

This foundation offers support to individuals receiving home parenteral and enteral nutrition therapy and to their families. It has patient/family support groups and publishes a quarterly newsletter, *Lifeline Letter.* Services are provided free of charge to patients and families.

Options Unlimited

76 East Main St.
Huntington, NY 11743
516-673-1150

This group provides case management services for the coordination of care and services of patients with illnesses or injuries requiring long-term and critical medical care. It has a nationwide network of case management consultants, available on a fee basis, who coordinate a variety of services, including working with insurance companies on billings and settlements, preparing the home for patient care, and helping to find alternative financial assistance.

R.A. Bloch Cancer Foundation, Inc.

4410 Main St.
Kansas City, MO 64111
816-932-8453

This community cancer resource center offers a cancer information hotline that provides information regarding national resources, peer counseling, medical second opinions, and support groups.

Skin Cancer Foundation

245 Fifth Ave., Suite 2402
New York, NY 10016
215-725-5176

This foundation provides patient education materials, a newsletter, books, brochures, pamphlets, and slide and video presentations and supports research on skin cancer.

Spirit and Breath Association

8210 Elmwood Ave., Suite 209
Skokie, IL 60077
1-708-673-1384

This organization's goal is to assist those with lung cancer through a national telephone networking service (telephone counseling). It distributes the *Spirit and Breath Exercise Book.* For those living in the Chicago area, support groups, a visitor program, and newsletter are available.

Susan G. Komen Breast Cancer Foundation

5005 LBJ Freeway, Suite 370
Dallas, TX 75244
214-450-1777
214-450-1710 (fax)
800-IM-AWARE/800-462-9273

This national organization focuses on advocacy, research, screening, and treatment for breast cancer. It also funds research and programs for medically underserved women. The national hotline provides information and referral to treatment centers.

United Ostomy Association

36 Executive Park, Suite 120
Irvine, CA 92714
1-714-660-8624

This nonprofit organization provides speakers, literature, and monthly information meetings for people with ostomies. Volunteers, most of whom are ostomates, may visit patients with ostomies in the hospital or home with the consent of the patient's physician.

United Way of America

Mid-America Region
1400 East Touhy Ave.
Des Plaines, IL 60018-3305
1-707-6160
The staff of local offices of this organization are very knowledgeable about the support services available to cancer patients in the surrounding communities and can provide referrals to such resources.

US TOO International, Inc.

930 North York Rd., Suite 50
Hinsdale, IL 60521-7866
708-323-1002
708-323-1003 (fax)
800-80-USTOO/800-808-7866
This organization offers information, counseling, and educational programs related to prostate cancer, surgery, radiation, medicine, nutrition, and psychology. Chapters across the United States and Canada have monthly meetings for patients and their families.

Women's Cancer Network

2413 West River Rd.
Grand Island, NY 14072
This network provides support, referrals, and resources for women who have survived breast cancer. It offers programs to the public and health care professionals and individual, institutional, and agency consultations. Through this network women with cancer can share experiences, receive support, "recharge," learn from each other, and obtain skills and strategies for healing and surviving the health care system.

Y-Me National Organization for Breast Cancer Information and Support, Inc.

18220 Harwood
Homewood, IL 60430
800-221-2141 (patient hotline, 9-5, CT, weekdays)
708-799-8338 (general information)
708-799-8228 (patient 24-hour hot-line)
This organization provides information, telephone counseling, educational programs, and support groups for patients with breast cancer and their families and significant others. It maintains a "bank" of donated prostheses and wigs for patients with limited financial resources.

PEDIATRIC RESOURCES

Association for the Care of Children's Health

3415 Wisconsin Ave. NW
Washington, DC 20016
202-244-1801
This international organization for health care professionals and parents of children living with illnesses distributes booklets, including *Chronic Illness and Handicapping Conditions* and *Preparing Your Child for Repeated Hospitalization,* as well as other resource materials.

Association for Research of Childhood Cancer

PO Box 251
Buffalo, NY 14225-0251
716-689-8922
This organization consists of parents who have lost children to cancer and people who support cancer research. It funds expansion and continuation of research in pediatric centers and provides money for pilot programs in cancer research. This group meets six times a year to support parents of children with cancer and also publishes a quarterly newsletter and the *Parent/Child Handbook.*

Candlelighters Childhood Cancer Foundation

1901 Pennsylvania Ave. NW, Suite 1001
Washington, DC 20006
202-659-5136
A national organization of parents and families whose children have or have had cancer. Services include self-help and support groups, literature information, and referral to local and regional resources. Many local chapters exist, and services may vary by locality.

Children's Hospice International

703-684-0330
703-684-0228 (fax)
800-24-CHILD (hotline)
This organization provides support and information for children with life-threatening conditions and for their families.

Compassionate Friends Hotline

312-990-0010
This hotline provides a support service for bereaved parents and siblings.

Ever Forward Foundation, Inc.

1101 SW Washington, Suite 101
Portland, OR 97205-9694
800-869-2995
503-224-9207 (fax)
Children with cancer are eligible to become members of the Kangaroo Klub and receive a membership packet. Membership also includes the One Year Program, which includes a full year of age-appropriate communication and encouragement for the child (e.g., newsletters, cards) and gifts of encouragement, especially on holidays, birthdays, and other special occasions. The kangaroo is chosen as the organization's mascot because kangaroos cannot move backward, only "ever forward."

Federation for Children with Special Needs

95 Berkley St.
Boston, MA 02116
800-331-0688 (voice or telecommunications device for deaf persons)
617-482-2915
This organization is the headquarters of the National Parent Resource Center Project, with regional offices throughout the United States. The Project works to assist and ensure collaboration between health care professionals and parents. Health and education counseling and a free newsletter are available.

Make-A-Wish Foundation of America

2600 North Central Ave., Suite 936
Phoenix, AZ 85004
602-722-9474

This nonprofit organization strives to fulfill the favorite wish of a child with a life-threatening or terminal illness. The organization will consider the wish of any child under age 18 anywhere in the world and covers all expenses related to granting that wish.

Ronald McDonald Houses

Golin/Harris Communications, Inc.
c/o McDonald's Corp.
One Kroc Dr.
Oak Brook, IL 60521
708-575-7418
708-575-3994 (fax)

These facilities, run in cooperation with local children's hospitals and McDonald's restaurants, offer a home-away-from-home for children and their parents during children's hospital treatments. It is a homelike atmosphere at a reasonable cost.

SKIP (Sick Kids Need Involved People)

990 Second Ave., 2nd Floor
New York, NY 10022
1-212-421-9160

SKIP is a national organization with the goal of providing case management and advocacy services to families of children with complex health care needs. These services are free and include identifying the services needed, helping families access those services to bring a child home from a medical facility, and locating financial aid resources. SKIP has chapters throughout the United States. Contact this office for the chapter nearest you.

We Care Foundation/Camp Dream Street

3043 Strawberry Dr.
Fayetteville, AR 72703
501-442-1548

This organization provides normal life experiences for children with cancer, their siblings, and their families.

PROFESSIONAL ORGANIZATIONS AND RESOURCES

Agency for Health Care Policy and Research

AHCPR Publication Clearinghouse
PO Box 8547
Silver Spring, MD 20907
800-358-9295
301-495-3453

This government organization provides clinical practice guidelines, quick reference guides (adult and pediatric versions), patient's guides, and guideline reports that include supporting materials, background information, and bibliography. Material available includes acute, chronic, and cancer pain in addition to other topics.

American Association of Cancer Education (AACE)

University of Texas
M.D. Anderson Cancer Center-189
1515 Holcombe Blvd.
Houston, TX 77030
713-792-2030
713-792-0807 (fax)

This multidisciplinary organization provides education and training programs for professionals involved in cancer care. Annual meetings are held, and members receive the AACE handbook on joining. The organization publishes the *Journal of Cancer Education.*

American Association for Cancer Research

Public Ledger Bldg., Suite 816
150 South Independence Mall, West
Philadelphia, PA 19106-3483
215-440-9300
215-440-9313 (fax)

The focus of this organization is to facilitate communication and dissemination of knowledge among scientists. This organization publishes four journals: *Cancer Research; Cancer Epidemiology, Biomarkers and Prevention; Cell Growth and Differentiation;* and *Clinical Cancer Research.*

American College of Oncology Administrators

30555 Southfield Rd., Suite 150
Southfield, MI 48076
810-540-4310
810-645-0590 (fax)

This organization promotes the professional standing of its members by offering continuing education in oncology management, research, strategic planning, and program development.

American Pain Society

5700 Old Orchard Rd., First Floor
Skokie, IL 60077
708-966-5595

This multidisciplinary organization, a national chapter of the International Association for the Study of Pain, has members from many specialties in the fields of medicine, dentistry, psychology, nursing, other health professions, and the basic sciences. Members include both investigators and clinicians in the field of pain and its treatment. One of the major goals is to promote education and training in the field of pain. Annual meetings are held.

American Society of Clinical Oncology

435 North Michigan Ave., Suite 1717
Chicago, IL 60611
312-644-0828

This society promotes and fosters the exchange of information relating to neoplastic diseases, with particular emphasis on human biology, diagnosis, and treatment. It publishes the *Journal of Clinical Oncology.*

American Society of Pain Management Nurses

PO Box 2162
Tucker, GA 30085

This nonprofit professional organization of nurses promotes and provides education, professional development of pain management nurses, scientific investigation in pain management, delivery of high standards of care, advocacy for nurses in legislation and government programs, and communication among health care professionals.

Association of Community Cancer Centers

11600 Nebel St., Suite 201
Rockville, MD 20852
301-984-9496

This organization provides a mechanism for the exchange of information among health professionals who believe high-quality cancer care should be available in the community. It publishes *Community Cancer Care Programs in the United States* and *Oncology Issues: The Journal of Cancer Program Management.*

Association of Nurses in AIDS Care

1555 Connecticut Ave. NW, Suite 200
Washington, DC 20036
202-462-1038
202-234-3587 (fax)

This professional organization supports professional development of nurses involved in all aspects of HIV care and promotes the health, welfare, and rights of patients with HIV disease.

Association of Oncology Social Work

1910 E. Jefferson St.
Baltimore, MD 21205
410-614-3990
410-614-3991 (fax)

This professional organization for social workers in oncology focuses on development of sound public and professional programs and policies for cancer patients.

Association of Pediatric Oncology Nurses

6728 Old McLean Village Dr.
McLean, VA 22101
703-556-9222

A professional organization open to all registered nurses with an interest in pediatric oncology. It offers a quarterly journal, annual meeting, and local chapter activities.

CancerNet

NCI International Cancer Information Center
9030 Old Georgetown Rd.
Bethesda, MD 20814-1519
800-NCI-7890 (United States)
301-486-7600 (international)
301-231-6941 (fax)
E-mail: cancernet@icicc.nci.nih.gov (type HELP in body of mail message for information and instructions)

This center provides access for the public and professionals to state-of-the-art treatment summaries, information on cancer screening, supportive care, patient publications, investigational drugs, and other NCI information services. Available 24 hours a day, 7 days a week.

Catalog of Resources on Medicine, Biomedical Research, and Mental Health

U.S. Superintendent of Documents
Stop SM
Washington, DC 20401
202-512-1656 (fax)

More than 100 valuable print or electronic information products are available for health care providers. Write for a free copy or fax your request.

Hospice Nurses Association

5512 Northumberland St.
Pittsburgh, PA 15217-1131
412-687-3231
412-687-9095 (fax)

This professional nursing organization promotes the exchange of information, experiences, and ideas; the understanding of the specialty of hospice nursing; and study and research.

International Society of Nurses in Cancer Care

Adelphi University School of Nursing
Box 516
Garden City, NY 11530
516-663-1001

The purpose of this society is to advance the knowledge and understanding of cancer nursing and to foster dissemination. Nurses who are working in cancer care and who subscribe to the journal *Cancer Nursing* are eligible for membership.

Internet Resources

J.A. Majors
214-247-2929

On-line service that provides a list of all recent medical and health care publications through the Internet.

Intravenous Nurses Society

Fresh Pond Square
10 Fawcett St.
Cambridge, MA 02138
617-441-3008 (phone)
617-441-3009 (fax)

A professional organization open to all registered nurses with an interest in IV therapy. It publishes guidelines and standards for IV therapy and practice. The *Journal of Intravenous Therapy* and INS newsline are provided to members. A national meeting is held annually, and local chapters exist in more than 30 states.

League of Intravenous Therapy Education

PO Box 3102
McKeesport, PA 15134-3102
412-678-5025

This nonprofit, multidisciplinary organization consists of nurses, pharmacists, and other health professionals active in IV therapy, offering educational programs, seminars, and newsletters.

National Alliance of Breast Cancer Organizations (NABCO)

9 East 37th St., 10th Floor
New York, NY 10016
212-719-0154
(NOTE: NABCO prefers written inquiries.)
This nonprofit information resource offers up-to-date information regarding the latest developments on detection, treatment, support, advocacy, and legislation to the public, professionals, and the media, as well as an annually updated resource list.

National Association of Physicians for the Environment

6401 Rockledge Dr., Suite 412
Bethesda, MD 20817
301-571-9791
301-530-8910 (fax)
This organization provides information to physicians, patients, and the public about the impact of pollutants and the personal and public health steps required to reduce or eliminate these pollutants. It is currently working with the Environmental Protection Agency (EPA) to promote the UV index, which predicts daily solar ultraviolet radiation exposure.

National Hospice Organization

1901 North More St., Suite 901
Arlington, VA 22209
703-243-5900
703-525-5762 (fax)
800-658-8898
This organization provides general information about hospice programs and referrals and publishes *Sourcebook,* which is a catalog of print and video materials available for purchase, including *The Guide to the Nation's Hospices, Hospice Volunteer Training Curriculum, A Consumer Guide to Hospice Care,* and *About Hospice Under Medicare.*

Oncology Nursing Society (ONS)

501 Holiday Drive
Pittsburgh, PA 15220-2749
412-921-7373 (phone)
412-921-6563 (fax)
A professional nursing organization whose purpose is to promote the highest professional standards in oncology nursing. It provides support to oncology nurses; encourages study, research, and exchange of information; and publishes guidelines and standards for oncology nursing practice and education. A journal, *Oncology Nursing Forum,* and newsletter, *ONS News,* are provided to members. A national congress is held annually, and local chapters exist throughout the United States. The ONS is also an ANA-accredited approver and provider of continuing education credits.

Resource Center for State Cancer Pain Initiatives

3671 Medical Sciences Center
1300 University Ave.
Madison, WI 53706
608-265-4013
608-265-4014 (fax)
This resource center for nationwide state initiatives involves a multidisciplinary effort aimed at improving the management of cancer pain. It is a cooperative effort of clinical care facilities, higher education, government, and many health care professionals, including physicians, nurses, pharmacists, social workers, and others with the goal of providing information, professional assistance, communications support, referrals, and other services.

The Senior Wellness Letter
716-437-1650
This monthly publication is directed at health care professionals who are providers for people over age 65.

GENERAL PUBLIC INFORMATION

Bereavement Magazine
Bereavement Publishing
8133 Telegraph Drive
Colorado Springs, CO 80920-7169
719-282-1948
719-282-1850 (fax)
This magazine, an outgrowth of Compassionate Friends, is based on the convictions that (1) bereaved persons can benefit from additional support that covers a broad range of grief concerns, helping professionals need and appreciate direct feedback from bereaved persons, and (2) nonbereaved persons can become more informed about how to provide support to bereaved individuals.

Center for Public Representation

121 S. Pinckney St.
Madison, WI 53703
1-800-369-0388
This organization is a nonprofit law firm, training center, and publishing house for unrepresented persons that publishes easy-to-read, practical self-help books on topics such as guardianship, senior citizens and the law, health care for children with chronic illnesses, power of attorney, planning for long-term care, and uninsured persons. Call or write for catalog and ordering information.

Choice in Dying

200 Varick St., 10th Floor
New York, NY 10014-4810
212-366-5540
800-989-WILL/800-989-9455
212-366-5337 (fax)
A national nonprofit organization committed to serving the needs of dying patients and their families. This organization deals broadly and practically with end-of-life issues, provides free public and professional education and counseling about advance directives, and offers educational videotapes, programs, speakers, and published materials to the public, health care professionals, and lawmakers. List of available materials is available on request.

Combined Health Information Database

National Institutes of Health
Box CHID
9000 Rockville Pike
Rockville, MD 20892
301-770-5164 (fax)
This is a computerized bibliographic data base developed and managed by federal health-related agencies that contains extensive references to health information and health education resources. The data base also includes resources and materials relating to education of patients with cancer, cancer prevention, cancer control, and other cancer-related issues.

Consumer Information Center
U.S. General Services Administration
Consumer Information Center-2D
PO Box 100
Pueblo, CO 81002
This governmental agency provides free or low-cost federal publications of consumer interest, including food and nutrition, health, drugs, health aids, medical problems, nursing home selection, and federal programs and benefits. A catalog is available for $1.

Coping Magazine
PO Box 682268
Franklin, TN 37068-2268
615-790-2400
615-791-4719 (fax)
The only nationally distributed consumer magazine for people whose lives have been touched by cancer. The magazine provides insights and knowledge concerning the day-to-day management of the disease and encourages development of coping skills and strategies.

Food and Drug Administration (FDA)
U.S. Office of Consumer Affairs
HFE-885600
Fishers Lane
Rockville, MD 20857
301-443-3170
A consumer source for publications concerned with food-related subjects, FDA regulations, cosmetics, general medical drug information, medical devices, radiologic health, and health fraud.

Head and Neck Cancer Information Service
Rush Cancer Institute
Rush-Presbyterian-St. Luke's Medical Center
1725 West Harrison St., Suite 863
Chicago, IL 60612
312-563-2322
312-563-2354
This information service answers questions and reviews problems pertaining to head and neck cancer. Calls are answered by a masters-prepared oncology nurse, and a team of physicians is available to address questions related to specialized care involving surgery, radiation, and medical oncology.

The Health Resource
Janice Guthrie
564 Locust St.
Conway, AR 72032
501-329-5272
The owner and founder of this resource provides a service to persons with cancer and physicians by conducting diligent and meticulous research of scientific journals, medical libraries, data bases, and newsletters. The goal is to make people aware of all the choices for treatment available, particularly to those who are locked into HMOs, where often the treatments offered are not all those available.

National Cancer Survivors Day Foundation, Inc.
PO Box 682285
Franklin, TN 37068-2285
615-794-3006
615-794-0179 (fax)
America's nationwide, annual celebration of life for cancer survivors, their families, friends, and oncology teams. This holiday is celebrated the first Sunday in June of each year in communities in the United States and Canada.

National Marrow Donor Program
Coordinating Center
3433 Broadway St. NE, Suite 400
Minneapolis, MN 55413
612-627-5844
800-627-7692/800-MARROW2
612-627-5877 and 612-627-5899 (fax)
This is a computerized registry of unrelated potential volunteer marrow donors. The program provides information on how to be listed as a potential donor and about transplants for patients with leukemia, aplastic anemia, or any other life-threatening disease.

Office of Minority Health Resource Center
U.S. Department of Health and Human Services
PO Box 37337
Washington, DC 20013-7337
800-444-6472
This governmental office provides information about health-related resources that target Asians, Pacific Islanders, black Americans, Hispanics/Latinos, and Native Americans at the federal, state, and local levels. It also provides a computer data base of minority health publications/programs, information on minority health funding, and a community resource network.

U.S. Department of Health and Human Services
Public Health Service
Agency for Health Care Policy and Research
2101 East Jefferson St., Suite 501
Rockville, MD 20852
1-800-952-7664
This governmental agency distributes health care literature for the general public, patients and their families, and health care professionals. Call or write for more information.

U.S. Department of Labor, Occupational Safety and Health Administration (OSHA)

Directorate of Technical Support
200 Constitution Ave. NW
Washington, DC 20210
1-202-523-7047

OSHA is involved in the development and enforcement of occupational safety health standards and strives to ensure safe and healthful working conditions for every worker in the U.S. The directorate of technical support can provide information regarding work related hazards and occupational injuries and illnesses.

HEREDITARY CANCER SCREENING PROGRAMS

(This is a partial listing.)

Alta Bates Comprehensive Cancer Center

5730 Telegraph Ave.
Oakland, CA 94609
510-204-4286

Cancer Prevention Clinic

University of Wisconsin Comprehensive Cancer Center
1300 University Ave.-7C
Madison, WI 53706
608-263-2118

Cleveland Clinic–Florida

3000 W. Cypress Creek
Ft. Lauderdale, FL 33309
800-359-5101

Hereditary Cancer Center

Saint Joseph Hospital
601 N. 30th St.
Omaha, NE 68131
402-280-4364/402-280-4367

Johns Hopkins Hospital

600 N. Wolfe St.
Baltimore, MD 21205
410-550-5405

M.D. Anderson Hospital and Tumor Institute

University of Texas
Department of Genetics, Section of Human Genetics
Houston, TX 77030
713-792-2575

Roswell Park Cancer Institute

Elm and Carlton Sts.
Buffalo, NY 14236
212-845-8983

Strang Clinic

320 E. 15th St.
New York, NY 10003
212-475-6066

University of Alabama at Birmingham Cancer Control Office

1824 Sixth Ave. South, Room 237
Birmingham, AL 35294-3300
205-934-5077

REIMBURSEMENT PROGRAMS AND FINANCIAL ASSISTANCE

Many pharmaceutical companies and related companies offer programs to assist with reimbursement, some of which are listed below.

Amgen, Inc.

800-272-9376
800-637-6698 (in Washington, DC area)
Amgen provides those who use or administer Neupogen with insurance billing guidance and information about Amgen's Safety Net Program, designed to provide Neupogen free of charge to medically needy patients.

Baxter Biotech N.A.

800-548-IGIV
202-637-6696 (Washington, DC area)
Gammagar S/DIGIV Reimbursement Hotline for providers and patients gives information regarding coverage, coding, and reimbursement issues and on prevention of bacterial infections for patients with chronic lymphoblastic leukemia.

Berlex, Inc.

800-473-2239
Hotline provides health professionals with information on claims assistance programs for indigent patients.

Bristol-Myers Oncology Division

800-872-8718
Reimbursement specialists provide assistance with reimbursement issues.

Bristol-Myers Squibb Oncology Access Program

800-272-4878
Program provides free products to patients who have no insurance, are not eligible for government assistance programs, and are unable to pay.

Burroughs Wellcome Co.

800-423-6869
A service provides information about coverage and reimbursement issues for all company products, assistance with claims submissions, appeals, and prior authorization for selected oncology products. The Patient Assistance Program for Oncology Products (800-722-9294) provides rapid access to any Burroughs Wellcome prescription medicine at no cost for patients who are financially disadvantaged.

Cerenex Pharmaceuticals

800-745-2967
Hotline assists providers with insurance coverage and problem claims.

Chiron Therapeutics

800-775-7533 (Proleukin)
800-939-4242 (Aredia)
Hotline provides assistance with payment, coverage, claim submissions, and appeals.

Genentech, Inc.

800-530-3083
Hotline provides information on reimbursement on Genentech products and helps patients maximize their coverage. Information about uninsured patient assistance programs is also available.

Immunex Corporation

800-321-4669
Program assists providers with all aspects of insurance verification, claims filing, and appeals.

Medi-Physics, Inc., Amersham Healthcare

800-204-5678
Service provides information to providers and patients regarding coverage, coding and reimbursement policies, and assistance with claims submission and troubleshooting.

Ortho Biotech, Inc.

800-553-3851
Hotline provides assistance with claims submissions and appeals and free carrier intervention services ("letters of medical necessity"). Company also offers reimbursement assurance program, financial assistance program, and cost-sharing program.

Roche Laboratories

800-443-6676
Company provides reimbursement support program, access to NCI data bases, biomedical literature searches, and cost assistance program, which will reimburse patients and third-party payers for costs in excess of $9800 for Roferon-A.

Rhone-Poulenc-Rorer Pharmaceuticals, Inc.

800-996-6626
Hotline provides assistance with coding, patient insurance verification, precertification/predetermination, claim support documents, claim submissions appeal strategies, payer education/negotiation, and payer policies/procedures.

Sandoz Pharmaceuticals Corp.

800-772-7556
Company provides information regarding insurance coverage by various insurers, including Medicare, Medicaid, and private insurers, as well as coverage criteria, coding, reimbursement levels, appeals, and referrals to indigent programs.

Schering Sales Corp.

800-521-7517
Hotline provides information on billing and determination of patient eligibility for one of three additional plans to provide drug or financial assistance.

TAP Pharmaceuticals Inc.

800-453-8438
Service provides information and assistance to professionals and patients with reimbursement issues.

Therabite Corp.

800-322-9500
Hotline provides information regarding coverage, reimbursement, appeals, and prior authorization.

U.S. Bioscience

800-887-2467
Company offers reimbursement assistance and will provide Hexalen or NeuTrexin free of charge to medically needy patients with no insurance or means to pay.

Seneca Pharmaceuticals

800-767-4424
Insurance reimbursement advice and a physician office guide is available for Zoladex.

Additional toll-free numbers of pharmaceutical companies that have indigent patient programs:
Abbott/Ross Laboratories: 800-922-3255
Adria Laboratories: 800-795-9759
Allergan prescription: 800-347-4500 (X6219)
Astra FAIR Program: 800-488-3247
Boehringer Ingleheim: 203-798-4131
Boots: 800-323-1817
Cetus Corp.: 800-755-7533
Ciba-Geigy Pharmaceuticals: 800-257-3273
DuPont Merck: 302-992-4240
Fisons: 800-234-5535
Fujisawa: 707-317-8638 (NebuPent assistance program); 800-366-6323 (gallium nitrate assistance) 800366-6323
Genentech: 800-879-4747
Glaxo: 800-GLAXO77
Hoechst-Roussel: 800-PROKINE; 800-422-4779
Hoffman-LaRoche: 800-443-6676 (Oncoline reimbursement); 800-526-6673 (indigent patient program); 800-227-7448 (cost assistance program)
IMRE Corp.: 800-635-4673
Janssen Pharmaceuticals: 800-253-3683
Janssen Pharmaceuticals #2: 908-524-9409 (Ergamisol)
Knoll Pharmaceuticals: 800-526-0710
Lederle Laboratories: 800-533-2273
Eli Lilly & Co.: 317-276-2950
Marion Merrell Dow, Inc.: 800-362-7466
McNeil Pharmaceuticals: 215-628-7803
Merck, Sharp & Dohme: 800-637-2579
Miles: 800-998-9180
Norwich-Eaton Pharmaceuticals: 800-447-3437
Parke, Davis & Co.: 210-540-2000
Pfizer Labs, Roerig Division: 212-573-3954
Purdue Frederick: 203-853-0123 (X4800)
Reed and Carnrick/Block Drug: 908-981-0070
Roxane Laboratories, Inc.: 800-848-0120
Snofi Winthrop Pharmaceuticals: 212-907-2000
G.D. Searle & Co.: 800-542-2526
Sigma-Tau Pharmaceuticals: 800-999-6673

SmithKline Beecham: 800-866-6273 (Eminase/Triostate program); 215-751-5760 (all other products)
Syntex Laboratories, Inc.: 800-444-4200 (provisional assistance); 800-822-8255 (indigent patient program)
Upjohn Co.: 616-323-6004
Wyeth-Ayerst Laboratories: 800-568-9938
Zeneca Pharmaceuticals: 800-456-5678

INFUSION PUMPS

Infusaid, Inc.
800-451-1050
Preauthorization and general assistance for infusion pump implants

Medtronic, Inc.
800-328-0810
Full-service assistance and prior authorization service for infusion pump implants

Sims Deltec, Inc.
800-433-5832
Assistance for customers and health care professionals and a wide range of other services, including legislative lobbying for oncology reimbursement, financial models for growth partnering, and billing seminars for branch offices and professional associations

PERSONAL CARE RESOURCES

About Faces Permanent Cosmetics
1001 Bridgeway Blvd., Suite 432
Sausalito, CA 94965
415-331-0663
This company specializes in permanent cosmetic application, a tattoo process in which pigments are applied to the eyelids, eyebrows, and lips to match skin tone. This process is used for alopecia areata (loss of facial and body hair), and loss of hair from chemotherapy.

Airway
3960 Rosslyn Dr.
Cincinnati, OH 45209
800-888-0458
This company manufactures a line of breast prosthesis called The Portrait Group along with fitting aids, bras, and swimsuits. Call company to identify a local dealer.

Alkin Hair Co.
254 West 40th St.
New York, NY 10018
212-719-3070
This company matches hair samples, which can then be braided, woven, or used for extensions. Call for information.

Caring Touch Division
International Hairgoods, Inc.
6811 Flying Cloud Dr.
Eden Prairie, MN 55344
800-424-7567
This company manufactures and distributes cranial hair prostheses for men, women, and children; eyebrow and mustache prostheses; and turbans and related supplies to a network of trained Caring Touch service centers. The company also offers patient educational materials on hair loss and the available appearance options. Call for information.

Designs for Comfort, Inc.
PO Box 8229
Northfield IL 60093
800-443-9226
This company has developed a combination cap and hairpiece called the Headliner as an alternative to wigs. The Headliner is available in a variety of colors and fabrics. This product may be reimbursed by individual insurance companies as a hair prosthesis. Call to order by mail or locate a local dealer.

Fairs' OPS, Inc.
PO Box 5760, Greenway Station
Glendale, AZ 85306
602-978-4435
This company distributes ostomy prothesis support (OPS) undergarments. These undergarments are available for both men and women. Call for information.

Frends Beauty Supply
5270 Laurel Canyon
N. Hollywood, CA 91607
818-769-3834
This company offers cosmetics, camouflage makeup, eyelashes, and eyebrows. For mail order catalog, send $3.75. You will receive $3 credit toward your first purchase.

Holly Cosmetics/Medical Image Products
4947 Brownsboro Rd.
Louisville, KY 40220
800-222-3964
This company offers a line of corrective cosmetics. Information about the Holly Cosmetics line and a video are available by mail. Call to order information and the video or to find a local consultant. This company is involved in the Look Good, Feel Better program.

Intimacies By Alice
3 Hudson Watch Dr.
Ossining, NY 10562
914-923-2010
This company manufactures a line of sleepwear and daywear, including lounging wear, sportswear, and lingerie, for women who have had breast surgery. These are available in specialty boutiques or by mail order. Call for more information.

Jodee
5085 West Park Rd.
Hollywood, FL 33021
800-821-2767
305-987-7274
This company provides mastectomy products. Call to request a catalog that includes bras, prostheses, and accessories.

Mary Catherine's

1914 N.E. 42nd Ave.
Portland, OR 97213
800-843-3215
A boutique for intimate apparel for women who have had breast surgery. Call or write for a catalog that includes bras, prostheses, and swimwear.

Nearly Me

316 W. Florence Ave.
Inglewood, CA 90301
310-330-7500 (Los Angeles)
800-421-2322
This company offers a line of breast prostheses, mastectomy swimwear, and accessories. Prostheses are available for all types of surgeries in a wide range of prices. Call for more information and a local dealer.

Worldwide Home Health Center, Inc.

926 E. Tallmadge Ave.
Akron, OH 44310
800-621-5938 (in Ohio)
800-223-5938
This company is a distributor for health care products and services. A free catalog is available that includes breast prostheses, skin care products, and ostomy products.

EDUCATIONAL RESOURCES

ABLEDATA

Adaptive Equipment Center
Newington Children's Hospital
181 E. Cedar St.
Newington, CT 06111
203-667-5405
800-344-5405
This is a continually updated product information data base with entries for more than 17,000 commercially available products from more than 2000 manufacturers. Detailed information is included on products for use in all aspects of independent living, including personal care, transportation, communication, and recreation. A printed copy of the data base will be provided in response to an inquiry specifying the type of product desired or type of activity or function to be achieved. The data base is also available through direct on-line searching or in a CD format for microcomputers. You can receive up to eight pages of information free.

American Cancer Society (ACS)

1559 Clifton Road NE
Atlanta, GA 30329
404-320-3333 (general information)
404-329-7616 (department of nursing)
The ACS offers printed and audiovisual materials as well as educational programs for nurses and other health care professionals. Scholarships are available for master's degree and doctoral students in cancer nursing.

American Pain Society (APS)

5700 Old Orchard Rd., First Floor
Skokie, IL 60077
708-966-5595
The APS, a national chapter of the International Association for the Study of Pain, is a not-for-profit educational and scientific organization. One of the APS's major goals is to promote education and training in the field of pain. It has developed a handbook, *Principles of Analgesic Use in the Treatment of Acute Pain and Chronic Cancer Pain: A Concise Guide to Medical Practice* (2nd edition). For more information, call or write the APS.

CancerFax

NCI International Cancer Information Service
9030 Old Georgetown Rd.
Building 82, Room 219
Bethesda, MD 20892
301-402-5874 (on fax machine handset)
301-496-8880 (for technical assistance)
The NCI has combined computer with fax technology and now offers to any health care professional with a fax machine current data on cancer treatment from NCI's comprehensive data base. Two types of summaries are available: (1) written to meet the informational needs of the health care provider and (2) written in language geared toward the general public. There is no charge for the service, only the cost of the telephone call. This service is available 24 hours a day, 7 days a week.

Cancer Information Service

800-4-CANCER
This service is available to answer questions by telephone from the general public, patients and their families, and health professionals. Printed materials on many topics related to cancer are available to callers without charge.

Disability Resources, Inc.

Disability Information at Your Fingertips
516-585-0290
This newly revised and expanded guide to toll-free telephone services for people with disabilities is a valuable resource.

National Cancer Institute (NCI)

Bethesda, MD 20205
301-496-7403
The *Cancer Information Clearing House* is an information service for organizations that use or develop materials for public and professional information and education. The Clearing House provides information exchange, either through bibliographic services or through custom searches of its collection of 7000 citations of cancer informational and educational materials and services.

The *International Cancer Information Center* sponsors CANCERLINE, which includes (1) 400,000 citations and abstracts of articles published since 1963 on all aspects of cancer, (2) descriptions of 10,000 ongoing cancer research projects, and (3) 4500 summaries of clinical investigations of new anticancer agents and treatment modalities.

The *Physician Data Query* (PDQ) is a computer data base for retrieval of cancer treatment information. Providing easy access to state-of-the-art cancer information, the data base has three interlinked files, organized and internally arranged to allow interactive searching and retrieval of information.

National Rehabilitation Information Center

8455 Colesville Rd., Suite 935
Silver Spring, MD 20910-3319
1-800-346-2742
This organization distributes a bibliographic data base, REHABDATA, covering disability and rehabilitation research literature, including citations to research reports from the National Institute on Disability and Rehabilitation Research, sponsored centers, and other sources, such as scholarly papers, selected journal articles, audiovisual materials, and reference documents.

Office of Cancer Communications

NCI Building 31, Room 10A16
Bethesda, MD 20892
1-301-496-5583
This office, a branch of the National Cancer Institute, provides services for the public and health care professionals, including information and publications on a variety of cancer topics.

University of Texas M.D. Anderson Cancer Center

Patient Education Office
1515 Holcombe, Box 21
Houston, TX 77030
ATTN: Patient Education Clearinghouse
713-792-7128
The center's Patient Education Office staff work with multidisciplinary committees to assess, implement, and evaluate educational activities for patients and their families. Teaching plans, printed materials, and audiovisual aids are available at a nominal cost to reinforce the instructions and information provided by individual members of the health care team. The Patient Education Materials Clearinghouse serves as a distribution center for printed patient education materials. Call or write to obtain ordering information.

RECOMMENDED BOOKS/PAMPHLETS

Access Device Guidelines
ONS Publications Dept.
1016 Greentree Rd.
Pittsburgh, PA 15220
412-921-7373
These guidelines, published as a series of three modules, are related to the use of catheters, implanted ports and reservoirs, and pumps. Available for a nominal fee.

Bereavement Booklets
Bereavement Publishing, Inc.
8133 Telegraph Rd.
Colorado Springs, CO 80920
719-282-1948
A bimonthly magazine and 14 educational booklets on a variety of bereavement/loss issues are available to professionals and the public for a nominal fee.

The Caregivers Guide
C. Rale and J. Reynolds
Houghton Mifflin, Boston
A book written for caregivers by caregivers. It has 15 chapters with useful information and caregiving techniques. A very good resource for home health aide training programs as well as informal caregivers.

Case Management Resource Guide
Center for Consumer Healthcare Information
PO Box 16067
Irvine, CA 92713-9950
800-627-2244
This 4-volume community resource guide is very comprehensive and contains information on available resources for a variety of health care needs, including home care, rehabilitation, support agencies, counseling, and medical equipment and supplies. Call or write for more information.

Cetus Oncology Resource Guide
Cetus Corp.
500 W. 8th St., Suite 100A
Vancouver, WA 98660
1-800-466-0701
This guide was created to support oncology teams and their patients. It is intended as an informational directory on adjunctive support services available locally, regionally, and nationally.

Domiciliary Palliative Terminal Care: A Handbook for Doctors and Nurses
Derek Doyle
Churchill Livingstone, New York
This handbook, recently updated in 1994, is a useful guide for health care professionals providing terminal care in the home setting.

Dying at Home: A Family Guide for Caregiving
Andrea Sankar
Johns Hopkins University Press, Baltimore
This book, published in 1991, is a helpful guide for families wanting to care for their loved one at home during the terminal stages of illness.

A Guide for the Bereaved Survivor
Robert Baugher and Marc Calija
Centering Corp.
1531 North Saddle Creek Rd.
Omaha, NE 68104
402-533-1200
This 1995 revised edition is clearly and concisely written and offers much support. It is an excellent resource for both male and female survivors and provides suggestions for the stages of grief.

Helping Yourself Help Others: A Book for Caregivers
R. Carter and S. Golant
Times Books, New York
This 1994 book is a good resource for caregivers.

HIV/AIDS: A Guide to Nursing Care (2nd edition)
J.H. Flaskerud and P.J. Ungvarski (eds)
Saunders, Philadelphia
This 1992 book is clear and concise and presents a framework for providing care to HIV/AIDS patients.

The Hospice Handbook
by Larry Beresford
Little, Brown; Boston
This 1993 book is an excellent resource for hospice volunteers, staff orientation, and the general public. It is a complete guide to all aspects of hospice and is not oversimplified.

The Illustrated Directory of Handicapped Products
Trio Publications
497 Cameron Way
Buffalo Grove, IL 60089
This unique publication has about 700 illustrations with detailed descriptions of products designed to help physically disabled patients. It is a good resource to help patients identify the products or services that will help them work or live better with their limitations.

Living with Dying: a Guide for Relatives and Friends
G. Davidson
Augsburg Fortress, Minneapolis
This 1990 book is the author's attempt to help relatives, friends, health care personnel, and clergy gain insight to the patient's perspectives on living and dying in order to provide better care and support to dying persons. The material is based on interviews with more than 600 patients, families, friends, and professional caregivers.

Mastering the Medicare Maze
Center for Public Representation
121 S. Pinckney St.
Madison, WI 53703
800-369-0388
This book provides easy-to-read information and practical advice about Medicare and how to appeal its decisions.

Palliative Care of the Terminally Ill
J.F. Hanratty
Radcliffe Medical Press, Oxford
This 1989 handbook is also a handy reference for health care professionals providing terminal care in the home.

Questions and Answers About Pain Control: A Guide for People with Cancer and their Families
Developed by the NCI, Bethesda, MD; distributed by the ACS, New York
This booklet is a very good, straightforward resource for patients experiencing cancer pain and for their families. To receive a copy, call the ACS, 800-ACS-2345.

The Role of the Oncology Nurse in the Office Setting
Susan B. Baird
Presented as a professional service by Adria Laboratories
Division of Erbamont, Inc.
Columbus, OH 43215
This publication is a useful guide for nurses working in the ambulatory setting. Professional and patient care issues are discussed.

Write Now: Maintaining a Creative Spirit While Homebound and Ill
609-299-0862
This book, the result of a nonprofit project, identifies the positive effects of writing when one is confined. The book provides numerous exercises as well as insights from others living with long-term illness.

NOTE: Literature for professional and patient education is also available through the support service organizations, pharmaceutical companies, and professional organizations listed earlier.

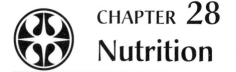

CHAPTER 28

Nutrition

LINDA ANDERSON
DEBORAH WARD

Cancer and its treatment may affect the nutritional status of the patient in a variety of ways. Besides being subject to metabolic effects, patients are emotionally stressed when nutritional intake is impaired. Because eating is a basic body function and often a social activity, inability to eat or difficulty in eating may have a profound physical and psychologic impact on the individual with cancer and the family.

Weight loss is present in half of patients at diagnosis and two thirds of patients with advanced cancer. It negatively impacts the ability to tolerate cancer treatment and has been associated with decreased survival and quality of life. Malnutrition is reported as the cause of death in as many as 20% of cancer patients.[67] Early assessment of nutritional status and interventions as needed are basic components of oncology nursing care.

EFFECTS OF CANCER ON NUTRITIONAL STATUS
Nutritional Components and Their Functions

Cancer may affect the metabolism of the nutritional components necessary to sustain life: carbohydrates, proteins, fatty acids, vitamins, minerals, and electrolytes. An alteration in the metabolism of these components affects the nutritional status of an individual, that is, the degree to which an individual's need for nutrition is met by his or her intake.

Carbohydrates are the sugars that provide energy for immediate use. They are converted to glycogen or fat for long-term storage or are converted to other molecules in the body. Carbohydrates can be divided into three classes: monosaccharides, disaccharides, and polysaccharides. *Monosaccharides* are simple one-molecule sugars; examples are fructose and dextrose (glucose). *Disaccharides* are two-molecule sugars; an example is sucrose (table sugar). *Polysaccharides* are complex sugars characterized by many molecules; examples are starch and dextran.

Glucose is the fuel for most of the cells of the body. It is metabolized rapidly in the presence or absence of oxygen. Each gram of glucose provides 3.4 kilocalories (kcal). Carbohydrates are also a long-term source of energy. When glucose intake exceeds demand, it is converted into glycogen or fat. Both sources of energy are stored in the body and used when a glucose shortage occurs. When metabolized by certain processes, the glucose molecule can be used as the basis for other molecules, including amino acids and fatty acids.

Amino acids are the building blocks of the body. *Proteins* are many amino acids joined into one molecule. Amino acids are divided into two categories: essential and nonessential. *Essential* amino acids must be supplied from the diet because the body is unable to synthesize them from glucose or other amino acids. *Nonessential* amino acids need not be supplied from the diet because the body is able to synthesize them.

Functions of amino acids include maintenance and growth. When tissue breakdown exceeds synthesis or when glucose for energy is lacking, the result is wasting of protein from muscles and loss of mass. Amino acids assist in the regulation of body processes and make up many enzymes found throughout the body. Enzymes are the chemical regulators of many of the synthetic processes in the body. During starvation the body uses proteins as a source of energy. Each gram provides 4 kcal.

Lipids and fatty acids serve many roles in the body. *Fatty acids* are basic molecules, and *lipids* are long chains of fatty acids. Lipids may be saturated or unsaturated, depending on the number of double-bonded carbons in their structure. Lipids are an excellent source of energy, supplying 9 kcal per gram. They are also the long-term storage form of glucose. Fat-soluble vitamins are transported by lipids. Many fat-soluble vitamins (A, D, E, and K) are transported throughout the body bound to fatty acids. The fat content of food is responsible for the taste of many foods and the feeling of fullness that results from eating. Lipids also provide insulation and padding. The fatty acids are precursors to many hormones, including testosterone and estrogen. They are also the basis for cholesterol.

Vitamins are compounds used in a number of enzymatic steps that regulate many processes. Normal amounts of the adult daily requirements (ADRs) of vitamins are obtained by consuming a balanced diet. Vitamins can be divided into two groups: fat-soluble and water-soluble. *Fat-soluble vitamins* are stored by the body in fat. Deficiencies take a long time to develop because these vitamins are stored. Vitamin A is important in maintaining vision and in tooth and skeletal development, and it acts as a precursor to cholesterol. Vitamin D acts to regulate protein and calcium metabolism. Vitamin E is an antioxidant; that is, it prevents or lessens damage to body tissue caused by atmospheric oxygen. Vitamin K helps maintain the clotting ability of blood.

Water-soluble vitamins are not stored in the body and are readily eliminated in the urine. Deficiencies may develop quickly if inadequate quantities are consumed. Vitamin C is used in the formation of collagen, enhances iron absorption, and serves as an antioxidant. B-complex vitamins are cofactors in many enzymatic reactions.

Macro elements, or *electrolytes,* maintain osmotic pressure and water balance, facilitate nerve conduction and muscle contraction, and perform other functions. The macro elements are sodium, potassium, chloride, calcium, magnesium, phosphorus, and sulfur.

Trace elements are so named because they are needed by the body in small quantities. Deficiencies can develop quickly, but clinical signs of deficiency may not be apparent for a long time. Trace elements include zinc, manganese, copper, chromium, selenium, iron, and cobalt, among others.

Systemic Effects of Cancer

The *anorexia-cachexia syndrome* of advanced cancer is a complex response of the body to the presence of tumor. It is thought to be caused by the body's production of inflammatory *cytokines,* which orchestrate a series of changes that result in increased metabolism, decreased intake, and wasting. The changes are similar to those produced in normal inflammatory responses to invasion, such as in sepsis. In this case, however, the invading substance is tumor.[47] Alterations in the normal metabolism of carbohydrates, proteins, and fats result in increased energy expenditures. A normal body's response is to increase appetite and therefore intake, but the person with cancer experiences anorexia and has further decline in ability to meet demands. The process can be exacerbated by psychologic responses: anxiety about cancer, its possible progression, depression, anticipatory phenomena, and learned food aversions.[49]

The body of the person with cancer responds to the increased demand for glucose required by cancer cells and normal body cells with a high rate of gluconeogenesis. *Gluconeogenesis* is the synthesis of glucose by the liver and renal cortex from noncarbohydrate sources such as lactate and amino acids. When protein is broken down to provide amino acids for this process, muscle wasting results. Progressive wasting is called *cachexia.*[5,51,91]

Fat metabolism is affected in individuals with cancer. Stored fat in the form of fatty acids is mobilized from adipose tissues and released into the bloodstream for use as fuel for energy production. This process is controlled by the inhibitory effects of insulin. These inhibitory effects are compromised in individuals with cancer. Body stores of fat are depleted as the disease progresses.[22,76]

Vitamin deficiencies observed in cancer patients include a deficiency of vitamin A in many individuals with cancer of the lung and alimentary tract. Thiamine and vitamin C deficiencies have also been reported in various malignancies. Iron deficiency may result from the unavailability of iron in the diet, malabsorption, or chronic bleeding.

Fluid and electrolyte imbalances may result from direct and indirect effects of tumors. Parathyroid, lung, kidney, and colon tumors may produce an ectopic parathyroid-like hormone that deposits calcium in the renal tubules and may result in renal failure. Hypercalcemia may also cause a concentrating effect that leads to polyuria and water depletion. Leukemia and lymphomas may induce hyperuricemia, hyperphosphatemia, and hyperkalemia as a result of electrolytes released by cellular breakdown. A common presentation of bronchiogenic carcinomas, such as small cell cancer, is the *syndrome of inappropriate secretion of antidiuretic hormone* (SIADH). This syndrome is characterized by urinary loss of sodium and excessive retention of water by the renal tubules. Renal tumors may secrete renin and in turn cause increased secretion of aldosterone, resulting in hypokalemia.[88] Treatment with platinum-based chemotherapeutic agents may deplete magnesium and potassium.

Patients who are nutritionally depleted can have decreased immunocompetence, which becomes more severe as the disease progresses. Malnutrition decreases the size of the lymphoid tissues. Lymphatic structures such as the spleen, lymph nodes, and thymus participate directly in the immune response, and a decrease in their size contributes to immunosuppression. Decreased function of B-cell and T-cell lymphocytes will also result from malnutrition. Fewer T cells, especially helper T cells, and phagocyte dysfunction are common. The greater the malnutrition, the greater is the deficiency of T lymphocytes. This produces a delayed hypersensitivity response. The immune system works with cancer treatment to destroy tumor cells. Preservation of both nutritional status and immune system function are thus important considerations in cancer therapy.[13,48]

Local Effects of Cancer

Several local effects of cancer may alter the nutritional intake of the affected individual. Impaired ingestion may be caused by mechanical and anatomic alterations. Patients with cancer of the head and neck area, esophageal cancers, and brain tumors may have trouble with opening the mouth, chewing, and swallowing as well as with peristalsis. Obstruction of the esophagus can inhibit the passage of food. Gastric tumors often cause pain and distention. Cancers along the alimentary tract may cause obstructions, and they often inhibit the absorption of nutrients. Cancer of the small intestine affects the digestion and absorption of food. A fistula of the bowel may develop as a result of tissue necrosis from a gastrointestinal (GI) tract tumor and induce electrolyte imbalance and malabsorption.

NUTRITIONAL CONSEQUENCES OF CANCER TREATMENT, ASSESSMENT, AND INTERVENTIONS

Effects of Various Modes of Treatment

Surgical alterations in any area of the alimentary tract from the mouth to the anus may cause temporary or occasionally permanent alterations in nutritional intake or absorptive capabilities. Surgical procedures that alter the patient's ability to chew or swallow may prompt the need for soft or blenderized foods, and tube feedings may be required. Assessment and correction of malnutrition have led to improvements in the preoperative and postoperative management of patients with head and neck cancers over the past 20 years.[90] Partial or total gastrectomy can cause severe nutritional problems. When the greater portion of the stomach is removed, the intrinsic factor is not produced in quantities sufficient for the absorption of vitamin B_{12}, and pernicious anemia develops. With resection of the stomach, the quantity of food that can be consumed at one time is limited, and frequent, small feedings are necessary. *Dumping syndrome* may also appear after gastrectomy; a few minutes after ingestion, food is dumped into the jejunum, and nausea, cramping, and diarrhea follow. Malabsorption of fat occurs in patients who have undergone a gastrojejunostomy. The duodenum is bypassed, and pancreatic insufficiency results. Malabsorption of fat impairs absorption of fat-soluble vitamins and calcium. Iron absorption is also decreased, and anemia occurs.[79]

Radiation therapy may affect the normal tissues surrounding the treatment areas. Patients with cancer of the head and neck have both acute and chronic symptoms. Specifically, the normal tissues of the salivary gland, oral mucosa, muscle, and occasionally bone may be affected. In the acute phase, inflammation and swelling of tissues with resulting discomfort may affect nutritional intake. Stomatitis can be complicated with candidiasis (monili-

asis), an oral infection with *Candida albicans* that requires antifungal medications. Taste changes, such as a diminished sense of taste or metallic taste when eating red meats, may cause aversion to food and decreased intake. *Xerostomia,* or diminished production of saliva, is a long-term side effect of radiation therapy. Pain and difficulty swallowing often occur. Saliva substitutes and topical anesthetics for oral use may be helpful, and eating moist foods is recommended.[43,68] Dental caries may occur as a late effect of head and neck radiation. Radiation therapy to the mediastinum for lung or esophageal cancer can cause esophagitis. Dysphagia usually begins within 2 weeks of treatment and can continue for several months afterward. Interventions include topical anesthetics such as liquid antacid mixed with lidocaine viscous, nonsteroidal antiinflammatory drugs (NSAIDs), systemic analgesics, and histamine blockers to reduce stomach acid reflux. Dietary modifications, such as soft, bland food and liquid supplements, may help maintain intake.[25] Enteral feeding is sometimes necessary during the acute phase if symptoms are severe. Long-term strictures of the esophagus may require periodic dilation.

Irradiation of the stomach and small intestine produces vomiting, anorexia, diarrhea, and gastric distention. Antiemetics taken 30 minutes before treatment, a low-residue and lactose-free diet, and adequate hydration may alleviate or minimize these side effects. Antidiarrheal medications may be necessary to minimize fluid loss and permit oral intake. Generally, these acute effects resolve with the completion of therapy.[82] Long-term side effects of radiation to the intestines that affect nutrition may be chronic obstruction, malabsorption, and fistula formation.[25]

Chemotherapy may produce side effects that impair the patient's nutritional status. Chemotherapy causes nutritional deficiencies by promoting anorexia, stomatitis, taste alterations, and alimentary tract disturbances. Deficiencies of vitamins B_1, B_2, and K and of niacin, folic acid, and thymine may also result from chemotherapy. Taste alterations, such as an aversion to red meat, are common with platinum-based products. Cool foods with little aroma and bland foods are often tolerated well. Topical application of analgesics often minimizes the discomfort of stomatitis.[26]

Other common side effects of chemotherapy are nausea and vomiting. The severity of symptoms and their effect on nutritional status varies from patient to patient. Use of antiemetics and dietary measures may help. Newer antiemetics have significantly reduced acute effects of nausea and vomiting, but delayed reactions may persist.[69] Nausea and vomiting may have a psychogenic component; anticipatory nausea and vomiting before a chemotherapy treatment may occur. Odor, sight, and even thought of food may produce emesis in some patients. Relaxation and diversion therapy is sometimes indicated. Aversions to specific foods may occur as a result of the association of those foods with nausea and vomiting. One intervention is the use of "scapegoat" foods or beverages not usually taken that are intentionally introduced before the treatment period to block formation of food aversion to other favorite foods.[54,64]

The side effects of *biotherapy* are generally less severe than those of chemotherapy. Anorexia is a common complaint, and nausea and vomiting occur occasionally. Long-term low-dose treatment may result in fatigue that is intense enough to preclude fixing meals and eating. Interventions may include meal planning for quick, small meals and shopping assistance.[41] Diarrhea may occur, depending on the agent used. Short courses of high-dose biotherapy can cause profound diarrhea with fluid and nutrient loss; however, patients are usually able to regain weight between treatment courses.

Nutritional Assessment

A nutritional assessment can screen for potential or existing problems in nutritional status, provide a data base for individuals at high risk, and determine response to treatment or dietary interventions. Although all patients should be assessed, particular attention should be given to the elderly patient. Older adults experience physiologic effects of aging that impair their nutritional status. For instance, one in five older adults experiences xerostomia. Assessment of the patient's eating patterns, nutrient intake, and supplement use and influences on eating habits should be completed before initiation of cancer treatment.[24,39,75]

Several methods can be used to estimate or quantify the patient's nutritional status (see box at right). A simple method is clinical observation. A thorough nursing history will identify concurrent health problems that may affect nutrition, such as diabetes, hypertension, and malabsorption. Psychosocial factors, including the home environment, food preparation methods, and the patient's body image, should be noted. Ability to purchase food and supplements should be addressed. A physical assessment will reflect the patient's overall nutritional status. Specifically, examination of the hair, teeth, gums, and general muscle tone may provide an early indication of nutritional deficiencies.[42] Poorly fitting dentures after weight loss may impair ability to chew. A functional assessment will determine patients' ability to prepare meals and feed themselves. Uncontrolled pain can significantly impair appetite and should be addressed.[36] Fatigue should be assessed for its impact on the ability to obtain food and eat.

Dietary evaluation is a simple and effective tool for assessing nutritional intake. A 24-hour food diary, a complete dietary history with notations of food allergies and preferences, and direct observation of intake coupled with evaluation of nutrient composition are methods for

---

COMPONENTS OF NUTRITIONAL ASSESSMENT

NURSING HISTORY

Date diagnosed
Type of cancer
Type and duration of therapy
Concurrent medications
Concomitant medical conditions
Surgical procedures
Side effects of therapy
Allergies

PSYCHOSOCIAL ASSESSMENT

Home environment
Family support
Coping abilities
Self-image
Perceptions of role of nutrition
Cultural/religious considerations

PHYSICAL ASSESSMENT

General overall appearance
Hair texture
Skin turgor and integrity
Condition of mouth and gums
Performance status
Alterations in elimination, comfort, etc.

DIETARY EVALUATION

24-hour recall of intake
Food preferences
Food allergies
Use of vitamin supplements
Changes in diet or eating on life-style patterns
Observation of intake
Evaluation of nutrient composition

BIOCHEMICAL MEASUREMENTS

Serum albumin
Hemoglobin, hematocrit
Serum transferrin
Total lymphocyte count
Creatinine
Urine urea nitrogen
Creatinine-height index
Skin testing

ANTHROPOMETRIC DATA

Height
Weight
Weight change over time (actual weight compared with ideal body weight)
Triceps skin fold thickness
Midarm muscle circumference
Subscapular skin fold thickness

dietary evaluation. Much of this information can be collected from the patient; however, the patient may not report accurately. Direct observation of the patient's intake by a consistent nurse or dietitian is more precise but has limitations for patients who are not hospitalized.[79] Family members can be enlisted to help keep a record at home.

Biochemical measurements include laboratory values such as serum albumin, which is used to estimate visceral protein levels; serum transferrin, which reflects the body's ability to make serum proteins; and total lymphocyte count, which tests immunocompetence. Skin testing can reveal T-cell–mediated immunocompetence, and urine urea nitrogen may be measured to estimate skeletal muscle mass. Serum prealbumin level is a sensitive indicator of changes in nutritional status. Albumin levels take longer to respond to increased intake.[79]

Anthropometric measurements are the patient's midarm muscle circumference (MAMC), triceps skin fold thickness (TSF), subscapular skin fold thickness (SST), and weight for height as compared with reference standards. The measurements estimate subcutaneous fat stores, energy reserves, and skeletal muscle protein mass. Moreover, measuring weight and comparing it with the patient's ideal body weight and monitoring changes in weight over time will assist in identifying any downward trend in nutritional status. The nurse must adjust for obvious changes from edema or effusions. Weighing the patient weekly can help assess changes. Daily weights are more appropriate to assess changes in fluid status.

Nutritional Intervention

The extent of nutritional intervention depends on the cause of weight loss and the overall goals of the patient and health care team. It may be palliative or quite aggressive.[34] The oral route is always preferred when available. Enteral feedings may be considered when a mechanical defect precludes ingestion of food. Total parenteral nutrition (TPN) is indicated only when the gut is not suitable to provide nutrients. Research has demonstrated that intense nutritional support may provide some weight gain or lessen weight loss, but long-term benefits have not been realized. Survival and remission rates did not differ significantly with TPN treatment in a review of numerous research trials.[52] In fact, evidence suggests that atrophy of the gut occurs with TPN,[66] and catheter-related infection increases morbidity. Supplemental feeding has been shown to be of value in specific instances when providing nutrition increases the patient's ability to withstand treatment, such as radiation for head and neck tumors or surgery.[14]

Enteral or parenteral nutrition should be considered only for patients who demonstrate most of the following conditions: (1) inability to eat for a long period, (2) weight loss from inability to eat rather than tumor-

induced metabolic changes, (3) availability of professional support to reduce complications of therapy, and (4) cancer that can be expected to respond to treatment.[52]

NUTRITIONAL SUPPORT
Oral Nutrition

After the need for nutritional support has been established, the next step is to determine the method of delivery. The oral route is most desirable. The degree of intervention is based on the severity and etiology of the nutritional deficiency.

Individuals with mild anorexia often respond to *dietary counseling*. They may benefit from frequent small meals and snacks. Foods high in protein, such as cheese, fish, and poultry, and foods high in calories are recommended. Family members and caregivers should offer a variety of foods; foods not appealing at one time may be favorites at another. Milkshakes, peanut butter on crackers, and prepackaged puddings are snacks that are not only nutritious, but also easy to prepare. Supplements such as Instant Breakfast (Carnation) can be taken between meals. Adding dry milk powder to cream soups or milk can increase calorie and protein content. Providing lists of recommended foods or prepared booklets can give caregivers concrete ideas to implement at home. Teaching may be necessary to overcome previous avoidance of high-calorie foods. If indicated, caregivers should provide high-calorie, high-protein supplements such as Sustacal (Mead Johnson), Ensure (Ross), or Citrotein (Sandoz). The nurse should monitor for alterations in elimination when using lactose-based products; some patients experience diarrhea and do not tolerate these formulas. Fruit-flavored supplements may be well tolerated by patients who do not like milk.

Consideration needs to be given to *cultural issues* in our increasingly diverse society, since some hospitalized patients may find standard American food not suited to their taste. Family members may be encouraged to bring in favorite foods. Written materials may need to be developed in languages other than English and should include food choices familiar to the targeted population.

Individuals who have a mild weight loss because of alterations in skin integrity of the oral mucosa (*stomatitis*) or taste alterations may benefit from a high-calorie bland diet. Avoidance of seasoning and experimentation with alternative flavorings such as vanilla may be beneficial. Use of a topical analgesic for stomatitis may reduce discomfort. Good mouth care cannot be overlooked; slight modifications may be needed. Substitution of baking soda or use of a toothpaste specifically for sensitive mouths may be indicated. Patients should avoid commercial mouthwashes, since they contain additives and flavorings that are often painful for those with altered oral mucosal integrity. Cold foods, particularly popsicles, ice cream, and frozen yogurt, often have a numbing effect and may be well tolerated. Liquids that are known to have high acidity, such as orange and lemon juice, should be avoided.[74] Patients experiencing xerostomia may encounter difficulties maintaining adequate nutritional intake. The addition of liquids, particularly sauces and gravies, may be helpful.[71]

Psychosocial support is indicated in addition to dietary interventions. Ineffective individual and family coping often occurs when the patient begins to lose weight. Efforts by family members to encourage a better intake are sometimes met with resistance. Frustration for both patient and family results as the patient perceives the relatives to be unsympathetic and lacking in understanding. Family members often perceive a lack of effort by the patient and become frustrated at their inability to do more. Nurses should listen to problems with nutrition and provide guidance and instruction when indicated. It may be helpful to teach families about biologic causes of anorexia to increase understanding of why the patient finds eating so difficult.

Nondietary interventions for patients with a mild weight loss include varying surroundings, eating at the table with family and friends, and arriving at the table immediately before meals to minimize the effect of food odor on appetite. Using small plates and eating more often may be helpful. Relaxation techniques may be useful for some patients.

Medications may be necessary to control the side effects of the disease or treatment that may be affecting intake. Serotonin (5HT3) blockers such as ondansetron have been shown to reduce emesis significantly after cisplatin administration, especially when given in combination with dexamethasone.[73] Antiemetics given 30 minutes before meals and use of artificial saliva to control the symptoms of xerostomia are other examples of pharmacologic interventions. Several randomized, controlled studies have also suggested that use of megestrol acetate with a dose range of 320 to 1600 mg/day improves appetite and food intake in patients with anorexia and advanced cancer.[83] Dronabinol, δ-9-tetrahydrocannabinol (THC), the active ingredient in marijuana, has also been found to be an effective appetite stimulant in selected patients with advanced cancer and human immunodeficiency virus (HIV) infection. It has been used as an antiemetic for chemotherapy-associated nausea and vomiting.[65,80]

It should be noted that narcotics used to treat pain can decrease appetite, especially if constipation becomes an issue. Care should be taken to maintain bowel function.

Enteral Nutrition

Although oral nutrition is preferred, adequate intake may not be possible for patients who have a mechanical impairment. For these patients, it may be necessary to use a feeding tube (enteral nutrition). The enteral route is preferable because it uses the GI tract. Using the gut for feeding maintains the GI tract's digestive and absorptive capabilities and assists in maintaining GI motility. Metabolic comparisons show a more nearly normal use of some nutrients with the enteral route than with the parenteral route.

A thorough assessment is essential for determining which patients are candidates for enteral nutrition. Generally, patients with functioning GI tracts who are unable to ingest adequate nutrients to meet their metabolic demands are likely to benefit from tube feedings. They should have a reasonable expectation for improvement through increasing delivery of nutrients, a good support system to help with feedings at home, and reasonable life expectancy. Parenteral (intravenous) feeding is indicated only for patients who have totally nonfunctioning GI tracts, who require bowel rest, or who are intolerant of enteral nutritional support.[59]

Tube feedings can be administered by the nasogastric, nasoduodenal, nasojejunal, esophagostomy, gastrostomy, and jejunostomy routes (Figure 28-1). Passage of the feeding tube through the nose into the stomach or intestine is indicated for short-term feeding. It is best tolerated when a small, flexible feeding tube is used. Larger, stiffer tubes may damage the mucosa of the GI tract and

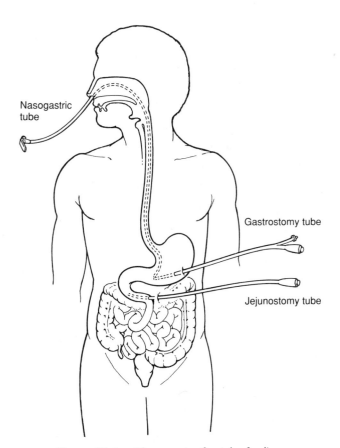

Nasogastric tube

Gastrostomy tube

Jejunostomy tube

Figure 28-1   Three routes for tube feeding.

irritate the nose. A feeding ostomy is indicated for long-term therapy, whenever obstruction makes insertion through the nose impossible, or after GI surgery. Ostomy tubes eliminate nasal irritation and are more cosmetically acceptable to the patient. Possible complications include infection or skin irritation around the feeding tube site; however, this risk is lessened with appropriate skin care.[55] Percutaneous endoscopic gastrostomy (PEG) or jejunostomy (PEJ) tubes are inserted by GI endoscopy and require a patent esophagus. It is a relatively simple procedure, with the tube being threaded through the abdominal and stomach or jejunal wall over a guide wire. The tube can be used soon after placement. Recovery time is short. It may be possible to place a button gastrostomy into a mature gastrocutaneous fistula and thereby eliminate the need for a protruding tube.[78] If GI endoscopy is not possible, placement is more complicated, requiring laparotomy and a longer recovery time.

Nasogastric, esophagostomy, and gastrostomy feedings allow the digestive process to begin in the stomach. Aspiration may occur more easily with gastric feedings than with intestinal feedings because only the gastroesophageal sphincter is functioning to prevent gastric reflux. Alteration of the gastroesophageal sphincter by tumor or surgery may increase the risk of aspiration. Nasoduodenal, nasojejunal, and jejunostomy feedings, which are delivered directly into the small intestine, may be preferred in these selected patients because they then have the pyloric sphincter to prevent reflux. Tube selection is based on several factors, including the duration of therapy, history of abdominal procedures, GI function, level of debilitation, and the discharge plan. Adequate digestion and absorption occur in the small intestine; however, when feedings are improperly selected or administered, nausea, diarrhea, and cramps can result.[30,32,57,70]

A cervical esophagostomy is a surgically created, skin-lined canal extending from the border of the neck to the area below the cervical esophagus. The feeding tube is passed through this opening to the stomach for each feeding and removed after the feeding is finished.

Administration of tube feeding. The size of the tube selected for enteral feedings should be the smallest through which the food will flow. A variety of tubes are available. Most are made of soft, flexible material such as polyurethane or silicone rubber. These tubes do not stiffen when exposed to gastric juices and are more comfortable for the patient than are stiff tubes. The tubes are available in different French sizes and lengths, and most are radiopaque.[92]

The volume and concentration of nutriment delivered by tube feeding should meet the individual's specific needs. A patient who has been without adequate food intake before tube feeding requires a period of adaptation before full volume and strength can be tolerated. Isotonic formulas are more easily tolerated than hypertonic formulas and do not require dilution. The duodenum and jejunum are more sensitive than the stomach to both volume and osmolality. Therefore duodenal or jejunal feeding should be low in osmolality and delivered by continuous drip or pump.[56]

Consultation with the dietary department is usually done to determine the caloric needs and most suitable formula. Water requirements are also calculated. Generally, patients need at least 1 ml of fluid per calorie. Formulas range from 75% to 85% water (check exact amount on can or literature). It is usually adequate to presume about 80% for most formulas. Additional water needs to be given to meet demands. For instance, a patient with 1800 calories delivered by formula needs at least 1800 ml of water, 1440 of which will be delivered in the formula (80% of 1800). The remainder must be given as flushes or extra boluses of water. Dehydration is known to occur with tube-fed patients. Additional fluid may be needed to replace fluid losses from diarrhea, sweating, or wound drainage. Patients who cannot swallow their own saliva because of obstruction may also require extra fluid replacement.

Feedings into the stomach can be done by bolus, gravity, or pump methods. Bolus feedings of enteral formulas are usually administered at 250 to 400 ml over a few minutes, five to eight times daily. Patients who are intolerant of bolus feedings may have nausea, diarrhea, aspiration, abdominal distention, and cramps.[56,61] Generally, only relatively healthy individuals can tolerate bolus feedings.

Gravity feedings may be intermittent or continuous. Gravity flow rates may be inconsistent and thus must be assessed frequently. Even if checks are made as frequently as every half hour, accidental bolus delivery is possible. Ideally, the tube position should be checked two to three times daily, and gastric residual should be checked every 2 to 4 hours.

Continuous feedings may be given during the night over 10 to 12 hours or around the clock. Feedings to the distal duodenum or jejunum should be given by continuous pump infusion to prevent dumping syndrome. They should be started at 50 ml or less and advanced only if the patient shows no diarrhea, cramping, or other signs of intolerance. When the desired rate has been reached, the strength can be increased as tolerated. Generally, an isotonic or nearly isotonic formula can be started at full strength; hypertonic or concentrated formulas are usually started at half strength (half formula, half water) or at half speed. Adding water or other liquids such as dye can contaminate feedings and should be done as carefully as possible. Table 28-1 compares oral supplements and tube-feeding formulas.

Various feeding sets, containers, and pumps are available for tube feeding. Selection of equipment and supplies is based on the formula to be given, rate and fre-

Table 28-1   Common Supplements and Tube-Feeding Formulas

	Ensure (Ross)	Ensure Plus (Ross)	Pulmocare (Ross)	Instant Breakfast (Carnation)	Jevity (Ross)	Glucerna (Ross)	Peptamen (Clintec)
Calories (kcal/ml)	1.06	1.5	1.5	0.93	1.06	1.0	1.0
Protein (g) (liter/can)	37.2/8.8	55/13	62.6/14.8	58/15	44.4/10.5	41.8/9.9	40/10
Fat (g) (liter/can)	37.2/8.8	53.3/12.6	92.1/21.8	35/8	36.8/8.7	55.7/13.2	39/9.2
CHO (g) (liter/can)	145/34.3	200/47.3	106/25	136/35	151.7/35.9	97.3/22.2	127/32
Sodium (mEq/L)	36.8	49.6	57	11.3/8 oz	40.4	40	21.7
Potassium (mEq/L)	40	54	48.6	18.7/8 oz	40	40	32.1
Osmolality	470	690	475	720	300	375	270-380
Similar to:	Sustacal (Mead Johnson) Resource (Sandoz)	Sustacal Plus (Mead Johnson) Resource Plus (Sandoz)	NutriVent (Clintec) Respalor (Mead Johnson)	—	ProBalance (Clintec) FiberSource (Sandoz)	Glytrol (Clintec)	Vivonex (Sandoz)
Comments	Lactose free, low residue	Lactose free, low residue, high calorie	55% fat, 28% carbohydrates Good for pulmonary patients, reduced carbon dioxide production	Contains lactose Above analysis mixed with whole milk	Contains fiber, lactose and glucose free	Low carbohydrates for abnormal glucose tolerance, contains fiber, lactose free	Elemental for easy digestion
Route	Tube/oral	Tube/oral	Tube/oral	Oral	Tube	Tube/oral	Tube

quency of feedings, tube site, and other considerations, including the caregiver's preference. Most feeding bags and administration sets are large enough to accommodate 500 to 1000 ml of formula. To prevent bacterial contamination when a large container is used, the amount of formula in the bag should approximate that which can be given over 8 hours. In warm environments a feeding bag with a pouch for an ice bag is desirable to prevent curdling of the formula and bacterial growth. New formula should not be added to formula that has already been hanging for 8 hours at room temperature. The container and tubing should be rinsed well before adding formula. With very careful cleaning, a feeding bag may be used for 2 days; however, discarding the bag after 24 hours is recommended.[20,56]

Ready-to-hang enteral feedings can be used for patients who are on stable regimens. They can provide approximately 1000 to 1500 ml of formula in a container that is stable for 24 hours and are as cost-effective as using a bag and multiple cans of formula. They are available in screw-top or spikable prefilled bottles or bags, which decrease the chance for bacterial contamination.

Several enteral pumps can provide a controlled rate of administration. Most have internal batteries to allow limited mobility and have alarm systems that indicate problems or completion of feeding. Most pumps have occlusion and low-battery alarms and are simply designed to allow easy troubleshooting. An enteral pump is usually indicated if the patient is being fed by the small intestine, if the feedings are given continually around the clock, or if the desired rate is less than 200 ml/hour.

Psychologic impact of tube feeding. Recognition of the psychologic and social needs of the patient receiving tube feedings is an important component of nursing care. Patients facing long-term feedings must adapt to the loss of control over food selection and consumption. Because eating is a social, cultural, and sometimes religious activity, adaptation may be difficult. In addition, alterations of body image related to the presence of a nasogastric or percutaneously inserted feeding tube may cause distress.[44]

Table 28-2   Common Complications of Enteral Nutrition

Complication	Etiology
MECHANICAL	
Nasal irritation and erosion	Use of rigid, large-bore tubes
Esophagitis, pharyngitis	Use of rigid, large-bore tubes
Tube dislocation	Coughing or pulling on tube, tube migration
Tube occlusion	Kinked tube, inadequate irrigation, formula incompletely crushed, incompatible medications
GASTROINTESTINAL	
Abdominal distention	Rapid infusion rate, delayed gastric emptying, formula intolerance
Nausea, vomiting	Rapid infusion rate, delayed emptying, formula intolerance, malabsorption, electrolyte imbalance, contaminated formula
Diarrhea	Rapid infusion rate, formula intolerance, malabsorption, contaminated formula
Constipation	Long-term use of low-residue solutions, inadequate fluid intake
RESPIRATORY	
Aspiration pneumonia	Gastric reflux of aspiration (especially with large-bore tubes), improper tube placement, large gastric residuals, patient's head elevated less than 30 degrees
METABOLIC	
Hyperglycemia	Underlying diabetes, sepsis, stress, intolerance to infusion rate
Hypokalemia	Concurrent diuretic, insulin, or antibiotic therapy
Hyperkalemia	Metabolic acidosis, renal insufficiency, excessive potassium in formula
Hypernatremia, dehydration	Insufficient water (especially if hyperosmolar, high-protein formulas used)

Thirst, taste deprivation, and inability to satisfy the appetite are common complaints of tube-fed patients. Patients may feel self-conscious surrounded by the equipment and supplies needed for formula administration and may find mobility limited by the feeding pump and pole. Limiting tube feedings to night hours or using gravity administration may enhance adaptation.

An assessment of the patient's life-style, home environment, body image, and motivation for tube feeding is critical before implementing therapy. Exploration of the patient's perceptions of the importance of food and eating will assist in identifying areas of concern and is a good starting point for teaching. Involvement of the patient and family in the tube feedings is helpful. The rationale for all procedures should be described, and the patient and family should be encouraged to assist in the feeding.

Occasionally, patients are allowed some oral intake, usually fluids and soft, bland foods. Patients receiving all their nutrition from tube feedings may be permitted to chew gum or suck on hard candies, thus satisfying their sense of taste and their desire to chew. Some patients may satisfy a craving for a particular food by chewing and then spitting it out if they cannot swallow.

Patients requiring long-term enteral therapy may benefit from meeting with other tube-fed patients. The support and role models provided often ease the transition to tube feeding.

Monitoring the patient. The patient's weight is a simple test for assessing whether caloric and fluid needs are met. Weighing the patient every 2 or 3 days to start will alert the caregiver to a deviance from the anticipated weight gain or maintenance. If the patient loses weight during tube feeding, adjustments in the rate, formula, or calorie content may be made quickly.

Serum proteins may also be monitored, usually every 7 to 10 days to start. In the presence of malnutrition, decreased albumin synthesis occurs. With optimal enterally provided nutritional support, serum prealbumin and protein levels may increase as the patient receives adequate calories and protein; however, abnormal metabolism of nutrients in patients with advanced cancer may preclude significant gains.

Nasal tube placement should be verified by aspirating gastric contents and by listening to the area over the stomach while injecting air through the tube. Gastric contents should be checked for residual and feeding delayed if more than 100 ml is obtained (see second box, p. 737).

Complications of tube feeding. Many of the complications of tube feedings are preventable through appropriate selection of formula and tubes, proper administration, and frequent monitoring. Complications may be mechanical or metabolic and may affect the GI and respiratory systems (Table 28-2).[4,8,17,45,60]

A common complication is tube clogging as a result of inadequate flushing or improper administration of medication. As a rule, tubes should be flushed with 30 to 60 ml of water at these times: before and after intermittent feedings, every 4 hours during continuous feedings, before and after medication administration, after checking tube placement, and after checking gastric residual and returning contents.[6] Patency of clogged tubes can often be restored by irrigating the tube with carbonated beverages, such as colas and ginger ale. No syringe larger than 50 ml should be used to apply pressure to a plugged tube because larger syringes may cause the tube to rupture. See box below on medication delivery via enteral tubes.

Diarrhea is a common problem in tube-fed patients, especially when first begun. If the patient has not been eating, the gut may be intolerant of feeding and feeding should be started slowly. Isotonic formulas (near 290 mOsm) begun at half rate and slowly increased may be well tolerated. The use of fiber-containing formulas can help provide more normal intestinal function. Infection may occur from contaminated feeding or *Clostridium difficile* infection if the patient has been taking antibiotics. Stool culture can help rule out infectious causes of diarrhea.

Home enteral therapy. An estimated 65,000 patients per year receive enteral nutrition at home.[78] Patients with advanced head and neck or esophageal cancer are frequently candidates for home enteral support. In one study, home enteral nutrition was given for a median of 94 days, resulting in stable nutritional indices for the patients studied.[9]

Once it is determined that a patient needs enteral therapy and discharge is anticipated, the patient is assessed. A caregiver is selected if the patient is unable to perform self-care. The capabilities of the caregiver are assessed, the home environment is discussed, and the caregiver is trained until he or she can independently care for the tube-fed patient. A home care referral for nursing

visits to continue teaching and supervise care should be made. General care of the tube-fed patient at home includes tube care, feeding, and assessment of complications and goal achievement (see box below).[93]

Parenteral Nutrition

Parenteral nutrition therapy supplies all of the essential nutrients by means of the intravenous (IV) route. Parenteral therapy may be called *hyperalimentation* and may be partial or total. Many patients receive partial parenteral nutrition in the form of dextrose solutions as part of their usual care. Total parenteral nutrition (TPN) supplies all the daily requirements for protein and calories directly into the bloodstream. Parenteral nutrition is indicated for patients who have totally nonfunctioning GI

DELIVERY OF MEDICATIONS VIA FEEDING TUBE

Use liquid preparation when possible.

Crush medications as finely as possible and mix with warm water.

Check with pharmacist if in doubt or for sustained-release products.

Flush tube with warm water before and after administering medications.

Do not mix medications; flush between administration of each drug.

Do not mix medications with formula.

Hold feeding 2 hours before and 1 hour after medications that need to be given on an empty stomach (e.g., phenytoin).

Do not crush or open enteric-coated preparations.

Blood levels may need to be checked with certain medications (e.g., theophylline, warfarin) because drug absorption may differ with various enteral formulas.

CARE OF THE TUBE-FED PATIENT AT HOME

TUBE CARE
Nasogastric

1. Change tape every other day.
2. Clean edges of both nostrils at least once a day. Lubricate with K-Y Jelly if desired.
3. Brush teeth and tongue twice daily.
4. Use lanolin-based cream to moisturize lips.

Gastrostomy

Perform gastrostomy care daily:
1. Inspect skin.
2. Observe for tube migration.
3. Clean with soap and water, starting at tube and moving outward.
4. Place transparent or hypoallergenic tape dressing.

FEEDING ADMINISTRATION

1. Elevate patient's head at least 30 degrees during feeding and for 1 hour after feeding.
2. Check tube placement. Listen with stethoscope while injecting air into tube or aspirate gastric contents.
3. Check amount of gastric residual before each intermittent feeding or approximately every 2 to 4 hours during continuous feeding. If residual is more than 100 ml, delay feeding for 1 hour and check again.
4. Flush tube with 20 to 30 ml of room-temperature water or carbonated drink before and after each intermittent feeding or every 3 to 4 hours during continuous feeding.

ASSESSMENT OF COMPLICATIONS

1. Observe for signs of complications, including nausea, cramps, diarrhea, and aspiration.
2. Inspect hands and feet for signs of fluid retention.

ASSESSMENT OF GOAL ACHIEVEMENT

1. Weigh daily or every other day.
2. Report weight loss of 2 or more pounds to physician.

tracts, require bowel rest, or are intolerant of enteral therapy. Cancers of the GI tract and related obstructions are often indications for TPN. Because absorption of nutrients is impaired in such patients, TPN is often the only option available. The effects of cancer therapy, including radiation enteritis and intractable diarrhea, are also indications for TPN.[18,23,37]

The delivery routes for TPN are peripheral and central veins. Peripheral administration of TPN solutions is accomplished by using the veins of the arm. The external jugular vein in the neck may also be used. With the peripheral route the following factors should be considered[27,84]:

- Peripheral administration provides limited calories, generally fewer than 2500 kcal/day, as well as a limited amount of protein, less than 100 g/day.
- Solutions administered peripherally can be very irritating to the vein, especially if dextrose is more than 10%.
- Solutions may be stopped quickly; tapering and weaning are not needed.
- Peripheral administration is useful for short-term nutritional support.

Administration of TPN via the central route is done using a central venous access device placed into a major vein such as the superior vena cava. Central venous access devices used for TPN include ports; triple-lumen catheters; Broviac, Hickman, and Groshong catheters; and occasionally Swan-Ganz lines.[7,85] With the central route the following factors should be considered:

- Central administration can provide a large amount of calories and protein.
- Final dextrose concentrations can be as high as 35% and final amino acid concentrations more than 5%.
- These solutions cannot be discontinued suddenly. Abrupt cessation may induce profound hypoglycemia. Tapering down the rate and concentration is the most effective method for discontinuation.

Components. The three main components of TPN are glucose, amino acids, and fats. The glucose content of TPN, usually in the form of dextrose 50%, provides both immediate and long-term energy. Amino acids or proteins are provided with or without electrolytes and are usually ordered in concentrations of 5.5% or 8.5%. The lower concentration is indicated for patients with hepatic or renal dysfunction or failure. Administration of fats with TPN is required because the TPN solution stimulates the production of insulin, which in turn prevents fat from being metabolized. A fatty acid deficiency may result. Fat is provided through lipid emulsions formulated from safflower and soy bean oils emulsified with egg phospholipid. Therefore lipids are not administered to patients with a history of allergy to eggs.[86] Lipid emulsions usually come in a concentration of 10% or 20% and may be "piggybacked" or added to the TPN solution. Exact formulations are specific to the patient; they

depend on individual requirements, tolerances, body chemistry, and disease processes (Table 28-3).

A TPN formula that combines the dextrose, amino acids, and fat emulsion in one container is often called a *three-in-one* or *total nutrient admixture*. Eliminating the need for piggybacking lipids allows for a closed system that reduces the risk of infection, minimizes manipulations, and cuts waste. Often, three-in-one solutions are ordered for patients receiving TPN at home because they are convenient and easy to administer. If lipids are piggybacked, they generally are given two or three times per week.[10,29]

Many patients receiving TPN have a multilumen central venous catheter inserted. The additional lumens provide access for drug administration and blood sampling. Patients with single-lumen catheters who require medications must either have the line flushed before and after administration of medication or have the medication added to the TPN bag.[7,89] Several drugs have been tested to be compatible with TPN formulas for at least 12 hours[9,32] (see box below).

Administration. TPN solutions may be given continuously or by cycling the infusion over 12 to 20 hours per day. Cycling is most often used for patients receiving TPN at home during the night because it allows them to be mobile during the day. The disadvantage of cycling TPN is that patients must be able to tolerate a high-volume load. Cyclic TPN may be increased slowly at the start and then tapered at the end of the cycle. Programmable pumps are widely used to prevent or minimize hyperglycemia and hypoglycemia as blood sugars rise and fall. Compact, portable TPN pumps are also available

---

DRUGS TESTED TO BE COMPATIBLE WITH TOTAL PARENTERAL NUTRITION (TPN) FORMULAS FOR AT LEAST 12 HOURS

Aminophylline
Antibiotics
  Cephalothin
  Clindamycin
  Erythromycin
  Gentamicin
  Methicillin
  Oxacillin
  Penicillin G
  Tetracycline
  Tobramycin
Antineoplastics
  Cyclophosphamide
  Cytarabine
  Fluorouracil
  Methotrexate

Corticosteroids
H₂-receptor antagonists
  Cimetidine
  Ranitidine
Heparin
Insulin
Iron dextran
Metoclopramide
Narcotic analgesics
  Hydromorphone
  Meperidine
  Morphine

Table 28-3 Adult and Pediatric Parenteral Solution Formulas

Formula	Amount	Formula	Amount
ADULT		**PEDIATRIC**	
Base solution		**Base solution**	
40%-50% dextrose in water	500 ml	40% dextrose in water	500 ml
8.5%-10% crystalline amino acids	500 ml	8.5% crystalline amino acids	500 ml
Additives to each unit		**Additives to each unit**	
Sodium chloride, acetate, or lactate	40-50 ml	Sodium chloride	3-4 mEq/kg wt/daily
Potassium chloride	20-30 mEq	Potassium acid phosphate	2-3 mEq/kg wt/daily
Potassium acid phosphate (10-20 mM phosphorus)	15-30 mEq	Magnesium sulfate	0.25-0.5 mEq/kg wt/daily
Magnesium sulfate	15-18 mEq	Calcium gluconate	0.5-1 mEq/kg wt/daily
Multivitamin infusion	10 ml	Multivitamin infusion	
A	3300 IU	A	2300 IU
D	200 IU	D	400 IU
E	10 IU	E	7 IU
Ascorbic acid	100 mg	K	200 μg
Folic acid	400 μg	Ascorbic acid	80 mg
Niacin	40 mg	Folic acid	140 μg
Riboflavin	3.6 mg	Niacinamide	17 mg
Thiamine	3 mg	Riboflavin	1.4 mg
B_6 (pyridoxine)	4 mg	Thiamine	1.2 mg
B_{12} (cyanocobalamin)	5 μg	B_6 (pyridoxine)	1 mg
Pantothenic acid	15 mg	B_{12} (cyanocobalamin)	1 μg
Biotin	60 μg	Dexpanthenol	7 mg
Additive to any one unit twice weekly		Biotin	20 μg
Vitamin K	10 mg	Intravenous fat emulsion 10%, 3-7 times weekly	50-75 ml/kg
Intravenous fat emulsion 10% or 20%		**INFUSION RATE**	115 ml/kg/day
500 ml 2-7 times weekly	50-100 g		115 kcal/kg/day
Carbohydrate calories	850 kcal		3 g protein/kg/day
Protein calories	150 kcal		
Fat calories	1000-2000 kcal		
Nitrogen	6.5-8 g		
Amino acids	40-50 g		

with programmable functions. The portable pump, worn in a backpack-type carrying bag, is best suited for the ambulatory patient.

Patients requiring long-term parenteral nutrition face different challenges than those needing TPN for only a short time. Long-term therapy is most often accomplished in the home; the patient or designated caregiver performs many of the procedures.[72] Patients must be motivated to receive TPN at home and must be able to provide competent self-care. Assessment of capabilities before implementing home TPN is critical, since many patients are extremely anxious about performing highly technical procedures. Anxiety usually resolves with education and time.

Many patients note an altered self-image with long-term TPN. Their self-perceptions are undermined by being underweight or even cachexic, and this is com-

pounded by the presence of a central venous access device connected to the TPN formula and equipment. Sleep disturbances may be induced by depressive illness, anxiety, nocturnal urination, and occasionally pump alarms.

When TPN is given to those requiring complete bowel rest, the absence of food intake may be traumatic. Eating is a major social and cultural event, and prohibiting food for several weeks disrupts the patient's life.

Patients may voice concerns about the cost of TPN therapy. Although usually covered by insurance and Medicare, home TPN may cost $400 or more per day. In the hospital, TPN is a third more costly, and long-term inpatient TPN is financially prohibitive. Often the patient is facing loss of income because of cancer and its treatment and may incur large medical bills. Patients with limited financial resources may find that anxiety related to the cost of care compounds the adjustment process.

NURSING MANAGEMENT

The additional nursing interventions listed below and stated as directed to the patient can be made depending on the specific alteration in intake or the patient's digestive abilities.

NURSING DIAGNOSIS

• *Nutrition, altered: less than body requirements, related to taste/olfactory changes, dysphagia, dyspepsia, anorexia, gastrointestinal mucositis, nausea and vomiting*

OUTCOME GOALS

Patient will be able to:
• Maintain or improve nutritional intake, as evidenced by maintaining or gaining weight, depending on stage of disease or response to treatment.
• Safely receive enteral or parenteral support when appropriate.

INTERVENTIONS: Taste/Olfactory Changes

• Use tart food to stimulate taste buds.
• Use extra seasoning.
• Try sauces and flavor additives.
• Substitute fish and chicken for red meat.

INTERVENTIONS: Dysphagia

• Eat soft or liquid foods.
• Use sauces and gravies.
• Eat small meals frequently.
• If eating is painful, eat bland foods.

INTERVENTIONS: Dyspepsia

• Avoid fatty and spicy foods.
• Avoid gas-producing foods.
• Use antacids.
• Avoid lying down after meals.

INTERVENTIONS: Anorexia

• Vary surroundings.
• Eat with family and friends.
• Try new foods and recipes.
• Use smaller plates.
• Eat high-calorie snacks.
• Drink high-protein shakes.
• Try hard candy.
• Use distraction: radio, TV, etc.

INTERVENTIONS: Gastrointestinal Mucositis

• Avoid acidic fruits and juices.
• Eat cool foods.
• Use a topical analgesic before eating.

INTERVENTIONS: Nausea and Vomiting

• Drink clear liquids and advance diet as tolerated.
• Drink flat beverages.
• Avoid sweet, rich, and fatty foods.
• Try dry foods (e.g., toast, crackers).
• Try easily digested foods (e.g., rice).
• Avoid food odors.
• Eat cool foods.
• Eat small, frequent meals.
• Use antiemetics 30 minutes before meals.

NURSING DIAGNOSIS

• *Constipation*

OUTCOME GOALS: Constipation

Patient will be able to:
• Identify factors that influence elimination.
• Demonstrate adequate nutritional/fluid intake.
• Maintain appropriate level of physical mobility.

INTERVENTIONS

• Drink adequate fluids.
• Eat high-fiber foods.
• Exercise regularly.
• Avoid cheese and concentrated foods.

NURSING DIAGNOSIS

• *Diarrhea*

OUTCOME GOALS: Diarrhea

Patient will be able to:
• Verbalize signs and symptoms of diarrhea.
• Identify potential causes of diarrhea.
• Demonstrate adequate nutritional/fluid intake.
• Eliminate foods/medications that cause/increase diarrhea.

INTERVENTIONS

• Drink adequate amounts of fluid.
• Drink fluids providing electrolytes.
• Avoid milk products.
• Avoid fatty, gas-producing foods.
• Avoid high-fiber foods.
• Eat high-potassium foods.

INTERVENTIONS: Dumping Syndrome

• Avoid fatty foods.
• Avoid concentrated foods.
• Eat small, frequent meals.
• Drink liquids 30 minutes before and after meals.

An assessment of the patient's life-style, home environment, family and support systems, body image, and perceptions about TPN should be conducted when it is started. During hospitalization, frequent assessments are needed to assist in identifying patients who are candidates for TPN at home.[46]

Monitoring the patient and complications of therapy. Patients beginning TPN must be monitored frequently to assess side effects and complications of the treatment. Daily monitoring of vital signs, weight, and laboratory values may indicate metabolic changes requiring the adjustment of TPN formula or its rate of administration. The metabolic and technical problems sometimes associated with TPN are numerous. Some are related to the insertion of the central venous access device. Other problems include electrolyte imbalance, infection, and volume overload (Table 28-4). *Refeeding syndrome,* characterized by a rapid drop in levels of potassium, magnesium, and phosphorus, may be precipitated by the introduction of TPN in the severely malnourished patient. Excess amino acid intake can cause elevations in blood urea nitrogen (BUN) and creatinine levels. *Cracking* of the solution can occur in TPN/lipid formulas with a high content of calcium or phosphorus or those containing salt-poor albumin. An oily layer or oily globules within the solution indicate cracking has occurred, and the infusion should not be used.[86] With frequent monitoring by an experienced staff or well-educated patient performing self-care, the risk of complications is greatly reduced.

Home parenteral nutrition. Since the late 1960s, TPN has been administered successfully in patients' homes. It is estimated that 3000 patients currently receive home TPN, and an increased rate is predicted as technologic advances continue.[27] Even in rural areas, home parenteral nutrition has become commonplace.[58] Home TPN has been particularly beneficial for pediatric oncology patients.[4]

Screening patients for home TPN includes assessment of the home environment, availability of a caregiver, learning abilities or disabilities, physical limitations, and motivation to learn procedures. Ideally, education of the caregiver is begun before discharge. Teaching sessions over several days are best for teaching the complex procedures of TPN home administration (see box, p. 742). Provision of a take-home booklet is recommended, and return demonstrations performed by the caregiver are often beneficial. One key aspect of at-home care is assessment of the central venous access device and dressing change procedure.[70]

Infectious complications of long-term central venous catheters include infections of the tunnel and exit site, catheter-related bacteremia, and septic thrombophlebitis.[16] Standardization of dressing change procedures currently is lacking in the home setting. One study suggests that transparent dressings on central venous catheters are associated with an increased risk of catheter tip infection.[38] Astute assessment and meticulous dressing change technique by the caregiver minimize this complication.[11,77]

Table 28-4 Common Complications of Parenteral Nutrition

Complication	Etiology
NONMETABOLIC	
Allergy or sensitivity	Sensitivity to either amino acid solution or lipid emulsion
Infection	Catheter-related sepsis
Volume overload	Improper pump rate
Catheter placement	Puncture of or injury to nearby organs or vessels
Pneumothorax	
Arterial puncture	
Hematoma	
Thoracic duct puncture	
Brachial plexus injury	
Pulmonary embolism	
METABOLIC	
Hyperglycemia/hyperosmolarity	Inability to metabolize high glucose concentration of formula
Hypoglycemia	When TPN is abruptly discontinued, high insulin levels cause rebound drop in blood sugar
Vitamin or mineral deficiencies	Administration of formulas lacking sufficient vitamins or micronutrients
Fatty acid deficiencies or overload	Insufficient or excessive administration of lipids
Hyponatremia	Formulas without sufficient sodium content
Hypokalemia, hyperkalemia	Insufficient or excessive potassium content
Hypocalcemia, hypercalcemia	Insufficient or excessive calcium content
Hypomagnesemia	Insufficient magnesium or increased metabolism of magnesium

---

CARE OF THE PATIENT RECEIVING PARENTERAL NUTRITION AT HOME

CATHETER CARE

1. Change dressing and assess venous access device per frequency ordered by physician or institution or agency policy.
2. Flush with saline or heparin if cyclic schedule.

PREPARATION OF MEDICATION

1. Inject additives (e.g., vitamins) into premixed bags.
2. Assemble bag and connect tubing.

OPERATION OF EQUIPMENT

1. Connect and disconnect pump.
2. Program pump if cyclic schedule or enter rate, volume, and other data.
3. Perform equipment troubleshooting.

ASSESSMENT OF COMPLICATIONS

1. Assess for electrolyte imbalance and presence of hyperglycemia.
2. Observe feet and fingers for edema.
3. Monitor temperature and urine for sugar and acetone.

ASSESSMENT OF GOAL ACHIEVEMENT

Weigh daily or every other day.

Follow-up visits in the home are essential. Although many patients may appear quite competent in the hospital, a home visit ensures that procedures are followed appropriately. A home assessment also provides the opportunity to determine whether TPN formulas and supplies are stored correctly and whether infection control measures are observed (see Chapter 27).

Patients vary in the number of teaching sessions and follow-up visits required to assess compliance. Many need a visiting nurse to obtain blood samples and monitor on a schedule. The frequency of clinic visits for evaluation by the physician varies according to the patient's needs, ranging from once a week to every 6 months.

ETHICAL CONSIDERATIONS

Recently, increased attention has been given to evaluating the use of supportive nutritional therapies. The widespread use of home parenteral therapy has raised several ethical issues, including potential overutilization and inequitable access because it is primarily the well-insured patient who receives TPN.[35,53] The use of inpatient TPN has also come under scrutiny. Preoperative TPN in well-nourished patients appears to be unwarranted at this time; however, efficacy of preoperative TPN in malnourished

surgical patients has been established.[14] Further research is needed to determine how nutritional support influences nutritional status, abnormal host metabolism, GI symptoms, and/or tumor growth.[15]

Nutritional support of the terminally ill patient with cancer remains controversial. Frequently, family members insist on feeding their loved one. Nurses should advocate for the patient by teaching that loss of appetite often occurs.[2,81] Helping the patient and family understand that it is an unfortunate but inevitable part of many cancer experiences can relieve stress. Nursing interventions should be directed at structural or functional deficits, such as stomatitis, nausea, and vomiting, and managing concurrent symptoms, such as pain, fatigue, and dyspnea.[21] The use of IV hydration may be helpful in loosening pulmonary secretions, decreasing gastric secretions, and correcting fluid and electrolyte imbalances in select patients who are not imminently terminal. However, the potential benefits of IV hydration must be carefully weighed against the potential risk of infection, the effect of the therapy on the patient's quality of life, and the cost of IV therapy. In terminal patients, dehydration decreases pulmonary secretions and level of consciousness, acting as a natural anesthetic. Maintaining moisture of oral tissues with ice chips and lubricants reduces the most distressing side effect of dehydration. Termination of nutritional support should occur when the patient, family, physician, and nurse judge that the patient no longer benefits from the nutritional support.[1,40,50] The decision must be made in accordance with accepted community standards of care and in compliance with applicable law.[1]

More than half of all patients with malignant disease eventually attempt unorthodox treatment. Nutritional therapies are often used, particularly by patients with advanced disease.[12] Teaching regarding the need for balanced nutrition (i.e., refer to the Food Guide Pyramid) in any diet can help patients and families evaluate the adequacy of nutritional therapies. Ongoing communication with patients and their families about nutritional concerns is essential.

CONCLUSION

Cancer and its treatment affect nutritional status to varying degrees. Patients with local and systemic effects require ongoing assessment and prompt intervention. Nutritional support ranges in complexity depending on needs, and those needs change over time. Oral supplementation, the simplest type of support, is most effective when the patient is highly motivated, has manageable or temporary side effects, and can ingest and digest nutrients. Enteral and parenteral nutrition may be required for individuals with more severe symptoms and for those with demonstrated physical impairments of the gastrointestinal tract. Despite their complexity, enteral nutrition and parenteral nutrition are often administered in the home, with family members as caregivers. Advances in home therapies and nutritional support have enabled individuals with cancer and nutritional deficiencies to remain at home and have promoted an improved quality of life.

■ CHAPTER QUESTIONS

1. Anorexia in the patient with cancer is exacerbated by:
   a. Anxiety about cancer
   b. Depression
   c. Learned food aversions
   d. All the above
2. Progressive muscle wasting results when protein is broken down to provide amino acids for use as a noncarbohydrate source of glucose for gluconeogenesis. This progressive muscle wasting is called:
   a. Synthesis
   b. Metabolism
   c. Cachexia
   d. Anorexia
3. Enteral nutrition should be considered for patients who demonstrate which of the following conditions?
   a. Mild anorexia
   b. Mechanical impairment that interferes with oral intake
   c. Loss of GI tract motility
   d. Six-week life expectancy from advanced cancer
4. A simple test to assess whether calorie and fluid intake needs are being met is:
   a. Three-day calorie count
   b. Daily laboratory values to assess electrolytes
   c. Anthropometric measurements
   d. Daily weights
5. Parenteral nutrition is indicated for patients who:
   a. Have totally nonfunctioning GI tracts
   b. Require bowel rest
   c. Are intolerant of enteral therapy
   d. All the above
6. All these can be causes of diarrhea in tube-fed patients *except:*
   a. Intolerance to bolus feeding
   b. Bacterial contamination
   c. *Clostridium difficile* infection
   d. Hanging formula for 6 hours in a clean bag
7. Dehydration in a terminally ill patient may result in:
   a. Loss of appetite
   b. Decreased level of consciousness
   c. Increased pulmonary secretions
   d. Increased urination

BIBLIOGRAPHY

1. American Society for Parenteral and Enteral Nutrition: Standards for home nutrition support, *Nutr Clin Pract* 7(2):65, 1992.
2. Barnie DC: Percutaneous endoscopic gastrostomy tubes: the nurse's role in a moral, ethical, and legal dilemma, *Gastroenterol Nurse* 12:250, 1990.
3. Bendorf K, Meehan J: Home parenteral nutrition for the child with cancer, *Issues Compr Pediatr Nurs* 12:171, 1989.
4. Benya R, Mobarhan S: Enteral alimentation: administration and complications, *J Am Coll Nutr* 10:209, 1991.
5. Beutler B: Cachexia: a basic biochemical mechanism, *Nutrition* 5:129, 1989.
6. Bockus, S: When your patient needs tube feeding, *Nursing '93* 23(7):34, 1993.
7. Brendel V: Catheters utilized in delivering total parenteral nutrition, *NITA* 7:488, 1984.
8. Campbell SM: Adult enteral nutrition. In Young LY, Koda-Kimble MA, editors: *Applied therapeutics: the clinical use of drugs,* Vancouver, Wash, 1988, Applied Therapeutics.
9. Campos AC, Butters M, Meguid MM: Home enteral nutrition via gastrostomy in advanced head and neck cancer patients, *Head Neck* 12(2):137, 1990.
10. Campos AC, Paluzzi M, Meguid MM: Clinical use of total nutrient admixtures, *Nutrition* 6:347, 1990.
11. Capka MB and others: Nursing observations of central venous catheters: the effect on patient outcome, *J Intrav Nurs* 14:243, 1991.
12. Cassileth BR, Berlyne D: Counseling the cancer patient who wants to try unorthodox or questionable therapies, *Oncology* 3(4):29, 1989.
13. Chandra RK: Protein-energy malnutrition and immunological responses, *J Nutr* 122(3 suppl):597, 1992.
14. Chen MK, Souba WW, Copeland EM: Nutritional support of the surgical oncology patient, *Hematol Oncol Clin North Am* 5:125, 1991.
15. Chlebowski RT: Nutritional support of the medical oncology patient, *Hematol Oncol Clin North Am* 5:147, 1991.
16. Clarke DE, Raffin TA: Infectious complications of indwelling long-term central venous catheters, *Chest* 97:966, 1990.
17. Cogen R, Weinryb J: Aspiration pneumonia in nursing home patients fed via gastrostomy tubes, *Am J Gastroenterol* 84:1509, 1989.
18. Copeland EM: Total parenteral nutrition in the cancer patient: the present as viewed from the past, *Nutrition* 6(4 suppl):2, 1990.
19. Crocker KS: Planning for home parenteral and enteral nutrition, *Contin Care* 8:18, 1989.
20. Curtas S and others: Bacteriological safety of closed enteral nutrition delivery systems, *Nutrition* 7:340, 1991.
21. D'Agostino NS: Managing nutritional problems in advanced cancer, *Am J Nurs* 89(1):50, 1989.
22. Daly JM, Torosian MH: Nutritional support. In DeVita VT Jr, Hellman S, Rosenberg SA, editors: *Cancer: principles and practice of oncology,* ed 4, Philadelphia, 1993, Lippincott.
23. Daly JM and others: Nutritional support of patients with cancer of the gastrointestinal tract, *Surg Clin North Am* 71:523, 1991.
24. Davies L, Knutson KC: Warning signals for malnutrition in the elderly, *J Am Diet Assoc* 91:1413, 1991.
25. Dow KH, Hilderly LJ: *Nursing care in radiation oncology,* Philadelphia, 1992, Saunders.
26. Dreizen S and others: Nutritional deficiencies in patients receiving cancer chemotherapy, *Postgrad Med* 87:163, 1990.
27. Drescher M: Advances in peripheral vein nutrition, *NITA* 6:533, 1985.
28. Dudrick SJ and others: 100 patient years of ambulatory home total parenteral nutrition, *Ann Surg* 199:770, 1984.

29. Ebbert-Sauer ML: Adult parenteral nutrition. In Young LY, Koda-Kimble MA, editors: *Applied therapeutics: the clinical use of drugs,* Vancouver, Wash, 1988, Applied Therapeutics.

30. Eisenberg PG: Pulmonary complications from enteral nutrition, *Crit Care Nurse Clin North Am* 3:641, 1991.

31. Fay DE and others: Long-term enteral feeding: a retrospective comparison of delivery via percutaneous endoscopic gastrostomy and nasoenteric tubes, *Am J Gastroenterol* 86:1604, 1991.

32. Filibeck D: A review of the stability and compatibility problems associated with total parenteral nutrition solutions, *Nutr Supp Serv* 5:67, 1985.

33. Frey AM: Taking the confusion out of multiple infusion: IV medications and TPN, *NITA* 6:460, 1986.

34. Fry ST: Ethical aspects of decision-making in the feeding of cancer patients, *Semin Oncol Nurs* 2:59, 1986.

35. Fry ST: Ethical issues in total parenteral nutrition, *Nutrition* 6:329, 1990.

36. Feuz A, Rapin CH: An observational study of the role of pain control and food adaptation of elderly patients with terminal cancer, *J Am Diet Assoc* 94, 767, 1994.

37. Grant JP: Proper use and recognized role of TPN in the cancer patient, *Nutrition* 6(4 suppl):6, 1990.

38. Hoffman KK and others: Transparent polyurethane film as an intravenous catheter dressing: a meta-analysis of the infection risks, *JAMA* 267:2072, 1992.

39. Horwath CC: Nutrition goals for older adults: a review, *Gerontologist* 31:811, 1991.

40. Jansson L, Norberg A: Ethical reasoning concerning the feeding of terminally ill cancer patients: interviews with registered nurses experienced in the care of cancer patients, *Cancer Nurs* 12:352, 1989.

41. Jassak PF: Biotherapy. In Groenwald S, editor: *Cancer nursing: principles and practice,* ed 3, Boston, 1993, Jones and Bartlett.

42. Jeejeebhoy KN, Detsky AS, Baker JP: Assessment of nutritional status, *J Parenter Enteral Nutr* 14(5 suppl):193, 1990.

43. Johnson J and others: Reducing the negative impact of radiation therapy on functional status, *Cancer* 61:46, 1988.

44. Kittelberger-Bockus SB, Cataldo CB, Steinbaugh ML: Tube feedings: clinical application, Columbus, Ohio, 1986, Ross Laboratories.

45. Kohn CL, Keithley JK: Enteral nutrition: potential complications and patient monitoring, *Nurs Clin North Am* 24:339, 1989.

46. Koithan M: Home total parenteral nutrition complications, *NITA* 8:231, 1985.

47. Langstein HN, Norton JA: Mechanisms of cancer cachexia, *Hematol Oncol Clin North Am* 5:125, 1991.

48. Lehmann S: Immune function and nutrition: the clinical role of the intravenous nurse, *J Intrav Nurs* 14:406, 1991.

49. Lesko LM: Psychosocial issues in the diagnosis and management of cancer cachexia and anorexia, *Nutrition* 5:114, 1989.

50. Lin EM: Nutrition support: making the difficult decisions, *Cancer Nurs* 14:261, 1991.

51. Lindsey AM: Cancer cachexia: effects of the disease and its treatment, *Semin Oncol Nurs* 2:19, 1986.

52. Lipman TO: Clinical trials of nutritional support in cancer, *Hematol Oncol Clin North Am* 5:125, 1991.

53. Mahmood T, Rubin AD: Home-based intravenous therapy for oncology patients, *NJ Med* 89(1):43, 1992.

54. Mattes RD: Prevention of food aversions in cancer patients during treatment, *Nutr Cancer* 21(1):13, 1994.

55. Meguid MM, Eldar S, Wahba A: The delivery of nutritional support: a potpourri of new devices and methods, *Cancer* 55:279, 1985.

56. Metheny NM: Twenty ways to prevent tube-feeding complications, *Nursing '85* (15):47, 1985.

57. Monturo CA: Enteral access device and selection, *Nutr Clin Pract* 5(5):207, 1990.

58. Morley JE: Anorexia in older patients: its meaning and management, *Geriatrics* 45(12):59, 1990.

59. Muggia-Sullam M and others: Postoperative enteral versus parenteral nutrition support in gastrointestinal surgery, *Am J Surg* 49:106, 1985.

60. Mullan H, Roubenoff RA, Roubenoff R: Risk of pulmonary aspiration among patients receiving enteral nutrition support, *J Parenter Enteral Nutr* 16:160, 1992.

61. Murphy JI: Tube feeding problems and solutions, *Adv Clin Care* 5(2):7, 1990.

62. Murphy LM, Lipman TO: Central venous catheter care in parenteral nutrition: a review, *J Parenter Enteral Nutr* 11:190, 1987.

63. Murray ND, Vanderhoof JA: Home TPN in sparsely populated areas, *Nutr Clin Pract* 4(2):62, 1989.

64. Nahikian-Nelms ML: General feeding problems. In Bloch AS, editor: *Nutrition management of the cancer patient,* Rockville, Md, 1990, Aspen.

65. Nelson K and others: A phase II study of delta-9-tetrahydrocannabinol for appetite stimulation in cancer associated anorexia, *J Palliative Care* 10(1):14, 1994.

66. Ng EH, Lowey SF: Nutritional support and cancer cachexia, *Hematol Oncol Clin North Am* 5:125, 1991.

67. Ottery FD: Cancer cachexia: prevention, early diagnosis and management, *Cancer Pract* 2(2):123, 1994.

68. Padilla GV: Gastrointestinal side effects and quality of life in patients receiving radiation therapy, *Nutrition* 6:367, 1990.

69. Pisters KM, Kris MG: Management of nausea and vomiting caused by anticancer drugs: state of the art, *Oncology* 6(2 suppl):99, 1992.

70. Ponsksy JL and others: Percutaneous approaches to enteral alimentation, *Am J Surg* 149:102, 1985.

71. Rhodus NL, Brown J: The association of xerostomia and inadequate intake in older adults, *J Am Diet Assoc* 90:1688, 1990.

72. Ricour C: Home TPN, *Nutrition* 5:345, 1989.

73. Riola F and others: A double-blind multicenter randomized crossover study comparing the antiemetic efficacy and tolerability of ondansetron vs ondansetron plus dexamethasone in cisplatin treated patients, *J Clin Oncol* 9:675, 1991.

74. Robuck JT, Fleetwood JB: Nutritional support of the patient with cancer, *Focus Crit Care* 19(2):129, 1992.

75. Roe DA: Geriatric nutrition, *Clin Geriatr Med* 6:319, 1990.

76. Ropka ME: Nutrition. In Johnson BL, Gross J, editors: *Handbook of oncology nursing,* New York, 1985, Wiley & Sons.

77. Segura M, Sitges-Serra A: Clinical predictors of infection of central venous catheters used for parenteral nutrition, *Infect Control Hosp Epidemiol* 12:407, 1991.

78. Shike M: Percutaneous endoscopic stomas for enteral feeding and drainage, *Oncology* 9(1):39, 1995.

79. Skipper A, Szeluga DJ, Groenwald S: Nutritional disorders. In Groenwald S, editor: *Cancer nursing: principles and practice,* Boston, ed 3, 1993, Jones and Bartlett.

80. Spaulding M: Recent studies of anorexia and appetite stimulation in the cancer patient, *Oncology,* special suppl, August 1989, p 17.

81. Stephany TM: Nutrition for the terminally ill, *Home Healthcare Nurse* 9(3):48, 1991.

82. Strohl RA: The nursing role in radiation oncology: symptom management of acute and chronic reactions, *Oncol Nurs Forum* 15:429, 1988.

83. Tchekmedyian NS, Hickman M, Heber D: Treatment of anorexia and weight loss with megestrol acetate in patients with cancer or acquired immunodeficiency syndrome, *Semin Oncol* 18(1 suppl 2):35, 1991.

84. Timmer JG: Use of peripheral veins for TPN, *Nutrition* 5:346, 1989.

85. Viall CD: Daily access of implanted venous ports: implications for patient education, *J Intrav Nurs* 13:294, 1990.

86. Viall CD: Taking the mystery out of TPN. Part I, *Nursing '95* 25:34, 1995.

87. Viall CD: Taking the mystery out of TPN. Part II, *Nursing '95* 25:57, 1995.

88. Vokes TJ, Robertson GL: Disorders of antidiuretic hormone, *Endocrinol Metab Clin North Am* 17:281, 1988.

89. Watson D: Piggyback compatibility of antibiotics with pediatric parenteral nutrition solutions, *J Parenter Enteral Nutr* 9:220, 1985.

90. Williams EF, Meguid MM: Nutritional concepts and considerations in head and neck surgery, *Head Neck* 11:393, 1989.

91. Wilmore DW: Catabolic illness: strategies for enhancing recovery, *N Engl J Med* 325:695, 1991.

92. Wright B, Robinson L: Enteral feeding tubes as drug delivery systems, *Nutr Supp Serv* 6:33, 1986.

93. Young CK, White S: Preparing patients for tube feeding at home, *Am J Nurs* 92(4):46, 1992.

CHAPTER 29
Pain Management

CAROL J. SWENSON

Pain has an element of blank;
It cannot recollect
When it began, or if there were
A day when it was not.

"Pain Has an Element of Blank"
Emily Dickinson

Nurses play a major role in the successful management of the person who is experiencing cancer pain by preventing the situation of pain that Emily Dickinson describes—to not be able to remember when the pain was not there. One of the Oncology Nursing Society's position statements on cancer pain is that *"nurses are responsible and accountable for implementation and coordination of the plan for management of cancer pain."* [109] In all health care settings this is important, because the nurse is the professional person who most often conducts the assessment on an on-going basis and therefore can determine whether the pain has increased, whether side effects are being managed effectively, and, most important, whether the patient and family are satisfied with the pain relief provided. Nurses must accept the responsibility and accountability for the plan of care in the management of cancer pain.

With the pharmacologic agents and technology currently available, it is unfortunate when untreated cancer pain causes patients to suffer unnecessarily. It is estimated that 90% to 95% of pain can be relieved in the highly-controlled settings of hospices or palliative care units, yet the question remains whether medications and technology are being adequately used to control cancer pain. Pain affects a person's sleeping pattern, family, work, and social relationships. Ultimately, it affects a patient's quality of life and possibly the will to live.

DEFINITIONS

Pain—"Whatever the experiencing person says it is, existing whenever the experiencing person says it does" [73] is the most global and patient-centered pain description.

The American Pain Society[8] and the ONS position paper on pain[108] both use Merskey's definition of pain: "an unpleasant sensory and emotional experience associated with actual or potential tissue damage, or described in terms of such damage." [80] From these two descriptions of pain, it becomes apparent that pain is multidimensional and subjective. Because pain is a subjective experience, the patient is the only authority on its existence—not the health care professional.

Other definitions that assist in understanding the pain experience are suffering, tolerance, addiction, and dependence.

• *Suffering*—a physical or mental experience, that the person dislikes (e.g., adversity, agony, anguish, torment, trouble). Suffering is more global than pain, because pain implies only the physical sphere, whereas suffering may be spiritual, emotional, or social as well as physical. Suffering is distinct from pain and can occur with or without the presence of pain.

• *Drug tolerance*—the involuntary need for increasing doses of analgesic to achieve the same level of pain relief. The actual incidence of tolerance is not known, and many people will never develop it. When an increase of medication is required, it is most often an event of disease progression, but tolerance must be considered. According to Cherny,[19] "concerns about tolerance should not impede the use of opioids early in the course of disease." The use of non-opioids together with opioids will help to delay the possible onset of tolerance. Weissman and colleagues[124] state that "tolerance will develop more rapidly following IV or intraspinal administration than after oral or rectal administration." When drug tolerance develops, first the duration of relief decreases and then the level of pain relief decreases. If tolerance is suspected, another opioid can be used. When another opioid is used, one third to one half of the equianalgesic dose should be given because cross-tolerance between narcotics is incomplete and the person may otherwise be overmedicated.[8]

- *Addiction*—the use of narcotics for the psychologic euphoric effect and not for the analgesic effect; there is overwhelming involvement with obtaining and using drugs for other than approved medical reasons. Addiction as a result of medically prescribed narcotics is rare (less than 1:1000). Porter and Jick[96] report that of 11,882 hospitalized patients who had received at least one opioid injection during hospitalization, there were only four cases of documented addiction in patients with no previous history of addiction. Most often health care professionals overestimate the incidence of addiction after prescribed opioids for medical purposes. The lay public are often also frightened of potential addiction and need education about the appropriate use of opioids and assurance that addiction is a nonissue in cancer pain management.
- *Physical dependence*—the body's adaptation to the use of opioids without which abstinence syndrome (or withdrawal symptoms) will occur based on physiologic changes. The person with cancer who uses opioids for longer than 3 to 4 weeks will be physically dependent but is not addicted.[8,116] The physically dependent person will not have the craving for the euphoric effect and will not be engaging in drug-seeking behaviors. (See p. 760 for directions on "weaning" the physically dependent person from opioids.)

According to McCaffery's definition, nurses must believe every patient who says that he or she has pain in order not to inadvertently miss treatment of pain. Lack of observable pain does not mean lack of pain.

PHYSIOLOGY OF PAIN TRANSMISSION

The complex neurophysiologic activity that results in pain comprises four steps[115]:

1. *Transduction* is the process by which noxious (i.e., painful) stimuli lead to electrical activity in the endings of the primary afferent fibers. The stimulus may be mechanical, thermal, or chemical,[78] causing the release of biochemical substrates that lead to the generation of an action potential (influx of sodium, efflux of potassium, change in the charge along cellular membrane) and electrical changes in the neuron. The primary afferent pain fibers are[45,87]:

    A—large myelinated fibers that have
    rapid conduction
    C—small unmyelinated fibers that have
    slower conduction

2. *Transmission* is the relay by which impulses are sent from the primary afferent nerves to the dorsal horn of the spinal cord. The primary afferent nerve terminates, and the spinothalamic tract neuron carries the message across to the contralateral side of the spinal cord, where it joins a group of fibers that carry pain messages.

3. *Perception* is the translation of neural response into sensation in the cerebral cortex; the person recognizes the feeling as pain.

4. *Modulation* is the control of pain transmission and may include both inhibition and enhancement of nociceptive stimuli.[128] Modulation involves opiate receptors in the cortex, midbrain, spinal cord, gastrointestinal tract, bladder, and uterus. They bind endogenous and exogenous opiates to block pain transmission.

In the past, theories of pain were developed because of the lack of the capability to determine precisely what occurs physiologically during the pain experience. Some of the past theories were as follows:

- *Specificity*—the intensity of nociceptive stimulus and perception of pain are directly correlated and travel along specific pathways from the pain receptors to the spinal cord.
- *Gate control theory*—nociceptive impulses are transmitted via the spinothalamic tract but can be modulated in the spinal cord, brain stem, or cerebral cortex. Two types of afferent fibers have been identified: thinly myelinated A-delta fibers and unmyelinated C fibers. The substantia gelatinosa in the dorsal horn of the spinal cord is the proposed site of the "gating" mechanism. McGuire and Sheidler[77] state that "activity in the large fibers can 'open' the gate, while activity in the small fibers can 'close' it." Melzack and Wall, as well as others, have modified their theory over the past 30 years.
- *Endorphins and enkephalins*—in the mid-1970s these "morphine within" opioid-like substances in the brain and spinal cord were discovered.

Today studies are involved with the exact physiology of pain and people are researching the neurodynamics of pain. Paice[86] writes of "unraveling the mystery of pain" and describes the primary afferent fibers, dorsal horn of the spinal cord, spinothalamic tract, cortex, and modulatory systems and their interactions in the transmission and interpretation of pain.

Science may have progressed beyond the theory stage, but much is yet to be learned of this complex phenomenon called *pain*.

TYPES OF PAIN

Some of the ways that pain can be categorized are as follows (Table 29-1):

Acute pain—acute pain is brief in duration (less than 3 to 6 months), the cause is usually known, the inten-

Table 29-1   Characteristics of Acute and Chronic Pain and Chronic Cancer Pain

Acute pain	Chronic pain	Chronic cancer pain
Identifiable cause	Cause hard to find	Usually identifiable cause
Short duration	Lasts longer than several months	Duration varies
Sudden onset	Begins gradually and persists	Onset varies
Well defined	May or may not be well defined	May or may not be well defined
Limited	Unlimited	Unlimited
Decreases with healing	Persists beyond healing time	May persist beyond healing
Reversible	Exhausting and useless	Exhausting and useless
Objective signs and symptoms	Objective signs absent	Objective signs absent
Anxiety	Depression and fatigue	Depression, fatigue, and anxiety
Mild to severe	Mild to severe	Mild to severe
Presence of autonomic responses:	Absence of autonomic responses	Absence of autonomic responses
↑ Heart rate		
↑ Blood pressure		
↑ Pupillary dilation		
↑ Muscle tension		
↓ GI motility		
↓ Salivary flow		

sity may range from mild to severe, and the treatment is aimed at elimination of the cause.

Chronic pain—chronic pain extends beyond 3 months, the cause may or may not be known, it has not responded to treatment, or it does not subside after the injury heals. The intensity may range from mild to severe, and treatment varies.

Chronic cancer pain—cancer pain may be both acute and chronic. There is the time element of chronic pain, the intensity may be severe, the pain can be described as "intractable" (i.e., cannot be relieved), and it may be have several etiologies.

Breakthrough pain—sometimes referred to as *incident pain,* breakthrough pain is "characterized as a transient increase in pain to greater than moderate intensity."[44] This pain may occur when the patient moves, coughs, or even with flatulence.

INCIDENCE OF CANCER PAIN

Not all people with cancer experience pain. The incidence of cancer pain is difficult to determine, but several experts agree that the figure is 40% to 80% when considering all types and stages of cancer.[124] Foley[45] states that 70% to 90% of patients with advanced cancer experience moderate to severe pain. In 1996 the American Cancer Society (ACS) estimates cancer deaths at 554,740, which means that between 332,844 and 499,266 people in the United States may experience pain related to their diagnosis of cancer during 1996. Recent surveys show that 40% to 50% of patients fail to achieve adequate relief of cancer pain.[17,18,108,117] Despite more knowledge about pain and a wider dissemination of such knowledge, Hill[55] notes that cancer pain relief is still inadequate.

Whether pain occurs in cancer depends on several factors. The major factors include the following:

- *Location* of the primary or metastatic site of cancer. If there is bony involvement (as occurs with spinal metastases) or neural involvement (by direct tumor invasion or compression of any nerve tissue), the pain will be more severe than pressure caused by organ involvement.
- *Stage* of the tumor activity. A patient in a later stage of cancer experiences pain more often and at a more severe intensity than a person who is in an early stage of disease. Spross[107] states that 79% to 90% of people with advanced disease report pain.

ETIOLOGIES OF CANCER PAIN

There may be many causes for pain in the person with cancer.

Direct Tumor Involvement

Direct tumor involvement (e.g., proliferation of malignant cells within bone, nerves, viscera, soft tissue) is a cause for pain. The site of the pain produces different sensations and intensities. Also, the location of the site impacts on the type of analgesic indicated. A Memorial Sloan Kettering Cancer Center (MSKCC) survey found direct tumor involvement as the source of 78% and 62% of inpatients and outpatients, respectively.[46] The types of pain produced by direct tumor involvement may include the following:

- *Somatic pain (nociceptive)*—results from stimulation of afferent nerves in the skin, connective tissue, muscles, joints, or bones. It is usually localized and described as throbbing, sharp, or aching and is localized. The response to analgesics is usually good.

- *Visceral pain (nociceptive)*—involves organs in the thoracic or abdominal area. It can be caused by infiltration, pressure, or distention. The pain is more diffuse and is often described as gnawing, crampy, constant, aching, or deep. This type of pain may be referred to cutaneous areas. Visceral pain may be seen in advanced pancreatic or liver cancer.
- *AIDS patients* may experience specific pain caused by retroperitoneal adenopathy or bowel wall invasion (e.g., Kaposi's sarcoma).[53]
- *Neuropathic pain (deafferentation)*—results from peripheral or central sensory nerve trauma injury causing abnormal firing. It is usually described as burning, shooting, lancinating, or tingling. Several neuropathic pain syndromes originate in the central or peripheral nerves. Response to analgesics is usually poor.
- *Cancer pain syndrome*—by definition, a syndrome is a number of different types of pain, different etiologies of pain, and different methods of treatment. Some of the known pain syndromes caused by direct tumor involvement are the following:
- *Bone involvement*—"multiple bony metastases are by far the most common cause of generalized bone pain," according to Portenoy.[94] In the case of vertebral involvement, it is imperative that the nurse report this occurrence, since pain alone will precede nerve compression and prompt intervention may prevent neurologic deficit formation.
- *Peripheral nerves*—sites where this may occur include the chest wall and retroperitoneal space, which may produce pain in the back, abdomen, or legs.
- *Brachial plexus*—this is usually a result of a primary lung tumor (Pancoast syndrome), and aching is present in the shoulder and upper back. According to Portenoy,[94] as many as 50% of patients with Pancoast syndrome will go on to develop cord compression if left untreated. Again, it is imperative that pain is assessed thoroughly, reported accurately, and treated promptly.
- *Epidural spinal cord compression*—"over 95% of patients with epidural spinal cord compression report pain, which may be focal or referred."[94] The pain will precede any sensory or motor deficit, and again it is mandatory that any new back pain be communicated immediately.

Cancer Treatment

Surgery, radiation therapy, or chemotherapy may exacerbate pain. A MSKCC survey found that treatment was the source of pain in 19% and 25% of inpatients and outpatients, respectively.[46] Some of the syndromes that may follow cancer treatment include the following:

- *Postthoracotomy pain syndrome*—the intercostal nerve may be damaged at the time of surgery. This will usually be described as a burning pain (neuropathic).
- *Postmastectomy pain syndrome*—the intercostobrachial nerve may be damaged at the time of surgery. This is usually described as a burning pain (neuropathic) and may occur soon after surgery or months later. Foley[46] estimates that 4% to 10% of all women undergoing a breast surgical procedure are at risk to develop this syndrome. Stevens and others[111] found a prevalence rate of 20% in a study of 95 women who had undergone breast cancer surgery; of this group 78.9% had a mastectomy and 21.1% had a lumpectomy. Kwekkeboom[67] reviewed eight studies (1974-1993) on postmastectomy pain and found incidence rates of 8% to 100%; presence of pain was correlated with the extent of surgery (i.e., lumpectomy, modified radical mastectomy, traditional radical mastectomy), whether the intercostobrachial nerve was spared, and the number of axillary lymph nodes removed. There was a minor decrease of the incidence of pain over time; although for many it did persist for years.
- *Postamputation syndrome*—this may be caused by the formation of a neuroma that has both lancinating (shooting) and "burning" components, or it may be a phantom sensation that exhibits both continuous dysesthesia and "shooting" pain.[94]
- *Multiple neural involvement*—several neural areas may be affected by chemotherapy (principally the vinca alkaloids [e. g., vincristine] or cisplatin). This paresthesia or dysesthesia tends to be dose-related and will generally improve over 6 to 12 months.
- *Mucositis*—the inflammation of the oral mucosa as a side effect of some of the chemotherapeutic agents (especially the antimetabolites) can produce intensely painful ulcerations. It is not uncommon for patients to require opioids to relieve pain during this period.
- *Postradiation pain*—there may be unintentional damage to the spinal cord, mucosa, or bone as a result of radiation fibrosis.

The pain associated with cancer therapies may occur immediately or long after the therapy is started, making it more difficult to determine whether the pain is the result of a complication of therapy or recurrent disease.

Pain Unrelated to Cancer

Conditions unrelated to cancer (e.g., arthritis, decubitus, tension headache, diabetic neuropathy) can cause pain for the cancer patient. A MSKCC survey found 3% and 10% of inpatients and outpatients, respectively, had pain unrelated to their cancer.[46]

If someone is immunocompromised, it is not unusual for the person to develop herpes zoster (shingles). After the treatment and healing phase, a postherpetic neuralgia can remain that can be difficult to manage and needs to be addressed as a neuropathic pain in origin.

Any pain usually has special significance for the patient with cancer. Whether it is a "routine" headache or gastritis, the fear is that the pain represents an extension of the cancer. All reports of pain must be evaluated.

When there is obvious trauma to a body part, the

source of one's pain is evident, but with cancer it is often difficult to determine the anatomic injury that may be occurring, and full assessment and evaluation is warranted.

FACTORS AFFECTING RESPONSE TO PAIN

An individual's response to pain is influenced by several factors, which helps explain why pain is such a complex experience.

Anxiety

Anxiety is considered to be the most important factor affecting an individual's response to pain because it affects a person's ability to tolerate and cope with pain. Because increased anxiety increases pain, any strategy nurses can use to decrease a patient's anxiety will help control pain.

Measures to decrease anxiety (e.g., distraction, relaxation) will be covered in a later section of this chapter. It is important to ask the patient and family members what has helped control the patient's anxiety in the past. Many of these measures can be incorporated into the patient's individual plan of care.

Past Experience of Pain

In general, the more experience of pain one has in childhood, the greater the perceptions of pain in adulthood. It is important for the nurse to discuss past pain with the patient. The nurse should also determine what measures have helped relieve pain in the past. Even though some measures may seem unlikely to help, if they are not harmful or contraindicated, they may aid the patient's pain treatment plan. The nurse should also determine what measures have not helped relieve pain in the past.

Culture and Religion

Acceptable responses to pain are learned at a very early age. Cultural and religious practices in one's family play an important role in the pain experience. Some cultures may view the expression of pain or suffering as a weakness, so they tend to minimize pain. Other cultures expect expression of pain, so they may have greater overt manifestations of pain. The issue of ethnicity and its relation to pain is not resolved.[100]

In a multicultural study of beliefs about reporting cancer pain and using analgesics, Ward and others[122] identified cultural barriers to pain management. The three top fears among three cultures were found to be as follows:

Non-Hispanic Caucasian	Hispanic	Taiwanese
Addiction	Tolerance	Tolerance
Disease progression	Disease progression	Disease progression
Side effects	Addiction	Addiction

It is of interest that the Non-Hispanic Caucasian group was the only group to identify side effects as a fear and that all groups identified addiction as a fear.

It is important to realize that not all people manifest pain in the same way and that there is no right or wrong way. The nurse should accept all patients' expressions of pain, regardless of their cultural or religious backgrounds.

BARRIERS TO ADEQUATE CANCER PAIN MANAGEMENT
Lack of Knowledge

It is well documented that there is a lack of professional health care education regarding pain management that has resulted in less than optimal pain management for the person with cancer.[16,21,38,56,61] When 28 nursing textbooks were reviewed,[38] it was found that only one book accurately described the differences between physical dependence and addiction. McCaffery and Beebe[73] describe health care professionals as often unaware of their lack of knowledge about pain control despite the fact that 81% of baccalaureate nursing programs accredited by the National League for Nursing include some class content on pain.

Whether in basic or continuing educational opportunities, nurses traditionally have not been taught how to assess pain or to use different treatment modalities, especially medications, appropriately. Many nurses are not familiar with the pharmacokinetics of analgesics, the types of analgesics available, equianalgesic dosages, novel routes of delivery, or principles of scheduling administration. In a survey conducted at the fourth annual meeting of the American Society of Pain Management Nurses (ASPMN), pharmacology was identified as the number one information provided most frequently for colleagues.[75] McCaffery and Ferrell[74] report that although the percentage of nurses knowing that the risk of addiction is less than 1% has increased (i.e., an improvement), in a 1988 to 1989 survey of 2459 nurses, 21.6% still thought that at least 25% of patients receiving opioids for pain relief would become addicted. Portions of this study were replicated in Canada and reported in 1995; Brunier and others[16] found that 30% of the nurses believed that 25% of patients with pain become addicted to opioids.

A 1995 study of nurses in four states reported by Wallace and others[120] found that nurses rated their educational preparation midway between inadequate and adequate and their knowledge of financial issues of pain management as inadequate. One of the factors affecting patient compliance is the cost of medication. Hoffman and others[57] reported a study of physicians' knowledge of retail medication costs. It was found that 75% of physicians could not estimate correctly at least one half of the common medications in a list of prices, although a substantial range was given.

The Minnesota Cancer Pain Initiative conducted a study of physicians in six communities. Significant knowledge deficits were found in 9 of 14 Cancer Pain Management principles. One inappropriate attitude was found with an increased concern about opioid adverse effects.[37]

According to Hill,[56] cancer pain management has had only limited and unsatisfactory results. He proposes that pain education should be included in undergraduate curriculum and not be left to the postgraduate level. He describes undergraduate nursing as "more effective," because they are more intimately involved with patients and are present on an ongoing basis.

There is a call for reeducation of all health care team members so that adequate pain control can be achieved. Positive advances have been made in recent years, and nurses have been instrumental in the development of the hospice movement, oncology nursing's focus on symptom management (i.e., pain), and individual state cancer pain initiatives.

With today's knowledge and technology, nurses can assist the patient and family to achieve better pain management outcomes.

Regulatory Issues

Misconceptions also exist about narcotic regulations, both nationally and in many states that promote limiting prescription of narcotics even when needed for successful pain management. Von Roenn and others[119] conducted a study among Eastern Cooperative Oncology Group (ECOG) physicians and found that 18% identified excessive state regulation of analgesics as a barrier to cancer pain management. Weissman,[124] in an article on the history of narcotic control in the United States, explores the development of legal issues. He concludes with the statement that "physicians need to work with their state regulatory agencies" to identify impediments to patient care. Many states allow advanced-practice nurses to prescribe analgesics[61] but some do not permit this and others have multiple restrictions. Each state's practice act must be studied.

Myths and Misconceptions

The lay public and some health care professionals have held many myths and misconceptions about cancer pain management that are now beginning to be addressed. Some of these myths and misconceptions follow:

- The person taking pain medications will easily become addicted.
- Cancer pain cannot really be relieved; it is part of the disease.
- The "strong stuff" must be saved for later when the pain gets "really bad," or nothing will be available.

- "Shots" are stronger than pills.
- If opiates are administered routinely, death will be hastened as a result of respiratory depression.

Denying the existence of pain may function as a coping mechanism because any presence of pain may be viewed as disease progression. This must be evaluated in light of other factors (e.g., personality trait of stoicism, cultural beliefs, attitudes). Myths and misconceptions must be addressed by the health care professional in the initial assessment of pain and in subsequent reassessments.

DEVELOPMENTS IN CANCER PAIN MANAGEMENT

During the 1970s the hospice movement established itself in the United States. Throughout the country in large and small communities, home-care, free-standing, hospital-based, or agency-affiliated programs started serving the population who had a life-expectancy of 6 months or less. With this focus of care delivery, pain became one of the central symptom management issues. Hospice nurses were leading the way in recognizing the uniqueness of cancer pain and became the nursing profession's experts through hands-on practice.

The International Association for the Study of Pain (IASP) was formed in 1974. The American Pain Society (APS) is a national chapter of IASP.

In 1982 the World Health Organization (WHO) established a program in the cancer unit to study the incidence of cancer pain and to provide guidelines for cancer pain management. A 1984 meeting resulted in the publication of the booklet *Cancer Pain Relief* in 1986. The international WHO three-step analgesic ladder has been implemented in a number of countries (Figure 29-1). This ladder provides logical steps of progression of analgesics to treat the needs of the person who has pain. A revised edition, *Cancer Pain Relief and Palliative Care,* was published by the WHO in 1990.

In 1986 the WHO established the Wisconsin Cancer Pain Initiative as the demonstration project site of the United States to "develop a comprehensive program to reduce cancer pain in the state of Wisconsin." In 1991 there were 21 states with Cancer Pain Initiative Programs, and by 1996 there were 43 states with cancer pain initiative programs and the other 7 states were working to organize programs. Dahl[29] describes the Initiatives as based on a collaborative approach that depends on mutual respect and listening. Jacox[61] states that nurses should participate actively in interdisciplinary organizations as a means of influencing pain management policy making. All of the established state cancer pain initiative programs have nurse involvement, and some state programs are led by a nurse. State cancer pain initiatives address the issues of government regulations, myths and

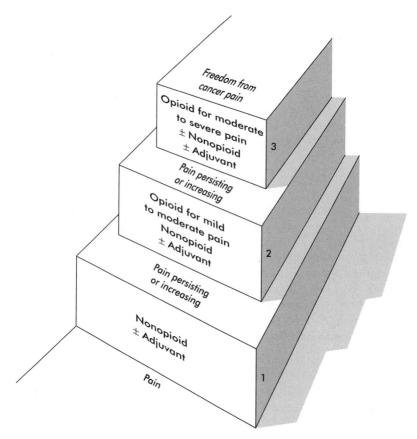

Figure 29-1　The World Health Organization (WHO) three-step analgesic ladder. (From Report of a WHO Expert Committee: *Cancer pain relief and palliative care,* Geneva, 1990, World Health Organization [WHO Technical Report Series, No. 804], p. 9.)

misconceptions of lay people and professionals, and professional education of pain management strategies. In addition, Blanchard and Seale[13] cite Spross as urging that professional and lay education also include assertiveness and conflict negotiation skills. A cancer pain role model education program has been implemented by the Wisconsin Cancer Pain Initiative. Weissman and Dahl[126] found that interdisciplinary team participants demonstrated a significant improvement in cancer pain knowledge as a result of the 1-day conference and that the teams had completed 227 educational or clinical practice projects. Dahl[28] describes the state initiatives as "dedicated to making relief of cancer pain a reality." (See Figure 29-2 for a map and Appendix B at end of chapter [Organizations].)

In 1990 the American Pain Society published its Standards on Acute and Cancer Pain. This interdisciplinary professional pain organization recognized that there was a means of setting criteria against which quality of practice could be measured. (See Section on Quality Assessment and Improvement.)

In 1990 the Oncology Nursing Society published its detailed document, "Oncology Nursing Society Position Paper on Cancer Pain,"[107-109] which includes the following:
- Introductory material
- Scope of nursing practice regarding cancer pain
- Ethics
- Practice (problem identification, assessment, planning, implementation and coordination, evaluation)
- Education (basic, graduate, continuing, patient, public)
- Research
- Resources
- Nursing administration
- Social policy
- Pediatric cancer pain

This document is a thorough and concise paper on quality pain management and nursing's role in providing this management.

The American Nurses Association (ANA) published a Statement on Promoting Comfort and Relieving Pain in Dying Patients on September 5, 1991. This position statement underscores the difference between relieving pain and mercy killing.[22] It stresses the vital role and responsibilities of the professional nurse in the management of pain.

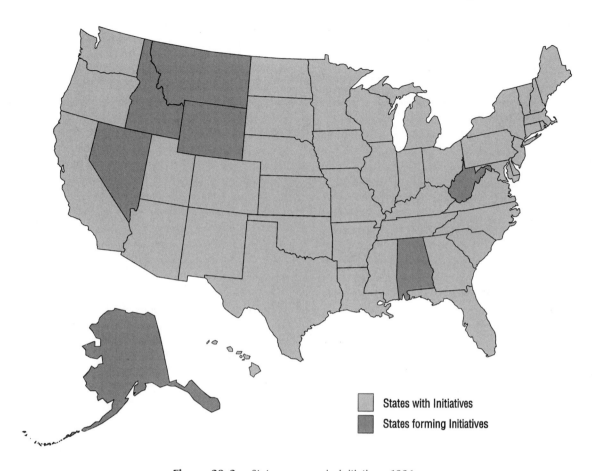

Figure 29-2   State cancer pain initiatives, 1996.

In 1991 the governmental Agency on Health Care Policy and Research (AHCPR) formed an expert panel to develop guidelines on pain management. The AHCPR was established in 1989 to enhance the quality, appropriateness, and effectiveness of health care services and access to those services.[61] It was decided that there would indeed be the need for two separate documents: one on acute operative and trauma pain and one on cancer pain. In 1992 the acute pain guideline was published, and the cancer pain guideline followed in 1994.

In 1992 the Ad Hoc Committee on Cancer Pain of the American Society of Clinical Oncology (ASCO) published "Cancer Pain Assessment and Treatment Curriculum Guidelines," which can guide systematically designed educational programs.[90]

In 1992 the Joint Commission on Accreditation for Healthcare Organizations (JCAHO) included pain management as one of its standards. (See Section on Quality Assessment and Improvement.)

Much time and effort have been spent studying the problem of cancer pain, identifying barriers, and establishing practice guidelines and standards. It is time to implement what is already known and make an impact on patients who experience cancer pain. Nurses do have

an active role in pain teams. Coluzzi and others[23] report on a survey of the NCI-designated cancer centers that identified that 67% of the centers that had pain management services had a nurse on the team.

PHARMACOLOGIC INTERVENTIONS

Portenoy [91,94] states that with optimal pharmacologic management alone, 70% to 90% of cancer pain can be adequately relieved.

Non-Opioid Analgesics

The non-opioids work primarily at the peripheral nervous system level and are used for mild to moderate pain, especially of bone metastases, soft-tissue infiltration, or arthritis (i.e., somatic pain). The categories of non-opioids include aspirin, acetaminophen, and the nonsteroidal antiinflammatory drugs (NSAIDs).

Most NSAIDs block the production of prostaglandins, which are chemicals that are produced when cells are damaged.[25,127] NSAIDs have potential gastrointestinal (GI) side effects, and this may limit their use over time. Inturrisi,[59] Wilkie,[127] and Cherny[19] note that all NSAIDs except choline magnesium trisalicylate (Trilisate) will in-

Table 29-2 Non-opioid Analgesics

Drug	Recommended dose and interval	Comments
PARA-AMINOPHENOL DERIVATIVE		
Acetaminophen (Tylenol, Panadol, Anacin-3, Excedrin, Midol, Sine-Aid)	500-1000 mg q 4-6 hours	Similar to aspirin in analgesic and antipyretic effects, but only slight antiinflammatory effects;[20] may not have effect on platelet aggregation; may cause liver toxicity in doses >6 gm/day.[20,84]
Nabumetone (Relafen)	500 mg q 12 hours	Time-release preparation; usually for arthritis.
ACETYLSALICYLIC		
Acetylsalicylic acid (aspirin)	500-1000 mg q 4-6 hours	Standard antiinflammatory; increased bleeding time caused by inhibition of platelet aggregation.
NONACETYLATED SALICYLATE		
Choline magnesium Trisalicylates (Trilisate)	1000-1500 mg q 8-12 hours	Minimal effect on platelet aggregation (platelet-sparing); available in liquid; minimal gastrointestinal (GI) toxicity.
Diflunisal (Dolobid)	500-1000 mg q 8-12 hours	Minimal antipyretic effect; minimal GI side effects.
Salsalate (Disalcid, Salsitab)	750-1000 mg q 8-12 hours	Minimal GI side effects; may have minimal effect on platelet aggregation.
NSAID (NONSTEROIDAL ANTIINFLAMMATORY DRUG) **Propionic acid derivatives**		
Ibuprofen (Motrin, Nuprin, Advil, Medipren)	400-600 mg q 6 hours	Available as oral suspension; may require escalation.
Fenoprofen (Nalfon)	200-400 mg q 4-6 hours	May require escalation.
Naproxen (Naprosyn)	250-500 mg q 6-8 hours	Available as oral liquid.
Naproxen Sodium (Anaprox)	275-550 mg q 6-8 hours	Faster onset than naproxen. Aleve® is available in a 220 mg dose taken q 12 hrs.
Ketoprofen (Orudis)	25-50 mg q 6-8 hours	
Acetic acid derivative		
Indomethacin (Indocin)	25-50 mg q 8-12 hours	Available as oral suspension and rectal suppository; high incidence of GI side effects.
Sulindac (Clinoril)	150-200 mg q 8-12 hours	GI side effects common; lower incidence of renal toxicity.
Tolmetin (Tolectin)	200 mg q 6-8 hours	Weak analgesic effect.
Ketorolac (Toradol)	30 mg q 6 hours IM 10 mg q 6 hours PO	Only injectable NSAID; not recommended for use longer than 7 days; equivalent to 10 mg parenteral morphine.
Fenamate		
Mefenamic acid (Ponstel)	250 mg q 6 hours	Not recommended for use longer than 7 days.
Meclofenamate (Meclomen)	50-100 mg q 6-8 hours	Diarrhea may occur as well as other GI side effects.
Oxicam		
Piroxicam (Feldene)	10-30 mg q 6 hours or 20 mg q day	Not recommended for patients with renal or liver dysfunction; effect may not be seen for 7-12 days.

Data from Agency for Health Care Policy and Research (AHCPR): *Management of cancer pain,* 1994, Publication No. 94-0592; American Pain Society: *Principles of analgesic use in the treatment of acute pain and chronic cancer pain,* ed 3, 1992; Weissman DE and others: *Handbook of cancer pain management,* ed 4, 1994, Wisconsin Cancer Pain Initiative.

terfere with platelet aggregation and therefore may not be appropriate for someone who is thrombocytopenic.

The NSAIDs' mechanism of action is believed to be inhibition of cyclooxygenase activity[97] and prostaglandin synthesis, but other mechanisms may exist. Food decreases the rate of absorption and may delay the time to reach peak levels; therefore NSAIDs should be taken between meals.

Non-opioids are often given together with opioids, and therefore a lower dose of opioid may be effective[101] (Table 29-2).

An analgesic that does not fit the usual categories is capsaicin (Zostrix). It is derived from the Hungarian red pepper[24] and is an antagonist that acts by depleting substance P. It is theorized that it may reduce the central transmission of information about pain and has been used in postmastectomy and postherpetic syndromes.[24] The 0.025% topical ointment is applied 3 or 4 times per day for several weeks. It does cause a burning sensation upon application, and for some people this is distressing enough for them to stop the treatment.

Opioid Analgesics

The opiates work primarily at the central nervous system (CNS) level. Those opioids used for mild to moderate pain often have acetaminophen or aspirin together with the opiate. The nurse should be aware of the total dosage of aspirin/acetaminophen consumed per 24 hours. The maximum dose of either should not exceed 6000 mg per 24 hours. If two tablets containing 500 mg each are taken every 3 hours, the total is 8000 mg per 24 hours. (See Table 29-3 and Table 29-4 for specifics for those weighing more than 50 kg and those weighing less than 50 kg).

It has been found that there is no ceiling effect of morphine,[60] which means that the dose can continue to be escalated to provide analgesia with increased pain levels. Some drugs have a ceiling, and beyond that ceiling dose there is no added analgesic benefit. There are exceptional instances in which patients may require 1000 to 2000 mg of morphine, or even more, per 24 hours, and the person will be alert, ambulatory, and participating in activities of daily living.

Table 29-3 Dose Equivalents for Opioid Analgesics in Opioid–Naive Adults >50 Kg*

Drug	Approximate equianalgesic dose		Usual starting dose for moderate to severe pain		Comments
	Oral	Parenteral	Oral	Parenteral	
OPIOID AGONIST†					
Morphine‡	30 mg q 3-4 hr (repeat around-the-clock dosing) 60 mg q 3-4 hr (single dose or intermittent dosing)	10 mg q 3-4 hr	5-10 mg q 3-4 hr††	10 mg q 3-4 hr	Standard of comparison for narcotic analgesics; 3- to 4-hour duration; the metabolite morphine-6-glucuronide may accumulate in patients with renal insufficiency[84]

Data from Agency for Health Care Policy and Research (AHCPR): *Management of cancer pain,* 1994, Publication No. 94-0592; American Pain Society: *Principles of analgesic use in the treatment of acute pain and chronic cancer pain,* ed 3, 1992; Weissman DE and others: *Handbook of cancer pain management,* ed 4, 1994, Wisconsin Cancer Pain Initiative.

*Caution: Recommended doses do not apply for adult patients with body weight less than 50 kg. For recommended starting doses for adults <50 kg body weight, see Table 29-4.

†Caution: Recommended doses do not apply to patients with renal or hepatic insufficiency or other conditions affecting drug metabolism and kinetics.

‡Caution: For morphine, hydromorphone, and oxymorphone, rectal administration is an alternate route for patients unable to take oral medications. Equianalgesic doses may differ from oral and parenteral doses because of pharmacokinetic differences. Note: A short-acting opioid should normally be used for initial therapy of moderate to severe pain.

§Transdermal fentanyl (Duragesic) is an alternative option. Transdermal fentanyl dosage is not calculated as equianalgesic to a single morphine dosage. See the package insert for dosing calculations. Doses above 25 μg/h should not be used in opioid-naive patients.

‖Not recommended. Doses listed are for brief therapy. Switch to another opioid for long-term therapy.

¶Caution: Doses of aspirin and acetaminophen in combination opioid/NSAID preparations must also be adjusted to the patient's body weight.

**Caution: Codeine doses above 65 mg often are not appropriate because of diminishing incremental analgesia with increasing doses but continually increasing nausea, constipation, and other side effects.

††Wisconsin Cancer Pain Initiative communication regarding starting dose, 1995.

‡‡Hanks GW, Fallon MT: *Transdermal fentanyl in cancer pain: conversion from oral morphine, J Pain Symptom Manage* 10(2):87, 1995.

Note: Published tables vary in the suggested doses that are equianalgesic to morphine. Clinical response is the criterion that must be applied for each patient; titration to clinical responses is necessary. Because there is not complete cross-tolerance among these drugs, it is usually necessary to use a lower than equianalgesic dose when changing drugs and to retitrate to response.

q, Every; *N/A,* not available; *R,* rectally; *NR,* not recommended.

Continued.

Table 29-3 Dose Equivalents for Opioid Analgesics in Opioid-Naive Adults >50 Kg—cont'd

Drug	Approximate equianalgesic dose		Usual starting dose for moderate to severe pain		Comments
	Oral	Parenteral	Oral	Parenteral	
OPIOID AGONIST†—cont'd					
Morphine controlled-release‡,§ (MS Contin, Oramorph SR)	90-120 mg q 8-12 hr	N/A	15-30 mg q 12 hr††	N/A	12-hour sustained-released preparation; available in 30, 60, 100, and 200 mg tablets
Hydromorphone‡ (Dilaudid)	7.5 mg q 3-4 hr	1.5 mg q 3-4 hr	2-4 mg q 3-4 hr††	1.5 mg q 3-4 hr	Available R; high concentration is available for parenteral use
Methadone (Dolophine)	20 mg q 6-8 hr	10 mg q 6-8 hr	5-10 mg q 6-8 hr††	10 mg q 6-8 hr	Good oral potency; long plasma half-life; accumulates with repetitive dosing
Levorphanol (Levo-Dromoran)	4 mg q 6-8 hr	2 mg q 6-8 hr	2 mg q 8 hr††	2 mg q 6-8 hr	Long plasma half-life
Oxycodone (Roxicodone)	30 mg q 3-4 hr	N/A	5-10 mg q 3-4 hr	N/A	No ceiling effect; is available as 5 mg tablet and as 5 mg/ml and 20 mg/ml solution
(OxyContin)	30 mg q 12 hr	N/A	30 mg q 12 hr	N/A	12-hour sustained-released tablet; available in 10 mg, 20 mg, and 40 mg tablets; food has no significant effect on absorption; oral oxycodone is equal to morphine PO
Oxymorphone‡ (Numorphan)	N/A	1 mg q 3-4 hr	N/A	1 mg q 3-4 hr	5 mg R suppository = 5 mg parenteral morphine
Meperidine‖ (Demerol)	300 mg q 2-3 hr	100 mg q 3 hr	N/R	100 mg q 3 hr	Shorter acting than morphine (2-3 hours); toxic metabolite (normeperidine) accumulates with repeated dosing, causing central nervous system (CNS) excitation, which can lead to seizures; avoid use in patients on monoamine oxidase (MAO) inhibitors because of potential adverse reaction that mimics malignant hyperthermia and may lead to cardiovascular collapse

Table 29-3   Dose Equivalents for Opioid Analgesics in Opioid-Naive Adults >50 Kg—cont'd

Drug	Approximate equianalgesic dose		Usual starting dose for moderate to severe pain		Comments
	Oral	Parenteral	Oral	Parenteral	
Fentanyl (Sub-limaze) (Duragesic)	N/A	0.1 mg	N/A		Transdermal patch; 8- to 12-hour delay[40] in on-set and offset of patch; fever increases dose delivery rate
	Transdermal conversion‡‡				
	Morphine PO (24 hours)	*Morphine par-enteral (24 hours)*	*Patch*		
	5-20 mg	15-60 mg	25 mcg		
	25-35 mg	75-105 mg	50 mcg		
	40-50 mg	120-150 mg	75 mcg		
	55-65 mg	165-195 mg	100 mcg		
COMBINATION OPIOID/NONSTEROIDAL ANTIINFLAMMATORY DRUG (NSAID) PREPARATION¶					
Codeine (with aspirin or acetaminophen)**	180-200 mg q 3-4 hr	130 mg q 3-4 hr	60 mg q 3-4 hr	60 mg q 2 hr IM/SC	
Hydrocodone (in Lorcet, Lortab, Vicodin, others)	30 mg q 3-4 hr	N/A	10 mg q 3-4 hr	N/A	
Oxycodone (Roxicodone, also in Percocet, Percodan, Tylox, others)	30 mg q 3-4 hr	N/A	10 mg q 3-4 hr	N/A	
MIXED AGONIST-ANTAGONIST					
Pentazocine (Talwin)	180 mg q 3-4 hours	60 mg q 3-4 hours			May cause psychomi-metic effects at high dose; may precipitate withdrawal in opioid-dependent patients; not recommended for can-cer patients
Nalbuphine (Nubain)	N/A	10 mg q 3-4 hours			Not available orally; inci-dence of psychomi-metic effects lower than that associated with pentazocine
Butorphanol (Stadol)	N/A	2 mg q 3-4 hours			Not available orally; inci-dence of psychomi-metic effects lower than that associated with pentazocine; nasal spray is available
Dezocine (Dalgan)		10 mg			Same profile of effects as that associated with nalbuphine
PARTIAL AGONIST					
Buprenorphine (Buprenex)	N/A	0.3-0.4 mg q 6-8 hours			May precipitate with-drawal in opioid-dependent patients; not readily reversed by naloxone

Table 29-4 Dose Equivalents for Opioid Analgesics in Opioid-Naive Adults <50 kg

Drug	Approximate equianalgesic dose		Usual starting dose for moderate to severe pain		Comments
	Oral	Parenteral	Oral	Parenteral	
OPIOID AGONIST*					
Morphine†	30 mg q 3-4 hr (repeat around-the-clock dosing) 60 mg q 3-4 hr (single dose or intermittent dosing)	10 mg q 3-4 hr	0.3 mg/kg q 3-4 hr	0.1 mg/kg q 3-4 hr	Standard of comparison for narcotic analgesics; 3- to 4-hour duration; the metabolite morphine-6-glucuronide may accumulate in patients with renal insufficiency[84]
Morphine, controlled-release†,‡ (MS Contin, Oramorph SR)	90-120 mg q 12 hr	N/A	N/A	N/A	12-hour sustained-released preparation; available in 30, 60, 100, and 200 mg tablets
Hydromorphone† (Dilaudid)	7.5 mg q 3-4 hr	1.5 mg q 3-4 hr	0.06 mg/kg q 3-4 hr	0.015 mg/kg q 3-4 hr	Available R; high concentration is available for parenteral use
Levorphanol (Levo-Dromoran)	4 mg q 6-8 hr	2 mg q 6-8 hr	0.04 mg/kg q 6-8 hr	0.02 mg/kg q 6-8 hr	Long plasma half-life
Meperidine§ (Demerol)	300 mg q 2-3 hr	100 mg q 3 hr	N/A	0.75 mg/kg q 2-3 hr	Shorter acting than morphine (2-3 hours); toxic metabolite (normeperidine) accumulates with repeated dosing, causing central nervous system (CNS) excitation, which can lead to seizures; avoid use in patients on monoamine oxidase (MAO) inhibitors because of potential adverse reaction that mimics malignant hyperthermia and may lead to cardiovascular collapse
Methadone (Dolophine, others)	20 mg q 6-8 hr	10 mg q 6-8 hr	0.2 mg/kg q 6-8 hr	0.1 mg/kg q 6-8 hours	Good oral potency; long plasma half-life; accumulates with repetitive dosing

*Caution: Recommended doses do not apply to patients with renal or hepatic insufficiency or other condition affecting drug metabolism and kinetics.

†Caution: For morphine, hydromorphone, and oxymorphone, rectal administration is an alternate route for patients unable to take oral medications. Equianalgesic doses may differ from oral and parenteral doses because of pharmacokinetic differences. Note: A short-acting opioid should normally be used for initial therapy of moderate to severe pain.

‡Transdermal fentanyl (Duragesic) is an alternative option. Transdermal fentanyl dosage is not calculated as equianalgesic to a single morphine dosage. See the package insert for dosing calculations. Doses above 25 μg/h should not be used in opioid-naive patients.

§Not recommended. Doses listed are for brief therapy. Switch to another opioid for long-term therapy.

‖Caution: Doses of aspirin and acetaminophen in combination opioid/NSAID preparations must also be adjusted to the patient's body weight.

¶Caution: Some clinicians recommend not exceeding 1.5 mg/kg of codeine because of an increased incidence of side effects with higher doses.

Note: Published tables vary in the suggested doses that are equianalgesic to morphine. Clinical response is the criterion that must be applied for each patient; titration to clinical responses is necessary. Because there is not complete cross-tolerance among these drugs, it is usually necessary to use a lower than equianalgesic dose when changing drugs and to retitrate to response.

q, Every; N/A, not available; R, rectally; N/R, not recommended.

Table 29-4   Dose Equivalents for Opioid Analgesics in Opioid-Naive Adults <50 kg–cont'd

Drug	Approximate equianalgesic dose		Usual starting dose for moderate to severe pain		Comments
	Oral	Parenteral	Oral	Parenteral	
COMBINATION OPIOID/NONSTEROIDAL ANTIINFLAMMATORY DRUG (NSAID) PREPARATION‖					
Codeine¶ (with aspirin or acetaminophen)	180-200 mg q 3-4 hr	130 mg q 3-4 hr	0.5-1 mg/kg q 3-4 hr	N/A	
Hydrocodone (in Lorcet, Lortab, Vicodin, others)	30 mg q 3-4 hr	N/A	0.2 mg/kg q 3-4 hr	N/A	Only available with acetaminophen
Oxycodone (Roxicodone, also in Percocet, Percodan, Tylox, others)	30 mg q 3-4 hr	N/A	0.2 mg/kg q 3-4 hr	N/A	Elixir available 5 mg/ml and 20 mg/ml; caution with impaired ventilation, asthma, increased intracranial pressure, and liver failure
Dihydrocodeine 16 mg + acetaminophen 356.4 mg + caffeine 30 mg (DHC Plus)			1-2 tabs q 4 hr	Is a schedule III product	

After many years of experience with meperidine (Demerol), caution is now being expressed in two areas. First, it should never be used on a continuous basis for cancer pain treatment because the metabolite (normeperidine) is a central nervous system stimulator[60,66] and this hyperexcitability can lead to tremors or seizure activity with repeated dosing. Second, the AHCPR Clinical Practice Guidelines include the warning against the use of meperidine for people who are taking monoamine oxidase inhibitors. "Severe adverse reactions, including death through mechanisms that mimic malignant hyperthermia, have been reported when these drugs are used together."[2,3]

Oxycodone is an agonist that at one time was available only in combination with acetaminophen or aspirin. It is now available as a single agent in a 5 mg tab, solutions of 5 mg/ml and 20 mg/ml and as a time-release 12-hour preparation in 10 mg, 20 mg, and 40 mg tablets. As a single agent there is no ceiling-effect, and the equianalgesic conversion is 1:1 to oral morphine.[48]

The question as to the efficacy of heroin over morphine has been studied with the conclusion that heroin does not offer any advantage over morphine when an equianalgesic conversion is done.[65,116] Heroin (diamorphine) is metabolized to morphine before it reaches the opiate receptors of the brain. Before the studies were done, heroin was most often the narcotic of choice in the Brompton's Cocktail in hospice programs in England; now oral morphine is routinely used.

Mixed agonist-antagonists may also be used for moderate to severe pain. Using mixed agonist-antagonists to manage cancer pain should be done with caution for the following reasons:

- After using agonists (e.g., morphine), withdrawal-like symptoms can be precipitated when a mixed agonist-antagonist is given.
- If given with an agonist, the mixed form will antagonize and give poor pain relief with possible increase in psychomimetic effects.

Special Issues of Opioids

Titration/escalating doses. Most often an increasing need for medication is indicative of progressive disease or a developing complication, and thorough assessment is warranted. When it is determined that more medication is needed to manage an individual's pain, the safe plan of increasing the dose is to *increase 25% to 50% of the previous dose.*[19,93]

Example:
Current dose: 60 mg PO morphine q 4 hr;
Add: 15-30 mg PO morphine q 4 hr; thus
New Prescription: 75 to 90 mg PO morphine q 4 hr.

Continue assessment to determine whether additional increases are needed.

Rescue doses. An order should be obtained for an immediate-release analgesic to offer every 1 to 2 hours for breakthrough pain. The "rescue" medication should be the same drug (e.g., morphine) as the scheduled analgesic; a liquid immediate-release formula will act more rapidly than a tablet form. This dose should equal 33% to 50% of the regularly scheduled every-4-hour dose or 10% of the total 24-hour requirement. According to Cherny,[19] Coyle,[24] and Portenoy,[91,94] the rescue dose may be 5% to 15% of the 24-hour baseline dose; Hanks[53] recommends 5% to 10% of the baseline 24-hour dose.

Example:

If 180 mg oral morphine is required per 24 hours, at 10% the rescue dose would be 18 mg.

If 30 mg oral morphine is scheduled q 4 hr, at 50% the rescue dose would be 15 mg.

If greater than or equal to 3 rescue doses are required per 24 hours, an order should be obtained that includes that amount in the around-the-clock (ATC) dosing. The order for rescue dosing should be maintained. (See General Principles of Analgesic Administration, no. 4, p. 765.)

Decreasing doses. If a person's pain decreases (e.g., after palliative radiation to bone metastases, nerve block), the opioid requirements may indeed decrease dramatically. According to the American Hospital Formulary Service,[6] abstinence syndrome (withdrawal) will occur if someone has required 240 mg or more of morphine per day for 30 days although the "Management of Cancer Pain" AHCPR guideline states that abstinence syndrome may occur after 2 weeks of opioid therapy and does not indicate a specific dosage range.

S & S withdrawl during 1st 24 hours:

• Restlessness	• Perspiration
• Lacrimation	• Gooseflesh
• Rhinorrhea	• Restless sleep
• Yawning	• Mydriasis

S & S withdrawl during 24 to 72 hours:

- Twitching/muscular spasms
- Kicking movements
- Severe aches in back, abdomen, and legs
- Nausea, vomiting, diarrhea
- Coryza and severe sneezing
- Increase in all vital signs (temperature, pulse, respiration, and blood pressure)

To safely "wean" the person from the opioids and prevent abstinence syndrome from occurring, the following formula is used:

Give 50% of the previous order for 48 hours and then reduce by 25% every 48 hours until less than 10 to 15 mg (parenteral morphine equivalent) per 24 hours.[3]

Example: Patient has been receiving 180 mg morphine sulfate PO/24 hours (at a 3:1 ratio, this is 60 mg parenteral morphine/24 hours)

Days 1 and 2: 90 mg PO morphine sulfate/24 hours
Days 3 and 4: 70 mg PO morphine sulfate/24 hours
Days 5 and 6: 50 mg PO morphine sulfate/24 hours
Days 7 and 8: 40 mg PO morphine sulfate/24 hours

Days 9 and 10: 30 mg PO morphine sulfate/24 hours (all preceding doses are 10 mg parenteral morphine equivalents)
Day 11: nothing

Duration of opioids. Not all opioids have the same duration of effectiveness; some opioids are short-acting, some are long-acting, and some are in the middle. Scheduling must be according to how long the medication is actually lasting, or pain will occur.

Short-acting opioids

Fentanyl (Sublimaze) ½ hr

Intermediate-acting opioids

Meperidine (Demerol) 2 to 3 hr
Morphine 3 to 4 hr
Hydromorphone (Dilaudid) 3 to 4 hr
Codeine 3 to 4 hr
Oxycodone 3 to 4 hr
Propoxyphene (Darvon) 3 to 4 hr

Long-acting opioids

Methadone (Dolophine) 6 to 8 hr
Levorphanol (Levo-Dromoran) 6 to 8 hr

Controlled-release oral formulations allow an extended schedule. Current formulations now available include morphine (MS Contin, Oramorph SR) q 12 hr, oxycodone (Oxycontin) q 12 hr, and fentanyl transdermal (Duragesic patch) q 3 days.

Equianalgesia is the conversion of one route to another or of one opioid to another in an equivalent amount. Converting from one route of administration to another or from one opioid to another must be done in such a manner as to not undermedicate or overmedicate the patient. The parenteral morphine equivalent of the combination analgesics (e.g., acetaminophen with codeine) is approximately 2.5 to 3.0 mg.[112] When switching from one opioid to another opioid, one half of the analgesic drug dose of the new opioid should be given as the initial starting dose.[44,60,94] This concept is just beginning to be realized, and nurses can do much to educate other health care professionals in the process of equianalgesic conversion.

Opioid side effect management. With the administration of opioids, side effects may occur. According to Inturrisi,[60] "Patients with renal impairment are more sensitive to morphine and liable to develop toxic effects, as a result of delayed elimination of the active metabolite morphine-6-glucuronidel." In addition, patients with severe hepatic dysfunction require decreased doses, and caution must be used with opioids because CNS signs and symptoms may be exacerbated. Concerns about the control of side effects were identified by 65% of physicians in an ECOG study.[119] An interesting procedure to manage opioid side effects is the rotation of medications. de Stoutz and others[31] found that a dose significantly lower than the equianalgesic amount could manage the pain with decreased side effects. The questions then become: Are expected side effects being managed effectively? Are there any unexpected side effects?

A discussion of the expected side effects follows.

Constipation. Constipation does not diminish over time. The opioid effects on the gastrointestinal system produce a decrease in intestinal secretions and peristalsis.[60] All patients on opioids should be given stool softeners and agents to increase bowel motility to prevent constipation as opioids inhibit peristalsis in the GI tract.[8,121] Glare and Lickiss[47] describe 90% of patients in a palliative care program as experiencing constipation. Preventing severe constipation requires treating consistently and prophylactically. Often the discomfort of constipation is more distressing to the patient than other pain. If there are not orders for a bowel regimen, the nurse should obtain them immediately (see interventions for constipation, p. 762). Walsh[121] offers the SOS plan:

1. Stool softener (docusate sodium—Colace)
2. Osmotic laxative (Milk of Magnesia) if stool softener does not work
3. Stimulant laxative (bisacodyl—Dulcolax)

Nausea/vomiting. In a study conducted by Campora, Merlini, and Pace,[18] 18% of patients on morphine had moderate to severe nausea and 28% experienced emesis. Approximately 40% of patients receiving narcotics will develop mild to moderate nausea. The intensity of nausea and/or vomiting in patients receiving opioids varies from patient to patient and from opioid to opioid. The etiology of the nausea/vomiting appears to be the result of the effect of opioids on the chemoreceptor trigger zone in the medulla, increased vestibular sensitivity, and delayed gastric emptying. This side effect generally decreases after 2 to 3 days of repeated dosing[72,121] as tolerance to the side effect develops. The side effect should be treated aggressively; it may require ATC management for 1 to 2 weeks. Antiemetic trials are warranted if nausea/vomiting is a problem.

Sedation. Because opioids have a depressant effect on the central nervous system, some drowsiness can be anticipated. Once pain management is achieved, normal extended sleep patterns should not be confused with sedation; the person may have been exhausted from interrupted sleep patterns caused by previous pain and may, in fact, sleep for extended periods initially just to "catch up." The questions to ask follow:

• Is the person alert and oriented when awake?
• Has the person established a good nighttime sleep pattern?
• Is the person arousable from sleep?

If sedation persists for more than 3 to 5 days, possible added stimulation might be required; methylphenidate counteracts sedation related to opioids.[118]

Confusion and hallucinations. These are most often temporary, lasting a few days to a week or two.[24]

The nurse should be aware of impaired renal function (because it will have an impact on the clearance of the narcotics); some other possible causes of confusion to be ruled out are cerebral metastases, hypercalcemia, and sepsis. Because the source of the impaired mental status (IMS) may be multicausal, all possible causes must be evaluated. The active morphine metabolite, morphine-6-glucuronide (M-6-G) has been implicated in both IMS and myoclonus in patients receiving morphine. A study reported in 1995 by Tiseo and others[114] found that neither IMS nor myoclonus was significantly associated with M-6-G/morphine ratio when adjusted for other variables. The study did confirm the correlation between decreased renal function and increasing M-6-G/morphine ratio. Active metabolites of opioids can be a source of IMS, and Bruera and others[14] demonstrated a lower incidence of IMS with hydration of one liter and opioid rotation in terminal cancer patients. Tolerance to these side effects usually develops within 48 to 72 hours. Foley[45] states that haloperidol is the drug of choice to treat drug-induced psychosis. Haloperidol in low doses (0.5 to 1.0 mg PO) is often used[24,45] because of its efficacy and low incidence of cardiovascular and anticholinergic effects.

Pruritus. This intense itching is more often observed with the administration of intraspinal narcotics and is not frequently seen with the other routes of administration. The person will exhibit this first on the face and may be unconsciously rubbing or scratching at the nose or cheeks. This can be managed with an antihistamine or with even a dilute infusion of a mixed agonist/antagonist or naloxone. Pruritus is not life-threatening but is certainly bothersome. Rapid nursing intervention will enhance the comfort level of the patient.

Respiratory depression. Tolerance to this potential side effect develops rapidly (see box below). The Texas

---

GUIDELINES FOR RESPIRATORY DEPRESSION

1. Always have a baseline respiratory rate.
2. Respiratory depression is usually slow in onset and preceded by sedation.
3. Respiratory depression usually occurs:
   7 minutes after IV
   30 minutes after IM
   90 minutes after SC
4. Use a flow sheet to record respiratory rate and pain relief.
5. Dilute Narcan 0.1 to 0.4 mg in 10 ml saline and administer intravenously over 2 to 4 minutes.

Data from McGuire L: Pain. In Beare PG, Myers JL: *Principles and practice of adult health nursing,* ed 2, St. Louis, 1994, Mosby.

NURSING MANAGEMENT

NURSING DIAGNOSIS

• *Constipation*

OUTCOME GOALS

Patient will be able to:
• Verbalize understanding of constipation as a continuous side effect of opioids.
• Report bowel activity.
• Drink 2-3 L of fluids per day.
• Verbalize understanding of dietary bulk and exercise needs.
• Take medication as prescribed.

INTERVENTIONS

• Assessment at regular intervals:
—Are bowel sounds present?
—What is the normal elimination pattern?
—Is there an established bowel elimination pattern of every ≤3 days?
—Number of stools per day?
—Character of stool?
—Absence of stool elimination?
• Action:
—Treat prophylactically.
—General nursing measures:
   Promote adequate fluid intake of 2-3 L/day.
   Encourage high-fiber diet.
   Promote exercise/activity as tolerated.
• Obtain orders for medications and administer as needed:
—Docusate sodium (e.g., Colace, Modane Soft)
   range: 1-2 tablets TID
—Senna (e.g., Senokot)
   range: 2-4 tablets BID
—Docusate sodium + senna (e.g., Senokot-S)
   range: 2-4 tablets BID
—Bisacodyl (e.g., Dulcolax; a bisacodyl enema = Fleet)
   range: 2-3 tablets HS
—Colyte
   range: 8 oz QD or BID

RATIONALE

• The opiate side effect of diminished neural stimulation resulting in constipation will *not* diminish over time.

• Provide hydration to bowel contents.
• Increase bulk.
• Improve general tone and stimulation.
• Routine administration required if equivalent of 30 mg PO morphine per 24 hr.
• Stool softener that lowers surface tension, permitting water and fats to penetrate and soften stools.
• Mild natural laxative derivative from the Cassia plant; it induces peristalsis.
• Stool softener plus mild laxative (see above).

• A contact laxative that stimulates sensory nerves to produce parasympathetic reflexes resulting in increased peristaltic contractions of the colon.
• An electrolyte lavage; a glycol acts as an osmotic agent, and there is virtually no net ion absorption or loss.

NURSING DIAGNOSIS

• *Nutrition, altered: less than body requirements related to nausea and/or vomiting*

OUTCOME GOALS

Patient will be able to:
• Verbalize understanding of temporary nature of nausea/vomiting.
• State techniques to reduce impediments to nutritional intake.
• Take antiemetics as prescribed, based on need.

INTERVENTIONS

- Monitor and record I & O.
- Weigh every 3-5 days, if appropriate.
- Record number of episodes of emesis per 24 hours.
- Teach patient/family techniques to improve nutritional intake:
  —Small, frequent meals.
  —Reduce odors.
  —Eat in pleasant surroundings.
  —Do not lie flat immediately after a meal.
- Administer antiemetics as needed:
  —Hydroxyzine (e.g., Vistaril, Atarax)
      range: 25-50 mg q 4-6 hr
  —Prochlorperazine (e.g., Compazine)
      range: 10 mg q 4-6 hr
  —Thiethylperazine (Torecan, Norzine)
      range: 10 mg q 8 hr
  —Chlorpromazine (e.g., Thorazine)
      range: 10-25 mg q 4 hr
  —Metoclopramide (e.g., Reglan)
      range: 10-20 mg q 6 hr
  —Haloperidol (Haldol)
      range: 0.5-1.0 mg q 4-8 hr

NURSING DIAGNOSIS

- *Sleep pattern disturbance related to sedation*
- *Thought processes, altered, related to confusion*

OUTCOME GOALS

Patient will be able to:
- Verbalize understanding of the temporary nature of sedation and confusion.
- Take stimulants as prescribed, based on need.

INTERVENTIONS

- Assess and document:
  —Patient's ability to communicate and comprehend.
  —Patient's disorientation/confusion, agitation, or impaired memory.
- Interview patient/family:
  —Are they comfortable with the level of alertness, or is it troublesome in any way?
- Discuss other possible causes with other members of the health care team.
- Administer stimulants as needed:
  —Caffeine
      range: 65 mg (to 200 mg/day)
  —Methylphenidate (e.g., Ritalin)
      range: 10-15 mg (divide between early AM and noon)
  —Dextroamphetamine (e.g., Dexedrine)
      range: 5-10 mg AM[82]; 2.5-10 mg[5]
- Orient to person, place, and time prn.

RATIONALE

- The side effect of nausea/vomiting is usually transitory and will subside within 3-7 days.

- Has antiemetic, analgesic, and mild sedative activity[8] as well as being an antihistamine.
- Antiemetic.

- Antiemetic.

- Antiemetic; use if sedation is desired, may reduce hiccups.
- Promotes gastric emptying.

- Antiemetic; use if patient is too sedated.

RATIONALE

- Sedation and/or confusion caused by opiates will decrease with repeated dosing.

- The individuality of each person is to be respected.

- Impaired renal function, hypercalcemia, or brain metastases can be the cause of confusion/sedation rather than the opiates.
- Stimulant; has been shown to increase analgesia when given with aspirin-like drugs[5]
- Stimulant; has analgesic properties; low toxicity (4%) includes hallucinations and paranoia; tolerance may develop within 1 month and dose require escalation.[9]
- Stimulant; side effects may include anxiety, anorexia, or nervousness.
- Confirm reality.

Continued.

NURSING DIAGNOSIS

• *Breathing pattern, ineffective, related to respiratory depression secondary to use of opiates*

OUTCOME GOALS

Patient will be able to:
• Verbalize understanding of the rare occurrence of respiratory depression with ongoing use of opioids.
• Exhibit absence of true respiratory depression.

INTERVENTIONS	RATIONALE
• Assess rate, depth, and quality of respirations, especially after dose escalation: —Respiratory rate ≥10 —Breathing pattern is even and unlabored	• True respiratory depression related to opiates is rare in the person who is not opiate-naive because the body develops a tolerance to the side effects.
• If respiratory depression is questioned, assess for hypoxia: —Labored respirations —Tachypnea —Tachycardia —Cyanosis —Position is semi- or high-Fowler's.	• Physiologic changes that occur with hypoxia.
• Distinguish between respiratory depression caused by opiates and a natural change if patient is terminal.	• A natural change in respiratory pattern (Cheyne-Stokes) occurs as death approaches.
• Administer naloxone (Narcan) *only after determination of true respiratory depression.*	• Opiate antagonist; use with caution to avoid profound withdrawal, seizures, and severe pain. The APS[8] recommends a dilute solution (0.4 mg in 10 ml saline) administered as 0.5 ml IV push every 2 minutes.
• Discuss rare occurrence of true respiratory depression with patient/family.	• Provide education and support to reduce fears of causing death rather than providing pain relief.

Cancer Plan states that there is an inordinate fear of respiratory depression.[51] Pain is a natural antagonist to the respiratory depressant effects of opiates, and therefore pain provides a natural stimulant. "When respiratory depression occurs, it is usually in opioid-naive patients."[60] Pasero and McCaffery[88] identify the rate of clinically significant respiratory depression in hospitalized adults receiving opioids as 0.09%. A sleeping rate of six to eight respirations per minute may be normal in the totally relaxed person. The "arousable factor" is a satisfactory guide: Can the person be aroused rather quickly from sleep? This will stimulate respirations. "New respiratory symptoms are virtually never a primary drug effect in those receiving stable doses of narcotics."[89] When doses are escalated, respirations should be monitored for any drastic change even though it is unlikely. The patient/family should understand that respiratory depression is a rare occurrence with continued use of opioids and that death is not being promoted.

Naloxone (Narcan) is an opiate antagonist but must be used with caution to avoid profound withdrawal, seizures, and severe pain. The APS[8] recommends diluting 0.4 mg in 10 ml of saline and giving 0.5 ml IV push every 2 minutes.

Potentiators

By definition, to potentiate is to endow with power or make potent. A word of caution is required regarding what is referred to as the use of "potentiators" to increase the effectiveness of an analgesic. Medicine and nursing have long taught that when the phenothiazine promethazine (Phenergan) is added to a narcotic, it will intensify (or potentiate) the analgesic effect of the narcotic. Studies by McGee and Alexander[76] and Dundee and Moore[34] show that, in fact, promethazine may only increase the intensity of one's pain. McCaffery calls this an antianalgesic effect. What is observed in the patient is more a potentiation of the side effects: increased sedation, hypotension, and respiratory depression. The American Pain Society[8] states that "except for methotrimeprazine (Levoprome 10-20 mg. available in parenteral formulation only), *phenothiazines neither relieve pain nor po-*

tentiate opioid analgesia". Hydroxyzine (Vistaril, Atarax) does have analgesic properties and may be a useful adjunct for the patient who is also anxious or nauseated.[8]

GENERAL PRINCIPLES OF ANALGESIC ADMINISTRATION

1. *Choose the analgesic appropriate to the type and level of pain.* The choice of a non-opioid or weak, moderate, or strong opioid should be based on pain intensity that is determined through careful assessment (See Figure 29-1). The concept of an orderly progression from the occurrence of pain to its successful management can be visualized as the rungs of a ladder in the following sequence:
   - Pain exists.
   - Use a non-opioid with or without an adjuvant drug.
   - If pain persists or increases . . .
     Use an opioid for weak to moderate pain, with or without a non-opioid, and with or without an adjuvant drug
   - If pain persists or increases . . .
     Use an opioid for moderate to strong pain, with or without a non-opioid, and with or without an adjuvant drug. The top rung of this ladder is freedom from cancer pain. This orderly progression allows for trials of various medications at all levels and ensures that everything is being attempted to control the pain across the spectrum.

2. *Choose the easiest and most cost-effective route of administration.* Based on the KISSING principle (Keep It Sanely Simple In Narcotic Giving)—use the oral route whenever possible! If nausea and/or vomiting prohibit this route, try the rectal route. Consider the following progression of routes:
   - Oral
   - Rectal
   - Transdermal
   - Subcutaneous
   - Intramuscular
   - Intravenous
   - Intraspinal (epidural or intrathecal)

3. *Schedule administration.* ATC dosing is mandatory to achieve a steady state of analgesia and avoid the peaks and valleys that produce cycles of pain periods alternating with sedation. A PRN schedule should never be used because the pain level then escalates and the patient must spend time just to "catch up" to prior levels of analgesia. The important feature here is to stay ahead of the pain, and this principle requires teaching and reinforcement by nurses because it differs from usual pain management to which patients are accustomed.

4. *Be prepared for breakthrough pain.* Whatever the medication, route, or frequency of administration, an order should be available for "breakthrough" pain. This is a sudden, and sometimes brief, increase in pain that may be the result of increased activity or a particular motion. This "rescue dose" is administered over and above the regularly scheduled ATC medication. If three to four analgesic doses are required each 24 hours, the ATC regularly scheduled doses should be increased to include the amount used for previous breakthrough pain while still maintaining a PRN dose for future breakthrough pain.

5. *Plan treatment of side effects.* Management of side effects must be done aggressively and often should be prophylactic. Be aware that the following side effects may occur with the repeated administration of opioids:
   - Constipation (does *not* decrease over time)
   - Nausea/vomiting (usually temporary, lasting about 1 week)
   - Sedation (usually temporary)
   - Respiratory depression (rarely occurs)
   - Other (confusion/hallucinations, dizziness, urinary retention)

6. *Never use placebos.* Placebos have no place in the oncology patient population. As McCaffery states, "Pain is whatever the client says it is, whenever he says it does."[73]

Adjuvant (Co-analgesic) Drugs

Several medications have been found to be analgesic for particular types of pain. These drugs may be ordered for other than their usual indications (Table 29-5). They should be used only after an adequate trial of opioids has proven ineffective.[92] See Table 29-6 for drugs and routes of administration not recommended for treatment of cancer and pain.

Antidepressants. These can produce analgesia in particular circumstances and are appropriate despite a lack of emotional depression; they seem to act by increasing the serotonin level. Indications are neuropathic pain (especially burning), depression, or insomnia. Gonzales[49] describes the use of amitriptyline for postherpetic neuralgia. Foley[45] states that there may be some response within 1 week but that it may take 2 to 3 weeks for full effect.

The analgesic therapeutic dose of antidepressants is only one eighth to one sixth of the dose required to treat clinical depression.

Anticonvulsants. Indications are for neuropathic pain (especially shooting or stabbing), lancinating pains (e.g., postherpetic pain), tics, or myoclonic jerks. The mechanism of action is presumably suppression of paroxysmal neural discharges.[92]

Stimulants. Indications are to increase analgesic effect of other medications or to reduce the sedative effect of opioids.

Table 29-5 Adjuvant Co-analgesics

Drug	Dose	Indications	Comments
TRICYCLIC ANTIDEPRESSANT			
Amitriptyline (Elavil)	25-150 mg daily (hs); start at low dose and titrate upward to effect	Neuropathic and postherpetic neuralgia (especially burning pain)	Side effects include dry mouth, urinary retention, sedation, orthostatic hypotension, delirium; may potentiate narcotics by blocking re-uptake of serotonin (a neurotransmitter)
Nortriptyline (Pamelor, Aventyl)	25-100 mg	Same	Same; less orthostatic hypotension; available in liquid form
Desipramine (Norpramin)	25-150 mg	Same	Same; less sedation and anticholinergic effects
Imipramine (Tofranil)	25-100 mg	Same	
Doxepin (Sinequan)	25-150 mg	Same	

The analgesic therapeutic dose of antidepressants is ⅛ to ⅙ of dose required to treat clinical depression.

Drug	Dose	Indications	Comments
ANTIHISTAMINE			
Hydroxyzine (Vistaril, Atarax)	25-50 mg PO or IM q 4-6 hr	Pain together with nausea, anxiety	Has analgesic effects (50 mg IM = 5 mg morphine) as well as antianxiety, antiemetic, and antihistamine effects; irritating to tissue
ANTICONVULSANT			
Carbamazepine (Tegretol)	100 mg q 6-8 hr	Neuropathic lancinating pain (shooting/stabbing) (e.g., postherpetic neuralgia, tic-like pain caused by nerve injury)	Side effects include vertigo, sedation, confusion, and bone marrow suppression; contraindicated in leukopenia
Clonazepam (Klonopin)	0.25 mg q 12 hr	Same	
Phenytoin (Dilantin)	3-5 mg/kg/day	Same	Side effects include ataxia, skin rash, liver dysfunction; plasma levels should be monitored
Valproic acid (Depakene)	15 mg/kg/day	Same	Hepatotoxic; available in liquid form
STEROID			
Dexamethasone (Decadron)	10-20 mg × 1; then 4 mg q 6 hr; up to 96 mg if spinal cord compression	Neuropathic pain caused by infiltration or compression (e.g., brachial or lumbosacral plexus); increased intracranial pressure; spinal cord compression	Reduces edema in tumor and nerve tissue; chronic use may cause weight gain, Cushing's syndrome, increased risk of GI bleed with NSAIDs
Prednisone	20-80 mg/day		
BENZODIAZEPINE			
Diazepam (Valium)	5-10 mg PO or IV TID	Acute anxiety or muscle spasm associated with acute pain	Side effects: sedation, respiratory depression (also used in terminal dyspnea); not effective analgesic except for muscle spasm

Data from Agency for Health Care Policy and Research (AHCPR): *Management of cancer pain,* 1994, Publication No. 94-0592; American Pain Society: *Principles of analgesic use in the treatment of acute pain and chronic cancer pain,* ed 3, 1992; Weissman DE and others: *Handbook of cancer pain management,* ed 4, 1994, Wisconsin Cancer Pain Initiative.

hs, Bedtime; *PO,* by mouth; *IM,* intramuscular; *TID,* three times a day; *IV,* intravenous; *GI,* gastrointestinal; *NSAIDs,* nonsteroidal antiinflammatory drugs.

Table 29-5 Adjuvant Co-analgesics—cont'd

Drug	Dose	Indications	Comments
Lorazepam (Ativan)	1-2 mg PO or IV TID	Same	
STIMULANT			
Caffeine	65 mg	Lethargy; counteract sedative effect of opioids	Side effects: insomnia, tachycardia, palpitations, anorexia; may produce additive analgesia
Dextroamphetamine (Dexedrine)	2.5-7.5 mg AM & noon	Same	Same
Methylphenidate (Ritalin)	5-15 mg/day	Same	Same; tolerance may develop over 1 month, requiring dose escalation
LOCAL ANESTHETIC			
Mexiletine (Mexitil)	150 mg q 8 hr	Neuropathic pain	Clinical trials done in diabetic neuropathy; is a cardiac dysrhythmic agent
Flecainide (Tambocor)	50 mg q 12 hr	Neuropathic pain	Survey of cancer patients with malignant infiltration of nerves[83]; is a cardiac dysrhythmic agent
Tocainide (Tonocard)	20 mg/kg/day[54]	Neuropathic pain	Is a cardiac dysrhythmic agent
Lidocaine 2.5% and prilocaine 2.5% (EMLA)	Topical cream applied thickly	Postherpetic neuralgia; before procedure	Must be applied 1 hour before procedure; use only on *intact* skin
RADIOPHARMACEUTICAL			
Strontium-89 (Metastron)	4 mCi	Prostatic and breast metastasis to bone; osteoblastic sites	Administered IV; effect lasts several months; side effects include myelosuppression and pain flares[88]
BIPHOSPHONATE			
Pamidronate (Aredia)	60 mg over 4 hr; 90 mg over 24 hr	Bone metastases	Inhibits osteoclastic activity; effect lasts 2 weeks

Corticosteroids. Indications are for nerve infiltration or compression, bone pain, increased intracranial pressure, anorexia, or mood disorders.

Local anesthetics. Local anesthetics may be injected locally, applied topically, or taken orally. They block sodium channels and therefore block the action potential and impede the transduction of pain. All oral local anesthetics must be used cautiously in patients with cardiac diagnoses. The use of Eutectic Mixture of Local Anesthetics (EMLS) was demonstrated by Taddio and others[113] to significantly lower pain scores in infants on whom it was applied before immunization.

Radiopharmaceuticals. Specifically used in metastatic osteoblastic bone lesions related to prostate or breast cancer, Strontium-89 provides pain relief in as many as 80% of patients, with a median response of 6 months.[95] It is administered intravenously over 2 min-

utes by radiation oncologists. One side effect to monitor is bone marrow suppression, which may temporarily result in 20% to 30% reductions in leukocyte and thrombocyte counts, according to Robinson and others.[98] This agent does not appear to affect tumor activity, and therefore the current objective is pain palliation with an improvement in quality of life.

Routes of Administration

The box on p. 769 presents the routes of administration. Each of these routes is described in the discussion that follows.

Oral. Oral the route of choice for economy, safety, and ease in pain management. Even severe pain requiring high doses of narcotics can be managed orally as long as the patient is able to swallow medication without difficulty. Several studies have shown that 70% to 90% of

Table 29-6 Drugs and Routes of Administration Not Recommended for Treatment of Cancer Pain

Class	Drug	Rationale for not recommending
Opioid	Meperidine	Short (2-3 hr) duration; repeated administration may lead to central nervous system (CNS) toxicity (tremor, confusion, or seizures); high oral doses required to relieve severe pain, and these increase the risk of CNS toxicity.
Miscellaneous	Cannabinoids	Side effects of dysphoria, drowsiness, hypotension, and brady-cardia preclude its routine use as an analgesic.
	Cocaine	Has demonstrated no efficacy as an analgesic or co-analgesic in combination with opioids.
Opioid agonist-antagonist	Pentazocine	Risk of precipitating withdrawal in opioid-dependent patients; analgesic ceiling.
	Butorphanol	
	Nalbuphine	Possible production of unpleasant psychomimetic effects (e.g., dysphoria, hallucinations).
Partial agonist	Buprenorphine	Analgesic ceiling; can precipitate withdrawal.
Antagonist	Naloxone	May precipitate withdrawal; limit use to treatment of life-threatening respiratory depression.
	Naltrexone	
Combination preparation	Brompton's cocktail	No evidence of analgesic benefit to using Brompton's cocktail over single opioid analgesics.
	DPT (meperidine, promethazine, and chlorpromazine)	Efficacy is poor compared with that of other analgesics; high incidence of adverse effects.
Anxiolytic alone	Benzodiazepine (e.g., alprazo-lam)	Analgesic properties not demonstrated except for some instances of neuropathic pain; added sedation from anxiolytics may limit opioid dosing.
Sedative/hypnotic drug alone	Barbiturates	Analgesic properties not demonstrated; added sedation from sedative/hypnotic drugs limits opioid dosing.
	Benzodiazepine	

ROUTES OF ADMINISTRATION		**RATIONALE FOR NOT RECOMMENDING**
Intramuscular (IM)		Painful; absorption unreliable; should not be used for children or patients prone to develop dependent edema or for patients with thrombocytopenia.
Transnasal		The only drug approved by the FDA for transnasal administration at this time is butorphanol, an agonist-antagonist drug, which generally is not recommended. (See opioid agonist-antagonists above.)

Jacox A and others: *Management of cancer pain: clinical practice guideline,* No. 9, AHCPR Publication No. 94-0592, Rockville, Md, March 1994, Agency for Health Care Policy and Research, U.S. Department of Health and Human Services, Public Health Service.

pain experienced by cancer patients can be controlled by oral administration of analgesics.[53,123] It is very important to convert the parenteral to oral doses correctly because they are different and the amounts cannot be interchanged (see Tables 29-3 and 29-4). Education may be required to convince the patient/family that they do not need "shots" to control the pain and that parenteral administration does not mean stronger medication. As long as the equianalgesic amount is the same, the analgesic effect will be the same. Sustained-release morphine is now available, which makes 12-hour dosing effective.

The buccal or sublingual surface may be used for absorption of liquid analgesics in small quantities. Data from controlled clinical studies are not available, but anecdotes from practice support the idea[44,73]:

• *Buccal*—the space between the cheek and gum of the

upper molars; this does not stimulate salivation. Foley[45] states that the tablet must remain in contact with the gum for 1 to 2 hours.

• *Sublingual*—beneath the tongue; administration guidelines are 1 ml every 3 minutes. According to Stanley and Ashburn,[110] the highest permeability occurs sublingually, but Foley[45] states that morphine is poorly absorbed sublingually but anecdotally is reported to be effective. Robison and others[99] reviewed the absorption, bioavailability, and tolerance of sublingual versus oral morphine. They state that there is no significant advantage of sublingual over the oral route and that nurses must continue to evaluate their actions through comprehensive pain assessment and base their decisions on the individual response of patients (i.e., efficacy and tolerance to taste). Coyle[24] states that the sublingual route has limited value in cancer pain manage-

ROUTES OF ADMINISTRATION

ORAL

- Preferred route for analgesics; patients maintain control
- Allows greater mobility
- Drug levels peak in 1 to 2 hours
- Ease in administration
- Cost efficient

TRANSMUCOSAL

- Indicated only for hospital setting: (1) preanesthetic; (2) conscious sedation
- Unit is constructed as a "lollipop" to suck (not chew)
- Available as fentanyl
- For short-term use only

RECTAL

- Good for patients who are NPO, nauseated, or unable to swallow
- May be more expensive than oral route and more difficult to obtain
- Most often a 1:1 ratio with oral

TRANSDERMAL

- Good for patients who are NPO, nauseated, or unable to swallow
- Takes 14-24 hours to peak initially; lasts approximately 17 hours after removal
- A fentanyl patch lasts 2-3 days
- Ease in administration
- Difficult to titrate
- Local anesthetics (2.5% lidocaine and 2.5% prilocaine [EMLA]) can be used for cutaneous and mucosal lesions (e.g., postherpetic neuralgia, ulcers)
- Capsaicin (0.025%) may cause a burning sensation after application; apply four times per day

SUBCUTANEOUS INFUSION

- Provides prolonged parenteral administration of narcotics and/or intermittent bolus
- Avoids repetitive injections
- Avoids peaks and valleys in bloodstream
- Avoids need for intravenous access
- Readily managed at home
- Recommended for cancer patients who cannot take anything by mouth
- Requires use of infusion pump with alarms

PATIENT-CONTROLLED ANALGESIA (PCA)

- Allows patient to receive a predetermined intravenous bolus of a narcotic by a pump mechanism
- Gives patient sense of control, less anxiety
- Provides quick pain relief
- Patient may require less narcotic
- Eliminates the need for repeated injections

IV CONTINUOUS INFUSION

- Provides constant narcotic intravenous infusion to maintain constant blood levels
- No peaks and valleys in blood levels
- Recommended when unable to achieve pain control through oral or rectal routes with high dosages of narcotics or unable to use oral/rectal route
- Requires use of infusion pump with alarms

IV BOLUS

- Good for acute pain and/or procedures
- Provides most rapid onset but shortest duration
- Not recommended for constant pain because of peaks and valleys in bloodstream

IM INJECTION

- Should be used mainly for acute short-term pain
- Painful administration; rotate sites
- Not recommended for chronic long-term pain—especially cancer pain
- Not recommended for use with children, emaciated patients, or patients with a decrease in muscle mass

SPINAL ADMINISTRATION
Epidural

Dose: 5-10 mg morphine
Pain relief: 12-24 hours

Intrathecal (subarachnoid)

Dose: 0.5-1.0 mg morphine
Pain relief: up to 36 hours

- Narcotic (usually morphine) administered through catheter into epidural or intrathecal space
- May be intermittent bolus or by continuous infusion pump
- Careful selection of the patient necessary as procedure is expensive and may be risky
- Side effects include nausea, vomiting, pruritus, sedation, urinary retention, respiratory depression
- Possible complication of infection and/or meningitis

ment because of poor absorption of most drugs, inability to deliver high doses, and the lack of specific sublingual formulations.

• *Transmucosal*—a convenient unit of fentanyl is prepared as a lollipop for children to suck preoperatively. Although contraindicated for a child 15 kg or less, the recommended dose above that weight is 5 to 10 mcg/kg.

Rectal. If oral administration is not possible because of the presence of nausea/vomiting, if the person is unable to swallow, or if dysphagia is present, the same dose of oral medication administered rectally can also achieve pain relief. Controlled studies are not available to support the practice fully, but it appears that the rectal mucous membrane absorbs equally to the oral cavity (thus a 1:1 ratio) and may prevent the necessity of changing to a parenteral route. The limitations for this route include the presence of diarrhea, anal/rectal fissures, or thrombocytopenia.

Available prepared suppositories include[22,73]:

Morphine (5, 10, 20, or 30 mg)
Hydromorphone (Dilaudid) (3 mg)
Oxymorphone (Numorphan) (5 mg)

Transdermal. Now on the market in the form of a controlled-release "patch." Duragesic is fentanyl, a short-acting narcotic, which is available as a 72-hour continuous-release product and patients/families can manage this with ease. There will be a delay of approximately 12 to 24 hours[59,64,84] until the peak serum level of fentanyl is reached; therefore supplemental medications will be required. A trial period may be needed to make certain that the dose is correct and that the product does indeed provide analgesia for a 72-hour duration for the patient; a subset of patients will require patch exchange every 48 hours instead of 72 hours. After removing the patch, it takes an average of 17 hours for the fentanyl serum concentration to fall by 50%; therefore the patient should be monitored for 24 to 36 hours after discontinuation.

Subcutaneous. This is an often overlooked route since intravenous administration has become customary. The ratio of dosing for subcutaneous versus IM/IV is 1:1. A small gauge (25 or 27 gauge) butterfly needle can be placed anywhere there is adequate subcutaneous tissue (e.g., abdomen or even thigh if the individual is not ambulatory), and the line may be used continuously or intermittently. The site should be inspected every 8 hours for redness, edema, and tenderness, but the butterfly needle can be left in place for 5 to 7 days without changing sites if there are no complications. Ideally, the medication should be concentrated so that there is 1 ml or less infused per hour, but it is possible to administer even larger amounts if absorption is adequate. Bruera and others[15] describe the successful subcutaneous infusion of

narcotics and fluids at the rate of 20 to 100 ml/hr with the addition of hyaluronidase and potassium chloride (KCl). Any medication with a parenteral formulation can be used for subcutaneous infusion.

Moulin and others[82] compared the efficacy of subcutaneous and intravenous routes and found no statistically significant differences in pain intensity, pain relief, mood, or sedation between the two routes. Johanson[63] reports a cost savings of $350 per week with subcutaneous administration rather than intravenous.

Intravenous. For home use, a permanent central venous access device would probably be required. Unless the patient requires the access for other purposes (e.g., hydration, nutrition, antibiotics), it adds considerable cost (the device, surgeon's fee, surgical suite costs, maintenance) without additional benefit over other routes for pain management. If the patient cannot swallow, has diarrhea, and has inadequate subcutaneous tissue, this may be the route of choice. It can be used intermittently (with a flushing schedule) or continuously via a patient-controlled analgesia (PCA) system.

Patient-controlled analgesia (PCA). This method of pain control involves a machine-delivery system that is programmed by the nurse and can deliver a basal (continuous) amount with an incremental/bolus (intermittent) amount, or a combination of both. Ideally, a PCA system will be programmed to have a continuous (basal) infusion that covers the usual analgesic requirements and a bolus option available to treat breakthrough pain incidences. This type of technology can be used either subcutaneously or intravenously and allows the patient to have control over this area of life, namely pain management.

Intramuscular. Although this route has been used over time for pain management, it is least preferred for the person with cancer, who may require medications for an extended period. Sites may become limited, absorption may become erratic, and, more important, it requires the added pain of an injection when the intent is to relieve pain.

Direct central nervous system (CNS) administration. When the other methods of analgesic administration have been tried and they are not effective (e.g., intolerable side effects, high dose levels), a route that may indeed provide relief is via the opiate receptors of the spinal column. The analgesia is produced by the direct effect on the opiate receptors in the dorsal horn of the spinal column. According to Lamer,[68] the major advantage of spinal opioids is pain relief with minimal side effects. The sites may be the following:

• *Epidural*—a catheter is placed between the vertebral column and the dura. The patient will require about one tenth the amount of narcotic as required parenterally. According to Lamer,[68] the major advantage of spinal opioids is pain relief with minimal side effects.

• *Intrathecal*—a catheter is placed in the subarachnoid region. The patient will require about one hundredth of the narcotic as required parenterally.

The placement of the catheter requires strict aseptic technique by a skilled physician. The epidural or intrathecal catheter may be tunneled to the exterior for intermittent injection, or a port/pump may be implanted for continuous infusion with a bolus option. Pain relief is extended (12 to 24 hours) after a single injection, but for some individuals a continuous infusion may be more efficacious.

Direct CNS analgesia is a relatively new area in nursing practice, and it requires that each state determine what its nurse practice act allows in regard to an intraspinal catheter (e.g., inject [and if nurses may inject, which medications may be injected?]). Nurses working with spinal administration of narcotics must have documentation of adequate educational preparation for care. The agency/institution must have policies and procedures to govern practice.

Wilkie[127] advocates the use of preservative-free solutions until current research determines whether preservatives are harmful. One other area of question is whether to use alcohol or povidone-iodine to cleanse the injection port. Most of the guidelines specify povidone-iodine because of the known toxic effect of alcohol to the spinal cord.[7]

Because this pain management modality is costly, it is usually not considered unless life expectancy is at least 3 months. It falls into the category of "high-tech," and the other modalities warrant trials first.

NONPHARMACOLOGIC PAIN RELIEF TECHNIQUES

Nurses can teach the patient/family many activities that aid in the reduction of pain. These interventions are most effective when the pain level is low, but they can also be used as an adjunct to medications when the pain is moderate. Research to support many of these mechanical or psychosocial interventions is lacking, but in many instances they have merit and warrant a trial basis.

Most of the interventions are inexpensive and easy to perform. As Spross[106] states, "They may appear too simple or too 'low tech' to be of use in the 'high tech' settings in which cancer patients receive care." Most have low risks and few side effects, and, very important, they provide the ability for the patient to have some control over this aspect of their pain management.

Noninvasive pain relief techniques can be useful alone or as adjuncts to the management of pain. The mechanical techniques consist of cutaneous stimulation (therapeutic touch, pressure, heat, cold, massage, and transcutaneous electrical nerve stimulation [TENS]). Behavioral pain relief techniques include distraction, imagery/

visualization, music, humor, prayer, education, play therapy, biofeedback, and hypnosis.

Mechanical interventions	Behavioral interventions
Cutaneous stimulation	Relaxation
Therapeutic touch	Distraction
Pressure	Imagery/Visualization
Massage	Music
Heat/cold	Humor
TENS	Prayer
	Education
	Play therapy
	Biofeedback
	Hypnosis

Noninvasive Mechanical Interventions

Cutaneous stimulation. Cutaneous stimulation is any activity that stimulates the skin for the purpose of relieving pain. Massage is one form of this intervention.

Heat and cold. Because applications of heat and cold are so common and because they have been used for so long, nurses may underestimate their value in pain control. Heat may provide comfort and relaxation, whereas cold may produce numbness and decrease pain-causing substances (e.g., bradykinin, potassium, lactic acid).[106] Both heat and cold decrease pain and muscle spasm. Deciding which therapy to use should be based on the physiologic effects desired (Table 29-7).

Important factors that the nurse should remember when using heat or cold therapy are the age of the patient, medical history, condition of the skin, and any discomfort. Some patients may benefit from alternating heat and cold therapy. However, if the patient cannot tolerate heat or cold therapy, it should be discontinued.

Transcutaneous electrical nerve stimulation (TENS). TENS consists of a pocketsize, battery-operated device that provides a continuous mild electrical current to the skin via electrodes. The electrodes are generally placed on or near the painful site. The stimulation is again of the large nerve fibers, which will "close" the gate.

TENS units have different dials so that the patient can adjust the intensity, rate, and pulse width (duration) to achieve a soothing, pleasant sensation.

Table 29-7   Effects of Heat and Cold

	Heat	Cold
Pain	Decreased	Decreased
Muscle spasm	Decreased	Decreased
Inflammation	Increased	Decreased
Blood flow	Increased	Decreased
Hemorrhage	Increased	Decreased
Edema	Increased	Decreased

Data from McGuire L: Pain. In Beare PG, Myers JL: *Principles and practices of adult health nursing,* ed 2, St. Louis, 1994, Mosby.

The nurse plays an important role in teaching these techniques, in assessing whether they are being done correctly, and in evaluating whether they are indeed effective.

Behavioral Interventions

Behavioral interventions focus the person's mind on something other than the pain sensation. They may be effective because they assist to decrease the person's anxiety. These techniques are very individual as to the person's preference and will be effective only when the person believes that they will work.

For behavioral interventions to be effective, the nurse must explore the interest areas of the patient, determine which areas may have meaning for the patient, and determine if the patient believes the approach will make a difference in relieving pain. Each technique requires time to teach and practice in order to become effective. Briefly, the techniques are described below:

Relaxation. Relaxation is the state of relative freedom from both anxiety and skeletal tension. Some examples include distracting thoughts, rhythmic breathing, peaceful images, quiet environment, and repetition.[73]

Distraction. Distraction is focusing on stimuli other than the pain sensation. This is often done without realizing that it is a form of analgesia and is reducing the sensation of pain. Distraction helps alter the patient's ability to tolerate pain. Some examples include music (auditory distraction), tapping (tactile distraction), television or flowers (visual distraction), people, and humor. Each of these activities may easily be employed with little or no cost and used as an adjunct to medications, but distraction has a short duration and does not replace pharmacologic analgesics.[73]

Imagery/visualization. Mentally creating a picture is the use of one's imagination. This may be a focus on a close person, a place of enjoyment, a past event, or anything that is thought to bring pleasure. Examples of imagery include emptying the sandbag, breathing out pain, and a ball of healing energy. The mind is occupied, and therefore the pain is reduced in focus.[73]

Music. Music (tapes, records, CDs, live performances) is used to take the thoughts away from the painful sensation. This is very individual as to the person's preference, and the patient's choice must be explored. A teenager's choice of music would probably not be the choice of the person over 70, and the person trained in classical music may not be a country/western fan.[73]

Humor. Laughter is used as a distraction. Humor can provide immediate distraction, but it also can provide prolonged pain relief even up to 2 hours. Does the person have a favorite comedian? Are there audio or visual recordings available of that person performing? Is there a joke book that would match the person's sense of humor? Encourage the use of humor because many people who experience an ongoing pain find that they have little to laugh about.[73]

Prayer. Prayer is the use of communication with a higher power. Obviously the patient's religious beliefs need to be explored. Is the person a Christian and accustomed to talking with God? Is the person a Hindu for whom there are many gods? Is the person a Moslem who prays to Allah? Is the person an atheist for whom there is no god or higher power and for whom this would not be an option?

Play therapy. Play therapy is the use of games or toys. This can be especially useful for children, but it is also for adults. To play is to involve the person physically and mentally in an activity and thus provide distraction. To a child, dolls can become the object taking on the pain. To an adult, a board game may provide a scene of competition and focus from which they are not otherwise involved.

Biofeedback. Biofeedback is the ability to alter the body functions (e.g., heart rate, blood pressure, muscle relaxation) by intentional mental focusing. This requires the skill of a professional person who is trained in the technique; it may be more difficult in the home setting, but the person may have used this approach in the past and it is worth exploring as an adjunct during this time of pain.

Hypnosis. Hypnosis is the use of psychotherapy to alter the affective component as well as the sensory component of pain; the patient's perception of pain is modified. Hypnosis has been used to decrease stress, but studies on its efficacy in pain control are lacking. Hypnosis requires a professional who is skilled in teaching hypnosis, and again, it may not be feasible for the home setting. Ahles[4] questions how effective this technique might be for patients with other than mild to moderate pain. More research is required in this area.[73]

Invasive Techniques

"In a substantial minority of patients, estimated at 1% to 15%, the use of these invasive procedures is necessary."[62] A discussion of invasive procedures follows.

Nerve blocks. The nerve block is an injection of an anesthetic agent into or near a nerve to numb pain pathways. The nerve block can be performed with either a local temporary anesthetic agent or a permanent neurolytic agent. Local anesthetic agents provide pain relief for several hours to days. The celiac plexus block can be used for pain arising from the pancreas, upper retroperitenum, liver, gallbladder, and proximal small bowel. Response rates in pancreatic cancer are 50% to 90% and response lasts 1 to 12 months, according to Cherny.[19] In a meta-analysis of celiac plexus blocks by Eisenberg and others,[35] good to excellent response rates were identified in 89% of patients during the first 2 weeks and in 90%

of patients alive at 3 months. The pain source determines the appropriate nerve block:

Pain source	Block
Perineum	Sacral
Chest	Intercostal
Abdominal viscera	Celiac plexus or splanchnic nerve
Pelvic viscera	Hypogastric plexus

Neurosurgical procedures. Neurosurgical procedures for pain relief are surgical or chemical (alcohol) interruption of pain pathways. It is essential that patients be carefully selected for these procedures and that they completely understand the potential risks and benefits.

Acupuncture. Acupuncture, the insertion of needles at various points into the body to relieve pain, comes from the Latin words *acus,* needle, and *pungere,* puncture. This invasive technique is based on an ancient Chinese theory of two opposing forces, *yin* and *yang;* the Chinese theory says that pain and illness are caused by an imbalance of yin and yang. It is theorized that acupuncture works because it stimulates large nerve fibers to close the gate in the spinal cord to pain impulses. It is also postulated that acupuncture causes the release of endorphins.

QUALITY ASSESSMENT AND IMPROVEMENT

Pain, as well as other aspects of health care, must be assessed for quality management. A basic first step is the development of policies and procedures related to pain. Coluzzi[23] found that 62% of NCI-designated cancer centers had written pain policies and procedures. Accurate evaluation of improvement of pain management must incorporate measurement of outcomes, which for pain includes patient satisfaction. Several groups have addressed this issue and have set standards that can be applied to an individual health care agency.

1. The Oncology Nursing Society (ONS) together with the American Nurses Association (ANA) in 1987 published the "Standards of Oncology Nursing Practice." The "standards are primarily intended to help nurse generalists provide effective care and pursue professional development."[107-109]
2. The Joint Commission on Accreditation of Healthcare Organizations (JCAHO) has included in their 1992 Manual for Hospitals the following section under Patient Rights:
   • The organization supports the rights of each patient.
   —Organizational policies and procedures describe the mechanism by which the following rights are protected and exercised:
   —The care of the dying patient optimizes the comfort and dignity of the patient through
   Effectively managing pain
   This is the first time that pain has been included in JCAHO standards and signifies the importance of ad-

dressing pain management as an individual patient's right.
3. The American Pain Society (APS) has developed "Standards for Monitoring Quality of Analgesic Treatment of Acute Pain and Cancer Pain." (See Appendix A.) Each of the standards is identified as structure, process, or outcome and can be used in an agency's Quality Assessment and Improvement program. The document includes a patient interview tool to measure patient satisfaction. The APS Quality of Care Committee[10] conducted studies of the implementations of the guidelines at three medical centers and identified five key elements of quality improvement pain programs.
   • Assuring that a report of unrelieved pain raises a "red flag" that attracts clinicians' attention
   • Making information about analgesics convenient where orders are written
   • Promising patients responsive analgesic care and urging them to communicate pain
   • Implementing policies and safeguards for the use of modern analgesic technologies
   • Coordinating and assessing implementation of these measures
4. The Agency for Health Care Policy and Research (AHCPR), an interdisciplinary federal panel of health care experts, in 1992 released the Guidelines on Acute Pain Management: Operative or Medical Procedures and Trauma.
5. In 1994 the Agency for Health Care Policy and Research (AHCPR) published Cancer Pain Management.

The implementation of any of the guidelines/standards requires an interdisciplinary collaborative effort. Duncan and Otto[33] describe the process starting with a task force consisting of four physicians, four nurses and one pharmacist with a nurse facilitator.

Thus there are now a national accrediting body, national professional organizations, and the federal government that have developed and published information that asks the basic questions:
• Is pain being addressed as a symptom?
• How well is pain being managed?
   . . . from the patient's point of view?
   . . . from the health care professional's point of view?
Quality Assessment and Improvement (QAI) audits are important to be able to document current status and future improvements in pain management. Coluzzi and others[23] found that 50% of NCI-designated facilities performed pain audits. One outcome which can be monitored is readmission for pain. Grant and others[50] report a study in which 12.8% of 804 unscheduled readmissions were for pain. Of the 103 unscheduled readmissions related to pain, 54% of those were within 12 days of discharge. After implementing a pain edu-

cation program, identifying pain as a quality improvement focus, and providing additional personnel, the total percent of admissions for uncontrolled pain was reduced from 4.4% to 3%.

- Is there adequate documentation? Siehl[104] states "only when our documentation of specific pain interventions is complete, then so is the application of our knowledge in relieving pain for our patients."
- What education is needed (professional and lay)? Max[71] proposes that education alone may not be sufficient to change behaviors and that guidelines and tools need to be developed to ease assessment and communication between and among patients and health care professionals. Dalton and others[30] describe an educational program for rural nurses in North Carolina. The interactive program was conducted 1 day per week for 6 weeks. There were demonstrated improvements in documentation, descriptions of pain, use of pharmacologic and nonpharmacologic treatment, follow-up evaluation, and use of pain-related consultants. This program incorporated didactic and practice experiences and used guidelines for documentation that were updated during the course.

The issue of the effectiveness (or the lack of effectiveness) of pain management has also become a legal issue. Angarola and Donato[11] report that a jury awarded $15 million in damages to a family as a result of nursing actions that caused increased pain and suffering through withholding narcotics during the terminal illness of a man with prostate cancer metastasized to the spine and femur. Cushing[27] and Shapiro[103] state that the jury award was later resolved, and an undisclosed amount was settled among the parties. Yes, pain management is becoming a quality of care issue.

THE NURSING ROLE IN PAIN MANAGEMENT

Although the care of patients with pain is multidisciplinary, in most cases nursing care is the cornerstone.[72] Pain management is a challenge that every nurse must face when caring for a patient with cancer. Regardless of the setting, the nurse has a vital role in pain management because the nurse has the ongoing contact with the patients in pain. Nurses must be vocal in the area of cancer pain. A nurse who is an advocate for cancer pain management need not be a pain expert, but rather one who is dedicated to the problem of cancer pain relief. An algorithm (decision-making tree) for the progression of pain management through the WHO ladder has been developed by Hudzinski.[58]

Assessment Issues in Pain Management

Nursing is involved in obtaining a detailed quantitative and qualitative assessment of the patient's pain experience. Pain is a subjective experience, and it is only the person who has the pain who is able to legitimately de-

scribe the event in detail. In a study reported by Yeager and others,[130] there were several differences found between patients and their caregivers, with caregivers viewing the experience more negatively than the patients. Family caregivers reported the following:

1. Patients had significantly higher levels of pain than patient reports
2. Patients experienced significantly greater distress than the patients reported
3. The caregivers experienced greater distress from the patients' pain than the patients reported.

Ferrell and others[43] found that an educational intervention by homecare nurses was effective in supporting patients and families in pain management.

Again, the most meaningful and accurate assessment of pain is directly from the patient.[62]

As early as 1987, the NIH Consensus Development Conference stated that "nurses have well-established pivotal roles in the assessment and management of pain."[83] The importance of a thorough pain assessment was emphasized in the ECOG cancer pain study, in which 76% of the physicians identified inadequate pain assessment as a barrier to cancer pain management.[119]

Nursing's qualitative assessment includes observations of behavior and appearance and the patient's description of sensations and personal impact of the pain. The quantitative assessment includes the patient's description of the intensity of the pain and the analgesic requirements over time. Many assessment tools are available, but care must be taken to select one that the patient can use. Shannon and others[102] recommend (1) beginning pain assessment while the patient is able to respond and (2) monitoring behaviors specific to that person that indicate pain. This study found that 44.8% of patients were unable to use the McGill-Melzack Pain Questionnaire, the Memorial Pain Assessment Card, or the Faces Pain Rating Scale because of cognitive impairment, a communication barrier, or other reasons.

Qualitative assessment includes the following:
- Reported symptoms associated with moderate to severe pain[68]:
  —Mood disturbances: anxiety, depression, anger, and irritability
  —Decreased ability to concentrate/communicate
  —Loss of appetite, nausea, and vomiting
  —Sleep disturbances/sleep deprivation
  —Sexual dysfunction/lack of interest
  —Splinting, limited mobility, disuse syndromes
  —Fatigue
  —Behavioral changes
- Classification of pain
  —Acute: less than 3 to 6 months
  —Chronic: longer than 3 to 6 months
- Location
  —Is it confined to one area, or does it radiate?

—Has it changed from a previous location or extended beyond a previous site?
- Quality—Because the source of pain can vary, it is imperative that the nurse elicit a description that describes the pain most accurately. Use the patient's own words for what the pain feels like. Keep in mind that the following descriptors may indicate a particular type of pain:
  —Burning: possibly neuropathic pain
  —Stabbing: possibly neuropathic pain
  —Dull or sharp: possibly somatic pain
  —Constant or deep: possibly visceral pain
- Duration
  —Onset: when did it start?
  —Intermittent: does it last briefly after movement?
  —Constant: does it never go away?
- Aggravating and Relieving Factors
  —What makes the pain worse? . . . better?
  —Does it help to lie down, stand, sit up?
  —What has person tried?
     Analgesics?
     Type?
     Dose?
     Frequency?

     Positioning
     Heat/cold
     Massage
  —Does the pain interfere with activities of daily living (ADLs)? Is sleep affected (awakens because of pain)? Is sociability limited?
  —What is the expectation for pain relief?
     An acceptable level that is tolerable
     No pain
Quantitative assessment includes the following:
- Intensity—0 to 10 with "0" being no pain and "10" the worst pain imaginable. The intensity may be a verbal or visual identification. (See Figure 29-3 for assessment scale.) A conversion of numbers into word descriptors for the levels may include the following:
  — 0 = None
  — 2 = Mild—pain unnoticed with activity
  — 4 = Discomforting—sometimes interferes with activities or sleep
  — 6 = Distressing—usually interferes with activities or sleep
  — 8 = Severe—severely "restricts" person
  —10 = Excruciating—unable to tolerate

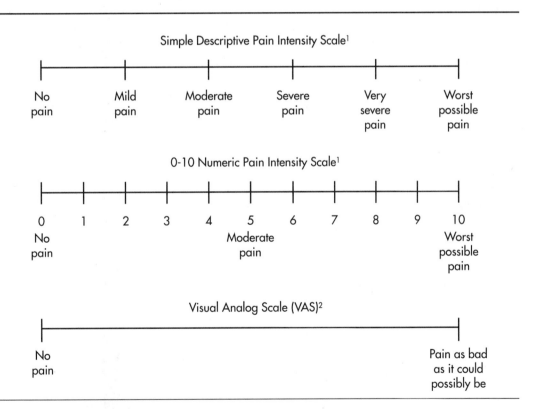

Simple Descriptive Pain Intensity Scale¹

| No pain | Mild pain | Moderate pain | Severe pain | Very severe pain | Worst possible pain |

0-10 Numeric Pain Intensity Scale¹

0 1 2 3 4 5 6 7 8 9 10
No pain   Moderate pain   Worst possible pain

Visual Analog Scale (VAS)²

No pain   Pain as bad as it could possibly be

¹If used as a graphic rating scale, a 10-cm baseline is recommended.
²A 10-cm baseline is recommended for VAS scales.

Figure 29-3   Examples of pain intensity scales. (From Agency for Health Care Policy and Research [AHCPR]: *Management of cancer pain: adults, clinical practice guideline,* Rockville, Md, March 1994, Agency for Health Care Policy and Research, U.S. Department of Health and Human Services, p. 26.)

- Equianalgesic amounts per 24 hours—it is important for the nurse to calculate what the total amount of analgesics required per 24 hours has been and convert this into the common language of morphine equivalents. (See Tables 29-3 and 29-4 for details.) Figure 29-4 is an example of a pain assessment chart that contains both qualitative and quantitative elements. The continuing assessment portion allows for a graphic display of pain intensity over time, which is valuable information for all members of the health care team.

GERIATRIC PAIN ISSUES

A segment of our population that has been often overlooked in the management of pain is the elderly. With the increase in longevity and the resultant "aging population," health care professionals must develop a more acceptable attitude toward administering pain medications and controlling pain in the elderly. Ferrell[40] reports of two reviews of geriatric textbooks and their sparse content on pain management. Of 11 medical textbooks, only 2 had chapters addressing pain, and of 5000 pages of nursing geriatric texts, fewer than 18 pages dealt solely with pain. In addition, little pain research has been designed specifically for the elderly.

McCaffery and Beebe[73] have a chapter devoted to this topic with explanations and recommendations. Some of the myths that impede health care professionals in adequately managing pain in the elderly are the following:

- Pain is a natural outcome of growing old.
- Pain perception, or sensitivity, decreases with age.
- The potential side effects of narcotics make them too dangerous to use to relieve pain in the elderly.
- If the elderly patient appears to be occupied, sleeps, or can be otherwise distracted from pain, he or she does not have much pain.
- If the older person is depressed, especially if there is no known cause for the pain, depression is causing the pain. Pain is a symptom of depression and would subside if the depression were effectively treated.
- Narcotics are totally inappropriate for all patients with chronic nonmalignant pain.

With so many myths regarding pain in the elderly, what physiologic realities does the nurse need to keep in mind when addressing pain in the elderly?

Nursing Issues Related to the Care of Geriatric Patients

- Distribution of drugs—there are changes in the body composition (an increase of fat and decrease in heart, kidney, and muscle mass) as aging occurs; therefore usual adult doses may need to be decreased to avoid toxic drug levels in the blood and tissue. Decreased circulating proteins as a result of serum proteins, malnutrition, or chronic disease potentially result in greater

drug effect from higher concentrations of unbound drug, with a greater risk of toxic effect.
- Metabolism of drugs—there is limited research in the area of hepatic metabolic rates in relation to aging, but it may be safer to allow for longer intervals between doses in the elderly.
- Excretion of drugs—a decrease in renal mass, renal blood flow, glomerular filtration rate, and tubular secretion can all occur in the kidney because of aging. With reduced function, the drugs or their active metabolites may remain in the body longer.

For an elderly population, analgesics are appropriate for pain management with the following considerations:

- The dose may need to be decreased.
- The interval between doses may need to be lengthened.
- The frequency of assessment and evaluation is increased.
- The responses cannot be predicted or generalized.

PEDIATRIC PAIN ISSUES

Hester[54] states that pain in children is underaddressed. She also reports on several studies that have shown that pain is often a presenting symptom when children are diagnosed with cancer; more than half of the cases of leukemia, lymphoma, and soft tissue sarcomas and *all* of the cases of Ewing's sarcoma, osteosarcoma, and neuroblastoma presented with pain.

Banos and Barajas[12] noted in a letter to the editor that there are now a number of pain assessment tools with established validity and reliability. The question then becomes, Are the current assessment tools being used?

See Table 29-4 for medications and doses for people <50 kg.

Guideline
Older than 12 years: full adult dose
7 to 12 years: 50% of adult dose
2 to 6 years: 20% to 25% of adult dose

Vetter[117] reports a study of morphine versus meperidine patient-controlled analgesia (PCA) systems in 50 pediatric patients. There was no difference in side effect occurrence, but there was a statistically significant difference in pain scores; the morphine group had better (lower) scores.

Nursing Issues Related to the Care of Pediatric Patients

- Assess accurately
- Approach preventively
- Titrate to effect

In other words, intervene exactly as you would for other age-groups; the analgesics are the same, but the doses, based on body weight, are different.

When a child in the family has cancer, it is difficult for everyone. Ferrell and others[42] reported a study of

Text continued on p. 781.

Pain Assessment Chart (For Admission and/or Follow-up) _____

1. Patient _____ 2. DX _____

Assessment on Admission

Date _____ / _____ / _____   Pain ☐   No Pain ☐   Date of Pain Onset _____ / _____ / _____

1. Location of Pain (indicate on drawing)

2. Description of Predominant Pain (in patient's words) _____

   _____

   _____

3. Intensity [Scale 0 (no pain) – 10 (most intense)] _____

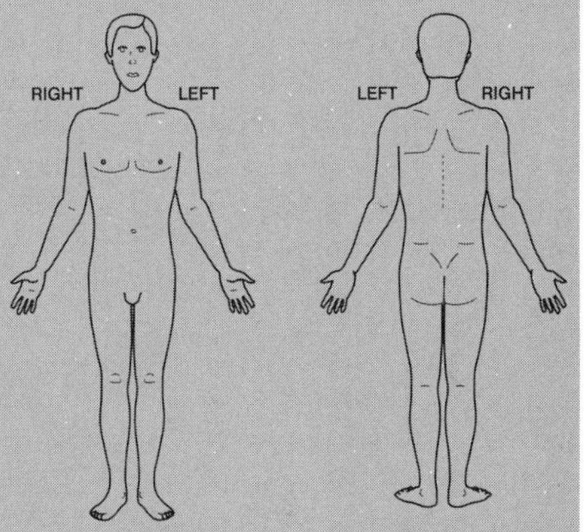

   _____

4. Duration & when occurs _____

   _____

5. Precipitating Factors _____

   _____

6. Alleviating Factors _____

   _____

7. Accompanying Symptoms

   GI: Nausea ☐   Emesis ☐   Constipation ☐   Anorexia ☐

   CNS: Drowsiness ☐   Confusion ☐   Hallucinations ☐

   Psychosocial: Mood _____   Anger _____

   Anxiety _____   Depression _____

   Relationships _____

   _____

8. Other Symptoms

   Sleep _____   Fatigue _____

   Activity _____   Other _____

9. Present Medications _____

   _____

   _____

   Doses and times medicated last 48 hours _____

   _____

10. Breakthrough Pain _____

    _____

Signature: _____

Figure 29-4   Pain Assessment Chart. (From The Purdue Frederick Company, 1991. Prepared in consultation with Carol P. Curtiss, RN, MSN, OCN; Betty Ferrell, PhD, FAAN; and Alfred L. McKee, MD.)   _Continued._

Continuing Pain Assessment and Interventions

Date/ Time														
Med(s)/ Dose														

Most Intense Pain — No Pain Sensation, scale 10 to 0

Blood Pressure														
Respiration														
Nausea														
Emesis														
Constipation														
Anorexia														
Drowsiness														
Confusion														
Hallucination														
Sleep														
Activity														
Mood														

INSTRUCTIONS: Ask patient to rate the intensity of his/her pain. Plot this rating on the graph and connect the dots.

Figure 29-4—cont'd. For legend see p. 777.

NURSING MANAGEMENT

NURSING DIAGNOSES

Once the assessment of pain is completed, appropriate nursing diagnoses may include the following:
• *Alterations in:*
  —*Comfort (pain, sleep, and/or pruritus)*
  —*Mobility, impaired physical*
  —*Coping*
  —*Constipation*
  —*Diarrhea*
  —*Protection, altered*
• *Knowledge deficit related to action of analgesics, schedule of administration, potential side effects*
• *Anxiety*
• *Fear*
• *Fatigue*
• *Spiritual distress*
• *Social isolation*
• *Hopelessness*[107]

OUTCOME GOALS: *Qualitative Components*

Patient will be able to:
• Participate in ongoing pain assessment.
• Identify qualitative components of pain.
• State the quality of the pain in descriptive terms.
• Identify previous aggravating and alleviating factors.
• State expectation of pain relief.

INTERVENTIONS: *Qualitative Components*

• Assessment:
  —Conduct on a systematic, ongoing basis.
  —Use a tool that addresses *qualitative* components:
    Reported symptoms
    Mood disturbances (anxiety, depression, anger, irritability)
    Decreased ability to concentrate/communicate
    Loss of appetite, nausea, and vomiting
    Sleep disturbances/sleep deprivation
    Sexual dysfunction/lack of interest
    Splinting, limited mobility, disuse syndromes
    Fatigue
    Behavioral changes
    Interference with activities of daily living (ADLs)[68]
    Location (one or more sites)

    Quality:
      Burning (neuropathic)
      Stabbing (neuropathic)
      Dull or sharp (somatic)
      Constant or deep (viseral)

RATIONALE

• For accurate knowledge of patient's pain status and outcome of previous analgesic interventions.

A change in location may be a new pain or a referred pain.
Particular descriptor may indicate a specific type of pain.
Use the patient's own words for what the pain feels like.

Continued.

Duration:
  Onset
  Intermittent or constant
Aggravating and relieving factors:
  Standing, sitting, lying down
  What has the person tried (analgesics, heat/cold, massage, positioning)?
  Expectation for pain relief (an acceptable level or no pain)?

Incorporating previously effective methodologies into the plan of care recognizes the past involvement of patient and family, strengthening a sense of personal control.

If the patient's expectations are not realistic (i.e., total pain relief and no side effects), disappointment in the health care system could arise.

OUTCOME GOALS: *Quantitative Components*

Patient will be able to:
- Use a consistent method of quantifying pain intensity.
- Identify effective pain relief strategies.
- Accept pain medication as prescribed.
- Participate with members of the interdisciplinary pain management team.
- Discuss documentation tools and be aware of their content.
- Report accurately whether pain relief has occurred.

INTERVENTIONS: *Quantitative Components*

RATIONALE

- Assessment:
  —Conduct on a systematic, ongoing basis.
  —Use a tool that addresses *quantitative* components:
    Intensity (0-10 scale)

  Equianalgesic amount required per 24 hours

Consistency in measurement gives a measurable means to determine an increase or decrease in severity.
A common base of amounts (i.e., morphine) provides a consistent measurement of analgesic requirements.

• • •

- Planning (qualitative and quantitative):
  —Determine whether current treatment is adequate and whether patient is satisfied with the pain relief.
- Interventions (qualitative and quantitative):
  —Administer analgesics according to pain requirements and based on the principles of cancer pain management.
  —Investigate the possible use of behavioral interventions in addition to analgesics.
  —Instruct patient on behavioral pain management interventions.
  —Collaborate with other health care professionals (e.g., physician, pharmacist, social worker) to use team approach to care.
- Evaluation and documentation (qualitative and quantitative):
  —Use tools to measure:
    Intensity
    Satisfaction
    Quality of life
  —Conduct evaluation at intervals appropriate for severity of pain as a problem.

See analgesic tables (29-2 to 29-4) for specific medication information.

Active participation in pain relief measures will increase the sense of personal control.

An interdisciplinary team approach will address the total spectrum of pain.

Written information is available to the interdisciplinary team.

The evaluation frequency is dependent upon whether pain is an active patient problem.

PLANNING: *Qualitative and Quantitative*

- Where is the patient on the World Health Organization (WHO) stepladder of pain management? (See Figure 29-1.)
- Is current treatment adequate?
- Does physician need to be contacted for additional orders?
- Do the patient and family understand (and agree with) the current treatment plan?
- Is the patient satisfied with pain relief, or is more pain relief desired?

EVALUATION: *Qualitative and Quantitative*

Once assessment, planning, and interventions have been implemented, evaluation then proceeds to determine effectiveness of pain management. Evaluation includes keeping a daily pain diary in which the patient/family record the following data on an ongoing basis:

- Intensity—is the pain rating score lower than it was before?
- Analgesic intake (per 24 hours)
- Satisfaction—is the patient/family pleased with the effect of the analgesic therapy? What more can be done?
- Quality of life—is the patient doing what she or he wants to do? Is pain interfering in any way with activities or personal interactions?

See box on right for patient teaching priorities.

PATIENT TEACHING PRIORITIES
Pain Management

Nurses play a major role in the teaching process. It may be spontaneous and informal or a lengthy session with resources (see Appendix B for available printed materials.) Some of the areas of patient education are the following:
Cause of pain
Anticipated outcome (pain relief)
  Is the patient expecting no pain or manageable pain?
What to report to MD/RN
  Unmanaged side effects
  Uncontrolled pain
Medication information (schedule, dose, refills, drug interactions)
Side effects of medications and what to do to prevent or treat them (e.g., patient may be drowsy the first few days of narcotic use, but this effect will pass)
Information to restructure attitudes and beliefs regarding addiction, medications, etc.
Plan for follow-up and who to call for emergency assistance
Patient's and providers' responsibilities for pain management plan

According to Jacox and others,[62] patients should receive a written pain management plan of care whenever possible and this does reinforce verbal instructions. The public is receiving more information about pain management. Lay literature has articles addressing the myths and misconceptions and where to call for information (e.g., NCI, APS, ACS).[69] Hill[56] strongly states that successful pain management may depend on empowering patients to demand adequate pain treatment and that empowerment requires teaching the public about pain.

families with a child who had cancer. They found that the experience of pain was distressing to family members (x = 79.03 on a 0-100 scale) and that there was a need for basic knowledge of pain principles.

CONCLUSION

Nurses are central to the successful management of cancer pain. As Spross[104] stated in her ONS/Schering Clinical Lecture, "Pain is an emergency for the person with cancer and, because of the distress it causes, nurses should respond with the same sense of urgency that exists when nurses respond to spinal cord compression or hypercalcemia." *Not only can you make a difference in successful cancer pain management for the patient who is experiencing pain, you do make the difference.*

■ CHAPTER QUESTIONS

1. When considering all types and stages of cancer, the incidence of pain is:
   a. 10%-50%
   b. 20%-60%
   c. 40%-80%
   d. 50%-90%
2. The side effect of opioid administration that does *not* diminish with repeated dosing is:
   a. Nausea
   b. Sedation
   c. Constipation
   d. Pruritus
3. All of the following *except* one may be used as adjuvant or coanalgesics for neuropathic pain. The exception is:
   a. Dextroamphetamine
   b. Amitriptyline

 b. Carbamazepine
 c. Dexamethasone
4. The equianalgesic conversion from the oral to rectal route of morphine administration is:
 a. 1:1
 b. 1:3
 c. 1:4
 d. 1:6
5. The nursing assessment of pain includes both qualitative and quantitative aspects. A qualitative assessment includes:
 1. nature of pain 2. 24-hour analgesic requirement
 3. location of pain 4. intensity
 a. 1, 2
 b. 1, 3
 c. 2, 3
 d. 2, 4
6. The most accurate evaluation of pain and/or the efficacy of an analgesic regimen is:
 a. Nurse
 b. Physician
 c. Significant other
 d. Patient
7. The complex neurophysiologic activity that results in pain comprises four steps:
 a. Transduction, transmission, sensation, modulation
 b. Transduction, transmission, perception, modulation
 c. Transduction, transmission, perception, sensation
 d. Transduction, transmission, perception, communication
8. Behavioral interventions for pain management include:
 a. Relaxation, distraction, imagery, music, opioids
 b. Distraction, imagery, music, biofeedback, TENS
 c. Distraction, humor, visualization, TENS, prayer
 d. Relaxation, imagery, music, prayer, play therapy

BIBLIOGRAPHY

1. Ad Hoc Committee on Cancer Pain of the American Society of Clinical Oncology: Cancer pain assessment and treatment guidelines, *J Clin Oncology* 10(12):1976, 1992.
2. Agency for Health Care Policy and Research (AHCPR): *Management of cancer pain,* Rockville, MD: U.S. Department of Health and Human Services, Publication No. 94-0592, 1994.
3. Agency for Health Care Policy and Research (AHCPR): *Acute pain management: operative or medical procedures and trauma: clinical practice guideline,* Rockville, MD: U.S. Department of Health and Human Services, Publication No. 92-0032, 1992.
4. Ahles T: Psychological techniques for the management of cancer-related pain. In McGuire DB, Yarbro CH, editors: *Cancer pain management,* Orlando, Fla, 1987, Grune & Stratton.
5. American Cancer Society: *Cancer statistics 1996, CA Cancer J Clin* 46(1):8, 1996.
6. American Hospital Formulary Service: *Opiate agonists,* Bethesda, Md, 1991, American Society of Hospital Pharmacists.
7. American Nurses Association Position Statement on the Role of the Registered Nurse in the Management of Analgesia by Catheter Techniques, *Am Nurse,* 67(2):7, 1992.
8. American Pain Society: *Principles of analgesic use in the treatment of acute pain and chronic cancer pain,* ed 3, 1992. (Copies available through the American Pain Society, 4700 West Lake Ave., Glenview, IL 60025).
9. American Pain Society Subcommittee on Quality Assurance Standards: Standards for monitoring quality of analgesic treatment of acute pain and cancer pain, *Oncol Nurs Forum* 17(6):952, 1990.
10. American Pain Society Subcommittee on Quality of Care Committee, *JAMA* 274:1874, 1995.
11. Angarola RT, Donato BJ: Inappropriate pain management results in high jury award (letter), *J Pain Symptom Manage* 6(7):407, 1991.
12. Banos J, Barajas C: Assessment of pediatric pain: time for an agreement, *J Pain Symptom Manage* 10(3):181, 1995.
13. Blanchard JS, Seale DD: Lessons from the first year of a state cancer pain initiative, *J Oncol Manage* 2(6):22-28, 1993.
14. Bruera E and others: Changing pattern of agitated impaired mental status in patients with advanced cancer: association with cognitive monitoring, hydration, and opioid rotation, *J Pain Symptom Manage* 10(4):287, 1995.
15. Bruera E and others: Hypodermoclysis for the administration of fluids and narcotic analgesics in patients with advanced cancer, *J Pain Symptom Manage* 5(4):218, 1990.
16. Brunier G, Carson MG, Harrison DE: What do nurses know and believe about patients with pain? Results of a hospital survey, *J Pain Symptom Manage* 10(6):436, 1995.
17. Cahill C, Panzaulla C, Spross JA: Pediatric cancer pain. In Oncology Nursing Society Position Paper on Cancer Pain—Part III, *Oncol Nurs Forum* 17(6):948, 1990.
18. Campora E and others: The incidence of narcotic-induced emesis, *J Pain Symptom Manage* 6(7):428, 1991.
19. Cherny NI, Portenoy RK: The management of cancer pain, *CA Cancer J Clin* 44(5):262, 1994.
20. Cleeland CS and others: Pain and its treatment in outpatients with metastatic cancer, *N Engl J Med* 330(9):392, 1994.
21. Cohen FL: Postsurgical pain relief: patients' status and nurses' medication choices, *Pain* 9:265, 1980.
22. Cole L, Hanning CD: Review of the rectal use of opioids, *J Pain Symptom Manage* 5(2):118, 1990.
23. Coluzzi PH and others: Survey of the provision of supportive care services at National Cancer Institute–designated centers, *J Clin Oncol* 13(3):756, 1995.
24. Coyle N, Cherny N, Portenoy RK: Pharmacologic management of cancer pain. In McGuire DB, Yarbro CH, Ferrell BR, editors: *Cancer pain management,* ed 2, Boston, 1995, Jones & Bartlett.
25. Cross SA: Pathophysiology of pain, *Mayo Clin Proc* 69:375, 1994.
26. Curtin LL: Promoting comfort and relieving pain in dying patients, *Nurs Manage* 26(8):64, 1995.
27. Cushing M: The legal side: pain management on trial, *Am J Nurs* 92(2):21, 1992.
28. Dahl JL: State cancer pain initiatives, *J Pain Symptom Manage* 8(6):11, 1993.
29. Dahl JL: State cancer pain initiatives: a progress report, *APS Bulletin,* 12(3):5, 1995.
30. Dalton JA and others: Managing cancer pain: content and scope of an educational program for nurses who work in pre-

dominantly rural areas, *J Pain Symptom Manage* 10(3):214, 1995.

31. de Stoutz ND, Bruera E, Suarez-Almazor M: Opioid rotation for toxicity reduction in terminal cancer patients, *J Pain Symptom Manage* 10(5):378, 1995.

32. Donovan MI: An historical view of pain management: how we got to where we are! *Cancer Nurs* 12(4):257, 1989.

33. Duncan SK, Otto SE: Implementing guidelines for acute pain management, *Nurs Manage* 26(5):40, 1995.

34. Dundee JW, Moore J: The myth of phenothiazine potentiation, *Anesthesiology* 16:95, 1961.

35. Eisenberg E, Carr DB, Chalmers TC: Neurolytic celiac plexus block for treatment of cancer pain: a meta-analysis, *Anesth Analg* 80:290, 1995.

36. Eland JM: The child who is hurting, *Semin Oncol Nurs* 1(2):116, 1985.

37. Elliot TE and others: Physician knowledge and attitudes about cancer pain management: a survey from the Minnesota cancer pain project, *J Pain Symptom Manage* 10(7):94, 1995.

37a. Enck RE: Parenteral narcotics for pain control in the home care environment, *Caring* 9(5):38, 1990.

38. Ferrell BR, McCaffery M, Rhiner M: Pain and addiction: an urgent need for change in nursing education, *J Pain Symptom Manage* 7(2):117, 1992.

39. Ferrell BR, Ferrell BA: Easing the pain, *Geriatr Nurs* 11(4):175, 1990.

40. Ferrell BR, Ferrell BA: Pain in elderly persons. In McGuire DB, Yarbro CH, Ferrell BR, editors: *Cancer pain management,* ed 2, Boston, 1995, Jones & Bartlett.

41. Ferrell BR and others: Pain management as a quality of care outcome, *J Nurs Qual Assur* 5(2):50, 1991.

42. Ferrell BR and others: The family experience of cancer pain management in children, *Cancer Practice* 2(6):441, 1994.

43. Ferrell BR and others: The impact of cancer pain education on family caregivers of elderly patients, *Oncol Nurs Forum* 22(8):1211, 1995.

44. Foley KM: Pain and its management. In Wyngaarden JB, Smith LH, Bennett JC, editors: *Cecil textbook of medicine,* ed 19, Philadelphia, 1992, Saunders.

45. Foley KM: Management of cancer pain. In Holland JF and others, editors: *Cancer medicine,* Philadelphia, 1993, Lea & Febiger.

46. Foley KM: Pain assessment and cancer pain syndromes. In Doyle D, Hanks CWC, MacDonald N, editors: *Oxford textbook of palliative medicine,* New York, 1993, Oxford University Press.

47. Glare P, Lickiss JN: Unrecognized constipation in patients with advanced cancer: a recipe for the therapeutic disaster, *J Pain Symptom Manage* 7(6):369, 1992.

48. Glare PA, Walsh TD: Dose-ranging study of oxycodone for chronic pain in advanced cancer, *J Clin Oncol* 11(5):973, 1993.

49. Gonzales GR: Postherpes simplex type 1 neuralgia simulating postherpetic neuralgia, *J Pain Symptom Manage* 7(2):320, 1992.

50. Grant M and others: Unscheduled readmissions for uncontrolled symptoms: a health care challenge for nurses, *Nurs Clin North Am* 30(4):673, 1995.

51. Guidelines for treatment of cancer pain: final report of the Texas Cancer Council's Workgroup on Pain Control in Cancer Patients, Texas Cancer Council, Austin, 1991.

52. Hanks GW, Fallon MT: Transdermal fentanyl in cancer pain: conversion from oral morphine, *J Pain Symptom Manage* 10(2):87, 1995.

53. Hanks GW and others: Difficult pain problems. In Doyle D, Hands GWC, MacDonald N, editors: *Oxford's textbook of palliative medicine,* New York, 1993, Oxford University Press.

54. Hester NO: Integrating pain assessment and management into the care of children with cancer. In McGuire DB, Yarbro CH, Ferrell BR, editors: *Cancer pain management,* ed 2, Boston, 1995, Jones & Bartlett.

55. Hill CS: The barriers to adequate pain management with opioid analgesics: the management of pain in the cancer patient, *Semin Oncol* 20(2) Suppl 1:1, 1993.

56. Hill CS: When will adequate pain treatment be the norm? *JAMA* 274(23):1881, 1995.

57. Hoffman J, Barefield FA, Ramamurthy S: A survey of physician knowledge of drug costs, *J Pain Symptom Manage* 10(6):432, 1995.

58. Hudzinski DM: An algorithmic approach to cancer pain management, *Nurs Clin North Am* 30(4):711, 1995.

59. Inturrisi CE: Management of cancer pain: pharmacology and principles of management, *Cancer* 63(11):2308, 1989.

60. Inturrisi CE, Hanks G: Opioid analgesic therapy. In Doyle D, Hanks GWC, MacDonald N, editors: *Oxford textbook of palliative medicine,* New York, 1993, Oxford University Press.

61. Jacox AD: Health policy and its relation to cancer pain. In McGuire DB, Yarbro CH, Ferrell BR, editors: *Cancer pain management,* ed 2, Boston, 1995, Jones & Bartlett.

62. Jacox AD, Carr DB, Payne R: New clinical practice guidelines for the management of pain in patients with cancer, *N Engl J Med* 330(9):651, 1994.

63. Johanson GA: IV versus SQ opioid infusions for cancer pain, *Am Hospice Palliative Care* July/August:6, 1991.

64. Johanson GA: New routes of opiate administration, *Am Hospice Palliative Care,* 9(4):4, 1992.

65. Kaiko RF: Heroin: facts and comparisons, *PRN Forum* 4:1, 1985.

66. Kaiko RF and others: Central nervous system excitatory effects of meperidine in cancer patients, *Ann Neurol* 13:180, 1983.

67. Kwekkeboom K: Postmastectomy pain syndromes, *Cancer Nurs* 19(1):37, 1996.

68. Lamer TJ: Treatment of cancer-related pain: when orally administered medications fail, *Mayo Clin Proc* 69:473, 1994.

69. Lang SS: Suffer no more. *Good Housekeeping,* Nov:90, 1994.

70. Marks R, Sachar E: Undertreatment of medical inpatients with narcotic analgesics, *Ann Intern Med* 78:173, 1973.

71. Max MB: Improving outcomes of analgesic treatment: is education enough? *Ann Intern Med* 114(4):342, 1991.

72. McCaffery M: Managing your patients' adverse reactions to narcotics, *Am J Nurs* 89(10):166, 1989.

73. McCaffery M, Beebe A: *Pain: a clinical manual for nursing practice,* St. Louis, 1989, Mosby.

74. McCaffery M, Ferrell BR: Opioid analgesics: nurses' knowledge of doses and psychological dependence, *J Nurs Staff Develop* 8(2):77, 1992.

75. McCaffery M and others: Informational needs of nurses, *AS-PMN Pathways* 4(3):1, 3, 1995.

76. McGee JL, Alexander MR: Phenothiazine analgesia: fact or fantasy? *Am J Hosp Pharm* 36:633, 1979.

77. McGuire DB, Sheidler VR: Pain. In Groenwald SL and others, editors: *Cancer nursing: principles and practice,* ed 2, Boston, 1990, Jones & Bartlett.

78. McGuire L: Administering analgesics: which drugs are right for your patients? *Nursing* 90:34, 1990.

79. McLaughlin-Hagan M: Continuous subcutaneous infusion of narcotics, *J Intrav Nurs* 13(2):119, 1990.

80. Merskey H: Classification of chronic pain: description of chronic pain syndrome and definitions of pain terms, *Pain* 3:217, 1986.

81. Miaskowski C, Donovan M: Implementation of the American Pain Society quality assurance standards for relief of acute pain and cancer pain in oncology nursing practice, *Oncol Nurs Forum* 19(3):411, 1992.

82. Moulin DE and others: Comparison of continuous subcutaneous and intravenous hydromorphone infusions for management of cancer pain, *Lancet* 337:465, 1991.

83. NIH Consensus Development Conference: The integrated approach to the management of pain, *J Pain Symptom Manage* 2(1):35, 1987.

84. Niles R: Pharmacologic management of cancer pain, *Nurs Clin North Am* 30(4):745, 1995.

85. Paice JA: The phenomenon of analgesic tolerance in cancer pain management, *Oncol Nurs Forum* 15(4):455, 1988.

86. Paice JA: Unraveling the mystery of pain, *Oncol Nurs Forum* 18(5):843, 1991.

87. Paice JA, Williams AR: Intraspinal drugs for pain. In McGuire DB, Yarbro CH, Ferrell BR, editors: *Cancer pain management,* ed 2, Boston: 1995, Jones & Bartlett.

88. Pasero CL, McCaffery M: Avoiding opioid-induced respiratory depression, *Am J Nurs* 94(4):25, 1994.

89. Portenoy RK, Coyle N: Controversies in the long-term management of analgesic therapy in patients with advanced cancer, *J Pain Symptom Manage* 5(5):307, 1990.

90. Portenoy RK: Cancer pain: from curriculum to practice change, *J Clin Oncol* 10(12):1830, 1992.

91. Portenoy RK: Cancer pain management: the management of pain in the cancer patient, *Semin Oncol* 20(1)suppl 1:19, 1993a.

92. Portenoy RK: Adjuvant analgesics in pain management. In Doyle D, Hanks GWC, MacDonald N, editors: *Oxford's textbook of palliative medicine,* New York, 1993b, Oxford University Press.

93. Portenoy RK: Pharmacologic management of cancer pain. In Yarbro JW, Bornstein RS, Mastrangelo MJ, editors: Chemotherapeutic and nonchemotherapeutic palliative approaches in the treatment of cancer, *Semin Oncol* 22(2)suppl 3:112, 1995.

94. Portenoy RK: Cancer pain: epidemiology and syndromes, *Cancer* 63(11):2298, 1989.

95. Porter AT, Ben-Josef E: Strontium-89 in the treatment of bony metastases. In DeVita VT, Helman A, Rosenberg SA, editors: *Important Adv Oncol* 5:87, 1995.

96. Porter J, Jick H: Addiction rate in patients treated with narcotics (letter), *New Engl J Med* 302(2):123, 1980.

97. Rawlins MD: Non-opioid analgesics. In Doyle D, Hanks GWC, MacDonald N, editors: *Oxford's textbook of palliative medicine,* New York, 1993, Oxford University Press.

98. Robinson RG and others: Clinical experience with strontium-89 in prostatic and breast cancer patients, *Semin Oncol* 20(3)suppl 2:44, 1993.

99. Robison JM, Wilkie DJ, Campbell B: Sublingual and oral morphine administration, *Nurs Clin North Am* 30(4):725, 1995.

100. Schmitt Fink R, Gates R: Cultural diversity and cancer pain. In McGuire DB, Yarbro CH, Ferrell BR, editors: *Cancer pain management,* ed 2, Boston, 1995, Jones & Bartlett.

101. Schug SA and others: A long-term survey of morphine in cancer pain patients, *J Pain Symptom Manage* 7(5):259, 1992.

102. Shannon MM and others: Assessment of pain in advanced cancer patients, *J Pain Symptom Manage* 10(4):274, 1995.

103. Shapiro RS: Liability issues in the management of pain, *J Pain Symptom Manage* 9(3):146, 1994.

104. Siehl S: The need for quality assurance in pain management, *J Pain Symptom Manage* 5(4):215, 1990.

105. Spross JA: Cancer pain and suffering: clinical lessons from life, literature and legend, *Oncol Nurs Forum* 12(4):23, 1985.

106. Spross JA, Burke MW: Nonpharmacological management of cancer pain. In McGuire DB, Yarbro CH, Ferrell BR, editors: *Cancer pain management,* ed 2, Boston, 1995, Jones & Bartlett.

107. Spross JA, McGuire DB, Schmitt RN: Oncology Nursing Society position paper on cancer pain. Part I: Scope of nursing practice regarding cancer pain, ethics and practice, *Oncol Nurs Forum* 17(4):595, 1990.

108. Spross JA, McGuire DB, Schmitt RN: Oncology Nursing Society position paper on cancer pain. Part II: Education, research and list of cancer pain management resources, *Oncol Nurs Forum* 17(5):751, 1990.

109. Spross JA, McGuire DB, Schmitt RN: Oncology Nursing Society position paper on cancer pain. Part III: Nursing administration, pediatric cancer pain and appendices, *Oncol Nurs Forum* 17(6):943, 1990.

110. Stanley TH, Ashburn MA: Novel delivery systems: oral transmucosal and intranasal transmucosal, *J Pain Symptom Manage* 7(13):163, 1992.

111. Stevens PE, Dibble SL, Miaskowski C: Prevalence characteristics and impact of postmastectomy pain syndromes: an investigation of women's experience, *Pain* 61:61, 1995.

112. Swenson CJ and others: Narcotic oral equivalents, *Oncol Nurs Forum* 18(5):942, 1991.

113. Taddio A and others: A revised measure of acute pain in infants, *J Pain Symptom Manage* 10(6):456, 1995.

114. Tiseo PJ and others: Morphine-6-glucuronide concentrations and opioid-related side effects: a survey of cancer patients, *Pain* 61:47, 1995.

115. Twycross RG, Lack SA: *Oral morphine: information for patients, friends and families,* Beaconsfield, Bucks, England, 1983, Beaconsfield Publishers, Ltd.

116. Twycross RG, Lack SA: *Oral morphine in advanced cancer,* ed 2, Beaconsfield, Bucks, England, 1983, Beaconsfield Publishers Ltd.

117. Vetter TR: Pediatric patient-controlled analgesia with morphine versus meperidine, *J Pain Symptom Manage* 7(4):204, 1992.

118. Vigano A, Watanabe S, Bruera E: Methylphenidate for the management of somatization in terminal cancer patients, *J Pain Symptom Manage* 10(2):167, 1995.

119. Von Roenn JH and others: Physician attitudes and practice in cancer pain management, *Ann Intern Med* 119(2):121, 1993.

120. Wallace KG and others: Staff nurses' perceptions of barriers to effective pain management, *J Pain Symptom Manage* 10(3):204, 1995.

121. Walsh TD: Prevention of opioid side effects, *J Pain Symptom Manage* 5(6):362, 1990.

122. Ward SE, Lin CC, Hernandez L: Beliefs about reporting cancer pain and using analgesics: patients' concerns and misconceptions, *APS Bulletin* 12(1):15, 1995.

123. Warfield CA: Guidelines for routine use of controlled-release oral morphine sulfate: the management of pain in the cancer patient, *Semin Oncol* 20(1)suppl 1:36, 1993.

124. Weissman DE: Doctors, opioids, and the law: the effect of controlled substances regulations on cancer pain management: the management of pain in the cancer patient, *Semin Oncol* 20(1)suppl 1:53, 1993.

125. Weissman DE and others: *Handbook of cancer pain management,* ed 4. From the Medical College of Wisconsin and the University of Wisconsin Medical School in conjunction with The Wisconsin Pain Initiative, 1994.

126. Weissman DE, Dahl JL: Update on the cancer pain role model education program, *J Pain Symptom Manage* 10(4):292, 1995.

127. Wilkie DJ: Cancer pain management: state-of-the-art nursing care, *Nurs Clin North Am* 25(2):331, 1990.

128. Wilkie DJ: Neural mechanisms of pain: a foundation for cancer pain assessment and management. In McGuire DB, Yarbro CH, Ferrell BR, editors: *Cancer pain management,* ed 2, Boston, 1995, Jones & Bartlett.

129. World Health Organization (WHO): *Cancer pain relief and palliative care,* Geneva, Switzerland, 1990, World Health Organization.

130. Yeager KA and others: Differences in pain knowledge and perception of the pain experience between outpatients with cancer and their caregivers, *Oncol Nurs Forum* 22(8):1235, 1995.

131. Zhukovsky DS and others: Unmet analgesic needs in cancer patients, *J Pain Symptom Manage* 10(2):113, 1995.

APPENDIX A

STANDARDS FOR MONITORING QUALITY OF AN-
ALGESIC TREATMENT OF ACUTE PAIN AND CANCER
PAIN

AMERICAN PAIN SOCIETY SUBCOMMITTEE ON
QUALITY ASSURANCE STANDARDS

[From American Pain Society Subcommittee on Quality Assurance Standards: Standards for monitoring quality of analgesic treatment of acute pain and cancer pain, *Oncol Nurs Forum* 17[6]:952-954, 1990.]

Summary

Hospital and chronic care facilities in the United States
have active "quality assurance committees" that monitor
selected outcomes of care, working toward steady improvement in results. In order to harness these existing mechanisms to improve pain treatment, the American Pain Society
has drafted a set of standards that embody five key elements
for favorably influencing behaviors of patients and clinicians:
(1) ensuring that a report of unrelieved pain raises a "red
flag" that clinicians cannot ignore; (2) putting information
about analgesics conveniently at hand where orders are
written; (3) promising patients responsive analgesic care and
urging them to communicate pain; (4) providing policies and
safeguards for the use of modern analgesic technologies; and
(5) monitoring the facility's success in implementing these
measures.

Introduction

Undertreatment of acute pain and chronic cancer pain persists despite decades of efforts to provide clinicians with information about analgesics.[32,55,83] Traditional educational approaches, we believe, must be complemented by interventions
that more directly influence the routine behaviors of clinicians
and patients to ensure that pain is communicated and that treatment is rapidly adjusted to provide relief.[10,71,108]

In the United States, virtually all healthcare facilities have
"quality assurance committees" composed of physicians,
nurses, pharmacists, other clinicians, and administrators. Each
committee chooses a number of clinical objectives that it considers important to monitor. They examine process, that is,
whether the appropriate personnel follow the proper procedures
in dealing with the clinical problem, and outcome, the result
for the patient. Outside organizations, most notably the Joint
Commission on Accreditation of Healthcare Organizations
(JCAHO),[61] make regular inspections of facilities to assess
how well they are monitoring care. Because the economic viability of facilities often depends on successful accreditation,
administrators provide strong incentives for professionals to
comply.

To support individual clinicians who wish to make pain relief a targeted outcome in their facilities,[83] the American Pain
Society has developed the following draft standards with the
informal advice of JCAHO staff. The standards will be disseminated through publication in medical and nursing journals
and through mailings to hospitals. Some facilities also may
wish to examine treatment of chronic pain not due to cancer
or nonpharmacological treatments. We have focused, however,

on the drug treatment of acute pain and cancer pain because
there is already a consensus regarding treatment methods.

To facilitate their use, a number of other materials will
be distributed along with these standards, such as the American Pain Society's pamphlet, Principles of Analgesic Use
for the Treatment of Acute Pain and Chronic Cancer Pain[8];
a brief questionnaire, included in the appendix, to assess
patient satisfaction with analgesic care (Standard IC); and
a patient education brochure, still in preparation, that de-
clares the facility's commitment to responsive analgesic
care.

American Pain Society Quality Assurance Standards for Treatment of Acute Pain and Cancer Pain in Hospitals and Chronic Care Facilities

PREFACE (TO BE INCLUDED WITH STANDARDS).
In the majority of patients with acute pain and chronic cancer pain, comfort can be achieved with the attentive use of
analgesic medications. Historically, however, the outcomes
of analgesic treatment often have not been satisfactory,
largely because clinical care units have had no systems in
place to ensure that the occurrence of pain is recognized and
that when pain persists, there is rapid feedback to modify
treatment. These suggested standards are offered as one
approach to developing such a system. Individual facilities
may wish to modify these standards to suit their particular
needs.

The guidelines are intended both for clinical facilities in
which only conventional analgesic methods are used (e.g., intermittent parenteral or oral analgesics) as well as in those using the most modern technology for pain management. In either case, the quality of pain control will be enhanced by a
dedicated pain management team whose personnel acquire special training in pain relief. Newer, more aggressive methods
of pain control, such as patient-controlled analgesic infusion,
epidural opiate administration, and regional anesthetic techniques, may provide better pain relief than intermittent parenteral analgesics in many patients, but they carry their own risks.
Should institutions choose to use these methods, they must be
delivered by an organized team with frequent follow-up and
titration and with adequate briefing of the primary caregivers.
Such teams should be organized under one of the recognized
medical departments of the facility. Specific standards for such
methods, monitored by that department, might well augment
the general guidelines articulated here.

I. ACUTE PAIN AND CHRONIC CANCER PAIN ARE RECOGNIZED AND EFFECTIVELY TREATED

Required Characteristics (Process)

IA.

A measure of pain intensity and a measure of pain relief
are recorded on the bedside vital sign chart or on a similar
record that facilitates regular review by members of the healthcare team and is incorporated in the patient's permanent record.

IA1.

The intensity of pain/discomfort is assessed and documented
on admission, after any known pain-producing procedure, with

each new report of pain, and routinely, at regular intervals that depend upon the severity of pain. A simple, valid measure of intensity will be selected by each clinical unit. For children, age-appropriate pain intensity measures will be used.

IA2.

The degree of pain relief is determined after each pain management intervention, once sufficient time has elapsed for the treatment to reach peak effect (e.g., 1 hour for parenteral analgesics, 2 hours for oral analgesics). A simple, valid measure of pain relief will be selected by each clinical unit.

IB.

Each clinical unit will identify values for pain intensity rating (e.g., greater than the midpoint on the pain intensity scale) and pain relief rating (e.g., less than 50% at its maximum) that will elicit a review of the current pain therapy, documentation of the proposed modifications in treatment, and subsequent review of their efficacy. This process of treatment review and follow-up should include participation by physicians and nurses involved in the patient's care. As the general quality of treatment improves, the clinical unit will upgrade this standard to encourage a continuous process of improvement.

Required Characteristics (Outcome)

IC.

At regular intervals (to be defined by the clinical unit and the quality assurance committee), each clinical unit will assess a randomly selected sample of patients who have had surgery within the past 72 hours, have another acute pain condition, and/or have a diagnosis of cancer. Patients will be asked whether they have had pain during the current admission. Those who have experienced pain will then be asked about:
1. Current pain intensity.
2. Intensity of the worst pain experienced within the past 24 hours (or other interval selected by the clinical unit).
3. Degree of relief obtained from pain management interventions.
4. Satisfaction with responsiveness of the staff to reports of pain.
5. Satisfaction with relief provided.

II. INFORMATION ABOUT ANALGESICS IS READILY AVAILABLE (PROCESS)

Information about analgesics and other methods of pain management, including charts of relative potencies of analgesics, is situated on the unit in a way that aids writing and interpreting orders. Nurses and physicians can demonstrate the use of this material. Appropriate training to treat patients' pain is available to health professionals and included in continuing education activities.

III. PATIENTS ARE PROMISED ATTENTIVE ANALGESIC CARE (PROCESS)

Patients are informed on admission, verbally and in a printed format, that effective pain relief is an important part of their treatment, that their communication of unrelieved pain is essential, and that health professionals will respond quickly to their reports of pain. Pediatric patients and their parents will receive materials appropriate to the age of the patient.

IV. EXPLICIT POLICIES FOR USE OF ADVANCED ANALGESIC TECHNOLOGIES ARE DEFINED (PROCESS)

Advanced pain control techniques, including intraspinal opioids, systemic or intraspinal patient-controlled opioid infusion (PCA) or continuous opioid infusion, local anesthetic infusion, and inhalational analgesia, must be governed by policy and standard procedures that define the acceptable level of patient monitoring and the appropriate roles and limits of practice for all groups of healthcare providers involved. Such policy should include definitions of physician accountability, nurse responsibility to patient and physician, and the role of pharmacy.

V. ADHERENCE TO STANDARDS IS MONITORED (PROCESS)

Required Characteristics (Structure and Process)

VA.

An interdisciplinary committee, including representation from physicians, nurses, and other appropriate disciplines (e.g., pharmacy), monitors compliance with the above standards, considers issues relevant to improving pain treatment, and makes recommendations to improve outcomes and their monitoring. Where a comprehensive pain management team exists, its activities are monitored through the parent department's quality assurance body, which also may serve as the facility's quality assurance committee for pain relief. In a nursing home or very small hospital where an interdisciplinary pain management committee is not feasible, one or several individuals may fulfill this role.

VB.

At least the chair of the committee has experience working with issues related to effective pain management.

VC.

The committee meets at least every 3 months to review process and outcomes related to pain management.

VD.

The committee interacts with clinical units to establish procedures for improving pain management where necessary and reviews the results of these changes within 3 months of implementation.

VE.

The committee provides regular reports to administration and to the medical, nursing, and pharmacy staffs. Example of

Patient Outcome Questionnaire (Standard IC) (To be filled out by Interviewer).

1. Have you experienced any pain in the past 24 hours?
   Yes No

2. On this scale, how much discomfort or pain are you having right now? (Category, numerical [0-10], or VAS scales may be used for questions 3-5.)
   (record rating)

3. On this scale, please indicate the worst pain you have had in the past 24 hours.
   (record rating)

4. On this scale, please indicate the average level of pain you have had in the past 24 hours.
   (record rating)

5. Circle the number below that describes how, during the past 24 hours, pain has interfered with your:
   A. General activity
      0 1 2 3 4 5 6 7 8 9 10
   B. Mood
      0 1 2 3 4 5 6 7 8 9 10
   C. Walking ability
      0 1 2 3 4 5 6 7 8 9 10
   D. Relations with other people
      0 1 2 3 4 5 6 7 8 9 10
   E. Sleep
      0 1 2 3 4 5 6 7 8 9 10
   F. (For postoperative patients) Other activities that are needed to recover from illness (e.g., coughing and deep breathing after surgery; clinician should specify activity). _____
      0 1 2 3 4 5 6 7 8 9 10
   G. (For outpatients with chronic pain) Normal work, including housework
      0 1 2 3 4 5 6 7 8 9 10
   H. (For patients with chronic pain) Enjoyment of life
      0 1 2 3 4 5 6 7 8 9 10
      Does not interfere   Completely interferes

6. Select the phrase that indicates how satisfied or dissatisfied you are with the results of your pain treatment overall.
   Very dissatisfied   Slightly satisfied
   Dissatisfied   Satisfied
   Slightly dissatisfied   Very satisfied

7. Select the phrase that indicates how satisfied you are with the way your nurses responded to your reports of pain.
   Very dissatisfied   Slightly satisfied
   Dissatisfied   Satisfied
   Slightly dissatisfied   Very satisfied

8. Select the phrase that indicates how satisfied or dissatisfied you are with the way your physicians responded to your reports of pain.
   Very dissatisfied   Slightly satisfied
   Dissatisfied   Satisfied
   Slightly dissatisfied   Very satisfied

9. When you asked for pain medication, what was the longest time you had to wait to get it?
   <10 minutes   >60 minutes
   11-20 minutes   Asked for medication, but never
   21-30 minutes   received it
   31-60 minutes   Never asked for pain medication

10. Was there a time that the medication you were given for pain didn't help and you asked for something more or different to relieve the pain?
    Yes   No
    If your answer is "yes," how long did it take before your physician or nurse changed your treatment to a stronger or different medication and gave it to you?
    <1 hour   5-8 hours
    1-2 hours   9-24 hours
    3-4 hours   >24 hours

11. Early in your care, did your physician or nurse make it clear to you that we consider treatment of pain very important and that you should be sure to tell them when you have pain?
    Yes No

12. Do you have any suggestions for how your pain management could be improved?
    Modified from the Consensus Statement of the American Pain Society Quality of Care Committee, *JAMA*, December 20, 1995, p. 1878.

APPENDIX B   RESOURCES

ORGANIZATIONS

American Cancer Society, National Office (ACS)
1599 Clifton Road
Atlanta, GA 30329
404-320-3333

American Pain Society (APS)
A national chapter of the International Association for the Study of Pain
4700 West Lave Avenue
Glenview, IL 60025
708-966-5595

American Society of Pain Management Nurses (ASPMN)
2755 Bristol Street, Suite 110
Costa Mesa, CA 92626
714-545-1305

International Association for the Study of Pain (IASP)
A multidisciplinary professional organization
909 NE 43rd Street, Suite 306
Seattle, WA 98105-6020
206-547-6409

National Cancer Institute (NCI)
Office of Cancer Communications
NCI/NIH
Bethesda, MD 20892
800-4-CANCER

National Hospice Organization (NHO)
Publishes Hospice magazine (professional orientation) and The Hospice Journal (research orientation)
1901 North Moore Drive, Suite 901
Arlington, VA 22209
703-243-5900

Oncology Nursing Society (ONS)
501 Holiday Drive
Pittsburgh, PA 15220-2749
412-921-7373

WHO Cancer Pain Relief Program
American Association for World Health
1129 20th Street N.W., Suite 400
Washington, DC 20036
202-466-5883

Wisconsin Cancer Pain Initiative
3675 Medical Science Center
University of Wisconsin Medical School
1300 University Avenue
Madison, WI 53706
608-262-0978

PROFESSIONAL PUBLICATIONS

"Acute Pain Management: Operative or Medical Procedures and Trauma" (Clinical Practice Guideline). Agency for Health Care Policy and Research (AHCPR) Publication No. 92-0032.
"Acute Pain Management in Adults: Operative Procedures" (Quick Reference Guide for Clinicians). AHCPR Publication No. 92-0019.
"Acute Pain Management in Infants, Children and Adolescents: Operative and Medical Procedures" (Quick Reference Guide for Clinicians). AHCPR Publication No. 92-0020.
Center for Research Dissemination and Liaison AHCPR Publication Clearinghouse
P.O. Box 8547
Silver Spring, MD 20907
800-358-9295 or 301-495-3453

APS Journal
Official Journal of the American Pain Society
Churchill Livingstone Inc.
5 S. 250 Frontenac Road
Naperville, IL 60563
800-553-5426

Journal of Pain and Symptom Management
A multidisciplinary publication that supports research and education in all areas of palliative care
Elsevier Publishing Co., Inc.
Subscription Customer Service
655 Avenue of the Americas
New York, NY 10010
212-633-3950

"Cancer Pain Release"
A publication of the World Health Organization Collaborating Center for Symptom Evaluation
634 WARF
610 Walnut Street
Madison, WI 53705
608-262-0727

"Cancer Pain Relief and Palliative Care" (1990)
76-Page handbook for pain management compiled by international experts
WHO Publications Center—USA
49 Sheridan Avenue
Albany, NY 12210
518-436-9686
$8.10 per copy plus $3.00 postage and handling

"Current Trends in the Treatment of Cancer Pain" monograph (1993) by KM Foley
Upjohn Company
Kalamazoo, MI 49001

"Handbook of Cancer Pain Management" (ed 4, 1994) by DE Weissman, SL Burchman, PA Dinndorf, JL Dahl:
Wisconsin Pain Initiative
3671 Medical Sciences Center
1300 University Avenue
Madison, WI 53706
608-262-0978
($3.00 per copy, plus postage)

"Innovations in Cancer Pain Management" (1992)
40-Page booklet written by national experts
Janssen Pharmaceutica Inc.
40 Kingsbridge Road
Piscataway, NJ 08855
908-524-9378

"Management of Cancer Pain: Clinical Practice Guideline"
Agency for Health Care Policy and Research (AHCPR)
Publication No. 94-0592, March 1994
"Management of Cancer Pain: Adults. Quick Reference Guide for Clinicians"
Publication No. 94-0593, March 1994
U.S. Department of Health and Human Services
Agency for Health Care Policy and Research
Executive Office Center Suite 501
2101 East Jefferson Street
Rockville, MD 20852
800-4-CANCER

"Oncology Nursing Society Position Paper on Cancer Pain Monograph"
Oncology Nursing Society (1990)
501 Holiday Drive
Pittsburgh, PA 15220-2749
412-921-7373
($7.00 per copy for non-member; $6.00 for member)

"Oral Morphine in Advanced Cancer" (ed 2., 1989) by R Twycross, S Lack
Bath, England: Bath Press
(Available through Roxane Laboratories)
P.O. Box 16532
Columbus, OH 43216
800-848-0120

"Principles of Analgesic Use in the Treatment of Acute Pain and Chronic Cancer Pain: A Concise Guide to Medical Practice" (ed 3., 1992)
41-Page booklet
American Pain Society
4700 West Lake Avenue
Glenview, IL 60025
708-966-5595

"Pain: Clinical Manual for Nursing Practice" (1989) by M McCaffery, A Beebe
C.V. Mosby Company
11830 Westline Industrial Drive
St. Louis, MO 63146

"3-Step Analgesic Ladder for Management of Cancer Pain" (1991)
A summary pocket guide of pharmaceutical review by RK Portenoy
(Available through Roxanne Laboratories)
P.O. Box 16532
Columbus, OH 43216
800-848-0120

"The Network News"
A newsletter
Memorial Sloan Kettering Cancer Center
Box 421
1275 York Avenue
New York, NY 10021
212-639-3164

PATIENT INFORMATION
Booklets
"Cancer Pain Can Be Relieved" (1988)
"Children's Cancer Pain Can Be Relieved" (1989)
"Jeff Asks About Cancer Pain" (1990)
(Addresses the adolescent with cancer pain)
Wisconsin Cancer Pain Initiative
3675 Medical Sciences Center
University of Wisconsin Medical School
1300 University Avenue
Madison, WI 53706
608-262-0978
($0.50 plus postage each for non-Wisconsin residents)

"How to Talk to Your Doctor About Acute Pain" (1987) by Ronald Melzak, Paul Paris, Ada Rogers
DuPont Pharmaceuticals Biomedical Department
E.I. DuPont de Nemours & Co., Inc.
Wilmington, DE 19898
800-543-8693

"Managing Cancer Pain" (Consumer version)
Publication No. 94-0595, March 1994
U.S. Department of Health and Human Services
Agency for Health Care Policy and Research (AHCPR)
Executive Office Center, Suite 501
2101 East Jefferson Street
Rockville, MD 20852
800-4-CANCER

"Oral Morphine: Information for Patients, Families and Friends" (1990) by Robert G. Twycross, Sylvia Lack
Roxanne Laboratories
P.O. 16532
Columbus, OH 43216
800-848-0120

"Questions and Answers About Pain Control: A Guide for People with Cancer and Their Families"
National Cancer Institute and the American Cancer Society
(Available through local ACS offices)
"Up-to-Date Answers to Questions About Measuring Pain"
(To help patients living with cancer) (1991)
Purdue Frederick Company
Norwalk, CT 06850-3590
203-853-0123

"You Don't Have to Suffer: A Complete Guide to Relieving Cancer Pain for Patients and Their Families" (1994) by SS Lang, RB Patt
Oxford University Press
New York, NY

Groups
International Pain Foundation
Supports public education about pain disorders and their treatment through literature and information.
909 N.E. 43rd Street, Room 306
Seattle, WA 98105-6020
206-547-2157

American Society of Pain Management Nurses (ASPMN)
2755 Bristol Street
Costa Mesa, CA 92626
714-545-1305

VIDEOTAPES
"Cancer Pain Control: Winning the Battle"
"Cancer Pain Control: Controlling Your Cancer Pain"
(Both are client-oriented with "Controlling Your Cancer Pain" being more specific on the "how-to")
Marshfield Video Network
Marshfield Clinic
1000 North Oak Avenue
Marshfield, WI 54449

"No Fears . . . No Tears: Children with Cancer Coping with Pain"
Canadian Cancer Society
(Professionally oriented)
Available through local ACS offices

SLIDE SET
"Cancer Pain *Can* Be Relieved"
Illinois Cancer Pain Initiative
P.O. Box 6794
Villa Park, IL 60181
800-DUL-PAIN
cost is $35.00 (24-slide set with script designed for presentation to the general public)

CANCER RESOURCES ON THE INTERNET

Roxane Pain Institute   Educational material on cancer and AIDS pain management from the Roxane Laboratories and the Roxane Pain Institute are now accessible by entering the side address (http//www.Roxane.com). Users can obtain newsletters, clinical articles, presentation slides on cancer pain management, a schedule of upcoming pain management seminars, and the Agency for Health Care Policy and Research cancer pain management guidelines.

ONCOPAIN   The purpose of Oncopain is to facilitate networking among clinicians regarding cancer pain assessment and management. It will allow for assistance with a clinical problem, or networking research opportunities. To subscribe, send an E-mail message to listserv%med.ucalgary.ca. In the 'body' of your message to listerv, write: subscribe Oncopain and then write your name (e.g., subscribe Oncopain John Doe).

USENET   is a distributed computer information service used by some computer "hosts" on the Internet. The USENET newsgroup named *alt.support.cancer* provides a forum for cancer patients and some physicians to exchange information and advice.

ONCOLINK   is accessible using both gopher and World Wide Web software. To access OncoLink using World Wide Web, the address is http://cancer.med.upenn.edu/; to access OncoLink via gopher, point your gopher client software to gopher://cancer.med.upenn.edu:80.

CANCERNET   provides full, extensive cancer information. To use CancerNet, send an electronic mail message to cancernet%icicb.nci.hih.gov with the word "help" in the body of the message. Further instructions and a complete contents list will be mailed back within about 10 minutes from the CancerNet computer. CancerNet information is also available on several gopher servers, including the National Institutes of Health gopher at gopher.nih.gov, and through several World Wide Web servers.

PDQ   The NCI's comprehensive cancer database, contributes much of the information on CancerNet. In addition to full-text information statements, PDQ contains an extensive register of ongoing and closed clinical trials and directories of physicians and organizations active in cancer care. PDQ is available both online and via CD-ROM from a number of vendors. For further information, call 800-NCI-7890.

(The computer online information is from "The Network News," Memorial Sloan Kettering Cancer Center, Winter 1995, p 9.)

CHAPTER 30

Protective Mechanisms

SUZANNE SHAFFER

Numerous mechanisms protect humans from foreign substances and invading organisms. This chapter looks at these mechanisms and their importance to the person with cancer, the nursing process, related nursing diagnoses, and nursing interventions.

IMMUNITY

Immunity is a protective mechanism that maintains the integrity of the body against foreign substances or agents. The study of immunity was based on the study of infectious diseases but cannot be limited to such and now encompasses the areas of organ transplantation, blood transfusion, cancer, and autoimmunity.

Four main functions of the immune system include (1) defense against invading organisms; (2) homeostasis—removal of dead "self" cells; (3) surveillance—removal of mutant cells; and (4) regulation—augmentation and depression of immune response.

The major purpose of a fully functional immune system is to distinguish self from nonself. The ability of the body to develop tolerance of self-produced antigens is a part of this function. The two basic types of immunity are *innate* and *acquired*. Innate immunity is a nonspecific immune system function. Acquired immunity is specific and depends on the recognition of self and nonself.[35,38,50]

Innate Immunity

Innate immunity is a nonspecific response to any breach of the skin and mucous membranes. This type of immunity is present at birth and is species specific. Innate immunity provides initial protection against foreign substances and invading organisms. The four mechanisms of innate immunity are *mechanical barriers, chemical barriers, fever,* and *inflammation.*[1,38]

Mechanical barriers. Mechanical barriers include epithelial surfaces, such as skin and mucous membranes, and their projections along the gastrointestinal, respiratory, and genitourinary tracts. Intact skin and mucous membranes present an effective physical barrier to the entrance of organisms and toxins. Epithelial surfaces carry receptors for specific antigens on the cell surfaces. These receptors are essential for maintaining the skin and mucous membranes' normal microorganism flora. Secretory IgA, an antibody, prevents the attachment of pathogenic organisms to epithelial cells. Routine exfoliation of epithelial cells, with loss of adherent organisms, also serves to limit invasion by organisms.[1,38]

Chemical barriers. Chemical barriers include such substances as saliva, mucus, tears, sweat, gastric juices, sebum, cerumen, lysozyme products, and numerous other substances secreted by the body. These prevent entry of potentially harmful substances and organisms by various mechanisms such as pH, viscosity, and the presence of other substances with antimicrobial activity that physically inhibits attachment and invasion by organisms.[1,21]

Fever. Fever (elevated body temperature) is a protective mechanism directed against temperature-sensitive organisms such as bacteria and viruses. These organisms secrete substances that act as pyrogens, elevating body temperature in response to their presence. Temperature-sensitive organisms such as these rarely survive sustained body temperature elevations in excess of 102.2° F (39° C). Warm-blooded animals elevate body temperature by internal means in response to pyrogens such as bacterial toxins and leukocyte products (cytokines) when inflammation or immune response occurs.[47,54,70] Fevers of 100.8° F (38.2° C) to 103.1° F (39.5° C) are generally well tolerated.

Fever is a defense mechanism that has a positive effect on the survival of patients with life-threatening infections. Recent investigations have identified the immune-enhancing effect of fever on antigen recognition and sensitization.[70] There appears to be increasing support for the positive effects of fever and that aggressive antipyresis for low-grade temperature elevations may be detrimental.[40,54,70,74]

Inflammatory response. The inflammatory response is a local reaction initiated when mechanical or chemical barriers of the body are invaded by organisms. This limited, nonspecific response is initiated and mediated by phagocytic white blood cells (WBCs) such as neutrophils, eosinophils, basophils, monocytes, and macrophages. It does not require recognition of self. The process of inflammation is not complete until all invading organisms, dead and dying phagocytic cells, and necrotic cellular debris are removed by macrophages (histiocytes) and tissue damage is repaired by fibroblasts.[49]

Acquired Immunity

Acquired immunity is the body's specific neutralizing response to foreign invaders and their products. This type of immunity is not fully functional at birth. It may take 6 to 7 years for the immune system to mature, and as a person reaches late middle age, its level of functioning begins to decline,[60,73] as evidenced by increased incidence of autoimmune disorders and cancers.[82]

The two main mechanisms of acquired immunity are cell-mediated immunity and humoral immunity. Both employ lymphocytes as effector cells.[73]

Lymphocytes. Lymphocytes are small, round, mononuclear cells, which make up approximately 30% of the peripheral circulating leukocyte population. Lymphocytes are derived from pleuripotential stem cells found in the bone marrow. Two major subtypes of lymphocytes have been identified: thymus-derived or thymus-dependent lymphocytes (T cells) and bursa-derived or bursa-dependent lymphocytes (B cells [beta cells, B lymphocytes]).[73]

Cell-mediated immunity. Cell-mediated immunity (CMI) uses T cells as the primary effector cells. T cells function as immunoregulatory and cytotoxic cells. CMI provides defense against intracellular bacteria such as *Mycobacterium tuberculosis* and *Listeria monocytogenes,* fungi, viruses, and protozoa (see box below). Delayed hypersensitivity reactions are a type of CMI. Transplantation rejection, by both graft and host, is caused in part by the T cell and its ability to distinguish self from nonself. Immune surveillance, or the body's inherent ability to prevent cancers, is also thought to be a function of CMI with the natural killer cell (NK cell or large, granular lymphocyte) being the primary effector cell of surveillance.[42]

Cell-mediated immune deficiencies may be congenital or acquired (see box below). Congenital anomalies include children born without thymus glands and those with poorly functioning thymus glands. Death usually occurs in the first years of life and is caused by infection. Secondary or acquired causes of diminished T-cell function are more common and include acquired immu-

---

INFECTING ORGANISMS ASSOCIATED WITH CELLULAR IMMUNE DEFICIENCY

INTRACELLULAR BACTERIA

Mycobacterium tuberculosis
Atypical *mycobacterium*
Listeria monocytogenes

FUNGI

Candida albicans
Cryptococcus neoformans
Aspergillus species
Histoplasma capsulatum

VIRUSES

Herpes simplex
Herpes zoster
Cytomegalovirus
Epstein-Barr
Hepatitis B

PROTOZOA

Pneumocystis carinii
Cryptosporidium
Toxoplasma gondii
Giardia lamblia
Isospora belli

CELL-MEDIATED IMMUNE DEFICIENCIES

PRIMARY IMMUNE DEFICIENCIES
Predominantly T cell

Chronic mucocutaneous candidiasis
Nezelof syndrome
DiGeorge syndrome (thymic-parathyroid aplasia)

Combined T cell and B cell

Ataxia-telangiectasia
Severe combined immunodeficiency
Severe combined immunodeficiency with adenosine
    deaminase deficiency
Short-limbed dwarfism
Wiskott-Aldrich syndrome

SECONDARY IMMUNE DEFICIENCIES
Malignant disease

Acute lymphoblastic leukemia
Chronic lymphocytic leukemia
Hairy cell leukemia
Hodgkin's disease
Mycosis fungoides and Sézary syndrome
Non-Hodgkin's lymphoma
Advanced carcinomas

Therapeutic

Cytotoxic drugs
Immunosuppressive agents
Radiation therapy

Infections

Human immunodeficiency virus
Cytomegalovirus
Epstein-Barr virus
Non-A/Non-B hepatitis
Leprosy
Tuberculosis
Histoplasmosis
Cryptococcosis
Toxoplasmosis

nodeficiency syndrome (AIDS), Hodgkin's disease, organ transplantation immunosuppression, and some autoimmune disorders. Persons who have defects in cell-mediated immunity, regardless of cause, are susceptible to opportunistic infections from a host of bacteria, viruses, fungi, and protozoa and to the development of cancers, particularly those arising from lymphoid tissue.[73]

Humoral immunity. Humoral immunity is the part of acquired immunity that involves the production of antibodies. *Antibodies* are substances produced by plasma cells (sensitized B cells) in response to specific recognition of an antigen (foreign substance). They are serum proteins called *immunoglobulins*. The five major categories of immunoglobulins are IgG, IgM, IgA, IgD, and IgE. The body has an unlimited ability to produce different antibodies against specific antigens. Antibodies function by neutralizing toxins, agglutinating and lysing microorganisms and other cells, and serving as opsonins (coating organisms and making them more palatable to phagocytic cells).

Defects in humoral immunity, like those of cell-mediated immunity, may be congenital or acquired (see box below). Agammaglobulinemia and some types of hypogammaglobulinemia may be congenital. These produce lifelong susceptibility to severe bacterial infections. Secondary humoral immune deficiencies, most com-

monly hypogammaglobulinemias, are often related to lymphoproliferative disorders such as chronic lymphocytic leukemia, non-Hodgkin's lymphomas, and plasma cell dyscrasias such as multiple myeloma and Waldenström's macroglobulinemia. Acquired idiopathic hypogammaglobulinemias occur without known cause. Regardless of cause, the person with a defective humoral immune system is susceptible to infection by high-grade (nonopportunistic) encapsulated bacteria, both gram-positive and gram-negative. These infections are often life-threatening and recurrent.[40]

Interactions. The specific immune response requires complex interaction between cell-mediated and humoral immunity. The macrophage (a phagocytic WBC) is necessary for the proper functioning of this response. The macrophage processes and presents the antigen to the T cell for recognition and elicitation of response. The primary responsibility of the T cells is recognition of self. In the presence of nonself antigens, a number of processes are elicited. Among these is the production of lymphokines. Lymphokines, part of a larger group called *cytokines,* are soluble chemical mediators that facilitate intercellular communication among T cells, B cells, macrophages, and other phagocytic cells. Particular lymphokines (see box below) may cause activation of macrophages, sensitization of other T cells, and conversion of B cells to plasma cells with resultant production of antibodies. T cells are also regulatory cells of the immune system. Helper/inducer T cells (T4 or CD4 lymphocytes) stimulate and promote immune system function, whereas suppressor T cells (T8 or CD8 lymphocytes) inhibit or

---

HUMORAL IMMUNE DEFICIENCIES[44,62]

PRIMARY ANTIBODY DEFICIENCIES

X-linked hypogammaglobulinemia
X-linked hypogammaglobulinemia with growth hormone deficiency
Transient hypogammaglobulinemia of infancy
Common variable unclassifiable hypogammaglobulinemia
Selective immunoglobulin deficiencies (IgA, IgG-subclass)
Autosomal recessive hypogammaglobulinemia

PRIMARY MIXED T- AND B-CELL DEFICIENCIES

(See cell-mediated immune deficiencies listed in the second box, p. 793.)

SECONDARY ANTIBODY DEFICIENCIES

Chronic lymphocytic leukemia
Acute lymphoblastic leukemia
Non-Hodgkin's lymphoma—B-cell origin
Multiple myeloma
Heavy-chain disease
Waldenström's macroglobulinemia
Thymoma
Nephrotic syndrome
Protein-losing enteropathies
Burns
Splenectomy

EXAMPLES OF CYTOKINES

MONOKINES

Interleukin-1 (IL-1) or endogenous pyrogen (EP)
Tumor necrosis factor (TNF)
Interferon alfa-2a (leukocyte) (IF)
Granulocyte-colony stimulating factor (G-CSF)
Granulocyte/macrophage–colony-stimulating factor (GM-CSF)
Interleukin-6 (IL-6)

LYMPHOKINES

Macrophage activating factor (MAF)
Macrophage inhibition factor (MIF)
Interferon, gamma (immune) (IF)
Interleukin-2, T-cell growth factor (IL-2)
Interleukin-3, multi-CSF growth factor (IL-3)
Interleukin-6, B-cell differentiation factor (IL-6)
Chemotactic factor (CF)
B-cell growth factor (BCGF)
Tumor necrosis factor (TNF)
Lymphotoxin (LT)

prevent immune system functioning. T8 or CD8 lymphocytes may also become T cells capable of "cell-to-cell" combat. These cells are "killer" or cytotoxic T cells.[73]

SKIN
Anatomy and Physiology

The skin is one of several mechanical barriers that can prevent the entrance of invading organisms and toxins and maintain homeostasis. The skin is composed of the epidermis, dermis, and assorted derivatives of epidermal/dermal origin, which include hair, nails, cutaneous glands, and teeth.[34]

The epidermis, or topmost epithelial layer, functions primarily to conserve water. Pigment-forming cells called *melanocytes* reside within this layer. Constant mitotic activity replaces dead cells. Repair and replacement occur from the bottom up; old cells are lost through wear and tear of daily living and are replaced by new cells developing underneath.[34]

The dermis, or inner layer of skin, determines skin thickness. It is thickest on dorsal surfaces of the body, palms of hands, and soles of feet and thinnest on ventral surfaces including the abdomen and genitalia. The dermis contains blood vessels, lymphatics, and sensory nerve endings.[64] The skin is a multifunctional organ. Its recognized functions include the following[1,34]:

- Distinguishes between pain, temperature, and touch
- Regulates loss of water and electrolytes
- Regulates body temperature by vasoconstriction and vasodilation
- Absorbs substances applied directly to the skin
- Excretes excess water and electrolytes
- Prevents entrance of external gases, liquids, and pathogens as long as intact and so protects the internal body
- Provides nutrition to underlying structures through abundant blood supply

Pathophysiology

A person with cancer may experience multiple disruptions of skin integrity.

Disease-related causes. Disease-related causes of skin integrity disruption include primary skin malignancies such as malignant melanoma, basal cell carcinoma, squamous cell carcinoma, Kaposi's sarcoma, and mycosis fungoides. Metastatic tumors of the skin, such as chest wall recurrence in breast cancer, and leukemic and lymphomatous infiltrates (leukemia cutis and lymphoma cutis respectively) may also disrupt skin integrity. Cutaneous manifestations associated with remote effects of malignancy, such as acanthosis nigricans, acquired ichthyosis, dermatomyositis, and exfoliative dermatitis, may cause disruption of skin integrity secondary to scratching and cracking of skin. Thrombocytopenia with resultant petechiae, purpura, and ecchymoses may lead to increased fragility of the skin.[34]

Treatment-related causes. Treatment-related causes of skin impairment include those associated with chemotherapy such as drug extravasation, alopecia, hyperpigmentation, hyperkeratosis, photosensitivity, ulceration, and radiation recall reactions. Skin reactions associated with nonantineoplastic agents include allergic skin eruptions, Stevens-Johnson syndrome, and erythema multiforme. Radiation therapy skin reactions may progress to wet or dry desquamation. Surgical incisions and other invasive procedures such as needle biopsies and placement of vascular access devices also disrupt skin integrity.[34,62,75,80]

Complicating factors. Complicating factors that may interfere with the maintenance of skin integrity include immobility, malnutrition, obstruction, infection, incontinence, and pruritus.

Assessment. Skin assessment should include a thorough inspection of all skin surfaces with attention focused on the following: color, vascularity, bleeding (location, type, and amount), lesions (appearance, number, location, distribution, and ulceration), edema, moist areas, and general condition of hair and nails. If lesions are present, the nurse should assess for general characteristics, morphologic structure (nodularity, scaling, crusting, erosions, and fissures), size (measure), drainage (color, character, amount, and odor), associated pain and tenderness, depth of lesions (measure) and presence of vital structures within the lesion (i.e., carotid artery). High risk areas (chest, abdomen, neck, and scalp) should be palpated with palms of hands for presence of "silent" lesions. Metastatic lesions are generally hard and immovable. Assessment should include attention to any history of allergies, medications, and past and present skin disorders. Risk assessment for pressure ulcers using a reliable instrument such as the Norton scale or the Braden scale is an integral part of the nursing process. Reassessment of skin integrity and risk factors should occur periodically.[13,65]

Medical Management

Treatment of skin complications may include the administration of antibiotics, antifungals, and antivirals for infection; surgical procedures for incision and drainage, débridement, and skin grafting; radiation therapy for obstructive phenomena; chemotherapy to treat the underlying disease for relief of pruritus; and management of disfiguring, nonhealing, or ulcerating malignant skin lesions.

MUCOUS MEMBRANES
Anatomy and Physiology

The oral mucosa provides a mechanical barrier to inhibit the invasion of microorganisms. The oral mucosa is composed of three layers: an outer layer of stratified, squamous epithelium; a middle layer, the lamina propria, consisting of fibrous fingerlike projections that extend into the epithelium and contain blood vessels, nerves, and glandular tissue; and an inner submucosal layer that varies in thickness with the function at specific anatomic locations. The lamina propria and epithelium are separated by basement membrane. Stem cells of the basement membrane divide and differentiate into the various cells of the surface epithelium. These cells have an estimated life span of 3 to 5 days. It is estimated that the surface epithelial layer of the oral mucosa is replaced every 7 to 14 days. When loss exceeds the rate of replacement, shallow ulcerative lesions occur. Repair continues at a fixed rate, which may leave large areas of mucous membrane denuded of surface epithelium. Intact mucous membranes provide an effective mechanical barrier against harmful exogenous and endogenous organisms. The normal oral flora, mainly consisting of gram-positive bacteria, gram-negative bacteria, and fungi, serve to inhibit the growth of pathogenic organisms. When these barriers are disrupted, bacterial translocation of more pathogenic organisms may occur. Other mucous membrane–covered surfaces exhibit similar function and growth and replacement patterns.[10,25]

Pathophysiology

The following terms are defined for the purpose of this discussion:

- *Stomatitis*—a general term referring to the inflammatory reaction and shallow ulcerative lesions occurring on the mucosal surfaces of the mouth and oropharynx 7 to 14 days after administration of certain chemotherapeutic agents and after radiation therapy to the head and neck.[10-12,31,32]
- *Mucositis*—a general term referring to the inflammatory reaction and shallow ulcerative lesions occurring on mucosal surfaces, not limited to the mouth and oropharynx, frequently associated with the administration of certain chemotherapeutic agents and after radiation therapy to mucous membrane–bearing sites. Stomatitis, esophagitis, gastritis, enteritis, colitis, proctitis, and vaginitis are examples of treatment-related mucositis.[23,37]

Disease-related causes. Disease-related causes of the disruption of mucous membranes include primary tumors of the head, neck, gastrointestinal tract, respiratory tract, and genitourinary tract; agranulocytic oral ulcers; gingival hypertrophy and infiltration associated with acute leukemia; non-Hodgkin's lymphoma or acute leukemia involving Waldeyer's ring; and Kaposi's sarcoma among others. Disease-related immunosuppression may lead to superinfection with herpes simplex virus (HSV), *Candida albicans,* and other opportunistic agents.[10,25]

Treatment-related causes. Treatment-related causes of mucous membrane disruption include chemotherapy-induced mucositis (see box above), radiation-associated

---

ANTINEOPLASTIC AGENTS TOXIC TO MUCOUS MEMBRANES

ANTIMETABOLITES

Cytosine arabinoside
Fludarabine
Fluorouracil
Mercaptopurine
Methotrexate
Thioguanine

PLANT ALKALOIDS

Etoposide
Paclitaxel
Teniposide
Vinblastine
Vincristine
Vinorelbine

ABLATIVE DOSES

All antineoplastics

ANTIBIOTICS

Bleomycin
Dactinomycin
Daunorubicin
Doxorubicin
Mitomycin
Mitoxantrone
Plicamycin

MISCELLANEOUS

Hydroxyurea
Procarbazine

BIOLOGICALS

rIL-2/LAK cells
Levamisole

---

mucositis, xerostomia (dry mouth), parotitis (inflamed and swollen salivary glands), osteoradionecrosis of the bone (late destruction of irradiated bone and subsequent loss of teeth), and surgical procedures. Chemotherapy effects are systemic and may be widespread. Radiation-associated effects are site specific and involve only the areas within the treatment port. Persons undergoing bone marrow transplantation are at greater risk for oral complications, related to the intensity of the preparative therapy and manifestations of graft-versus-host disease.[30,33,75,80]

Complicating factors. Complicating factors include infections, which may become systemic; bleeding from nonintact mucosal surfaces; poor nutritional status; and pain secondary to the lesions. Preexisting dental and periodontal diseases predispose to more severe complications of disease- and treatment-related mucositis as does chronic exposure to oral mucosal stressors such as chemical and physical irritants (alcohol, heat, and tobacco), other medications associated with drying mucosal surfaces, and oxygen administration.[10,25] Other risk factors include age older than 65 or younger than 20 years, inadequate self-care abilities, and altered fluid or nutritional status.

Assessment. Numerous oral assessment tools are available in the nursing literature. Most assess the lips, tongue, mucous membranes, gingiva, teeth, saliva, voice, and ability to swallow. The use of an oral assessment tool provides the ability to assign numerical (objective and comparative) scores to the examination. It also provides a common base (language) for ongoing physical assessment and evaluation of patient outcomes.[10,25,27,32]

Oral assessment requires the use of readily available tools including a pair of examination gloves, gauze sponges, flashlight, and tongue depressor. Oral assessment should be done at least twice daily and the findings documented in the patient record. The patient and family should be taught the techniques of assessment so that they can follow the progress when the patient is home. The patient and family should also be instructed to report any changes in oral sensation or taste and the appearance of lesions.[32,61]

Rectal and vaginal mucosal assessment in the neutropenic patient should be limited to visual inspection only. This prevents trauma to ulcerated mucosa and decreases the potential for dissemination of infection through manipulation of the rectal and vaginal tissue. The patient should be questioned about the presence or absence of rectal or vaginal bleeding, pain, itching, discharge, drainage, and other discomfort or changes in sensation.[23,85]

Medical Management

Treatment of complications involving nonintact mucous membranes includes antibiotics, antifungals, and antivirals for superinfections; platelet transfusion and antifibrinolytic agents for bleeding from mucous membranes; topical and systemic analgesics for pain; and dilation of strictures involving the esophagus and vagina.

BONE MARROW SUPPRESSION
Anatomy and Physiology

The bone marrow is the production site for all formed blood elements: erythrocytes, granulocytes, monocytes, lymphocytes, and megakaryocytes. During early fetal development, hematopoiesis (production of blood) occurs in the liver and yolk sac. By the 20th week of gestation the bone marrow begins to produce blood cells, and by the 30th week the bone marrow has achieved normal cellularity. At birth, active bone marrow is found in all bones of the body. With age the functional marrow space contracts, so that by adulthood active marrow is found primarily in the axial skeleton, sternum, ribs, vertebral bodies, pelvis, skull, and the proximal ends of the long bones.[35,38]

Bone marrow is a spongy organ made up of a fibrous network of connective tissue called *stroma*. The stroma is supported within the marrow cavity by spicules of bone radiating to the center of the bone marrow cavity from cortical bone. The bone marrow is a highly vascular organ with numerous nutrient arteries and interconnecting venous sinusoids. Poorly understood regulatory mechanisms prevent immature blood cells from entering the venous sinusoids and circulating blood until they reach maturity.[35,38]

All blood cells arise from a common progenitor cell called the *stem cell*.[38,83] The stem cell probably re-

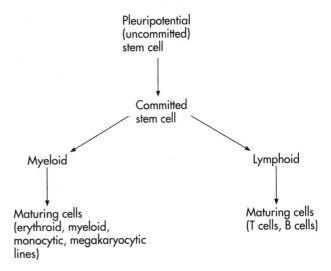

Figure 30-1 Stem cell differentiation and maturation.

sembles and cannot be distinguished by sight from the small mature lymphocyte. The stem cell pool is self-renewing; for every stem cell that enters the differentiation and maturation pool, another cell returns to the stem cell pool. Conditions causing destruction of the stem cell pool lead to the development of marrow aplasia. Stem cells may be either pleuripotential (uncommitted) or unipotential (committed) (Figure 30-1).

Stem cells, having entered a designated cell line, mature under the influence of specific hematopoietic growth factors. The first to be identified and the best known of these growth factors is erythropoietin (EPO), a glycoprotein hormone produced by the kidney. EPO is necessary for proper differentiation and maturation of erythrocytes (RBCs). EPO levels are regulated by tissue oxygen levels. EPO production reflects need for oxygen-carrying capacity via hemoglobin. Current research has led to the identification of several other hematopoietic growth factors. Recombinant deoxyribonucleic acid (DNA) technology has made it possible to produce large quantities of these growth factors, allowing increased clinical trials. Growth factors undergoing trials include, but are not limited to, recombinant erythropoietin (rEPO), granulocyte/macrophage–colony-stimulating factor (rGM-CSF), granulocyte–colony-stimulating factor (rG-CSF), interleukin-3 (rIL-3) or multi-CSF, stem cell factor (rSCF), and macrophage–colony-stimulating factor (rM-CSF). The target cells of the growth factors both vary and overlap. rGM-CSF, rSCF, and rIL-3 are multilineage in that they stimulate and regulate most of the cell lines of the myeloid series (i.e., granulocytes, monocytes, macrophages, erythrocytes, megakaryocytes), whereas rEPO, rG-CSF, and rM-CSF are lineage restricted (affecting only the erythrocyte, neutrophil, or monocyte/macrophage lines, respectively). rEPO, rGM-CSF, and rG-CSF have received approval from the Food

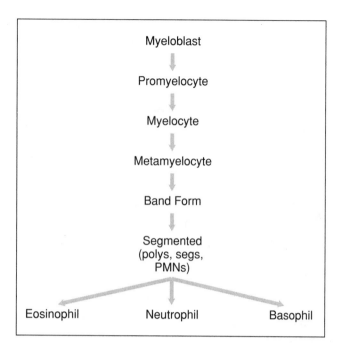

Myeloblast

↓

Promyelocyte

↓

Myelocyte

↓

Metamyelocyte

↓

Band Form

↓

Segmented
(polys, segs,
PMNs)

Eosinophil   Neutrophil   Basophil

Figure 30-2   Myeloid maturation.

and Drug Administration as supportive therapy for patients undergoing treatment for cancer, marrow transplantation, and HIV infection. Neither rGM-CSF or rG-CSF stimulates platelet production to any great extent. It is hoped that, through the development of other growth factors or combinations of growth factors, prolonged myelosuppression will be a thing of the past.[42,58,71,78]

Once a stem cell has entered a particular cell line, differentiation and maturation occur in a manner characteristic of erythroid, myeloid, lymphoid, or megakaryocytic cells (Figure 30-2). Residence (maturation) time within the marrow varies from cell line to cell line and with the body's need for the cell type. Some cell lines have storage pools. Once the cells are released into circulation, life span ranges from 6 to 8 hours for the neutrophil to 120 days for the erythrocyte. The marrow is able to respond to increased need for particular cells by permitting early release from the maturation and storage pools.[49]

Pathophysiology

Pathologic bone marrow conditions arise from a defect in the stem cell or the marrow microenvironment. The stem cell defect may be intrinsic, as in the leukemias, or extrinsic, as in exposure to stem cell toxins such as benzene or chloramphenicol. Microenvironment problems may occur intrinsically, as in myelofibrosis, a myeloproliferative disorder characterized by replacement of the marrow cavity with fibrous tissue, or extrinsically, as when a nonhematologic malignancy metastasizes to the marrow. Replacement followed by marrow failure may

occur. Treatment of malignant disorders by chemotherapy or radiation therapy may alter the stem cell pool and its environment permanently.[42,71]

Definition of terms. The following terms are defined for the purpose of this discussion:

- *Leukopenia*—a condition said to occur when the total leukocyte complement is reduced. Leukopenia is a nonspecific finding and usually reflects a decrease in all WBCs (Table 30-1).
- *Granulocytopenia*—a condition said to occur when the absolute granulocyte complement is reduced. When granulocytopenia occurs, there is a decrease in neutrophils, eosinophils, and basophils.
- *Neutropenia*—a condition that exists when there is an absolute decrease in the number of circulating neutrophils, usually less than 1000/mm^3. The absolute neutrophil count (ANC) is calculated as follows:

Segs (%) + Bands (%) × White blood cell count = ANC
0.10   +   0.10   ×   2000   = 400/mm^3

Neutropenia is associated with a profound impairment in the inflammatory response, leading to lack or minimization of the usual signs and symptoms of infection such as erythema, swelling, heat, and pain.[14,16] Purulence is not present. Neutropenia is the single most important predisposing factor to infection in the person with cancer:

ANC >1500/mm^3 = normal risk
ANC <1000/mm^3 = moderate risk
ANC <500/mm^3 = severe risk
ANC <100/mm^3 = extreme risk

Neutropenia may be related to basic disease processes such as acute nonlymphocytic leukemia or aplastic anemia. Neutropenia may occur also as a result of myelosuppressive treatment for malignant disease such as chemotherapy or radiation therapy.

- *Immunosuppression*—a condition that exists when lymphocyte function or interaction is suppressed. Immunosuppression may result from either disease process or treatment. Selective immunosuppression may inhibit either cell-mediated or humoral immunity. Immunosuppression may be primary or secondary; secondary immunosuppression is the most common.

  Immunosuppression secondary to corticosteroid therapy is the most common secondary or acquired suppression. Acquired immunodeficiency syndrome (AIDS) resulting from depletion of immunoregulatory T cells occurs after infection with the human immunodeficiency virus (HIV). Primary lymphoid malignancies such as chronic lymphocytic leukemia and non-Hodgkin's lymphoma may also cause immunosuppression.[6]

- *Anemia*—a condition characterized by a decrease in hemoglobin level or circulating erythrocytes. Anemia oc-

Table 30-1 Types of Circulating Leukocytes

Type of WBC	% of WBC	Function
Neutrophil	50-70	Phagocytosis, inflammation
Eosinophil	1-4	Chemotaxis, allergies
Basophil	0-4	Anaphylaxis, allergies
Monocyte	2-9	Phagocytosis, inflammation, differentiation into macrophages
Macrophage	—	Circulating and fixed, phagocytosis, antigen processing and presenting cell for the T cell
Lymphocyte	20-40	Specific immune response, cell-mediated immunity and humoral immunity

curs when loss or destruction exceeds production of RBCs. This may occur from acute hemorrhage, replacement of normal marrow elements with abnormal cells, loss of the stem cell pool, decreased or ineffective production of RBCs, and accelerated destruction of RBCs. Anemia may result from both basic disease process and treatment.[6]

• *Thrombocytopenia*—a condition characterized by decreased numbers of circulating platelets or thrombocytes.[9,39] Thrombocytopenia may result from decreased or ineffective production of platelets secondary to marrow replacement by tumor, exposure to marrow toxins or infectious agents, and ionizing radiation. Thrombocytopenia may result also from increased destruction secondary to immune-mediated conditions, such as immune thrombocytopenia purpura (ITP) and heparin-induced thrombocytopenia or thrombosis syndrome (HITTS),[56] or coagulopathies such as disseminated intravascular coagulation (DIC). In some instances platelet numbers may be normal or increased and a bleeding tendency still exist. This abnormal bleeding may result from a qualitative platelet defect.[39] The most common causes of qualitative platelet defects are (1) ingestion of aspirin or similar drugs that interfere with normal platelet function and (2) the presence of abnormal platelets secondary to myeloproliferative disorders.[9,39]

• *Pancytopenia*—a term used when there is a deficiency of all the cell elements of the blood (erythrocytes, platelets, and all the white blood cells [neutrophils, eosinophils, basophils, monocytes, macrophages, and lymphocytes]).

Complicating factors. Complications associated with bone marrow suppression include increased susceptibility to infection secondary to neutropenia, fatigue associated with anemia, and increased risk of bleeding secondary to low platelet counts.

Assessment

Infection. Daily assessment of the cancer patient should include identification of risk factors for the development of infection, such as neutropenia, lymphopenia, immunosuppressive therapy, nonintact skin or mucous membranes, and the presence of vascular access devices. Close observation for the usual signs and symp-

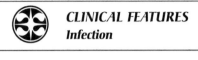

CLINICAL FEATURES
Infection

Temperature > 100.4° F (38° C)
Flushed skin, diaphoresis
Shaking chills
White, cream-colored lesions in mouth
Erythema, swelling, or pain in skin, throat, eyes, joints, perineal or rectal areas
Cough, chest pain, tachypnea, or dyspnea
Changes in character or color of sputum, urine, or stools
Dysuria or frequency of urination
Malaise, lethargy, myalgias, or arthralgias
Skin rash
Confusion, mental status change

toms of infection is necessary because neutropenic patients may exhibit little or no inflammatory response[5,14] (see box above). Fever and, occasionally, hypothermia represent serious infection in immunocompromised individuals.[40,44,47]

Changes in usual respiratory pattern (rate, depth, breath sounds, sputum production), in gastrointestinal tract functioning (nausea, vomiting, dysphagia, hiccoughs, abdominal pain, cramping, diarrhea, rectal pain or itching), and in the genitourinary system (dysuria, oliguria, anuria, pelvic pain, vaginal or urethral discharge) are frequently associated with infection.[16,22] Breaks in the integrity of the skin (head and neck, axillae, intertriginous areas, buttocks, and perineum) and mucous membranes (oral, anal, vaginal) represent portals of entry for infectious organisms and should be duly noted. Sepsis, or blood-borne systemic infection, produces significant morbidity and mortality. Assessment for and early detection of sepsis is important in caring for the severely neutropenic patient[55,69] (see box, p. 800).

Bleeding. Assessment for bleeding should include the following: a check of daily laboratory values for hemoglobin and platelet count; a check of medications that may alter platelet production or function; assessment for the presence of petechiae and ecchymoses, prolonged bleeding from venipunctures, minor cuts, or scratches,

CLINICAL FEATURES
Impending Septic Shock (Hyperdynamic or Warm Shock)

Mental confusion
Chills and fever
Skin flushed and dry
Blood pressure normal or slightly low
Pulse pressure widened
Tachycardia
Tachypnea
Hypoxemia
Urine output normal to slightly increased

INFECTING ORGANISMS ASSOCIATED WITH NEUTROPENIA

GRAM-NEGATIVE BACTERIA

Pseudomonas aeruginosa
Klebsiella and *Enterobacter* species
Escherichia coli

GRAM-POSITIVE BACTERIA

Staphylococcus aureus
Streptococcus pyogenes

FUNGI

Candida albicans
Aspergillus species
Mucorales species

LONG-TERM VASCULAR ACCESS DEVICES

Staphylococcus epidermidis
Corynebacterium JK

---

frank bleeding from any body orifice, and occult blood in excreta and vomitus.[39]

Anemia. Assessment for anemia and its resultant fatigue should include the following: a check of daily laboratory values for hemoglobin and platelet count, a check for presence of occult blood in the excreta of the thrombocytopenic patient, a check for the presence of frank bleeding from any body orifice, and assessment of the pattern of fatigue and its impact on activities of daily living and life-style.[39]

Medical Management

Infection. The medical management of suspected infection in the neutropenic or otherwise immunocompromised patient includes its prompt recognition with a workup including cultures, radiologic studies, a thorough physical assessment, and the immediate institution of broad-spectrum, empiric, intravenous antibiotics. Blood cultures should be obtained from both peripheral and central venous access sites, if present, for aerobic and anaerobic bacteria, fungi, and viruses if indicated. Cultures from body orifices, other body fluids, and any suspicious lesions should be obtained before initiating antibiotic therapy.[16,17,53,66,84] Sites of infection in the neutropenic patient are the following:

- Lungs
- Skin
- Oral cavity
- Gastrointestinal tract
- Genitourinary tract
- Blood

The choice of antibiotics is based on the prevalence and sensitivities of organisms commonly cultured at the health care facility[66] (see second box above). Controversy surrounds the best therapy for suspected infection in the neutropenic patient. This is particularly true concerning whether to use monotherapy with a single broad-spectrum antimicrobial (newer approach) or a combination of an aminoglycoside and a broad-spectrum β-lactam (more traditional approach). Factors to consider include severity of neutropenia, presence of suspected focus of infection, and clinical picture (i.e., presence of unstable vital signs, sepsis, acute respiratory distress syndrome [ARDS], and mucositis). Antibiotic coverage may be narrowed when the culture results are available. Antibiotic therapy usually continues for a minimum of 10 to 14 days or until the patient's neutrophil count recovers to between 500/mm^3 and 1500/mm^3 (another point of controversy). If the patient continues febrile for longer than 72 hours, it is advisable to reculture and, depending on previous culture results, change antibiotic therapy. If the patient has a vascular access device and the current antibiotics do not have good coagulase-negative staphylococcus coverage, therapy may need to be changed to include a drug such as vancomycin. If the patient's clinical course deteriorates or there is reason to suspect the infecting agent may be either fungal or viral, amphotericin B (an antifungal) or acyclovir (an antiviral) or both may be added empirically.*

Bleeding. Bleeding related to thrombocytopenia may be manifested as petechiae, purpura, ecchymoses, bleeding from a hollow viscus (GI tract, lungs, or GU tract), intracranial hemorrhage, or occult bleeding identified through routine testing of excreta.[39,52] Workup of a suspected bleed should include a thorough physical examination, radiologic examination as indicated by the clinical presentation, and laboratory evaluation, including a complete blood count (CBC), prothrombin time (PT) and partial thromboplastin time (PTT), and fibrinogen and fi-

---

*References 17, 36, 48, 53, 59, 66, 79.

brin degradation products (FDPs) if indicated.[2] Treatment depends on the cause of the bleeding. If the bleeding is secondary to thrombocytopenia or a qualitative platelet defect, platelet transfusions will be of value. If the bleeding results from a coagulopathy such as DIC, platelets and coagulation factors may be replaced, using concentrates, cryoprecipitate, or fresh frozen plasma. Aminocaproic acid (Amicar) may be added to inhibit lysis of the clot by the fibrinolytic system.[9,39,52]

Anemia. Symptoms of anemia may occur at variable levels of hemoglobin, depending on the rapidity with which it has occurred, age of the patient, and status of the cardiorespiratory system.[72] Findings may include the following: palpitations, shortness of breath, orthopnea, congestive heart failure with pulmonary edema, angina, fatigue, weakness, intolerance of cold, tinnitus, digestive complaints, difficulty in concentration, and numerous other nonspecific findings.[72,73] The workup should include a thorough physical assessment looking for the site of bleeding and the level of cardiorespiratory compensation. Laboratory examination should include CBC, reticulocyte count, lactic dehydrogenase and bilirubin values, and a hemolysis screen if indicated.[73] A trial of rEPO may be administered to improve hemoglobin levels. Transfusion of RBCs is indicated if there is evidence of cardiac decompensation or if low hemoglobin levels are combined with low platelet counts. Transfusion of whole blood is not indicated unless there is massive bleeding and volume replacement cannot be accomplished by other means. Replacement of circulating red cell mass to improve oxygen-carrying capacity should be accomplished by transfusion of packed RBCs. This provides for more efficient use of blood components and less risk of volume overload.[57]

TRANSFUSION THERAPY

The use of blood component therapy is one of the more common supportive therapies employed in the care of the person with myelosuppression. Even so, transfusion therapy must be used with care. Although major mismatch transfusion reactions are rare and usually result from management systems error (the patient received the wrong unit of blood because of improper identification of blood and/or patient), febrile transfusion reactions are quite common. Febrile reactions are caused by the recipient reacting to donor leukocyte antigens. This can be discomforting for the patient and may accelerate alloimmunization or sensitization to transfused blood.

Historically, febrile reactions have been dealt with by the use of premedications that may suppress the response or by the administration of leukocyte-poor blood products. Saline-washed RBCs provided significantly reduced numbers of leukocytes although this is costly in time, money, and loss of RBCs. Early leukodepletion filter required extra processing and cooling of the RBCs. Leukocyte-poor platelets were rarely provided. Recent technologic advances have produced more efficient filters that are both user friendly and available for platelets. The provision of leukocyte-poor blood components is more important for those persons who are expected to require transfusion support for prolonged periods and alloimmunization prevention.[7] Other potential benefits from leukodepletion include (1) decreased risk of blood-borne pathogens that reside in leukocytes, such as cytomegalovirus (CMV), and (2) possible decreased risk of transfusion-associated graft-versus-host disease.[3,7,46,57]

CMV infection, especially CMV pneumonitis, carries a significant risk for morbidity and mortality in patients who are severely immunosuppressed. CMV transmission may occur when a CMV-negative (CMV−) recipient is transfused with blood from a CMV-positive (CMV+) donor. The virus may remain dormant in lymphocyte for years after active infection. CMV+ persons with normal immune system function are unaffected by the virus, since their immune system keeps the virus in check. Interest is great regarding methods of reducing risk for the CMV− person. Leukodepletion of blood components may help decrease the risk by removing potentially infectious leukocytes.[7] Another method that is showing promise is the development/identification of a CMV− blood donor pool. This necessitates screening and designation of CMV− donors. Not in widespread use, this method is costly, time-consuming, and removes potential donors from the general blood donor pool.

Since the mid-1980s when HIV transmission via blood transfusion was confirmed, potential blood transfusion recipients have shown a great interest in directed donations (the personal selection of one's blood donors). It has been assumed that directed donors would be safer than donors from the volunteer pools, when in fact it has been shown that the incidence of infectious disease markers is higher in directed donor population. A more recent problem with directed donations is transfusion-associated graft-versus-host disease (TA-GvHD).[7] Although its occurrence is exceedingly rare, TA-GvHD carries a mortality rate approximating 100%. The high mortality rate is associated with bone marrow failure. TA-GvHD has been associated most frequently with directed donations from first-degree relatives such as parents or siblings. TA-GvHD occurs when the transfusion recipient has two nonidentical HLA haplotypes and the transfusion (lymphocyte) donor is homozygous for either of the HLA haplotypes of the recipient. The recipient is unable to recognize the donor lymphocytes as "nonself" while the donor (transfused) lymphocytes are able to recognize the recipient as "nonself." The lymphocyte reaction is essentially the same as that seen after allogeneic marrow transplantation. The exception is that the recipient marrow stem cells are a target organ for the graft-versus-host (GvH) reaction, whereas in BMT-associated GvHD, the marrow stem cells are of donor origin and therefore "self" and are not reacted against. The potential for TA-GvHD after directed donation is such that it is recommended that all blood components from first-degree relatives be irradiated before transfusion. Irradia-tion of blood components before transfusion is standard procedure for marrow transplant recipients and premature or other immunocompromised neonates. It is possible that leukodepletion filtration may decrease the risk of TA-GvHD, but it is not as effective as ionizing radiation.[3,7,46]

Text continued on p. 813.

NURSING MANAGEMENT

SKIN INTEGRITY

NURSING DIAGNOSES[19,45,48,62,64]

- *Skin integrity, impaired, risk for/actual, related to immobility, malignant skin lesions, infectious skin lesions, nonspecific rashes, irritation from urinary or fecal incontinence, abrasions resulting from scratching and shearing forces, invasive therapeutic procedures, radiation skin reactions, "recall" skin reactions, chemotherapy extravasations, lymphatic or vascular obstruction, decubiti, malnutrition*
- *Infection, risk for, related to impairment of skin integrity secondary to any of the contributing factors just listed, surgical incision, presence of long-term venous access device*
- *Pain related to any of the contributing factors just listed, postherpetic neuralgia, pruritus secondary to basic disease process or adverse drug reaction*
- *Body image disturbance related to malignant skin lesions, extremity edema, alopecia*

OUTCOME GOALS

Patient will be able to:
- Identify/demonstrate measures to maintain/promote skin integrity.
- Identify/demonstrate measures to prevent infection related to impaired skin integrity.
- Achieve adequate control of pain related to impaired skin integrity.
- Show evidence of effective coping with body image disturbance related to impaired skin integrity.

Intact Skin

INTERVENTIONS: Assessment

- Inspect high-risk skin areas for color, vascularity, edema, injuries, scars, lesions, nodules.
- Document assessment at least once a shift.

INTERVENTIONS: Preventive Measures to Maintain Intact Skin

- Reposition, at least every 2 hours, any individual in bed who is assessed to be at risk for developing pressure ulcers.
- Use draw sheet for turning and positioning.

- Elevate head of bed to maximum of 30 degrees except for mealtimes, at which time bed may be elevated more.
- Use footboard to prevent sliding.
- Provide over-bed trapeze to assist in position change.
- Lift patient to change position rather than pulling or sliding.
- Use devices to decrease pressure areas, such as mattress overlays or alternating pressure mattresses (see Table 30-2).
- Use heel and elbow protectors.
- Provide meticulous skin hygiene—mild soap, thorough rinsing, patting dry (not rubbing), air drying when feasible, applying lotions to skin over bony prominences.

INTERVENTIONS: Malnourishment

- Follow general preventive measures.
- Provide adequate nutritional support.
- Assess risk daily.

INTERVENTIONS: Incontinence

- Follow general preventive measures.
- Offer bedpan and urinal every 2 hours.
- Wash buttocks and perineum after each incontinence; pat or air dry.
- Place waterproof pads between draw sheets rather than next to patient's skin.
- Evaluate need for bowel and bladder retraining program.

INTERVENTIONS: Immobility

- Follow general preventive measures.
- Use splints and braces to prevent contractures.
- Use dietetic and nutrition consultants.
- Initiate referrals to rehabilitation medicine, social services, and vocational rehabilitation.
- Institute bowel program with stool softeners and laxatives to prevent constipation.
- Provide diversionary activities to prevent boredom.

INTERVENTIONS: Pruritus

- Follow general preventive measures.
- Maintain hydration of the skin by increasing fluid intake, applying water-soluble emollients to damp skin, and providing a humidified environment.

Table 30-2 Pressure Reduction Devices/Specialty Beds

Indications for use	Support surfaces	Manufacturer	Intended use
Low risk/prevention: Stages 0-I ulcer	Foam overlay	Bio Clinic Mason Span-America	Used on top of existing mattress; single patient use; least expensive.
	Water/gel-filled overlay	Flotation Systems Mason	Durable; easy to clean; heavy; both may cause high pressure at heels.
Medium risk: Stages I-III ulcer	Static air-filled pressure pad	Gaymar Kinetic Concepts Mason	Redistributes pressure to areas of less pressure.
	Dynamic air-filled pressure pad	Bio Clinic Gaymar Grant Hill-Rom HNE Healthcare Mason	Also called *alternating pressure pads;* pump constantly changes pressure points; requires constant monitoring.
Medium/high risk: Stages I-IV ulcer	Foam mattress; gel and foam mattress	Bio Clinic Hill-Rom Kinetic Concepts Mason Span-America	Provide support and conformity; reduce pressure and shear; may be hospital replacement mattress.
	Low air-loss mattress	Bio Clinic Gaymar Kinetic Concepts	Calibrated to patient's weight; air not cycled—shifts in response to movement.
	Active mattress overlay system	Gaymar Hill-Rom HNE Healthcare Kinetic Concepts	Air cycles continuously; used with standard hospital bed frame and mattress.
High risk: Stage IV ulcer	Dynamic flotation mattress	Bio Clinic Gaymar Hill-Rom HNE Healthcare Kinetic Concepts Mason	Sensor pad continuously monitors the system.
	Low air-loss bed	Bio Clinic Hill-Rom Kinetic Concepts	On special frame—scales, or CPR quick-release lever.
Ultra high risk: Stage IV ulcer	Air-fluidized bed	Hill-Rom Kinetic Concepts	For small group of patients who cannot tolerate any pressure.

Modified from Carroll P: *RN* 58(5):44, 1995.

Bed manufacturers may be contacted as follows: Bio Clinic, (800) 388-4083; Floatation Systems Inc, (800) 888-8529; Gaymar Industries Inc, (800) 828-7341; Grant Airmass Corp, (800) 243-5237; Hill-Rom, (800) 638-2546; HNE Healthcare, (800) 223-1218; Kinetic Concepts Inc, (800) 531-5346; Mason Medical Products, (800) 233-4454; Span-America Medical Systems Inc, (800) 888-6752.

- Keep fingernails short and smooth.
- Wash hands frequently.
- Use alternative methods of skin stimulation such as pressure, massage, vibration, and cold compresses.
- Avoid inciting agents and tight, irritating, nonabsorbable clothing.
- Prevent vasodilation by providing a cool environment and cool baths and showers, avoiding alcohol- and caffeine-containing foods and beverages, and decreasing anxiety level through use of distraction.
- Institute medical treatment as prescribed, which may include treatment of the underlying malignancy, antihistamines, corticosteroids, tranquilizers, and topical agents.

• • •

Maintenance of normal skin integrity should be a major emphasis of nursing management. This includes continued assessment, evaluation of risk, prevention of skin breakdown, and specific interventions if impaired skin integrity occurs. Systematic protocols or care plans should be implemented to ensure continuity of care.

Continued.

PATIENT AND FAMILY EDUCATION

Patients and families need to be taught the importance
of maintaining intact skin, the fundamentals of assessing
skin, and how to prevent breakdown by proper positioning
and padding to prevent pressure points. Patients
and families should be taught the signs and symptoms
of infection and when and whom to notify on the health
care team.

Nonintact Skin
INTERVENTIONS: Assessment

• Inspect skin lesions and document: general character,
location and distribution, configuration, size (measure),
morphologic structure (nodularity, scaling, crusting,
erosions, fissures), drainage (color, amount, character,
odor), depth of lesion, presence of vital structure in lesion
(carotid artery).
• Use National Pressure Ulcer Advisory Panel (NPUAP)
staging system for pressure ulcers (Table 30-3).
• Monitor for signs and symptoms of infection (elevated
temperature, tachycardia, tachypnea, change in color
and odor of drainage, erythema).
• Evaluate for associated signs and symptoms (pain and
tenderness).
• Evaluate patient's physical and psychologic responses
to lesions.
• Assess patient's and family's ability to care for problem
in the home.

Table 30-3   Staging of Pressure Ulcers

Stage	Description
I	Nonblanchable erythema of intact skin—the heralding lesion of skin ulceration. Should not be confused with reactive hyperemia, which may be expected to be present for one-half to three-fourths as long as pressure occludes blood flow to the area.
II	Partial-thickness skin loss involving epidermis and/or dermis. The ulcer is superficial and presents clinically as an abrasion, blister, or shallow crater.
III	Full-thickness skin loss involving damage or necrosis of subcutaneous tissue that may extend down to, but not through, underlying fascia.
IV	Full-thickness skin loss with extensive destruction, tissue necrosis or damage to muscle, bone, or supporting structures. Undermining and sinus tracts may be associated with stage IV ulcers.

Data from National Pressure Ulcer Advisory Panel: Pressure ulcers in
adults: protection and prevention, US Dept of Health and Human Services,
Public Health Service, Agency for Health Care Policy and Research,
Rockville, Md, AHCPR Pub. No. 92-0047, May, 1992.

INTERVENTIONS: General Maintenance

• Follow general preventive measures.
• Implement infection control measures.
• Implement measures to prevent bleeding and trauma.
• Provide adequate pain control.
• Obtain enterostomal therapy/skin care specialist consult.
• Obtain home health referral well in advance of discharge.

INTERVENTIONS: Nonulcerating Lesions

• Follow general preventive measures.
• Use dry dressings to protect against irritation and
trauma.
• Use occlusive dressings with topical medications for increased
penetration.

INTERVENTIONS: Ulcerating Lesions

• Cleanse area with antibacterial soap using gentle motion.
Rinse well. Prevent cross-contamination if local
infection is present.
• Follow recommended protocol for débridement (i.e.,
cotton swabs, wet-to-dry soaks, continuous soaks, or
proteolytic enzymes).

INTERVENTIONS: Prevention and Management of Local Infection

• Irrigate with antibacterial agent as prescribed.
• Use sterile technique.
• Administer systemic antibiotics as prescribed.
• Obtain specimens for culture as ordered or if fever is
present.
• Apply dry, sterile, nonadherent dressing. Change and
cleanse every 8 hours or more often as needed.

INTERVENTIONS: Hemostasis

• Use silver nitrate sticks or styptic pencils as prescribed
for mild oozing.
• Apply 1:1000 epinephrine or topical thrombin to areas
with moderate oozing as prescribed. Local radiation or
application of hemostatic dressings may be used.
• Administer platelet transfusions as ordered for bleeding
associated with thrombocytopenia.

INTERVENTIONS: Drainage

• Change dressing as frequently as necessary (as soon as
it is wet).
• Use absorbent dressings for small to moderate amounts
of drainage or on areas too large to pouch.
• Apply drainage bag or ostomy pouch for copious
amounts of drainage. Apply skin protectant to surrounding
skin to prevent irritation and breakdown.
• Secure sterile dressings with Montgomery straps,
stretchable gauze, or Stomahesive.

INTERVENTIONS: Odor

- Cleanse wound and change dressing as frequently as necessary.
- Obtain culture and sensitivities of wound.
- Apply commercial deodorizing agents to outside of dressings.
- Administer agents such as metronidazole (orally or topically) to control odor caused by anaerobes.
- Place shallow tray of activated charcoal in patient's room.
- Place commercial room deodorizer in room (if room deodorizer is not more offensive than wound odor).

PATIENT AND FAMILY EDUCATION

In addition to teaching general preventive measures to maintain intact skin, the nurse should teach the patient/family the signs and symptoms of infection and who and when to notify if they occur. Treatments and procedures should be discussed: clean or sterile technique, hand-washing technique, disposal of used/soiled materials and dressings, environmental and personal hygiene practices, measures to prevent cross-contamination, application and expected effects of medications, measures to maintain hydration and nutrition, and measures to control bleeding. The primary caregiver must be instructed how to change the dressing in the home.

NURSING MANAGEMENT

ORAL MUCOUS MEMBRANES

NURSING DIAGNOSES*

- *Oral mucous membranes, altered, related to side effects of chemotherapy or radiation therapy, local infection, tumor*
- *Infection, risk for, related to side effects of systemic chemotherapy or radiation therapy to the head and neck*
- *Knowledge deficit regarding good oral hygiene techniques, side effects of cancer therapy and radiation therapy*
- *Pain related to oral/esophageal mucositis as evidenced by patient's complaints of discomfort, excess or viscous oral secretions, oral lesions leading to discomfort, stimulation of the gag reflex*
- *Nutrition, altered: less than body requirements, related to oral discomfort as evidenced by decreased caloric intake, weight loss of more than 10% of preillness weight, weakness*
- *Communication, impaired verbal, related to oral discomfort, increased or decreased salivation*

OUTCOME GOALS

Patient will be able to:
- Exhibit oral cavity, gums, and lips free of irritation or ulceration.
- Demonstrate knowledge and competency related to prescribed oral hygiene measures.
- Demonstrate relief of pain related to oral mucositis.
- Identify/Demonstrate measures to prevent nutritional deficit.
- Achieve adequate verbal communication through the use of pain medications and frequent oral care measures.

*References 6, 10-12, 19, 23, 24, 31, 32, 60, 61.

INTERVENTIONS: Measures to Decrease Inflammation of Mucous Membranes

- Avoid exposure to chemical or physical irritants such as commercial mouthwashes, alcohol, tobacco, and hot, spicy, or coarse foods.
- Encourage adequate fluid intake (>3 L/day).
- Use a systematic oral care protocol, which includes oral hygiene measures before and after each meal and at bedtime as a minimum and every 2 hours around the clock when oral mucositis is present.

INTERVENTIONS: Measures to Increase Comfort

- Use topical protectant and analgesic agents.
- Use systemic analgesics when pain is uncontrolled by topical agents.
- Use safe, effective agents for oral care, which include normal saline (1 tsp/1 L of water) and sodium bicarbonate (1 tsp/1 L of water) alone or in combination (1:1).
- Facilitate brushing and flossing as the best defense against plaque build-up, but should be discontinued when the absolute neutrophil count (ANC) is less than 1000/mm^3, the platelet count is less than 50,000 mm^3, or mucositis is present. Toothettes or a gauze-wrapped finger may be used instead.[81] Low pressure irrigation set-ups, such as a gavage bag or an IV solution bag with tubing (using 500 ml normal saline), or a bulb syringe may be used to soften and remove debris. Suction equipment should be available for those patients at risk for aspiration.
- Water soluble lubricants may be used for dry, cracked lips.
- Dentures should be cleaned with a denture brush and an antimicrobial detergent such as chlorhexidine gluconate when oral care is done. Dentures should be rinsed with normal saline or water.

Continued.

- Dentures should be removed while sleeping and as often as possible to give mucosa a rest. When dentures are not in use, they should be soaked in commercial denture cleanser. Solution should be changed daily.
- Dentures should not be worn except for meals when mucositis is present or when ANC is less than 1000 mm^3 or platelet count is less than 50,000 mm^3 even when no oral pathology is present.
- For mild to moderate mucositis, implement oral care protocol every 2 hours while awake and every 4 hours during night.
- For severe mucositis, implement oral care protocol every 1 to 2 (not to exceed 2) hours during day and every 2 to 4 (not to exceed 4) hours during night.

INTERVENTIONS: Measures to Minimize Complications

- Modify dietary intake to include bland, soft, or liquid food (avoiding acidic foods and liquids) high in calories and protein, served at room temperature or cool—not hot or cold.
- Encourage use of oral hygiene measures before eating.
- Administer topical or systemic analgesics before meals.
- Provide calorie-containing liquids of choice for patient to sip frequently.
- For xerostomia (dry mouth), provide artificial saliva at bedside for patient use. Encourage patient to rinse mouth with water at least every 2 hours while awake. Provide beverages and sauces with meals to help alleviate difficulty swallowing.
- Identify alternative means of communication such as magic slates, notes, cards, and direct, short-response questions.

INTERVENTIONS: Medical Treatment

- Administer antibiotics, antifungals, and antivirals as prescribed.
- Administer analgesics as needed. Patient may require around-the-clock systemic analgesia.

- Administer dietary supplements, enteral nutrition, or parenteral nutrition as prescribed.
- For bleeding from oral mucosa, administer antifibrinolytics and platelets as prescribed, and/or apply topical thrombin and Gelfoam.
- Obtain swabs (specimens) for bacterial, fungal, and viral cultures and sensitivities.

• • •

Nursing management of oral and esophageal mucositis includes systematic assessment and documentation of condition of oral cavity at least once a day, informing the physician of any abnormalities, and using a consistent and safe systematic oral care plan around the clock.* Promote comfort through the use of topical anesthetics and systemic analgesics, maintain optimal nutritional status, teach patient/family to use interventions to prevent/minimize oral mucositis, and use precautions when caring for the unresponsive patient to prevent aspiration while administering oral care.

PATIENT AND FAMILY EDUCATION

Teaching should include emphasis on the following:
- Importance and technique of daily oral assessment
- Signs and symptoms of mucositis and infection
- Importance of continuing use of a systematic oral care protocol at home
- Importance of fluids and adequate nutrition
- Necessity of dietary changes secondary to the presence or absence of oral and esophageal lesions
- Avoidance of trauma to mucous membranes secondary to smoking, smokeless tobacco, alcohol, extremes of temperature, chemical irritants such as commercial mouthwashes, and physical irritants such as highly seasoned or hard- or sharp-textured foods and poorly fitting dentures.

*References 10, 25-27, 30-33, 51, 68, 76.

NURSING MANAGEMENT

VAGINAL/RECTAL MUCOSITIS
NURSING DIAGNOSES[19,37,45,83,85]

- *Tissue integrity, impaired, related to side effects of chemotherapy and/or radiation therapy as evidenced by signs and symptoms of mucositis*
- *Infection, risk for, related to nonintact vaginal and/or rectal mucosa*
- *Knowledge deficit regarding safe sexual practices, good personal hygiene, side effects of mucositis related to cancer therapy*

- *Pain related to mucositis evidenced by the patient's complaints of painful urination, defecation, sexual intercourse*
- *Diarrhea related to gastrointestinal mucositis*
- *Pain related to painful defecation secondary to rectal mucositis*
- *Sexuality patterns, altered, related to decreased energy, potential fear of trauma or infection*

OUTCOME GOALS

Patient will be able to:

- Demonstrate health practices to prevent further impairment and promote integrity of vaginal and rectal mucous membranes.
- Remain infection-free related to impaired vaginal or rectal mucositis.
- Achieve adequate pain relief related to vaginal/rectal mucositis.
- Demonstrate measures to control or correct diarrhea.
- Identify/Demonstrate strategies to manage or correct alteration in sexuality.

INTERVENTIONS: *Measures to Decrease Inflammation of Mucous Membranes*

- Avoid exposure to chemical and physical irritants such as tampons, deodorant-containing vaginal pads or liners, deodorant-containing personal hygiene sprays, douches, rectal thermometers and suppositories, and vaginal and anal intercourse.
- Encourage adequate fluid intake.
- Wash perineum with soap and water after each urination and defecation; pat or air dry.

INTERVENTIONS: *Measures to Increase Comfort*

- Use sitz baths.
- Avoid standing or sitting for long periods.
- Avoid irritating, constricting, nonabsorbent underclothing.

INTERVENTIONS: *Measures to Minimize Complications*

- Modify dietary intake to minimize diarrhea and constipation.
- Encourage frequent perineal hygiene measures.
- Instruct female patients to wipe from front to back after urination and defecation.
- Avoid trauma to either vaginal or rectal mucosa.
- Monitor patient for signs and symptoms of vaginal infection or rectal cellulitis/abscess; culture as needed; notify physician.

PATIENT AND FAMILY EDUCATION

Teaching should include emphasis on the following:

- Personal risk factors for development of mucositis secondary to chemotherapy, radiation therapy.
- Signs and symptoms of mucositis, such as pain, itching, and discharge or drainage, which should be reported.
- Measures to prevent complications.
- Situations that require professional interventions, such as fever, diarrhea, and uncontrolled pain.

Nursing management of vaginal and rectal mucositis includes frequent, indirect assessment of signs and symptoms of mucositis, prevention of diarrhea and constipation, encouragement of bathing of perineal and rectal areas after each urination and defecation, teaching female patients to wipe front to back to prevent contaminating vaginal and urethral areas with fecal organisms, and teaching sexual practices that minimize trauma and risk of infection.

Teaching should include the signs and symptoms of mucositis and infection, whom and when to call, and sexual and elimination practices that prevent or minimize the risk of trauma and infection. Vaginal intercourse should be avoided while platelet and neutrophil counts are low and if mucosal ulcerations are present. Intercourse should be permitted and encouraged after recovery of blood counts and mucosa. This may help prevent development of vaginal strictures and webbing, which may occur after pelvic irradiation. Women who are not sexually active may need to use vaginal dilators to maintain vaginal patency after pelvic irradiation. Condoms should be worn by the male partner to prevent transmission of organisms through nonintact mucosa. Adequate lubrication should be obtained using a water-soluble, not a petroleum-based, product. Anal intercourse should be avoided.[23]

NURSING MANAGEMENT

INCREASED SUSCEPTIBILITY TO INFECTION

NURSING DIAGNOSES[2,21,60,83-85]

- *Infection, risk for, related to disease entity; side-effects of treatment; neutropenia, immune suppression, etc.; disruption of mucous membranes or skin; presence of long-term venous access device*
- *Body temperature, altered, risk for, related to infection secondary to neutropenia, immunosuppression, nonintact skin or mucous membranes*
- *Knowledge deficit regarding basic disease process, treatment, signs and symptoms of infection, neutropenic precautions*
- *Sexuality patterns, altered, related to decreased energy and potential fear of trauma or infection*
- *Social isolation related to therapeutic environment or fear of acquiring an infection*
- *Anxiety related to knowledge of diagnosis, treatment, prognosis*
- *Fear related to discharge concerning home management, self-care, uncertainty about long-term outcome*

Continued.

OUTCOME GOALS

Patient will be able to:

- Remain infection-free during hospitalization or illness.
- Demonstrate knowledge about diagnosis and disease process, therapy, signs and symptoms of infection, survival skills.
- Report a desire to resume sexual activity.
- Identify reasons for feelings of isolation and identify appropriate diversional activities.
- Relate an increase in psychologic and physiologic comfort.
- Express desire for discharge and demonstrate competency in performing self-care activities.

Preventive Measures

Prevention of infection in susceptible individuals is an important nursing measure. Hand-washing is the single most important action for the health care professional, the patient, the patient's family, and visitors. The importance of adequate hand-washing using running water, soap, and friction cannot be overstated. The health care professional must use good hand-washing technique before and after any direct patient contact. Gloves are not to be used as a substitute for good hand-washing.[16,18,22]

Protective isolation techniques vary from institution to institution. The Centers for Disease Control and Prevention no longer recognizes or recommends protective isolation for persons who are immunosuppressed or neutropenic. Protective isolation can be thought of more as a "mind set" than an actual category of isolation.[29,63] It must become second nature for the nurse caring for the neutropenic or immunosuppressed patient to be aware of the patient's increased risk and the risk the nurse represents to the patient.[16,18] Most institutions advocate the use of a private room, good hand-washing practices, and an infection-free staff to care for the patient. Dietary restrictions for the neutropenic patient may include an order for "cooked diet" only. Raw fruits and uncooked vegetables are often excluded because of soil contact and repeated handling by dietary personnel during storage and preparation.[16,18,21]

INTERVENTIONS: *General Preventive Measures*

- Wash hands with soap, water, and friction before and after all direct patient contact.
- Provide private room if possible; if unavailable, ensure uninfected roommate.
- Provide infection-free staff to care for patient.
- Give nursing care to neutropenic patient first to decrease risk of cross-contamination.
- Provide meticulous skin and oral hygiene for patient.
- Provide cooked diet only—no raw fruits or vegetables.
- Do not allow live plants or cut flowers in standing water in room.

- Avoid all sources of stagnant water in room such as water pitchers, denture cups, humidifiers, and respiratory therapy equipment; change daily.
- Screen visitors for illnesses.
- Avoid overcrowded areas such as waiting rooms.
- Use Universal Precautions when caring for all patients.

INTERVENTIONS: *Prompt Recognition of Suspected Infection*

- Assume that any change from the ordinary is infection until proven otherwise.
- Assess patient's risk of infection by calculating ANC and reviewing patient history for predisposing factors such as basic disease process, myelosuppressive therapies, immunosuppressive therapies, and antibiotic therapy.
- Assess skin and mucous membranes each shift and document in patient record.
- Assess vital signs including temperature at least every 4 hours and document in patient record.
- Notify physician of temperature elevation greater than 100.8° F (38.2° C), changes in skin and mucous membrane integrity, lesions, or rashes and any altered level of consciousness.
- Facilitate workup of suspected infection by obtaining ordered cultures, blood specimens, and radiologic studies in a timely manner.
- Initiate and administer antibiotics as prescribed in a timely manner.
- Observe and assess patient for adverse effects of antibiotic administration.

• • •

Nursing management of the infected cancer patient is a complex and challenging task. Infection is the most common cause of death for the person with cancer. Nurses represent a crucial and constant part of the care team—and frequently the difference between life and death for the patient.[84]

Nursing management of infection demands its prompt recognition, which requires the health care professional to maintain a high index of suspicion. Literally anything out of the ordinary could be infection. The nurse's intuitive feelings are frequently helpful in the absence of objective findings of infection. Physician notification and documentation of the nursing assessment in the patient record are essential parts of the nursing process.[16,22,41]

The nurse's assistance in the workup of suspected infection will include timely retrieval of specimens for culture, coordination of radiologic studies, and facilitation of physical assessment by the physician and nurse.[8,16,53]

Empiric antibiotic therapy should be instituted within 4 hours of an initial temperature spike, as well as obtaining cultures. It is the nurse's responsibility to provide for timely and safe administration of antibiotics.

Table 30-4   Nursing Implications of Antibiotic Administration

Drugs	Side effects	Implications
AMINOGLYCOSIDES		
Amikacin Gentamicin Tobramycin Vancomycin	Nephrotoxicity, ototoxicity	Monitor renal function carefully. Monitor for signs of hearing loss, tinnitus, and vertigo. Observe for signs of superinfection. Follow infusion guidelines carefully.
PENICILLINS (β-lactam)		
Azlocillin Carbenicillin Mezlocillin Piperacillin Ticarcillin	Skin rashes, drug fever, anaphylaxis, hypokalemia, abnormal platelet function	Monitor renal function carefully. Elicit allergy history. Be prepared for possible allergic reaction. Monitor CBC and liver function tests carefully. Monitor serum electrolytes (potassium [K^+] and sodium [Na^+]). Observe for signs of superinfection.
CEPHALOSPORINS (β-lactam)		
Cefoperazone Cefotaxime Ceftazidime Ceftriaxone	Skin rashes, drug fever	Monitor renal function carefully. Observe for phlebitis if given peripherally. Observe for signs of superinfection.
MONOBACTAMS		
Aztreonam (β-lactam)	Seizures, altered taste, diarrhea, nausea, vomiting, skin rash, superinfection, anaphylaxis	Elicit history of allergies. Monitor liver function. Monitor renal function. Monitor coagulation. Monitor neurotoxicity. Observe for signs of superinfection.
CARBAPENEM		
Imipenem/cilastin	Seizures, somnolence, hypotension, nausea, diarrhea, vomiting, rash, phlebitis, anaphylaxis	Elicit allergy history. Monitor renal function. Monitor liver function. Monitor CBC and Coombs' test. Observe for signs of superinfection.
QUINOLONES		
Ciprofloxacin	Nausea, vomiting, diarrhea, headache, rash, anaphylaxis, nephrotoxicity, phlebitis	Monitor liver function tests. Restrict caffeine intake. Avoid excess sun exposure. Monitor renal function tests. Observe for phlebitis. Observe for signs of superinfection.
ANTIFUNGAL AGENTS		
Amphotericin B Liposomal ampho B (Abelcet)	Hypokalemia, fever, rigors, phlebitis, nausea, vomiting, headache, nephrotoxicity, ototoxicity, elevated liver enzymes	Monitor renal function carefully. Monitor serum electrolytes carefully. Monitor liver function tests carefully. Premedicate with diphenhydramine, acetaminophen, and meperidine. Administer additional meperidine IV as ordered for relief of rigors. Monitor patient's temperature at baseline and during infusion. Infuse slowly, preferably with infusion pump. Drug is a colloid; administer with nonfiltered tubing; agitate bag frequently to maintain in suspension; keep out of direct sunlight.

Continued.

Scheduling, timing of infusions, and knowledge of drug toxicities and interactions are also the responsibility of the nurse (Table 30-4).[48,52,59,66]

Frequent assessment of the patient with suspected infection is essential. Vital signs including temperature should be measured no less frequently than every 4 hours. Other key points of assessment should include auscultation of breath sounds, auscultation and palpation of abdomen, observation of skin and mucous membranes, and assessment of level of consciousness.[16,47]

Fever management includes administration of antipyretics and the use of tepid baths, cooling blankets, ice packs, and other nonpharmacologic methods of reducing elevated body temperature. Once antipyretics have been instituted and fever recurs, it is often less physiologically stressful to administer them on an around-the-clock schedule to avoid the see-saw pattern of hyperthermia and hypothermia. It is important to prevent shivering, which increases body temperature. Parenteral meperidine or morphine or both may be administered to alleviate rigors.[40,44,47,74]

Early recognition of septic shock is essential to patient survival. Impending sepsis is frequently suggested by the findings of tachycardia, tachypnea, widened pulse pressure, elevated body temperature, hot, dry skin, and al-

tered mental status. Survival is improved if sepsis is recognized before circulatory collapse occurs.*

PATIENT AND FAMILY EDUCATION

Educational efforts should center on teaching the patient and family the signs and symptoms of infection, which may include any of the following: fever, cough, dysuria, shortness of breath, oral ulcers, diarrhea, nausea, and vomiting. Because of the risk of septic shock associated with neutropenia, it is imperative that the patient and family take any fever seriously and notify the appropriate health care professional. Teaching should be explicit about when and whom to call and include a list of telephone numbers giving the patient and family 24-hour access to the health care setting.[28]

"Survival teaching" should be individualized to each patient, taking into consideration readiness to learn and ability to take charge of his or her life and illness. Content may include laboratory test interpretation; calculation of an absolute neutrophil count; keeping a journal of dates, drugs, dosages, blood counts, and side effects; neutropenic precautions; hand-washing technique; personal hygiene practices; activity; diet; and sexual practices.[28]

---

*References 8, 15, 17, 22, 41, 43, 55, 67, 69.

NURSING MANAGEMENT

INCREASED RISK OF BLEEDING

NURSING DIAGNOSES[2,9,19,39,45]

- *Injury, risk for, bleeding related to decreased platelet count, basic disease process, cancer treatment*
- *Knowledge deficit regarding thrombocytopenia and increased risk of bleeding, signs and symptoms of bleeding*
- *Sexuality patterns, altered, related to decreased energy, potential fear of trauma or infection*
- *Anxiety related to knowledge of diagnosis, treatment, prognosis*
- *Fear related to discharge concerning home management, self-care, uncertainty about long-term outcome*

OUTCOME GOALS

Patient will be able to:
- Remain free from injury related to bleeding.
- Demonstrate knowledge of signs and symptoms of bleeding.
- Report desire to resume sexual activity.
- Relate an increase in psychologic and physiologic comfort.

- Express desire for discharge and demonstrates competency in performing self-care activities.

Preventive Measures

Bleeding should be prevented in the thrombocytopenic patient. Measures should include those that maintain skin and mucous membrane integrity.[2,9]

Provision of a safe environment falls within the confines of nursing practice. In severely thrombocytopenic patients, bed rails should be up at all times, the patient should be up with assistance only, and the patient who is weak or showing signs of bleeding should be on complete bed rest.

All excreta and vomitus should be tested for the presence of occult blood. The results of each test should be entered in the patient record and the physician notified if the results vary significantly from previous testing.

Laboratory tests should be done as ordered. The nurse should know results and how they are related to the patient's risk for bleeding. The nurse should be able to interpret laboratory results in terms of platelet disorder, coagulation factor deficiency, mixed coagulopathy, and lack of vascular integrity.[39,52]

INTERVENTIONS: *General Preventive Measures*

- Limit invasive procedures.
- Provide safe environment (e.g., side rails up, assistance with ambulation).
- Avoid intramuscular injections.
- Avoid aspirin-containing medications or nonsteroidal antiinflammatories.
- Suppress menses in premenopausal female patients by hormonal manipulation as ordered by the physician.
- Avoid tooth flossing and hard toothbrushes.
- Avoid use of rectal thermometers, suppositories, enemas, and rectal examinations.
- Avoid alcohol-containing beverages.

INTERVENTIONS: *Assessment of Bleeding*

- Check laboratory values for platelet count, hemoglobin and hematocrit, and any other coagulation studies, such as prothrombin time (PT), partial thromboplastin time (PTT), fibrinogen, and fibrin degradation products (FDP) to assess patient's risk of bleeding.
- Assess skin and mucous membranes for presence of petechiae, purpura, and ecchymoses, document in patient record, and notify physician of any evidence of bleeding.
- Assess for any evidence of frank bleeding (e.g., epistaxis, hemoptysis, hematemesis, hematochezia, melena, hematuria, vaginal bleeding), document in patient record, and notify physician if present.
- Quantitate amount of frank bleeding as accurately as possible, document, and report.
- Hemetest all stools, urine, and emesis for the presence of occult blood whenever the platelet count is less than 50,000/mm^3.
- Apply pressure and/or pressure dressings to venipunctures, bone marrow aspiration and biopsy sites, and other sites of invasive procedures until hemostasis occurs.
- Observe sites of invasive procedures, such as vascular access device placement, for continued hemostasis and notify physician if bleeding is present or recurs.
- Administer appropriate medications to prevent activities that raise intracranial pressure such as vomiting, coughing, sneezing, and straining in stool.
- Report any complaints of headache with or without change in level of consciousness or vital signs.
- Administer platelet transfusions and other blood component therapy as ordered.
- Obtain physician order and administer premedications of diphenhydramine, acetaminophen, and/or corticosteroids to patient with history of transfusion reaction.
- Monitor patient for signs and symptoms of transfusion reaction and take appropriate measures (Table 30-5).

INTERVENTIONS: *Patient and Family Education*

- Assess skin and mucous membranes daily for evidence of bleeding.
- Assess personal risk of bleeding by knowing current platelet count and other pertinent laboratory values.
- Assess for and report any evidence of frank bleeding including petechiae, purpura, and ecchymoses.
- Avoid all aspirin-containing compounds. Read the label. Do not take any medications unless prescribed by your physician.
- Report any feelings of increased weakness, change in stool color and consistency, emesis, headache, and change in level of consciousness. For nosebleed, apply ice pack across bridge of nose and pressure to nostrils below bridge of nose. If bleeding does not stop within 5 minutes or bleeding is profuse, notify physician. Anterior or posterior nasal packs may be required.

• • •

Nursing management of the bleeding patient depends on prompt recognition of the problem so that definitive therapy can be undertaken. Bleeding precautions should be initiated when the platelet count drops below 50,000/mm^3. Frequent assessment should be made of vital signs, mental status, skin and mucous membranes, sites of invasive procedures, and all excreta and vomitus for occult blood. Signs of intracranial hemorrhage include decreased level of consciousness, headache, seizures, unequal pupil size and reaction, hypertension, and bradycardia. Administration of antiemetics, cough suppressants, and stool softeners and laxatives when indicated may help lower the risk of intracranial hemorrhage by preventing the sudden raising of intracranial pressure while retching, coughing, and straining at stool.

Platelet transfusion is generally the treatment of choice for bleeding secondary to thrombocytopenia. Indications for platelet transfusion are not always clear. Some physicians may prefer to wait for signs of bleeding before transfusing platelets; others may opt to transfuse with platelets prophylactically when the platelet count drops below 20,000/mm^3. Platelet transfusions may be random donor (obtained from multiple units of fresh whole blood), single donor (obtained by platelet pheresis), or single donor, human leukocyte antigen (HLA) matched (obtained by platelet pheresis from a related, matched donor). Transfusion reactions occur most frequently with random donor platelets and usually consist of febrile reactions, urticaria, or both. This type of transfusion reaction is most likely to be related to leukoagglutinins and may be alleviated by premedication or leukocyte-poor platelets. Alloimmunization (development of antiplatelet antibodies) occurs after exposure to platelet transfusions. When this occurs, optimal response to platelet transfusions fails to occur and the platelet count remains the same or drops lower. With alloimmunization it may be necessary to reserve platelet transfusions for times of active bleeding.[2,52,57]

Continued.

Table 30-5 Transfusion Reactions

Type of reaction	Signs and symptoms	Interventions
Hemolytic	Fever, chills, back pain, substernal tightness, dyspnea, circulatory collapse, urticaria, vomiting, diarrhea, hemoglobinuria, renal shutdown, bleeding diathesis	Prevent by proper identification of patient and blood for transfusion. Discontinue the transfusion; send to blood bank and obtain urine and blood specimens per hospital policy for transfusion reaction workup. Administer saline diuresis, furosemide, and mannitol to prevent acute renal tubular necrosis.
Allergic	Urticaria, itching, bronchospasm, anaphylactoid reactions	Elicit history of prior allergic reactions. Premedicate with diphenhydramine and/or corticosteroids. If reaction occurs, stop the transfusion; follow hospital policy for suspected transfusion reaction; for anaphylactoid reaction, administer epinephrine, maintain airway and perfusion; administer additional emergency measures as needed.
Febrile (leukocyte antigens)	Fever with or without rigors, tachycardia, tachypnea, hypotension, cyanosis, fibrinolysis, leukopenia	Elicit history of febrile reactions. Premedicate with acetaminophen. If reaction occurs, stop the transfusion and follow hospital policy for suspected febrile reaction. Administer saline-washed or leukocyte-poor red blood cells.
Bacterial (gram-negative organisms and endotoxin release)	Fever, rigors, circulatory collapse, mental confusion, septic shock	Maintain proper blood storage and administration conditions. Stop the transfusion immediately. Obtain blood for cultures; return blood to laboratory for culturing. Administer emergency treatment as needed. Administer antibiotics as ordered.

PATIENT AND FAMILY EDUCATION

The educational process for the patient and family should include practical guidelines for the prevention of bleeding, such as using acetaminophen instead of aspirin, always checking the ingredients of over-the-counter medications, not taking any medications unless prescribed by the physician, avoiding trauma, what to do for ecchymoses, when to call the physician if bleeding occurs or is suspected, what is serious bleeding, and how to recognize intracranial hemorrhage.[28]

NURSING MANAGEMENT

FATIGUE ASSOCIATED WITH ANEMIA

NURSING DIAGNOSES[19,45,57,72]

• *Activity intolerance, risk for/actual, related to anemia secondary to bone marrow suppression; related to decreased tissue perfusion secondary to anemia as evidenced by fatigue, motor weakness, and inability to perform activities of daily living*

• *Gas exchange, impaired, related to decreased oxygenation secondary to anemia (decreased hemoglobin)*
• *Sexuality patterns, altered, related to decreased energy secondary to anemia*
• *Mobility, impaired physical, related to decreased strength and endurance*
• *Knowledge deficit related to basic disease process, signs and symptoms of anemia*

OUTCOME GOALS

Patient will be able to:

- Demonstrate an increase in activity tolerance and a decrease in subjective complaints of fatigue.
- Demonstrate knowledge of relationship of red blood cells, hemoglobin, and availability of oxygen to fulfill needs of body tissue for normal functioning.
- Relate desire to resume sexual activity.
- Identify measures necessary to reduce the risks of injury related to decreased strength and endurance.
- Demonstrate knowledge of signs and symptoms of decreased oxygen availability to tissue.

Preventive Measures

Preventive measures include the following: frequent assessment of skin and mucous membranes for pallor; frequent assessment of cardiovascular system for signs of decompensation such as irregular rhythms, murmurs, changes in blood pressure and pulse rate, peripheral edema, and dyspnea; pulmonary examination for changes in rate and depth of respirations and rales; and neurologic examination for altered levels of consciousness and inability to concentrate. Nurses should be aware of current laboratory values for hemoglobin, hematocrit, reticulocyte count, and platelet count. Persons known to be anemic should be encouraged to monitor their activity closely to prevent overtiring.

INTERVENTIONS

Nursing management of the patient with fatigue associated with anemia should include teaching energy conservation techniques, helping the patient cope with the changes in life-style that severe fatigue may dictate, providing the time and opportunity for the patient to ventilate anger, frustration, and feelings of depression, monitoring patient activity, planning activities to prevent overtiring, and transfusing packed red blood cells as ordered by the physician. The nurse must be aware of safe trans-fusion practices, signs and symptoms of transfusion reactions, and indications for premedication and administration of leukocyte-poor blood[7,57] (see Table 30-5).

PATIENT AND FAMILY EDUCATION

Teaching plans should include the following instructions[2,72]:

- Rest when tired—anemia and fatigue are expected and temporary side effects of treatment for cancer.
- Develop a progressive ambulation plan—do not try too much at one time.
- Pace your activities—try to maintain as normal a life-style as possible; plan periods of exercise and rest.
- Seek assistance with such things as child care, meal planning and preparation, laundry, and house-cleaning.
- Eat a nutritionally balanced diet.
- Maintain usual patterns of sleep.

See box below.

 PATIENT TEACHING PRIORITIES
Protective Mechanisms

Discuss normal functions of immune system, bone marrow, and barrier defenses.

Discuss relationship between disease process, treatment, and impaired host defenses.

Discuss signs and symptoms to report to physician/nurse.

Plan for management of impaired protective mechanisms.

Obtain culture-sensitive teaching materials.

Discuss complementary therapies and need for communicating with physician.

Discuss availability of community resources—financial, nursing care, durable medical equipment, transportation, support groups.

CONCLUSION

Protective mechanisms such as skin, mucous membrane, and bone marrow protect the body from foreign substances and invading organisms. The patient with cancer undergoing the various treatment modalities becomes at risk for breakdown of one or all of these protective mechanisms. Nursing management requires prompt recognition of the signs and symptoms of infection, bleeding, and skin breakdown so that definitive therapy can be implemented. Nurses caring for these patients are key members of the health care team at this crucial time.

■ CHAPTER QUESTIONS

1. Which of the following is not considered to be a major function of the immune system?
   a. Defense
   b. Homeostasis
   c. Excretion
   d. Regulation

2. Immunosuppression may involve a defect in cell-mediated immunity, humoral immunity, or a combination of both. Combined cell-mediated and humoral immune deficiency occurs in the patient:
   a. Who is 3 months status postallogeneic bone marrow transplantation for acute nonlymphocytic leukemia

b. Who has been diagnosed with non-Hodgkin's lymphoma and is receiving chemotherapy

c. Who is receiving high-dose corticosteroid therapy for autoimmune hemolytic anemia

d. Who is undergoing surgical resection for a renal cell carcinoma

3. Life-threatening infections are most frequently associated with:
   a. Leukopenia
   b. Neutropenia
   c. Leukocytosis
   d. Thrombocytopenia

4. A 43-year-old patient received remission induction chemotherapy for acute nonlymphocytic leukemia 7 days ago. Today the patient is febrile, tachycardic, tachypnec, and disoriented. The first thing the nurse caring for the patient should do is:
   a. Notify the physician immediately
   b. Draw blood cultures from the central venous catheter only
   c. Initiate empiric antibiotics before obtaining cultures
   d. Administer acetaminophen and retake the temperature after 2 hours

5. A recombinant hematopoietic growth factor used to stimulate RBC production in the person undergoing therapy for cancer is:
   a. rG-CSF
   b. rEPO
   c. rGM-CSF
   d. rIL-2

6. Symptoms of anemia are related to all of the following except:
   a. Decreased oxygen-carrying capacity of the blood
   b. Compensatory increase in heart rate and respiratory rate
   c. Shunting of blood away from nonvital organs
   d. Decreased production of cytokines by erythroid precursers

7. Pressure reduction devices are used for both prevention and treatment of decubitus ulcers. Your patient has a stage IV ulcer. An appropriate choice of pressure reduction device would include:
   a. A foam overlay
   b. A static air-filled pressure pad
   c. An active mattress overlay system
   d. A hard innerspring mattress

8. Oral care for the person with chemotherapy-associated mucositis should include:
   a. Brushing and flossing before meals, after meals, and at bedtime
   b. Sponge swabs dipped in commercial mouthwash every 4 hours
   c. Rinse with normal saline every 2 to 4 hours
   d. Rinse with 1:1 hydrogen peroxide/water every 4 hours

9. Bleeding precautions for the patient with thrombocytopenia (platelet count <100,000/mm^3) include all of the following except:
   a. No ASA-containing compounds
   b. No intramuscular injections
   c. No shaving with blades
   d. No pheresis-obtained platelets

BIBLIOGRAPHY

1. Adams A: External barriers to infection, *Nurs Clin North Am* 20(1):145, 1985.

2. Alexander EJ: Injury, potential for, related to thrombocytopenia. In McNally JC and others, editors: *Guidelines for oncology nursing practice,* ed 2, Philadelphia, 1991, Saunders.

3. Anderson KC, Weinstein HJ: Transfusion-associated graft-versus-host disease, *N Engl J Med* 323:315, 1990.

4. Andrews MM, Boyle JS: *Transcultural concepts in nursing care,* ed 2, Philadelphia, 1995, Lippincott.

5. Baird SB: *Decision making in oncology nursing,* Toronto, 1988, Decker.

6. Baird SB, McCorkle R, Grant M: *Cancer nursing,* Philadelphia, 1991, Saunders.

7. Baranowski L: Filtering out the confusion about leukocyte-poor blood components, *J Intrav Nurs* 14:298, 1991.

8. Barry SA: Septic shock: special needs of the patient with cancer, *Oncol Nurs Forum* 16(1):31, 1989.

9. Bavier AR: Alterations in hemostasis. In Johnson BL, Gross J, editors: *Handbook of oncology nursing,* New York, 1985, John Wiley & Sons.

10. Beck S: Impact of the systematic oral care protocol on stomatitis after chemotherapy, *Cancer Nurs* 2:185, 1979.

11. Beck S: Prevention and management of oral complications in the cancer patient, *Curr Issues Cancer Nurs Pract* 6:1, 1992.

12. Beck S, Yasko J: *Guideline for oral care,* ed 2, Crystal Lake, Ill, 1993, Sage.

13. Bergstrom N and others: The Braden scale for predicting pressure sore risk, *Nurs Res* 36:205, 1987.

14. Bodey GP: Quantitative relationship between circulating leukocytes and infection in patients with acute leukemia, *Ann Intern Med* 64:328, 1966.

15. Bone RC: The pathogenesis of sepsis, *Ann Int Med* 115:457, 1991.

16. Brandt B: Nursing protocol for the patient with neutropenia, *Oncol Nurs Forum* 17(1s):9, 1990.

17. Carlisle PS, Gucalp R, Wiernik PH: Nosocomial infections in neutropenic cancer patients, *Infec Control Hosp Epidemiol* 14:320, 1993.

18. Carlson AC: Infection prophylaxis in the patient with cancer, *Oncol Nurs Forum* 12(3):56, 1985.

19. Carpenito LJ: *Handbook of nursing diagnosis,* ed 6, Philadelphia, 1995, Lippincott.

20. Carroll P: Bed selection—help patients rest easy, *RN* 58(5):44, 1995.

21. Carter LW: Bacterial translocation: nursing implication in the care of patients with neutropenia, *Oncol Nurs Forum* 21:857, 1994.

22. Chernecky CC, Ramsey PW: *Critical care of the client with cancer,* Norwalk, Conn, 1984, Appleton-Century-Crofts.

23. Clark JC: Mucous membrane integrity, impairment of, related to vaginal changes. In McNally JC and others, editors: *Guidelines for oncology nursing practice,* ed 2, Philadelphia, 1991, Saunders.

24. Cunningham M: Dental prosthetics: physiologic and microbial insults, *Oncol Nurs Forum* 11:78, 1984.

25. Daeffler RJ: Oral hygiene measures for patients with cancer, Part I, *Cancer Nurs* 3:347, 1980.

26. Daeffler RJ: Oral hygiene measures for patients with cancer, Part II, *Cancer Nurs* 3:427, 1980.

27. Daeffler RJ: Oral hygiene measures for patients with cancer, Part III, *Cancer Nurs* 4:29, 1981.

28. Derdiarian A: Informational needs of recently diagnosed cancer patients, *Nurs Res* 35(5):276, 1986.

29. Donovan C: Protective isolation, *Oncol Nurs Forum* 9(3):50, 1982.

30. Dose AM: The symptom experience of mucositis, stomatitis, and xerostomia, *Semin Oncol Nurs* 11:248, 1995.

31. Dudjak LA: Mouth care for mucositis due to radiation therapy, *Cancer Nurs* 10:131, 1987.

32. Eilers J, Berger AM, Peterson MC: Development, testing and application of the oral assessment guide, *Oncol Nurs Forum* 15:325, 1989.

33. Ezzone S and others: Survey of oral hygiene regimens among bone marrow transplant centers, *Oncol Nurs Forum* 20:1375, 1993.

34. Gallagher J: Management of cutaneous symptoms, *Semin Oncol Nurs* 11:239, 1995.

35. Gallucci BB: The immune system and cancer, *Oncol Nurs Forum* 14(6s):3, 1987.

36. Giamarellou H: Empiric therapy for infections in the febrile, neutropenic, compromised host, *Med Clin North Am* 70:559, 1995.

37. Goodman M, Stoner C: Mucous membrane integrity, impairment of, related to stomatitis. In McNally JC and others, editors: *Guidelines for oncology nursing practice,* ed 2, Philadelphia, 1991, Saunders.

38. Grady C: Host defense mechanisms: an overview, *Semin Oncol Nurs* 4(2):86, 1988.

39. Griffin JP: Be prepared for the bleeding patient, *Nursing* 16(6):34, 1986.

40. Griffin JP: Fever, when to leave it alone, *Nursing* 16(2):57, 1986.

41. Griffin JP: Nursing care of the critically ill immunocompromised patient, *Crit Care Nurs Q* 9(1):25, 1986.

42. Haeuber D: Future strategies in the control of myelosuppression: the use of colony-stimulating factors, *Oncol Nurs Forum* 18(2s):16, 1991.

43. Hall KV: Detecting septic shock before it's too late, *RN* 44(9):29, 1981.

44. Henschel L: Fever patterns in the neutropenic patient, *Cancer Nurs* 8(6):301, 1985.

45. Herberth L, Gosnell DJ: Nursing diagnoses for oncology nursing practice, *Cancer Nurs* 10(1):41, 1987.

46. Holland PV: Prevention of transfusion-associated graft-versus-host disease, *Arch Pathol Lab Med* 113:285, 1989.

47. Holtzclaw BJ: The febrile response in critical care: state of the science, *Heart Lung* 21:482, 1992.

48. Hughes WT: Empiric antimicrobial therapy in the febrile granulocytopenic patient, *Infect Control Hosp Epidemiol* 11:151, 1990.

49. Jett MF, Lancaster LE: The inflammatory-immune response: the body's defense against invasion, *Crit Care Nurs* 3(9):63, 1983.

50. Kemp D: Development of the immune system, *Crit Care Nurs Q* 9(1):1, 1986.

51. Kenny SA: Effect of two oral care protocols on the incidence of stomatitis in hematology patients, *Cancer Nurs* 13:345, 1990.

52. King NH: Controlling bleeding when the platelet count drops, *RN* 47(8):25, 1984.

53. Klastersky J: Febrile neutropenia, *Support Care Cancer* 1:233, 1993.

54. Kluger MJ: Fever: role of pyrogens and cryogens, *Physiol Rev* 71:93, 1991.

55. Lamb LS: Think you know septic shock? *Nursing* 12(1):34, 1982.

56. Lapka DMV, Wild LD, Barbour LA: Heparin-induced thrombocytopenia and thrombosis: a case study and clinical overview, *Oncol Nurs Forum* 21:871, 1994.

57. Lichtiger B, Huh YO: Transfusion therapy for patients with cancer, *CA Cancer J Clin* 35(5):1, 1985.

58. Lieschke GJ, Burgess AW: Granulocyte colony-stimulating factor and granulocyte-macrophage colony factor, *N Engl J Med* 327:28, 1992.

59. Link DL: Antibiotic therapy for the cancer patient: focus on third generation cephalosporins, *Oncol Nurs Forum* 14(5):35, 1987.

60. McNally JC, Stair J: Potential for infection. In McNally JC and others, editors: *Guidelines for oncology nursing practice,* ed 2, Philadelphia, 1991, Saunders.

61. Malkiewicz J: What assessing the mouth can tell you, *RN* 45(5):65, 1982.

62. Montrose PA: Extravasation management, *Semin Oncol Nurs* 3(2):128, 1987.

63. Nauseef WM, Maki DG: A study of the value of simple protective isolation in patients with granulocytopenia, *N Engl J Med* 304:448, 1981.

64. Owen P: Skin integrity, impairment of, related to malignant skin lesions. In McNally JC and others, editors: *Guidelines for oncology nursing practice,* ed 2, Philadelphia, 1991, Saunders.

65. Panel on the Prediction and Prevention of Pressure Ulcers in Adults: *Pressure ulcers in adults: prediction and prevention.* Rockville, Md, 1992, Agency for Health Care Policy and Research, Public Health Service, US Dept of Health and Human Services.

66. Pizzo PA: Management of fever and infection in the patient with cancer, *Mediguide Infect Dis* 2(4):1, 1983.

67. Rackow EC, Astiz ME: Pathophysiology and treatment of septic shock, *JAMA* 266:548, 1991.

68. Ransier A and others: A combined analysis of a toothbrush, foam brush, and a chlorhexidine-soaked foam brush on maintaining oral hygiene, *Cancer Nurs* 18:393, 1995.

69. Rice V: The clinical continuum of septic shock, *Crit Care Nurs* 4(9):86, 1984.

70. Roberts NJ: Impact of temperature elevation on immunologic defenses, *Rev Infect Dis* 13:462, 1991.

71. Rostad M: Current strategies for managing myelosuppression in patient with cancer, *Oncol Nurs Forum* 18(2s):7, 1991.

72. Rostad M: Injury, potential for, related to anemia. In McNally JC and others, editors: *Guidelines for oncology nursing practice,* ed 2, Philadelphia, 1991, Saunders.

73. Smith SL: Physiology of the immune system, *Crit Care Nurs Q* 9(1):7, 1986.

74. Styrt B: Antipyresis and fever, *Arch Intern Med* 150:1589, 1990.

75. Tenebaum L: Cancer chemotherapy and biotherapy, a reference guide, ed 2, Philadelphia, 1994, Saunders.

76. Tombes MB, Gallucci B: The effects of hydrogen peroxide rinses on normal oral mucosa, *Nurs Res* 42:332, 1993.

77. Varricchio C: Cultural and ethnic dimensions of cancer nursing care: introduction, *Oncol Nurs Forum* 14:57, 1987.

78. Vose JM, Armitage JO: Clinical application of hematopoietic growth factors, *J Clin Oncol* 13:1023, 1995.

79. Walsh TJ and others: Empiric therapy with amphotericin B in febrile granulocytic patients, *Rev Infect Dis* 13:496, 1991.

80. Wilkes GM, Ingwerson K, Burke MB: *Oncology nursing drug reference,* Boston, 1994, Jones & Barlett.

81. Williams LT, Peterson DE, Overholser CD: Acute periodontal infection in myelosuppressed oncology patients: evaluation and nursing care, *Cancer Nurs* 5(6):465, 1982.

82. Workman ML: Immunological late effects in children and adults, *Semin Oncol Nurs* 5(1):36, 1989.

83. Workman ML, Ellerhorst-Ryan J, Hargrave-Koertge V: *Nursing care of the immunocompromised patient,* Philadelphia, 1993, Saunders.

84. Yeager KA, Miaskowski C: Advances in understanding the mechanisms and management of acute myelogenous leukemia, *Oncol Nurs Forum* 21:541, 1994.

85. Yeomans AC: Rectal infections in acute leukemia, *Cancer Nurs* 9(6):295, 1986.

CHAPTER 31
Psychosocial and Quality-of-Life Issues

NOELLA DEVOLDER McCRAY

I wanted a perfect ending so I sat down to write the book with the ending in place before there even was an ending. Now I've learned the hard way that some poems don't rhyme, and some stories do not have a clear beginning, middle and end. Like my life, this book has ambiguity. Like my life, this book is about not knowing, having to change, taking the moment and making the best of it without knowing what is going to happen next.[62]

INTRINSIC FACTORS
The Personal Meaning of Cancer

Individual response. Living with uncertainty, as poignantly described by the late comedienne Gilda Radner, is the major challenge that faces individuals diagnosed with cancer, as well as those with whom they share significant relationships. The future, which once may have seemed to hold unlimited potential, immediately becomes limited when viewed within the context of a cancer diagnosis. As noted by Weisman, "cancer is not just another chronic disease, it evokes many of the deepest fears of mankind."[63] The meaning a cancer diagnosis holds for a particular individual is highly personal and is derived from numerous sources, including past experiences with cancer, cultural biases, and information gained from the media. Each of these sources may or may not be accurate, may or may not be helpful, and may or may not lead to positive coping and adaptation. The individual and those with whom significant relationships are shared have all had different experiences, which influence their interpretation and expectations. Thus, although similar behaviors or response patterns may emerge and be observed by the nurse, it is crucial to remember that each individual diagnosed with cancer experiences a unique situation framed by highly personal life experiences.[57]

The specific kind of cancer and necessary treatment present unique challenges to be faced and influence potential responses. Visible physical changes can accentuate the personal and social impact. Crucial differences in response also arise from the extent of altered daily functioning. With time and experience, the meaning and implications of the diagnosis evolve but adaptation and uncertainty remain as haunting challenges.

The initial diagnosis may have been preceded by varying levels of concern, ranging from a low level of suspicion associated with routine examinations to the steadily increasing anxiety and suspicion associated with sequential diagnostic procedures. The individual and family initially experience the shock of an unexpected diagnosis or the pain of having their worst fears confirmed. The personal meaning of cancer then evolves over time.[18,55]

Timing and role strain. The timing of a cancer diagnosis in terms of the developmental level of the individual and the individual's family may exacerbate or mitigate the feelings produced by the diagnosis.[32,57] Age and stage of life affect perceptions, understanding, and acceptance. The diagnosis of a malignancy in a child, young adult, or person experiencing a productive middle age is often viewed as more devastating than in the older individual who has seemingly completed significant life events.

Timing is significant not only in terms of development, but also in relation to other stressors. Periods of life transitions, such as marriage, childbirth, retirement, or death in the family, can intensify responses. The point in time influences the degree of role strain incurred by each individual involved. Perceived burdens of care can lead family members to struggle with feelings of guilt, resentment, or anger. Roles may change dramatically. Partial or full unemployment can drain financial resources and change roles. These changes can be accompanied by altered communications in relationships.

Nurses are cautioned not to consider an initial response as permanent or representative of the way the individual and family will cope in the future. Weisman and Worden have described the initial response as that of the existential plight.[63] During approximately the first 100 days after diagnosis, the individual attempts to address some of the existential issues related to the diagnosis, including those related to dying, the future, and the meaning life has had. During this same time, the individual is presented with a treatment plan and therefore must simultaneously begin to learn to cope with recovery from surgical procedures and side effects of cancer therapies.

The significance of the initial diagnosis period cannot be overemphasized. A wide range of responses are observed as the individual and family attempt to adapt to an overwhelming situation. It is particularly important to refrain from labeling a particular response as abnormal or maladaptive. There is nothing normal about being diagnosed with a life-threatening disease, nor is there a right way to face the threatened loss of a loved one. Because all individuals have the potential to learn, to grow, and to change, the foundations of their psychosocial care and respect is a nonjudgmental attitude. A major determinant of their coping success can be a nurse's ability to coach, teach, and support them through this tumultuous time.[62]

Spiritual distress. The person with cancer and those with whom significant relationships are shared may experience some degree of spiritual distress as they struggle with the effects of the diagnosis and its meaning. The perceived misfortune or tragedy uncovers concerns about the unfair distribution of suffering in the world. This often begs a confrontation with the concept of a kind and loving God. Attempts to explain or transform bad into good and pain into privilege are often used to defend God.[30]

Questions may outnumber answers. "Why me?" may never be satisfactorily answered. Whereas some feel enriched by their faith at this time, others may feel robbed by it. This may be a time for the nurse to assist in a values clarification process.

The nurse can be supportive by being aware of and showing respect for differing religious beliefs. More important, the nurse provides support through nonjudgmental listening, providing an opportunity for the individual to tell his or her story, and identifying the individual's values. Through such listening, the appropriateness of a referral to clergy and other resources can be ascertained. Whereas some are comforted by displays of faith, others are best served by supportive listening. An assessment of spiritual distress can guide the nurse, but such an assessment can be effectively done only after the nurse has reconciled a personal spirituality and accepts ambiguity and differences in values.[45,51]

Psychosocial Adjustment and Quality of Life

Complex psychologic and social issues are interwoven aspects of the response to a diagnosis of a chronic disease process. Recognition of this fact has led professional caregivers to establish concurrent care goals—disease control and quality of life. As the medical understanding and management of cancer have progressed steadily, so have the understanding and management of quality of life. Psychosocial oncology has become a distinct field of study and practice. An emerging theoretic base provides the pathways for intervention.[31]

Interdisciplinary team approach. As the aspects of care are interwoven, so are the roles of professional caregivers. Interdisciplinary team care is the standard in quality care delivery. Some aspects of psychosocial care are best suited to the psychologist, psychiatrist, clergy, social worker, or counselor. Another potential team member is the lay volunteer or another cancer survivor who is trained and matched with a patient to provide special support. Each team member can contribute to altering perceptions of the situation, improving coping abilities, and altering the overall response to the situation. Nurses in various settings contribute to psychosocial care, either directly or indirectly through referrals and coordination of care. Each interdisciplinary team member serves the patient and family best when working together in an interdisciplinary manner.[17,32]

Structured assessment. Nurses and all health care professionals benefit from a structured assessment or data base from which they can determine the capacity of the patient and family to manage their situation.[55] Symptom and well-being inventories can be used to measure anxiety, depression, hostility, somatization, and general distress or well being.[55] This assessment requires time and is best accomplished after the establishment of a trusting relationship.

Data can be collected over time and should be recorded in a systematic way. Published guides are available for conducting a psychosocial assessment.[63,69] The system adopted should be one that is workable within the constraints of the setting yet complete enough to form an objective base for establishing priorities and reasonable care goals.

The data base should then be available to all plan-of-care providers in various settings throughout the care continuum.

As a result of nursing and other team members' assessments, numerous nursing diagnoses or problems related to psychosocial care can be identified[43] (see box, p. 819). Each diagnosis must be substantiated by a data base and followed with a plan of care. The plan of care should document the mutual goals of the patient and interdisciplinary team in partnership.

Adaptation process. The goals of cancer therapy range from disease cure to palliation of symptoms. Thus the degree of personal threat experienced by the individual and the subsequent ability to adapt or cope will vary over time. The process of adapting is characterized

---

NURSING DIAGNOSES RELATED TO PSYCHOSOCIAL CARE

Adjustment, impaired	Communication, impaired verbal
Anxiety	Knowledge deficit (specify)
Body image disturbance	Parenting, altered
Coping, defensive	Parenting altered, risk for
Coping family: potential for growth	Powerlessness
Coping, ineffective family: compromised	Protection, altered
Coping, ineffective family: disabling	Role performance, altered
Coping, ineffective individual	Self-esteem, chronic low
Decisional conflict (specify)	Self-esteem, situational low
Denial, ineffective	Sleep pattern disturbance
Family processes, altered	Social interaction, impaired
Fear	Social isolation
Grieving, anticipatory	Spiritual distress (distress of the human spirit)
Grieving, dysfunctional	Thought processes, altered
Health maintenance, altered	Violence, risk for: self-directed or directed at others
Hopelessness	

Data from North American Nursing Diagnoses Association: Taxonomy I Revised, 1995-1996.

by a series of transitions in terms of knowledge of the disease process, emotional responses on the part of the individual and significant others, and the need to negotiate changes in life-style patterns to adjust to the demands of treatment. Although individuals diagnosed with cancer share many issues of common concern, these issues may vary according to the position the individual occupies on the cancer care continuum.[18,57]

Adaptation to cancer can be addressed from several time frames: initial diagnosis, treatment, recurrence, advanced disease, and death or long-term survival. The needs of the individual differ at each point on the continuum. Artificially dividing the cancer experience into such phases can be helpful in describing human responses. However, the potential then exists of failing to recognize that human emotional responses do not have artificial boundaries.

Initial diagnosis and treatment. The common experience is that of being told the diagnosis. Immediately after the disclosure of a cancer diagnosis, each person sets out on a unique path characterized by highly individual physical and psychosocial responses to a situation marked by uncertainty. The primary concern of the newly diagnosed person is life versus death.[63,69] Family and friends also share these initial concerns. They experience an acute grief reaction to the diagnosis itself and the uncertainty of the outcome. Grief reactions as a response to chronic illness can be viewed from the framework of attachment theory.[63,69] Attachment theory is based on the premise that the level of distress experienced is directly related to the significance the individual places on the body function or part that is threatened.[32] This theoretic framework can serve as a basis for a nursing assessment. When treatment is initiated, the individual who values

physical appearance may find coping with threatened alopecia most difficult and the individual who is career-focused may be highly distressed by therapy-related fatigue and subsequent loss of function. The nurse must therefore also consider the impact the potential loss will have on the individual's body image (see Chapter 32).

During the initial diagnostic and treatment stage, the individual and family are often overwhelmed and have trouble comprehending all that is said. A study of newly diagnosed cancer patients provided valuable information regarding the process of informing the patient of the diagnosis.[32] Half of the individuals studied were initially told of their diagnosis when they were alone or with only other medical personnel. Greater distress was reported by those told in a recovery room or by telephone. Many individuals reported feeling numb or shocked and particularly vulnerable in instances when they were alone. They reported a need to have their sense of personal tragedy acknowledged.[32]

Although further study of ways to minimize the trauma of presenting the diagnosis is needed, this preliminary study has implications for nurses in recovery rooms, physicians' offices, and all settings where a diagnosis is confirmed. The physician who makes treatment recommendations, often a consulted oncologist, is in the position of reexplaining the diagnosis a second or third time. Thus, by the time the individual is presented with a specific treatment plan, he or she may be overwhelmed with the information given and not understand the diagnosis or treatment plan. The nurse who is present at this time is in the best position to assess the response and level of understanding. The nurse who anticipates this situation may recommend that the patient come accompanied by a friend or family member and use a tape recorder to enhance understanding and retention of information. The nurse can repeat information, validate understanding, and gently encourage participation in treatment decisions and goal setting.[35,36]

The process of clarifying information and reducing confusion can be facilitated by various nursing interventions. Paper and pencil can be provided to encourage the individual to write down questions that come to mind and record answers received. Questions and concerns may then be prioritized and can serve as the basis of further discussion with physicians and other care providers. Information can then be reviewed by the patient or family at their convenience. By such coaching and teaching, the nurse promotes patient and care provider partnership.[25,29,54]

Recurrence. Although an ever-increasing number of individuals diagnosed with cancer achieve long-term control and are eventually considered cured of their disease, a significant proportion of individuals do not achieve such a goal. When cure is not feasible, the goal of therapy is control, or the longest possible disease-free period. This goal presents the patient and family with the double-edged sword of hope and fear. The hope of defying the odds is bound by the fear of recurrence. Statistics may predict life expectancy based on diagnosis, pathology, and stage of disease but do not consider the individual's response.[44,55] Each individual's experience is physically and psychosocially unique and somewhat unpredictable.

Fear of recurrence and lack of predictability have been cited as a source of decreased personal control. This sense of uncertainty can be manifested in a variety of behaviors. The patient and family may blame health care providers or each other as they review the events leading to diagnosis, treatment, and recurrence. The nurse can show support by allowing the individual to retell their story, thus acknowledging their pain and grief and validating their feelings.[59,62]

When initial therapy is completed, the individual may experience a fear of abandonment by health care providers. Less frequent appointments and examinations can become a source of anxiety for patient and family. Minor physical changes raise concerns over potential recurrence. Heightened concern over new symptoms may affect the return to usual routines and family life. These concerns may be manifested through frequent phone calls to review symptoms or, paradoxically, nonreporting or minimizing concerns.

Family members may find themselves emotionally drained. The immediate need to support the loved one diminishes, and they are left with their own anxieties. The patient's complaints of fatigue, a cough, or gastrointestinal disturbances may all be interpreted by the family as proof that the cancer is recurring. Nurses can assist the individual and family by acknowledging their concerns as real and assessing physical findings to determine the need for further evaluation.[63]

When recurrence is documented, the nurse can assist the patient and family by providing an understanding of its significance. The recurrence signifies an increased tumor cell burden occurring at an interval of time related to the growth rate of the specific cancer cell line. The return of clinically evident disease indicates an inadequate response to initial therapy. The recurrence does not necessarily mean there is no chance for cure. In some instances reinstitution of the same therapy or a second line therapy can achieve a second remission or a cure.[31,63,69]

The psychosocial response to a recurrence depends on several variables. A study of a large number of patients with a wide variety of malignancies revealed surprising findings.[63] Of the population studied, 30% found the experience of recurrence less traumatic than the initial diagnosis. This group reported their initial treatment experience as smooth or uneventful. Individuals who experienced greater emotional distress were most often physically debilitated and experiencing a decrease in function. The study also noted that individuals who lived with a realistic expectation of recurrence were much less distressed than those who believed the disease was completely eradicated. Individuals who had completed therapy but were in remission less than 1 year were the most concerned about relapse. Those who experienced longer periods of remission began to allow themselves the hope of a cure, so recurrence was more emotionally distressing to this group.[8,10,18,21] It is important to note that the individuals who lived with the realistic possibility of recurrence were not, as a group, pessimistic about their future. Rather, they were hopeful that they would experience another remission. Although the concerns of individuals experiencing recurrent cancer deserve greater study, the nurse is cautioned not to assume that patients who experience a recurrence are universally overwhelmed or depressed. Current symptoms, functional status, previous experience with cancer therapy, and ongoing expectations since initial diagnosis are important variables in determining how one copes with recurrence. The nurse remains in a central supportive role at this time.[47,62]

Long-term survival. When the individual's disease-free period extends, the fear of recurrence seems to decrease.[35,64] Professionals must note that the publicly regarded milestone of a 5-year disease-free survival period may no longer be considered appropriate in certain diseases.[51] A vital component of the care of people experiencing disease-free status is to provide them with current, appropriate information regarding the significance of the length of the disease-free interval in relation to their particular situation and the important role of follow-up. When disease control is not an attainable goal and palliative care is given, the challenge of creating a vision of hope still exists.[59,64] The caregiver's provision of measures to relieve physical and psychosocial distress can foster the hope for comfort and peace.

Patient and Family Coping Strategies

Alterations in coping. The personal meaning a cancer diagnosis holds for individuals and their loved ones and possible outcomes of cancer therapies are the source of multiple and complex issues faced by the individual and family for the balance of life. Nurses are cautioned to avoid labeling any behavioral responses as permanent or ineffective. The nursing diagnosis accepted by NANDA (see box, p. 819) for this process is "Ineffective coping related to." The determination of ineffective or effective coping is more often the nurse's judgment call than the patient's own determination.[21]

Measurement of effectiveness relies on patient self-report. Studies of such reports by large numbers of cancer patients have formed the basis of lists that identify coping strategies as ineffective, effective, or positive.

The goal of coping is problem resolution. Coping may be simplistically viewed as what one does about any problem to feel better. This involves recognition of a problem and some degree of action followed by a personal evaluation of the efficacy of the action. The person diagnosed with cancer brings to this new situation a coping history.

Positive coping strategies have been characterized by several different types of behaviors. The following list provides examples of some strategies, identified by specific behaviors[21,62,63,69]:

- Avoidance behaviors are minimal. Denial of the potential problem is minimized by gaining appropriate information, including referrals to appropriate health care providers.
- Realities are confronted. The possible outcomes of cancer therapies are realistically acknowledged and addressed.
- Problems are redefined into a solvable form, such as scheduling therapy to minimize disruptions in work and family activities.
- Alternatives are considered, such as having a backup plan for needed child care arrangements.
- Open and mutual communication with significant others is maintained. The feelings, concerns, and anxieties of the individual and significant others are addressed with honesty by both parties.
- Constructive help, including adequate medical care, is sought. The individual seeks a second opinion or actively searches for health care providers with whom he or she feels comfortable.

- Support is accepted when offered and assertive behavior is used when necessary. The individual accepts support that is helpful and recognizes behaviors that are not helpful.
- Morale is enhanced through self-reliance or the use of available resources. The individual pursues activities that are personally meaningful and recognizes that compromises may need to be made, such as working part-time or reducing the amount of time spent in volunteer activities.
- Self-concept is as important as symptom relief, and the individual who, while living with compromise, maintains a sense of control and does not behave as if powerless, continues to value self as a functioning being.
- Hope is self-pride, not self-deception. The ability to hope for a cure, increased life expectancy, or an inevitable peaceful death does not indicate a lack of knowledge or understanding of the situation. Hope may include time-focused activities, such as the desire to witness the birth of a first grandchild.[40]

Weisman also reports behaviors described by patients as not helpful when used consistently.[63,69] Ineffective coping strategies include withdrawal, suppression, excessive use of alcohol or other drugs, passive acceptance, and reckless, impulsive behaviors. It is important to note that the individual or family may use an ineffective style in an isolated situation, usually in response to extreme stress. Some of these behaviors are understandable in the context of an individual's background. Withdrawal to prepare one's questions or explanations to family members may be quite effective for the normally quiet, self-reliant individual. Passive acceptance may be culturally related or based on a fear of being labeled a "bad" patient or a "difficult" family. The length of time such behaviors are used is more important than their use in an individual situation. Individuals and their families who choose to consistently engage in impulsive behaviors, substance abuse, or suppression of symptoms may require the assistance of a clinical nurse specialist, social worker, or physician.[12,29,40]

The nurse's role in fostering coping begins with an assessment of previous stressors and coping responses. Many individuals clearly assert that no matter how successfully they have coped with previous experiences, they are now overwhelmed by the cancer diagnosis.

The needs of the individual, family, and friends change over time, and all coping strategies are not needed simultaneously. A flexible and resourceful style can emerge in response to change.

Nonjudgmental Support

In aiding the patient and family through the adaptation process, the nurse contributes the most when offering nonjudgmental support. The nursing focus can be to assist the individual in building on past successes and learning from those experiences in which the individual's self-assessment of coping was that of needing improvement. By focusing on learning from experiences, the nurse conveys nonjudgmental support and teaches the patient a reframing technique that supports positive change.

It may be helpful for the individual and family to engage in education programs that teach coping skills. The American Cancer Society's program "I Can Cope" encourages the development and mastery of skills that facilitate an understanding of cancer as a chronic disease, self-care management of common therapy-related side effects, and the recognition and acceptance of emotional concerns. Family members and friends are also encouraged to attend "I Can Cope" sessions to recognize and cope with their own concerns. The success of such programs has been well documented.[26,54]

EXTRINSIC FACTORS
The Nurse's Self-Assessment

Personal meaning. To render quality psychosocial care to the individual with cancer and the family, the impact of the disease must also be viewed from the perspective of the nurse. The nurse and other caregivers can experience a wide range of emotional responses. The meaning a cancer diagnosis holds for a particular nurse is framed within the nurse's own life experience.

Professional experience. The care brought to each situation builds on previous experiences and influences expectations. An individual newly diagnosed with cancer may remind the nurse of similar patients or the nurse may be reminded of personal experiences with family or close friends who have faced cancer.

Such memories may be positive or negative, helpful or not helpful. Patients' families may also serve as a reminder of positive or negative experiences. The challenge for the nurse is to realize that similarities, unless consciously recognized, may hinder an accurate assessment of the actual needs of an individual and family.

Cancer patients' and nurses' perceptions of caring behaviors have been identified and compared.[12,13] In two different studies, the patient's initial perception of the most important nurse-caring behaviors were the technical components of good physical care delivery. Patients initially did not report valuing aspects of a trusting relationship as highly as did the nurse. This discordance should be viewed carefully by nurses. Nurses can appreciate that through the provision of quality physical care they can establish a trusting relationship for psychosocial care. The nurse can also appreciate that the strain of facing never-ending physical and psychosocial needs can lead to exhaustion. The literature supports the fact that constant caregiving demands can lead to such exhaus-

tion.[67,69] Nurses then must reevaluate strategies for self-care.

Theoretic Psychosocial Models

Crisis theory. Crisis is a state provoked when a person faces an important obstacle in relation to life goals and for a time finds it insurmountable through the use of customary problem-solving methods.[69] Not every untoward event results in crisis or illness, but it does present an upset in the steady state.[31] Crisis occurs as an emotional response to a threatening situation.

Crisis theory describes three phases of response. In the *precrisis phase* the individual seeks to maintain equilibrium by adapting to physical and psychosocial changes within the context of normal life events. Problems arise. The problem itself is not the crisis. Crisis occurs as a response to a problem. Within the context of cancer, the perceived degree of threat associated with the discovery of a breast lump, for example, may initiate a crisis response in a woman with a strong family history of breast cancer. The important factor is the individual's perception of threat. The expectations and fears are derived from the family history of cancer. The crisis response is initiated not by a confirmed diagnosis, but by the perceived threat.[31,35,36]

The *crisis phase* is characterized by disorganization. Attempts are made to solve the problem, which may or may not be successful. In the example of a woman with a newly discovered breast lump, several possibilities emerge. The woman may respond by attempting to ignore the lump yet be haunted by an anxiety about progressive disease because of her delayed action in seeking care. She may minimize her findings and delay seeking attention while busying herself with other activities. Or she may alleviate her distress by seeking immediate medical evaluation and becoming proactively involved in her treatment planning.

In the *postcrisis phase,* several possibilities can emerge. Successful problem resolution reduces the crisis and can influence the individual's functioning in future crisis situations. If the postcrisis period is marked by deterioration in physical and emotional function, the individual may function at a level lower than in the precrisis state. If new skills are learned and personal growth occurs, future functioning may be at a higher level of coping.

Oncology nurses can use the crisis intervention model to foster personal growth. The nurse can assist the individual through the initial difficulty by teaching problem-solving skills that aid in regaining personal control. Such teaching and support can assist individuals and families to achieve a higher level of postcrisis functioning.[63]

Areas of predominant concern. Studies of large numbers of cancer patients have yielded data regarding psychosocial impact. The issues patients and families reported they "frequently worried about" have been clustered and identified by Weisman and Worden as seven areas of predominant concern[63,67,69]:

- *Health concerns*—level of worry is related to the individual's interpretation of disease spread and significance of therapy-associated symptoms.
- *Self-appraisal*—changes in physical appearance or employment status influence self-esteem and body image.
- *Work and finances*—physical disability, temporary or permanent job changes, questions of insurance coverage, or any change in financial status can be a great source of emotional distress.
- *Family and significant others*—general mood swings or specific sexual concerns can strain relationships.
- *Religion*—the regularity of church attendance does not always indicate the depth of a belief system. Some feel comfort from a religious belief, whereas others feel abandonment.
- *Friends and associates*—the kindness of friends and associates is appreciated, but the limitations of such relationships are acknowledged. Specific expectations may be absent.
- *Existential concerns*—regardless of the prognosis given, the individual struggles with finite existence and the possibility of early death.

Psychosocial staging. As goals of therapy are adjusted to the stage of disease progression, likewise supportive care is adjusted to various psychosocial stages of response to the disease process. Weisman and Worden described four psychosocial stages that can be considered in conjunction with the physical stage of disease[63,69]:

- *Stage I: Existential Plight*—the first 100 days after diagnosis have been described as the period of existential plight. The initial period, when the diagnosis has been confirmed, is described as that of impact distress. As time progresses, the initial shock becomes focused on coping with treatment plans and therapy side effects. Regardless of prognosis, the fear of death during this time is recurrent. In general, emotional distress parallels the degree of physical change.
- *Stage II: Mitigation and Accommodation*—this stage encompasses the issues faced during remission or the time after which cure is designated. Adjustments are related to long-term side effects and the fear of recurrence. Successful adjustment includes living with minimal emphasis on disease-related changes and achieving preillness function and autonomy. Reinvestment in life occurs as plans for the future are again made.
- *Stage III: Decline and Deterioration*—recurrence signals a time-limited prognosis. The realization of disease return may be related to the degree of symptoms experienced. The actual life expectancy may remain unclear. This stage may last for a long time or progress rapidly to preterminality.

- *Stage IV: Preterminality and Terminality*—this stage acknowledges the beginning of the dying process. Symptom control and personal choices should guide care. From preterminality to death, caregivers can provide safe conduct or passage for the dying.

Death and dying. The landmark work that facilitated much of our understanding of the dynamics of dying was done by Kübler-Ross. She identified five stages associated with the dying process: denial, anger, bargaining, depression, and acceptance.[30] Some professionals later misinterpreted these data and believed it was important to progress through the stages in an orderly series from diagnosis until death. Some believed it was important to help the individual move from stage to stage. Professionals sometimes reported feelings of inadequacy when their patients did not die in a stage of acceptance. In reality, the stages are to be understood as fluid and changing. The fluid nature of individual responses can make the assessment difficult.[4,52]

Kavanaugh built on the research of Kübler-Ross and described two major tasks to be accomplished in the dying process.[30,52] The first task is for the dying person to receive permission to die from every important person who will be left behind. This task may be accomplished for some, all, or none of the family or friends of the dying. When accomplished, it may be in an open, direct manner or very subtly. The second task is for the dying person to voluntarily let go of every important person and possession held dear. This task is also very highly individualized. At any given time the dying person, family, and friends (including health care professionals) may be struggling with different stages or tasks. Nurses have a supportive role in the midst of these individual responses.

Professional rewards come from recognition of efforts in this process. Nurses can recognize that family members who do not abandon the dying, in the face of their own discomfort, may silently be granting permission for the death. The individual who acknowledges the joy and difficulties experienced in life may be able to picture the world without his or her presence and voluntarily let go of life.[4,52]

Common Misconceptions

Denial and hope. Denial and hope are often misunderstood and can therefore lead to inaccurate assessments. The term *denial* is sometimes used by health care providers to describe individuals who do not verbalize or display an understanding of the severity of their situation. Denial may also be described as minimization of physical or psychosocial distress, withdrawal, or distortion of information. Denial is a process rather than a fixed style.[69] Specific aspects of the disease situation, such as the prognosis, may be denied. Prognosis may be acknowledged only to certain individuals and then not consistently. Selection of limited situations or relation-ships for open disclosure is often based on the perceived safety of the situation or relationship. Caregivers can feel shut out and therefore misconstrue the response as de-nial.[29,40,62]

Denial can be a helpful mechanism. Staying consis-tently in touch with all of the emotional aspects of a life-threatening situation is neither realistic nor helpful. In the midst of apparent denial, the individual may be strug-gling with a competing increased awareness. This pro-cess can therefore be adaptive rather than maladaptive. Concern over a maladaptive response may be appropri-ate when an individual consistently engages in self-destructive behaviors or refuses therapy that offers long-term control or cure.

There may be a confusing period in the patient's ad-justment and response that is also confusing to the wit-ness. It may be seen when the emotional distress of ad-vanced disease or impending death is so painful that es-cape routes are sought. Individuals who have previously articulated knowledge of their prognosis suddenly em-bark on a course of behaviors or statements that seem to reflect little knowledge or acceptance of reality. Patients or families may say "when I am better" or "we are plan-ning a trip to Europe in a couple of months when he is stronger," or there may be a sudden avoidance of ques-tions about their condition. This phenomenon has been described as a *period of middle knowledge*.[21] During this period caregivers may best respond by gently refocusing the individual toward reality. Statements such as "I hope you are able to go, but it may not be possible" do not support unrealistic expectations but rather support the concept of hope.

The concept of hope is elusive. It is a highly personal experience that represents one's imagined future. Hope has been defined as an emotion, an expectation, an illu-sion, and a disposition.[21,51] It has been characterized as having two distinct subsets: *generalized hope,* which is a positive view of life or the world, and *particularized hope,* which is directed toward a specific outcome with a personal meaning.[21,51] A study addressing the relation-ship between hope and coping in individuals diagnosed with cancer found a positive correlation between hope and effective coping.[21,51,60] In this study, subjects still receiving therapy were more hopeful than those to whom only supportive care was given. The ability to perform self-care or carry out family responsibilities was also noted as significant to the degree of hope. A strong reli-gious faith showed a positive correlation. Another study noted that being hopeful requires energy.[40,45] The latter study identified as hopeful those individuals who de-scribed meaningful lives and were peaceful regarding their situation.

Nursing assessment of psychosocial adjustment can be hampered by misconceptions of denial and hope. Hope-ful attitudes can initially appear to be a denial of a grave situation. Strong religious beliefs can also be misinter-preted as false hope or maladaptive denial. The ability to differentiate comes from a strong nurse-patient-family relationship and a systematic assessment. The relation-ships and assessment evolve over time and are charac-terized by openness and a nonjudgmental approach that enables hope to exist.

Sadness and depression. Another challenging psy-chosocial assessment involves the distinction between sadness and depression. Sadness is a normal human re-sponse to a potential or real loss. Depression is a severe expression of normal sadness.[6,31] Sadness is uncomfort-able for both the cared for and the caregiver.

When confronted with the diagnosis or recurrence of cancer, a grief reaction normally ensues. The grief reac-tion may be manifested in numerous ways: anger, inabil-ity to concentrate, lapses in short-term memory, with-drawal, or tearfulness. Individual and cultural variances are also noted. When such responses lead to an inability to carry out self-care or a prolonged state of diminished self-esteem, supportive intervention is needed. An as-sessment of preillness relationships and crisis response patterns is necessary. A history of family discord, sub-stance abuse, or depression should be evaluated.[37]

A complete assessment of emotional states includes a search for potential physical causes. The fatigue associ-ated with cancer therapies, electrolyte abnormalities, or side effects of drugs may precipitate or aggravate depres-sive symptoms. When depressive symptoms persist, psy-chiatric consultation may be indicated.[31] Psychotherapy and pharmacologic intervention can help a subset of pa-tients. Nursing interventions should focus on fostering a supportive environment that accepts a variety of emo-tional responses as appropriate and valid. Caution should be observed with individuals who internalize rather than verbalize feelings. Although catharses may be helpful for some, it must be recognized that a safe environment for catharsis demands a skillful therapeutic relationship. When individuals feel forced to verbalize feelings, they will subsequently feel awkward in the presence of the individual perceived to be responsible.[31,69] A team ap-proach may be most helpful in assessing and managing sadness and depression.

MAXIMIZING AND MEASURING QUALITY OF LIFE

The myriad psychosocial issues that are a part of cancer nursing care stem from the individual response of the pa-tient, family, friends, and society to a diagnosis and prog-nosis. Maximizing quality of life is the goal regardless of disease outcome. Both supportive care and survivorship involve specific issues that must be addressed successfully to maximize quality of life.[7]

Quality of life encompasses physical, social psychologic, and spiritual well-being. Physical well-being is determined by functional activity, strength or fatigue, sleep and rest, pain, and other symptoms. Social well-being is determined by roles and relationships, affection and intimacy, appearance, leisure enjoyment, isolation, work and finances, and family distress. Psychologic well-being relates to control, anxiety and fear, depression, cognition, and distress of illness and treatment. Spiritual well-being encompasses meaning of illness, hope, transcendence, uncertainty, religiosity, and inner strength.[14,15,39]

Consideration of these multidimensional factors indicates a focus on quality of life and disruption to well-being. The subjective nature of these factors challenge our ability to measure our effectiveness. Some are able to tolerate severe impairment and still feel fortunate to receive therapy, whereas others with minimal dysfunction are extremely dissatisfied. Quality of life may therefore best be defined as *what the individual says it is*. Perception of illness includes more than physical disability. Some individuals are unable to express their values or define quality of life without some assistance in a values-clarification process.[28,61,65] There is no gold standard for measuring quality of life. Each situation poses unique concerns. In research settings, quality of life measures are often considered along with measurement of treatment efficacy. Major oncology study groups (e.g., SWOG, ECOG) include quality-of-life measures in their treatment protocol studies. When considering the evaluation instrument, content and length must be considered along with reliability and validity. The design or selection of a questionnaire is influenced by the setting, degree of data sophistication desired, and particularly the patient's expected treatment outcome—curative, life-extending, palliative, or phase 1 investigational. The sicker the patient, the less complex the measurement instrument must be.[6,7,70]

As we increase our emphasis on cost-effective care and cost-utility, palliative care in particular may come under scrutiny. This scrutiny promotes quality-of-life measurement.

Survivorship

From the time of diagnosis and for the balance of his or her life, an individual diagnosed with cancer is considered a survivor. During the experience the individual first fights to beat the disease and then to sustain disease-free survival.[41] The perception of survivorship has expanded and evolved. It was once viewed as the period of time when therapy was completed and one lived beyond the 5- to 10-year survival mark. Therapy-related complications and the need for long-term surveillance have

brought us to an expanded view. Survivorship brings with it many aspects of rehabilitation. The physical, psychosocial, vocational, and financial effects of cancer are receiving more attention than ever.[2,5,33,53]

A new group of survivors has emerged to address these concerns. These individuals come together through various forums to search, explore, and learn together. They attend meetings, share newsletters, and write books. They exchange "war" stories and work together to achieve quality time. They have found meaning and usefulness in the concept of survival rather than cure. The organization called the *National Coalition for Cancer Survivorship (NCCS)* was thus formed. The Coalition defines survivorship as a dynamic process of living with, through, and beyond cancer.[20,23]

An estimated 8 million Americans with a history of cancer share survivorship concerns. In an attempt to call public attention to the survivor's needs, the American Cancer Society put forth "The Cancer Survivor's Bill of Rights."[31,41] These rights address medical care, personal life adjustment, job opportunities, and insurance coverage. The aim is to have society foster a truly normal life span for cancer survivors.

In spite of progress in treatment, cancer continues to be associated with negative outcomes. With such a prevailing attitude, often too little thought is given to aggressive rehabilitation. The growing survivorship movement has refocused concern on life after treatment and the rehabilitation needs of cancer patients. The continued struggle of living with residual disease or treatment effects defines rehabilitation needs. The rehabilitation philosophy has become a component of survivorship and focuses on self-care and maximizing potential for wellness.[61,67]

Cancer rehabilitation. Cancer rehabilitation may be defined as the process of minimizing the physical, psychologic, social, and vocational dysfunction that may result from the disease or its treatment. Rehabilitation measures are aimed at restoration of function and prevention of further complications and include compensatory and supportive measures. When disabilities cannot be corrected, coping or adaptation must occur. Adaptation is an attempt to maintain sameness with a focus on altering to conform to demands and maintain the system.[2] The system may be the family, school, work, or community. Adaptation is not always achievable, and the broader concept of coping must then be explored. The goal of coping is problem resolution, which necessitates a change in both the person and the situation. With coping as a goal, the person uses a variety of resources to regain personal control. The problem may not be permanently solved, but the process can begin again.[16]

Rehabilitation is dynamic, since abilities and goals are continually changing.[16] Confrontation is an integral part of the strategies employed.[6,20] Such rehabilitation involves measures that enable individuals to feel at home with their bodies, self-image, emotional status, social setting, and work.[16,41]

Physical rehabilitation. Physical rehabilitation should begin as soon as the likelihood of disability is recognized. Loss or dysfunction of a body part requires various approaches to physical rehabilitation. Surgical amputation of a body part or limb may lead to the need for a prosthesis and techniques to aid in maintaining function and prevent further complications, such as lymphedema after breast surgery. Other examples of physical consequences include loss of voluntary bowel or bladder control, loss of energy, loss of appetite, inability to speak or swallow, deterioration in muscle strength, inability to ambulate, or unstable gait.[8] Functional restoration will depend on the degree of impairment, disability, or handicap experienced. Other physical changes, such as impaired fertility, may be the source of distress requiring psychosocial rehabilitation.

Nurses and physical therapists can work together with the patient and family employing techniques, such as upper extremity range of motion, arm and hand strength or endurance, coordination, splinting, and compensatory techniques for sensory loss. In aiding with the adjustment to a physical loss, there is no substitute for the support and role modeling that can come from a peer—someone who has experienced the same loss. Referrals to such groups as Reach to Recovery or laryngectomy clubs can complement the efforts of nurses and therapists and bolster the self-esteem of the patient.[8,41,47]

Psychosocial rehabilitation. Because of their complexity, psychosocial needs are best assessed in a systematic manner. The history should include information about the family makeup and relationships, work history, religious and community involvements, educational status, financial resources, and, when possible, clues to prior coping mechanisms. Emotional distress scales or similar types of measurements may be helpful in objectifying information.

Cancer survivors frequently perceive themselves as being treated differently by family, friends, and business associates. Myths, misconceptions, fear of recurrence, and poor communication may all contribute to the dissolution of such relationships. Patients soon decide with whom they can talk about their illness. They may seek those less likely to be frightened or overwhelmed with anxiety.

Conflicting data exist regarding the long-term impact of a cancer diagnosis on marital relationships. Changes in body image, impaired fertility, degree of unresolved conflicts, and preillness maturity within a relationship must all be considered.[33] The cancer survivor who is single also has special concerns. Anxieties over developing intimate relationships center on explaining the

cancer history, potential infertility, and body image changes.[64] These concerns should be clinically addressed proactively. A psychosocial data base can uncover such concerns and guide the caregiver in strengthening the adjustment process. A psychosocial plan of care should involve a team approach and consider developmental needs, realities of treatment, prognosis, and all aspects of rehabilitation.

When disease or treatment leaves the individual with residual impairment, specific rehabilitation goals aimed at restoration may be needed. Participation in activities of daily living can be the joint goal of patient, family, nurse, physical and occupational therapists, social worker, and psychologist. Techniques employed may include a life-style interview or checklist and providing information on energy conservation, pacing, work simplification, home adaptation, and adaptive equipment. Adaptive living techniques can foster the maintenance of self-esteem. The rehabilitation team can employ such techniques as stress management, relaxation, dealing with depression through activity, and making life-style changes to maximize independence.

Employment/vocational rehabilitation. Employment often means more than a source of income. A job or career may be a major part of feelings of identity and self-worth. Most successfully treated cancer patients are able to resume previous occupations with minor or no alteration in circumstances. Those who do face problems when returning to work cite the attitudes of employers and coworkers as a major concern.[21] Nurses should prepare patients for the possibility of such reactions. Some patients recognize their own attitudes as the obstacle. Fear of recurrence and fatalism about the disease may be at the root of the problem. Some cancer survivors describe a sense of being locked into a current position or employer.[64] They are hesitant to change positions because of specific concerns about obtaining insurance benefits. Actual discrimination may be difficult to prove since it can be subtle. The Americans With Disabilities Act (ADA) of 1990 requires equal opportunity in selection, testing, and hiring of qualified applicants with disabilities. Under the act, anyone who has had cancer is considered disabled. This law prohibits discrimination against workers with disabilities and is similar to the Civil Rights Act of 1964 and Title V of the Rehabilitation Act of 1973.[47]

The ADA covers discrimination that may occur in hiring, promotion, pay, job training, benefits, and firing. Since 1994 the law applies to any private employer with 15 or more employees, state and local government agencies, labor organizations, religious bodies that are employers, and Congress. A different law covers Federal government employees. The individual who is familiar with these laws can protect themselves from discrimination through preventive strategies. Unless the effects of disease or treatment directly affect the individual's ability to perform the essential functions of a job, there is no obligation to disclose information. It is important not to lie but also not necessary to volunteer information. The employee should be prepared to educate the employer and to stress specific job qualifications and abilities. The emphasis must be on present ability to perform the job, not on disability or medical history. The Equal Employment Opportunity Commission (EEOC) assumes the federal government role of enforcing the standard. Local government offices can assist in investigations or claims.

Any person with a history of cancer who meets specified job qualifications and can perform the essential functions of the employment position is protected under the Americans With Disabilities Act of 1990. The employer is required to provide reasonable accommodation, which includes retraining, special devices, or a change in part of the job such as flexible scheduling. Such accommodation makes the disabled enabled. When residual effects of disease or treatment alter the individual's ability to continue in the preillness job, vocational rehabilitation interventions may be necessary. Retraining, partial disability, or full disability may be the only alternative for some. In these situations a rehabilitation team is needed to establish specific and realistic goals.[2,8,10,31] Rehabilitation programs and services are needed to smooth transition from the brief encounters with acute care and ambulatory care settings to self-care in the home setting. Oncology nurses, along with rehabilitation specialists, can assist in successful reentry. The rehabilitation team can also assist in educating employers to dispel cancer myths and assist in transition back into the workplace.

Finances, Insurance, and the Law

An individual's insurance coverage and financial resources greatly influence access to care and quality of care. The uninsured and underinsured are limited to indigent care providers or state and federal programs with limited resources. Limited services and limits on coverage can place individuals in the compromised position of underreporting health problems. This situation fosters delayed diagnosis and treatment, increased acuity, and spiraling of health care cost.

The cost of care adds to the individual's and family's burden of living with cancer. They may be faced with the dilemma of forced choices: limited job mobility, paying medical bills versus living expenses, not reporting symptoms, seeking financial assistance, changing relationships, and insurance limitations as a subtle form of discrimination.[48,49]

Insurance companies can decide the type of insurance contract they will sell and to whom. Contracts are negotiated with employers and with individuals. The contract cost is determined by the coverage limits. The individual with evidence of persistent or recurrent disease may be considered a high risk to the insurance industry. The concept of excess mortality (observed death rates versus standard expected rates) is used in calculating premiums. Private insurance companies can establish waiting periods, deny coverage, and cancel policies based on the provision of each policy.

Currently no federal law guarantees a right to adequate health insurance. Cancer survivors do have the opportunity of keeping the health insurance obtained through their employer even after they are no longer employed. This opportunity is provided through The Comprehensive Omnibus Budget Reconciliation Act (COBRA) and The Employee Retirement and Income Security Act (ERISA). The COBRA plan can provide short-term coverage while the individual is seeking new employment or a new group plan. The ERISA law entitles the individual to file a claim when benefits are denied through discrimination. The ERISA law is enforced by the Pension and Welfare Benefits Administration of the United States Department of Labor. Nurses and other interdisciplinary team members can support the individual with financial concerns by sensitively assessing their situation and educating them about rights and resources.

Providing Comfort in Terminal Care

When cure or disease control are no longer attainable goals, there is a shift to palliative care in what is commonly referred to as the *terminal phase of illness*. The transition into this phase may be gradual, and the shift in care needs are not always recognized and acknowledged. As caregiving needs change, role strain may increase. The distinct needs of the patient and the caregiver must be recognized. The literature provides a systematic description and distinction between the needs of patient and primary caregiver.[66]

Nurses who recognize differing levels of need and need awareness in the patient and family can respond sensitively with supportive care. The nurse must be able to focus attention on the patient's goals, as stated by the patient, without neglecting the needs of the family. By asking questions and listening, the nurse can distinguish facts from feelings and ethical concerns. Clinical judgment suffices when dealing with the facts of disease progression and symptoms, but a more ethical decision-making process is required to deal with value-laden concerns. When values come in conflict, ethical dilemmas can arise.[13,49,68]

Advance directives. When addressing quality-of-life issues and clarifying values, the health care team approaches the subjects of hospice care, living wills, advance directives and durable power of attorney. The definition of each of these concerns must be clear to all involved in the care.

The two types of advance directives are *living will* and *durable power of attorney for health care* or *health care proxy.* They do not need to be prepared by or signed by an attorney. The living will is a treatment directive stating what medical therapies the patient chooses to omit or refuse. Durable power of attorney is a patient's written statement designating the appointment of an agent or proxy, usually a relative or trusted friend, to make decisions on their behalf when they can no longer decide for themselves in any illness or injury situation. It is recognized that the view of loved ones may differ greatly; therefore the written statement protects the patient's wishes.[42] (See box, Chapter 27, pp. 704-705, "Making Your Own Choices: A Guide to Help You Decide About Advance Directives.")

The cornerstone belief is that when death is inevitable, dignity is essential. Though not universally accepted, it is a common belief that it is not detrimental to tell a patient death is near. Honest communication should be tempered with sensitivity. In the context of such open communication, the wise physician may suggest that the patient prepare for the possibility of becoming unable to communicate and participate in treatment decisions.[10]

A Supreme Court ruling affirmed the constitutional right of liberty to refuse any medical treatment, including life-prolonging procedures and the right to name an agent/surrogate decision-maker for when the individual loses the personal capacity to do so. This ruling became law in the Patient Self-Determination Act of 1991.[10] These rights are proclaimed by enacting an advance directive that is a signed, dated, and witnessed legal document. Some states require notarization of the document. The individual who signs such a document must provide copies to their family, physician, and other appropriate individuals and discuss the specific details with these individuals.[10,42,52]

Right to die. Individuals, legislative bodies, and society as a whole continue to struggle with the right-to-die issue. Individual views are based on values and beliefs influenced by family, religion, education, and other unique forces. Legislative views are rooted in the principles of right to privacy, right to control one's own body, and the due process of liberty interest. The right to have control over one's own body is connected to the doctrine of informed consent and the right of a competent individual to refuse medical treatment. Society faces the issue with controversial responses determined by standards of care, legal precedence, religious and activist group influence, and geographic and cultural influences.

Major concerns center around the issue of competence, declared terminal state, cessation of medical or life-sustaining treatment, or affirmative steps to end life through active voluntary euthanasia or physician-assisted suicide.

When determining what constitutes an action and what constitutes an omission, moral judgments complicate decisions. Individuals and families struggle to come to a personal decision. Health care professionals seek to clarify their personal morality and professional ethics. Legislative bodies struggle with the issues on a case-by-case basis.[48] Few states have enacted definitive laws governing these decisions. Each of these individuals or groups may seek the counsel of medical ethicists.

The individual nurse serves the individual patient best when the nurse is clear about personal morality and professional ethics and is knowledgeable about institutional/agency ethics policies and current status of the law. Most important, the nurse serves patients best when he or she is aware of their wishes and guides them in expression of those wishes.

Hospice care. Discussion of care goals will lead to planning for a method of care delivery. When the focus of care is on the needs of the patient and family, attempts are made to leave as much control as possible in their hands. This approach serves to reaffirm life.[52] The setting and use of available health care agencies are determined by the individual situation. Regardless of the setting or agencies involved, the hospice approach or philosophy can serve the spectrum of needs. Hospice involves physical care, counseling services, volunteer assistance, respite care, support at the time of death, and bereavement follow-up. The coordination of care is based on stringent assessment of the resources, both internal and external, of the individual and family.[39,52]

Changes in health care reimbursement reward early discharge and home care. Home care and palliative needs require nursing assistance. The availability of a constant care provider is essential. Nurses coordinate the multidisciplinary care delivery. While delivering skilled care directly, they also teach family and friends how to deliver personal care. Hospice has therefore been described as primarily a nursing intervention.[52] Physical comfort is the priority. When physical symptoms are well managed, the dying may have the emotional energy to prepare themselves for death.

The dying individual has the right to choose which decisions to be involved in and which are of less concern.[4,39,52] Some individuals may wish to plan their own funeral and tell others of the plan, either verbally or in writing. Some may wish to make concrete arrangements for the family's financial and legal stability while avoiding conversation about feelings related to the dying process. During the dying process, less fear may be described than earlier in the disease process, yet a sense of disbelief may still be maintained.[39,52] The hospice nurse assesses the emotional position and lends gentle support without pressure to influence the response.

The needs of family members are unique to each member. Nursing assessment should identify the type of support family members are seeking.[53] The challenge of nursing is to prioritize the needs of patient and family members, noting the degree of congruence or discordance. The nurse can then more readily distinguish between reasonable and ideal psychosocial care.

Bereavement. The nurse who cares for the dying knows that grief does not begin with death or end with the funeral. With long-term illness, there is an opportunity to prepare for the actual loss by anticipating it. Anticipatory grief may or may not ease or shorten the bereavement process. The degree of emotional attachment and quality of communication within relationships influence the impact and outcome of grief. Constant pain, suffering, and a protracted death can increase the emotional pain. During the period of anticipation, the family may rehearse the impending death and feel depressed but also attempt to readjust their lives. At the time of death, there may be little display of emotion. Nurses and other caregivers may perceive a premature detachment. Therapeutic assessment throughout the illness and dying process can lessen the chance of misinterpreting the grieving process.[56]

Grief and mourning have many faces. Descriptions of normal grief come from reports of common symptoms. Crying, depressed mood, and sleep and eating disturbances are commonly reported. The sequence of events is reported as phases of shock and disbelief, developing awareness, and resolution.[69]

The time necessary for grief resolution is highly variable. Behavioral adaptation may be a response to societal expectation and not a barometer of emotional healing. Clear evidence of grief resolution may be the ability to speak of the lost relationship comfortably and realistically, recounting pleasures and disappointments of the relationship.[67,69]

Psychosocial management of the bereaved ideally begins with assessment of coping resources before the death. Helping the family know what to expect may ease the impact. Practical information and helpful acts convey compassionate support. The nurses' composure can create an atmosphere of control. When nurses' genuine feelings and emotional responses are controlled rather than denied, the bereaved are most therapeutically served. Extended care for the bereaved can take many forms: presence at funeral services, notes of sympathy, phone calls at specific intervals, support group offerings, or social gatherings. Such extension of care by health care professionals can be preventive medicine for the bereaved.

There are no timetables for grief and bereavement. The extent of follow-up must be individualized to the bereaved's needs and the constraints of the professional and institutional resources. Focus on high-risk needs and further referrals may be the priority.[67,69]

Spirituality. Pain and suffering can be overwhelming and deleterious, yet it can be viewed as positive. It can be positive when it serves to uncover meaning and hope, enhance coping, and foster personal growth and self-understanding. Both responses are often connected with an individual's spirituality.[22] A pain assessment and a spiritual assessment become vital tools for the nurse in reducing suffering. Persons at high risk for suffering have unrelieved pain, unresolved relationships issues, unresolved grief, or loss of autonomy.

Spirituality is the capacity to transcend self. This capacity is reflected in the need for self, based on meaning and purpose, and the need for relationship with others or a supreme other, characterized by unconditional love, trust, and forgiveness. This forms a basis for hope. Hope is the need to imagine and participate in enhancing a positive future.[22]

Psychospiritual intervention. Through education and counseling the nurse can address uncertainty, guilt, fear, anxiety, and hopelessness. Though fears may be well-founded, they may lessen when management strategies are explored and realities are carefully considered. Cognitive interventions, information and explanations, can be reassuring and thereby relieve psychospiritual distress. Uncertainty and powerlessness can be reduced through a process of realistic goal setting. The nurse can acknowledge small gains and affirm personal strengths, such as faith, courage, and a sense of humor. Through such affirmation the nurse offers caring support. Other cognitive interventions include imagery, distraction, and therapeutic storytelling. Environmental interventions can include modifying noise, heat, or light and using decorative or favorite objects, music, or "environmental" tapes. Encouraging the regulations of visitors and increasing the sensitivity of family and care providers can decrease powerlessness and increase comfort. Prayer, scripture reading, and visits from clergy may also provide comfort but should always be used with the patient's consent. The nurse must have personal comfort in these areas to be effective.[27,46]

Support for the Caregiver

Priority-setting. During the entire course of coping with cancer, there are psychologic and social effects on family functioning. The process can become destructive or turn in a positive direction toward personal growth. The direction taken at each crisis point may differ for each family member based on their unique perceptions of crises as threat or opportunity. Varied perceptions and expectations can lead to communication barriers. Such barriers can impede effective coping and personal growth. Nurturing can remove such barriers.[3,68] Therapeutic interventions by a nurse or other caregiver are critical at these susceptible times. Interventions can become therapeutic when preceded by careful assessment and mutual goal-setting. Each individual's goals or priorities must be considered.

In distinguishing between ideal and reasonable goals, priority-setting becomes of paramount importance. Priority-setting often parallels a hierarchy of needs. Physical needs must be met first. Emotional and social needs are more complex. The individual who successfully meets these needs may experience the personal growth that permits addressing spiritual needs. Care demands must be assessed in light of the priorities.[44] The clarification of goals and priorities fosters shared responsibilities. The level of communication needed to establish priorities can also aid in minimizing demands, making problems manageable, and preventing burnout.

Burnout is a syndrome of physical and personal exhaustion accompanied by negative attitudes and loss of concern for self and others. Family members and professional caregivers alike risk such a response when giving highly specialized care in emotionally charged situations. A cycle of frustration, helplessness, and cynicism can develop. The risk of burnout can be reduced by voicing frustration appropriately, developing a support system, setting priorities, and establishing reasonable expectations.[13,53,66]

Life-enhancement skills. High-quality care and avoidance of burnout can be achieved when life enhancement skills are developed. Life enhancement begins with self-care. Attending to the needs of others must be balanced with attending to one's own needs. A nutritious diet, adequate sleep, and physical exercise aid in physical self-care. Psychic and social comfort can be achieved through a variety of activities that provide a form of decompression. Prodromal signs of distress or inappropriate coping must be recognized and confronted. Life enhancement skills are developed from a philosophy of being true to self—a personal spirituality and commitment to caring for self and others. These skills can include such things as exercise, reading, writing, crafts, hobbies, music, dance, drama, and humor. Such skill development fosters resilience. With resilience, crisis can eventually be perceived as an opportunity for growth.

The crisis of cancer begins as a psychosocial response to a biologic growth but can become a psychosocial and spiritual growth process of life enhancement. This response is supported by nurses who have chosen a profession of life enhancement.[67,69]

NURSING MANAGEMENT

FACILITATING POSITIVE COPING
The Nurse's Role as Coach

Nursing interventions for psychosocial care are aimed at facilitating positive coping. The coach or teacher of positive coping skills must possess a number of competencies. First is the competency of *timing*. Timing is the art of capturing readiness to learn. Cancer nurses' competency is challenged here when information about disease, side effects of therapy, and self-care measures is to be taught at a time of high stress and overwhelming emotional responses. Teaching must be done progressively and repeatedly. Initial goals are to obtain informed consent, advise of immediate side effects, and assure safe self-care behaviors. The second competency is *integration*. Early rehabilitation is achieved when the nurse teaches self-care strategies that emphasize the healthy aspects of the individual and integration of the implications of illness and recovery into their life-style. The third competency is *understanding*. The nurse who skillfully listens to the patient's interpretation of information can mobilize appropriate psychologic and spiritual resources. Fourth is the competency of *interpretation*. Interpretation provides the patient with a rationale for treatments, procedures, and self-care measures. Skillful interpretation will reduce the sense of being overwhelmed. The fifth competency is *coaching*. The nurse coach assists the patient through difficult events such as bone marrow aspirations,

venipunctures, nausea and vomiting, and alopecia. The nurse who gently coaches the patient through stressful and unfamiliar situations, one step at a time, can provide maximum support and facilitate successful coping.[26,67]

Promoting Self-Care

Whether the goal be cure, control, or palliation, coping is most often facilitated when self-care is fostered. Situations and times will dictate the need for caregivers to assume aspects of care. Self-determination may then be more important than actual self-care. The skills needed for self-care and self-determination do not always come naturally. In many chronic diseases, model patient education programs have been developed to foster self-care and effective coping.[26,67]

The "I Can Cope" program, developed by Johnson and Norby and offered through the American Cancer Society, is a model cancer education program that teaches self-care and coping skills. The series of classes addresses learning about the disease and treatment, managing side effects, dealing with emotions, maintaining physical fitness, enhancing sexuality, and identifying and using resources. The class learning is enhanced by audiovisuals and printed materials that can later be used as reference guides for self-care. The self-help strategies taught in the classes are also described in a book of the same title, *I Can Cope*.[26,67]

The Patient's Sense of Maintaining Control

Studies suggest that cognitive information—that is, specific facts about the disease or treatment—is preferred by individuals during the initial phase of therapy. As treatment progresses, behavioral information is more readily assimilated. Determining individual learning needs is an important component of fostering self-care. The work of the "I Can Cope" program originators suggests that many individuals also respond to information that focuses on sensory experiences such as relaxation or massage.[26] Although research is needed to determine the type of information most beneficial to groups and individuals, the nurse can best meet any need by using professional experience and individualized assessment as a guide. The ultimate goal is to foster self-care and aid the patient in maintaining a sense of control in the situation.

Assisting the Patient with Goal-Setting

When the patient or family experiences episodes of feeling overwhelmed either physically or emotionally, goal-setting can be a helpful intervention. This process begins by asking the patient what outcome is desired. The nurse can help determine what goals are attainable within specific time frames. The nurse can provide assistance in establishing attainable goals within specific time frames. For example, this technique can be used to coach the individual through periods of inadequate fluid intake. Another attainable goal may be to come to the dinner table at least once a day rather than eating in one's room. Such small and attainable goals can build feelings of success. Periodic review of attained goals can be a morale booster for even the most withdrawn individual. Such coaching functions by the nurse aid in reaching the goal of positive coping.[34,47,68]

Referral for Counseling

Cancer patients rarely employ a maladaptive coping style in a consistent manner. However, there are occasions when particular behavioral patterns are a manifestation of an inability to cope effectively and require the intervention of an individual with advanced skills in psychosocial assessment. The experienced nurse is frequently in a position to recognize these patterns and to make a referral for further assessment. First it is important to observe for consistency, especially when dealing with a new diagnosis or recurrence. Some assessment techniques require advanced practice skills to determine the extent of maladaptive coping.[8,31] Maladaptive coping may manifest itself as three or more of the following behaviors:

- Poor eye contact and little facial expression; slow speech
- Nonfluctuating, generally negative mood
- Significantly depressed appetite; refusing adequate nutrition
- Sleep pattern characterized by early morning awakening, insomnia, or excessive daytime sleeping
- Lack of attention to hygiene and activities of daily living

The initial diagnosis or recurrence of cancer may initiate or exacerbate several of these behaviors. A complete assessment includes noting the persistence of such behaviors. Even in the absence of the symptomatology described, there may be indications for referral to specially skilled psychosocial caregivers.

Coping can be ineffective without being maladaptive. Many individuals are at risk of developing further problems if appropriate psychosocial assessment and intervention do not take place. Nurses may ask the patient or family to keep a log of feelings or responses during treatment or at critical times of change. Such a technique may aid in documenting negative thought or behavior patterns and confirm the need for a skilled counseling referral.[26,40,60]

Noncompliance can be a manifestation of ineffective coping and indicate the need for referral or a psychosocial consultation. Lack of compliance usually represents unmet needs or signifies a lack of understanding. Noncompliant behavior may also be a manifestation of anger, anxiety, or depression. Failure of an individual to follow a recommended treatment regimen may stem from other concerns, such as economics, a desire to avoid side effects, or a genuine lack of comprehension regarding the treatment regimen. To ensure continuity of care, patient compliance should be monitored continuously. Complex information should be tailored to meet individual needs, and specific behaviors that enhance compliance should be identified and reinforced. Caregivers often perceive noncompliant behavior as a conscious decision to annoy the caregiver. Adequate assessment can deter such a perception.[51,62,63,69]

BEHAVIORAL TECHNIQUES
Rationale

Specific behavioral interventions may be useful adjuncts in facilitating positive coping. Such interventions are particularly helpful in the management of anxiety, nausea and vomiting, and chronic pain. Behavioral techniques are most effective when combined with standard management approaches to specific problems. The comfort of patients receiving emetogenic chemotherapy may be enhanced by using relaxation therapy along with effective antiemetics. Distraction or the use of imagery along with appropriate analgesics may reduce pain perception. The use of rhythmic breathing during acutely painful procedures can reduce anxiety.

Behavioral techniques are to be taught, not imposed. Some individuals may resist behavioral approaches out of a fear of losing control or behaving in an embarrassing manner. An association with stage hypnosis may un-

Continued.

derlie such fear or reluctance. It is important to clarify concepts that are often misunderstood.[5,8,11,18,46] When presenting behavioral techniques as an option, it is important to point out that such techniques are successful because the person does remain in control of thoughts and functions.

Types of Behavioral Techniques

Relaxation, imagery, and hypnosis are three behavioral techniques that may be used individually or in combination. *Relaxation* is described as the absence of tension. Benson's relaxation response uses progressive muscle relaxation.[4] Reduction in tension can be physiologic or psychologic. *Imagery* has been described as the internal experience of an event without external stimuli.[37] A common imagery experience is that of a daydream. Imagery uses the imagination to visualize and sense an experience. *Hypnosis* is the induction of a trancelike state.[37] The trance is described as a wakeful dissociative state characterized by an increased receptivity to suggestion.

These techniques require varying degrees of training. After successful training, nurses can teach patients to do progressive relaxation alone or with the use of music or directed audio tapes. These techniques can be used as an adjunct in the management of chemotherapy-induced nausea.[37,38,58] Numerous scripts are available to assist nurses in implementing relaxation and imagery techniques.[58] Biofeedback is a technique that requires the use of monitoring instruments to assess muscle tension or thermoregulation. Some individuals are more attracted to such an approach than others and may benefit by a referral to someone qualified to implement such techniques. Although the goals of relaxation and hypnosis may be similar, the approaches and techniques are quite different. Hypnosis depends on the achievement of a trance state. Supervised training is necessary for the safe use of hypnotic techniques. After individualized assessment and mutual goal-setting have been completed by the nurse and patient, an appropriate technique may be selected.

CONCLUSION

The biologic disease process is unique for each individual, and the psychosocial response is equally individual. The psychosocial response extends to the family, friends, and professional caregivers. Meaningful support and therapeutic interventions can be difficult to deliver. A structured assessment and team approach can foster objective and complete data collection, support uniqueness, and aid in priority-setting. With such an approach, an open, evolving system is established and the potential arises for adaptation, positive coping, and holistic growth in the person with cancer and in family, friends, and caregivers.

■ CHAPTER QUESTIONS

1. Cancer patients rehabilitation needs are legally best addressed by:
   a. The Americans With Disabilities Act (1990)
   b. Title V Rehabilitation Act (1973)
   c. The Civil Rights Act (1964)
   d. The Patient Self-Determination Act (1991)
2. In an attempt to call public attention to survivor's needs, a bill of rights was put forth by:
   a. The National Coalition of Cancer Survivors
   b. The National Cancer Institute
   c. The American Cancer Society
   d. The National Hospice Organization
3. The reported sequence of events or phases of grief and mourning are:
   a. Denial, anger, bargaining
   b. Shock/disbelief, developing awareness, resolution
   c. Confronting the pain, bargaining, acceptance
   d. Denial, bargaining, acceptance
4. The Right to Die Legislation is rooted in the principles of Right to Privacy, Due Process of Liberty, *and:*
   a. Right to individual values and beliefs
   b. Justice
   c. Fidelity and veracity
   d. Informed consent doctrine
5. Psychosocial adjustment is related to the concurrent care goals of disease control *and:*
   a. Symptom control
   b. Insurance approval
   c. Quality of life
   d. Access to intensive counseling
6. The most significant aspect of care in meeting the needs of the person experiencing spiritual distress is:
   a. Knowledge of major religious beliefs
   b. Nonjudgmental listening
   c. Referral to clergy
   d. Exploring values and beliefs
7. The primary concern of the newly diagnosed person with cancer is:
   a. Pain
   b. Health care costs
   c. Role strain
   d. Life versus death
8. The Patient Self-Determination Act of 1991 affirms all the following rights *except:*
   a. To request an assisted death
   b. To name an agent/surrogate decision maker
   c. To name specific treatments allowed
   d. To refuse any medical treatment

BIBLIOGRAPHY

1. Baird SB: The impact of changing health care delivery on oncology practice, *Oncol Nurs,* 2(3):1, 1995.
2. Berry DL: Return-to work experiences of people with cancer, *Oncol Nurs Forum* 20(6):905, 1993.
3. Boland DL, Sims SL: Family care giving at home, *Image* 28(1):55, 1996.
4. Brescia FJ: Specialized care of the terminally ill. In DeVita V, Hellman S, Rosenberg S, editors: *Cancer principles and practice of oncology,* ed 4, Philadelphia, 1993, Lippincott.
5. Bushkin E: Signposts of survivorship, *Oncol Nurs Forum* 20(6):869, 1993.
6. Cella DF: Measuring quality of life in palliative care, *Semin Oncol* 12(2):74, 1995.
7. Cheson BD and others: Clinical trials referral resource: clinical trials assessing quality of life, *Oncology* 9(11):1171, 1995.
8. Christ GH and others: Providing community resources for cancer patients, In DeVita V, Hellman S, Rosenberg S, editors: *Cancer principles and practice of oncology,* ed 4, Philadelphia, 1993, Lippincott.
9. Devolder-McCray N: *Ratings by health professionals of effective coping strategies for cancer patients,* Master's thesis, University of Kansas, 1979.
10. Diamond EP: Two years of the self-determination act, *Oncology Nursing Patient Treatment and Support* 1(2):1, 1994.
11. Dodd M, Ahmed N: Preference for type of information in cancer patients receiving radiation therapy, *Cancer Nurs* 10(5):244, 1987.
11a. Eakes GC: Chronic sorrow: a response to living with cancer, *Oncol Nurs Forum* 20(9):1327, 1993.
12. Engelking C: A comforting presence, *Innovations in Breast Cancer Care* 1(1):1, 1995.
13. England M: Caregiver planning, *Image* 28(1):17, 1996.
14. Ferrans CE: Quality of life through the eyes of survivors of breast cancer, *Oncol Nurs Forum* 21(10):1645, 1994.
15. Ferrell B: Quality of life in breast cancer, quality of life and the cancer patient: a 20-year evolution, symposium presentation, April 1995, Anaheim, Calif.
16. Gerber LH and others: Evaluation and management of disability: rehabilitation aspects of cancer. In DeVita V, Hellman S, Rosenberg S, editors: *Cancer principles and practice of oncology,* ed 4, Philadelphia, 1993, Lippincott.
17. Glass BC: The role of the nurse in advanced practice in bereavement care, *Clin Nurs Spec* 7(2):62, 1993.
18. Hagopian GA: Cognitive strategies used in adapting to a cancer diagnosis, *Oncol Nurs Forum* 20(5):759, 1993.
19. Harper JM: Grief components. Part II. *Thanatos* 20(2):14, 1995.
20. Herbst S: Survivorship: redefining the cancer experience, *Oncol Nurs Forum* 22(3):527, 1995.
21. Herth K: The relationship between level of hope and level of coping response and other variables in patients with cancer, *Oncol Nurs Forum* 16(1):67, 1989.
22. Highfield MF: Spiritual health of oncology patients: nurse and patient perspectives, *Cancer Nurs* 15(1):1, 1992.
23. Hoffman B: Cancer survivors at work: job problems and illegal discrimination, *Oncol Nurs Forum* 16(1):39, 1989.
24. Hollen PJ, Hobbie WL: Risk taking and decision making of adolescent long-term survivors of cancer, *Oncol Nurs Forum* 20(5):769, 1993.
25. Jassak PF: Nursing considerations for patients receiving biological response modifiers, *Semin Oncol Nurs* 9(3):suppl 1, 32, 1993.
26. Johnson J, Klein L: *I can cope: staying healthy with cancer,* Minneapolis, 1988, DCI.
27. Johnston K, Rohaly-Davis J: An introduction to music therapy: helping the oncology patient in the ICU, *Crit Care Nurs Q* 18(4):54, 1996.
28. King CR: Latent effects and quality of life one year after marrow and stem cell transplantation, *Quality of Life—A Nursing Challenge* 4(2):40, 1995.
29. Kolcaba KY: The art of comfort, *Image* 27(4):287, 1995.
30. Kushner H: *When bad things happen to good people,* New York, 1981, Schocken Books.
31. Lederberg MS, Massie MJ: Psychosocial and ethical issues in the care of cancer patients. In DeVita V, Hellman S, Rosenberg S, editors: *Cancer principles and practice of oncology,* ed 4, Philadelphia, 1993, Lippincott.
32. Lind S and others: Telling the diagnosis of cancer, *J Clin Oncol* 7(5):583, 1989.
33. Loescher LJ and others: Surviving adult cancers. Part 1. Physiologic effects, *Ann Intern Med* 111(5):411, 1989.
34. Lynch HT, Lynch J: Genetic counseling for hereditary cancer, *Oncology* 10(1):27, 1996.
35. Mahon SM, Casperson D: Hereditary cancer syndrome. Part I. Clinical and educational issues, *Oncol Nurs Forum* 22(5):763, 1995.
36. Mahon SM, Casperson D: Hereditary cancer syndrome. Part II. Psychosocial issues, concerns, and screening—results of a qualitative study, *Oncol Nurs Forum* 22(5):775, 1995.
37. Massie M and others: Psychiatric complications in cancer patients. In Murphy GP, Lawrence W Jr, Lenhard RE Jr, editors: *American Cancer Society textbook of clinical oncology,* ed 2, Atlanta, 1995, American Cancer Society.
38. McCaffrey M, Beebe A: *Pain clinical manual for nursing practice,* St Louis, 1989, Mosby.
39. McMillan SC, Mahon M: A study of quality of life of hospice patients on admission and at week 3, *Cancer Nurs* 17(1):52, 1994.
40. Morse JM, Doberneck B: Concept of hope, *Image* 27(4):277, 1995.
41. Mullen F, Hoffman B: *An almanac of practical resources for cancer survivors charting the journey,* New York, 1990, Consumers Union.
42. Neumark DE: Providing information about advance directives to patients in ambulatory care and their families, *Oncol Nurs Forum* 21(4):771, 1994.
43. North American Nursing Diagnoses Association: *Conference Proceedings,* St Louis, 1994, The Association.
44. Oberst M and others: Caregiving demands and appraisal of stress among family caregivers, *Cancer Nurs* 12(4):209, 1989.
45. Owen D: Nurses' perspective on the meaning of hope in patients with cancer: a qualitative study, *Oncol Nurs Forum* 16(1):75, 1989.
46. Pope DS: Music, noise, and the human voice, *Image* 27(4):291, 1995.

47. Powel L, McFadden ME: Repercussions of cancer treatment: long-term physiologic and psychologic sequelae, *Quality of Life—A Nursing Challenge* 4(2):33, 1995.

48. Powell JA, Cohen AS: The right to die, *Issues Law Med* 10:169, 1994.

49. Quigley K: The adult cancer survivor: psychosocial consequences of cure, *Semin Oncol Nurs* 5(1):63, 1989.

50. Radner G: *It's always something,* New York, 1989, Simon & Schuster.

51. Raleigh EDH: Sources of hope in chronic illness, *Oncol Nurs Forum* 19(3):443, 1992.

52. Sammarino D: Dealing with the dying patient. In DeVita V, Hellman S, Rosenberg S, editors: *Cancer principles and practice of oncology,* ed 4, Philadelphia, 1993, Lippincott.

53. Scanlon C: Creating a vision of hope: the challenge of palliative care, *Oncol Nurs Forum* 16(4):491, 1989.

54. Scanlon C, Glover J: A professional code of ethics: providing a moral compass for turbulent times, *Oncol Nurs Forum* 22(10):1515, 1995.

55. Sneed N and others: Adjustment of gynecological and breast cancer patients to the cancer diagnosis: comparisons with males and females having other cancer sites, *Health Care Women Int* 13:11, 1992.

56. Solari-Twadell PA and others: Pinwheel model of bereavement, *Image* 27(4):323, 1995.

57. Sorenson DLS: Life event timing, *Image* 27(4):297, 1995.

58. Spross J: Pain, suffering and spiritual well-being: assessment and interventions, *Quality of Life—A Nursing Challenge* 2(3):70, 1993.

59. Taylor EJ: Factors associated with meaning in life among

60. Thorne SE: Helpful and unhelpful communications in cancer care: the patient perspective, *Oncol Nurs Forum* 15(2):167, 1988.

61. Webster JS: Survivorship issues in post-induction therapy, *Nursing Care Issues in Adult Acute Leukemia* 2(4):28, 1995.

62. Weekes DP, Kagan SH: Adolescents completing cancer therapy: meaning, perception, and coping, *Oncol Nurs Forum* 21(4):663, 1994.

63. Weisman AD, Worden WJ: The emotional impact of recurrent cancer, *J Psychosoc Oncol* 3(4):5, 1986.

64. Welch-McCaffrey D and others: Surviving adult cancers. Part 2. Psychological implications, *Ann Intern Med* 11(6):517, 1989.

65. Whedon M, Stearns D, Mills LE: Quality of life of long-term adult survivors of autologous bone marrow transplantation, *Oncol Nurs Forum* 22(10):1527, 1995.

66. Wingate A, Lackey N: A description of the needs of noninstitutionalized cancer patients and their primary caregivers, *Cancer Nurs* 12(4):216, 1989.

67. Wolfelt AD: *Understanding grief, helping yourself heal,* Muncie, 1992, Accelerated Development Inc.

68. Woods N, Yates B, Primomo J: Supporting families during chronic illness, *Image* 21(1):46, 1989.

69. Worden JW: *Grief counseling and grief therapy,* ed 2, New York, 1991, Springer.

70. Zacharias DR, Gilg CA, Foxall MJ: Quality of life and coping in patients with gynecologic cancer and their spouses, *Oncol Nurs Forum* 21(10):1699, 1994.

people with recurrent cancer, *Oncol Nurs Forum* 20(9):1399, 1993.

CHAPTER 32
Impact of Cancer on Sexuality

JUDITH A. SHELL

Human beings are sexual from the time of birth until their death, and being sexual is a primary part of being human. If this factor is dismissed by the nurse or physician, the patient may perceive himself or herself as less than human. Until recently, health care professionals were inclined to focus on the physical and emotional aspects of the human being while overlooking the psychosexual. This was especially true with patients who are disabled, chronically ill, or over the age of 62.

Williams and colleagues reported in the late 1980s that "sexuality remains a sensitive, infrequently addressed issue in our society for health professionals as well as for the lay population."[78] However, attitudes are beginning to change and sexual rehabilitation is more often part of cancer treatment. Reasons for this change in attitude may include (1) better education concerning human sexuality; (2) a more receptive attitude by society; and (3) an increased demand for open discussion of sexuality issues.[2] Sexuality is a term that can mean different things to different people. The definition Weiss offers best details male and female humanness[76]:

Sexuality isn't really about the things we've been taught to think it is. It isn't about pleasing others, nor is it about owning or controlling others. It isn't about intercourse or having babies. It isn't about competition and beauty contests or proving ourselves more beautiful or sexy than others. It isn't about giving others pleasure so we can feel loved by them, nor is it about trading our bodies for financial, material, or emotional security and comfort. It isn't even only about having orgasms and other pleasurable physical sensations. Sexuality is about connecting our head with our gut through our heart. It's about genuinely caring for ourselves, finding ecstasy in simply being alive, and giving creative voice to our ideas and feelings. It's about bridging physical pleasures with spiritual awareness and serenity. It's about opening ourselves to the sensations of the body and to the joys of the imagination and the heart. It's about sharing and enjoying our sexual selves with partners we feel affectionate and safe with, and it's about loving ourselves and others.

The author would like to express her appreciation to Cindy Wadlow for typing this manuscript.

Although nurses often feel a responsibility to address their patients' sexual concerns, many experience discomfort with this role. This discomfort may be because of (1) personal feelings of anxiety regarding sexual topics; (2) embarrassment about obtaining a sexual history; and (3) negative societal stereotypes about sexuality and chronic illness or disability.[18]

Even with expanded general knowledge of human sexuality, past studies have shown that the nurse's attitude concerning sexuality and illness has not altered significantly.[19,79] However, increased confidence in sexual assessment and intervention may be attained if specific information and "how-to's" are made available. The Oncology Nursing Society and American Nurses Association Outcome Standards for Cancer Nursing Practice have provided guidelines for the nurse, which include the area of sexuality, and this chapter expands on those guidelines with details of site-specific concerns.

PSYCHOSOCIAL DEVELOPMENT THROUGH THE LIFE CYCLE

Of the many patients faced with a diagnosis of cancer, most experience a life crisis. Although death is often the first fear, the potential for other stressors exists.[49] Surgery, adjuvant therapy (chemotherapy and radiation), the possible spread of malignancy, and an uncertain prognosis are all factors that necessitate life-style adjustments. Changes in role function and an altered body image or self-esteem often threaten the patient with loss of feelings of femininity or masculinity, as well as sexual functioning. As early as 1966, Masters and Johnson explained that almost half of all couples who are physically and psychologically "healthy" have had sexual problems at some time during their relationship.[39] It is reasonable to assume, then, that many cancer patients will have sexual concerns given the added stressors of their disease. And now, in the 90s, Masters, Johnson, and Koloday continue to espouse the fact that "in cases where passion has turned to indifference, or where a couple is having fundamental problems with unfulfill-

Table 32-1 Psychosexual Stages of Development

Stage	Basic psychosocial task	Sexual task
Infancy (0-2 years)	Acquiring basic trust; learning to walk, talk	Gender identity
Childhood (2-12 years)	Acquiring a sense of autonomy versus shame and doubt; entering and adjusting to school	Pleasure-pain associated with sexual organs and eliminative functions; masturbation takes place with resulting shame and acceptance; secondary sex characteristics become evident
Adolescence (13-20 years)	Acquiring sense of identity versus role confusion	Mastery over impulse control, acceptance of conflict between moral proscription and sexual urges, handling new physiologic functions (menses for girls and ejaculate for boys)
Young adulthood (20-45 years)	Acquiring a sense of intimacy versus isolation; vocational effectiveness; interpersonal security, "sexual adequacy"	Sexual adequacy and performance plus fertility concerns and questions related to parenting
Middle adulthood (50-70 years)	Acquiring a sense of self-esteem versus despair; adjusting to diminution of one's energy and competence; "empty nest syndrome" plus care of aging parents or their death; adjusting to change in physique and evidence of aging	For the female, menopause and resulting vasomotor changes, atrophy of breasts, clitoral size, and vaginal lubrication; for the male, delay on attaining an erection, reduced compulsion to ejaculate, episodic impotence, possible prostatitis
Old age	Adjusting to loss of friends, family, confrontations with old age and dying, painful joint conditions, reduced hearing and visual acuity; adjustment to social stigmatization of being "old"	Reduced vitality, fear of incompetence or injury (coital coronary); fear of being viewed as "dirty old person"; unavailability of a partner (widowhood); limited physical capacity and reduced options

From Schain W: Sexual problems of patients with cancer. In DeVita VT, Hellman S, Rosenberg SA, editors: *Cancer: principles and practice of oncology,* Philadelphia, 1985, Lippincott.

ing sex, it often takes careful orchestration to get things back in tune."[40]

A person's sexual expression varies throughout the life cycle. Although personal beliefs and values are influential, interference with the psychosexual stages of development by an event such as disease may cause sexual dysfunction (Table 32-1).[49] For the cancer patient, passage from one stage to the next may be precluded by the disease and its treatment or prognosis. Awareness of these stages will help the caregiver recognize patients at risk for possible sexual dysfunction.

In addition to these stages, various other factors of importance should be considered. The patient's personal reaction to his or her illness and previous experience with the disease should be explored. Where are they in the continuum between denial and acceptance? What are their expectations and fears? If the patient has a significant other or spouse, consideration should be given to the couple's prior strengths and the stability of the relationship. What were their feelings toward sexuality before the disease? If the partners were supportive before diagnosis, they tend to be supportive after diagnosis.[4,49,53] Marriage stability after cancer diagnosis and treatment is generally based on the precancer situation.

ANTICIPATION OF AND ADAPTATION TO THE EFFECTS OF CANCER

Once patients are assured of survival beyond the initial diagnosis, the quality of their life becomes a concern. Will they be able to function as "normal" people do? Taken-for-granted activities like work, recreation, travel, parenting, and sex take on a new importance. While undergoing treatment or in the recovery period, patients will experience fluctuating degrees of fatigue, anorexia and nausea, and discomfort and debilitation. These will affect their level of sexual interest and ability and their sense of adequacy and self-esteem. Depending on the type of cancer and therapy employed, specific physiologic and psychologic changes can impair normal sexual functioning and feelings of femininity or masculinity.

Sense of Adequacy

For some people, the mere process of being ill may cast doubt on their sexual identity and response, which in turn will reflect on their sense of adequacy. Because of the seriousness of their illness, cancer patients are often too embarrassed to raise questions about their sexual concerns. They may feel that worrying about such a relatively unimportant matter as sex is unjustified. It must be emphasized, however, that sexuality is physically and emotionally a source of satisfaction and great pleasure and also the most intimate way we share ourselves with others.

Male and female sexual response is normally integrated into the sexual response cycle (excitement, plateau, orgasm, and resolution). The *male sexual response* (desire, subjective arousal, erection, emission, ejaculation, and orgasm) has separate mechanisms of control and can therefore be affected independently.[68] Although cancer therapy may destroy the capability for an erection, the pleasure of sexual arousal and orgasm often remain intact. This factor is important because men are often worried about whether they can function as they did before. For an in-depth explanation of male and female sexual response during the cancer experience, see von Eschenbach and Schover.[73] Masters, Johnson, and Koloday also provide a thorough description of the physical changes during the sexual response cycle, a conceptual model of sexual desire, and detailed photographs of the internal and external changes of the penis, vagina, and breast during sexual intercourse.[40]

Female sexual response (desire, subjective arousal, vaginal expansion and lubrication, and orgasm) is less well understood. Women with cancer may lose sexual desire during debilitating treatment, especially if the therapy affects the structure or innervation of the clitoris or vagina. This, along with painful intercourse, are factors that tend to interfere with orgasm. In addition, emphasis is placed on perceived damage resulting from therapy, which women feel may lead to rejection from their partner.[2]

Because the capability of relating sexually is extremely important in our culture, some patients may declare a lost interest in sex just to protect themselves from the embarrassment of lost orgasmic function or erectile failure.

Sexual dysfunction apart from a disability may also be present. This can be caused by "special problems such as alcohol, drug abuse, a history of physical and sexual abuse, or a history of irresponsible sexual behavior."[16] Moreover, added sexual inadequacy that is the result of a potentially fatal disease then predictably often leads to a threatened self-image.

Sense of Self-Esteem

Even when there is no organic illness, feelings of unworthiness and incompetence lead to a negative body image. Cancer patients are at much greater risk of having a negative body image because of mutilating surgery and devastating side effects of therapy. Cancer and its treatment can produce considerable loss of economic independence, alter role behavior and significant relationships, and reduce sexual responsiveness. What follows is fear of abandonment, withdrawal, and sexual dysfunc-

---

MOTIVES FOR SEXUAL INTERCOURSE

- Desire for closeness
- Wish to conceive
- Attempt to control or manipulate one's partner
- Nonverbal expression of affection
- Defense against depression or anxiety
- Bid for attention
- Confirmation of worth
- Defense against intimacy

From Schain W: Sexual problems of patients with cancer. In DeVita VT, Hellman S, Rosenberg SA, editors: *Cancer: principles and practice of oncology,* Philadelphia, 1985, Lippincott.

---

tion. To enhance sexual self-esteem, resumption of the ability to function sexually one way or another becomes of paramount importance. This allows the patient to feel more desirable and retain the ability to relate intimately with others.[64]

Gratification and Performance

The feelings of belonging and receiving approval are closely associated with the process of giving and receiving sexual pleasure. Cancer patients often feel undesirable and unattractive and, because they are now typecast as "ill," feel they are not supposed to be sexual. It has been reported that these patients desire touch more than overt sexual activity.[33] The reason for this is unclear but may be related to side effects, fatigue, weakness, and pain, which all cause diminished libido. However, it is also postulated that they feel sexual desires but take it for granted that their partner does not desire them. The partner, in turn, worries that the patient may be too sick to want sexual activity and feels guilty about having a sexual interest in someone who is sick and under treatment. Unfortunately, if these misconceptions persist, patients and their partners are likely to avoid the intimate and/or sexual contact that might be possible.

Schain explains that sexual functioning is part of the reflection of an individual's coping mechanisms and that sexual activity may reflect different motives at different times during the health-illness continuum (see box above). The cancer diagnosis may change the motive for sexual acts, and the couple may need to change their focus from one of performance and orgasm to one of touching and general pleasuring.

Nurses must not fail to see alternatives to stereotypical sexual behavior and must acknowledge each patient's unique sexual identity.[10] It is the nurse's responsibility to be free of fixed ideas and to continue to discuss sexual concerns at all stages of cancer and its treatment, regardless of the patient's circumstances or age. It must never

HEAD AND NECK CANCER
INTERVENTIONS

- A gastrostomy tube may be placed to rid the patient of nasogastric feeding tube, which interferes with kissing and facial petting.
- Sugarless mints and artificial saliva help to freshen stale breath caused by a dry mouth (from radiation therapy).[32] Artificial saliva (Moi-Stir, Xerolube) also helps prevent tooth decay.
- The patient may have a decreased sense of smell, so that perfumes cannot be appreciated. Candles, scented or not, can provide a relaxed ambience for both patient and partner, though the fragrance is not appreciated by the patient.

- Tracheostomies should be cleaned of mucus and covered lightly during sexual activity. (For information on obtaining tracheostomy covers, see Resources at the end of this chapter.)
- Partners should be made aware that the patient's heavy breathing may sound different. If the larynx is removed, a sexy voice, whispered love talk, and other eroticisms will be eliminated.[26]
- Various positions may need to be tried for sexual activity because the partner may be fearful of cutting off the patient's air supply.
- Patients, especially females, may wish to wear a fancy nightgown with a high neck, or other erotic neckwear. Males may wish to wear a dickey.

be assumed that the patient who has raised no question has no concerns. Concentrated attention must be given to the issue of sexuality just as it is given to other aspects of cancer care, because sexuality is one of the most fundamental aspects of humanity.

SITE-SPECIFIC ISSUES AFFECTING SEXUALITY

The following nursing diagnoses apply to the nursing interventions that are discussed.[13]

Principal Nursing Diagnoses

- *Sexual dysfunction related to impotence, ineffective coping, lack of knowledge, change or loss of body part, and physiologic limitations*
- *Self-esteem disturbance related to change in body image, self-concept, role performance, and personal identity*

Secondary Nursing Diagnoses

- *Activity intolerance related to fatigue*
- *Pain which decreases sexual desire*
- *Communication, impaired verbal, related to tracheostomy*
- *Social isolation related to cancer (incontinence, disfiguring surgery, superstitions of others)*

Most discussions in the literature related to sexual problems of cancer patients begin with malignancies of the genital organs, because cancer in this area is most likely to cause sexual dysfunction. Consequently, head and neck cancers, sarcomas that result in amputation, hematologic malignancies, and lung cancers are frequently overlooked or barely mentioned. Therefore a nursing approach to these concerns will be addressed first.

Head and Neck Cancer

Physiologic and body image alterations. The social significance of youth and facial beauty continues to be profound and is exemplified through movies, television, and magazines. The few older people portrayed by the mass media are usually very attractive. Therefore the impact of head and neck cancer and its treatment can be particularly devastating, since the defects caused by the disease are immediately recognizable. The patient feels grossly unattractive and frequently has difficulty with life's most basic needs, such as talking, eating, and even breathing. Given these fundamental problems, it is not surprising that little or no attention is given to the need for closeness, touching, and genital sexual pleasures.

Sexual relationships may be influenced by the patient's age, smoking and drinking habits, and the general emotional impact of treatment. Many patients are more than 60 years of age at the time of diagnosis and are entering a period of adjustment to a decrease in frequency of sexual intercourse, although desire often remains about the same.[40] The patient may also be an alcoholic, which will influence treatment and the rehabilitation process. Metcalfe and Fischman explain that intimacy, trust, and open communication are frequently nonexistent in alcoholic relationships because intimacy is too threatening to the alcoholic individual.[43] Because alcoholic men and women are known to have a low sense of self-esteem, the nurse may have to focus on this issue before moving on to the patient's feelings of masculinity or femininity.[59]

Patients with head and neck cancer often require rehabilitation, which may be accomplished with reconstructive surgery or prostheses or both. It is important to remember that the expectations of the patient may differ from actual treatment results. Consequently, the patient may suffer one or more disappointments, as illustrated by the following anecdote[16]:

A woman had an oral prosthesis made. The match and the appearance were excellent, and she regained confidence and employment and she delighted in sociability. Her praise and gratitude were profuse. However, once when we had lunch together she said, "I have so much to be thankful for and yet . . . ," and she turned away and she touched the prosthesis. "When I laugh, this never laughs, and when I take it off I sometimes wonder if I can go on."

Head and neck cancer patients will necessarily face lingering cosmetic and functional impairments, which will impact on their body image and sexuality. Often, presurgical levels of function and aesthetics cannot be restored.[77] Although attempts at prosthetic rehabilitation are noble, the health care professional should remember that the patient's concept is often quite different from the medical concept. Rehabilitation will change the patient's practices and habits. To this patient, a kiss and a hug may be worth a thousand words.

Sarcomas of Bone and Soft Tissue and Limb Amputation

Physiologic and body image alterations. Little information is available regarding the sexual adjustment of upper or lower extremity amputees. Commonly, concentration is placed on the patient's functional problems during and after prosthetic rehabilitation and any reference to sexuality is omitted.

Major limb amputation creates emotional hurdles for patients' perception of themself, as well as acceptance by their partner (Figure 32-1). A decrease in self-esteem and a negative body image are common because of the presence of a gross defect that is obvious even when covered with clothes. The male may equate the loss of a limb to the loss of manhood. Some patients may view the surgery as a punishment for past transgressions.[28]

Cummings has discussed several potential sexual problems, which include the simple mechanics of body positioning during intercourse, immobility because of physical isolation, amputee fetishism, associated disease states that can alter sexual function, and phantom pain sensations.[15] Phantom limb pain can be quite disturbing and can in itself impair sexual functioning.

Amputees are admittedly apprehensive about their physical capabilities, but this fear often subsides once they begin prosthetic training, ambulation, or articulation. As patients become more independent, confidence in their sexuality usually returns.[48] Some patients fail to gain satisfaction from a prosthesis. Those patients then resort to using crutches rather than be restricted by the somewhat awkward movement of artificial limbs. They forfeit a better cosmetic appearance, however.

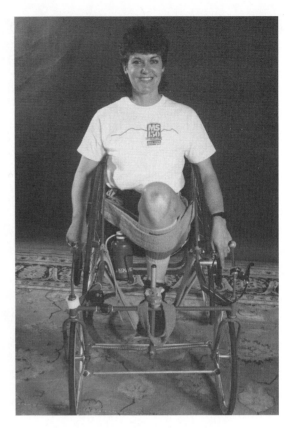

Figure 32-1   Lou Keyes, hemipelvectomy patient, in her racing wheelchair. Lou also uses a prosthetic device proficiently and crutches when she is in a hurry.

The life-style of amputees may be profoundly affected, especially if they have been independent and physically active. The range of problems usually depends on the extensiveness of the amputation. For example, a female with a shoulder disarticulation may find that simple tasks like styling hair and getting clothing to look good are difficult. Less dramatic upper extremity amputations allow for easier manipulation of a conventional hand prosthesis, a hook prosthesis, or a newer myoelectric powered hand (Figure 32-2).

Lower extremity amputees, especially those with hip disarticulations and hemipelvectomies, have a different set of uncertainties with prosthetics.[45] Most prevalent worries are socket discomfort, mobility, and energy expenditure. With an exoskeletal device, the socket area envelops the entire pelvis and adds to hip and waist measurements (Figure 32-3). One female patient stated that she couldn't tuck her blouses in and thought her clothes looked too big. Females often have difficulty wearing sanitary pads during menses and may wish to use double tampons. All amputees must deal with undesirable noises produced by prosthetic joints, and even buying a pair of shoes can be disconcerting.

For those patients without partners, there may be a

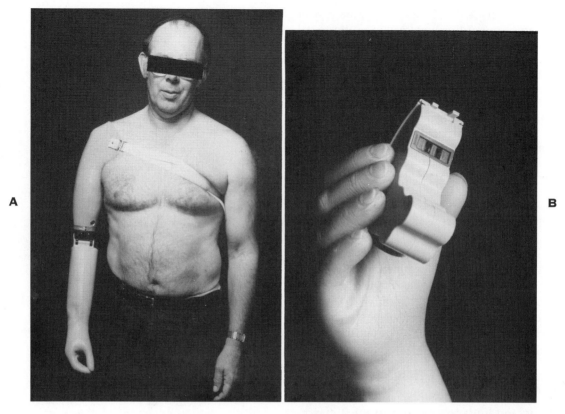

Figure 32-2 **A**, Above the elbow, myoelectric prosthesis. **B**, Myoelectric hand grasping object. (Courtesy American Medical Systems, Minnetonka, Minnesota.)

Figure 32-3 Prosthesis on left is a hip flexion bias system without a rotator knee and no flexibility in the socket—cost $11,000. Prosthesis on the right is a hip flexion bias system with a rotator knee and partially flexible socket—cost $13,000.

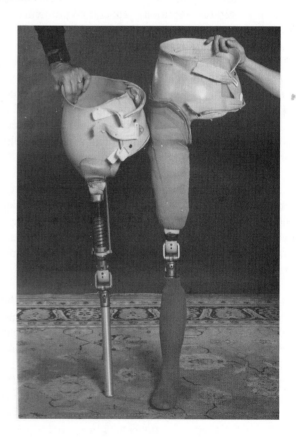

support group or sporting activities to become involved in, such as wheelchair racing. These are good opportunities to meet people and share like experiences. The more the patient gets out and regains self-confidence, the easier it will be to meet and interact with other people. (For more information, see Support Groups (LEAPS) at the end of this chapter.)

For those patients with partners, feelings of maleness or femaleness can be regained with the partner's love, support, and understanding. A loving and intimate relationship can help restore self-confidence and determination to adapt to their disability.

LIMB AMPUTATION
INTERVENTIONS

Not only is the amputee's body image and self-concept threatened, but often many taken-for-granted activities are either eliminated or severely hampered. Some suggestions that may be helpful to amputees in resuming an intimate relationship with their partners follow:

- After some experimenting, some amputees find that intercourse can be maintained without any modification or adjustment of positions.
- Some patients may expend slightly more energy, which may result in mild fatigue, but this rarely hampers sexual function.
- If balance and movement are a problem, pillows or other forms of support may be used to maintain a level pelvis.[51]

- Lovemaking does not always have to occur in the bedroom. A sofa or large chair can be used to balance on, or the female amputee can lean against a chair while her partner makes love from behind.
- The female may need to assume the superior position during coitus.
- An upper extremity amputee may wish to use a side-lying position with the existing arm free to balance.
- Hemipelvectomy patients may have extra folds of skin used to make their flaps. Because these patients may be uncomfortable exposing themselves to their partner, these skin folds can be held in place by a "compression sock." This sock compresses the folds into a hiplike shape, and the sock can then be modified with an opening in the crotch to allow for intercourse.

HEMATOLOGIC MALIGNANCIES
Impact of Therapy Side Effects on Body Image

Although the diagnosis of lymphoma/leukemia or multiple myeloma can be terrifying, treatment does not comprise surgery or amputation, which can cause disfigurement. What the individual may not realize, however, is that chemotherapy and radiation therapy can be just as devastating to sexuality. Except for multiple myeloma, these diagnoses are often made in young, active people who see themselves as infallible, and they often do not comprehend the impact of the illness until well into their therapy.

Most men and women experience reduced desire for sexual intercourse during chemotherapy treatments, particularly during the first few days after receiving the drugs. This is usually the result of increased weakness, fatigue, and intermittent nausea and vomiting. Also, whether the patient is young or old or male or female, defacement caused by hair loss can destroy self-confidence. Another problem for acute myelocytic leukemia patients is the prolonged hospitalization during chemotherapy with consequent lack of privacy.

Lack of sexual eagerness can also be induced by an effect on the testes or ovaries. Ovarian dysfunction is progressive, and women may experience symptoms such as amenorrhea or irregular menses, hot flashes, decreased libido, and vaginal dryness. Testicular dysfunction occurs more abruptly and results in oligospermia (decreased sperm) or azoospermia (absent sperm), as well as difficulty with erections.[6,66] Fortunately, these problems are often temporary and hormone levels and sexual desire

return to normal after chemotherapy or radiation therapy ends.

Myelosuppression and its consequences can cause fatigue and shortness of breath, which decrease sexual desire. Concern about bleeding and infection will be present because of low platelet and white blood cell/absolute neutrophil counts. A perfect environment for a vaginal yeast infection may be created, which inflames the lining of the vagina and causes itching and burning during intercourse. The male patient's ability to have an erection may also be affected. Creativity will be necessary to promote sexual intimacy.

Many patients will experience moments of anxiety and depression throughout their treatment, and therapy can last for as long as 3 years. The nurse should stress the importance of maintaining involvement in activities and relationships with their friends when they feel good. Patients should be advised on ways to ask for assistance with activities of daily living and should be reminded not to be ashamed to ask for help, as they have most likely often helped others.

A discussion may be needed to assess the feelings of the spouse or significant other. It is helpful to identify ways they can support the patient's feelings of self-worth and masculinity or femininity. They should be encouraged to reassure the patient that sexuality and lovability are not affected by appearance only.

One of the most stressful events for any patient is alopecia.[7] Some patients may feel that hair loss is even worse than amputation, and because of its effect on body image, sexual inadequacy can ensue. Sensitivity should

NURSING MANAGEMENT

HEMATOLOGIC MALIGNANCIES
INTERVENTIONS

- The patient who is neutropenic should be advised against oral, penile/vaginal, and anal sexual manipulation. Remind the patient and partner that gratification may be derived from simply touching and holding. The couple may bathe together. Bubbles, a little candlelight, romantic music, and some wine (in plastic glasses) make for an intimate experience. The couple can share each other intimately without performance anxiety, and the warm water may help ease some of the general aches and pains.
- Intercourse can be planned for after antiemetics are given and when the medications will be most effective.
- Advise patients to avoid the stress of heavy meals and liquor before intercourse.

- To avoid fatigue, a nap before intercourse may be helpful. The supine position or a side-lying position uses less energy. Also, avoid temperature extremes if possible.
- The importance of contraceptive measures during chemotherapy and radiation must be emphasized to all patients. Although chemotherapy will affect sperm count and ovulation, the patient cannot depend on this alone for contraception.[46] Teratogenic effects are seen during the first trimester of pregnancy, especially if the female is under treatment.[23,45,66] Studies are underway to determine possible effects on future generations.[23,36]
- Encourage sperm banking before initiation of chemotherapy.
- If the patient's complexion is pale because of decreased RBCs, encourage bright colors and the use of make-up to enhance appearance.

SUGGESTIONS FOR PATIENTS WHO EXPERIENCE ALOPECIA

- Use a mild, protein-based shampoo, cream rinse, and conditioner. Rinse the hair well and pat dry, *not* vigorously. Shampoo every 4 to 7 days.
- Avoid excessive brushing and use a wide-toothed comb/brush.
- Avoid hair spray and hair dye. Permanents are okay, but if hair loss is expected, it is best to wait until regrowth to perm the hair.
- Avoid electric hair dryers and curling irons, clips, bobby pins, barrettes, and pony tails.
- Many types of hats and caps are available. Purchase some kind of head wrap or turban, whether it is winter or summer, because the hair helps to keep the head warm. Even in warm weather, the head can get very cold if left uncovered in an air-conditioned environment.
- Use sunscreen on scalp when outside.

---

be used when explaining this side effect to any patient, male or female, and patients should be provided with the information presented in the box above.

BREAST CANCER
Physiologic and Body Image Alterations

Today's society has idealized the female breast to such an extent that it has become a "sociosexual" symbol of sexuality and femininity.[50] Physiologically, removal of a breast should not decrease sexual desire or activity, but in reality studies have demonstrated high levels of stress

in regard to sexual functioning among mastectomy patients.[4,53] Mastectomy makes an obvious change in the body's contour, which can lead to fears about loss of identity as a woman and a desirable sexual being. The partner's perceived importance of a breast can also impact the female's perspective should she choose mastectomy, even though reconstruction is more prevalent today. Anxiety is also present regarding the cancer diagnosis.

The patient who is treated with lumpectomy and radiation therapy has concerns about her sexuality as well. Although this patient's breast is preserved, she may experience a skin reaction and increased fatigue while receiving radiation treatment. This can last for several weeks and also lead to decreased desire for sexual activity. Long-term depression and maladjustment are not as likely in this population, but it is just as important to assist these patients with their doubts and anxieties.

A woman's response to treatment for breast cancer and its corresponding threat to sexuality will depend on several conditions[51]:
- Her feelings about her femininity
- The value she bestows on her missing breast
- Her physical discomfort
- The response of her significant other
- The reinforcement she receives from the nurse regarding her sexual identity
- Her sense of self-worth

The status of the patient's preoperative sexual relationships and her interpretation of sexual satisfaction must also be ascertained. Cultural and religious attitudes will also influence "acceptable" sexual practices.

Rarely addressed are the single, divorced, widowed, and lesbian population (to be discussed later). Years ago,

BREAST CANCER
INTERVENTIONS

Much information in the literature quotes Mildred H. Witkin and her personal and professional experience with mastectomy.[49] One of her recommendations is for the couple to experience the loss of the breast together in the hospital. The partner may wish to assist with dressing changes and caring for the mastectomy wound. For example, a few years ago, a lumpectomy and radiation patient had a skin reaction on her breast and had to have daily dressing changes. Her husband was a willing participant and even created a "cross your heart" bandage for his wife. The patient expressed several months later how much it meant to her to experience his care and interest during her treatment.

Another behavioral prescription from Witkin is that the couple stand nude together in front of a mirror and express the thoughts and feelings this elicits.[52] In this circumstance the patient is likely to feel less vulnerable, since she and her partner are both nude. Of course, not all couples will be able to accept or handle this type of exercise, and they should be encouraged to use their own coping strategies. Because coping mechanisms will vary from person to person and couple to couple, numerous behaviors will be exhibited. These will range from allowing the partner to participate in care and view the mastectomy scar immediately to not allowing anyone but the physician to see the wound. Support is continually needed to promote healthy adjustment by the patient and partner.

When making love, these suggestions may be incorporated:

- Until the woman is ready to disrobe or let her partner touch the wound area, she can wear a fancy camisole or short nightgown. This camouflages the area but is still sexually stimulating for the couple.
- To minimize a direct view of the woman's missing breast, the partner may assume the superior position (missionary position) or use a rear-entry position. *Joy of Sex,* edited by Dr. Alex Comfort, is an excellent reference for positions a couple may use to increase sexual pleasure.
- The couple may make love by candlelight to decrease the impact of the change in body contour.
- Concentration on a certain sexual task (sensate focus) may increase stimulation and reduce appearance concerns. One suggestion is a touching exercise, explained in depth in the American Cancer Society's book *Sexuality and Cancer: For the Woman Who Has Cancer, and Her Partner.* The focus is initially on massaging the extremities and back and ignoring the genital sexual organs, and the result is relaxation and sensual pleasure.[57]
- Since many women derive great pleasure from stroking, sucking, and manipulation of the breast during foreplay, the remaining breast can continue to be stimulated if the woman so desires. Reassure the patient that manipulation will not cause another breast cancer.

Lewis and Bloom made the assumption that these women may have a more difficult time adjusting to their new situation and resuming sexual relations.[35] An excellent resource for this population, as well as for married women, is the Reach to Recovery program (see Support Groups at the end of this chapter). This program tries to pair the patient with a volunteer mastectomy patient of the same race, side of mastectomy, social status (married, widowed, divorced), etc. The volunteer explains exercises for the affected side's arm, tells where to get prostheses and clothing, and gives emotional support.

Rehabilitation may consist of reconstructive surgery, which may be done immediately or several months after treatment is complete. Occasionally, surgical repair must be done before good reconstruction can be accomplished. Although the reconstructed breast will never look like the original breast, some women exercise this option because they feel it looks more natural. These women must be reminded that there is little to no sensation in this breast, which may be particularly disappointing during foreplay. A multitude of breast prostheses are also available; some of them are listed in the Resources at the end of this chapter.

FEMALE PELVIC AND GENITAL CANCER
Physiologic and Body Image Alterations

As in breast cancer, the surgery needed to cure female patients of cancers of the genital organs can be very threatening to a woman's sexuality.[4]

A threat to a woman's capability of being physically sexual can lead to a lost sense of femininity.[63] McDonald and colleagues report that as the patient progresses through treatment, fluctuations in self-esteem and body image occur.[41] The female sexual response cycle will most likely be affected if treatment affects the structure and innervation of the clitoris or the vagina.

Surgical resection or radiation therapy for cancer of the cervix, uterus, ovary, vulva, vagina (diethylstilbes-

FEMALE PELVIC AND GENITAL CANCER

The following nursing interventions apply to radical hysterectomy, partial or total pelvic exenteration, radical vulvectomy, cystectomy, and radiation therapy.

INTERVENTIONS

Radical Hysterectomy

As discussed in Chapter 10, in radical hysterectomy, the vaginal canal is shortened somewhat (up to one half) but is not believed to be sexually appreciable in all cases. Penile thrusting may be uncomfortable, since the trigone of the bladder and sigmoid colon may be closely associated with the new vaginal apex.

Donahue and Knapp suggest alternate methods of intercourse that can be most helpful (see box below).[17] Delayed resumption of bladder function introduces an embarrassing problem. If a long-term indwelling catheter is present, vaginal sexual relations can be impeded. Partners may change positions, and rear-entry intercourse can be practiced.[70] To prevent dislodgement, the catheter can be placed up over the lower abdomen and taped into place. Alternate ways of expressing physical love can also be fulfilling and can include oral, anal, and digital expressions.

Pelvic Exenteration

Several factors of adjustment may be generated by this particular surgery.[3] These can include adaptation to a urinary conduit, bowel conduit, or both, and this can cause worry about appearance and appliance fit, possible leakage, and odor. The vulva will be extensively denervated, which results in decreased erotic sensations. Creation of a neovagina may also be necessary. Clitoral swelling and pain may occur, requiring a clitoridectomy for relief.[71]

ALTERNATIVE COITAL POSITIONS AND COITAL EQUIVALENTS

- Angle of penile thrust can be altered by elevating the woman's hips on 1 or 2 pillows.
- Deeper vaginal barrel can be mimicked by enclosing the penis within one or both palms.
- Some patients find that vaginal penetration from behind between closely adducted thighs will increase pleasure.
- If coitus is not possible, the basic mechanics of cunnilingus (application of tongue or mouth to the vulva) and fellatio (sexual gratification by intromission of the penis into another individual's mouth) should be explained.

From Donahue V, Knapp R: Sexual rehabilitation of gynecologic cancer patients, *Obstet Gynecol* 49:118, 1977.

It is understandable that many patients report decreased frequency of sexual activity and satisfaction and a loss of sexual self-confidence.

To assure the most beneficial adjustment psychologically and sexually for the patient and her partner, it is necessary to provide specific alternatives and realistic information before surgery. Unfortunately, some women have been told that sexual intercourse will feel the same and be as good as before the surgery. Many women complain of the inability to voluntarily constrict the vaginal introitus, and for those women with a neovagina, some allege that it is too short or too large or associate it with an increased chronic discharge.[60] Some women maintain orgasm ability, but others lose it or achieve orgasm only with extra effort. Also, after reconstruction, vaginal sensation is usually decreased. To promote total healing and the ability to detect early recurrence, a waiting period of 6 weeks to 2 months is advised before resumption of sexual intercourse.[17]

Although much more rare today, young women who were exposed to DES during gestation and consequently develop vaginal cancer are treated in another way. This group also requires vaginal reconstruction and presurgical counseling and education. Once reconstruction has taken place, coitus is encouraged immediately, if possible and appropriate.[46] Because these women are often in their teens when diagnosed, intercourse is not always possible for moral or religious reasons or simply for lack of a partner. In this case, silastic stents are placed to maintain a patent vaginal canal. These young women understandably become easily discouraged because of the discomfort and peculiar stretching sensation caused by the stents.

An alternative to the stents is the use of a small- to medium-sized dildo. Young women have few objections to use of a dildo because it is flesh colored, soft plastic, more pliable, and more comfortable than a dilator.[63]

Positive encouragement and support are vital if these women are to feel as normal as possible. This support will be especially meaningful if it comes from other women who have experienced the same kind of reconstruction.

Alternatives to sexual intercourse available to women who have had vaginal reconstruction and to those not interested in such surgery may include nudity, cuddling, and general pleasuring; autoeroticism and mutual masturbation with a partner; oral-genital relations and anal love play; and fantasy.

Radical Vulvectomy and Cystectomy

Cancer of the vulva usually occurs in women who are well past menopause, and these older women are often reluctant to seek treatment until the disease has progressed. As a result, the therapy can have a particularly frightful impact on body image and sexual identity.[5]

For early stage disease, patients are usually treated with skinning vulvectomy, laser treatment, and/or wide local excision rather than simple vulvectomy. Skinning vulvectomy is a technique used by Rutledge, which "excises vulva skin and conserves fat, muscle and glandular structures below the skin."[46] A split-thickness graft from the inner thigh is then applied to cover the denuded area.[46] This procedure gives an optimal cosmetic and functional result. Laser treatment involves destruction of the lesion by vaporizing the tissue. Healing is excellent with this procedure, but there is not a thorough pathologic review of the diseased specimen.[46] Patients have few complaints of dyspareunia or decreased sexual responsiveness with laser therapy. Topical 5% fluorouracil cream used over a 2- to 3-month period is another treatment choice. It is advocated by some clinicians, but most find it impractical, since the cream must be applied until desquamation occurs.[46] This produces a significant degree of local discomfort, and intercourse can be painful until healing takes place. In radical vulvectomy, the fine sensory perception experienced during foreplay is destroyed and must be compensated for by excitement of other erogenous zones such as the earlobes, breasts, fingers, toes, and inner thighs.[31]

The patient's partner must be included in all education and counseling because of the radical nature of the treatment and long recuperative period after therapy. Patients comment that adequate information is rarely given so they can begin to alter their sexual expectations, and others state that the treatment is embarrassing and creates an isolated feeling.[2,5]

Little is mentioned in the literature concerning female patients undergoing cystectomy and the sexual problems that arise from excision of the bladder and more than one third of the vagina. Problems identified are vaginal tightness and dryness and self-conscious anxiety because of the ostomy. Scarring can develop, as well as numbness and lost sensation, because of impaired innervation of the perineum. Recommended remedies may include a vaginal estrogen cream and vaginal dilators to help decrease dyspareunia. Most women like to cover their ostomy appliance with a fabric cover, and feminine lingerie may also be worn during sexual activity. Kegel exercises are helpful to relieve tension and decrease dyspareunia.[62] Positive reinforcement and specific suggestions can make an important difference in the woman's achievement of a satisfying sexual adjustment.

Radiation Therapy

Both external therapy and internal radiation insertion can cause irritating side effects, which are disruptive to sexual activity. Diarrhea, skin reaction of the external genitalia, and especially vaginal irritation, stenosis, and dryness are the most troublesome.[29] To prevent a diminished sense of femininity, a discussion with pertinent facts and proposals should precede radiation therapy.

The vagina will react to radiation by becoming shorter and narrower, having adhesions and problems with lubrication. The nurse may suggest the following:

- Continued sexual intercourse during treatment is usually encouraged to decrease possible adhesions and prevent shortening. Sometimes tissues may become tender, or an external skin reaction may necessitate stopping sexual intercourse. It can be resumed when healing and comfort allow.
- A water-soluble lubricating jelly is always needed to decrease vaginal discomfort and can be applied privately or as part of foreplay.[63]
- During sexual activity, the hips may be elevated or the adducted thighs lubricated to emulate a deeper vaginal barrel and improve sexual stimulation for a male partner. The female superior position allows her more control but is usually not as comfortable. Rear entry is another alternative.[29]
- Vaginal dilators can be used if a woman does not have a sexual partner or is not sexually active. Sexually active women may also use dilators during treatment if intercourse is too exhausting. Normal sexual activity is preferred because some women hesitate to place foreign objects into their vagina, and some are concerned about implications of masturbation. Sometimes dilators are indeed necessary, and the patient's compliance will increase if she is made aware that complete vaginal stenosis will occur, obstructing the physician's view in follow-up, if not used.[46]

It is important to be sensitive to both the patient and her partner when explaining dilator use.

---

trol [DES] exposure), and bladder can be either simple or extensive. Women faced with this type of treatment have many apprehensions:

- Threat to life
- Feelings of lost femininity
- Concern about what their external region will look like
- Ability to have intercourse and, if so, whether it will be painful

- Fear that along with the loss of fertility will come loss of vitality and orgasmic potential
- Fear of physical aging, diminished libido, loss of vaginal lubrication, and dyspareunia

To prevent extensive morbidity and sexual dysfunction from the concerns just mentioned, early intervention with counseling is imperative for the gynecologic cancer patient.

Table 32-2 Effects of Surgery on Male Sexual Functioning

Surgery	Direct effect	Indirect effect
AP resection	Damage to sympathetic and parasympathetic nervous systems resulting in: 1. Varying degrees of impotence (erectile difficulties) 2. Ejaculatory problems 2.1. Retrograde ejaculation 2.2. Decreased amount ejaculate 2.3. Decreased ejaculatory force	Altered sexual expression as a result of: 1. Physical impairment 2. Body image change 3. Altered self-esteem 4. Fears 5. Pain
Radical cystectomy	As above but to a greater extent 1. May be 100% impotent 2. Retrograde or no ejaculation	As above
Pelvic exenteration	As with AP resection and radical cystectomy	As above
Radical prostatectomy	Stress incontinence (temporary) Varying degrees of impotence	As above
Orchiectomy	Loss of gonads and testosterone resulting in: 1. Sterility 2. Decreased libido	As above
Cord surgeries Paraplegia Quadriplegia (tumor removal, pain control)	As with AP resection	As above

From Shipes E, Lehr S: *Cancer Nurs* 5:375, 1982.

MALE PELVIC CANCER
Physiologic and Body Image Alterations

Men as well as women have stereotypical roles that society expects them to live by. They are supposed to be heroes and good providers, to hide their emotions and be strong, not to touch each other unless engaging in sports, and never to relate on an emotional level or be dependent on another.[68] Masculinity is also equated with activity and productivity; a man must never admit to possible physical problems and must always be in control.[68] Pertaining to sexuality, the state of a man's penis is always of utmost importance. Consequently, when the male patient experiences a malignancy in the pelvis or genital area, his entire self-image may be threatened. After diagnosis and treatment are complete and the fear of death is no longer uppermost in the patient's mind, he concentrates on the sequelae.[25] The impact on self-image will be even greater if his sexuality is threatened.

When the malignancy involves the prostate, testicle, or penis, there is a temporary or permanent disturbance in relation to erection, emission, and ejaculation. Orgasm is not as frequently affected and can actually be achieved even when genital function is lost. See Table 32-2 for an in-depth description of common cancer surgeries of the male pelvis and their effect on sexual functioning.[68] To promote adjustment and sexual rehabilitation, support and assistance for the patient and his partner are essential through knowledge care specific interventions.

COLORECTAL CANCER
Physiologic and Body Image Alterations

Surgery for colorectal cancer often has a profound effect on body image and sexual responsiveness. Because of the societal taboos centered around eliminative functions, many men and women feel disgusted that their feces now come from the front of their body.[27] Women undergo feelings of having been violated, whereas men experience the surgery as castration or mutilation.[27,51] Some patients report embarrassment because they equate the cleaning of their stomas with masturbation. Others are distressed because they have no "vacation" from stoma maintenance. They must always make sure that there are adequate facilities for cleaning themselves in private; consequently, leisure activities may be compromised.[51]

Regardless of the type of surgical diversion performed (colostomy, ileostomy, or urinary diversion), patients express many common reactions. These reactions may include (1) greater-than-expected fatigue and weakness; (2) feelings of fragility and vulnerability to harm; (3) despair at the initial viewing of the stoma; (4) feelings of invalidism and depression; (5) fear of accidents, odor, leakage, and staining; (6) excessive emotional investment in the stoma; and (7) feelings of lost personal control.[64] Understanding and support from the nurse are important for healthy recovery. If the nurse is not an ostomate herself, the patient may receive great reassurance from a fellow ostomate. Members of an ostomy organization usually visit

MALE PELVIC CANCER
INTERVENTIONS
Prostate

Surgery for prostate cancer has a definite impact on male sexual potency, depending on how extensive it is. When transurethral resection (TUR) is employed in early-stage disease, approximately 80% of these patients experience scanty or absent ejaculation, although they are still able to have an erection. Until recently, if radical prostatectomy was the treatment of choice, 85% to 90% of those patients experienced erectile impotence. Now with nerve-sparing surgical techniques, one study reported that 86% of a group of men could achieve erections 1 year after surgery although others have not had this much success.[56] Problems can occur when radiation is used in lieu of surgery because of probable fibrosis of the pelvic arteries.[54] Incidental reports of erectile impotence vary from 14% to 46% after treatment with external radiation. Interstitial treatment may be used if the tumor burden is small, and incidence of impotence is reported between 7% and 13%.[80]

Endocrine treatment (castration, estrogen, and/or a luteinizing hormone/regulatory hormone [LH/RH] antagonist [Lupron]) commonly causes difficult and embarrassing problems such as gynecomastia, phallic atrophy, loss of libido, and erectile impotence.[25] Many men experience physical debilitation, depression, anxiety, and pain, all of which may decrease sexual desire.

One of the most important issues in the area of male pelvic cancers may be to help the patient and his partner develop a change in attitude toward sexual intercourse if erection is no longer possible or if it is impaired. As Schain put it, it might "be necessary to learn alternative responses to the notion that intercourse (with an erect penis in the vagina) is the point at which all sexual encounters should be finalized."[51] Even if frequency drops, the potential for sexual arousal remains with the correct stimulus:
- Many men become sexually aroused with erotic books, pictures, or movies.
- Long periods of foreplay, including romantic dinners, showering or bathing together, and using different rooms for lovemaking, may be stimulating. A changed or strange environment such as a local motel may bring new excitement.
- If a full erection is not possible, mutual masturbation may allow the patient to reach orgasm and ejaculation. The partner should massage the penis by pushing down with pressure at the base of the penis. The penis should not be pulled up toward the abdomen or it can lose blood. A female partner can assist erection by inserting a partially erect penis into the vagina and flexing her perineal muscles.
- During ejaculation, semen may be propelled into the bladder, which may threaten the male's sense of masculinity. The partner, however, may enjoy oral stimulation more since she no longer has to taste or swallow semen.[55]
- If the patient has problems with urinary incontinence, he should empty his bladder before intercourse and perhaps wear a condom if this becomes worrisome to his partner. Remind the couple that urine is sterile and will not harm the partner.
- The risks and benefits of penile implants should be explained to the couple. Schover recommends waiting 6 months after surgery before installing a prosthesis.[55] The patient and partner may choose from several different types of prosthesis. A comparison of two of the types (Figure 32-4) is given in Table 32-3. An excellent resource is *Bio-Potency: A Medical Guide to Sexual Success* by Richard and Deborah Berg.
- Intracavernous injections into the penis using papaverine to stimulate erections is becoming a common treatment.[1,47]
- Finally, like other cancer patients, a male pelvic cancer patient may simply need physical closeness and intimacy. Sexual activity is not always what is needed to promote feelings of love and belonging.

Testicle

Not surprisingly, men with cancer of the testicle not only have problems with fertility, but also with their intimate relationships.[22] This population is generally young (15 to 34 years old) and in a crucial stage in life, and cancer treatment produces organic problems and sexual anxieties leading to dysfunction. When more treatment than unilateral orchiectomy is necessary, sexual dysfunction increases. Extensive surgery (retroperitoneal lymph node dissection [RLND]), radiation, and chemotherapy may cause erectile and orgasmic dysfunction.[34] To prevent sexual dissatisfaction, the couple should be educated and encouraged with the following information (this does not include fertility information):
- Stress the fact that normal sexual desire and pleasurable sensations, erection, and orgasm will probably continue. If sexual desire is lost, serum testosterone should be checked; replacement therapy may be needed.
- Alpha-adrenergic-stimulating drugs can increase ejaculation and occasionally the intensity of orgasm for some patients who have had retroperitoneal lymph node dissection.[35]
- Loss of a testicle can cause embarrassment; however,

Continued.

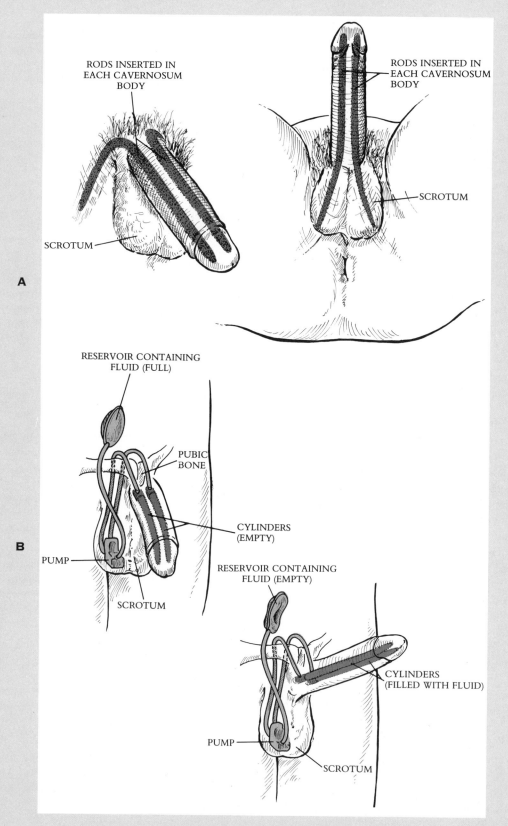

Figure 32-4 Penile prostheses can be of two types. **A**, In one type two semirigid silicone rods are implanted into the penis. **B**, In the second type two expandable cylinders are inserted into the penis and are connected by a tubing system to a fluid-filled bulb. (From Denney N, Quadagno D: *Human sexuality*, St Louis, 1988, Mosby.)

Table 32-3   A Comparison of Inflatable and Semirigid Penile Prostheses

Factor	Type of prosthesis	
	Semirigid	**Inflatable**
Ease of concealment	May need special briefs; noticeable in locker room or at public urinal	No problem, although self-contained version may not lie down completely
Size of erection	Some loss of length and thickness	Normal thickness, some loss of length (self-contained version cannot add thickness)
Function during sexual intercourse	80% to 90% of patients satisfied	80% to 90% of patients satisfied
Infection during healing	Occurs in 1% to 2% of patients	Occurs in 1% to 2% of patients
Prosthesis erodes through spongy tissue inside penis	In less than 5% of patients	No problems
Prolonged pain after healing	Rare	Rare
Need to repair prosthesis	Rare	5% to 15% reoperation rates
Usual hospital stay*	2 to 4 days	2 to 5 days
Total costs*	$6,000 to $10,000	$10,000 to $12,000

From Schover L: *Sexuality and cancer: for the man who has cancer, and his partner,* New York, 1988, American Cancer Society.
*Based on our experience in 1987 with surgery performed under a general anesthetic.

this can no longer be remedied by a silicone prosthesis because they have been removed from the market.

- Reinforce the fact that the cancer is not contagious through sexual activity and that radiation therapy will not contaminate the partner.
- For those patients with permanent erectile difficulties, see the suggestions under prostate cancer and penile implants.
- Encourage both partners to ask directly for the type of caressing and touching he or she prefers.[61]
- Remind the patient that often people feel awkward and anxious when resuming sexual activity, but sexual relations, if physiologically possible, may resume about 6 weeks after pelvic surgery.
- If retrograde ejaculation is a problem because of RLND and cannot be reversed, Schover and Fife describe a technique to harvest sperm after orgasm. "Postorgasmic urine is immediately voided into a sterile container. Viable sperm cells are centrifuged out and placed in a nutrient solution preparatory to use in artificial insemination."[58]
- Sperm banking may be an option worth exploring if the number and motility of the sperm are adequate. This is costly, and the success of future artificial insemination is not guaranteed. If the patient is interested, however, sperm banking must be done before chemotherapy begins or between the first and second treatments.

Penis

Penile cancer, although very rare, results in the greatest risk of sexual dysfunction. Partial or total penectomy is usually needed to control the cancer. If partial penectomy is done, the penile stump usually becomes erect with

stimulation and is long enough for intercourse with antegrade ejaculation.[52] If the entire glans penis is removed, a perineal urethrostomy is created behind the scrotum.[54] When it is stimulated to orgasm, ejaculation takes place through the perineal urethrostomy. Counseling for this man and his partner must include reassurance that both can be satisfied in several different ways:

- Some couples may wish to use a phallic-shaped vibrator as a substitute penis for partner satisfaction.
- If total penectomy has occurred, stimulation of the mons pubis, perineum, and scrotum can produce orgasms with pleasurable contractions in the remaining cavernous musculature.[54]
- If partial penectomy has occurred, men report erections and orgasms of normal or near normal intensity with the phallic stump.[55]
- Female partners must be advised (without instilling avoidance of sexual contact) to have a yearly Papanicolaou (Pap) smear, since they may be at increased risk for cervical cancer from exposure to the human papillomavirus.[55]

Cystectomy

Sexual dysfunction after cystectomy is similar to that after radical prostatectomy. The surgery is similar except that with radical cystectomy, urethrectomy may be included, which further damages penile innervation or blood flow. The other major difference is that a urinary diversion must be done, which can result in the need for an ostomy appliance. Many patients choose to have a continent internal urinary reservoir or ileocolonic neobladder, and those men are reported to remain more sexually active than men with appliances.[55]

Continued.

In addition to the interventions mentioned previously, following are a few ways to decrease anxiety from a urostomy:

- Before intercourse, the appliance should be emptied. Some patients secure the bag with a supportive belt.
- Like females, males may choose to wear a cover over their ostomy bag. Men may also wish to wear provocative underwear (silk boxer shorts) and expose only their genitalia during intercourse.
- To avoid friction on the stoma and pouch, other positions besides the missionary position may be tried.

- Some patients like to have their stomas touched during lovemaking, but they must be reminded that the stoma is fragile and too much rubbing may cause tearing. Objects should not be placed into the stoma.

Male pelvic cancer patients, like their female counterparts, must be treated with tenderness and understanding during the time of diagnosis, treatment, and long-term adjustment. Although many suggestions for mechanical aids and alternatives have been forthcoming, it is also important to remember the common expressions of affection and sexuality.

NURSING MANAGEMENT

COLORECTAL CANCER
INTERVENTIONS

Many patients with colon cancer are not ready to talk about their sexuality and sexual activity immediately after surgery. Many say that sex is one of the farthest things from their mind. The subject should at least be broached so patients will feel more comfortable thinking about their sexuality and will feel freer to ask questions at a later date.

Sexuality education is more readily available for ostomates and their partners than for many cancers (see Resources at the end of this chapter). The following methods may be useful:

- Prepare the pouch before sexual activity by emptying and assuring the seal. If the ostomy is dry or controllable with irrigation, a small cover or patch may be sufficient cover.
- Deodorize the pouch (1 or 2 drops of Banish is helpful) and avoid foods that cause gas.

- Test out comfortable positions (e.g., lateral scissors position, rear entry).
- Wear attractive camouflage like a cummerbund or cloth cover for the pouch.
- To protect from leakage, a rubber sheet may be placed under the sheet and a towel on top of the sheet.
- Underwear with an opening up the center is provocative and also provides a cover.
- Males may experience retrograde ejaculation after surgery and should be warned of this to prevent thoughts that "things aren't working quite right."
- As mentioned, penile implants are an option for men unable to have an erection.
- Most important, a good sense of humor is necessary, because accidents will happen. The couple may even consider rehearsing for when that time comes.

the patient both before and after surgery and substantially reduce anxiety and depression. Rehabilitation is of utmost importance to these patients, since they will probably have many productive years with an ostomy appliance.

LUNG CANCER
Physiologic and Body Image Alterations

Unlike many other malignancies discussed in this chapter, lung cancer has a dismal prognosis even when surgery has been performed, unless it is diagnosed in the very early stages. Little is realized in the literature in relation to psychosocial issues and the person with lung cancer, and no studies specific to sexuality and lung cancer are found. Reasons for this may be because these patients are often diagnosed with advanced disease that progresses rapidly and their performance status

is often very poor.[8] Quality of life is always an important factor in relation to the person with cancer and should be especially important to those with a shortened life expectancy. Because treatment for these people is often palliative rather than curative, it is important to consider their feelings of masculinity, femininity, and self-esteem, along with the basic aspects of care such as pain control. Because of the often rapidly fatal nature of lung cancer, the patient and partner must make significant decisions and adjustments, which often affects the patient's sense of self-esteem and worthiness: (1) if the patient has been a smoker, he or she will probably have tremendous feelings of guilt to overcome or deal with; (2) if the patient's performance status is poor and remains so as a result of fatigue and weakness, he or she will be unable to continue as a productive member of the family; (3) if the patient/partner

LUNG CANCER
INTERVENTIONS

The nurse should encourage lung cancer patients and their partners to experience sexual closeness that does not necessarily lead to intercourse, which can exacerbate excessive fatigue and dyspnea. Along with the other interventions mentioned in this chapter, the following suggestions may be helpful:

- When experiencing sexual closeness, the significant other should continue to treat the patient as a partner rather than an invalid. These are the few moments when the patient can feel like a real person again.

- Make sure the significant other can be near to the patient when in an office setting or in a hospital bed.
- Being physically close, hand holding, sharing an intimate moment will enhance feelings of maleness and femaleness, especially when the patient is getting treatment or is hospitalized.
- Soft caressing or light massage with oils or creams is sensual and can help reduce pain and discomfort.
- Mutual masturbation while watching adult movies promotes intimacy and conserves energy.
- Use strategies for managing dyspnea (see Chapter 14).

decide to take treatment (chemotherapy, radiation therapy), energy must be expended to cope with the side effects; and (4) if the patient/partner decide not to take treatment, there will be issues to resolve such as coping with an early death and caregiving. In regard to treatment decisions, Bernhard and others explain that, to the person with lung cancer, treatment is often associated with hope. "This allows active efforts in dealing with the course of disease and helps cancer patients manage free-floating anxiety."[9] Given all of the aforementioned anxiety-producing symptoms, side effects, and treatment regimens to deal with, it is not surprising that Bernhard and others report that lung cancer patients tend to withdraw socially.[9] All of these factors will have an effect on the relationship the patient has with his or her partner, and it is no wonder that there may be little time, energy, or desire for intimacy.

SPECIAL ISSUES INFLUENCING SEXUALITY
The Gerontologic Patient

Gendel reports an informal survey of one of her college psychology classes in which 75% of the class did not believe their parents were sexually active and 95% did not believe their grandparents could possibly be sexually active.[21] This small survey supports previous studies and documents beliefs that many hold, including health care professionals. Older people face a double bias about their sexuality: it is assumed that "old" people are (1) too ill to be thinking sexually and (2) incapable of sexual activity.[21] If attitudes such as these prevail, chances are few that sexual issues will be considered in these patients' general health care.[44,67]

We must reflect on our own attitudes about sexuality and the aging population and ask ourselves some questions. How do I feel about my elderly parents or grandparents having sex? If I see two elderly people kissing and fondling each other, how do I react?[70] (See Figure

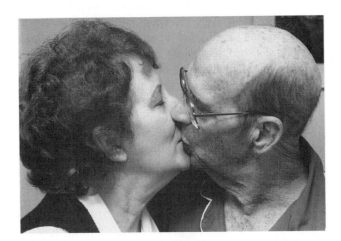

Figure 32-5 Henry and Margie share a tender moment.

32-5.) Frank-Stromborg tells us that there is "a misunderstanding of the normal physiologic changes in sexual capacities and functioning that occur with advancing age. These changes alter sexual performance; they do not destroy it."[20] One interesting note in Gendel's article points this out: "An 82-year-old male patient who was to have his left testicle removed, but who had already undergone other pelvic surgery resulting in loss of erectile function, was requesting a testicular prosthesis. His current sexual style with his partner was mutual genital stimulation to orgasm without erection, but he did not want her to fondle an 'empty sac'."[21]

When providing sexual counseling for the elderly, the nurse should be aware that all couples will not be interested in sexual activity. Respect for this option is necessary. However, the nurse should make sure that the couple is not abstaining because that is what is expected of them.

Various methods of sexual relating besides vaginal intercourse should be discussed with an elderly couple. For those patients who still have the desire for sexual involvement, the nurse may wish to encourage the following:

- A weak back and/or muscles can be helped by exercising those muscles. This will also make the person feel more sexually attractive.
- A nutritional diet using the Food Guide Pyramid can prevent depression and apathy, which may decrease sexual performance and interest.
- For the partners to achieve lubrication and erection, longer precoital stimulation may be needed to compensate for slowed physical response.
- Because of musculoskeletal changes, various positions for intercourse should be tried to promote comfort and save energy.[56,57]
- Both partners may not achieve orgasm; however, sexual pleasuring can still be enjoyed. Also the male may have little or no ejaculate.[40]
- During prolonged hospitalization or nursing home confinement, privacy should be provided for couples to hold, touch, fondle, and have intercourse if desired. This holds true for couples of any age.
- Warm baths, gentle massage, caressing and touching, masturbation, and fantasy all provide a sense of satisfaction and reassurance.
- Cleanliness, skin care (makeup, perfume, aftershave), hair care, mouth care, and attractive clothing can enhance feelings of masculinity and femininity.

The Gay/Lesbian Patient

It must never be assumed that all patients have or wish to have a partner or that all partners are of the opposite sex. It is the nurse's responsibility to be knowledgeable about the entire patient population and not to be judgmental. All patients are entitled to competence and a caring attitude. This is not always easy, however, because the literature that offers information concerning the gay/lesbian cancer population is limited and it is not always clear that the patient is homosexual.[65]

The sociocultural structure of gay relationships differs from that of lesbians. Six types of sociosexual relationships have been identified for the male, ranging from one-night stands to stable cohabitation or "marriage."[27] Less is known about lesbian relationships, but there is less promiscuity and more of them marry.[11] The gay/lesbian sexual repertoire and erotic positions are similar to those of heterosexuals except when limited by identical anatomy. Hogan explains that "the number of different sex roles and activities the homosexual is willing to engage in is directly related to age, length of homosexuality, the degree of acceptance of sexual impulses, and homosexual orientation."[27]

As with heterosexuals, the precancer sexual relationship has an important effect on the stability of the postcancer relationship. Those gays and lesbians involved in a permanent sexual relationship usually have fewer problems. If the patient has been diagnosed with cancer and still has to "cruise" (look for a sexual partner), it will be as difficult to deal with his or her new body image as it is for the heterosexual patient. Successful "scoring" may be substantially decreased.[27]

Because of inexperience in the area of sensitivity to behavioral cues, staff may be unsuccessful in obtaining information about sexual orientation because they do not ask the right questions. Rather than asking about a spouse, husband, or wife, the nurse can ask the patient whether he or she is sexually active or has a significant other.[38] Questions about sexual activity may deal with sexual preference such as "Do you prefer sexual activity with women, men, or both?"[39] Mapou tells us that ". . . most clients are not offended by such questions and those who are gay or lesbian are likely to appreciate the candor."[38] The nurse should treat the significant other as a spouse and involve him or her in the treatment process. This is likely to promote self-confidence and self-esteem in both members of the couple.[39]

In a group of gay patients with testicular cancer, one man expressed worry that his homosexuality caused his testicular cancer. Others were embarrassed at the lack of semen at ejaculation and did not know how to explain this to their partner.[61] Gay ostomates may wish to use their stomas as receptacles for intercourse, and they must be emphatically cautioned against this practice. The stoma is fragile and can tear and bleed.

The Patient Experiencing Spinal Cord Compression

All cancers have the propensity to metastasize to other areas of the body including the spinal cord, and most of the cancers dealt with in this chapter can cause problems of this nature. Because the literature on rehabilitative medicine and nursing has dealt extensively with the issue of sexuality and the paralyzed patient, this chapter will not address the topic. The reader is referred to the Resources at the end of this chapter for information.

STERILITY, INFERTILITY, AND PREGNANCY

It has been reported that 5% of new cancer cases occur in patients age 34 years or younger, and this means that approximately 5000 or more patients will be treated for cancer during their reproductive years.[6] The patient's age, gender, and stage of development and the type, dose, and duration of therapy are all integral factors in relation to reproductive tissue damage. Heiney[24] reports several concerns in relation to reproductive damage and future capacity; they include (1) abnormal sexual development, impaired sexual performance, and infertility; (2) potential damage to germ cells producing chromosomal changes; (3) transmission of the cancer-bearing gene to offspring; (4) problems with childbearing capabilities;

and (5) likelihood for marriage. Heiney found no conclusive evidence of congenital abnormality or cancer transmission except for genetic forms of cancer. She did find an increase in spontaneous abortion with combination (radiation and chemotherapy) therapy. The young cancer survivor tends to be less likely to marry than the average person.

Generally, male fertility is more susceptible to early damage than female fertility because of the constant mitotic cycles needed for spermatogenesis compared with the relative inactivity of the female oocyte. Testes are more susceptible to injury than are ovaries because rapidly dividing cells are most often affected by cancer therapies. Consequently, many chemotherapeutic agents alone, and especially in combination, can cause azospermia, oligospermia, or permanent sterility. Alkylating agents such as nitrogen mustard, cyclophosphamide, and chlorambucil cause sterility in the majority of treated males. However, depending on the drugs used, drug dose, and length of treatment, fertility may return, and the time frame can vary from 15 to 49 months after completion of therapy.[6,66] Comparisons of different chemotherapy combinations are reported by Averette and others, and one study showed that 3 of 21 patients in a nitrogen mustard, Oncovin, procarbazine, prednisone (MOPP) regimen had return of spermatogenesis, whereas all patients in an Adriamycin, bleomycin, vinblastine, dacarbazine (ABVD) group showed recovery.[6] "Several reports suggest decreased sensitivity to chemotherapy-induced gonadol toxicity in the prepubertal testes compared with the adult testes."[6] Successful pregnancy is often limited because of abnormalities of the pretreatment sperm specimen. However, with the advent of assisted reproductive technologies (ART) such as in vitro fertilization (IVF), gamete intrafallopian transfer (GIFT), and zygote intrafallopian transfer (ZIFT), men with lower than normal sperm concentration can take advantage of semen cryopreservation.[66]

Again, age plays a role for the female concerning possible ovarian dysfunction after treatment with chemotherapy because there are progressively fewer germ cells in the aging ovary. Averette and others reported on several studies that used multiagent chemotherapy such as MOPP.

> . . . 49% of patients experienced ovarian failure, and 34% had irregular ovarian activity, some of which progressed to complete ovarian failure. An age-dependent effect was noted since 89% of the patients with amenorrhea received treatment after age 25.[6]

As with boys, the ovarian function of prepubertal girls seems less susceptible to damage from chemotherapy. One other major concern for women is cancer and pregnancy. Harris reports that 1 in 1800 pregnant women will have cancer and all forms of neoplasms are found during pregnancy, with breast, cervical, ovarian, lymphoma, and colorectal occurring most frequently.[23] In making a decision whether to treat the patient during pregnancy, several factors should be considered: (1) "gestation age of the fetus; (2) maternal and fetal health at the time of diagnosis; (3) mother's prognosis and likelihood of future pregnancies after treatment; and (4) the known teratogenic effects of the drugs to be used."[75] If the administration of chemotherapy is initiated after the first trimester, surprisingly few complications are associated with treatment. Also, pregnancy after chemotherapy is not usually discouraged although some oncologists are concerned about recurrence facilitated by hormonal and immunologic changes. Because little scientific data support these worries, women should consider ultimate prognosis and the desire for children.

Finally, the children of patients treated with chemotherapy must be considered. No known studies are available that show an increase in congenital anomalies or other diseases in these children. One study did a chromosomal analysis of 24 children whose parents had been treated with chemotherapy and found 23 with normal karyotypes.[5] In addition, one other study that followed another subset of children up to 12 years (median follow-up, 2.5 years) showed growth, development, and school performance to be normal. If the parent is treated with a combination of chemotherapy and radiation therapy, there appears to be more complications of pregnancy. Wives of male patients have more spontaneous abortions, and female patients have more offspring with a variety of problems. Many scientists feel that prolonged observation must be done to better define the possible mutagenic nature of chemotherapy and radiation therapy in these children.

ASSESSING AND PRESERVING THE SEXUAL HEALTH OF THE CANCER PATIENT
Nursing Assessment Techniques

When performing a sexual health assessment, several elements can enhance both the nurse's and the patient's comfort during the discussion.[37] Key elements that will promote optimal patient teaching can be found in the box, p. 854.

There are several different approaches to sexual history-taking. Three sets of questions are presented here.

McPhetridge includes assessment of the effects of the illness on sexuality as a part of the nursing history. For our purposes, these questions might read as follows[42]:

- Has having cancer (or its treatment) interfered with your being a mother (wife, husband, father)?
- Has your cancer (or its treatment) changed the way you see yourself as a man (woman)?
- Has your cancer (or its treatment) caused any change in your sexual functioning (sex life)?

SEXUAL HEALTH ASSESSMENT

- Privacy is essential when doing the assessment. If the patient is not in a private room, move to another area if possible. An office, conference room, or a vacant patient room is preferable.
- Assure the patient of confidentiality. This tends to decrease the level of anxiety markedly. Usually it is good to include the partner, but it may be necessary to meet privately with the patient at first to establish rapport.
- Try to obtain a sexual history early in your association with the patient (see the approaches that follow). This implies that sexuality is an important and natural part of good health. Fatigue and how it can affect the patient's sexual activity may be included during an explanation of chemotherapy side effects. In this way one can introduce the concept, talk about it somewhat, and come back to it without making the patient uncomfortable.
- Avoid overreaction in your verbal and nonverbal communication. Wide eyes and an open mouth are not conducive to trust. Also try not to be bored. Listening with genuine interest helps to convey acceptance.
- Move from less sensitive to more sensitive issues.
- Determine the patient's goals for treatment.
- Realize when a problem is too complex to handle or when you do not know enough to be therapeutic and refer the problem on (e.g., clinical nurse specialist, psychologist, sexual rehabilitation counselor).

- Do you expect your sexual functioning (sex life) to be changed in any way after you leave the hospital?

Kolodny and others recommend general basic questions in the original contacts with patients when it is known that sexuality is likely to be affected by treatment. The focus in this brief sexual history is on sexual functions[30]:

1. Are you sexually active? (If "yes," then 2)
2. What is the approximate frequency of your sexual activity?
3. Are you satisfied with your sex life? (If "no," then proceed.) Why not?

For men:
4. Do you have difficulty obtaining or maintaining an erection?
5. Do you have difficulty with control of ejaculation?

For women:
6. Do you have difficulty becoming aroused?
7. Do you have any difficulty having orgasm?

For both men and women:
8. Do you have pain with intercourse?
9. Do you have any questions or problems?

VerSteeg describes an early assessment approach that is more comprehensive and addresses the following areas[72]:

- *Couple's relationship.* What kind of relationship is it?

What are its strengths, resources, coping abilities, degree of closeness, and importance of sexual aspects?
- *Understanding of cancer and its treatments.* What do they understand about the disease and its treatments? What is their understanding of the anatomy and physiology involved? What do they know about changes from therapy, its side effects, and their duration?
- *Impact on sexuality.* What do they understand about the impacts of cancer and its treatment—physically, psychologically, and socially? What do they understand about effects on sexuality and fertility?
- *Preparation for changes.* How do they want to prepare for expected changes? What kind of anticipatory guidance will help them be ready for common initial responses (anxiety and depression)? How can they explore alternatives, plan new responses, and communicate ideas and feelings?
- *Planning and participation in care.* How does the person being treated want to participate in planning for hospital care? What are the mutual expectations between patient and staff for self-care in the hospital and later at home? How will the partner be involved? What is his or her investment in various facets of care? What is the nature of support needed and how can the partner respond to that need?
- *Control and optimism will help.* What kinds of support will help the patient have a sense of control and optimism or hope regarding self, body, environment, and the unknowns involved in the situation?
- *Expansion of sexuality.* How does the couple want to expand their perceptions of sexuality and potential sexual activities? What are the best avenues of new learning for them, and in what order? Do they want information in printed form? Discussion with the nurse or with others who have had similar therapy? Do they want exercises to explore new behaviors together?

The PLISSIT is a model frequently used for sexuality counseling or a nursing intervention. Each step is taken depending on the nurse's knowledge and comfort level[14]:

- *P = permission.* This promotes discussion and encourages the couple to continue in their present pattern of sexual activity plus suggests some risk taking.
- *LI = limited information.* Includes the permission already given plus some new information specific to their sexuality concerns.
- *SS = specific suggestions.* May include new activities for the couple, which may entail "homework."
- *IT = intensive therapy.* This is when the couple is referred on to a therapist for more intense treatment.

A more complete model has been created by Schain.[53] Her model uses eight letters—PLEASURE—to cue the nurse to the topic area and to represent a good feeling. For a more in-depth explanation of this method, see Schain's article[53]:

- *P = partner.* Is there one, how many, what kind of relationship? Problems identified and recommendations will depend on whether there is a partner or not.

- *L = lovemaking.* What are the motives for being sexually active? Permission to engage in autoerotic behavior may be helpful.
- *E = emotions.* What is the patient's attitude about the illness and sexual problems? If underlying psychologic problems surface, referral may be appropriate.
- *A = attitude.* What is the "norm" of sexual activity for this patient and what are your own values?
- *S = symptoms.* An explicit explanation of the problems in regard to the three phases of the sexual response cycle is needed here.
- *U = understanding.* What are the etiologic factors (intrapsychic, physiologic, relationship) contributing to the problem?
- *R = reproduction.* What is the desire to have children, and if this ability is eliminated, how does that affect the patient's life goals?
- *E = energy.* How does the problem interfere with the individual's overall psychologic and sexual comfort, and do they want formalized sexual counseling?

PRESERVING INTIMACY

Today our patients survive longer after their treatment for cancer. Survivorship means that the nurse must look with the patient to rehabilitation. In sexual rehabilitation, the nurse's goal of helping to restore the patient's sexual function is followed closely by the goals of restoring self-image and self-esteem. Each patient's sexuality is unique and is reflected in touching, smelling, hearing, tasting, and visual stimulation. These create for the patient and partner their own special intimacy, sense of affection, and physical gratification. Many references have been made and suggestions given in this chapter, but when there are *no* acceptable alternatives within a relationship, it is the nurse's duty to help the couple use their own coping strategies and strengths. The values and beliefs of the couple are important to the use and success of various alternatives. What may be an acceptable expression for some may not be for others. Sometimes all they need is to be given permission to try something different. Encourage them to take the risk, and be there to support them.

CONCLUSION

As health care professionals continue to struggle to understand and be comfortable with their own sexuality, cancer patients continue to ask for help in dealing with disease and treatment related to sexual issues. In this situation it is important to extend our efforts beyond the disease and focus on the whole patient. For all of us, receiving sexual pleasure and closeness is linked to a sense of belonging and worthiness. Being accepted is intimately bound to self-esteem. As one author put it, "self-esteem is the sum total of all our feelings about ourselves . . . it is the reputation we share of ourselves with ourself."[12]

Resources

- —Headliner, Designs for Comfort, Inc., P.O. Box 8229, Northfield, IL 60093, 1-800-443-9226.
- —Sweetie Cap, Lan Care, Inc., 2747 17th Avenue Court, Moline, IL 61265, 1-309-762-4800.
- Literature on rehabilitation for the patient with spinal cord compression is as follows:
  - —Christina Mumma, editor: *Rehabilitation nursing: concepts and practice,* ed 2; available from Rehabilitation Nursing Foundation, 2506 Gross Point Road, Evanston, IL 60201.
  - —Kolodny R and others: *Textbook of Human Sexuality for Nurses,* Boston, 1979, Little, Brown & Co.
- Literature with reference to sexuality issues:
  - —Johnson J, Klein L: *I can cope: staying healthy with cancer,* Minneapolis, Minn, 1988, DCI Publishing.
  - —Noyes D, Mellody P: *Beauty and cancer,* Los Angeles, 1988, AC Press.
  - —Schover L: *Sexuality and cancer: for the woman who has cancer, and her partner,* Atlanta, Ga, 1988, American Cancer Society, Inc.
  - —Schover L: *Sexuality and cancer: for the man who has cancer, and his partner,* Atlanta, Ga, 1988, American Cancer Society, Inc.

Support Groups

- Support groups for head and neck cancer patients are often sponsored by the American Cancer Society, such as "The Lost Chord" for laryngectomies.
- One of the first support groups in the country for amputees was founded in the Kansas City area by Lou Keyes and is called LEAPS. This stands for Lower Extremity Amputees Providing Support; the telephone number is 1-816-361-3206. This group also has access to information about support groups nationwide.
- "Reach to Recovery" is a voluntary group of mastectomy patients sponsored and trained by the American Cancer Society (ACS). The ACS is located in most cities in the United States.
- Prostate cancer support groups (ACS).
- Tracheostomy covers may be obtained from Byram Health Care Center, Inc., Tracheo-stoma Bibs, 2 Armonk Street, Greenwich, CT 06380, 1-800-354-4054.
- Available breast prostheses include the following:
  - —Coloplast Corp., A thin, soft silicone gel; 1995 W. Oak Circle, Marietta, GA 30062, 1-800-995-9559.
  - —Spenco Medical Corp—manufacturer: "Nearly Me," Cloth, poly/foam, or silicone; 1-312-478-7701 or 1-800-421-2322.

—Bosom Buddy, thin glass beads cushioned by cotton, covered with nylon; 1-208-343-9696.

- Information on vaginal dilators is available from Syracuse Medical Devices, Inc., 214 Hurlburt Rd., Syracuse, NY 13224, 1-315-449-0657. Cost of dilator: extra small—$6.75; small—$6.40; medium—$7.40; large—$8.40.

- Literature on sexuality education for ostomates is available for a small charge from the United Ostomy Association, Inc., 36 Executive Park, Suite 120, Irvine, CA 92714, 1-714-660-8624.

- Options for men and women experiencing alopecia are as follows:
  —Great American Options, International Hairgoods, Inc., 6811 Flying Cloud Drive, Eden Prairie, Minn.

■ CHAPTER QUESTIONS

1. Once a patient is diagnosed with cancer, she or he may be concerned about several issues related to her or his *sexuality*. These issues will include which of the following:
   a. The possible spread of malignancy and death
   b. The number of chemotherapy treatments he or she must take
   c. An altered body image and self-esteem, which may impact on femininity or masculinity, and sexual function
   d. Denial of the disease

2. When people are ill, they begin to doubt their sexual identity. All of the following may impact this feeling *except:*
   a. Embarrassment to raise questions about sexual concerns because their illness is so serious
   b. The effect the illness will have on their ability to respond sexually (male and female sexual response)
   c. A wish to belong and receive approval, which is associated with receiving sexual pleasure
   d. Disinterest in sex because it is not important in our society

3. The person who has experienced limb amputation as a result of cancer may face several sexual problems. Which of the following may inhibit a sexual relationship?
   a. Amputee fetishism
   b. Phantom pain sensation
   c. Immobility resulting from physical isolation
   d. Body positioning during intercourse
   e. All the above

4. Patients with hematologic malignancies also face sexuality concerns. Which of the following is true about potential sexual concerns among this population?
   a. Myelosuppression can cause fatigue, shortness of breath, potential for infection, and bleeding, which preclude participation in sexual intercourse.
   b. Ovarian dysfunction is not a problem even though there may be irregular menses or hot flashes. The patient cannot get pregnant anyhow.
   c. Testicular dysfunction never occurs, so men need not be concerned.
   d. Chemotherapy causes few problems that impact this population's sexuality even though they may lose their hair.

5. All of the following will impact the patient with breast cancer and her sexuality *except:*
   a. The patient treated with lumpectomy and radiation may have just as many concerns as the patient treated with mastectomy.
   b. Even though the genital organs are not affected during treatment for breast cancer, many patients have a decreased sexual desire.
   c. The woman may express concern about showing her partner her wound and how to camouflage her wound during intercourse.
   d. Because a great deal of information is in the literature related to single, divorced, widowed, and lesbian breast cancer patients, we do not have to be as concerned about their support.

6. The sexual concerns of the geriatric patient are rarely, if ever, addressed by the nurse. Because an older couple is often still sexually active, which of the following is important to include in a discussion about sexuality?
   a. Longer precoital stimulation and various different positions for intercourse may need to be tried because of slowed physical response and musculoskeletal changes.
   b. Exercise and massage will not necessarily enhance a sexual relationship at this late life stage.
   c. Because either or both partners may not achieve orgasm, sex is no longer important.
   d. Privacy is not needed during hospitalization, since couples should behave themselves when ill.

7. Patients treated for head and neck cancers have sexual concerns that are often ignored by the nurse. To help this patient population, it would be appropriate to advocate which of the following?
   a. The use of artificial saliva or sugarless mints to freshen stale breath and prevent tooth decay.
   b. The use of scented candles, perfumes, and aftershaves to enhance sexual intimacy.
   c. The use of various positions during intercourse because of fear of cutting off the patient's air supply.
   d. The use of a fancy nightgown with a high neck or a dickey to cover the tracheostomy site.
   e. All the above.

8. Alternate methods to sexual intercourse may need to be tried after surgery for many of the female genital cancer patients, during and after the area has healed. All of the following may be included *except:*
   a. Close encounters such as cuddling, nudity (taking a bath together), and general pleasuring with massage.
   b. The best solution is to give up a sexual relationship with a partner and to masturbate if becoming sexually frustrated.
   c. New positions may need to be used, such as female on top to control penile thrusting and comfort.
   d. Oral-genital relations, mutual masturbation, and love-play or fantasy may be acceptable to some patients/couples.

9. Men who experience pelvic genital concerns often feel demasculinated and unlovable. The nurse can support which of the following to enhance the males' perspective on his masculinity?

a. Encourage arousal with erotic books, pictures, or movies.
b. If problems with incontinence occur, encourage the patient to empty his bladder before intercourse or to wear a condom.
c. Penile prosthesis, penile injection or vacuum devices to provide erection may be acceptable alternatives.
d. All the above.

BIBLIOGRAPHY

1. Al-Juburi A, O'Donnell P: Penile self-injection for impotence in patients after radical cystectomy-ileal loop, *Urology* 30(1):29, 1987.
2. Anderson B: Sexual functioning complications in women with gynecologic cancer: outcomes and direction for prevention, *Cancer* 60:1987.
3. Anderson B, Hacker N: Treatment for gynecological cancer: a review of the effects on female sexuality, *Health Psychol* 2:203, 1983.
4. Anderson B, Jochimsen P: Sexual functioning among breast cancer, gynecologic cancer, and healthy women, *J Consult Clin Psychol* 53:25, 1985.
5. Anderson B and others: Sexual functioning after treatment of in situ vulvar cancer: a preliminary report, *Obstet Gynecol* 71:13, 1988.
6. Averette H, Boike G, Jerrel M: Effects of cancer chemotherapy on gonadal function and reproductive capacity, *CA Cancer J Clin* 4:4, 1990.
7. Baxley K and others: Alopecia: effect on cancer patients' body image, *Cancer Nurs* 7:499, 1984.
8. Bernhard J, Ganz P: Psychosocial issues in lung cancer patients (Part 1), *Chest* 99:1, 1991.
9. Bernhard J, Ganz P: Psychosocial issues in lung cancer patients (Part 2), *Chest* 99:2, 1991.
10. Burt, K: The effects of cancer on body image and sexuality, *Nurs Times* 91(7):36, 1995.
11. Butler S, Rosenblum B: *Cancer in two voices,* Duluth, Minn, 1991, Spinsters Inc.
12. Cantor R: Self-esteem, sexuality and cancer-related stress, *Front Radiat Ther Oncol* 14:51, 1980.
13. Carpenito L: *Nursing diagnosis: application to clinical practice,* vol 4, Philadelphia, 1992, Lippincott.
14. Cooley M, Yeomans A, Cobb S: Sexual and reproductive issues for women with Hodgkin's disease: application of PLISSIT model, *Cancer Nurs* 9:248, 1986.
15. Cummings V: Amputees and sexual dysfunction, *Arch Phys Med Rehabil* 56:12, 1975.
16. Curtis T, Zlotglow I: Sexuality and head and neck cancer, *Front Radiat Ther Oncol* 14:26, 1980.
17. Donahue V, Knapp R: Sexual rehabilitation of gynecologic cancer patients, *Obstet Gynecol* 49:118, 1977.
18. Ducharma S, Gill K: Sexual values, training and professional roles, *J Head Trauma Rehab* 5:2, 1990.
19. Fisher S: The sexual knowledge and attitudes of oncology nurses: implications for nursing education, *Semin Oncol Nurs* 1:63, 1985.
20. Frank-Stromborg M: Sexuality and the elderly cancer patient, *Semin Oncol Nurs* 1:49, 1985.
21. Gendel E: Self-esteem and sexuality in older patients with cancer, *Front Radiat Ther Oncol* 20:166, 1986.
22. Gritz E and others: Long-term effects of testicular cancer on sexual functioning in married couples, *Cancer* 64(7):1560, 1989.
23. Harris B: Issues in nursing care of pregnant patients with cancer. In Lowdermilk D, editor: *NAACOGs clinical issues in perinatal and women's health nursing,* Philadelphia, 1990, Lippincott.
24. Heiney S: Adolescents with cancer: sexual and reproductive issues, *Cancer Nurs* 12:2, 1989.
25. Heinrich-Rynning T: Prostatic cancer treatments and their effects on sexual functioning, *Oncol Nurs Forum* 14:6, 1987.
26. Hoehm P, McCorkle R: Understanding sexuality in progressive cancer, *Semin Oncol Nursing* 1:56, 1985.
27. Hogan R: *Human sexuality: a nursing perspective,* Norwalk, Conn, 1985, Appleton-Century-Crofts.
28. Ingle R: Cancer and sexuality. In Fogel C, Lavver D, editors: *Sexual health promotion,* Philadelphia, 1990, Saunders.
29. Jenkins B: Sexual healing after pelvis irradiation, *Am J Nurs* 86:920, 1986.
30. Kolodny R and others: *Textbook of human sexuality,* Boston, 1979, Little, Brown.
31. Lamb M: Sexual dysfunction in the gynecologic oncology patient, *Semin Oncol Nurs* 1:9, 1985.
32. Larsen G: Rehabilitation for the patient with head and neck cancer, *Am J Nurs* 82:119, 1982.
33. Leiber L and others: The communication of affection between cancer patients and their spouses, *Psychosom Med* 38:379, 1976.
34. Levison V: The effect on fertility, libido, and sexual function of postoperative radiotherapy and chemotherapy for cancer of the testicle, *Clin Radiol* 37:161, 1986.
35. Lewis F, Bloom J: Psychosocial adjustment to breast cancer: a review of selected literature, *Int J Psychiatry Med* 9:1, 1978-79.
36. Li F: Genetic studies of survivors of childhood cancer, *Am J Pediatr Hematol Oncol* 9(1):104, 1987.
37. MacElveen-Hoehn P: Sexual assessment and counseling, *Semin Oncol Nurs* 1:69, 1985.
38. Mapou R: Traumatic brain injury rehabilitation with gay and lesbian individuals, *J Head Trauma Rehab* 5:2, 1990.
39. Masters W, Johnson V: *Human sexual response,* Boston, 1966, Little, Brown.
40. Masters W, Johnson V, Koloday R: *Heterosexuality,* New York, 1994, Harper Perennial.
41. McDonald T and others: Impact of cervical intraepithelial neoplasia diagnosis and treatment on self-esteem and body image, *Gynecol Oncol* 34(3):345, 1989.
42. McPhetridge L: Nursing history: one means to personalize care, *Am J Nurs* 68:73, 1968.
43. Metcalfe M, Fischman S: Factors affecting the sexuality of patients with head and neck cancer, *Oncol Nurs Forum* 12:21, 1985.
44. Mooradian A, Greiff V: Sexuality in older women, *Arch Internal Med* 150(5):1033, 1990.
45. Mulvihill J and others: Pregnancy outcomes in cancer patients: experience in a large cooperative group, *Cancer* 60(5):1143, 1987.

46. Perez C, Hoskins W, Young R: Gynecologic tumors. In De-Vita VT, Hellman S, Rosenberg SA, editors: *Cancer: principles and practices of oncology,* ed 3, Philadelphia, 1989, Lippincott.

47. Pierce A and others: Pharmacologic creation with intracavernosal injection for men with sexual dysfunction following irradiation: a preliminary report, *Int J Radiat Oncol Biol Phys* 21(5):677, 1991.

48. Reinstein L, Ashley J, Miller K: Sexual adjustment after lower extremity amputation, *Arch Phys Med Rehabil* 59:501, 1978.

49. Renshaw D: Sexual and emotional needs of cancer patients, *Clin Ther* 8:242, 1986.

50. Renshaw D: Beacons, breasts, symbols, sex and cancer, *Theor Med* 15:4, 1994.

51. Schain W: Sexual problems of patients with cancer. In DeVita VT, Hellman S, Rosenberg SA, editors: *Cancer: principles and practice of oncology,* ed 2, Philadelphia, 1985, Lippincott.

52. Schain W: *Sexual and reproductive issues in breast cancer: workshop on psychosexual and reproductive issues affecting patients with cancer,* San Antonio, Texas, American Cancer Society, Jan 1987.

53. Schain W: A sexual interview is a sexual intervention, *Innovations Oncol Nurs* 4:2, 1988.

54. Schover L: Sexual rehabilitation of urologic cancer patients: a practical approach, *CA Cancer J Clin* 34:66, 1984.

55. Schover L: *Sexual problems in men with pelvic or genital malignancies: workshop on psychosexual and reproductive issues affecting patients with cancer,* San Antonio, Texas, American Cancer Society, Jan 1987.

56. Schover L: *Sexuality and cancer: for the man who has cancer, and his partner,* New York, 1988, American Cancer Society.

57. Schover L: *Sexuality and cancer: for the woman who has cancer, and her partner,* New York, 1988, American Cancer Society.

58. Schover L, Fife M: Sexual counseling of patients undergoing radical surgery for pelvic or genital cancer, *J Psychosoc Oncol* 3:15, 1986.

59. Schover L, Jensen S: *Sexuality and chronic illness,* New York, NY, 1988, The Guilford Press.

60. Schover L, Schain W, Montague D: Psychologic aspects of patients with cancer: sexual problems of patients with cancer. In DeVita V, Hellman S, Rosenberg S, editors: *Cancer principles and practices of oncology,* ed 3, Philadelphia, 1989, Lippincott.

61. Schover L, von Eschenbach A: Sexual and marital counseling with men treated for testicular cancer, *J Sex Marital Ther* 10:29, 1984.

62. Schover L, von Eschenbach A: Sexual function and female radical cystectomy: a case series. *J Urol* 465:465, 1985.

63. Shell J: Sexuality for patients with gynecologic cancer. In Lowdermilk D, editor: *NAACOGs clinical issues in perinatal and women's health nursing,* Philadelphia, 1990, Lippincott.

64. Shell J: The psychosexual impact of ostomy surgery, *Progressions: developments in ostomy and wound care* 4(3):5, 1992.

65. Shell J: Do you like the things that life is showing you? The sensitive self image of the person with cancer, *Oncol Nurs Forum* 22(6):907, 1995.

66. Shell J, Bell K, Dougherty M: Gonadol toxicities. In Liebman M, Camp-Sorrell D, editors: *Multimodal therapy in oncology nursing,* St. Louis, 1996, Mosby.

67. Shell J, Smith C: Sexuality and the older person with cancer, *Oncol Nurs Forum* 21(3):553, 1994.

68. Shipes E, Lehr S: Sexuality and the male cancer patient, *Cancer Nurs* 5:375, 1982.

69. Sidi A and others: Intracavernous drug-induced erections in the management of male erectile dysfunction: experience with 100 patients, *J Urol* 135:704, 1986.

70. Steinke E, Bergen B: Sexuality and aging, *J Gerontol Nurs* 12:6, 1986.

71. Vera M: Quality of life following pelvic exenteration, *Gynecol Oncol* 12:355, 1981.

72. VerSteeg M: Options for sexual expression. In von Eschenbach P, Rodriguez D, editors: *Sexual rehabilitation of the urological cancer patient,* Boston, 1981, Hall.

73. von Eschenbach A, Schover L: The role of sexual rehabilitation in the treatment of patients with cancer, *Cancer* 54:2662, 1984.

74. Weaver S, Lange L, Vogts V: Comparison of myoelectric and conventional prosthesis for adolescent amputees, *Am J Occup Ther* 42:87, 1988.

75. Weeks D: Acute leukemia and pregnancy. In Lowdermilk D, editor. *NAACOGs clinical issues in perinatal and women's health nursing,* Philadelphia, 1990, Lippincott.

76. Weiss K: *Women's experience of sex and sexuality,* Center City, Minn, 1992, Hazolden Educational Materials.

77. Welty M and others: The patient with maxillofacial cancer: surgical treatment and nursing care, *Nurs Clin North Am* 8:137, 1973.

78. Williams H and others: Nurses' attitudes toward sexuality in cancer patients, *Oncol Nurs Forum* 13:37, 1986.

79. Wilson M, Williams H: Oncology nurses' attitudes and behaviors related to sexuality of patients with cancer, *Oncol Nurs Forum* 15:1, 49, 1988.

80. Zinreich E and others: Pre- and post-treatment evaluation of sexual function in patients with adenocarcinoma of the prostate, *Int J Radiat Oncol Biol Phys* 19:3, 1990.

Answers

CHAPTER 1

1. B	6. D
2. C	7. C
3. B	8. C
4. D	9. A
5. A	10. C

CHAPTER 2

1. B	6. D
2. A	7. C
3. D	8. A
4. D	9. A
5. B	10. C

CHAPTER 3

1. C	6. B
2. D	7. A
3. A	8. D
4. B	9. C
5. C	10. B

CHAPTER 4

1. C	6. C
2. D	7. D
3. A	8. A
4. C	9. D
5. D	10. B

CHAPTER 5

1. D	6. C
2. C	7. A
3. C	8. D
4. B	9. C
5. D	10. D

CHAPTER 6

1. C	6. C
2. D	7. B
3. B	8. C
4. D	9. D
5. A	10. A

CHAPTER 7

1. D	6. B
2. A	7. C
3. C	8. D
4. A	9. C
5. C	10. D

CHAPTER 8

1. B	6. D
2. A	7. D
3. C	8. B
4. D	9. D
5. A	10. A

CHAPTER 9

1. B	6. B
2. D	7. C
3. A	8. B
4. C	9. D
5. D	10. A

CHAPTER 10

1. C	6. A
2. B	7. C
3. D	8. A
4. A	9. C
5. C	10. D

CHAPTER 11

1. C	6. D
2. B	7. B
3. D	8. A
4. A	9. B
5. D	10. A

CHAPTER 12

1. A	6. A
2. C	7. A
3. D	8. B
4. B	9. D
5. D	10. C

CHAPTER 13

1. C	6. C
2. D	7. B
3. D	8. C
4. D	9. A
5. C	10. C

CHAPTER 14

1. B	7. B
2. D	8. E
3. A	9. C
4. D	10. B
5. A	11. A
6. C	12. B

CHAPTER 15

1. D	6. B
2. D	7. B
3. A	8. A
4. C	9. C
5. D	10. D

CHAPTER 16

1. B	3. D
2. C	

CHAPTER 17

1. C	6. C
2. D	7. A
3. A	8. C
4. B	9. B
5. D	10. D

CHAPTER 18

1. B	6. D
2. B	7. E
3. C	8. A
4. D	9. B
5. B	10. C

CHAPTER 19

1. C	7. C
2. B	8. A
3. D	9. B
4. A	10. A
5. B	11. C
6. D	12. D

CHAPTER 20

1. C	5. B
2. A	6. D
3. D	7. A
4. D	8. A

CHAPTER 21

1. B	7. B
2. A	8. C
3. C	9. C
4. A	10. A
5. D	11. D
6. B	12. B

CHAPTER 22

1. D	7. C
2. D	8. B
3. D	9. A
4. D	10. A
5. A	11. C
6. D	12. C

CHAPTER 23

1. C	8. C
2. A	9. B
3. B	10. B
4. B	11. C
5. D	12. A
6. A	13. D
7. C	

CHAPTER 24

1. A
2. A
3. C
4. D
5. A
6. D
7. D
8. B

CHAPTER 25

1. C
2. A
3. A
4. D
5. B

CHAPTER 26

1. B
2. C
3. D
4. C
5. B
6. D
7. D
8. D

CHAPTER 27

1. C
2. D
3. D
4. A
5. B
6. C
7. C
8. B

CHAPTER 28

1. D
2. C
3. B
4. A
5. D
6. D
7. B

CHAPTER 29

1. C
2. C
3. A
4. A
5. B
6. D
7. B
8. D

CHAPTER 30

1. C
2. A
3. B
4. A
5. B
6. D
7. C
8. C
9. D

CHAPTER 31

1. A
2. C
3. B
4. D
5. C
6. B
7. D
8. A

CHAPTER 32

1. C
2. D
3. E
4. A
5. D
6. A
7. E
8. B
9. D

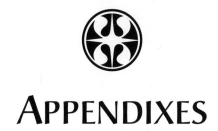

APPENDIXES

absolute risk   the number of specific cancer cases (breast) in a given population divided by the number of people (women) in the population—may be expressed as an average risk for every woman in that group.

acquired immunity   specific and depend on the recognition of self and nonself.

active immunotherapy   the administration of biologic or chemical products that stimulate the immune system of the host.

adjuvant chemotherapy   chemotherapy designed to eradicate microscopic foci of metastatic disease after local control with surgery, radiation therapy, or both.

adoptive immunotherapy (passive immunotherapy)   the direct transfer of cells or products of the immune system to a host.

allogenic   having cell types that are antigenically distinct.

allograft   a graft of tissue between individuals of the same species but of different genotype, called also *allogenic graft.*

anaphase   a stage of mitosis in which the chromosomes begin to move apart toward opposite poles of the spindle.

anaplasia   the loss of structural organization and useful function of a cell.

aneuploid   having more or less than the normal diploid number of chromosomes.

antibody   an immunoglobulin protein produced by plasma cells and B cells in response to antigen, which has the ability to combine with the antigen that stimulated its production.

antigen   a molecule that is specifically recognized by antibody and by cells of the adaptive immune system.

attributable risk   the number of cancer cases in a population that are associated with a given risk factor and that could potentially be prevented by alteration or removal of that factor.

autologous   related to self, designating products or components of the same individual organism.

azotemia   an excess of urea or other nitrogenous bodies in the blood.

B cells (B lymphocytes)   cells derived from bone marrow stem cell in humans, capable of responding to antigen by the production of antibody.

biological response modifier (BRM)   an agent that can modify host reactions against disease, with resultant potential to prevent progression of cancer or metastatic spread; includes, but not limited to, immunotherapy.

biotherapy   treatment with agents derived from biologic sources or affecting biologic response.

blast cell   an immature form of a blood cell or a normal embryonic cell.

cachexia   malnutrition with overall general poor health.

cancer in situ   early-stage cancer; before the invasion of surrounding tissue; usually implies total cancer removal with surgical incision or biopsy.

capillary leak syndrome   shift of fluid from the intravascular space resulting in accumulation of fluid in the extravascular space; symptoms include hypotension, tachycardia, and weight gain.

CD4 cell   cell expressing the CD4 protein on its surface, primarily cells of the immune system, particularly T helper cells (T4 cells) and monocytes/macrophages.

CD8 cell   cell expressing the CD8 protein on its surface, primarily a subpopulation of T cells, particularly cytotoxic T cells (T8 cells) and suppressor T cells.

cell-mediated immunity   involving specifically immune T cells and cells of the natural immune system (natural killer [NK] cells and monocytes/macrophages), particularly important to the body's defense against viral-infected cells and malignant cells.

cellularity   the ratio of hematopoietic (blood forming) tissue to adipose tissue in the marrow.

chemotactic   the movement of an organism or an individual cell, such as a leukocyte, in response to a chemical concentration gradient.

cocarcinogen   an agent that becomes carcinogenic when it interacts with a cancer-causing agent.

colony-stimulating factor (hematopoietic growth factor)   a group of hormonelike glycoproteins that are secreted by a wide range of cells in the body and on which the processes of hemopoiesis depend; substances that stimulates growth or orderly maturation of cells of the hematopoietic system.

commitment   process by which components of the hemopoietic hierarchy increasingly lose the potential to differentiate into alternative cell lines.

contact inhibition   the growth and movement of a normal cell stops when it comes in contact with another cell.

cytokine   a protein hormone of the immune system that is responsible for communication with other cells of the immune system or with cells outside of this system.

cytokinesis   the changes that take place in the cytoplasm during mitosis, meiosis, and fertilization.

cytostatic   suppresses cell proliferation.

cytotoxic   able to kill cells.

deafferentation   the elimination or interruption of afferent nerve impulses, as by destruction of the afferent pathways.

diaphanoscopy examination with the diaphanoscope; transillumination.

differentiation to develop a specialized shape, character, or function that differs from that of other cells or tissues; usually implies a loss of malignant nature.

diploid an individual or cell having two full sets of homologous chromosomes.

DNA a complex protein of high molecular weight, consisting of deoxyribose, phosphoric acid, and four bases (two purines, adenine and guanine, and two pyrimidines, thymine and cytosine). These are arranged as two long chains that twist around each other to form a double helix joined by bonds between the complementary system. Nucleic acid is present in chromosomes of the nuclei of cells and is the chemical basis of heredity and the carrier of genetic information for all organisms except the RNA viruses.

dysphonia difficulty or pain in speaking.

dysplasia disturbance in the size, shape, and organization of cells and tissues.

effector cells cells of the immune system that mediate an immune response.

ELISA (enzyme-linked immunosorbent assay) capable of detecting either antibody or antigen by the binding of an enzyme coupled to either anti-Ig or antibody specific to the antigen; used to detect HIV antibodies.

enzymes proteins that act as a catalyst to induce or speed up chemical reactions inside or outside the cell.

epidemiologic approach examines the frequency of the disease among relatives.

extravasation an inadvertent leakage of blood, drug, from a vessel into the tissues.

gene therapy insertion of a functioning gene into a human cell to direct the natural antiviral human cell response; provides a new function to the cell.

genetic approach studies the pattern of disease expression among relatives.

genetics the study of heredity and possible genetics factors influencing the occurrence of a pathologic condition.

genome the complete set of hereditary factors, as contained in the haploid assortment of chromosomes.

genotype the entire set of genes one inherits from both parents.

glycoprotein any of a class of conjugated proteins consisting of a compound of protein with a carbohydrate group.

haplotype the group of alleles of linked genes contributed by either parent.

hematopoiesis the process by which blood cells are produced in the bone marrow.

hematopoietic pertaining to or affecting the formation of blood cells.

hemolytic destruction of blood cells, resulting in liberation of hemoglobin from the red blood cell.

heterogeneous derived from a different source or species; xenograft.

homeostasis the condition in which the external and internal environment of a cell remains relatively constant.

homogeneous composed of similar elements or ingredients; of a uniform quality throughout.

humoral immunity specific immunity activated by antibody found in blood and lymph; particularly important in trapping viral and bacterial organisms that have not yet invaded cells of the body.

hybridoma technology process by which fusion cells, produced by myeloma plasma cells, are introduced into an immunized mouse.

hyperbaric characterized by greater than normal pressure or weight; applied to gases under greater than atmospheric pressure; as hyperbaric oxygen.

hyperplasia an increase in the number of cells in a tissue or organ.

hypoguesic abnormally diminished acuteness of the sense of taste.

idiotype an antigenic determinant present on and characteristic of a certain antibody molecule, usually located in the variable region.

immunity a protective mechanism that serves to maintain the integrity of the body against foreign substances or agents.

immunogenic capable of stimulating an immune response.

immunoglobulin a glycoprotein composed of heavy and light chains that functions as antibody; in humans, the five classes are designated as IgG, IgA, IgM, IgD, and IgE.

immunomodulation alteration of the immune response to induce up-regulation, suppression, or tolerance.

immunosuppression blocking or diminishing the functioning of the immune system.

immunosurveillance a theory that postulates that the immune system plays an important role in the prevention of development of detectable cancer.

incidence the number of newly diagnosed cases of cancer in a specified period of time (calendar year) in a defined population.

indolent slow-growing tumor.

initiation the first step in turning a normal cell cancerous as by drugs, chemicals, or other agents.

interferon (IFN) a class of cytokines originally identified for their ability to inhibit growth of viruses within cells; selectively inhibit the synthesis of viral RNA in infected cells; immunoregulatory functions, including enhancing the activities of macrophages and natural killer cells.

interleukin (IL) a class of cytokines produced by lymphocytes or macrophages in response to antigenic or mitogenic stimulation, which mediate communication among cells of the immune system.

interphase initial phase of mitosis; cells grow in size; chromosomes elongate; replication of DNA.

in vitro within a glass; observable in a test tube; in an artificial environment.

in vivo within the living body.

ionizing radiation a type of radiation that involves gamma rays that penetrate deeply into tissues; this form of radiation may have an enhanced biologic effect on tumors by degrading tumor DNA.

ipsilateral on the same side.

karotype the chromosomal constitution of the nucleus of a cell.

lentivirus any of a group of retroviruses, including those that cause maedi and visna in sheep.

leukoagglutinin an agglutinin directed against leukocytes.

leukocytosis a transient increase in the number of leukocytes in the blood, resulting from various causes such as hemorrhage, fever, infection.

lymphocytapheresis the selective removal of lymphocytes from withdrawn blood, which is then retransfused into the donor.

lymphokine activated killer cell—effector cell capable of killing tumor cells; activated by cytokines derived from lymphocytes (lymphokine), particularly interleukin-2; has broad activity.

lymphotoxin a product of lymphocytes; lymphotoxin is toxic for certain tumor cells and shares several properties with tumor necrosis factor.

metaphase the stage of mitosis in which the chromosome becomes aligned between the centrioles.

metaplasia one adult cell type is substituted for another type not usually found in the involved tissue (e.g., glandular for squamous).

metastasis the spread of cells from a primary tumor via the lymphatic system or venous system to distant body parts where such cells give rise to tumor mass.

monoclonal antibody (MAB) an antibody produced from a single clone of cells; MABs recognize a specific antigen.

monocytosis increase in the proportion of monocytes in the blood.

monokines cytokines such as tumor necrosis factor released by mononuclear phagocytes.

morbidity the condition of being diseased or morbid; the sick rate; the ratio of sick to well persons in a community.

morphology the science of the forms and structures of organisms.

mortality the number of deaths attributed to cancer in a specified time period in a defined population.

multipotent progenitor cell an early component of the hematopoietic hierarchy that has undergone some degree of differentiation but still has the potential to develop into any of several of the cell lines and has limited self-replicative ability.

murine pertaining to or affecting mice or rats.

mutagen a substance that alters DNA in a cell.

myelophthisis invasion of the bone marrow by neoplastic elements.

myeloproliferative pertaining to or characterized by medullary and extramedullary proliferation of bone marrow constituents.

neoadjuvant chemotherapy chemotherapy administered before other therapies.

neoplasm an abnormal mass of cells typically exhibiting progressive and uncontrolled growth; classified by the cell type from which they originate and their biologic behavior.

neuropathic functional disturbances or pathologic changes in the peripheral nervous system.

nociceptive receiving injury.

oncogene a gene involved in the transformation of a normal cell into a malignant cell, or a gene that increases neoplastic properties of a cell.

osteoradionecrosis necrosis of the bone after irradiation.

outcome the result of service delivery including patient, staff, and organizational performances.

passive immunotherapy the direct transfer of cells or products of the immune system to a host.

phenotype the entire physical, biochemical, and physiologic makeup of an individual as determined both genetically and environmentally as opposed to genotype.

pleiotropic the quality of a gene to manifest itself in multiple ways.

plexopathy any disorder of a plexus, especially of nerves.

ploidy the aggressiveness of a neoplasm by analyzing the cellular DNA content.

pluripotent stem cell the most primitive of the blood cells in the hematopoietic hierarchy; these cells, as yet unidentified in humans, are the forerunners of all of the cell lineages; the pluripotent stem cell is characterized by infrequent cell cycling and the ability to self-replicate.

precursor cell a nucleated cell that is morphologically recognizable as belonging to a specific lineage and that gives rise immediately to the mature components of the circulating blood.

prevalence measurement of all the cancer cases, both old and new, at a designated point in time.

primary prevention measures taken to ensure that cancer never develops (e.g., decreasing the number of new smokers).

process the manner in which service will be delivered; procedures, practice guidelines/protocols, action plans, and documentation systems describe process.

progenitor cells an early ancestor of the mature components of the blood; pluripotent stem cells are called also *common progenitor cells.*

prophase the second phase of mitosis, in which the DNA coils and the centrioles move to opposite poles.

provirus the genome of an animal virus integrated into the genetic material of a host cell.

radiobiology that branch of science that is concerned with the effect of light and ultraviolet and ionizing radiations on living tissue or organisms.

randomized to make random for scientific experimentation.

recombinant DNA technology process by which there is identification of a gene for a specific substance; the gene is then cloned and inserted into a bacterium that then serves as a factory to produce the desired substances (IL-2, TNF, IL-1).

refractory not readily yielding to treatment.

relative risk the incidence of cancer (breast) in a population (women) with a known or suspected risk factor (genetic) divided by the incidence rate of cancer (breast) in a population (women) without that risk factor (genetic).

reticuloendothelial pertaining to tissues having both reticular and endothelial attributes.

retinoid any derivative of retinal, whether naturally occurring or synthetic.

retrovirus a large group of RNA viruses that carry reverse transcriptase.

reverse transcriptase an enzyme that catalyzes RNA-directed polymerization of DNA.

RNA (ribonucleic acid) a part of the messenger system through which DNA controls protein production within the cell.

secondary prevention measures used for detecting and treating early diagnosed cancer while in its most curable stage.

sequestration isolation of a patient; the net increase in the quantity of blood within a limited vascular area.

seroconversion the change of serologic test from negative to positive, indicating the production of detectable, circulating antibodies.

simian pertaining to, characteristic of, or resembling an ape or monkey.

somatic growth factors substances that regulate growth of non-blood cells in the body; this is a more diverse and less well-understood system, with positive and negative regulation (insulin-like, epidermal, and platelet-derived growth factors).

standard a written value defining the rules, actions, results, or analyses that are related to the patient, staff, or system and that are sanctioned by an authority.

standard of practice a written value statement that defines the rules, actions, or conditions that direct patient care.

stem cell a cell with unlimited reproductive capacity; daughter cells may differentiate into other cells.

stereotactic pertaining to or characterized by precise positioning in space, said especially of discrete areas of the brain that control specific functions.

stratification the art or process of stratifying; developing different levels.

structure the circumstances under which a service will be delivered; the organization's mission, philosophy, goals, and policies define its structure.

suppressor T cells a subset of T lymphocytes that reduces the activity of other T and B cells.

syngeneic having identical matched cell type.

tachyphylaxis a rapidly decreasing response to a drug or physiologically active agent after administration of a few doses.

T cells (T lymphocytes) thymus-dependent cells that are involved in a variety of cell-mediated immune responses.

telangiectasis the spot formed most commonly on the skin by a dilated capillary or terminal artery.

telophase the final phase of mitosis, in which migration of chromosomes to cells is complete.

tenesmus straining, especially ineffectual and painful straining at stool or in urination.

teratogen a substance causing mutation in a developing fetus.

thermography a technique wherein an infrared camera is used to photographically portray the surface temperatures of the body, based on the self-emanating infrared radiation.

threshold (for evaluation) a preestablished level or pattern of performance related to an indicator at which further evaluation of the quality and appropriateness of an important aspect of care is initiated.

transcription the normal cellular response of turning a DNA gene copy into messenger RNA (mRNA).

translocation an interchange in which one segment of a chromosome is transferred to another chromosome, generally the result of breakage and abnormal reattachment.

trending analyzing the results of numerous studies on the same indicator to identify patterns that may influence the quality of outcomes related to the important aspect of care or service being monitored.

tumor marker a product produced by a cancer cell or in response to the presence of cancer, which may be released into the circulation or may remain associated with the cancer cell.

tumor necrosis factor (TNF) produced primarily by activated macrophages; TNF is cytostatic or cytotoxic for some neoplastic cells, induces hemorrhagic necrosis of some tumors, and has a range of activities similar to lymphotoxin.

unipotent progenitor cell early component of the hematopoietic hierarchy that has undergone further differentiation and is committed to one or two cell lines.

western blot an immunoassay used for measuring antiviral antibody responses, useful for distinguishing antibody responses to specific viral proteins; frequently used as a confirmatory test for HIV status.

window phase the time between the dates of actual exposure leading to infection and development of detectable serum antibodies.

APPENDIX B LABORATORY VALUES

Test	Purpose	Normal values (adult)	Nursing action
Arterial blood gases (ABGs)	Assess respiratory status, acid-base balance.	pH, 7.35-7.45; $Paco_2$, 35-45 mm Hg; Pao_2, > 70 mm Hg; HCO_3^-, 23-28; BE, 0 ± 3 mEq/L; Sao_2, >93% Fio_2	Mark laboratory slip as for any O_2 therapy at time sample collected. Send specimen on ice to laboratory immediately. Apply pressure on puncture site for 5 min. Include respiratory rate and O_2 therapy status when reporting ABG results to physician.
CHEMISTRY			
Electrolytes			
Calcium (Ca^{++})	Assess renal, neuromuscular bone status; parathyroid, thyroid function; increased levels with bone metastasis.	8.5-10.5 mg/dl	Observe for increased or decreased neuromuscular activity with Ca^{++} level <7 mg/dl or >13 mg/dl.
Ionized calcium	Serum ionized calcium level is *not* affected by changes in serum protein/albumin concentrations and it reflects calcium metabolism better than total calcium values.	4.4-5.9 mg/dl 2.2-2.5 mEq/L 1.1-1.24 mmol/L	
Chloride (Cl^-)	Assess renal status, acid-base balance.	95-100 mEq/L	Potassium replacement therapy should be accompanied by a 1:1 ratio of potassium to chloride.
Magnesium (Mg^{++})	Assess renal, metabolic, neuromuscular status, GI losses, alcoholism.	1.4-2.3 mEq/L	Assess antacid ingestion. If increased levels, observe and implement seizure precautions.
Phosphorus (P)	Assess renal, parathyroid function, bone status.	2.5-4.5 mg/dl	Assess dietary intake (e.g., starvation).
Potassium (K^+)	Assess renal status, endocrine, cardiac function, acid-base balance.	3.5-5.0 mEq/L	Monitor higher or lower level for potential cardiac toxicity; if increased level, metabolic acidosis.
Sodium (Na^+)	Assess renal status, endocrine function, acid-base balance.	135-145 mEq/L	Monitor fluid intake/output; implement precautionary safety measures if <120 mEq/L; decreased levels with metabolic alkalosis.
Albumin serum	Assess renal and nutritional status.	3.5-5.0 g/dl (20-day half-life)	
Prealbumin	Assess nutritional status.	17-42 mg/dl, short half-life	Provides an analysis of protein changes during previous 2 days.
Bilirubin	Assess hepatic, biliary tract, or hemolytic function; hemorrhage, drug toxicities, blood transfusion.	Total: 0.2-1.2 mg/dl Direct: 0.1-0.4 mg/dl Indirect: 0.1-0.8 mg/dl	
Calcitonin serum	Assess malignancy of thyroid.	50-500 pg/ml	
Cholesterol	Assess hepatic, pancreatic, biliary tract, thyroid function.	Age 40+: 150-300 mg/dl Age 30-39: 140-270 mg/dl Age 20-29: 120-240 mg/dl	High-fat, high-sugar diet may alter results.
Copper serum	Assess hepatic function.	70-165 μg/dl	
Creatinine serum	Assess renal and urinary tract function, bone status; ARF profile: Increased BUN, creatinine, potassium; decreased sodium.	0.7-1.4 mg/dl	

Continued.

APPENDIX B   LABORATORY VALUES—cont'd

Test	Purpose	Normal values (adult)	Nursing action
CHEMISTRY—cont'd			
Glucose serum	Assess pancreatic, liver, or endocrine status, diabetes mellitus, hypoglycemia, malabsorption, Cushing's syndrome.	Fasting (FBS) 65-110 mg/dl 2-hr postprandial (2-h PP) glucose level should be within normal limits	NPO past midnight before test. Report glucose levels of <40 mg/dl or >400 mg/dl immediately. Eating and specimen collection schedules must be coordinated.
Glycohemoglobulin (Hemoglobin A_{1c})	Assess pancreatic, liver, or endocrine status, diabetes mellitus.	4.3-6.1%	Provides steady state of blood glucose level over 4 to 6 weeks.
Urea nitrogen blood (BUN)	Assess renal function, hydration status.	10-20 mg/dl	A ratio of BUN to serum creatinine of >10:1 may be suggestive of dehydration, GI bleeding, or decreased cardiac output.
Uric acid serum	Assess renal function; hypercalcemia.	Female: 2.2-7.7 mg/dl Male: 3.9-9.0 mg/dl	Monitor intake and output; observe for elevations with rapidly dividing cell destruction; administer appropriate interventions.
Triglycerides lipid profile test	Assess risk of coronary and vascular disease.	Adult/elderly: Female: 35-135 mg/dl or 0.40-1.52 mmol/L (SI units) Male: 40-160 mg/dl or 0.45-1.81 mmol/L (SI units)	
Guaiac (fecal) or occult blood, Hemoccult	Determine presence of blood that is not visible.	Negative	Instruct patient to abstain from red meats for 48 to 72 hr before test.
HEMATOLOGY			
Complete blood count (CBC)	Assess clotting status, response to infection and inflammation.	RBC, WBC, platelets	Do not draw blood sample from same extremity as IV infusion.
Red blood cells (RBC)	Assess anemias, hydration, oxygen transport; RBC fragmentation, acute leukemia/myelodysplasia.	Female: 4.2-5.5 mil/mm³ Male: 4.4-6.0 mil/mm³ Older adult: 3.5 mil/mm³	
Hematocrit (Hct)	Assess blood loss, hydration, hematologic disorders.	Female: 37%-47% Male: 42%-52%	
Hemoglobin (Hgb)	Assess blood loss, anemias, dehydration.	Female: 12-16 g/dl Male: 14-18 g/dl	
RBC indices	Assess anemias and polycythemia.		
Mean corpuscular hemoglobin (MCH) (normal color)	Assess chronic blood loss, lead poisoning.	28-34 pg Older adult: 28-32 pg	
Mean corpuscular hemoglobin concentration (MCHC)		30%-40% Older adult: 29%-33%	
Mean corpuscular volume (MCV) (size of RBC)		82-101 µg³ Older adult: 90.5-105 µg³	

Test	Purpose	Normal value	Nursing considerations
Reticulocyte count	Assess anemia; bone marrow function.	Female: 0.5%-1.5% of erythrocytes Male: 0.5%-2.5% of erythrocytes	
White blood cell count (WBC)	Assess amount of infection, inflammation, and healing.	4,000-11,000/mm^3	Steroid drugs may suppress WBCs.
Differential neutrophils (poly-morphonuclears [polys] or segmentals [segs])	Determine presence of infection, inflammation, and stress.	42%-66% or 3000-7000/µl Older adult: 43% to 79%	Granulocytes include neutrophils, basophils, and eosinophils. Monitor for neutropenia; implement measures to prevent or minimize infectious process.
Band cells (stabs)	Assess presence of recent infection.	3%	
Basophils	Assess status of polycythemia vera, leukemias, Hodgkin's disease, allergic reactions, and stress.	0.4%-1.0% or 40-100/µl	
Eosinophils	Assess response to ACTH or epinephrine or status of allergy, leukemia, Hodgkin's disease.	1%-3% or 50-400/µl Older adult: 0%-0.3%	
Lymphocytes	Assess status of infection, especially viral, and stress.	25%-33% or 1000-4000/µl Older adult: 11%-48%	
Monocytes	Assess status of bacterial phagocytosis and healing.	0%-9% or 100-600/µl Older adult: 1%-5%	
Erythrocyte sedimentation rate (ESR)	Assess nonspecific inflammation and tissue injury; malignancy; rheumatic fever, and arthritis; acute and/or chronic infections.	Female: 0-30 mm/hr Male: 0-20 mm/hr	
Platelets	Assess bone marrow, clotting status; increases in advanced malignancy.	150,000-450,000/mm^3	Monitor for thrombocytopenia. Implement measures to prevent or minimize bleeding. Moderate risk <50,000 Severe risk <20,000; potential for CNS hemorrhage.
Platelet adhesion	Assess platelet function.	5,000-18,000/mm^3	
Platelet aggregation	Assess platelet function.	Visible <5 min	
Platelet volume	Determine platelet size; assess purpura, DIC, anemias.	8-10 fl 2.5 µm in diameter	
Ferritin serum	Assess hematopoietic status; increased levels with neuroblastoma.	Female: 5-100 ng/ml Male: 10-270 ng/ml	
Folic acid serum	Assess anemias.	4-16 ng/ml	
Iron serum	Assess anemias.	50-100µg/dl	
Total iron-binding capacity (TIBC)	Assess amount of iron that could be carried if transferrin were completely saturated: anemias, chronic blood loss, and liver disease.	250-400 µg/dl	
Ham (acid serum test)	Used to detect paroxysmal nocturnal hemoglobinuria.	10%-50% hemolysis of red blood cells	Contraindications: persons with recent blood transfusions. Report abnormal results.
Coagulation factors			
Factor I: fibrinogen	Assess clotting status, hemophilia.	60-100 mg/ml	
Factor II: prothrombin		10-15 mg/dl	
Factor V: proaccelerin		5-10 mg/dl	
Factor VII: proconvertin	Assess vitamin K deficiency.	5-20 mg/dl	
Factor VIII: antihemophilic globin	Assess von Willebrand hemophilia A.	30-35 mg/dl	

Continued.

APPENDIX B   LABORATORY VALUES—cont'd

Test	Purpose	Normal values (adult)	Nursing action
HEMATOLOGY—cont'd			
Coagulation factors—cont'd			
Factor IX: thromboplastin	Assess hemophilia B (Christmas disease).	30 mg/dl	
Factor X: Stuart-Prower		8-10 mg/dl	
Factor XI: morphilic		20-30 mg/dl	
Factor XII: Hageman	Assess for DIC.	0 mg/dl	
Factor XIII: fibrin stabilizing	Assess for bleeding tendency.	1 mg/dl	
Coagulation time (Lee-White, clotting time)	Assess coagulation; monitor heparin therapy.	5-15 min	Assess for potential bleeding. Pressure may be required on puncture site for 5 min.
D-dimer	Confirms DIC.	Negative (no D-dimer fragments present; <250 ng/ml or 250 mcg/L (SI units)	
Fibrin split products (FSPs)	Assess degree of coagulation.	<4 µg/ml	Monitor/report elevated levels of FSP.
Fibrin degradation products (FDPs)	Assess disorders (e.g., DIC).	<10	Monitor/report elevated levels of FDP.
Fibrinogen	Assess ability to form clots; to assess for leukemia, liver damage, DIC.	160-300 mg/dl Older adult: 470-485 mg/100 ml	DIC profile: decreased platelets, fibrinogen, plasminogen; increased PT, PTT, FDPs; report results STAT.
Prothrombin time (pro time PT)	Assess coagulant activity of the "extrinsic" system including factors V, VII, X, fibrinogen, and prothrombin.	100%; also reported in seconds, approximately 11-15; varies with laboratory	Assess for potential bleeding. Pressure may be required on puncture site for 5 min. Report results as ratio of patient to control rather than seconds.
Plasminogen	Assess DIC.	73%-122%	
Protamine sulfate	Assess coagulation, DIC.	Negative	
Activated partial thromboplastin time (APTT) or partial thromboplastin time (PTT)	Assess all plasma coagulation factors except VII and XII (e.g., stage II clotting disorders such as hemophilia).	APTT: 30-45 sec PTT: 16-25 sec	
Thrombin clotting time (thrombin time; TT)	Assess factor III clotting.	10-20 sec or within 3 sec of control	
Immunoglobulins	Assess immune system status.	Levels vary with age	Report abnormal results.
IgA	Assess for autoimmune disease.	65-650 mg/dl	
IgD	Assess for multiple myeloma.	0-30 mg/dl	
IgE	Assess for potential allergies.	0-200 ng/ml	
IgG	Assess for multiple myeloma.	600-1700 mg/dl	
IgM	Assess for hepatitis.	50-300 mg/dl	
ISOENZYMES			
Acid phosphatase serum	Assess prostate status, multiple myeloma, parathyroid, or renal function.	<4 ng/ml	Usually done on a serial basis for 3 days. Elevated in 75% of patients with bone metastases.

Test	Normal values	Purpose	Nursing considerations
Alkaline phosphatase (ALP) serum	30-115 mU/ml	Assess status of bone and of renal, hepatic, intestinal, and biliary tract; indicator for GVHD, osteogenic sarcoma.	NPO 8 hours before test; food can raise levels up to 25%.
Amylase serum	20-110 mU/ml	Assess pancreatic, renal, or salivary gland.	
CPK serum	CPK: total Female: <51 mU/ml Male: <82 mU/ml CPK-MB bands 3% indicate cardiac damage. CPK-MM bands 97%-100% indicate muscle damage. CPK-BB bands 0% indicate brain damage	Assess myocardial, muscle, and brain damage; infectious disease: HIV, hepatitis.	Elevation of MB bands 3-6 hr after onset of acute myocardial infarction; peaks in 24 hr.
Lactic dehydrogenase (LDH) serum	100-205 mU/ml	Assess hepatic, cardiac, renal, muscular, or RBC status.	Elevation seen 12-24 hr after onset of acute myocardial infarction; peaks in 2-6 days; elevation may indicate high-risk leukemia and lymphoma and/or relapse of these diseases. A flipped LDH_1/LDH_2 ratio with LDH_1 the highest indicates a myocardial infarction
LDH_1 cardiac	14%-26%		
LDH_2 cardiac	27%-37%		
LDH_3 pulmonary	13%-26%		
LDH_4 hepatic	8%-16%		
LDH_5 hepatic	6%-16%		
Lipase serum	0-190 U/L	Assess pancreas.	
Aspartate aminotransferase (AST) (formerly serum glutamic oxaloacetic transaminase [SGOT])	1-36 U/l 5-35 IU/L	Assess status of many organs (e.g., liver, heart); cellular death (chemotherapy and radiotherapy).	Elevation seen 8-12 hr after onset of acute myocardial infarction; peaks in 48 hr.
Alanine aminotransferase (ALT) (formerly serum glutamic pyruvic transaminase [SGPT])	8-20 U/L 5-40 IU/L	Assess status of many organs (e.g., liver); cellular death (chemotherapy and radiotherapy); hepatitis, cirrhosis, mononucleosis.	

OTHER TESTS

Test	Normal values	Purpose	Nursing considerations
Cerebrospinal fluid values	Albumin mean: 29.5 mg/dl + 112 SD: 11-48 mg/dl Bilirubin: 0 Cell count: 0-5 mononuclear cell per mm^3 Chloride: 120-130 mEq/L Glucose: 50-75 mg/dl IgG mean: 4.3 mg/dl + 112 SD: 0-8.6 mg/dl Protein Lumbar: 15-45 mg/dl Cisternal: 15-25 mg/dl Ventricular: 5-15 mg/dl	Assess cerebrospinal system; brain tumor, CVA, meningitis.	Sterile procedure for specimen collection; send specimen to laboratory immediately. *Do not* refrigerate specimen, because refrigeration may inhibit growth of meningococcus organisms and alter test accuracy.

Continued.

APPENDIX B LABORATORY VALUES—cont'd

Test	Purpose	Normal values (adult)	Nursing action
OTHER TESTS—cont'd			
Estrogen receptor assay	Useful in determining the prognosis and treatment of breast cancer.	Negative: <10 fmol/mg of protein Positive: >10 fmol/mg of protein	
Progesterone receptor assay	Useful in determining the prognosis and treatment of breast cancer.	Negative: <10 fmol/g of tissue Positive: >10 fmol/g of tissue	
Prostate specific antigen (PSA)	Assess prostate disease.	Normal: 0-4 ng/ml BPH: 4-19 ng/ml Prostate cancer: 10-120 ng/ml	
Gastric analysis	Assess gastric function; carcinoma of stomach, pernicious anemia, and gastric atrophy.	Basal Female: 2.0 + 1.8 mEq/hr Male: 3.0 + 2.0 mEq/hr Maximal (after histalog or gastrin) Female: 16 + 5 mEq/hr Male: 23 + 5 mEq/hr	NPO 8 hr before; requires nasogastric tube insertion to collect specimen. Assess gag reflex after procedure.
Duodenal drainage	Assess for duodenal ulcer status.	pH: 5.5-7.5 Amylase: over 1200 U total Trypsin: 35%-160% Viscosity: 3 min or less	
Blood cultures	Determine presence of pathogens.	Negative: usually drawn from different site to coincide with temperature elevation	Implement precaution measures for potential infection. Administer prescribed antibiotics.
Papanicolaou smear (Pap)	Assess cervical tissue for presence of disease.	Negative	Collect three separate slide specimens.
Urinalysis	Screening tool; assess renal, endocrine status, infection.	Color, turbidity: clear Negative for glucose, ketones, blood, bile, protein, bilirubin, crystals, RBC, WBC Casts: not waxy; few hyaline, epithelial, or granular	Urine sample must be fresh for accurate results.
Specific gravity		1.010-1.025 (urine osmolarity should always be higher than blood serum osmolarity)	
pH	Levels are affected by vegetarian, fruit, meat in diet.	5.0-7.5	
Acetone		Negative	
Amylase		24-76 µg/ml	
Bence-Jones protein	Assess oncologic status; multiple myeloma.	Negative	
Calcium	Assess parathyroid.	Negative	Keep urine container on ice.

Test	Normal Value	Clinical Use	Remarks
Catecholamine	Epinephrine: <20 µg Norepinephrine: <100 µg Metanephrine: <1.3 mg Vanillylmandelic acid: <6 mg	Assess renal system, Cushing's syndrome.	Collection container is kept on ice; collect all urine for 24 hr.
Creatinine clearance	75-125 ml/min Female: 0.8-1.8 g/24 hr Male: 1.0-2.0 g/24 hr	Assess renal status.	Usually drawn serially from different sites to coincide with temperature elevation. Collection container is kept on ice.
Culture	Negative or <10,000 organisms/ml	Determine presence of pathogens.	
Urobilinogen urine	Up to 1 mg in a 24-hr specimen	Assess GI malfunction.	
24-hour urine	Same as creatinine clearance	Assess renal status.	
Viruses		Determine presence of virus.	Implement infection precautions for positive virus results; report positive results for all viruses.

HTLV I	Negative	Detect T-cell leukemia.	HIV: 1—Seroconversion
			2—Lymph node involvement
			3—Progressive lymphadenopathy
			4—a—ARC fever; weight loss
			    b—Neuropathy changes
			    c—Infectious disease
			    d—Malignancy

HTLV II	Negative	Detect hairy cell leukemia.	
HTLV III	Negative	Detect retrovirus (HIV) AIDS.	
Herpes simplex	Negative	Detect herpes simplex virus I or II.	CD4—Normal findings: total count greater than 1000 cells/mm^3.
Varicella zoster	Negative	Detect chicken pox, shingles.	
Cytomegalovirus	Negative	Detect pneumonia.	
Epstein-Barr	Negative	Detect infectious mononucleosis.	
Rubella	Negative	Detect measles.	CD4 recommend monitoring every 3 to 6 months; as the CD4 measurements decrease, the percentage of persons developing AIDS increases. Forty-eight percent of patients can be expected to develop AIDS within 6 months when their CD4 count is ≥100 cells/mm^3.
Tumor markers are listed in Chapter 4.			
Hepatitis			
A—Anti-HAV, IgM	Negative	Infectious hepatitis.	
B—HBsAg, HBeAg	Negative	Serum hepatitis.	
C—Anti-HCV	Negative	Posttransfusion non-A, non-B hepatitis.	
D—Anti-HDV	Negative	Delta virus.	
E—No test available	Negative	Enteric non-A, non-B hepatitis.	

NORMAL TERM NEWBORN BLOOD VALUES

HEMATOLOGY

Hemoglobin	15-20 g/dl
Hematocrit	43% to 61%
WBC	10,000 to 30,000/mm^3
Neutrophils	40% to 80%
Immature WBCs	3% to 10%
Platelets	100,000-280,000/mm^3
Reticulocytes	3% to 6%
Blood volume	82.3 ml/kg (third day after early cord clamping)
	92.6 ml/kg (third day after delayed cord clamping)

CHEMISTRY

Sodium	124-156 mmol/L
Potassium	5.3-7.3 mmol/L
Chloride	90-111 mmol/L
Calcium	7.3-9.2 mg/dl
Glucose	40-97 mg/dl

IEM-PKU (inborn error of metabolism, phenylketonuria)	<4 mg	
Bilirubin (capillary heel stick)	4-6 mg/dl	(Bilirubin level peaks 3-5 days and should not exceed 13 mg/dl.)
Cord blood bilirubin	1.0-1.8 mg/dl	

URINALYSIS VALUES

Protein	<5-10 mg/dl
WBCs	<2-3
RBCs	Negative
Casts	Negative
Bacteria	Negative
Specific gravity	1.001-1.025
Color	Pale yellow

Breast-milk jaundice: Bilirubin rises the 4th day *after mature breast milk comes in;* bilirubin peak of 20-25 mg/dl is reached at 2-3 weeks of age.

APPENDIX C SELECTED DIAGNOSTIC TESTS

Diagnostic test	Purpose	Procedure/preparation	After procedure
Angiography	Used in various segments of the arterial system to determine vessel patency or the presence of an aneurysm, embolism, or arterial/venous malformations.	Assess for allergy to iodine preparation; NPO past midnight, sedation before procedure, local anesthesia before catheter insertion via fluoroscopy; contrast medium is infused via catheter; serial-timed radiographs are obtained.	A pressure dressing or sandbag may be applied to the entry site; monitor vital signs as ordered.
Barium studies	Assess for evidence of disease, anatomic abnormalities, malabsorption syndrome.	NPO status before test varies; 300-600 ml of contrast medium swallowed by patient for upper GI; lower GI preparation may include clear liquids, bowel prep of laxatives, suppositories, or enemas.	Large fluid intake is encouraged to promote barium excretion and minimize fluid loss.
Bone marrow biopsy	Examine the bone marrow for number, size, and shape of RBCs, WBCs, and megakaryocytes, estimation of cellularity, and determination of the presence of fibrotic tissue.	Aspiration of the marrow from the sternum, iliac crest, anterior and/or posterior iliac spine; proximal tibia in children; local anesthesia.	Apply pressure to puncture site; observe site for bleeding.
Bronchoscopy	Assess strictures, inflammation, or bleeding. Examine or remove pooled secretions and foreign bodies. Perform biopsy for analysis; place radiation beads for unresectable lung tumors.	NPO past midnight, sedation and atropine before procedure; fiberoptic bronchoscope inserted through nares.	Monitor vital signs; NPO status maintained until return of gag reflex.
Chest x-ray	Provide visualization of heart, lung, mediastinum, pulmonary vessels, trachea, bronchi, pleura, and diaphragm; assess response to therapy, location of monitoring catheters, pacemaker wires, etc., pleural effusions, neoplasms.	Optimal visualization requires that patient take in and hold a deep breath.	
Cholangiogram IV	Visualization of the biliary ductal system; assess inflammation; presence of stones and/or obstruction.	NPO past midnight; bowel preparation; IV infusion of iodine dye.	Assess that bilirubin level is <3.5 mg/dl so visualization is possible; if bilirubin is elevated, procedure may be cancelled; observe for allergic reaction from dye.
Colonoscopy	Examine the left, transverse, and right colon and sigmoid.	Clear liquid diet 1-3 days before; sedation and cathartics before exam, NPO past midnight; colonoscope inserted through anus.	Observe for unexpected bleeding.
Colposcopy	Provide direct visualization of the vagina, vulva, and cervical epithelium; to biopsy cervical tissue.	Colposcope is inserted into the vagina and advanced toward the cervix.	Monitor vital signs; observe for vaginal bleeding.
Computerized axial tomography (CT scan)	Noninvasive procedure to analyze tissue for density, assess for evidence of disease, inflammation, displacement, or enlargement.	May require NPO status; may be performed with or without a dye injection; CT scanning provides a cross-sectional image.	

Continued.

APPENDIX C   SELECTED DIAGNOSTIC TESTS—cont'd

Diagnostic test	Purpose	Procedure/preparation	After procedure
Culdoscopy	Permit observation of the uterus, fallopian tubes, ovaries, broad ligaments, rectal wall, and sigmoid colon from inside the cul-de-sac.	NPO past midnight; local, regional, or general anesthesia; surgical incision is made in the posterior vaginal wall; culdoscope is inserted into the vagina and passed through the incision into the cul-de-sac.	Monitor vital signs; observe for vaginal bleeding.
Cystoscopy	Permit direct examination of the urethra and bladder for strictures or bleeding sites; remove biopsy specimens of the prostate, bladder, and urethra; place ureteral catheters.	May require sedation or anesthesia before examination; cystoscope is inserted into the urethra and advanced into the bladder.	Monitor for urinary retention or bleeding and monitor vital signs.
Echocardiography	Assess congenital ischemic or acquired heart disease, presence of pericardial effusion, structure and mobility of heart.	Gel is applied to the skin, and the transducer is moved along the skin with some pressure. Heart valves and pericardial sac are examined.	
Electrocardiography (12-lead ECG)	Record electrical activity within the heart.	Electrodes are attached to patient's chest and to each of the four extremities.	
Electroencephalography (EEG)	Assess intracranial pathophysiology and organic brain syndrome and determine presence and type of epilepsy.	From 16 to 32 electrodes are applied to the head with electrode paste.	Assist with hair washing.
Endoscopic retrograde cholangiopancreatography (ERCP)	Assess suspected biliary duct pathology and pancreatic disease. Percutaneous transhepatic cholangiography (PTC) and ERCP are the only methods available to visualize the biliary tree in jaundiced patients.	NPO, sedative before procedure; IV line for medication administration; fiberoptic scope inserted for visualization.	Monitor vital signs; observe for bleeding; NPO status maintained until return of gag reflex.
Esophagoscopy with gastroscopy	Permit direct visualization of esophagus and stomach. Biopsy specimens, brushings, or washings may be obtained.	NPO, sedative before procedure; local anesthesia. Fiberoptic scope is inserted through the mouth.	Monitor vital signs; NPO status maintained until return of gag reflex.
I-125 fibrinogen uptake	Noninvasive test to identify suspected thrombus formation in the deep veins.	IV line for medication administration.	
Immunoscintigraphy	Detect recurrent metastatic colorectal or ovarian cancer.	No fasting required; injection with radiolabeled monoclonal antibody (radionuclide indium chloride-111) Images are obtained in 48 to 72 hours; the procedure takes approximately 1 hr each day for at least 1 to 4 days.	Same as nuclear scans. Encourage fluids
Intravenous pyelogram (IVP)	Provide visualization of the kidneys, ureters, and bladder to determine abnormalities, obstruction, and/or hematoma.	Assess for allergy to iodine preparation; contrast medium is injected IV and concentrates in the urine; NPO for 12 hours before examination; bowel prep may be required.	Monitor vital signs; encourage fluid intake.

Test	Purpose	Procedure	Nursing Care
Laparoscopy	Permit visualization of pelvis and intestines; ovarian biopsy or other surgical procedures may be performed as part of laparoscopy (e.g., lysis of adhesions, tubal ligation).	NPO past midnight; general anesthesia; a surgical incision is made and a trocar is inserted and then aspirated to ensure that intestine or large vessels have not been perforated; nitrous oxide or carbon dioxide may be inserted to create a pneumoperitoneum.	Monitor vital signs; observe for abdominal discomfort and bleeding.
Liver biopsy	Assess liver malfunction or disease.	NPO 6-8 hours before; sedative before procedure; local anesthetic; needle insertion to obtain specimen.	Apply pressure to biopsy site; turn patient on right side; observe for bleeding; give vitamin K injection; monitor vital signs.
Lumbar puncture	Assess diagnosis of brain or spinal cord neoplasm, hemorrhage, meningitis, encephalitis, autoimmune disorders of CNS, and/or degenerative brain disease.	Sterile procedure; place patient in lateral decubitus (fetal) position; local anesthetic; obtain 3 sterile specimens.	Explain to the patient that he or she MUST lie still during the procedure; rest in bed (flat position) for 1 hr after procedure.
Lymphangiography	Performed for staging purposes with lymphoma or to detect metastasis; to examine lymph vessels for obstruction.	Assess for allergy to iodine preparation: dye injected intradermally to test for allergy. If no apparent reaction, then give dye intravenously; serial-timed radiographs obtained.	Monitor vital signs; observe for respiratory distress.
Magnetic resonance imaging (MRI)	Noninvasive method for assessing tissue function and chemical composition of the body.	May require NPO status; contraindicated for patients with aneurysm clips or pacemakers because of magnetic field.	
Mammography	Determine presence of benign or malignant breast disease and cysts and to guide needle biopsy.	Breast is placed between the camera and film and compressed for a clear image.	
Mediastinoscopy	Allow visualization of mediastinum; potential biopsy of lymph nodes; to permit diagnosis and staging of cancer, infection, and sarcoidosis.	NPO past midnight; sedation before procedure; local or general anesthesia before insertion of mediastinoscope via incision at suprasternal notch.	Monitor vital signs; potential for bleeding and dyspnea; NPO status until return of gag reflex.
Myelography	Permit visualization of the subarachnoid space to detect abnormalities of the spinal cord and vertebrae and locate obstruction in the flow of cerebrospinal fluid (CSF).	NPO for 4 hours before procedure; local anesthetic; needle inserted into lumbar space; contrast medium injected with timed serial radiographs.	Monitor vital signs and neurologic status; follow postprocedure body position orders.
Nuclear medicine scans			
Bone	Detect focal defects in the bone, infection, fractures; to assess disease process.	Assess for previous reaction to contrast media; requires IV line for injection of dye; serial radiographs are obtained; NPO and sedation may be required.	Encourage fluid intake to aid in urinary excretion of radionuclide.
Brain	Delineate subdural hematoma, arteriovenous malformation, thrombosis, abscess, neoplasms, glioma, or other metastatic tumors.	Assess for previous reaction to contrast media; requires IV line for injection of dye; serial radiographs are obtained; NPO and sedation may be required.	Encourage fluid intake to aid in urinary excretion of radionuclide.
Gallium	Determine presence of neoplasms, lymphoma, bronchogenic cancer, Hodgkin's disease, or inflammation.	Assess for previous reaction to contrast media; requires IV line for injection of dye; serial radiographs are obtained; NPO and sedation may be required.	Encourage fluid intake to aid in urinary excretion of radionuclide.

Continued.

APPENDIX C SELECTED DIAGNOSTIC TESTS—cont'd

Diagnostic test	Purpose	Procedure/preparation	After procedure
Gastric emptying scan	Assess obstruction, (e.g., ulcer, malignancy); patency of surgical anastomosis.	Patient to ingest "test meal" containing a radionuclide technetium; stomach is scanned until gastric emptying is complete.	Encourage fluid intake to aid in urinary excretion of radionuclide.
Liver and spleen	Detect lesions (e.g., cysts, hematomas, abscesses, adenomas, lacerations, metastasis).	Assess for previous reaction to contrast media; requires IV line for injection of dye; serial radiographs are obtained; NPO and sedation may be required.	Encourage fluid intake to aid in urinary excretion of radionuclide.
Lung	Examine pulmonary vascular circulation and to locate pulmonary emboli.	Assess for previous reaction to contrast media; requires IV line for injection of dye; serial radiographs are obtained; NPO and sedation may be required.	Encourage fluid intake to aid in urinary excretion of radionuclide.
Multiple gated acquisition (MUGA)	Assess indices of ventricular effectiveness, ejection fraction, and ventricular volume of heart.	Assess for previous reaction to contrast media; requires IV line for injection of dye; serial radiographs are obtained; NPO and sedation may be required.	Encourage fluid intake to aid in urinary excretion of radionuclide.
Positron emission tomography (PET)	A unique technique that combines nuclear medicine with precise localization to penetrate body's metabolism by recording traces of nuclear annihilations in body tissue. Designed to measure blood flow and volume, protein metabolism.	Requires more than one IV access (infusion of radioisotope and serial blood samples); no restriction on diet or fluids; no sedatives or tranquilizers should be taken.	Encourage fluid intake to aid in urinary excretion of radionuclide.
Renal	Provide data on kidney size, shape, location, and perfusion.	Assess for previous reaction to contrast media; requires IV line for injection of dye; serial radiographs are obtained; NPO and sedation may be required.	Encourage fluid intake to aid in urinary excretion of radionuclide.
Thallium	Identify myocardial fibrosis and ischemia; perfusion imaging.	Assess for previous reaction to contrast media; requires IV line for injection of dye; serial radiographs are obtained; NPO and sedation may be required.	Encourage fluid intake to aid in urinary excretion of radionuclide.
Thyroid	Assess location, size, shape, and anatomic function of the substernal or enlarged thyroid glands.	Assess for previous reaction to contrast media; requires IV line for injection of dye; serial radiographs are obtained; NPO and sedation may be required.	Encourage fluid intake to aid in urinary excretion of radionuclide.
Oximetry	Assess arterial oxygen saturation (SaO_2); shock lung, pneumonia, asthma, mechanical ventilation status.	Place monitoring probe or sensor on the earlobe/fingertip.	Assure patient that test is noninvasive.
Paracentesis	Confirm presence of ascites; specimen analyzed for protein, amylase, RBC, WBC, fat, specific gravity, and cancer cells; fluid may be removed for palliative measures.	Local anesthetic; insertion of trocar, then catheter for drainage; may be continuous flow set-up.	Monitor vital signs; observe and record fluid loss.

Pericardiocentesis	Needle aspiration of fluid from pericardial sac; used for diagnostic or therapeutic purposes; ECG monitoring for localization and position of needle tip.	IV line for keep-vein-open rate; patient in supine position with head of bed elevated 60 degrees.	Observe and monitor vital signs, potential bleeding, and dyspnea.
Proctoscopy	Explore anus, rectum, and sigmoid colon.	Clear liquid diet, laxatives, NPO, enemas till clear before examination.	Observe for unexpected bleeding or sharp pain.
Sialography	Assess salivary ducts (parotid, submaxillary, submandibular, sublingual) and related glandular structures.	Ingestion of contrast medium; x-ray films are taken with the patient in various positions; patient is given a sour substance to stimulate salivary excretion.	
Sigmoidoscopy (flexible)	Examine left, transverse, right, and sigmoid colon with a flexible fiberoptic endoscope; biopsy and removal of polyps may be performed at this time.	Clear liquid diet 1-3 days before, NPO 6-8 hours before; cathartics before examination; fiberoptic endoscope inserted via anus.	Observe for unexpected bleeding or sharp pain.
Thermography	Technique by which differences in heat energy emanating from the skin of the breast are photographed using an infrared detector; hot spots may be a tumor, fibrocystic changes, or infection.	Thermoscope is placed over a small area of the breast to determine normal breast temperature; then both breasts scanned with infrared device; no discomfort is associated with the test.	
Thoracentesis	Obtain pleural fluid for analysis; therapeutic is performed to relieve intrathoracic pressure associated with excess fluid in the lung.	Local anesthesia before insertion of trocar, then chest tubes; needle insertion for biopsy may be guided by fluoroscopy.	Monitor vital signs; observe for respiratory distress, bleeding at entry site, and excessive blood in sputum.
Tomography	Assess nodules or calcification in pulmonary mass or infiltrate.	Radiographic imaging through a predetermined cross section of the body; optimal visualization requires that patient take in and hold a deep breath.	
Ultrasonography Doppler	Noninvasive procedure using sound waves to assess tissue function, abscess, trauma; determine blood flow velocity.	Gel is placed on the patient and the transducer is moved along the skin with some pressure.	
Venography	Demonstrate nonfilling of a vessel; assess for abnormal valves, thrombophlebitis, or hematoma.	Assess for allergy to contrast medium; inject contrast medium; serial-timed radiographs are obtained.	Monitor vital signs; observe for bleeding at entry site.
Ventriculography	Observe size, shape, and filling of ventricles; detect lesions and/or cerebral anomalies.	Serial x-ray of the skull after air or contrast material is injected via burr holes in the skull.	Requires general/local anesthesia, NPO status past midnight; monitor vital signs after procedure every 15 to 30 min for the initial 24 hr; head of bed elevated 10 to 15 degrees for 24 hr; observe scalp dressing; monitor pain and administer analgesics.

LABORATORY AND DIAGNOSTIC TESTS BIBLIOGRAPHY

1. Dickason EJ, Schult MO, Silverman BL: *Maternal and infant nursing care,* ed 2, St. Louis, 1994, Mosby.
2. Herreid JA: Hepatitis C: past, present, and future, *MEDSURG Nursing* 4(3):179, 1995.
3. Hoppe B: Taking the confusion out of calcium levels, *Nursing* 25(7):32kk, 1995.
4. Jackson MM, Rymer TE: Viral hepatitis: anatomy of a diagnosis, *Am J Nurs* 94(1):43, 1994.
5. Kee JL: *Laboratory & diagnostics tests with nursing implications,* ed 4, Norwalk, Conn, 1995, Appleton & Lange.
6. Ladewig PW, London ML, Olds SB: *Maternal-newborn nursing,* ed 3, Redwood City, Calif, 1994, Addison Wesley Nursing, Benjamin/Cumings.
7. Owen A: Tracking the rise and fall of cardiac enzymes, *Nursing* 25(5):35, 1995.
8. Pagana KD, Pagana TJ: *Mosby's diagnostic and laboratory test reference,* ed 2, St. Louis, 1995, Mosby.
9. Siconolfi LA: Clarifying the complexity of liver function tests, *Nursing* 25(5):39, 1995.

Clinical pathways are an interdisciplinary approach used to achieve high-quality care at a reduced cost. The pathway is determined prospectively by a team of health care professionals who are knowledgeable about the disease and the care component. The pathway describes the sequential patient care events, anticipated or actual, expected by each member of the health care team in all sites (acute care, ambulatory, physician's office, home, hospice, and extended care) for a specific diagnosis. Variances between the anticipated and actual patient care events are then determined, and measures are taken to remove the barriers and to facilitate the progression of the patient along the pathway.[3,5,6]

Clinical pathways for the patient with cancer are undergoing transformation. The pathway design (e.g., number of days and topics for each section) may vary with the specific patient population. Patients who are undergoing radiation therapy, chemotherapy, biotherapy, or surgical procedures will require treatment-related individualization to make the pathway more multidisciplinary "user friendly" (Figure 1). Components related to successful pathway implementation and ongoing use require strategic planning and a continual evaluation process.[1,2,4,7]

Factors to explore when developing, implementing, or evaluating clinical pathways include the following:

- *Leadership:* multidisciplinary participation is highly recommended (e.g., physicians, nurses, and staff from medical records, finance, quality improvement, social services, administration). Who will be involved and responsible for the development, design, documentation requirements, implementation, variance documentation, collecting and reporting, patient care outcomes, and practice guidelines changes?
- *Design format:* the team designing the clinical pathway should have representatives from all disciplines involved in relevant patient care activities. The patient population and clinical practice setting will influence the number of days on the pathway, the specific topics, documentation components, and where the clinical pathway will be located.[2,3,6]

- *Patient population:* patients for whom high costs are anticipated or costly services have already been provided; repeated inpatient admissions or those with disproportionately high usage outpatient; high-risk socioeconomic groups; those who encounter significant variances from the interventions or from expected outcomes associated with a clinical pathway; cases that involve multiple physicians or multiple disciplines; those identified as strategic case management priorities for the organization, and those for whom treatments fall into key product lines are the key patient population for clinical pathways.[3,5]
- *Implementation:* education and implementation are crucial elements for the success of the clinical pathway. Who will be responsible for the pathway implementation and agency personnel education regarding the clinical pathway usage? All users of the clinical pathway will require initial education and ongoing information regarding pathway use and patient care outcomes.
- *Variance reporting:* clinical pathways usually need automated tools to facilitate variance documentation, collection, and reporting. Guidelines need to be established regarding review of the pathway variances that require concurrent action.
- *Documentation:* the documentation system must be accessible, easy to use, have a multidisciplinary format, avoid duplication, and work in congruence with established clinical pathways used by the agency or organization. Multiple systems (e.g., computerized, charting by exception, manual documentation) are available in preprinted clinical pathway format.[2,5-8]
- *Risk and liability consideration:* the primary function of the medical record is to chronicle those facts on which diagnosis and treatment are based. Clinical pathways are a structured and systematic way to record all the events required to manage the patient during an illness episode. The agency or organization will need to determine documentation requirements for the clinical pathway as a permanent part of the medical record. Does the clinical pathway meet the agency's established practice and policy documentation guidelines?

Name: _____ **Diagnosis:** _____ **Physician:** _____

	Date: _____	Date: _____	Date: _____	Date: _____
Assessment	Vital signs Weight Pain N/V _____ Other: _____	Vital signs Weight Pain N/V _____ Other: _____	Vital signs Weight Pain N/V _____ Other: _____	Vital signs Weight Pain N/V _____ Other: _____
Consults	Social services Home care Physical therapy	_____ _____ _____	_____ _____ _____	_____ _____ _____
Medication IV Fluids	IV fluids Analgesia Antibiotic Antiemetic	IV fluids Analgesia Antibiotic Antiemetic	IV fluids Analgesia Antibiotic Antiemetic	IV fluids Analgesia Antibiotic Antiemetic
Treatments	Biotherapy Chemotherapy Radiation therapy Surgical procedure Dressing_____ Drains _____	_____ _____ _____ _____ _____ _____	_____ _____ _____ _____ _____ _____	_____ _____ _____ _____ _____ _____
Diagnostic Laboratory Tests	X-ray _____ CT scan _____ CBC, Hb, Hct, LDH, CEA, PSA	X-ray _____ CT scan _____ CBC, Hb, Hct, LDH, CEA, PSA	X-ray _____ CT scan _____ CBC, Hb, Hct, LDH, CEA, PSA	X-ray _____ CT scan _____ CBC, Hb, Hct, LDH, CEA, PSA
Diet	Clear liquids Soft Regular Weight Loss/Gain	_____ _____ _____ _____	_____ _____ _____ _____	_____ _____ _____ _____
Activity	Bedrest _____ Chair _____ Walk _____Day Progressive ambulation _____	Bedrest _____ Chair _____ Walk _____Day _____	Bedrest _____ Chair _____ Walk _____Day _____	Bedrest _____ Chair _____ Walk _____Day _____
Patient Education	Unit/office/ _____ Informed consent __ RX plan: _____ RX schedule: _____ RX side effects: ____	_____ _____ _____ _____ _____	_____ _____ _____ _____ _____	_____ _____ _____ _____ _____
Discharge Planning	Transportation _____ Consults _____ Community resources _____ Support group _____ Clothing/hair/devices _____	_____ _____ _____ _____ _____ _____ _____	_____ _____ _____ _____ _____ _____ _____	_____ _____ _____ _____ _____ _____ _____

N/V, Nausea/vomiting; *IV*, intravenous; *CT*, computed tomography; *CBC*, complete blood count; *Hb*, hemoglobin; *Hct*, hematocrit; *LDH*, lactate dehydrogenase; *CEA*, carcinoembryonic antigen; *PSA*, prostate specific antigen; *RX*, treatment.

Figure 1   Clinical pathway: cancer diagnosis

BIBLIOGRAPHY

1. Baird SB: The impact of changing healthcare delivery on oncology practice, *Oncology Nursing* 2(3):1, 1995.
2. Burke LJ, Murphy J: *Charting by exception: applications making it work in clinical settings,* Boston, 1995, Delmar.
3. Burns JM and others: Critical pathways for administering high-dose chemotherapy followed by peripheral stem cell rescue in the outpatient setting, *Oncol Nurs Forum* 22(8):1219, 1995.
4. Iyer PW, Camp NH: *Nursing documentation: a nursing process approach,* ed 2, St. Louis, 1995, Mosby.
5. Spath PL, editor: *Clinical paths tools for outcomes management,* Chicago, 1994, American Hospital Publishing.
6. Yasko JM: Clinical pathways: an interdisciplinary tool for high-quality, low-cost care, *Inn Breast Cancer Care* 1(2):25, 1995.
7. Zander K: Evolving mapping and case management for capitation, part I: the infrastructure solution, *The New Definition* 10(3):1, 1995.
8. Zander K: Evolving mapping and case management for capitation, part II: the problems and promises of databases, *The New Definition* 11(1):1, 1996.

Index

Page numbers in *italics* indicate illustrations.
Page numbers followed by a *t* indicate tables.

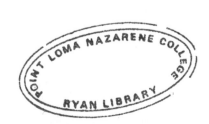